Transplantation of the Liver

Third Edition

Transplantation of the Liver
Third Edition

Edited by

Willis C. Maddrey, M.D., M.A.C.P., F.R.C.P.

Professor of Internal Medicine
The University of Texas Southwestern Medical Center at Dallas
Dallas, Texas

Eugene R. Schiff, M.D., F.A.C.P., F.R.C.P.

Professor of Medicine
Chief, Division of Hepatology
University of Miami School of Medicine
Center for Liver Diseases
Miami, Florida

Michael F. Sorrell, M.D., F.A.C.P.

Robert L. Grissom Professor of Medicine
Director, Liver Study Unit
University of Nebraska Medical Center
Omaha, Nebraska

LIPPINCOTT WILLIAMS & WILKINS
A **Wolters Kluwer** Company
Philadelphia · Baltimore · New York · London
Buenos Aires · Hong Kong · Sydney · Tokyo

Acquisitions Editor: Beth Berry
Developmental Editor: Delois Patterson
Surpervising Editor: Mary Ann McLaughlin
Manufacturing Manager: Benjamin Rivera
Production Editor: Janet Domingo, Compset, Inc.
Cover Designer: Christine Jenny
Compositor: Compset, Inc.
Printer: Maple Press

© 2001 by Lippincott Williams & Wilkins
530 Walnut Street
Philadelphia, PA 19106-3780 USA
LWW.com

Printed in the USA

Library of Congress Cataloging-in-Publication Data

Transplantation of the liver/edited by Willis C. Maddrey, Eugene R. Schiff, Michael F.
Sorrell.—3rd ed.
      p. ; cm.
   Includes bibliographical references and index.
   ISBN 0-7817-2039-7 (hard cover)
   1. Liver—Transplantation. I. Maddrey, Willis C. II. Schiff, Eugene R. III. Sorrell,
Michael F.
   [DNLM: 1. Liver Transplantation. WI 770 T772 2000]
   RD546 .T64 2000
   617.5'5620592—dc21
                                                    00-045341

Care has been taken to confirm the accuracy of the information presented and to describe generally accepted practices. However, the authors, editors, and publisher are not responsible for errors or omissions or for any consequences from application of the information in this book and make no warranty, expressed or implied, with respect to the currency, completeness, or accuracy of the contents of the publication. Application of this information in a particular situation remains the professional responsibility of the practitioner.

The authors, editors, and publisher have exerted every effort to ensure that drug selection and dosage set forth in this text are in accordance with current recommendations and practice at the time of publication. However, in view of ongoing research, changes in government regulations, and the constant flow of information relating to drug therapy and drug reactions, the reader is urged to check the package insert for each drug for any change in indications and dosage and for added warnings and precautions. This is particularly important when the recommended agent is a new or infrequently employed drug.

Some drugs and medical devices presented in this publication have Food and Drug Administration (FDA) clearance for limited use in restricted research settings. It is the responsibility of health care providers to ascertain the FDA status of each drug or device planned for use in their clinical practice.

10 9 8 7 6 5 4 3 2 1

Contents

Contributing Authors

Farin Amersi, MD *Postdoctoral Fellow, Liver and Pancreas Transplantation, UCLA School of Medicine, 10833 Le Conte Avenue, Suite 77-210 CHS, Los Angeles, California 90095*

Marina Berenguer, MD *Servicio de Medicina Digestiva, Hospital Universitaria La FE, Avda Campanar 21, Valencia 46009, Spain*

William Beschorner, MD *Professor of Surgery, Department of Surgery, University of Nebraska Medical Center, Swanson Hall 3029, 600 South 42nd Street, Omaha, Nebraska 68198-3285*

Henri Bismuth, MD *Hepato Biliary, Paul-Brousse Hospital, 14 AV P.V. Couturier, 94800 Villejuif, France*

Hartwig Bunzendahl, MD *Department of Surgery, School of Medicine, Campus Box 7210, University of North Carolina, Chapel Hill, North Carolina 27599*

Ronald W. Busuttil, MD *Professor and Chief, Division of Liver and Transplantation, Dumont Chair in Transplantation, UCLA School of Medicine, 10833 Le Conte, Room 77–120 CHS, Los Angeles, California 90095-7054*

E. Rolland Dickson, MD *Mayo Clinic, 200 First Street SW, Rochester, Minnesota 55905*

Jinwen Ding, MD *Multi-Organ Transplant Program, The Toronto General Hospital, University of Toronto, Toronto, Ontario, Canada*

David D. Douglas *Department of Medicine, Department of Surgery, Mayo Clinic Scottsdale, Scottsdale, Arizona*

Jean Emond, MD *Professor of Surgery, Surgical Director, Center for Liver Disease and Transplantation, Columbia University/Columbia-Presbyterian Medical Center, 622 West 168th Street, Suite PH 14 Center, New York, New York 10032*

Roger W. Evans, MD *Head, Section of Health Service Evaluation, Department of Health Science Research, Mayo Clinic, 200 First Street SW, Rochester, Minnesota 55905*

Gregory T. Everson, MD *Professor of Medicine, Director of Hepatology, Medical Director of Liver Transplantation, University of Colorado School of Medicine, 4200 East Ninth Ave., B-154, Denver, Colorado 80262*

Thomas W. Faust, MD *Assistant Professor of Medicine, Section of Gastroenterology, Department of Medicine, The University of Chicago, 5841 South Maryland Ave., Hospital MC 4076, Chicago, Illinois 60637*

Ira J. Fox, MD *Associate Professor of Surgery, Director of Transplant Research, Department of Surgery, 600 South 42nd Street, Omaha, Nebraska 68198-3285*

Jimmy R. Fulgham *Consultant, Department of Neurology, Mayo Clinic and Mayo Foundation; Assistant Professor of Neurology, Mayo Medical School, Rochester, Minnesota 55905*

Rafik M. Ghobrial, MD, PhD *Assistant Professor of Surgery, Liver and Pancreas Transplantation, UCLA School of Medicine, 10833 Le Conte, Room 77–120 CHS, Los Angeles, California 90095-7054*

Glenn A. Halff, MD *Department of Surgery, Organ Transplant Program, The University of Texas Health Science Center at San Antonio, San Antonio, Texas 78284*

Nigel D. Heaton, MD   *Consultant Surgeon-in-Charge, Liver Transplant Surgical Service, King's College Hospital, Denmark Hill, London SE5 9RS, United Kingdom*

Kishore Iyer, FRCS (Eng)   *Assistant Professor of Surgery, University of Nebraska Medical Center, Organ Transplantation Program, Omaha, Nebraska 68198-3285*

Sumodh Kalathil   *Department of Medicine, Department of Surgery, Mayo Clinic Scottsdale, Scottsdale, Arizona*

Igal Kam, MD   *Associate Professor of Surgery, Chief of Division of Transplant Surgery, 4200 East Ninth Ave., Denver, Colorado 80262*

Tomoaki Kato, MD   *Liver and Gastrointestinal Transplant Program, Division of Transplantation, University of Miami School of Medicine, Miami, Florida 33136*

Emmet B. Keeffe, MD   *Medical Director, Liver Transplantation Program, Chief of Gastroenterology, Stanford University Medical Center, 210 Welch Road, Suite 210, Palo Alto, California 94304-1509*

W. Ray Kim, MD   *Assistant Professor of Medicine, Mayo Medical School, Mayo Clinic, and Mayo Foundation, 200 First Street SW, Rochester, Minnesota 55905*

Michael J. Krowka, MD   *Consultant, Division of Pulmonary and Critical Care Medicine; Consultant, Division of Gastroenterology and Hepatology; Assistant Professor of Medicine, Mayo Medical School, Mayo Clinic, and Mayo Foundation, 200 First Street SW, Rochester, Minnesota 55905*

Alan Langnas, DO   *Professor of Surgery; Chief, Section of Transplantation; University of Nebraska Medical Center, Organ Transplantation, 983285 Nebraska Medical Center, Omaha, Nebraska 68198-3285*

Jay H. Lefkowitch, MD   *Department of Pathology, College of Physicians and Surgeons of Columbia University, 630 West 168th Street, New York, New York 10032*

John J. Lemasters, MD   *Laboratory of Hepatobiology and Toxicology, CB #7365, Faculty of Laboratory Office Building, Chapel Hill, North Carolina 27599*

David E. Levi, MD   *Liver and Gastrointestinal Transplant Program, Division of Transplantation, University of Miami School of Medicine, Miami, Florida 33136*

Gary A. Levy, MD   *Toronto Hospital, UN-10-151, 621 University Avenue, Toronto, Ontario M5G 2C4, Canada*

Leslie B. Lilly, MD   *Multi-Organ Transplant Program, The Toronto General Hospital, University of Toronto, Toronto, Ontario, Canada*

Jeffrey A. Lowell, MD   *Department of Surgery, University of Nebraska College of Medicine, 600 South 42nd Street, Omaha, Nebraska 68198-3208*

Michael R. Lucey, MD   *Associate Professor of Medicine, Director of Hepatology, Medical Director of Liver Transplantation, Hospital of the University of Pennsylvania, 3 Dulles, 3400 Spruce Street, Philadelphia, Pennsylvania 19104-6144*

Jurgen Ludwig, MD   *25007 Pinewater Cove Lane, Bonita Springs, Florida 34134*

Paul Martin, MD   *Director, UCLA School of Medicine, 10833 Le Conte Ave., 77-123D Center for Health Sciences, Los Angeles, California 90095*

Sue V. McDiarmid, MD   *Associate Professor of Pediatrics and Surgery, UCLA School of Medicine, Box 951752, Los Angeles, California 90095-1752*

David C. Mulligan   *Department of Medicine, Department of Surgery, Mayo Clinic Scottsdale, Scottsdale, Arizona*

José R. Nery   *Liver and Gastrointestinal Transplant Program, Division of Transplantation, University of Miami School of Medicine, Miami, Florida 33136*

James Neuberger, MD   *University Hospital Birmingham, The Liver and Hepatobiliary Unit, The Queen Elizabeth Hospital, Edgbaston, Birmingham B15 2TH, United Kingdom*

Antonio D. Pinna, MD   *Liver and Gastrointestinal Transplant Program, University of Miami School of Medicine, 603 Professional Arts Building, 1150 Northwest 14th Street, Miami, Florida 33136*

Jorge Rakela, MD   *University of Pittsburgh Medical Center, 201 Llormer Building, 200 Lothrop Street, Pittsburgh, Pennsylvania 15213-2582*

Mohamed Rela   *Consultant Surgeon and Honorary Senior Lecturer, Liver Transplantation; Institute of Liver Studies, King's College Hospital, Denmark Hill, Camberwell, London SE5 9RS, United Kingdom*

Hugo R. Rosen, MD   *Division of Gastroenterology/Hepatology, Oregon Health Sciences University, Portland Veterans Administration Medical Center, 3710 Southwest US Veterans Hospital Road, Portland, Oregon 97207*

Jayanta Roy-Chowdhury, MD, MRCP   *Professor of Medicine and Molecular Genetics, Albert Einstein College of Medicine, 1300 Morris Park Avenue, Bronx, New York 10461*

Robert H. Rubin, MD   *Chief of Surgical and Transplant, Infectious Disease, Massachusetts General Hospital, GRB 130, 55 Fruit Street, Boston, Massachusetts 02114*

Didier Samuel   *Hopital Paul Brousse, 94800, Villejuif, France*

Daniel F. Schafer, MD   *Associate Professor, Department of Internal Medicine, 600 South 42nd Street, Omaha, Nebraska 68198-3285*

Steven Schenker, MD   *Department of Medicine, University of Texas Health Science Center, 7703 Floyd Curl Drive, San Antonio, Texas 78284-7878*

Byers W. Shaw, Jr., MD   *Chairman, Department of Surgery, University of Nebraska Medical Center, 600 South 42nd Street, Omaha, Nebraska 68198-3285*

K. Vincent Speeg, Jr.   *Department of Medicine, Division of Gastroenterology and Nutrition, The University of Texas Health Science Center, San Antonio, Texas 78274*

Ashley St.J. M. Brown   *Institute of Hepatology, University College London, 69-75 Chenies Mews, London WC1E 4HX, United Kingdom*

Debra L. Sudan, MD   *Associate Professor of Surgery, University of Nebraska Medical Center, Organ Transplant Program, 983285 Nebraska Medical Center, Omaha, Nebraska 68198-3285*

Ronald G. Thurman, MD   *Laboratory of Hepatobiology and Toxicology, CB #7365, Faculty of Laboratory Office Building, Chapel Hill, North Carolina 27599*

Andreas G. Tzakis, MD   *Director, Liver and Gastrointestinal Transplant Program, University of Miami School of Medicine, 603 Professional Arts Building, 1150 Northwest 14th Street, Miami, Florida 33136*

William J. Wall, MD   *Director, Multi-Organ Transplant Program, London Health Sciences Centre-University Campus, 339 Windermere Road, London, Ontario N6A 5A5, Canada*

Roger Williams, CBE   *Director, Institute of Hepatology, University College London, Gower Street Campus, Harold Samuel House, 69-75 Chenies Mews, London WC1E 6HX, United Kingdom*

Laurel Williams-Todd   *Clinical Nurse Specialist, Department of Surgery, 600 South 42nd Street, Omaha, Nebraska 68198-3285*

Teresa L. Wright, MD   *Gastrointestinal Section (111BO Veterans Administration), 4150 Clement Street, San Francisco, California 94121-1598*

Zbigniew K. Wszolek, MD   *Senior Associate Consultant, Department of Neurology, Mayo Clinic Jacksonville, Jacksonville, Florida; Associate Professor of Neurology, Mayo Medical School, Rochester, Minnesota 55905*

Preface

The horizons for liver transplantation continue to evolve and expand. In this volume, many of the newer innovations are described and put into perspective. Issues of establishing liver transplantation as a therapy have given way to concerns regarding the availability of organs. The gap between the supply and demand of organs is an ever-increasing problem.

Living-related donor surgery is now being performed in several centers. Split-liver surgery is widely used. The focus now is shifting toward support of the use of genetically altered xenografts. There is undoubtedly a future for cloned organs and for hepatocyte transplantation. Liver transplantation will have a major place in the emerging area of gene therapy.

The advances over the past decade have been spectacular. Improved liver preservation made long-distance organ procurement and less time-sensitive transplant procedures feasible. There have been advances in the effective control of rejection, and evidence that even more effective agents are in the offing.

Issues regarding whether or not to perform transplantations in patients with alcohol-induced liver disease have been largely resolved in favor of proceeding in reasonably motivated suitable candidates. The remarkable additive liver injuries caused by alcohol and by hepatitis C have come to the fore and require more attention.

Efforts are underway to more effectively treat chronic viral hepatitis B and C, which are the major worldwide causes of chronic liver disease leading to candidacy for liver transplantation. The use of hyperimmune globulin and the nucleoside analogue lamivudine has changed the expectations regarding the outcome in patients with chronic hepatitis B to a favorable outlook. It is hoped that similar efforts to eradicate (or at least control) hepatitis C before and after transplantation will be increasingly successful. New information is emerging regarding disease recurrence after liver transplantation in a variety of disorders, including chronic hepatitis B and C, primary biliary cirrhosis, primary sclerosing cholangitis, autoimmune hepatitis, and alcohol-induced liver disease.

What we seek to achieve in the third edition of *Transplantation of the Liver* is a blend of the established and the innovative. Within this volume are comprehensive updates concerning such areas as histopathology, immunosuppressive therapy, and infectious problems in the patient who has received a liver transplant, and xenotransplantation, as well as protocols for the care of patients who have undergone (or will undergo) liver transplantation. The continued emphasis throughout this volume is that physicians caring for patients who are undergoing liver transplantation must act as an integrated team. Fortunately, prospects for the future are favorable and the possibilities extraordinarily exciting.

Transplantation of the Liver, edited by Willis C. Maddrey, Eugene R. Schiff, and Michael F. Sorrell. Lippincott Williams & Wilkins, Philadelphia © 2001.

CHAPTER 1

Liver Transplantation

Looking Back, Looking Forward

Daniel F. Schafer

For your own good reasons, you have opened a book on liver transplantation. In the subsequent (and substantive) chapters, you will find distillations of the knowledge and experience of several dozen experts on one of the most exotic and contentious areas of modern medicine. Liver transplantation is a classic half-way technology: It is expensive, resource intensive, and available to a limited number of those who are in need of it. In coming half-way, transplantation has forced physicians, patients, and even politicians to confront fundamental philosophical and ethical problems. These problems have had to be resolved in less-than-ideal circumstances by less-than-ideal individuals, sometimes under extreme time pressure. It is no wonder that the results have been less than perfect. The wonder and marvel is that we have results at all.

HISTORY

The best single primary source on the early history of liver transplantation is volume 15 of *Clio Chirurgica,* edited by Starzl, Groth, and Makowka.[1] This volume contains reprints of 40 important scientific reports with commentary by the editors. Another important source is *Experience in Hepatic Transplantation* by Starzl and Putnam.[2] This volume, published in 1969, contains references to virtually every experimental paper and every known clinical attempt at liver transplantation up to that time. Its pessimistic tone seemed justified by the poor survival rates among early patients.

Personal histories and remembrances of the early days of transplantation have been collected in two volumes by Paul Terasaki.[3,4] Although they contain some remarks on liver

transplantation, the bulk of the material concerns immunology and kidney transplantation. Two of the surgical founders of liver transplantation have published autobiographies. Thomas Starzl relates his life in *The Puzzle People,* and Roy Calne has produced a beautifully illustrated, nontechnical history in *Art, Surgery and Transplantation.*[5,6] Both these works stress the humane and social aspects of transplantation, which cannot be gleaned from the scientific reports.

Animal Studies

In 1955, C. Stuart Welch of Albany, New York, reported on his efforts to transplant an auxiliary liver into the right paravertebral gutter of nonimmunosuppressed mongrel dogs.[7] The livers withered quickly, a result Welch ascribed to rejection. The livers may well have atrophied in part due to lack of portal blood. The initial report of experimental liver replacement surgery was so short that neither the type of operation nor the species of the subject was mentioned.[8] The report does contain the following observation: "We have performed several 'successful operations' without survival of the 'patient.' "

In 1958, Francis Moore described the standard technique of canine liver orthotopic transplantation.[9] Thomas Starzl had been working on a similar model and performed over 200 canine transplants before his first attempt in a human.

Human Trials

The first human to undergo an orthotopic liver transplant was a 3-year-old boy who suffered from biliary atresia. He died before the operation was completed on March 1, 1963. Thomas Starzl, who performed the operation, gives the details of the patient's life and death in his memoir *Puzzle*

D. F. Schafer: Department of Internal Medicine, University of Nebraska Medical Center, Omaha, Nebraska, 68198-3285

People. As he relates, operating on a sick infant was shockingly different from operations on healthy dogs:

> Nothing we had done in advance could have prepared us for the enormity of the task. Several hours were required just to make the incision and enter the abdomen. Every piece of tissue that was cut contained the small veins under high pressure that had resulted from obstruction of the portal vein by the diseased liver. . . . His intestines and stomach were stuck to the liver in this mass of bloody scar. To make things worse, [the patient's] blood would not clot.

Success did not come quickly or easily. Over the next 10 years, perhaps 200 liver transplants were performed worldwide, about half of these by Starzl. The technical problems that began to be solved over this period included bile duct reconstruction, coagulation support, and refinement of the donor procedure (including the acceptance of the concept of brain death in 1968).

All the earliest liver transplant patients were treated with a drug regimen that had been developed for kidney grafts: azathioprine and steroids. At times, various antilymphocyte globulin preparations were added as well. These were inadequate drugs for the control of rejection. Long-term survival was seen in fewer than one-third of patients.

It was during this period (1963–1973) that a soil sample was gathered from Hardanger Vidda, Norway, by H. P. Frey.[10] A fungus from this sample was cultured in the laboratories of Sandoz, Inc. of Basel, Switzerland, and a metabolite isolated that became known as cyclosporin A. How this drug was developed at Sandoz is a matter of historical and economic interest. The credit for this triumph is generally given to Jean Borel, an important collaborator of Roy Calne of Cambridge. It is almost impossible to overestimate the importance cyclosporine had on liver transplantation. At countless meetings, Starzl and his trainees showed slides that depicted its pivotal position by dividing their survival curves into pre- and postcyclosporine eras. Cyclosporine transformed liver transplantation from a curiosity into a therapy.

For those who would enjoy a few hours investigating the birth of this drug, I recommend two references. The first is the transcript of a symposium honoring Jean Borel.[11] The second is a revisitation of the same historical ground by another (disgruntled) participant.[12] When finished, read them both again, noting the dates of publication. Your efforts will be rewarded.

How cyclosporin A was introduced into clinical medicine is also an extraordinary story.[13] The first animal trials in transplantation were performed in the laboratories of Roy Calne by a visiting Greek surgeon (Alkis Kostakis) and an immunologist (David White). Calne relates that Kostakis was worried that his professor in Greece would be upset if he didn't do some publishable experimental work. He learned to do ectopic heart transplants in rats and treated them with the experimental drug supplied by Sandoz and got remarkable results. In his second set of experiments, he improved the palatability of the lipid-soluble drug by dissolving it in olive oil sent to him by his mother. These experiments led to the first human trials.

THERAPY

The most important days in the history of liver transplantation were June 20 to 23, 1983. On those days, the National Institutes of Health (NIH) in Bethesda, Maryland, held a consensus development conference on liver transplantation. It had been 20 years since the first transplant was performed, and in the eyes of most physicians (and all insurance companies) the procedure was seen as dangerous and experimental. Four groups from four countries reported on their experience at the conference: 296 cases from the United States, 138 from England, 71 from Germany, and 26 from the Netherlands. The cumulative message from these 531 cases was that end-stage liver disease was no longer a death sentence. When the panel of experts declared that liver transplantation was a valid therapy for liver disease, the flood gates opened.

Five years after that NIH conference, there were 616 patients awaiting liver transplants in the United States. Ten years later, this number had ballooned to 12,056. Among the advances that made increased numbers of transplants possible was improved organ preservation. F. Belzer and coworkers deserve enormous credit for extending the life of preserved organs from a few hours to more than a day.[14] This allowed life-saving organs to be transported large distances.

In 1999, liver transplants were performed at 125 centers. This success has bred a swarm of difficulties. On average, an organ transplant (kidney, liver, heart, lung, etc.) was performed on an American every 30 minutes in 1998. Unfortunately, a name is added to an organ waiting list every 16 minutes. This disparity has resulted in 62,000 individuals currently awaiting transplantation. Many of these people are very ill; 4,000 of them die each year.[15]

THE CHALLENGES AHEAD

As you read the following chapters, weaving through the intricacies of uncommon phenomena and best guesses, take a moment to reflect on the edgy philosophical problems involved in transplantation.

What Is Death?

Death has never been easy to accept, define, or understand. Even the actual moment of death has been the subject of intense theological debate. In seventeenth-century Germany, the time of death held great moment for the parents of unbaptized infants. They felt that the souls of these infants would wander unsaved for eternity. Many of these dead infants were taken to sacred places where "children's signs of life" were watched for carefully. Feathers were placed on their lips to catch a faint breath. Perhaps an eye or finger would move. These miracles allowed the infant to be quickly baptized and buried.[16]

Now we watch for the earliest signs of death, so that Harvard criteria might be applied. Although the concept of "brain death" is accepted in the United States, this acceptance is not universal. For instance, in Japan, it is quite recent. In many countries, it is absent.

Who Decides?

Who decides what happens to donated organs? In February 2000 the governor of Kentucky signed a bill that prohibited organ procurement organizations in Kentucky from sending an organ anywhere before first offering it to a Kentucky transplant center. At least 13 states have considered similar legislation. In Colorado a representative has sponsored legislation to direct organs away from adults when they could be used by children. The neighboring (if not neighborly) states of Wisconsin and Illinois have fought a public battle over organ allocation.

In 2000, Congress must reauthorize the National Organ Transplant Act, the legislation that now governs organ sharing in the United States. By the time the next edition of this book arrives on your desk, it is likely that three or four transplantation cases will be before the Supreme Court because of the contentiousness of issues of allocation.

Who decides who is eligible for transplantation? As time has passed, indications for transplantation have changed. Patients with large, malignant tumors are less likely to be offered transplantation because the percentage of long-term survivors does not approach that of patients with nonmalignant disease. In fact, the pressure to provide transplantation to the "sickest" patients (who have longer hospitalizations and decreased rates of survival) may actually cause the overall survival rate of American transplant recipients to decrease for the first time in decades.

Can Donation Be Increased?

The current system of organ donation depends on the good will of individuals and their families to provide access to the dead. For the most part, in the United States you may decide what is done to your body until you are dead. At that point, your remains become part of your estate. The wish of those involved in organ donation and transplant medicine is to increase donation by public awareness. In some other countries, there is presumed consent for organ donation. But here in the capitalistic United States, the word "donation" irks some individuals. One such person has led a movement to allow Americans to sell their organs: free enterprise dispensing with free organs.[17]

What's Next?

The shortage of organs for transplantation has led to enlargement of the donor pool to the living and the healthy, the "living-related" organ donors. Because of the safety of left-lobe operations for the donor, this type of transplantation has become common to treat children with severe liver disease. More recently, right lobectomy has been used to allow adults to donate to adults. This procedure is more risky and as it becomes more common, deaths of healthy donors will be inevitable. Is this justifiable?

We may have to decide what "related" means. A friend? A sister-in-law? The gentleman who wants to sell his body parts? There are interesting days ahead.

REFERENCES

1. Starzl TE, Groth CG, Makowka L. *Liver transplantation.* Austin, TX: Silvergirl, 1988.
2. Starzl TE, Putnam CW. *Experience in hepatic transplantation.* Philadelphia: WB Saunders, 1969.
3. Terasaki PI, ed. *History of HLA: ten recollections.* Los Angeles: UCLA Tissue Typing Laboratory, 1990.
4. Terasaki PI, ed. *History of transplantation: thirty-five recollections.* Los Angeles: UCLA Tissue Typing Laboratory, 1991.
5. Starzl TE. *The puzzle people: memoirs of a transplant surgeon.* Pittsburgh: University of Pittsburgh Press, 1992.
6. Calne R. *Art, surgery and transplantation.* London: Williams & Wilkins Europe, 1996.
7. Welch CS. A note on transplantation of the whole liver in dogs. *Transplant Bull* 1955;2:54.
8. Cannon JA. Brief report. *Transplant Bull* 1956;3:7.
9. Moore FD, Wheeler HB, Demissianos HV, et al. Experimental whole-organ transplantation of the liver and spleen. *Ann Surg* 1960;152:374–381.
10. White DJG. *Cyclosporin A.* Amsterdam: Elsevier Biomedical Press, 1982.
11. Kahan BD, ed. The Jean Borel Symposium. *Transplant Proc* 1999;31(suppl 1/2A):3S–61S.
12. Stahelin HF. The history of cyclosporin A (Sandimmune) revisited: another point of view. *Experientia* 1996;52:5–13.
13. Calne R. Recollections from the laboratory to the clinic. In: Terasaki PI, ed. *History of transplantation: thirty-five recollections.* Los Angeles: UCLA Tissue Typing Laboratory, 1991;4:227–243.
14. Kalayoglu M, Sollinger HW, D'Alessandro AM, et al. Successful extended preservation of the liver for clinical transplantation. *Lancet* 1988;1:617–620.
15. Institute of Medicine. *Organ procurement and transplantation.* Washington, DC: National Academy Press, 2000.
16. Imhof AE. *Lost worlds: how our European ancestors coped with everyday life and why life is so hard today.* Charlottesville: University Press of Virginia, 1996.
17. http://www.organkeeper.com, February 2000.

Transplantation of the Liver, edited by Willis C. Maddrey, Eugene R. Schiff, and Michael F. Sorrell. Lippincott Williams & Wilkins, Philadelphia © 2001.

CHAPTER **2**

Selection of Patients for Liver Transplantation

Emmet B. Keeffe

Liver transplantation is widely accepted as an effective therapeutic modality for a variety of irreversible acute and chronic liver diseases for which no satisfactory therapy is available.[1-12] Following the first unsuccessful efforts at human liver transplantation in 1963,[13,14] development of the procedure evolved at first slowly and steadily for 20 years and then rapidly over the past two decades. The growth of liver transplantation was facilitated by the conclusion of the National Institutes of Health Consensus Development Conference in 1983 that liver transplantation is not an experimental procedure but an effective therapy that deserves broader application.[1]

The 1-year survival rate following liver transplantation was 30% to 50% prior to 1980;[1,2] however, the introduction of cyclosporine and continued refinement in surgical techniques and comprehensive patient care resulted in 1-year and 3-year survival rates of 74% and 67% in the first 1,000 recipients treated with cyclosporine at the University of Pittsburgh in the early 1980s.[15] By the late 1980s and early 1990s, similar results were duplicated at other U.S. transplant centers. Based on data from the United Network for Organ Sharing (UNOS), the 1-year, 4-year, and 10-year survival rates of 24,900 adult patients undergoing liver transplantations from October 1, 1987, through September 29, 1998, were 85%, 76%, and 61%, respectively.[4] Patients receiving a transplant in 1994 or later had a significantly better chance of survival than those receiving a transplant before 1994 (87% vs. 83% 1-year survival rates, respectively). Analysis of demographic characteristics from the UNOS database showed that males, Asians and African-Americans, and patients older than 60 years had poorer survival rates.[4] Analysis by the patient's primary liver disease showed the best survival among patients with cholestatic liver diseases (primary biliary cirrhosis and primary scle-

rosing cholangitis) and the worst survival in patients with hepatic malignancy (Table 2.1).

The performance of just over 4,000 liver transplantations in the United States in approximately 110 liver transplant centers in 1998 attests to the growth and expanded indications for liver transplantation.[4] The number of liver transplants increased 2.4-fold (from 1,713 to 4,058) from 1988 to 1996, but the number of patients on the UNOS liver list increased 12.1-fold (from 616 to 7,467); as would be expected, the number of deaths of listed patients increased 4.9-fold (from 195 to 954).[16] As of the beginning of 1999, approximately 12,000 potential liver transplant candidates were listed with UNOS.[17] The current supply of donor livers is insufficient to meet this need, and organ donation has been stagnant or increased by only a few percent in recent years. These facts underscore the importance of the appropriate selection of candidates for liver transplantation.

The overall goals of liver transplantation are to prolong life and improve the quality of life, and a recent

TABLE 2.1. *Survival after adult liver transplantation by diagnosis*

Diagnosis	Survival (%)		
	1 yr	4 yr	7 yr
Primary sclerosing cholangitis	91	84	78
Primary biliary cirrhosis	89	84	79
Autoimmune hepatitis	86	81	78
Chronic hepatitis C	86	75	67
Alcoholic liver disease	85	76	63
Cryptogenic cirrhosis	84	76	67
Chronic hepatitis B	83	71	63
Malignancy	72	43	34

UNOS database 1987–1998; n = 24,900 patients.
Adapted from Seaberg EC, Belle SH, Beringer KC, et al. Liver transplantation in the United States from 1987–1998: updated results from the Pitt-UNOS liver transplant registry. In: Cecka JM, Terasaki PI, eds. *Clinical transplants 1998.* Los Angeles: UCLA Tissue Typing Laboratory, 1999:17–37.

E. B. Keeffe: Division of Gastroenterology, Department of Medicine, Stanford University School of Medicine, Stanford, California, 94304–1509

meta-analysis of the English language literature documents that transplantation does indeed result in improved functional status in recipients.[18] The selection of appropriate patients for liver transplantation to achieve these goals is difficult and inexact, with no uniformly agreed upon national criteria. Even more troublesome is determination of the ideal timing of liver transplantation during the course of advanced chronic liver disease, a problem that has recently been accentuated by the prolonged time required on the waiting list for a donor organ. Most liver transplant centers have established guidelines for selecting liver transplant candidates, and there is now general agreement on the minimal listing criteria for liver transplantation adopted by transplant professionals and UNOS.[19] The two most common indications for liver transplantation in adult patients are chronic hepatitis C and alcoholic liver disease, and the usual indications for liver transplantation in pediatric patients are biliary atresia or α_1-antitrypsin deficiency. Since the initial review of the worldwide experience with liver transplantation,[2] the major change that has occurred in patient selection is that fewer patients undergo liver transplantation for hepatic malignancy whereas many more patients with alcoholic liver disease and fulminant hepatic failure undergo transplantation.[4]

In most transplant centers, a selection committee composed of transplant surgeons, hepatologists, psychiatrists, nurse coordinators, social workers, and others involved in the care of liver transplant patients determine the suitability of potential candidates and their priority for transplantation. The selection committees at major transplant centers are facing increasing challenges relating to the expansion of liver transplantation without a parallel increase in the supply of liver donors. The formulation of responsible criteria for patients with indications associated with recurrent disease or less favorable outcomes is becoming increasingly difficult.[7,8] Finally, the constriction in health care budgets is another motivation for refinement in the selection and timing of transplantation to achieve the most cost-effective outcome, realizing that sicker patients incur greater costs for transplantation.[20–22] This chapter reviews factors important in the identification and selection of adult patients for liver transplantation and in the determination of optimal timing of surgery. Several topics mentioned in this chapter will be discussed in greater detail in other chapters. The application of liver transplantation has evolved dramatically since its inception, and it is likely that indications and selection factors will continue to be refined in the coming years.

GENERAL SELECTION CRITERIA FOR LIVER TRANSPLANTATION

Table 2.2 lists the general criteria that should be considered in the selection of patients for liver transplantation. The clinical, biochemical, and psychosocial information available regarding any patient with advanced chronic liver disease or fulminant hepatic failure is first reviewed to determine

TABLE 2.2. *Patient selection for liver transplantation*

I. Accepted indications for liver transplantation
  A. Advanced chronic liver disease
  B. Fulminant hepatic failure
  C. Inherited metabolic liver disease
II. Controversial indications for liver transplantation
  A. Alcoholic liver disease
  B. Chronic hepatitis B
  C. Unresectable hepatic malignancy
III. No alternative form of therapy
IV. No absolute contraindication to the liver transplantation
V. Willingness and ability to accept liver transplantation and comply with follow-up care
VI. Ability to provide for the costs of liver transplantation and posttransplantation care

From Keeffe EB. Selection of patients for liver transplantation. In: Maddrey WC, Sorrell MF, eds. *Transplantation of the liver,* 2nd ed. Norwalk, CT: Appleton & Lange, 1995:13–60, with permission.

if these global selection criteria are met. This list of considerations should serve as a eligibility checklist for physicians considering referral of patients for evaluation at liver transplant centers.

The liver diseases for which liver transplantation has been performed in adults can be divided into the three broad categories of advanced chronic liver disease, fulminant hepatic failure, and unresectable hepatic malignancy, although the latter represents a controversial and less common indication for transplantation in current practice. An additional important but small category of diseases for which liver transplantation may be indicated is inherited metabolic liver diseases in which the inborn error of metabolism resides in the hepatocyte, such that liver transplantation is curative. A wide variety of these metabolic liver diseases have been treated with liver transplantation.[4] In the majority of patients with metabolic conditions that also cause parenchymal liver disease (e.g., α_1-antitrypsin deficiency or hemochromatosis), conventional indications for liver transplantation are based on the presence of liver failure or early development of a malignant hepatic tumor. However, anatomically normal livers have also been replaced solely to correct the metabolic defect, for example, in cases of type I hyperoxaluria and familial hypercholesterolemia.[23–25]

Within the broad category of indications for liver transplantation are specific liver diseases that stimulate controversy regarding whether individual patients should be approved for transplantation. In particular, whether patients with alcoholic liver disease, chronic hepatitis B, or unresectable hepatocellular carcinoma should receive transplants has provoked debate. The possibility of recurrent disease or reduction in long-term survival following liver transplantation in these three conditions fuels their controversial status.[7,8] Because donor organs are in short supply and the number of annual deaths on the waiting list has increased more than fivefold in recent years,[16] discussion in selection committees often focuses on whether or not donor livers might better be allocated to individuals on the waiting list expected to have good initial as well as long-term survival after liver transplantation. The arguments for and against liver transplantation for these diseases are outlined later in this chapter.

Other general patient selection criteria in Table 2.2 that are important when considering referral for liver transplantation are the absence of alternative forms of therapy that may reverse liver failure and defer the need for liver transplantation and the absence of any absolute contraindication to the procedure (contraindications are discussed later in this chapter). An important criterion, which is often subjective and difficult to determine, is that the patient should be willing and able to accept liver transplantation and to comply with longitudinal follow-up care. Finally, the substantial costs of liver transplantation mandate the necessity of patients being able to provide for the costs of liver transplantation as well as follow-up medical care and medications. Insurance coverage for transplantation is determined prior to referral, and is facilitated by the assistance of a financial counselor at the transplant center.

MINIMAL LISTING CRITERIA FOR LIVER TRANSPLANTATION

At a consensus conference at the National Institutes of Health organized by the American Society of Transplant Physicians and the American Association for the Study of Liver Diseases, minimal listing criteria for liver transplantation were developed and subsequently published.[19] The goal of this conference was to establish rational and uniform listing criteria so that patients at all transplant centers across the United States would be placed on the UNOS waiting list using standardized criteria.

The natural history of cirrhosis was the most important factor used for establishing uniform minimal criteria for listing patients with chronic liver disease for transplantation. The general listing principle for a patient with chronic liver disease of any etiology was an estimated 90% or less chance of surviving 1 year with supportive care, that is, a survival rate less than that expected with liver transplantation at most centers. Large natural history studies of patients with compensated chronic liver diseases of miscellaneous causes[26,27] or compensated cirrhosis secondary to chronic hepatitis C[28] showed that survival of patients with cirrhosis is significantly decreased after the development of decompensation with ascites, portal hypertensive bleeding, or encephalopathy. For example, in a seven-center study of the natural history of chronic hepatitis C with cirrhosis, the probability of decompensation after the diagnosis of cirrhosis was 18% at 5 years and 29% at 10 years, and the 5-year survival was 91% for patients without decompensation versus 50% for patients with decompensation of cirrhosis.[28] Decompensation with the development of ascites is associated with a poor prognosis in part because of the associated risk of spontaneous bacterial peritonitis and hepatorenal

TABLE 2.3. *Non-disease–specific minimal listing criteria*

Immediate need for liver transplantation
Estimated 1-yr survival ≤90%
Child-Pugh score ≥7 (Child-Pugh class B or C)
Portal hypertensive bleeding or a single episode of spontaneous bacterial peritonitis, irrespective of Child-Pugh score

Adapted from Lucey MR, Brown KA, Everson GT, et al. Minimal criteria for placement of adults on the liver transplant waiting list: a report of a national conference organized by the American Society of Transplant Physicians and the American Association for the Study of Liver Diseases. *Liver Transpl Surg* 1997;3:628–637.

syndrome, both of which further shorten survival. In a report from the University of Barcelona, the 1-year survival rate was 38% for patients with an episode of spontaneous bacterial peritonitis versus 66% for patients without one.[29] Hepatorenal syndrome is an even more ominous complication of ascites, with one center reporting a median survival after the onset of hepatorenal syndrome of only 1.7 weeks.[30]

The most ominous complication of cirrhosis with portal hypertension is variceal bleeding, and patients who bleed have a poor long-term prognosis irrespective of treatment. Available treatment to prevent recurrent variceal bleeding includes endoscopic ligation or sclerotherapy, beta-blockers (e.g., propranolol, nadolol), transjugular intrahepatic portosystemic shunt, and surgical shunts.[31] All of these treatment modalities reduce the incidence of rebleeding, and some may improve survival; however, the only definitive therapy for patients with variceal bleeding is liver transplantation.

In summary, a cirrhotic patient who is Child-Pugh class A is likely to remain stable for a considerable period of time, but once decompensation occurs, survival is poor. Thus, criteria for listing a patient for liver transplantation should be clinical decompensation of cirrhosis, particularly ascites or variceal bleeding, or combined clinical decompensation and biochemical deterioration of hepatic synthetic function that meet criteria for Child-Pugh class B or C. A non-disease-specific minimal listing criteria that was proposed based on analysis of the natural history of cirrhosis in light of the expected outcomes after liver transplantation is shown in Table 2.3.

BIOCHEMICAL AND CLINICAL INDICATIONS FOR LIVER TRANSPLANTATION

Chronic advanced liver disease and fulminant hepatic failure usually are associated with a parallel decrease in the quality of life and with abnormalities of biochemical liver tests compatible with impaired hepatic synthetic function. It has traditionally been helpful to identify threshold laboratory indices and specific characteristics of the complications of liver disease that should prompt referral for liver transplantation.[5–12]

Chronic Liver Failure

The most common indication for liver transplantation is progressive end-stage cirrhosis, which accounts for more than 80% of indications at most transplant centers (Table 2.4).[4] A major challenge is to identify potential candidates for liver transplantation at a time in the course of their disease when survival longer than 1 to 2 years is unlikely but when major complications that may increase the risk of transplantation have not yet occurred. The usual 12-month to 36-month time on the waiting list has prompted transplant physicians to encourage earlier referral and to list patients as soon as they meet minimal listing criteria.

Table 2.5 outlines the major manifestations of chronic liver disease that lead to a consideration of liver transplantation.[5,6] These general criteria may be divided into clinical and biochemical indications for proceeding with liver transplantation. The biochemical indices for considering liver transplantation differ in patients with chronic cholestatic liver diseases, such as primary biliary cirrhosis and primary sclerosing cholangitis, versus those with chronic hepatocellular diseases, such as chronic viral hepatitis and alcoholic cirrhosis. For example, patients with chronic cholestatic diseases should be considered for liver transplantation when the serum bilirubin level is greater than 10 mg/dL, whereas patients with chronic hepatocellular disease warrant evaluation for liver transplantation when the serum albumin level is less than 3 g/dL or the prothrombin time is greater than 3 seconds over control. Transient and reversible lowering of the serum albumin level may be related to complications such as gastrointestinal bleeding or spontaneous bacterial peritonitis, but fixed values less than 3 g/dL should prompt referral for liver transplantation.

TABLE 2.5. *Biochemical and clinical indications for liver transplantation in chronic liver disease*

I. Cholestatic liver disease
  A. Bilirubin >10 mg/dL
  B. Intractable pruritus
  C. Progressive bone disease
  D. Recurrent bacterial cholangitis
II. Hepatocellular liver disease
  A. Serum albumin <3.0 g/dL
  B. Prothrombin time >3 seconds above control
III. Both cholestatic and hepatocellular liver diseases
  A. Recurrent or severe hepatic encephalopathy
  B. Refractory ascites
  C. Spontaneous bacterial peritonitis
  D. Recurrent portal hypertensive bleeding
  E. Severe chronic fatigue and weakness
  F. Progressive malnutrition
  G. Development of hepatorenal syndrome
  H. Detection of small hepatocellular carcinoma

From Keeffe EB. Selection of patients for liver transplantation. In: Maddrey WC, Sorrell MF, eds. *Transplantation of the liver*, 2nd ed. Norwalk, CT: Appleton & Lange, 1995:13–60, with permission.

These biochemical parameters should serve as guidelines and should always be considered within the context of the clinical complications of advanced liver disease, which are typically also present. However, an occasional patient will have advanced cholestasis or significantly impaired hepatic synthetic function in the absence of clinically decompensated liver disease, and the biochemical indices will be the primary stimulus for listing patients for liver transplantation. Most patients with these degrees of laboratory abnormalities will develop clinical complications on short-term follow-up.

Specific clinical indications for liver transplantation that are common to the cholestatic liver diseases include intractable pruritus, progressive bone disease, or recurrent superimposed bacterial cholangitis in patients with primary sclerosing cholangitis (Table 2.5). Hepatic encephalopathy is a frequent clinical problem in end-stage hepatocellular disease, but also may affect patients with advanced cholestatic liver diseases. In both types of liver disease, refractory ascites, spontaneous bacterial peritonitis, recurrent variceal bleeding, severe and chronic fatigue and weakness, progressive malnutrition, early hepatorenal syndrome, and the detection of a small, incidental hepatocellular carcinoma are all reasons to proceed with transplantation.

A number of attempts to identify preoperative variables that predict outcome following liver transplantation have been made, and some of the patient characteristics that have been identified warrant consideration in determining referral and selection for liver transplantation. Child-Pugh classification provides a reliable estimate of surgical risk in cirrhotic patients undergoing portosystemic shunts.[32,33] A retrospective review of more than 200 liver transplant recipients demonstrated that Child-Pugh class C also predicted a higher

TABLE 2.4. *Liver disease of adult transplant recipients in the United States*

Primary liver disease	Number	Percentage
Chronic hepatitis C	5,155	20.7
Alcoholic liver disease	4,258	17.1
Alcoholic liver disease and hepatitis C	1,106	4.4
Chronic hepatitis B	1,368	5.5
Cryptogenic cirrhosis	2,719	10.9
Primary biliary cirrhosis	2,317	9.3
Primary sclerosing cholangitis	2,178	8.7
Autoimmune hepatitis	1,194	4.8
Acute liver failure	1,555	6.2
Hepatic malignancy	951	3.8
Metabolic diseases	923	3.7
Other	1,050	4.2
Unknown	126	5.0

UNOS database 1987–1998; n = 24,900 patients.
Adapted from Seaberg EC, Belle SH, Beringer KC, et al. Liver transplantation in the United States from 1987–1998: updated results from the Pitt-UNOS liver transplant registry. In: Cecka JM, Terasaki PI, eds. *Clinical transplants 1998.* Los Angeles: UCLA Tissue Typing Laboratory, 1999:17–37.

mortality from liver transplantation.[34] In this same study, patients who were in the intensive care unit immediately before transplantation and patients who had preoperative renal dysfunction had higher hospital mortality rates. Earlier studies had also noted a correlation between pretransplantation renal failure with an elevated serum creatinine level and posttransplantation sepsis and death.[35,36] Shaw et al. reported that survival at 6 months following liver transplantation was highly correlated with operative blood loss and also with the preoperative level of coma, degree of malnutrition, serum bilirubin level, and prothrombin time.[37] Ideally, therefore, patients should be referred and undergo transplantation prior to the development of these biochemical and clinical variables that predict a poorer outcome. Finally, there may be a future role for quantitative dynamic liver function tests, such as monoethylglycinexylidide (MEGX) formation from lidocaine and indocyanine green half-life, in the selection and timing of liver transplantation, because these tests have been shown to be superior to Child-Pugh score in assessing short-term prognosis in cirrhosis.[38]

Specific characteristics of the clinical indicators or complications of cirrhosis that should prompt referral of patients with chronic liver failure for consideration for liver transplantation are reviewed later in this chapter.

Hepatic Encephalopathy

Early, subclinical hepatic encephalopathy is often undetected but may be suspected by subtle decreased awareness of the environment, disturbances in sleep, depression, emotional lability, increased somnolence, and altered speech.[39,40] The diagnosis may be confirmed by physical examination showing the typical flapping tremor of asterixis, response to medical therapy, or laboratory demonstration of an elevated venous serum ammonia level, although the latter test is unreliable and more useful when done serially as a guide to therapy. Encephalopathy may occur spontaneously, but precipitating medical events are common and should be sought. Common precipitants include spontaneous bacterial peritonitis, gastrointestinal bleeding, azotemia, sedative and tranquilizer medications, constipation, or excessive dietary protein intake. The pathophysiology of hepatic encephalopathy remains uncertain, but ammonia intoxication from reduced hepatic metabolism or shunting of portal blood, alteration of serum amino acid pattern with increased aromatic amino acids and decreased branched-chain amino acids, or a circulating endogenous benzodiazepine receptor ligand have all been proposed.[41]

Mild hepatic encephalopathy alone is not an indication for liver transplantation, because it responds well to medical treatment with lactulose or neomycin and modest restriction of dietary protein.[41] The new onset of encephalopathy should prompt a search for a precipitating factor. On the other hand, recurrent or moderate to severe hepatic encephalopathy should prompt consideration of liver transplantation, which will reverse encephalopathy and may also improve the more serious hepatocerebral degeneration characterized by motor disturbances superimposed on hepatic encephalopathy.[42]

Refractory Ascites

Ascites itself is not an indication for liver transplantation, but increasing diuretic requirements or the need for alternative treatment such as large volume paracentesis should prompt referral for transplantation. The new development of ascites should be evaluated with diagnostic paracentesis, a safe procedure even in the presence of coagulopathy,[43] to exclude infection and malignancy. Patients with uncomplicated cirrhotic ascites associated with portal hypertension will have a serum-ascites albumin concentration gradient greater than 1.1 g/dL, a neutrophil count of less than 250/mL, a negative bacterial culture, and negative cytology.[44]

The initial approach to the management of ascites involves a sodium-restricted diet and diuretic therapy, most typically spironolactone 75 to 150 mg daily and, if diuresis is not satisfactory, furosemide 40 mg daily.[45] Doses may be titrated to 300 to 400 mg of spironolactone daily and 80 to 160 mg furosemide daily, while paying attention to the side effects of hyponatremia, hypokalemia, and azotemia. Patients who are intolerant of diuretic therapy may benefit from repeated 4- to 6-L large volume paracenteses; it is generally recommended that 25 to 50 g of serum albumin be administered intravenously to prevent impairment of renal function or development of electrolyte abnormalities from this maneuver.[46,47]

Peritoneovenous shunting may be effective in controlling advanced ascites and also may improve renal function, but morbidity and mortality are high and shunting offers few advantages over large volume paracentesis.[48,49] In addition to the complications of infection, disseminated intravascular coagulation, clotting, and congestive heart failure, peritoneovenous shunts can complicate the technical aspects of liver transplantation because the shunt becomes encased in fibrin and may be difficult to remove.[9] A better option for ascites refractory to diuretics and requiring frequent large volume paracenteses is transjugular intrahepatic portosystemic shunt (TIPS), which has been shown to be beneficial in the treatment of advanced ascites.[50,51] This procedure allows control of ascites with modest doses of diuretics by lowering portal pressure and improving renal excretion; however, progression of liver failure leading to death or disabling encephalopathy are potential complications.

Spontaneous Bacterial Peritonitis

Spontaneous bacterial peritonitis has a prevalence of 10% to 15% among hospitalized patients with advanced cirrhosis.[52] A single episode of spontaneous bacterial peritonitis should prompt referral for liver transplantation because this complication tends to be recurrent and has a mortality rate that approximates 50%. A presumptive diagnosis of spontaneous bacterial peritonitis is made when the ascitic fluid neutrophil count is greater than 250/mL and secondary causes of peritoneal infection are excluded. Anaerobic gram-negative bacteria account for 60% to 80% of cultured organisms, with gram-positive cocci accounting for the remainder. The pathogenesis probably involves several mechanisms, including seeding of ascitic fluid that has reduced bactericidal and opsonic activity.

The diagnosis of spontaneous bacterial peritonitis requires a high index of suspicion, because the classic features of fever, abdominal pain and tenderness, and elevated peripheral blood white cell count may all be absent.[53] As many as one-third of cases may be classified as monomicrobial nonneutrocytic bacterascites, defined as a positive ascitic fluid culture with a neutrophil count of less than 250/mL.[53] Once the diagnosis of infected ascites is suspected, antibiotic treatment with a third-generation cephalosporin such as cefotaxime should be instituted.[54] The previous antibiotic regimen of ampicillin and gentamicin has been abandoned because of frequent aminoglycoside toxicity and lesser efficacy. Most transplant programs will defer transplantation for at least 48 hours and sometimes for up to 5 days of antibiotic therapy after infection of peritoneal fluid is documented. A study employing serial paracenteses to determine the response of spontaneous bacterial peritonitis to antibiotic treatment demonstrated that 86% of patients were culture-negative 6 hours after a single dose of cefotaxime and 95% were culture-negative after 48 hours of therapy.[55] Moreover, 5 days of cefotaxime 2 g IV every 8 hours is associated with the same outcome in terms of mortality, bacteriologic cure, and recurrence of ascitic fluid reinfection as is 10 days of therapy.[56] Once a patient has had an episode of spontaneous bacterial peritonitis, the outcome following liver transplantation is not as favorable.[57] Approaches to the prevention of recurrent spontaneous bacterial peritonitis, which is a common problem, include diuresis and prophylactic antibiotic therapy with norfloxacin or trimethoprim/sulfamethoxazole.[58–60]

Portal Hypertensive Bleeding

A single episode of variceal bleeding in an otherwise stable cirrhotic patient meets the minimal listing criteria for liver transplantation.[19] This qualification for listing is based on published studies showing that patients who experience esophagogastric variceal bleeding have a poor long-term prognosis irrespective of treatment, and few survive more than 5 years.[61–64] Prospective studies have shown that the likelihood of developing varices in patients with cirrhosis ranges from 35% to 80% and that 25% to 30% of cirrhotic patients who have esophageal varices will experience bleeding.[61,62] The risk of recurrent variceal bleeding approaches 70% within 2 years of the index hemorrhage. For each bleeding episode, the mortality rate ranges from 35% to 50%.

In view of this poor prognosis, it is clear that urgent treatment of acute variceal bleeding and interval management, including prevention of rebleeding, is essential in the potential liver transplant candidate. A number of new medical, radiologic, and surgical therapies have been introduced in an attempt to not only decrease the morbidity and mortality of portal hypertensive bleeding but also prevent the first variceal bleed.

Patients with suspected bleeding from varices require hospitalization and immediate endoscopy, even if bleeding has stopped spontaneously, as it often does. Endotracheal intubation should be performed in patients with a major bleed or significant hepatic encephalopathy to protect the airway and prevent aspiration. If the diagnosis of variceal bleeding is reasonably certain, vasoactive drugs (octreotide or vasopressin) can be initiated prior to endoscopy. Pharmacotherapy for acute variceal bleeding decreases portal flow and hence portal pressure and reduces bleeding during resuscitation, thus providing improved visualization during endoscopy. Prospective, randomized trials have historically shown that sclerotherapy is effective treatment for the control of acute variceal bleeding, with success rates ranging from 70% to 90% for initial control.[62–64] Endoscopic variceal band ligation is a preferable alternative to sclerotherapy because it is associated with fewer complications, a lower rate of rebleeding, and a decrease in the number of sessions required to obliterate varices.[65,66] The role of sclerotherapy in the control of active gastric variceal bleeding is much less certain and is associated with a high incidence of early rebleeding.[67]

Pretransplantation sclerotherapy followed by corticosteroid therapy as part of an immunosuppression program after liver transplantation may put patients at higher risk for esophageal perforation.[9,68,69] One liver transplant center reported a very high complication rate of sclerotherapy in 172 patients with cirrhosis (stricture, 56%; bleeding esophageal ulcers, 10.5%; perforation, 2.9%) and recommended balloon tamponade followed by urgent liver transplantation rather than sclerotherapy.[69] Logistics, including adequate time for pretransplant evaluation and organ availability, and the development of new modalities to control variceal bleeding, such as TIPS, usually make this approach unnecessary. However, the feasibility and effectiveness of urgent liver transplantation for variceal bleeding not controllable by standard measures has been demonstrated.[70] Most studies show the greatest benefit of liver transplantation for Child's class C patients who have had successful control of variceal bleeding by the usual treatment measures and then undergo elective transplantation.[71] Previous esophageal variceal bleeding does not have an adverse effect on survival after liver transplantation.[72]

Other therapies for control of active variceal bleeding include balloon tamponade, vasoconstrictive agents, TIPS, and operations such as emergency portosystemic shunt or transection of the esophagus.[63,64,73] Balloon tamponade is seldom used as a primary treatment of acute variceal bleeding but is useful in the patient who is exsanguinating; emergent placement of the balloon with control of bleeding can stabilize a patient prior to endoscopy. The agents that have been studied the most extensively in patients with active variceal bleeding include vasopressin and its longer-acting analogue terlipressin (glypressin), and somatostatin and its longer-acting analogue octreotide. Vasopressin and terlipressin cause splanchnic arteriolar constriction, which decreases portal venous inflow and pressure. Vasopressin is usually administered as an intravenous infusion at a rate of 0.4 U/min or less, and control of variceal bleeding is achieved in 50% to 70% of patients.[62,63] Vasopressin administration is associated with side effects, particularly cardiac complications, that may be serious in 25% of patients and fatal in 5% of patients. A major advance in the pharmacologic therapy of acute variceal bleeding has been the combination of nitroglycerin with vasopressin, which has several advantages over vasopressin alone.[74] Nitroglycerin results in an additional reduction of portal pressure that further improves the control of bleeding in up to 85% of patients and also ameliorates the systemic vasoconstrictive side effects of vasopressin.[62-64] Nitroglycerin is most often given by continuous intravenous infusion (starting at 40 μg/min, and titrating up to 100–400 μg/min), but may also be given sublingually or as a paste.

Vasopressin has generally been replaced by somatostatin (half-life, 1–2 min) or its longer-acting analogue octreotide (half-life, 1–2 hours) for the control of bleeding due to portal hypertension. Octreotide has a dramatic impact on splanchnic hemodynamics and decreases portal pressure primarily by decreasing portal venous flow. In contrast to vasopressin, somatostatin and octreotide have minimal impact on systemic hemodynamics. Controlled trials have shown better control of bleeding with octreotide than placebo, vasopressin or terlipressin, and balloon tamponade, and equal control of acute bleeding compared with sclerotherapy.[62-64,75] Octreotide may be given as a 50 μg bolus intravenously, followed by an infusion of 50 μg/h.

An important innovation in the control of acute variceal hemorrhage is TIPS.[76,77] Technical success and control of bleeding occur in more than 90% to 95% of cases. Morbidity (20%) and early mortality (5%) are acceptable, and portal pressure can be reduced below the level at which recurrent hemorrhage will occur. Variceal rebleeding is almost always due to stenosis or occlusion of the shunt. Hepatic encephalopathy complicates TIPS in 30% to 40% of cases but is severe in only 5% of patients. Factors that have been associated with an increased risk of hepatic encephalopathy include older age, Child's class C, hepatopetal rather than stagnant or hepatofugal portal blood flow, and use of larger diameter shunts.

TIPS may be the ideal bridge to liver transplantation. TIPS is currently used for patients who fail endoscopic therapy with banding or sclerotherapy; it may obviate the need for a rescue surgical shunt procedure, which increases the technical problems during subsequent liver transplantation. Trials comparing TIPS with chronic sclerotherapy after initial control of hemorrhage show that TIPS is superior to endoscopic therapy in the prevention of variceal rebleeding over 1 to 2 years in Child's class A or B patients with an episode of severe bleeding but is associated with an increased risk of hepatic encephalopathy.[78-80] TIPS may be less attractive in patients with Child's class C cirrhosis, particularly if associated with less severe bleeding, and probably should be reserved for those who fail initial endoscopic therapy or have recurrent bleeding. The long-term utility of TIPS must also be evaluated in the context of shunt stenosis or occlusion, which is a management problem after TIPS.

Emergency surgical shunts continue to be a treatment option for variceal bleeding if all else fails, but mortality is high and patients who survive for subsequent liver transplantation must undergo what is often a technically more difficult procedure.[81] Patients who do require a shunt should receive a distal splenorenal shunt or mesocaval shunt, both of which avoid the porta hepatis and do not contraindicate later liver transplantation.[82] A jugular interposition shunt that preserves the portal vein has also been used.[83]

In addition to the modalities of banding or sclerotherapy, TIPS, and surgical shunts, nonselective β-adrenergic blocking agents (propranolol and nadolol) can also prevent recurrent variceal bleeding.[62-64] Analysis of eight controlled studies of beta-blockers in the prevention of rebleeding demonstrates that bleeding is significantly reduced in the treated group compared with untreated controls (45% vs. 66%) but that survival rates are the same.[62-64] Data from several studies have also shown that chronic sclerotherapy is effective in reducing the incidence of repeat hemorrhage in patients with portal hypertension; however, the overall effect of variceal sclerosis on long-term survival is not as clear.[84] Among patients who have already had a variceal bleed, evidence is mounting that a combination of sclerotherapy and propranolol is better than either alone.[85] Propranolol has also been shown to be effective in the prevention of recurrent bleeding from portal hypertensive gastropathy, an important cause of portal hypertensive bleeding.[86] The dose of propranolol or nadolol is titrated to achieve a 25% reduction in resting heart rate. Contraindications to the use of beta-blockers include peripheral vascular disease, chronic obstructive pulmonary disease, diabetes mellitus, and heart block. Isosorbide mononitrate plus a beta-blocker may be more effective than a beta-blocker alone in the prevention of recurrent bleeding. The initial dose of isosorbide mononitrate is 10 mg daily, with titration to 20 mg twice daily if there is no hypotension or severe headaches.

Another recent development in the treatment of portal hypertension is the ability to prevent a first episode of variceal bleeding with the use of beta-blockers or nitrates or both. Meta-analyses of the value of propranolol or nadolol in the prevention of an index variceal hemorrhage indicate that these beta-blockers are safe and effective (16% of treated patients bled from varices vs. 27% of untreated control patients); beta-blocker therapy also reduces the mortality associated with episodes of bleeding and rebleeding.[87,88] Beta-blockers are particularly beneficial for the subgroup of patients with large or medium varices and portal pressure greater than 12 mm Hg, and these drugs should be considered in the transplant candidate with such varices who is undergoing evaluation or waiting for transplantation.[89] Isosorbide mononitrate plus a beta-blocker is more effective than a beta-blocker alone for primary prophylaxis of variceal bleeding. Isosorbide mononitrate can also be given as monotherapy in those patients who cannot tolerate beta-blocker therapy. Unfortunately, prophylactic sclerotherapy to prevent the initial hemorrhage from varices is associated with increased mortality and demonstrates no significant benefit.[90]

In summary, endoscopic therapy with band ligation or sclerotherapy is the treatment of choice for the control of acute variceal bleeding. For the prevention of recurrent variceal bleeding, long-term beta-blockers, possibly in combination with isosorbide mononitrate, should be used in addition to band ligation or sclerotherapy until varices are obliterated. Failure of this treatment protocol with continued bleeding or rebleeding should lead to the performance of a TIPS procedure or, in special circumstances, a portosystemic shunt, and consideration of more urgent liver transplantation. Finally, patients with medium or large varices who have never bled should receive medical therapy with beta-blockers and isosorbide mononitrate to prevent the first variceal hemorrhage.

Severe Chronic Fatigue and Weakness

Severe and disabling fatigue may on occasion be the predominant manifestation of advanced chronic liver disease. The symptom may be severe enough to prevent employment or to interfere with the activities of daily living. When fatigue is out of proportion to other manifestations of advanced liver disease, all other potentially contributing medical conditions, such as depression or hypothyroidism, must be excluded. However, fatigue may be the primary reason for proceeding with liver transplantation, particularly when found in association with biochemical evidence of major impairment in hepatic synthetic function.

Progressive Malnutrition

Advanced chronic liver disease is typically accompanied by varying degrees of malnutrition that is frequently unrecognized.[91] The presence of muscle wasting with reduced strength and endurance should be determined by direct questioning; when wasting is present, the patient should be promptly referred for consideration of liver transplantation. Malnutrition has long been recognized as a risk factor for postoperative complications in surgical patients, and the impact of malnutrition on the prognosis of patients with cirrhosis was first emphasized by Child and Turcotte in 1964.[32] It has been difficult to precisely define the impact of malnutrition on survival following liver transplantation.[92,93] On the other hand, malnutrition is a potentially reversible problem in patients with advanced liver disease,

and therefore attempts to improve nutritional status should be undertaken. Rigid protein restriction should be avoided prior to transplantation, particularly when there is no history of encephalopathy. Small, frequent meals with a low fat content may facilitate improved nutrition.

Hepatorenal Syndrome

Hepatorenal syndrome, or functional renal failure, is characterized by azotemia and oliguria (<500 cc per day) in association with a low urine sodium concentration (<10 mEq/L) in a patient with advanced cirrhosis and ascites.[94] The urinary sediment is normal, and the kidneys have no major structural abnormalities. In patients with cirrhosis and ascites, the probability of developing hepatorenal syndrome on follow-up is 18% at 1 year and 39% at 5 years; low serum sodium concentration, high plasma renin activity, and small liver size are predictors of this complication.[94] The pathogenesis appears to be related to portal hypertension with sequestration of blood in the splanchnic circulation and in the periphery, resulting in decreased effective intravascular volume and alteration of many renal vascular control systems. These alterations lead to diminished renal blood flow and reduced glomerular filtration rate.

Hepatorenal syndrome is a common cause of renal insufficiency in patients with advanced chronic liver disease and often develops during hospitalization for treatment of other conditions. It may be precipitated by volume depletion from excessive diuresis or diarrhea associated with lactulose use, spontaneous bacterial peritonitis, or agents such as nonsteroidal anti-inflammatory drugs. The differential diagnosis includes acute tubular necrosis (which some investigators report to be more common than hepatorenal syndrome in patients with cirrhosis), aminoglycoside nephrotoxicity, and chronic intrinsic renal disease.[95,96] Management is dependent on early recognition and treatment of precipitating events, if possible.

Patients have often been approved for liver transplantation prior to the development of hepatorenal syndrome, which occurs late in the natural history of advanced cirrhosis; hospitalization with supportive care is necessary upon development of this syndrome, and patients should be assigned a higher priority for transplantation. If a patient had not previously been considered for liver transplantation, urgent referral and an expedited evaluation is required. Supportive therapy with hemodialysis or continuous arteriovenous hemofiltration may be beneficial.[97,98] However, the only effective treatment is liver transplantation, and recent large studies confirm the original claim that transplantation reverses hepatorenal syndrome.[99–101]

Small Hepatocellular Carcinoma

Patients with a variety of chronic liver diseases, particularly chronic hepatitis C, chronic hepatitis B, and hemochromatosis, are at substantial risk of developing hepatocellular carcinoma.[102,103] These patients may have small carcinomas that are discovered by the pathologist at the time of sectioning the explant, are found during the transplant operation, or are detected during pretransplantation evaluation on routine surveillance by imaging studies. These lesions are typically smaller than 3 or 5 cm in diameter and have been called "incidental." Patients found to have an incidental hepatocellular carcinoma in the explant have a good prognosis, in contrast to patients with larger and symptomatic lesions, who have long-term survival rates of 20% to 30%.[104–106] Whether detection of a small tumor by imaging studies prior to transplantation can result in a timely operation and an equally good prognosis as for patients with truly incidental tumors found in the explant remains to be determined.

Acute Liver Failure (Fulminant Hepatic Failure)

Liver transplantation represents a major advance in the management of severe acute liver failure. The published experience with the treatment of such patients with liver transplantation has demonstrated substantial improvement in survival over the past 10 years.[107,108] Factors that have facilitated these improved results, other than the overall improvements in the surgical and medical management of liver transplant patients, include the development of a national donor procurement network that allows rapid identification of donors and the development of a multidisciplinary approach to the intensive care management of these patients, with anticipation and treatment of complications such as infection, bleeding, and cerebral edema.

Various terms have been applied to severe acute liver failure, which refers to the rapid onset of hepatic synthetic dysfunction in a patient without previous liver disease. *Fulminant hepatic failure* is a term that was originally employed to define the presence of acute liver failure with superimposed hepatic encephalopathy developing within 8 weeks of the onset of illness.[109] Other investigators have suggested that this term should be applied to the development of hepatic encephalopathy within 2 weeks of the onset of jaundice, whereas the term *subfulminant hepatic failure* (or *late-onset hepatic failure*) should be applied to a syndrome developing from 2 weeks to 3 months.[110] The potential importance of the latter stratification of hepatic failure is that certain complications can be expected in these two subgroups, for example, cerebral edema in the fulminant groups, and portal hypertensive complications in the subfulminant patients.

The selection of patients with acute liver failure who are likely to die and therefore would benefit from liver transplantation is challenging but can be predicted by certain biochemical and clinical features, the most popular of which were established at King's College Hospital in London and by the Paris group at Villejuif (Table 2.6).[111,112] The major responsibility of the referring physician is to consider early referral of patients who may require liver transplantation, so that aggressive supportive care can be provided and transplant evaluation and listing for a donor can be expedited.

TABLE 2.6. *Criteria for liver transplantation in fulminant hepatic failure*

Criteria of King's College, London[a]
I. Acetaminophen toxicity patients
  A. pH <7.3, or
  B. Prothrombin time >6.5 (INR) and serum creatinine level >3.4 mg/dL
II. Other patients
  A. Prothrombin time >6.5 (INR), or
  B. Any three of the following variables:
    1. Age <10 yr or >40 yr
    2. Etiology: non-A, non-B hepatitis, halothane hepatitis, idiosyncratic drug reaction
    3. Duration of jaundice before encephalopathy >7 d
    4. Prothrombin time >3.5 (INR)
    5. Serum bilirubin level >17.6 mg/dL

Criteria of Hôpital Paul-Brousse, Villejuif[b]
Hepatic encephalopathy and
I. Factor V level <20% in patient younger than 30 years
II. Factor V level <30% in patient 30 years or older

INR, international normalized ratio.
[a]Adapted from O'Grady JG, Alexander GJ, Hayllar KM, et al. Early indicators of prognosis in fulminant hepatic failure. *Gastroenterology* 1989;97:439–445.
[b]Adapted from Bernuau J, Samuel D, Durand F, et al. Criteria for emergency liver transplantation in patients with acute viral hepatitis and factor V (FV) below 50% of normal: a prospective study [Abstract]. *Hepatology* 1991;14:49A.

Traditionally, the degree of hepatic coma had been touted as the best predictor of the outcome of fulminant hepatic failure.[113] More recently, investigators at King's College Hospital in London proposed specific criteria defining a poor prognosis and the need for liver transplantation based on experience with over 500 patients.[111] Separate criteria were established for patients with fulminant hepatic failure secondary to acetaminophen overdose and patients with fulminant hepatic failure caused by viral or drug-induced hepatitis (Table 2.6). These criteria were predictive of outcome irrespective of the grade of encephalopathy. The same investigators had previously demonstrated the importance of the underlying cause of fulminant hepatic failure in predicting prognosis, with survival rates as high as 67% for failure caused by hepatitis A, 53% for acetaminophen overdose, and 39% for hepatitis B, but considerably lower for failure caused by non-A, non-B hepatitis, halothane hepatitis, and idiosyncratic drug reactions.[114] At Villejuif, selection for liver transplantation is made on the basis of factor V levels.[112] A factor V level of less than 20% in patients who are younger than 30 years, or less than 30% in patients who are older than 30 years, if associated with hepatic encephalopathy, is the indication for listing for transplantation.[112] Use of these prognostic criteria and daily assessment of patients will usually allow early determination of the need for transplantation prior to the onset of grade 4 hepatic encephalopathy with its attendant risk of cerebral edema. These criteria are immensely helpful in deciding who should be listed and undergo liver transplantation.

Less common causes of fulminant hepatic failure that have responded well to liver transplantation include *Amanita phalloides* mushroom poisoning,[115,116] Wilson's disease,[117–120] and acute fatty liver of pregnancy.[121] Mushroom poisoning is a dramatic event, with poisoning often occurring in small groups of patients, and appears to behave similar to acetaminophen poisoning, with marked coagulopathy but lesser degrees of hepatic encephalopathy.[115,116] Wilson's disease should be considered in any young patient with unexplained fulminant hepatic failure. Potential clues to the diagnosis are disproportionately low levels of aminotransferases and alkaline phosphatase, high serum copper concentration, and coexistent hemolytic anemia.[117,119,120] The diagnosis may be confirmed by the finding of a low serum ceruloplasmin level, detection of Kayser-Fleischer rings, and the presence of an elevated 24-hour urinary excretion of copper, with the latter being the most reliable indicator.

Aggressive supportive care is necessary in patients with fulminant hepatic failure to prophylactically treat and prevent the complications of bleeding, infection, cerebral edema, renal failure, and respiratory failure.[107,108] These complications are the main reasons that transplantation may not be possible, and they may also contribute to postoperative morbidity and mortality. An assessment of the applicability of liver transplantation for acute liver failure noted that 34% of patients who met criteria for liver transplantation could not undergo transplantation because of contraindications, primarily complications of liver failure such as infection, or because of death before a donor organ became available.[122] Extradural monitoring of intracranial and cerebral perfusion pressures, not only before and during liver transplantation but also in the immediate postoperative period, in patients reaching stage 3 or stage 4 encephalopathy may be a valuable adjunctive tool to clinical assessment.[123,124] Many episodes of increased intracranial pressure are silent, and monitoring allows prompt treatment with mannitol to prevent brain damage. Specific contraindications to liver transplantation in patients with fulminant hepatic failure include uncontrolled sepsis, brainstem dysfunction, and refractory hypotension.

Alternative treatment strategies for fulminant hepatic failure include auxiliary hepatic support with filtration devices or hepatocyte transplantation, heterotopic auxiliary liver transplantation, and use of split livers or living related donors in pediatric patients.[107,108] Hepatic support devices are experimental but theoretically could serve either as a bridge to liver transplantation or as definite therapy.[125] Heterotopic liver transplantation presents a number of technical problems that limit its widespread application.[107] Living-related liver transplantation may play a role in pediatric patients or even small adults with fulminant hepatic failure.[126]

CONTRAINDICATIONS TO LIVER TRANSPLANTATION

As more experience has been gained with liver transplantation, the list of contraindications to transplantation has been refined and shortened. The contraindications to liver transplantation that are considered absolute are generally, but not universally, agreed upon by transplant centers (Table 2.7). The general criterion for establishing an absolute contraindication is that the outcome of transplantation, when it has been performed, was extremely poor. In other cases, contraindications are based more on medical judgment than on published data.

In the case of human immunodeficiency virus (HIV) disease and liver transplantation, a reasonable amount of information is available. Retrospective data from the University of Minnesota on 12 patients who were HIV negative at the time of liver transplantation but acquired HIV disease from an infected donor organ or blood products demonstrate that outcome following liver transplantation is poor.[127] After a mean follow-up of 37 months, acquired immunodeficiency syndrome (AIDS) developed in 3 patients, and 4 of the 12 patients died after transplantation. With further follow-up, the number of these HIV-positive patients developing AIDS would be expected to increase. Fortunately, current screening of organ donors and blood products has reduced the problem of HIV infection with liver transplantation to a very small risk. In the University of Minnesota review, 10 patients were known to be HIV positive when they underwent liver transplantation; 9 of these 10 patients died, the majority from AIDS-related causes.[127] Data from the University of Pittsburgh regarding liver transplantation in HIV-positive patients are similar, with AIDS being the leading cause of death posttransplantation.[128,129] On the basis of these data, it seems reasonable to exclude patients who are HIV positive from liver transplantation, whether or not they have AIDS.

Common sense dictates avoiding liver transplantation in the presence of extrahepatic malignancy. The only potential exception to this dictum is the performance of liver transplantation in patients with unresectable hepatic metastases from slow-growing neuroendocrine tumors, such as carcinoid or islet cell tumors.[130,131] In reviews of the literature, approximately 50% of patients with these tumors survived long term following transplantation.[130,131] On the other hand, the increasing donor shortage and lower survival rate may be arguments against liver transplantation in this group of patients. Finally, the results of liver transplantation are so poor with cholangiocarcinoma that most centers now consider the pretransplantation diagnosis of this tumor an absolute contraindication to transplantation.[104]

TABLE 2.7. *Contraindications to liver transplantation*

Human immunodeficiency virus (HIV) seropositivity
Extrahepatic malignancy
Cholangiocarcinoma
Active untreated sepsis
Advanced cardiopulmonary disease
Active alcoholism or substance abuse
Anatomic abnormality precluding liver transplantation

In general, active untreated sepsis should be controlled prior to proceeding with liver transplantation. A practical issue that often arises is how long to treat patients with spontaneous bacterial peritonitis before it is safe to proceed with transplantation. The general criteria at most transplant centers is to treat patients for 2 to 5 days, which appears to be associated with a high rate of bacteriologic cure,[54,56] and then proceed with transplantation if a donor organ becomes available.

The decision to exclude patients from liver transplantation because of advanced cardiac or pulmonary disease often rests on the consensus opinion of consulting physicians as well as members of the transplant team. When deciding on the cardiac status of patients, the low systemic vascular resistance and reduced afterload associated with advanced cirrhosis may result in difficulty in predicting posttransplantation cardiac performance from the preoperative evaluation.[132] Patients with advanced chronic obstructive pulmonary disease or pulmonary fibrosis are excluded from liver transplantation, but reversible conditions such as asthma and respiratory impairment from ascites or muscle weakness secondary to chronic liver failure should not prohibit referral for transplant evaluation.[9]

The challenges of alcoholism or substance abuse in the potential liver transplant candidate are discussed later in the chapter. However, nearly all transplant centers consider active alcoholism or substance abuse an absolute contraindication to liver transplantation.

Finally, a number of anatomic abnormalities preclude liver transplantation, such as thrombosis of the entire portal circulation, although aggressive and novel ways to reconstruct the portal vein have been reported.[133] Isolated portal vein thrombosis, previously considered an absolute contraindication, is now a relative problem because portal vein thrombectomy and reconstructive surgery is often feasible.[134,135]

FACTORS INCREASING THE RISKS OF LIVER TRANSPLANTATION

A large number of conditions negatively affect survival after liver transplantation and have been generally classified as relative contraindications to liver transplantation. The relative importance of such factors on the decision to proceed with transplantation vary considerably from one transplant center to another.

Advanced Age

Advanced age by itself is not a contraindication to liver transplantation. In fact, patients older than 60 years are undergoing transplantation with increasing frequency and experiencing a favorable outcome at many transplant centers.[136–144] In the initial 20-year experience with liver transplantation, an upper age limit of 45 to 55 years was the usual arbitrary rule. Survival data from 1987 through 1998 published by UNOS show a significantly reduced survival fol-

TABLE 2.8. *Survival after adult liver transplantation by age*

Age (yr)	No.	Survival (%)		
		1 yr	4 yr	7 yr
16–29	1,923	86	80	75
30–39	3,491	88	80	74
40–49	7,866	87	79	73
50–59[a]	7,395	84	74	65
60+[b]	4,225	80	67	56

UNOS database 1987–1998; n = 24,900 patients.
[a]Relative risk of death = 1.5 ($p < 0.001$).
[b]Relative risk of death = 2.1 ($p < 0.001$).
From Seaberg EC, Belle SH, Beringer KC, et al. Liver transplantation in the United States from 1987–1998: updated results from the Pitt-UNOS liver transplant registry. In: Cecka JM, Terasaki PI, eds. *Clinical transplants 1998.* Los Angeles: UCLA Tissue Typing Laboratory, 1999:17.

lowing liver transplantation in recipients aged 50 to 59 years (1.5-fold relative risk of death) and an even further reduction in recipients aged 60 and older (2.1-fold relative risk of death) (Table 2.8).[4] In contrast to this UNOS data, the survival of older patients following liver transplantation at individual transplant centers is often not different from survival in younger patients (Table 2.9).[136–144] More than two-thirds of older patients who survive liver transplantation are fully functional.[138] However, an analysis of data from the University of Nebraska demonstrates that the severity of liver disease has a greater impact on survival in older than in younger patients.[145] These investigators noted that older patients classified preoperatively as being high risk had a significantly poorer than expected outcome; for example, low-risk older transplant patients had a 95% survival compared with a 29% survival in high-risk older patients.

In summary, older patients who undergo transplantation in a timely fashion appear to be physiologically equal to younger transplant recipients and have a good outcome. The two major precautions regarding liver transplantation in older individuals are the poorer results seen in some centers in subjects older than 65 years and the reduced survival of patients receiving transplants in the late stages of liver failure.

There is evidence that advancing age is associated with diminished immune function, as demonstrated by a higher incidence of neoplasia and decreased response to immunizations.[146,147] This immunosenescence might improve the results of liver transplantation in older subjects by leading to less allograft rejection, but this hypothesis remains theoretical.[137] More important, reduction in immunosuppressive drug dosage can be achieved and is particularly beneficial in older patients.

The pretransplantation evaluation of the older liver transplant candidate is similar to that of a younger patient, except that the increased risks of subclinical cardiac and pulmonary disease and malignancy dictate that appropriate consultations and screening tests be carried out. Older female patients are

TABLE 2.9. *Results of liver transplantation in older compared with younger subjects*

Author (ref.) and institution	Year	No. patients (Age in years)	Patient survival (%)			
			Overall	1 yr	2 yr	3 yr
Zetterman et al. (136) LTD	1998	600 (<60)		90		
		135 (≥60)		81*		
Stieber et al. (138) U. Pittsburgh	1991	965 (18–60)		78		71.4
		156 (61–76)		71.3*		65.5
Shaw (139) U. Nebraska	1992	Low risk				
		52 (all adults)	90.5			
		18 (>60)	94.5			
		Medium risk				
		27 (all adults)	85.2			
		15 (>60)	60			
		High risk				
		22 (all adults)	44.5			
		7 (>60)	28.6			
Pirsch et al. (141) U. Wisconsin	1991	84 (18–59)			76	
		23 (60–72)			83	
Emre et al. (140) Mt. Sinai	1993	107 (<60)[a]		86.6		
		56 (<60)[b]		66		
		19 (>60)[a]		84.2		
		20 (>60)[b]		75		
Bromley et al. (142) King's College	1994	289 (18–59)	68			
		42 (>60)	72			
de la Pena et al. (143) Pamplona	1998	43 (<60)	88.3			
		18 (≥60)	85.6			
Annual report (144) UNOS	1990	1514 (19–44)		72.8		
		1657 (45–64)		69.7		
		78 (>64)		60*		
Box et al. (137) BUMC	1993	618 (20–59)		85	78	73
		83 (60–64)		76	74	71
		20 (>64)		51	51	51
Box et al. (137) CPMC	1993	228 (18–59)	81.3			
		45 (60–72)	82			
		255 (18–65)	81.3			
		18 (66–72)	83.3			

LTD, Liver Transplant Database of the National Institute of Diabetes and Digestive and Kidney Diseases; UNOS, United Network for Organ Sharing; BUMC, Baylor University Medical Center; CPMC, California Pacific Medical Center.
*Significant difference.
[a]UNOS status 3–4 (home).
[b]UNOS status 1–2 (hospitalized).

also at particular risk for osteoporosis, and preoperative hormonal replacement therapy for these individuals appears reasonable.

Renal Failure

Patients being considered for liver transplantation may have variable degrees and types of renal dysfunction, including hepatorenal syndrome.[95,96] It is important to distinguish among hepatorenal syndrome, reversible acute renal failure, and chronic renal failure. Transient deterioration in renal function may be related to intercurrent events such as spontaneous bacterial peritonitis, gastrointestinal bleeding, or overzealous use of diuretics and is usually not a problem unless complicated by the development of hepatorenal syndrome. Renal biopsy, imaging studies, and historical information are helpful in the differential diagnosis of chronic renal insufficiency in the cirrhotic patient.

Chronic renal failure secondary to intrinsic renal disease is not a contraindication to liver transplantation, but necessitates consideration of simultaneous liver and kidney transplantation.[148] A particular dilemma in the setting of moderate renal failure is to determine whether renal dysfunction is likely to be irreversible after liver transplantation, thereby making it necessary to proceed with a combined liver and kidney transplantation.[148] In general, a low glomerular filtration rate that is fixed requires the combined procedure, which typically has a favorable outcome. In one series of seven patients undergoing combined liver and kidney transplantation, six patients were alive with functioning grafts.[148] In addition, the rate of liver allograft rejection in these patients was only 37.5% compared with 59.3% in patients having liver transplantation alone. Obviously, a detailed pretransplantation evaluation with the assistance of transplant nephrologists is necessary in patients with renal insufficiency.

Prior Hepatic Surgery

Prior abdominal surgery is an important consideration for the operating surgeon, but problems of extensive adhesions with portal hypertensive vessels can usually be overcome by meticulous surgical technique, although at the expense of increased blood loss and longer operative time.[149,150] Problems may occur from major operations such as the creation of portosystemic shunts for refractory variceal bleeding or biliary operations in patients with primary sclerosing cholangitis. However, even a previous cholecystectomy may affect the amount of dissection and blood loss required for liver transplantation.

In view of these considerations, physicians providing long-term management of patients with chronic liver disease are encouraged to consider alternative management options for uncontrollable hypertensive bleeding, such as TIPS, or endoscopic or radiologic approaches to patients with dominant obstructing strictures of the common bile duct in the setting of primary sclerosing cholangitis.

IMPACT OF SYSTEMIC DISEASES ON LIVER TRANSPLANTATION

A number of common systemic diseases have an impact on the decision of whether an individual patient is an acceptable candidate for liver transplantation.

Cardiac Disease

A dilemma is posed when a patient with end-stage liver disease who is otherwise a good candidate for liver transplantation is found to have moderate or severe coronary artery disease.[10,151,152] The general consensus is to treat the coronary artery disease before transplantation because liver transplantation poses the risks of myocardial ischemia or infarction, particularly in patients with either three-vessel or left main coronary disease.[10] If coronary artery disease cannot be suitably treated by percutaneous transluminal coronary angioplasty, then coronary artery bypass grafting can be considered. However, it is recognized that patients with end-stage liver disease may experience hepatic deterioration after bypass surgery, including worsening of coagulopathy and portal hypertensive bleeding. For this reason, prophylactic use of TIPS has been proposed before performing coronary

artery bypass surgery.[10] A few patients have even had coronary artery disease and end-stage liver disease treated with both bypass surgery and liver transplantation immediately following one another.[153]

A recent retrospective study from the University of Pittsburgh reveals a sobering outcome in 32 patients with coronary artery disease undergoing liver transplantation, with an overall mortality of 50% and morbidity of 81%.[151] The morbidity and mortality rates were similar in the 20 patients who had bypass surgery 6 months to 12 years prior to transplantation. This outcome of liver transplantation in patients with coronary artery disease needs to be studied further; however, if these poor results are confirmed, health care policy issues of cost effectiveness and donor scarcity may discourage the performance of liver transplantation in patients with documented coronary artery disease, whether or not they were treated adequately with coronary artery bypass in the past.

Patients with advanced cardiac disease associated with poor ventricular function, such as cardiomyopathy in the patient with alcoholic cirrhosis or hemochromatosis, or pulmonary hypertension in the patient with severe valvular heart disease, are not candidates for a liver transplantation.[4,5,152] Patients with aortic stenosis must be carefully evaluated, because a significant gradient associated with poor left ventricular function is associated with an unfavorable outcome after liver transplantation. Pretransplantation cardiac evaluation may not accurately predict cardiac function following liver transplantation secondary to the low systemic vascular resistance seen in patients with end-stage liver disease.[132]

Pulmonary Disease

It has been traditionally thought that patients with end-stage liver disease and severe hypoxemia caused by the hepatopulmonary syndrome would not experience improvement in pulmonary function following liver transplantation.[153] More recent evidence, however, shows that patients with hepatopulmonary syndrome associated with moderate to severe hypoxemia may rapidly improve following liver transplantation.[154,155] This syndrome occurs in 13% to 24% of patients with cirrhosis and portal hypertension, and these patients may have cyanosis and clubbing.[155] The hypoxemia is not the result of a true right-to-left shunt but is caused by impaired diffusion of oxygen due to intrapulmonary vascular dilations.[154]

Patients with other functional respiratory diseases, such as asthma, frequently do well with liver transplantation. One report even suggests that patients undergoing transplantation for α_1-antitrypsin deficiency may have improved pulmonary function following surgery.[153] Patients with previous pulmonary tuberculosis are acceptable candidates for transplantation. Active tuberculosis should be treated for at least 2 to 3 weeks and preferably for several months prior to transplantation, and treatment should be continued up to 1 year after surgery.[156] Obviously, patients with advanced and severe lung disease, such as chronic obstructive lung disease or pulmonary fibrosis, should be excluded from transplantation.

Endocrine Diseases

Patients with miscellaneous endocrine disorders such as diabetes mellitus, adrenal disorders, and thyroid disease need not be excluded from transplantation.

Inflammatory Bowel Disease

Patients with primary sclerosing cholangitis often have underlying inflammatory bowel disease, particularly ulcerative colitis.[157,158] Patients with bowel disease have a substantial risk of developing colon cancer, particularly when the bowel disease involves the entire colon and is long standing.[159,160] Patients with long-standing ulcerative colitis should undergo screening colonoscopy with multiple biopsies to exclude dysplasia or unrecognized adenocarcinoma. It has been suggested that immunosuppression following transplantation may facilitate the development of colon cancer; therefore, prophylactic colectomy should be considered after recovery from transplant surgery.[161]

Infectious Diseases

Infectious problems often defer but typically do not contraindicate liver transplantation. The most common infection experienced by patients with advanced end-stage liver disease is spontaneous bacterial peritonitis.[52] Peritoneal fluid is usually sterile after 48 hours of antibiotic therapy, and thus it is unlikely that transplantation needs to be delayed much beyond this period of time.[54,56] On the other hand, respiratory infections require aggressive and intensive therapy prior to proceeding with liver transplantation. Chronic serious infectious diseases, such as osteomyelitis, chronic fungal disease, and abscesses are significant contraindications to liver transplantation unless these conditions can be effectively treated by medical or surgical therapy.[9]

Severe Obesity

The feasibility of liver transplantation in patients with severe obesity has been demonstrated,[162] in spite of the proclivity for excessive weight gain in obese subjects following liver transplantation.[163] In an analysis of 18 patients with severe or morbid obesity undergoing liver transplantation, the survival rate was 100% and no major problems with further weight gain were noted.[162] As expected, wound infections were particularly common (61%), and some unique complications associated with obesity were also noted. This retrospective analysis confirmed that liver transplantation is indeed feasible in patients with severe obesity, who should therefore not be excluded from consideration for transplantation. Two later studies confirmed that long-term survival

after liver tranplantation is not different for severely obese patients.[164,165]

Previous Malignancies

With an increasing number of older patients being considered for liver transplantation, more referred patients will have a history of previously treated tumors. Questions often arise regarding the impact of the specific tumor on posttransplantation outcome and regarding the reasonableness and timing of transplantation. In an experience with 939 preexisting malignancies in 913 renal transplant recipients, some general conclusions and recommendations were offered.[166] Low recurrence rates posttransplantation (0%–10%) occurred with incidentally discovered renal tumors; lymphomas; and testicular, uterine cervical, and thyroid carcinomas. Intermediate recurrence rates (11%–25%) occurred with carcinomas of the uterine body; Wilm's tumors; and carcinomas of the colon, prostate, and breast. High recurrence rates (26%) occurred with carcinomas of the bladder, sarcomas, malignant melanomas, symptomatic renal carcinomas, nonmelanomatous skin cancers, and myelomas. It was concluded that a 2-year waiting period between the treatment of cancer and transplantation is appropriate for most cancers, with a few exceptions, and that more than 2 years is necessary for malignant melanomas, breast carcinomas, and colorectal carcinomas.[166]

Hemophilia

Patients with hemophilia may have advanced cirrhosis secondary to chronic hepatitis B or chronic hepatitis C acquired from transfusion of blood products. Both hemophilia A and hemophilia B have been corrected by liver transplantation.[167–169] Other bleeding disorders, including platelet dysfunction and Von Willebrand's disease, are not contraindications to transplantation but require special coagulation support.

TIMING OF LIVER TRANSPLANTATION

Timely referral and performance of liver transplantation early in the natural history of decompensated advanced liver disease is associated with a smoother operative and perioperative course, improved survival, and reduced costs. In an analysis of approximately 1,500 liver transplantations at the University of Pittsburgh, the 1-year survival rate for patients who were not dependent on hospital care at the time of transplantation was 86%, compared with approximately 70% for patients who were in the intensive care unit at the time of transplantation.[15] However, the 15% to 25% 1-year mortality rate associated with liver transplantation at various centers dictates waiting for unresponsiveness to medical therapy, decreased quality of life, the appearance of major complications of cirrhosis, or biochemical evidence of severe hepatic synthetic dysfunction before proceeding with transplantation. Ideally, patients should be referred when survival longer than 1 to 2 years is unlikely, but prior to progressive complications that increase the risks and costs of liver transplantation. The general biochemical and clinical indications for liver transplantation that were reviewed earlier have been established for patients with chronic cholestatic liver diseases, chronic hepatocellular diseases, and fulminant hepatic failure (Tables 2.5 and 2.6). The guidelines for referral or performance of liver transplantation in patients with chronic liver diseases, particularly the hepatocellular diseases, are broad and need better definition. As was noted previously, it is possible that quantitative tests of liver function will play a more important role in the future in helping decide the optimal timing of transplantation.

The best application of prognostic survival models to the timing and outcome of liver transplantation in chronic liver disease has been in the case of primary biliary cirrhosis, a disease with a predictable natural history.[170–173] In these models, age, serum bilirubin level, serum albumin level, and histology are commonly employed variables. The application of the Mayo model has demonstrated that liver transplantation improves survival as compared with supportive therapy in patients with primary biliary cirrhosis.[173] The Mayo model includes five independent prognostic variables predictive of survival, including serum levels of bilirubin and albumin, age, prothrombin time, and the presence of peripheral edema. Primary sclerosing cholangitis has a less predictable natural history because of a fluctuating course and the possibility of developing cholangiocarcinoma.[174,175] However, age, bilirubin level, histologic stage, hemoglobin level, and the presence or absence of inflammatory bowel disease were found to be independent predictors of prognosis in a large cohort of patients.[174]

Analysis of the natural history of other specific chronic liver diseases and the development of additional prognostic models will likely lead to more precise determination of the optimal timing for liver transplantation. It is unlikely, however, that any model will be perfect. Clinical judgment and assessment of the patient's quality of life, an important factor not found in any of the current models, will remain the cornerstone for deciding the timing of liver transplantation.

ACCEPTED INDICATIONS FOR LIVER TRANSPLANTATION

As shown in Table 2.4, the most common indications for liver transplantation are various causes of cirrhosis, including the chronic cholestatic liver diseases, which together account for more than 80% of all referrals for liver transplantations. This chapter's discussion of the diseases leading to transplantation has been arbitrarily divided into those that are generally accepted indications for transplantation, those that are controversial and changing, and those that represent uncommon but usually accepted indications for transplantation. The issues that most often trouble trans-

plant physicians regarding patients with the accepted indications for liver transplantation are not whether an individual patient should undergo transplantation but the proper timing of transplantation and the impact of coexistent systemic diseases, when present.

Primary Biliary Cirrhosis

Patients with primary biliary cirrhosis are generally good candidates for liver transplantation because the majority are middle-aged without other serious systemic diseases.[5,6,8–12] In contrast with most of the other liver diseases that may require liver transplantation, the natural history of primary biliary cirrhosis is reasonably well known and facilitates patient selection and the timing of liver transplantation.[170–172,176,177] The 5-year survival for patients with primary biliary cirrhosis ranges from 60% to 80% in several large series.[170–172,177] The easiest and most important variable to monitor, which is common to several prognostic models that define the natural history of this disease, is the serum bilirubin level.[170,176] Shapiro et al. noted that primary biliary cirrhosis is characterized by a long, stable phase with normal serum bilirubin concentration, followed by an accelerated phase of hyperbilirubinemia.[170] The mean survival of patients with a serum bilirubin level over 10 mg/dL is 1.4 years.

A number of studies from different institutions have been conducted using Cox proportional hazards regression models to determine independent risk factors to estimate survival.[176] The most widely used prognostic index formula was developed at the Mayo Clinic and involves age, serum bilirubin level, serum albumin level, prothrombin time, and the presence or absence of edema.[172] Although a single risk value does not dictate whether liver transplantation is needed, serial measurements may be helpful. In one report from New York, an abrupt change in the value of the risk factor calculated from the Mayo formula predicted a poor prognosis and supported proceeding with transplantation.[178]

Early reports of the results of liver transplantation in patients with primary biliary cirrhosis were favorable. In a large series of 97 liver transplantations performed in 76 patients, the projected 5-year survival was 66% and nearly all of the recipients were rehabilitated.[179] The Mayo survival model was used to evaluate the efficacy of liver transplantation in 161 patients undergoing transplantation at the University of Pittsburgh and Baylor University Medical Center.[173] In this study, application of the model showed that liver transplantation improved survival following transplantation as compared with the estimated survival with conservative therapy alone.

Bone disease may be particularly severe in primary biliary cirrhosis.[180,181] Transplantation is warranted, irrespective of the prognostic risk score, when pain or recurrent fractures, particularly vertebral collapse, occur. Osteopenia and reduced bone mineral density are generally present in patients with advanced primary biliary cirrhosis, but these complications are often not recognized until fractures occur. Bone mineral density should be assessed pretransplantation and followed serially posttransplantation. There is evidence that the bone disease associated with primary biliary cirrhosis worsens in the initial 3 to 6 months following transplantation but then improves to baseline by 1 year.[181] Bone mineral density in patients with primary biliary cirrhosis progressively improves after 1 year, and the incidence of fractures decreases. The potential pre- or posttransplantation role of therapy with calcitonin, biphosphonates, and estrogens, all of which are effective for postmenopausal osteoporosis, is uncertain but undergoing study.[181]

Finally, it should be noted that some but not all centers have reported that primary biliary cirrhosis may be recurrent after transplantation.[179,182] This debate is confused by the similar histologic appearances of primary biliary cirrhosis and chronic allograft rejection and by the persistence of the antimitochondrial antibody posttransplantation, albeit in lower titer. The possibility of recurrence in the transplanted organ should not influence decisions about the value of liver transplantation in advanced primary biliary cirrhosis.

Primary Sclerosing Cholangitis

The natural history of primary sclerosing cholangitis is not as well defined as for primary biliary cirrhosis. The disease usually progresses insidiously, but may be punctuated by episodes of superimposed bacterial cholangitis or jaundice from dominant strictures. Early reports suggested an overall poor prognosis.[157,158] However, studies from Yale University and the Mayo Clinic have suggested a more favorable course, with the latter institution reporting the median time of survival from diagnosis to be 11.9 years.[174,183] The Mayo survival model was recently expanded and revised based on further analysis of survival of patients from additional medical centers.[184] In this revised model, multivariate analysis revealed the following variables to be independent predictors of survival: serum bilirubin level, age, histologic stage, and the presence or absence of splenomegaly.

Approximately two-thirds of patients with primary sclerosing cholangitis have inflammatory bowel disease, usually ulcerative colitis. This bowel disease adversely affects allograft function posttransplantation, and the course of colitis is unchanged following surgery.[185] However, one report suggested that patients with both ulcerative colitis and primary sclerosing cholangitis are at increased risk for developing dysplasia or DNA aneuploidy, or both.[186] The development of colon cancer may be accelerated by liver transplantation and chronic immunosuppression.[161] In general, liver transplantation takes precedence over colectomy; the latter can be more safely performed posttransplantation in the presence of normal hepatic function without coagulopathy.[6,11]

Another unique feature of concern in primary sclerosing cholangitis is the risk of superimposed cholangiocarcinoma.[175,187,188] Clues to the diagnosis of cholangiocarcinoma include the rapid onset of persistent jaundice, pruritus, and weight loss with a marked rise in alkaline phosphatase and serum bilirubin levels. Cholangiography often shows segmental dilation of intrahepatic ducts. Repeated attempts at brushing for cytology by percutaneous or endoscopic approaches should be employed to distinguish benign from malignant dominant strictures.[189] Most centers consider the demonstration of a cholangiocarcinoma to be an absolute contraindication to transplantation.

In general, patients with primary sclerosing cholangitis should be referred early for consideration of liver transplantation, because the results of liver replacement are often good; transplantation should be performed before the development of cholangiocarcinoma or advanced cholestasis with liver failure.[190,191] For this reason, aggressive surgical approaches to relieve extrahepatic biliary tract obstruction prior to transplantation are not warranted.[192]

Autoimmune Hepatitis

Autoimmune hepatitis can usually be distinguished from chronic viral hepatitis and other etiologies of histologic chronic hepatitis (e.g., Wilson's disease) by clinical evaluation combined with immunologic and serologic testing. Autoimmune hepatitis is subdivided on the basis of immunologic testing into three subtypes (Table 2.10).[193,194] Hyperglobulinemia, female gender, and the presence of other autoimmune diseases characterize all three types. Type 1 is classic autoimmune hepatitis with positive antinuclear or smooth muscle antibodies, or both. Type 2 autoimmune hepatitis occurs more commonly in the pediatric age range and is characterized by the presence of antibody to a liver and kidney microsomal antigen (anti-LKM1). Type 3 autoimmune hepatitis is the least well characterized clinically, but is diagnosed by the presence of antibodies to soluble liver antigen (anti-SLA) or liver-pancreas antigen (anti-LP), or both. Patients with any of the three types are treated with immunosuppressive drugs, usually corticosteroids with azathioprine, and are candidates for liver transplantation when medical treatment fails and decompensated liver disease occurs.

TABLE 2.10. *Etiology, diagnosis, and treatment of autoimmune hepatitis*

Type	Diagnosis	Treatment
Type 1 (classic)	1a: ANA ±SMA 1b: SMA only	Corticosteroids, azathioprine
Type 2	Anti-LKM1, (−) ANA, (−) SMA	Corticosteroids, azathioprine
Type 3	Anti-SLA, anti-LP, (−) ANA, (±) SMA, (±) AMA	Corticosteroids, azathioprine

ANA, antinuclear antibody; SMA, smooth muscle antibody; anti-LKM, liver and kidney microsomal antibody; anti-SLA, antibody to soluble liver antigen; anti-LP, antibody to liver-pancreas antigen; AMA, antimitchondrial antibody.

Patients with autoimmune hepatitis and cirrhosis often develop late liver failure and represent good candidates for liver transplantation.[6,9–11] Immunosuppressive therapy has been proven to prolong life but not to prevent the development of cirrhosis.[193] Only a small number of patients enter a permanent remission; the majority require long-term immunosuppressive drug therapy. Liver failure usually develops very insidiously in these patients, but failing synthetic function and clinical decompensation are the indicators that transplantation is required. In one retrospective analysis, failure to achieve remission within 4 years of immunosuppressive drug therapy and the presence of the human leukocyte antigens A1 and B8 were associated with a poor prognosis.[195] Liver transplantation improved the survival of patients with treatment failure and was not associated with recurrent disease.

Chronic Hepatitis C

Chronic hepatitis C is a frequent cause of end-stage liver disease requiring liver transplantation.[196] A common dilemma in the determination of the etiology of liver disease prompting liver transplantation is the occurrence of hepatitis C virus (HCV) infection in patients with alcoholic liver disease as well as those classified as having cryptogenic cirrhosis.[197] Most patients have had HCV infection for many years to several decades prior to the onset of liver failure.

Following liver transplantation, HCV reinfection occurs in nearly all patients.[198] Fortunately, the infection appears to be benign in 80% to 85% of patients on short-term and medium-term follow-up. Whether significant chronic hepatitis and cirrhosis will occur with long-term follow-up remains uncertain. The mild hepatitis seen on liver biopsies posttransplantation, when hepatitis B virus (HBV) and cytomegalovirus (CMV) infections are excluded, is nearly always explained by HCV infection.[198,199] The overlapping histologic features of HCV infection and rejection, which include portal and parenchymal mononuclear cell infiltrates, fatty change, swollen hepatocytes with necrosis, and occasional bile duct damage, make distinguishing between these two entities difficult.[196]

Hepatitis C virus infection can also be acquired via transplantation from infected donor organs or from blood products.[196] Whether or not anti-HCV–positive donor organs should be transplanted is controversial, because the rate of infection in the recipient is uncertain. The policy of most organ banks is to restrict the use of anti-HCV–positive donor organs to patients with chronic hepatitis C or for lifesaving transplantation of liver, heart, and lung.

Drug-Induced Liver Disease

The diagnosis of drug-induced liver disease is always one of exclusion in the setting of recent use of a new medication. This cause of liver disease is relatively more common in the elderly, who are less likely to have viral hepatitis and often use a large number of medications. Patients with drug hepatotoxicity often develop fulminant or, more commonly, subfulminant liver failure, but may also develop chronic liver disease, such as methotrexate-induced cirrhosis or isoniazid chronic hepatitis.[200,201]

Cryptogenic Cirrhosis

The etiology of most cases of chronic hepatitis and cirrhosis will be apparent after clinical evaluation, immunologic and virologic testing, and liver biopsy. However, a small percentage of patients have true cryptogenic chronic liver disease that does not appear to be autoimmune or viral, even after thorough evaluation.[202] In the UNOS analysis of etiologies of cirrhosis leading to liver transplantation, 10.9% of the 58.0% of cases diagnosed as cirrhosis were unspecified in terms of etiology (Table 2.4).[4] How many of these were truly cryptogenic and had thorough evaluation is uncertain. As in other types of chronic hepatitis and cirrhosis, patients with cryptogenic chronic liver disease generally represent good candidates for liver transplantation.

Hemochromatosis

Hereditary hemochromatosis is a recessive disorder of iron metabolism with a disease frequency of 5 per 1,000 population.[203,204] The disease is characterized by increased intestinal iron absorption with deposition of parenchymal iron in the liver, heart, pancreas, pituitary, and joints. Hepatic iron accumulation may result in cirrhosis, which may be complicated by hepatocellular carcinoma.[103] The diagnosis of hemochromatosis is established by a transferrin saturation index greater than 62%, a hepatic iron index greater than 2.0, and homozygosity for the C282Y gene.[203–205]

The reported experience with liver transplantation for hemochromatosis is limited.[206–208] Investigators from the University of Pittsburgh initially described good results following liver transplantation for hemochromatosis complicated by liver failure,[206] but more recent reports from the same institution and from California Pacific Medical Center demonstrated a less favorable outcome, with 1-year and actuarial survivals of 52% and 53%, respectively.[207,208] Both reports emphasized the impact of infection and coexistent hepatocellular carcinoma on postoperative morbidity and mortality, and heart disease with congestive heart failure and arrhythmias was common in the series from California Pacific Medical Center. A recent multicenter compilation of the results of liver transplantation in patients with hemochromatosis confirmed the high frequency of hepatocellular carcinoma.[103] Both reports noted reaccumulation of iron in posttransplantation allograft biopsies.[207,208]

In conclusion, the survival of patients undergoing liver transplantation for hemochromatosis is decreased compared with other transplant recipients. Posttransplantation infectious, malignant, and cardiac complications account for this reduced survival. Anticipation of the infectious and cardiac problems, and possibly the initiation of pretransplantation phlebotomy to unload myocardial iron, might lead to improved survival following liver transplantation.

Wilson's Disease

Patients with Wilson's disease may be considered for liver transplantation for fulminant hepatic failure or for cirrhosis with decompensated liver disease.[6,9–11,117] Liver transplantation in the setting of fulminant liver disease secondary to Wilson's disease was discussed earlier in this chapter.

Wilson's disease is an autosomal recessive disorder of copper metabolism characterized by accumulation of copper in the liver, central nervous system, eyes, and other organs.[209] Liver disease is usually evident in late childhood or early adolescence and is manifested by acute hepatitis, fulminant hepatitis, or chronic hepatitis. When the disease is not recognized until adult life, the usual presentation is that of cirrhosis with various complications. The diagnosis can be made by the finding of a low serum ceruloplasmin level (<20 mg/dL), increased urinary excretion of copper (>100 mg/ 24 h), and Kayser-Fleischer corneal rings on slit lamp examination. A liver biopsy showing increased quantitative copper deposition is confirmatory. Therapy with D-penicillamine or trientine will arrest further progression of disease and may be associated with some reversibility of the clinical manifestations. However, once advanced liver disease has developed, liver transplantation is required.

Sternlieb described three groups of patients who should be considered for liver transplantation: patients presenting with fulminant hepatitis, cirrhotic patients who fail to respond to 2 to 3 months of D-penicillamine therapy and supportive therapy for decompensated cirrhosis, and patients who have severe hepatic insufficiency and hemolysis following discontinuation of D-penicillamine.[117]

The prognosis following liver transplantation appears to be good, with no evidence for reaccumulation of hepatic copper.

α_1-Antitrypsin Deficiency

Most patients with clinical liver disease from α_1-antitrypsin deficiency have the Pi (protease inhibitor) ZZ phenotype.[210] α_1-Antitrypsin deficiency is usually evident in early childhood, with decompensated liver disease occurring in adolescence; however, liver disease may not present or be diagnosed until middle or late adult life.[211] More than 50% of adult patients have coexistent pulmonary disease associated with α_1-antitrypsin deficiency, but fortunately lung disease is usually mild. The diagnosis of α_1-antitrypsin deficiency is made by the finding of significant lowering of the serum α_1-antitrypsin level, Pi ZZ phenotype, and diagnostic liver biopsy with periodic acid-Schiff–positive, diastase-resistant cytoplasmic globules. One report documented a high prevalence of viral hepatitis in patients with both homozygous and heterozygous α_1-antitrypsin deficiency, and

thus diagnostic evaluation of these patients should be thorough.[212] There is no replacement therapy that will favorably affect the liver disease. Liver transplantation is indicated for the usual biochemical and clinical findings of decompensated liver disease and should be performed before advancing lung disease complicates or prevents transplantation.[213,214] Following liver transplantation, the patient takes on the Pi phenotype of the donor, and the α_1-antitrypsin level returns to normal.

CONTROVERSIAL INDICATIONS FOR LIVER TRANSPLANTATION

Probably the most controversial indications for liver transplantation over the past several years have been alcoholic liver disease, chronic hepatitis B, and primary hepatic malignancies. All three of these conditions raise concern regarding recurrent disease, and published data suggest that long-term survival is substantially reduced following liver transplantation in the latter two conditions compared with other transplant recipients. Probably the least controversial of these three conditions is alcoholic liver disease, although selection criteria remain a subject of debate.

Alcoholic Liver Disease

The initial worldwide experience with liver transplantation for alcoholic liver disease demonstrated that results were poor,[2] and there was major concern regarding the likelihood that patients would return to alcoholism after transplantation. However, the attitude regarding liver transplantation for alcoholic liver disease changed in 1988 when a report from the University of Pittsburgh demonstrated that the survival of 42 patients who received transplants for alcoholic cirrhosis was not different from survival of patients undergoing transplantation for other causes of cirrhosis and that only 2 of 35 patients surviving more than 6 months returned to abusing alcohol.[215] Subsequently, published survival data from several other transplant centers confirmed these results and demonstrated that long-term survival for alcoholic cirrhosis after liver transplantation is not different from that of other types of cirrhosis.[216–218] In addition, these centers showed that the rate of recidivism averaged 15%, and patients who drank usually did so only transiently and did not resume troublesome drinking. Recent UNOS data indicate that alcoholic cirrhosis, either alone or with chronic hepatitis C, now accounts for approximately 21.5% of the cases referred for liver transplantation (Table 2.4).[4]

What has remained most controversial regarding liver transplantation for alcoholic cirrhosis is the specific selection criteria. Some centers have developed a comprehensive, structured approach that involves evaluation by a multidisciplinary team, including medical, surgical, and psychiatric members, to predict compliance with medical follow-up and long-term sobriety.[216,217] At the University of Michigan, an alcoholism prognosis scale was utilized based on factors such as acceptance of alcoholism by the patient and family; prognostic indices such as substitute activities, social relationships, and self esteem; and indicators of social stability and functioning such as employment, permanent residence, and marriage.[216] The actuarial survival of alcoholic patients who received transplants at this center was not different from the survival of nonalcoholic patients.

At our transplant center, a conceptually similar approach was used in which patients were ranked by a multidisciplinary team as low risk, moderate risk, or high risk for recidivism and noncompliance (Table 2.11).[217,218] Patients who were classified as high risk were denied transplantation. Moderate-risk patients fell into an intermediate category and were typically followed by their referring physicians and transplant team to confirm compliance prior to listing for transplantation. Low-risk patients were approved and listed for transplantation. Retrospective analysis of this multidisciplinary approach supported the predictive reliability of this type of stratification: 16% of patients who were classified as low risk drank alcohol (all transiently), whereas 80% to 100% of patients classified as moderate risk or high risk drank or were noncompliant. Other liver transplant programs require a specific period of abstinence as the primary criterion for consideration of liver transplantation. In one institutional review, multivariate analysis showed that sobriety for less than 6 months was the only factor associated with recidivism after liver transplantation.[219]

TABLE 2.11. *Criteria employed to assign patients with alcoholism into risk groups for recidivism and noncompliance*

Low-risk patients
Long documented period of abstinence (>6 months)
No previous failure at alcohol rehabilitation
Never been told that alcohol was affecting health
Signed "Alcohol Rehabilitation Contract"
Good social support system
No psychiatric disorder

Moderate-risk patients
Intermediate period of abstinence (1 to 6 months)
One or more previous failures at alcohol rehabilitation
Signed "Alcohol Rehabilitation Contract"
Willing to enter alcohol rehabilitation program (if medically stable)
Minimal social support system
Relative psychiatric contraindications to liver transplantation

High-risk patients
Undocumented or short period of abstinence (<1 month)
Multiple failures to remain abstinent in spite of medical complications of liver disease
Refusal to sign "Alcohol Rehabilitation Contract"
Poor or absent social support system
Absolute psychiatric contraindications for liver transplantation

Adapted from Gish RG, Lee AH, Keeffe EB, et al. Liver transplantation for patients with alcoholism and end-stage liver disease. *Am J Gastroenterol* 1993;88:1337–1342.

Investigators in France have designed a successive, proportional hazards prognostic model for alcoholic cirrhosis and reported a case-control study in which each transplant patient with alcoholic cirrhosis was matched to a control patient.[220] The actual survival of patients with alcoholic cirrhosis after transplantation was compared with the survival of simulated and matched controls. The probability of surviving 2 years for transplant patients with alcoholic cirrhosis was 73%, compared with 67% for the matched controls and 67% for the simulated controls. Patients with severe alcoholic cirrhosis benefited most, with a 2-year survival of 64% versus 41% in the matched controls and 23% in the simulated controls, but there were no differences for patients at low or medium risk. The plea was made that further studies are needed regarding the benefit of liver transplantation in patients with less severe forms of alcoholic cirrhosis.

In summary, although the specific selection criteria for liver transplantation for alcoholic liver disease continue to be debated, the performance of liver transplantation in these patients has become much less controversial. Medicare and most state Medicaid programs, and nearly all insurance carriers, approve funding for liver transplantation in carefully selected abstinent patients with alcoholic cirrhosis who have not drunk for a period of time, typically more than 6 months, and have psychosocial predictors for long-term compliance and sobriety.

Chronic Hepatitis B

A controversial, but rapidly evolving, area in patient selection for liver transplantation is whether to perform transplants in patients with hepatitis B virus (HBV) infection. Historically, patients positive for hepatitis B surface antigen (HBsAg) have been regarded as poor candidates for liver transplantation based on data from the University of Pittsburgh showing that the actuarial survival of patients undergoing liver transplantation for chronic hepatitis B was 45% to 50%, which was 25% to 30% less than survival following liver transplantation for other etiologies of advanced cirrhosis.[221] The reduced survival following liver transplantation in patients with chronic HBV infection is related to graft reinfection, which is associated with a broad spectrum of disease ranging from an HBsAg carrier state to (much more commonly) progressive chronic hepatitis with cirrhosis and liver failure.[221–223] HBV reinfection appears to reproduce the original viral disease over an accelerated time course. There is even a report of hepatocellular carcinoma developing after liver transplantation for chronic hepatitis B.[224]

A rapidly progressive and usually fatal form of liver disease associated with HBV reinfection after liver transplantation is fibrosing cholestatic hepatitis, or fibrosing cytolytic hepatitis.[222,223] The histologic findings in this syndrome are characterized by ballooning degeneration of pericentral hepatocytes, a relative paucity of inflammatory cells, and periportal fibrosis. *In situ* hybridization studies performed on liver biopsy specimens from patients with this syndrome indicate that enhanced HBV transcription with strong expression of viral proteins (hepatitis B core antigen [HBcAg] and HBsAg) is present, supporting direct cytopathic injury by HBV in the pathogenesis.[225] Immunosuppression with corticosteroids and cyclosporine likely plays a role in the pathogenesis of fibrosing cholestatic hepatitis. In addition, fibrosing cholestatic hepatitis has been reported in association with variant viruses ("e minus" or "precore" mutants) characterized by active viral replication with production of HBcAg but not HBeAg.[226,227]

An important retrospective study of 17 European centers performing 372 consecutive liver transplantations for patients with HBV infection between 1977 and 1990 was reported.[228] Recurrence of HBV infection, defined as the reappearance of HBsAg in serum, varied according to a number of pretransplantation variables. The highest risk of recurrence occurred in patients undergoing transplantation for HBV cirrhosis (67%), and was higher in those who were HBV DNA positive (by dot hybridization) (83%) than in those who were HBV DNA and HBeAg negative (58%). A lower risk of recurrence was found in patients who had fulminant hepatitis B (17%) and cirrhosis related to coinfection with HBV and hepatitis D virus (HDV) (32%).

In this review of European centers, the overall 1-year and 3-year survival rates were 75% and 63%, respectively. However, patients who remained HBsAg negative had 1-year and 3-year survivals of 90% and 83%, respectively, which were significantly higher than patients reinfected with HBsAg (73% and 54%, respectively). Most important, the use of passive immunoprophylaxis with hepatitis B immune globulin (HBIG) significantly affected the risk of HBV recurrence, which was 74% to 75% in patients given short-term or no immunoprophylaxis but only 36% among those treated with HBIG for 6 months or longer. The presumed mechanism of HBIG immunoprophylaxis is to neutralize circulating HBV and minimize reinfection of the graft. Although expensive (approximately $20,000 annually), most U.S. centers have now adopted protocols based on the European experience that involve long-term administration of HBIG by the intravenous route.[229,230] Therapy with HBIG is monitored by maintenance of the anti-HBs level at more than 100 to 200 mIU/mL or, in some cases, by a more aggressive regimen to achieve levels greater than 500 mIU/mL,[231] although administration using a fixed dosing schedule is effective and may be more practical.[230] It appears that HBIG therapy must be provided long term, and probably indefinitely, to be effective.

Although the European experience suggests that the degree of viral replication is an important determinant of the incidence and severity of recurrent HBV infection after liver transplantation, data from some centers suggest that the efficacy of HBIG therapy may outweigh the factor of viral replication.[229–231] Some U.S. transplant centers are only willing to transplant patients who are HBeAg or

HBV DNA negative, or both. Insurance carriers have variable policies; for example, Medicare until recently excluded liver transplantation for all patients who are HBsAg positive, whereas the California state Medicaid program recently revised its former policy of paying for HBsAg-positive patients only if they were HBeAg negative to paying for HBeAg-positive patients as well. Finally, studies are underway evaluating the role of lamivudine, an oral nucleoside analogue that potently inhibits HBV replication, for prophylaxis of HBV infection after liver transplantation as a more convenient and potentially cheaper alternative to HBIG therapy.

A provocative paper was published suggesting that the outcome of liver transplantation for Asian patients with chronic hepatitis B is worse than for non-Asians.[232] In this study, Asian patients experienced higher early mortality (31% vs. 3%), more frequent HBV reinfection (72% vs. 32%) and higher mortality associated with recurrent HBV infection (87% vs. 22%) than non-Asian patients. Data from our institution confirmed the increased mortality in Asian patients, which appeared to be related to late referral and more advanced liver disease at the time of transplantation, but did not confirm a higher HBV reinfection rate or worse late mortality in Asians.[233]

Management of patients with recurrent HBV infection remains a challenge. Analysis of a multicenter experience by questionnaire found very poor results in patients undergoing retransplantation for liver failure associated with HBV recurrence, although HBIG was seldom used in these patients.[234] Of 38 patients undergoing retransplantation, 20 had the procedure performed for recurrent HBV infection; 9 patients (55%) died within 60 days, with only a single patient (5%) surviving long term. By contrast, patients undergoing retransplantation for other reasons, such as poor graft function or technical problems, had a better survival rate, with 11 of 18 patients (61%) alive at a mean of 21 months posttransplantation. Thus, retransplantation in HBV patients for graft failure associated with recurrent HBV infection historically has a poor outcome when HBIG is not used, although evidence suggests that retransplantation in combination with HBIG therapy can be successful.[231]

Medical management of patients with recurrent HBV reinfection is also challenging. Intravenous and oral prostaglandin E treatment was associated with a sustained favorable response accompanied by improvement in histology and reduction of viral antigen staining in 8 of 10 patients.[235] Famciclovir is a nucleoside analogue that inhibits HBV replication and has been shown to reduce or eliminate serum HBV DNA in patients with recurrent hepatitis B after liver transplantation.[236] This success with the use of oral famciclovir confirms our studies using intravenous ganciclovir to suppress viral replication and improve histology in patients with recurrent HBV infection after liver transplantation.[237] Multicenter studies of lamivudine, another oral nucleoside analogue that is an even more potent inhibitor of HBV replication, demonstrated reduction of serum HBV DNA to undetectable or low levels within weeks of initiation of therapy.[238]

Hepatic Malignancy

The primary malignant hepatic tumors for which liver transplantation has been performed are hepatocellular carcinoma and cholangiocarcinoma. In the early experience with liver transplantation, particularly from European centers, as many as one-third of patients undergoing transplantation had malignant disease.[105,239] However, there has been a steady shift away from transplantation for hepatic malignancy, and neoplasms now account for only approximately 3.8% of liver transplantation in the United States (Table 2.4).[4] Among the uncommon primary hepatic malignancies treated by liver transplantation, the results are reasonably good for epithelioid hemangioendotheliomas and hepatoblastomas but quite poor for hemangiosarcomas and lesions metastatic to the liver, with the possible exception of slowly growing neuroendocrine tumors.[240]

Results of liver transplantation for cholangiocarcinoma are particularly poor, and many transplant centers now consider this diagnosis an absolute contraindication for transplantation. This decision is based on the results of large institutional reviews[105,239] as well as the confirmation of poor results even with an aggressive posttransplantation protocol that includes adjuvant chemotherapy with 5-fluorouracil in combination with radiotherapy.[241] In the latter institutional experience, survival remained poor, with a 1-year survival rate of 53% and disease-free survival rate of only 40%.

A particular dilemma arises in the patient with primary sclerosing cholangitis who is at risk for the development of superimposed cholangiocarcinoma. It has been suggested that patients with this underlying hepatobiliary disease should proceed to transplantation somewhat earlier in their natural history, because survival after transplantation is so poor once cholangiocarcinoma has developed. The aggressive use of endoscopic and radiologic approaches to diagnosis with brushings and biopsy is warranted so that ineffective, unnecessary transplantation is not carried out on the patient with a known preoperative diagnosis of cholangiocarcinoma.[189]

A much more common malignancy is hepatocellular carcinoma, which complicates a number of underlying chronic liver diseases, particularly chronic hepatitis B and chronic hepatitis C.[105,239,240,242,243] An unusual variant of hepatocellular carcinoma, fibrolamellar hepatocellular carcinoma, is a clinicopathologic variant that may have a more favorable outcome after liver transplantation.[244] This tumor typically occurs in younger patients who do not have preexisting liver disease, and a precise pathologic diagnosis can be made on the basis of histologic features. In general, this variant has a more prolonged

natural history than nonfibrolamellar hepatocellular carcinoma and thus is more often resectable.[242,244] In the experience of the University of Pittsburgh, patients with fibrolamellar hepatocellular carcinoma who underwent subtotal hepatic resection had significantly better 5-year survival than patients undergoing resection for nonfibrolamellar hepatocellular carcinoma.[242] However, the 5-year survival rates of patients with standard and fibrolamellar hepatocellular carcinomas were not different following liver transplantation and averaged only slightly better than 35%.[242] In contrast to this institutional experience, a review of transplant centers around the world demonstrated that patients with fibrolamellar hepatocellular carcinomas had the same tumor recurrence rate but better survival rates at 2 and 5 years when compared with patients with ordinary hepatocellular carcinomas.[240] Another type of hepatocellular carcinoma, the incidental lesion found in the explant, is associated with a much lower recurrence rate and better survival than the usual hepatocellular carcinoma.[240,242]

In an international review, the Cincinnati Transplant Tumor Registry collected data between 1968 and 1991 from 637 patients, including 365 patients with ordinary hepatocellular carcinomas.[240] Tumor recurrences occurred in 141 patients (39%), and the 2-year and 5-year overall survival rates were 30% and 18%. These survival rates were worse than those of patients with incidental hepatocellular carcinomas (57% at 2 and 5 years) or patients with fibrolamellar tumors (60% and 55% at 2 and 5 years). A retrospective review from the University of Pittsburgh compared resection to transplantation for hepatocellular carcinomas and showed no differences in short-term and long-term survival rates overall, but a better outcome in patients with cirrhosis and tumor compared with patients with hepatocellular carcinoma and no cirrhosis.[242]

Data from several transplant centers have defined risk factors that predict recurrence of standard hepatocellular carcinoma following liver transplantation. Risks for recurrence include lymph node involvement, gross vascular invasion evident by angiography or computed tomography (CT), microscopic invasion of blood vessels in the specimen, tumor size greater than 5 cm, multiple lesions, infiltrating rather than circumscribed lesions, involvement of more than one lobe, and pTNM staging.[105,239,240,242] It has become clear that patients with small (variously defined as less than 2 cm, less than 3 cm, or less than 5 cm diameter), coincidental (diagnosed by imaging pretransplantation) or incidental lesions (found in the explant) have a reasonably good prognosis following liver transplantation. However, reports indicate that radiographic staging of early hepatocellular carcinomas is suboptimal.[245,246] In the Mayo Clinic experience, the 2-year disease-free survival rate was suboptimal for seven patients with small (1.0–3.5 cm diameter) incidental lesions (69%), primarily related to understaging of the disease.[245] In another study, which included ultrasonography, CT, and hepatic angiography, all imaging studies had a poor sensitivity (range, 17% to 58%) in detecting satellite lesions.[246]

A number of adjuvant therapeutic modalities are undergoing study for the prevention of recurrent hepatocellular carcinoma, particularly when the tumors are small and few in number.[247] Intravenous doxorubicin given preoperatively, intraoperatively, and postoperatively[248] and pretransplantation chemoembolization with doxorubicin, mitomycin-C, and cisplatinum[249] both show promise in improving the outcome of liver transplantation for hepatocellular carcinoma. In a report from the University of Milan, 48 patients were selected for transplantation on the basis of the hepatocellular carcinoma being less than 5 cm in diameter or consisting of three lesions each less than 3 cm in diameter; the actuarial survival rate was 75% at 4 years.[250] Patients who had tumors that did not meet the entrance criteria at the time of transplantation had a reduced survival (50%). In a similar report from Stanford University, the actuarial survival of 26 consecutive patients with hepatocellular carcinoma of all sizes was 65% at 3 years.[251] In this study, traditional prognostic factors for recurrent disease were not predictive of survival. In both studies, a substantial percentage of patients had adjuvant chemotherapy, including chemoembolization, either before or after liver transplantation, and this therapy as well as selection factors likely influenced a more favorable outcome.

A thorough evaluation for possible liver transplantation is warranted for patients with hepatocellular carcinoma. The tumor must be confined to the liver as confirmed by abdominal, pelvic, and chest CT scans as well as bone scan. Patients are often entered into experimental protocols to undergo adjuvant therapy pending transplantation. The long waiting time for a donor organ in many areas in the United States significantly interferes with the goal of adjuvant chemotherapy and prompt liver transplantation. Patients are often brought to the hospital along with a potential backup recipient; if intra-abdominal metastases are found at the time of abdominal exploration, transplantation is abandoned and the donor organ is used for the backup recipient.

In summary, the treatment of hepatocellular carcinoma is partial hepatic resection if a single tumor is present in a noncirrhotic liver in a location amenable to safe and complete resection. However, patients with unresectable tumors or tumors and significant cirrhosis (Child's class B and C) should be considered for liver transplantation. Unfortunately, there are no data to determine whether resection versus liver transplantation should be performed for the patient with Child's class A cirrhosis and a small hepatocellular carcinoma. The poor long-term survival with liver transplantation alone for hepatocellular carcinoma (i.e., 20% to 30%) necessitates that patients be carefully screened for the absence of predictors of recurrence as well as undergo adju-

vant chemotherapy, which may increase survival rates to the 60% to 70% range.

UNCOMMON INDICATIONS FOR LIVER TRANSPLANTATION

There is a relatively long list of uncommon indications for liver transplantation, including a large number of rare metabolic diseases. In general, liver transplantation for these indications is accepted, although the published experience with any one disease is often scant. The complete list of potential indications for liver transplantation reads much like the table of contents of any standard textbook of hepatology. A few selected unusual indications for liver transplantation are noted in this section.

Budd-Chiari Syndrome

Budd-Chiari syndrome is characterized by thrombotic or nonthrombotic occlusion of the large hepatic veins, inferior vena cava, or both.[252] The most common etiology of Budd-Chiari syndrome is a myeloproliferative syndrome, which is often latent and only diagnosed by bone marrow or peripheral blood mononuclear cell cultures showing erythroid colony formation in the absence of erythropoietin. Other etiologies include oral contraceptives, pregnancy, polycythemia rubra vera, paroxysmal nocturnal hemoglobinuria, tumors, and vena caval webs. The natural history of this syndrome is typically but not invariably progressive, with ultimate hepatic decompensation caused by outflow block with centrilobular necrosis, fibrosis, and ultimately a cardiac-type cirrhosis.[252]

The management of Budd-Chiari syndrome includes both medical and surgical modalities. Medical approaches are limited and involve treatment of the underlying hematologic disorder and management of ascites. Therapeutic approaches focus on the selection and timing of decompressive shunt surgery versus liver transplantation.[253–255] Portosystemic shunt operations can relieve hepatic sinusoidal congestion by creating an outflow tract; a side-to-side portacaval or mesocaval shunt is used when the inferior vena cava is patent, and a mesoatrial shunt when it is obstructed. Good long-term results are reported in selected patients undergoing early shunt surgery before advanced hepatic decompensation.[256]

Liver biopsy may be helpful in choosing between shunt surgery and liver transplantation.[253–255] Obviously, patients with advanced fibrosis or cirrhosis on biopsy warrant consideration for liver transplantation, as do patients with severe hepatic synthetic dysfunction. Liver transplantation is effective therapy for Budd-Chiari syndrome,[244,253–255,257,258] and reports of recurrent venous thrombosis are unusual.[259] Some physicians prefer to treat patients with long-term anticoagulation therapy, but this may not be necessary in most patients.

Metabolic Liver Diseases

A large number of metabolic liver diseases have been treated by liver transplantation.[260] The clinical presentation of metabolic liver diseases is variable and includes fulminant hepatic failure (e.g., Wilson's disease), cirrhosis (e.g., α_1-antitrypsin deficiency), hepatocellular carcinoma (e.g., tyrosinemia), life-threatening extrahepatic conditions (e.g., Crigler-Najjar syndrome, type 1), and nonhepatic organ failure (e.g., primary hyperoxaluria, type 1). The metabolic defect may reside in the liver, with the liver primarily affected by the disease (e.g., Wilson's disease) or with extrahepatic organs primarily affected (e.g., familial hypercholesterolemia). The metabolic defect may reside in extrahepatic organs, but with the liver the primarily affected organ (e.g., protoporphyria). Finally, there may be a generalized metabolic disorder in which the liver and other organs are involved (e.g., cystic fibrosis). The indications for liver transplantation in these various disorders are liver failure (as defined previously) when there is hepatic involvement, development of an early hepatocellular carcinoma, or beginning failure of a second organ. Because the majority of these diseases affect pediatric patients, further details will not be provided in this review but can be found in standard sources.[260]

Alagille Syndrome

Alagille syndrome, or arteriohepatic dysplasia, is a chronic cholestatic liver disease that is often associated with syndromatic features including a characteristic facies, vertebral and cardiovascular anomalies, ophthalmologic abnormalities, growth and mental retardation, and hypogonadism.[261] Some patients have a benign course, but most patients progress to liver failure. Hepatocellular carcinoma may also complicate Alagille syndrome.[262] Liver transplantation is efficacious in this syndrome, but the survival rate is somewhat lower than in other indications for transplantation because associated cardiopulmonary disease in Alagille syndrome results in significant posttransplantation morbidity and mortality.[263]

Polycystic Kidney Disease

Hepatic cysts are relatively common in patients who have autosomal dominant polycystic kidney disease.[264,265] The prevalence of hepatic cysts increases with advancing age. Other factors that may modify the expression of hepatic cystic disease are female gender, pregnancy, the degree of renal cystic disease, and the extent of renal functional impairment.[264,265] Patients with adult polycystic kidney disease have an increased life expectancy on the basis of general improvements in the management of end-stage renal disease. As a result, complications associated with hepatic cysts may be more commonly recognized. Most patients with multiple liver cysts are asymptomatic, but complications that have been reported include hemorrhage, infection, biliary tract obstruction, portal hypertension, and rare malignant transformation. A few patients have undergone liver transplantation, or combined liver and kidney transplantation if kidney failure is present, for massive liver size associated with either hepatic complications or intractable abdominal pain.[11]

Hepatic Trauma

Major and severe hepatic trauma typically results in mortality from exsanguination. Thus prompt and effective control of hemorrhage is the most essential step in the operative management of these patients. The range of surgical procedures includes packing around the liver, limited hepatic resection, and major hepatic segmental resection. Most recently liver transplantation was added to the spectrum of treatment options.[266–268] In one report, a patient with massive hepatic trauma that was not amenable to other surgical procedures underwent total hepatectomy followed by liver replacement 14 hours later.[266] Obviously, donor availability is critical to the success of liver transplantation in the setting of hepatic trauma and uncontrollable hemorrhage.

Systemic Diseases

Amyloidosis is a disease of protein metabolism in which insoluble protein fibers are deposited in the extracellular matrix and cause structural and functional damage of organs.[269] Familial amyloid polyneuropathy is the most common hereditary form of amyloidosis and affects the heart, kidneys, and eyes, as well as causing a peripheral neuropathy.[269,270] A number of mutations in the transthyretin gene have been described, but the Met-30 variant is by far the most common. In a follow-up report of four patients undergoing liver transplantation for treatment of familial amyloid polyneuropathy, the variant transthyretin was replaced by the wild type, and three of the four patients improved in terms of general well-being, ability to walk, and bowel function. However, there was little objective improvement of the peripheral neuropathy on long-term follow-up. Selection factors for liver transplantation in areas where familial amyloid polyneuropathy is prevalent are certainly critical because of the potential excessive demand for donor organs.

Sarcoidosis is a systemic granulomatous disease that primarily affects the lungs and lymph nodes but also involves the skin, eyes, and liver. The majority of patients with sarcoidosis have granulomas on liver biopsy, but symptoms of hepatic functional impairment are uncommon.[271] Unusual hepatic manifestations of sarcoidosis include chronic intrahepatic cholestasis, jaundice, liver failure, and portal hypertension with variceal bleeding. In addition, sarcoidosis may coexist with other diseases, such as primary biliary cirrhosis.[271] In an experience with nine patients undergoing liver transplantation for sarcoidosis, patient and graft survival were good and the doses of immunosuppressive agents required to prevent allograft rejection resulted in a remission of systemic sarcoidosis.[272]

FINAL CANDIDATE SELECTION AND LISTING FOR LIVER TRANSPLANTATION

Before final selection and listing for liver transplantation, the prospective candidate undergoes a pretransplantation evaluation, which can usually be completed on an outpatient basis over 2 to 3 days. The transplant coordinator and transplant hepatologist are the key individuals who facilitate this evaluation and educate the patient and family members. A comprehensive evaluation is required to determine if absolute or relative contraindications are present and to define the current status of systemic diseases. All outside medical records and liver biopsy materials are reviewed.

Routine evaluation includes hematologic and blood bank studies, complete chemistry profile, viral serology (HBV, HCV, HIV, CMV), chest radiograph, and computed tomography of the abdomen or abdominal ultrasound with examination of blood flow in hepatic vessels. Patients also have an electrocardiogram and undergo pulmonary function testing if there is a history of lung disease. Purified protein derivative (PPD) testing for tuberculosis is routinely performed. Renal function is assessed by creatinine clearance. Transplant candidates over the age of 60, candidates over the age of 50 with risk factors for coronary artery disease, and patients with a history of cardiac disease undergo cardiology consultation with appropriate cardiac studies, often including stress thallium and cardiac catheterization. Doppler echocardiography of carotid or peripheral vessels may also be appropriate. Consultations with a social worker, financial counselor, and psychiatrist are routine in most centers. Cancer screening with Papanicolaou test, mammogram, fecal occult blood testing, and flexible sigmoidoscopy, depending on age and gender, is completed.

Once the pretransplantation evaluation is complete, the patient is presented to the liver transplantation selection committee made up of the entire transplant team, including consultants, for categorization and prioritization. Patients are generally assigned to one of four categories: suitable and ready, with listing for a donor organ; suitable but too well, with placement on inactive status and continued follow-up with the referring physician; potentially reversible current contraindication, with treatment and recategorization at a later date; and absolute contraindication, with denial of transplantation.

Patients who are approved for liver transplantation by the selection committee are then listed for a donor organ with UNOS, and final approval by the insurance carrier or third-party payer is sought. Livers are donated in the spirit of altruism and are a limited national resource; thus, it is only right that donor livers be allocated in a fair manner. Federally designated local Organ Procurement Organizations fa-

cilitate equitable distribution of donor livers and act as a bridge between a donor hospital (a hospital with a patient who is an organ donor) and the local transplant center(s). It is the policy of UNOS that all potential recipients of organ transplants must be listed on the national UNOS computer waiting list, with the priority for a donor organ determined by factors discussed below.

UNOS establishes policies regarding organ distribution and allocation based on broad consensus and periodically amends these policies. The historical allocation scheme has been that the sickest patient who has waited the longest receives the next available liver. In general, a donor is matched to a potential recipient on the basis of several factors: ABO blood type, body size, time waiting, and degree of medical urgency. UNOS uses a computerized point system to distribute organs in a fair manner. Recipients are chosen primarily on the basis of medical urgency and time waiting within each ABO blood group. The policies regarding medical urgency or disease severity have undergone revision on a regular basis; the classification system as of early 1999 is given in Table 2.12.

The average waiting time for a patient to receive a liver once he or she is listed with UNOS has increased and may be as long as 12 to 36 months. The waiting time varies according to the blood type; for example, patients with O blood type wait longer on average, and patients with B blood type wait for a shorter period of time. Ob-

TABLE 2.12. *UNOS liver status classification for patients older than 18 years according to disease severity*

Status 1	Fulminant liver failure with life expectancy <7 days
	• Fulminant hepatic failure as traditionally defined
	• Primary graft nonfunction <7 days of transplantation
	• Hepatic artery thrombosis <7 days of transplantation
	• Acute decompensated Wilson's disease
Status 2A	Hospitalized in ICU for chronic liver failure with life expectancy <7 days, with a Child-Pugh score of ≥10 and one of the following:
	• Unresponsive active variceal hemorrhage
	• Hepatorenal syndrome
	• Refractory ascites/hepatic hydrothorax
	• Stage 3 or 4 hepatic encephalopathy
Status 2B	Requiring continuous medical care, with a Child-Pugh score of ≥10, or a Child-Pugh score ≥7 and one of the following:
	• Unresponsive active variceal hemorrhage
	• Hepatorenal syndrome
	• Spontaneous bacterial peritonitis
	• Refractory ascites/hepatic hydrothorax Or, presence of hepatocellular carcinoma
Status 3	Requiring continuous medical care, with a Child-Pugh score of ≥7, but not meeting criteria for status 2B
Status 7	Temporarily inactive

From the United Network for Organ Sharing (http://www.unos.org), with permission. Initially implemented in July 1997; later modified in January 1998 and August 1998.

viously, the waiting time for status 3 patients who are at home is longer than the wait for status 2B patients at home or status 2A and 1 patients who are hospitalized. Status 1 and 2A are status-dependent categories irrespective of time spent waiting; patients in these categories receive available organs before patients who are listed as Status 2B or 3. Unfortunately, many more patients today who are referred and selected at an appropriate time in the natural history of their disease will deteriorate during the long wait for a donor organ. Local referral physicians and transplant center personnel together support patients approved and listed for transplantation during this crucial waiting period.

REFERENCES

1. National Institutes of Health consensus development conference statement: liver transplantation, June 20–23, 1983. *Hepatology* 1984; 4:107S–110S.
2. Scharschmidt BF. Human transplantation: analysis of data on 540 patients from four centers. *Hepatology* 1984;4:95S–101S.
3. Starzl TE. History of liver and other splanchnic organ transplantation. In: Busuttil RW, Klintmalm GB, eds. *Transplantation of the liver.* Philadelphia: WB Saunders, 1996:3–22.
4. Seaberg EC, Belle SH, Beringer KC, et al. Liver transplantation in the United States from 1987–1998: updated results from the Pitt-UNOS liver transplant registry. In: Cecka JM, Terasaki PI, eds. *Clinical transplants 1998.* Los Angeles: UCLA Tissue Typing Laboratory, 1999:17–37.
5. Maddrey WC, Friedman LS, Munoz SJ, et al. Selection of the patient for liver transplantation and timing of surgery. In: Maddrey WC, ed. *Transplantation of the liver.* New York: Elsevier Science, 1988:23–58.
6. Keeffe EB. Selection of patients for liver transplantation. In: Maddrey WC, Sorrell MF, eds. *Transplantation of the liver,* 2nd ed. Norwalk, CT: Appleton & Lange, 1995:13–60.
7. Keeffe EB, Esquivel CO. Controversies in patient selection for liver transplantation. *West J Med* 1993;159:586–593.
8. Yoshida EM, Lake JR. Selection of patients for liver transplantation in 1997 and beyond. *Clin Liver Dis* 1997;1:247–261.
9. Wiesner RH. Current indications, contraindications, and timing for liver transplantation. In: Busuttil RW, Klintmalm GB, eds. *Transplantation of the liver.* Philadelphia: WB Saunders, 1996:71–84.
10. Rosen HR, Shackleton CR, Martin P. Indications for and timing of liver transplantation. *Med Clin North Am* 1996;80:1069–1102.
11. Fabry TL, Klion FM. Liver transplantation: selection of patients for referral. In: Fabry TL, Klion FM, eds. *Guide to liver transplantation.* New York: Igaku-Shoin Medical Publishers, 1992:79–101.
12. Donovan JP, Zetterman RK, Burnett DA, et al. Preoperative evaluation, preparation, and timing of orthotopic liver transplantation in the adult. *Semin Liv Dis* 1989;9:168–175.
13. Starzl TE, Marchiori TL, Von Kaulla KN, et al. Homotransplantation of the liver in humans. *Surg Gynecol Obstet* 1963;117:659–676.
14. Starzl TE, Marchiori TL, Rowlands DT Jr, et al. Immunosuppression after experimental and clinical homotransplantation of the liver. *Ann Surg* 1964;160:411–439.
15. Iwatsuki S, Starzl TE, Todo S, et al. Experience in 1,000 liver transplants under cyclosporine-steroid therapy: a survival report. *Transplant Proc* 1988;20:498–504.
16. Keeffe EB. Summary of guidelines on organ allocation and patient listing for liver transplantation. *Liver Transpl Surg* 1998;4(suppl 1): S108–S114.
17. U.S. Scientific Registry (UNOS). Richmond, VA: United Network for Organ Sharing, 1999. http://www.unos.org.
18. Bravata DM, Olkin I, Barnato AE, Keeffe EB, Owens DK. Health-related quality of life after liver transplantation: a meta-analysis. *Liver Transpl Surg* 1999;5:318–331.
19. Lucey MR, Brown KA, Everson GT, et al. Minimal criteria for placement of adults on the liver transplant waiting list: a report of a national conference organized by the American Society of Transplant Physicians and the American Association for the Study of Liver Diseases. *Liver Transpl Surg* 1997;3:628–637.
20. Evans RW, Kitzmann DJ. The "arithmetic" of donor liver allocation. In: Cecka JM, Terasaki PI, eds. *Clinical transplants 1996.* Los Angeles: UCLA Tissue Typing Laboratory, 1997:338–342.
21. Showstack J, Katz PP, Lake JR, et al. Resource utilization in liver transplantation: effects of patient characteristics and clinical practice. *JAMA* 1999;281:1381–1386.
22. Gilbert JR, Pascual M, Schoenfeld DA, et al. Evolving trends in liver transplantation: an outcome and charge analysis. *Transplantation* 1999;67:246–253.
23. Bilheimer DW, Goldstein JL, Grundy SM, et al. Liver transplantation to provide low-density-lipoprotein receptors and lower plasma cholesterol in a child with homozygous familial hypercholesterolemia. *N Engl J Med* 1984;311:1658–1664.
24. McDiarmid SV. Liver transplantation for metabolic disease. In: Busuttil RW, Klintmalm GB, Eds. *Transplantation of the liver.* Philadelphia: W.B. Saunders, 1996:198–215.
25. Cochat P, Scharer K. Should liver transplantation be performed before advanced renal insufficiency in primary hyperoxaluria type 1? *Pediatr Nephrol* 1993;7:212–218.
26. Ginès P, Quintero E, Arroyo V, et al. Compensated cirrhosis: natural history and prognostic factors. *Hepatology* 1987;17:122–128.
27. Propst A, Propst T, Zangerl G, et al. Prognosis and life expectancy in chronic liver disease. *Dig Dis Sci* 1995;40:1805–1815.
28. Fattovich G, Giustina G, Degos F, et al. Morbidity and mortality in compensated cirrhosis type C: a retrospective follow-up study of 384 patients. *Gastroenterology* 1997;112:463–472.
29. Andreu M, Sola R, Sitges-Serra A, et al. Risk factors for spontaneous bacterial peritonitis in cirrhotic patients with ascites. *Gastroenterology* 1993;104:1133–1138.
30. Ginès A, Escorsell A, Ginès P, et al. Incidence, predictive factors, and prognosis of the hepatorenal syndrome in cirrhosis with ascites. *Gastroenterology* 1993;105:229–236.
31. D'Amico G, Pagliaro L, Bosch J. The treatment of portal hypertension: a meta-analytic review. *Hepatology* 1995;22:332–354.
32. Child CG III, Turcotte JG. Surgery in portal hypertension. In: Child CG III, ed. *The liver and portal hypertension.* Philadelphia: WB Saunders, 1964:50–64.
33. Pugh RNH, Murray-Lyon IM, Dawson JJ, et al. Transection of the oesophagus for bleeding oesophaeal varices. *Br J Surg* 1973;60: 646–649.
34. Baliga P, Merion RM, Turcotte JG, et al. Preoperative risk factor assessment in liver transplantation. *Surgery* 1992;112:704–711.
35. Cuervas-Mons V, Millan I, Gavaler JS, et al. Prognostic value of preoperatively obtained clinical and laboratory data in predicting survival following orthotopic liver transplantation. *Hepatology* 1986; 6:922–927.
36. Danovitch GM, Wilkinson AH, Colonna JO, et al. Determinants of renal failure in patients receiving orthotopic liver transplants [Abstract]. *Kidney Int* 1987;31:195.
37. Shaw BW Jr, Wood RP, Gordon RD, et al. Influence of selected patient variables and operative blood loss on six-month survival following liver transplantation. *Semin Liv Dis* 1985;5:385–393.
38. Oellerich M, Burdelski M, Lautz HU, et al. Assessment of pretransplant prognosis in patients with cirrhosis. *Transplantation* 1991;51: 801–806.
39. Gitlin N, Lewis DC, Hinkley L. The diagnosis and prevalence of subclinical hepatic encephalopathy in apparently healthy, ambulant, non-shunted patients with cirrhosis. *J Hepatol* 1986;3:75–82.
40. Rikkers L, Jenko P, Rudman P, et al. Subclinical hepatic encephalopathy: detection, prevalence and relationship to nitrogen metabolism. *Gastroenterology* 1978;75:462–469.
41. Mullen KD. Hepatic encephalopathy. In: Rector WG Jr, ed. *Complications of chronic liver disease.* St. Louis: Mosby-Year Book, 1992: 127–160.
42. Powell EE, Pender MP, Chalk JB, et al. Improvement in chronic hepatocerebral degeneration following liver transplantation. *Gastroenterology* 1990;98:1079–1082.
43. Runyon BA. Paracentesis of ascitic fluid: a safe procedure. *Arch Intern Med* 1986;146:2259–2261.
44. Hoefs JC. Diagnostic paracentesis: a potent clinical tool. *Gastroenterology* 1990;98:230–236.
45. Runyon BA. Care of patients with ascites. *N Engl J Med* 1994;330: 337–342.
46. Kellerman PS, Linas SL. Large volume paracentesis in treatment of ascites. *Ann Intern Med* 1990;112:889–891.

47. Ginès P, Titó L, Arroyo V, et al. Randomized comparative study of therapeutic paracentesis with and without albumin in cirrhosis. *Gastroenterology* 1988;94:1493–1502.
48. Moskovitz M. The peritoneovenous shunt: expectations and reality. *Am J Gastroenterol* 1990;85:917–929.
49. Ginès P, Arroyo V, Vargas V, et al. Paracentesis with intravenous infusion of albumin as compared with peritoneovenous shunting in cirrhosis with refractory ascites. *N Engl J Med* 1991;325:829–835.
50. Ochs A, Rössle M, Haag K, et al. The transjugular intrahepatic portal-systemic stent-shunt procedure for refractory ascites. *N Engl J Med* 1995;332:1192–1197.
51. Lebrec D, Giuily N, Hadengue A, et al. Transjugular intrahepatic portosystemic shunt (TIPS) vs paracentesis for refractory ascites: results of a randomized trial. *J Hepatol* 1996;25:135–144.
52. Runyon BA. Spontaneous bacterial peritonitis: an explosion of information. *Hepatology* 1988;8:171–175.
53. Runyon BA. Monomicrobial nonneutrocytic bacterascites: a variant of spontaneous bacterial peritonitis. *Hepatology* 1990;12:710–715.
54. Felisart H, Rimola A, Arroyo V, et al. Cefotaxime is more effective than is ampicillin-tobramycin in cirrhotics with severe infections. *Hepatology* 1985;5:457–462.
55. Akriviadis EA, Runyon BA. Utility of an algorithm in differentiating spontaneous from secondary bacterial peritonitis. *Gastroenterology* 1990;98:127–133.
56. Runyon BA, McHutchison JG, Antillon MR, et al. Short-course versus long-course antibiotic treatment of spontaneous bacterial peritonitis: a randomized controlled study of 100 patients. *Gastroenterology* 1991;100:1737–1742.
57. Ukah FO, Merhav H, Kramer D, et al. Early outcome of liver transplantation in patients with a history of spontaneous bacterial peritonitis. *Transplant Proc* 1993;25:1113–1115.
58. Runyon BA, Van Epps DE. Diuresis of cirrhotic ascites increases its opsonic activity and may help prevent spontaneous bacterial peritonitis. *Hepatology* 1986;6:396–399.
59. Schubert ML, Sanyal AJ, Wong ES. Antibiotic prophylaxis for prevention of spontaneous bacterial peritonitis? *Gastroenterology* 1991;101:550–552.
60. Ginès P, Rimola A, Planas R, et al. Norfloxacin prevents spontaneous bacterial peritonitis recurrence in cirrhosis: results of a double-blind, placebo-controlled trial. *Hepatology* 1990;12:716–724.
61. Graham DY, Smith JL. Course of patients after variceal hemorrhage. *Gastroenterology* 1981;80:800–809.
62. Lebrec D. Portal hypertension. In: Rector WG Jr, ed. *Complications of chronic liver disease*. St. Louis: Mosby–Year Book, 1992:24–67.
63. Roberts LR, Kamath PS. Pathophysiology and treatment of variceal hemorrhage. *Mayo Clin Proc* 1996;71:973–983.
64. Stanley AJ, Hayes PC. Portal hypertension and variceal hemorrhage. *Lancet* 1997;350:1235–1239.
65. Laine L, Cook D. Endoscopic ligation compared with sclerotherapy for treatment of esophageal variceal bleeding: a meta-analysis. *Ann Intern Med* 1995;123:280–287.
66. Slosberg EA, Keeffe EB. Sclerotherapy versus banding in the treatment of variceal bleeding. *Clin Liver Dis* 1997;1:77–84.
67. Trudeau W, Prindville T. Endoscopic injection sclerosis in bleeding gastric varices. *Gastrointest Endosc* 1986;32:264–268.
68. Keeffe EB. Response—sclerotherapy and corticosteroids: a word of caution [Letter]. *Gastrointest Endosc* 1990;36:541.
69. Pilay P, Starzl TE, Van Thiel DH. Complications of sclerotherapy for esophageal varices in liver transplant candidates. *Transplant Proc* 1990;22:2149–2151.
70. Egawa H, Keeffe EB, Dort J, et al. Liver transplantation for uncontrollable variceal bleeding. *Am J Gastroenterol* 1994;89:1823–1826.
71. Henderson JM. Liver transplantation for portal hypertension. *Gastroenterol Clin North Am* 1992;21:197–212.
72. Ho KS, Lashner BA, Emond JC, et al. Prior esophageal variceal bleeding does not adversely affect survival after orthotopic liver transplantation. *Hepatology* 1993;18:66–72.
73. D'Amico G, Pagliaro L, Bosch J. The treatment of portal hypertension: a meta-analytic review. *Hepatology* 1995;22:332–354.
74. Bosch J, Groszmann RJ, Garcia-Pagan JC, et al. Association of transdermal nitroglycerin to vasopressin infusion in the treatment of variceal hemorrhage: a placebo-controlled clinical trial. *Hepatology* 1989;10:962–968.
75. Sung JJY, Chung SCS, Lai CW, et al. Octreotide infusion or emergency sclerotherapy for variceal haemorrhage. *Lancet* 1993;342:637–641.
76. LaBerge JM, Ring EJ, Gordon RL, et al. Creation of transjugular intrahepatic portosystemic shunts with the Wallstent endoprosthesis: results in 100 patients. *Radiology* 1993;187:413–420.
77. Rössle M, Haag K, Ochs A, et al. The transjugular intrahepatic portosystemic stent-shunt procedures for variceal bleeding. *N Engl J Med* 1994;330:165–171.
78. Sanyal AJ, Freedman AM, Luketic VA, et al. Transjugular intrahepatic portosystemic shunts compared with endoscopic sclerotherapy for the prevention of recurrent variceal hemorrhage. *Ann Intern Med* 1997;126:849–857.
79. Cello JP, Ring EJ, Olcott EW, et al. Endoscopic sclerotherapy compared with percutaneous transjugular intrahepatic portosystemic shunt after initial sclerotherapy in patients with acute variceal hemorrhage. *Ann Intern Med* 1997;126:858–865.
80. Kowdley KV. Evaluating TIPS trials: the devil is in the details? *Gastroenterology* 1998;114:847–849.
81. Langnas AN, Marujo WC, Stratta RJ, et al. Influence of prior portasystemic shunt on outcome after liver transplantation. *Am J Gastroenterol* 1992;87:714–718.
82. Esquivel CO, Klintmalm G, Iwatsuki S, et al. Liver transplantation in patients with patent splenorenal shunts. *Surgery* 1987;101:430–432.
83. Crass RA, Keeffe EB, Pinson CW. Management of variceal hemorrhage in the potential liver transplant candidate. *Am J Surg* 1989;157:476–478.
84. Infante-Rivard C, Esnaola S, Villeneuve JP. Goal of endoscopic variceal sclerotherapy in the long-term management of variceal bleeding: a meta-analysis. *Gastroenterology* 1989;96:1087–1092.
85. Vinel J, Lamouliatte H, Cales P, et al. Propranolol reduces the rebleeding rate during endoscopic sclerotherapy before variceal obliteration. *Gastroenterology* 1992;102:1760–1763.
86. Perez-Ayuso RM, Pique JM, Bosch J, et al. Propranolol in prevention of recurrent bleeding from severe portal hypertensive gastropathy in cirrhosis. *Lancet* 1991;337:1431–1434.
87. Poynard T, Cales P, Pasta L, et al. Beta-adrenergic-antagonist drugs in the prevention of gastrointestinal bleeding in patients with cirrhosis and esophageal varices: an analysis of data and prognostic factors in 589 patients from four randomized clinical trials. *N Engl J Med* 1991;324:1532–1538.
88. Pagliaro L, D'Amico G, Sörensen TIA, et al. Prevention of first bleeding in cirrhosis: a meta-analysis of randomized trials of nonsurgical treatment. *Ann Intern Med* 1992;117:59–70.
89. Merkel C, Marin R, Enzo E, et al. Randomized trial of nadolol alone or with isosorbide mononitrate for primary prophylaxis of variceal bleeding in cirrhosis. *Lancet* 1996;348:1677–1681.
90. The Veterans Affairs Cooperative Variceal Sclerotherapy Group. Prophylactic sclerotherapy for esophageal varices in men with alcoholic liver disease: a randomized, single-blind, multicenter clinical trial. *N Engl J Med* 1991;324:1779–1784.
91. O'Keefe SJD, El-Zayadi AR, Carraher TE, et al. Malnutrition and immuno-incompetence in patients with liver disease. *Lancet* 1980;2:615–617.
92. Reilly J, Mehta R, Teperman L, et al. Nutritional support after liver transplantation: a randomized prospective study. *JPEN J Parenter Enteral Nutr* 1990;14:386–391.
93. Jenkins RL, Benotti P, Bothe AA, et al. Liver transplantation. *Surg Clin North Am* 1985;65:103–122.
94. Ginès A, Escorsell A, Ginès P, et al. Incidence, predictive factors, and prognosis of the hepatorenal syndrome in cirrhosis with ascites. *Gastroenterology* 1993;105:229–236.
95. McCauley J, Van Thiel DH, et al. Acute and chronic renal failure in liver transplantation. *Nephron* 1990;55:121–128.
96. Arroyo V, Ginès P, Navasa M, et al. Renal failure in cirrhosis and liver transplantation. *Transplant Proc* 1993;25:1734–1739.
97. Wilkinson S, Weston M, Parsons V, et al. Dialysis in the treatment of renal failure in patients with liver disease. *Clin Nephrol* 1977;8:287–292.
98. Golper TA. Continuous arteriovenous hemofiltration in acute renal failure. *Am J Kidney Dis* 1985;6:373–386.
99. Iwatsuki S, Popovtzer MM, Corman JL, et al. Recovery from "hepatorenal syndrome" after orthotopic liver transplantation. *N Engl J Med* 1973;289:1155–1159.

100. Gonwa TA, Morris CA, Goldstein RM, et al. Long-term survival and renal function following liver transplantation in patients with and without hepatorenal syndrome—experience in 300 patients. *Transplantation* 1991;51:428–430.

101. Seu P, Wilkinson AH, Shaked A, et al. The hepatorenal syndrome in liver transplant recipients. *Am Surg* 1991;12:806–809.

102. Tsukuma H, Hiyama T, Tanaka S, et al. Risk factors for hepatocellular carcinoma among patients with chronic liver disease. *N Engl J Med* 1993;328:1797–1801.

103. Kowdley KV, Hassanein T, Kaur S, et al. Primary liver cancer and survival in patients undergoing liver transplantation for hemochromatosis. *Liver Transpl Surg* 1995;1:237–41.

104. O'Grady JG, Polson RJ, Rolles K, et al. Liver transplantation for malignant disease: results in 93 consecutive patients. *Ann Surg* 1988; 207:373–379.

105. Ringe B, Pichlmayr R, Wittekind C, et al. Surgical treatment of hepatocellular carcinoma: experience with liver resection and transplantation in 198 patients. *World J Surg* 1991;15:270–285.

106. Iwatsuki S, Starzl TE, Sheahan DG, et al. Hepatic resection versus transplantation for hepatocellular carcinoma. *Ann Surg* 1991;214: 221–228.

107. Mutimer DJ, Elias E. Liver transplantation for fulminant hepatic failure. In: Boyer JL, Ockner RK, eds. *Progress in liver diseases*, vol 10. Philadelphia: WB Saunders, 1993:349–367.

108. Lidofsky SD. Liver transplantation for fulminant hepatic failure. *Gastroenterol Clin North Am* 1993;22:257–269.

109. Trey C, Davidson CS. The management of fulminant heptic failure. In: Popper H, Schaffner F, eds. *Progress in liver disease*, vol 3. New York: Grune & Stratton, 1970:282–298.

110. Bernuau J, Rueff B, Benhamou JP. Fulminant and subfulminant liver failure: definition and causes. *Semin Liv Dis* 1986;6:97–106.

111. O'Grady JG, Alexander GJ, Hayllar KM, et al. Early indicators of prognosis in fulminant hepatic failure. *Gastroenterology* 1989;97: 439–445.

112. Bernuau J, Samuel D, Durand F, et al. Criteria for emergency liver transplantation in patients with acute viral hepatitis and factor V (FV) below 50% of normal: a prospective study [Abstract]. *Hepatology* 1991;14:49A.

113. Tygstrup N, Ranek L. Assessment of prognosis in fulminant hepatic failure. *Semin Liv Dis* 1986;6:129–137.

114. O'Grady JG, Gimson AES, O'Brien CJ, et al. Controlled trials of charcoal hemoperfusion and prognostic factors in fulminant hepatic failure. *Gastroenterology* 1988;94:1186–1192.

115. Pinson CW, Daya MR, Benner KG, et al. Liver transplantation for severe *Amanita phalloides* mushroom poisoning. *Am J Surg* 1990; 159:493–499.

116. Klein AS, Hart J, Brems JJ, et al. *Amanita* poisoning: treatment and the role of liver transplantation. *Am J Med* 1989;86:187–193.

117. Sternlieb I. Wilson's disease: indications for liver transplants. *Hepatology* 1984;4:15S–17S.

118. Stampfl DA, Munoz SJ, Moritz MJ, et al. Heterotopic liver transplantation for fulminant Wilson's disease. *Gastroenterology* 1990; 99:1834–1836.

119. McCullough AJ, Fleming CR, Thistle JL, et al. Diagnosis of Wilson's disease presenting as fulminant hepatic failure. *Gastroenterology* 1983;84:161–167.

120. Berman DH, Leventhal RI, Gavaler JS, et al. Clinical differentiation of fulminant Wilsonian hepatitis from other causes of hepatic failure. *Gastroenterology* 1991;100:1129–1134.

121. Ockner SA, Brunt EM, Cohn SM, et al. Fulminant hepatic failure caused by fatty liver of pregnancy treated by orthotopic liver transplantation. *Hepatology* 1990;11:59–64.

122. Castells A, Salmerón JM, Navasa M, et al. Liver transplantation for acute liver failure: analysis of applicability. *Gastroenterology* 1993; 105:532–538.

123. Lidofsky SD, Bass NM, Prager MC, et al. Intracranial pressure monitoring and liver transplantation for fulminant hepatic failure. *Hepatology* 1992;16:1–7.

124. Keays R, Potter D, O'Grady J, et al. Intracranial and cerebral perfusion pressure changes before, during and immediately after orthotopic liver transplantation for fulminant hepatic failure. *Q J Med* 1991;79:425–433.

125. Cao S, Esquivel CO, Keeffe EB. New approaches to supporting the failing liver. *Ann Rev Med* 1998;49:85–94.

126. Emond JC, Heffron TG, Kortz EO, et al. Improved results of living-related liver transplantation with routine application in a pediatric program. *Transplantation* 1993;55:835–840.

127. Erice A, Rhame FS, Heussner RC, et al. Human immunodeficiency virus infection in patients with solid-organ transplants: report of five cases and review. *Rev Infect Dis* 1991;13:537–547.

128. Dummer JS, Erb S, Breinig MK, et al. Infection with human immunodeficiency virus in the Pittsburgh transplant population. *Transplantation* 1989;47:134–139.

129. Tzakis AG, Cooper MH, Dummer JS, et al. Transplantation in HIV⁺ patients. *Transplantation* 1990;49:354–358.

130. Alsina AE, Bartus S, Hull D, et al. Liver transplant for metastatic neuroendocrine tumor. *J Clin Gastroenterol* 1990;12:533–537.

131. Lehnert T. Liver transplantation for metastatic neuroendocrine carcinoma. *Transplantation* 1998;66:1307–1312.

132. Seifert RD, Yang YG, Begliomini B, et al. Baseline cardiac index does not predict hemodynamic instability during orthotopic liver transplantation. *Transplant Proc* 1989;21:3523–3524.

133. Castaldo P, Langnas AN, Stratta RJ, et al. Successful liver transplantation in a patient with a thrombosed portomesenteric system after multiple failed shunts. *Am J Gastroenterol* 1991;86:506–508.

134. Shaw BW Jr, Iwatsuki S, Bron K, et al. Portal vein grafts in hepatic transplantation. *Surg Gynecol Obstet* 1985;161:66–68.

135. Lerut J, Tzakis AG, Brown K, et al. Complications of venous reconstruction in human orthotopic liver transplantation. *Ann Surg* 1987;205:404–414.

136. Zetterman RK, Belle SH, Hoofnagle JH, et al. Age and liver transplantation: a report of the Liver Transplantation Database. *Transplantation* 1998;66:500–506.

137. Box TD, Keeffe EB, Esquivel CO. Liver transplantation in elderly patients. *Pract Gastroenterol* 1993;17:22–27.

138. Stieber AC, Gordon RD, Todo S, et al. Liver transplantation in patients over 60 years of age. *Transplantation* 1991;51:271–272.

139. Shaw BW Jr. Liver transplantation in patients over 60 years of age. *Liver update: function and disease.* Cedar Grove, NJ: American Liver Foundation 1992;5:3–4.

140. Emre S, Mor E, Schwartz ME, et al. Liver transplantation in patients beyond age 60. *Transplant Proc* 1993;25:1075–1076.

141. Pirsh JD, Kalayoglu M, D'Alessandro AM, et al. Orthotopic liver transplantation in patients 60 years of age and older. *Transplantation* 1991;51:431–433.

142. Bromley PN, Hilmi I, Tan KC, et al. Orthotopic liver transplantation in patients over 60 years of age. *Transplantation* 1994;58:800–803.

143. de la Pena A, Herrero JI, Sangro B, et al. Liver transplantation in cirrhotic patients over 60 years of age. *Rev Exp Enferm Dig* 1998; 90:3–14.

144. Annual report of the U.S. Scientific Registry for Organ Transplantation and the Organ Procurement and Transplantation Network, 1990. Richmond, VA: UNOS; Bethesda, MD: Division of Organ Transplantation, Health Resources and Services Administration.

145. Castaldo P, Langnas AN, Stratta RJ, et al. Liver transplantation in patients over 60 years of age [Abstract]. *Gastroenterology* 1991;100: A727.

146. Weigle WO. Effects of aging on the immune system. *Hosp Pract* 1989;24(12):112–119.

147. Ershler WB. Biomarkers of aging: immunologic events. *Exp Gerontol* 1988;23:387–389.

148. Gonwa TA, Nery JR, Husberg BS, et al. Simultaneous liver and renal transplantation in man. *Transplantation* 1988;46:690–693.

149. AbouJaoude MM, Grant DR, Ghent CN, et al. Effect of portasystemic shunts on subsequent transplantation of the liver. *Surg Gynecol Obstet* 1991;172:215–219.

150. Langnas AN, Marujo WC, Stratta RJ, et al. Influence of a prior portasystemic shunt on outcome after liver transplantation. *Am J Gastroenterol* 1992;87:714–718.

151. Plotkin JS, Scott VL, Pinna A, et al. Morbidity and mortality in patients with coronary artery disease undergoing orthotopic liver transplantation. *Liver Transpl Surg* 1996;2:426–430.

152. Keeffe EB. Comorbidities of alcoholic liver disease that affect outcome of orthotopic liver transplantation. *Liver Transpl Surg* 1997;3: 251–257.

153. Morris JJ, Hellman CL, Gawey BJ, et al. Three patients requiring coronary artery bypass surgery and orthotopic liver transplantation. *J Cardiothorac Vasc Anesth* 1995;9:322–332.

154. Krowka MJ, Cortese DA. Pulmonary aspects of chronic liver disease and liver transplantation. *Clin Chest Med* 1989;10:593–616.

155. Scott V, Miro A, Kang Y, et al. Reversibility of the hepatopulmonary syndrome by orthotopic liver transplantation. *Transplant Proc* 1993; 25:1787–1788.

156. Chaparro SV, Montoya JG, Keeffe EB, et al. Risk of tuberculosis in tuberculin-positive liver transplant patients. *Clin Infect Dis* 1999;29: 207–208.

157. Wiesner RH, LaRusso NF. Clinicopathologic features of the syndrome of primary sclerosing cholangitis. *Gastroenterology* 1980;79: 200–206.

158. Chapman RWG, Marbough BA, Rhodes JM, et al. Primary sclerosing cholangitis: a review of the clinical features, cholangiography, and hepatic histology. *Gut* 1980;21:870–877.

159. Ekbom A, Helmick C, Zack M, et al. Ulcerative colitis and colorectal cancer: a population-based study. *N Engl J Med* 1990;323: 1228–1233.

160. Nugent FW, Haggitt RC, Gilpin PA. Cancer surveillance in ulcerative colitis. *Gastroenterology* 1991;100:1241–1248.

161. Higashi H, Yanaga K, Marsh JW, et al. Development of colon cancer after liver transplantation for primary sclerosing cholangitis associated with ulcerative colitis. *Hepatology* 1990;11:411–480.

162. Keeffe EB, Gettys C, Esquivel CO. Liver transplantation in patients with severe obesity. *Transplantation* 1994;57:309–311.

163. Palmer M, Schaffner F, Thung SN. Excessive weight gain after liver transplantation. *Transplantation* 1991;51:797–800.

164. Braunfeld MY, Chan S, Pregler J, et al. Liver transplantation in the morbidly obese. *J Clin Anesth* 1996;8:585–590.

165. Sawyer RG, Pelletier SJ, Pruett TL. Increased early morbidity and mortality with acceptable long-term function in severely obese patients undergoing liver transplantation. *Clin Transplant* 1999;13: 126–130.

166. Penn I. The effect of immunosuppression on pre-existing cancers. *Transplantation* 1993;55:742–747.

167. Lewis JH, Bontempo FA, Spero JA, et al. Liver transplantation in a hemophiliac. *N Engl J Med* 1985;312:1189–1190.

168. Merion RM, Delius RE, Campbell DA Jr, et al. Orthotopic liver transplantation totally corrects factor IX deficiency in hemophilia B. *Surgery* 1988;104:929–931.

169. Delorme MA, Adams PC, Grant D, et al. Orthotopic liver transplantation in a patient with combined hemophilia A and B. *Am J Hematol* 1990;33:136–138.

170. Shapiro JM, Smith H, Schaffner F. Serum bilirubin: a prognostic factor in primary biliary cirrhosis. *Gut* 1979;20:137–140.

171. Roll J, Boyer JL, Barry D, et al. The prognostic importance of clinical and histologic features in asymptomatic and symptomatic primary biliary cirrhosis. *N Engl J Med* 1983;308:1–7.

172. Dickson ER, Grambsch PM, Fleming TR, et al. Prognosis in primary biliary cirrhosis: model for decision making. *Hepatology* 1989;10: 1–7.

173. Markus BH, Dickson ER, Grambsch PM, et al. Efficacy of liver transplantation in patients with primary biliary cirrhosis. *N Engl J Med* 1989;320:1709–1713.

174. Weisner RH, Grambsch PM, Dickson ER, et al. Primary sclerosing cholangitis: natural history, prognostic factors, and survival analysis. *Hepatology* 1989;10:430–436.

175. Wee A, Ludwig J, Colley RJ Jr, et al. Hepatobiliary carcinoma associated with primary sclerosing cholangitis and chronic ulcerative colitis. *Hum Pathol* 1985;16:19–26.

176. Wiesner RH, Porayko MK, Dickson ER, et al. Selection and timing of liver transplantation in primary biliary cirrhosis and primary sclerosing cholangitis. *Hepatology* 1992;16:1290–1299.

177. Christensen E, Neuberger J, Crowe J, et al. Beneficial effect of azathioprine and prediction of prognosis in primary biliary cirrhosis: final results of an international trial. *Gastroenterology* 1985;89: 1084–1091.

178. Klion FM, Fabry TL, Palmer M, et al. Prediction of survival of patients with primary biliary cirrhosis. *Gastroenterology* 1992;102: 310–313.

179. Esquivel CO, Van Thiel DH, Demetris AJ, et al. Transplantation for primary biliary cirrhosis. *Gastroenterology* 1988;94:1207–1216.

180. Maddrey WC. Bone disease in patients with primary biliary cirrhosis. In: Popper H, Schaffner F, eds. *Progress in liver diseases,* vol 9. Philadelphia: WB Saunders, 1990:537–554.

181. Hay JE. Bone disease in liver transplant recipients. *Gastroenterol Clin North Am* 1993;22:337–349.

182. Polson RJ, Portmann B, Neuberger J, et al. Evidence for disease recurrence after liver transplantation for primary biliary cirrhosis: clinical and histologic follow-up studies. *Gastroenterology* 1989;97:715–725.

183. Helzberg JH, Peterson JM, Boyer JL. Improved survival with primary sclerosing cholangitis. *Gastroenterology* 1987;92:1869–1875.

184. Dickson ER, Murtaugh PA, Wiesner RH, et al. Primary sclerosing cholangitis: refinement and validation of survival models. *Gastroenterology* 1992;103:1893–1901.

185. Shaked A, Colonna JO, Goldstein L, et al. The interrelation between sclerosing cholangitis and ulcerative colitis in patients undergoing liver transplantation. *Ann Surg* 1992;215:598–605.

186. Broomé U, Lindberg G, Löfberg R. Primary sclerosing cholangitis in ulcerative colitis—a risk factor for the development of dysplasia and DNA aneuploidy? *Gastroenterology* 1992;102:1877–1880.

187. Rosen CB, Nagorney DM. Cholangiocarcinoma complicating primary sclerosing cholangitis. *Semin Liv Dis* 1991;11:26–30.

188. Miros M, Kerlin P, Walker N, et al. Predicting cholangiocarcinoma in patients with primary sclerosing cholangitis before transplantation. *Gut* 1991;32:1369–1373.

189. Rabinovitz M, Zajko AB, Hassanein T, et al. Diagnostic value of brush cytology in the diagnosis of bile duct carcinoma: a study of 65 patients with bile duct strictures. *Hepatology* 1990;12:747–752.

190. Langnas AN, Grazi GL, Stratta RJ, et al. Primary sclerosing cholangitis: the emerging role for liver transplantation. *Am J Gastroenterol* 1990;85:1136–1141.

191. Marsh JW, Iwatsuki S, Makowka L, et al. Orthotopic liver transplantation for primary sclerosing cholangitis. *Ann Surg* 1988;207:21–25.

192. Ismail T, Angrisani L, Powell JE, et al. Primary sclerosing cholangitis: surgical options, prognostic variables and outcome. *Br J Surg* 1991;78:564–567.

193. Czaja AJ. Natural history of chronic active hepatitis. In: Czaja AJ, Dickson ER, eds. *Chronic active hepatitis: the Mayo Clinic experience.* New York: Marcel Dekker, 1986:9–24.

194. Johnson PJ, McFarlane IG, Eddleston AL. The natural course and heterogeneity of autoimmune-type chronic active hepatitis. *Semin Liv Dis* 1991;11:187–196.

195. Sanchez-Urdazpal L, Czaja AJ, Van Hoek B, et al. Prognostic features and role of liver transplantation in severe corticosteroid-treated autoimmune chronic active hepatitis. *Hepatology* 1991;15:215–221.

196. Pessoa MG, Wright TL. Hepatitis C infection in transplantation. *Clin Liver Dis* 1997;1:663–690.

197. Brown J, Dourakis S, Karayiannis P, et al. Seroprevalence of hepatitis C virus nucleocapsid antibodies in patients with cryptogenic chronic liver disease. *Hepatology* 1992;15:175–179.

198. Wright TL, Donegan E, Hsu HH, et al. Recurrent and acquired hepatitis C viral infection in liver transplant recipients. *Gastroenterology* 1992;103:317–322.

199. Poterucha JJ, Rakela J, Lumeng L, et al. Diagnosis of chronic hepatitis C after liver transplantation by the detection of viral sequences with polymerase chain reaction. *Hepatology* 1992;15:42–45.

200. Gilbert SC, Klintmalm G, Menter A, et al. Methotrexate-induced cirrhosis requiring liver transplantation in three patients with psoriasis. *Arch Intern Med* 1990;150:889–891.

201. Centers for Desease Control and Prevention. Severe isoniazid-associated hepatitis—New York, 1991–1993. *MMWR* 1993;42: 545–547.

202. Greeve M, Ferrell L, Kim M, et al. Cirrhosis of undefined pathogenesis: absence of evidence for unknown viruses or autoimmune processes. *Hepatology* 1993;17:593–598.

203. Edwards CQ, Kushner JP. Screening for hemochromatosis. *N Engl J Med* 1993;328:1616–1620.

204. Tavill AS, Bacon BR. Hemochromatosis: iron metabolism and the iron overload syndromes. In: Zakim D, Boyer TD, eds. *Hepatology,* 2nd ed. Philadelphia: WB Saunders, 1990:1273–1299.

205. Burke W, Thomson E, Khoury MJ, et al. Hereditary hemochromatosis: gene discovery and its implications for population-based screening. *JAMA* 1998;280:172–178.

206. Pillay P, Tzoracoleftherakis E, Tzakis AG, et al. Orthotopic liver transplantation for hemochromatosis. *Transplant Proc* 1991;23:1888–1889.

207. Farrell FJ, Nguyen M, Woodley S, et al. Outcome of liver transplantation in patients with hemochromatosis. *Hepatology* 1994;20: 404–410.

208. Fagiuoli S, Hassanein T, Gurakar A, et al. Liver transplantation for hereditary hemochromatosis (HHC) [Abstract]. *Gastroenterology* 1993;104:A898.

209. Sternlieb I. Perspectives on Wilson's disease. *Hepatology* 1990;12:1234–1239.

210. Perlmutter DH. The cellular basis for liver injury in α_1-antitrypsin deficiency. *Hepatology* 1991;13:172–185.

211. Rakela J, Goldschmiedt M, Ludwig J. Late manifestations of chronic liver disease in adults with alpha-1-antitrypsin deficiency. *Dig Dis Sci* 1987;12:1358–1362.

212. Propst T, Propst A, Dietze O, et al. High prevalence of viral infection in adults with homozygous and heterozygous α_1-antitrypsin deficiency and chronic liver disease. *Ann Intern Med* 1992;117:641–645.

213. Hood JM, Koep LJ, Peters RL, et al. Liver transplantation for advanced liver disease with alpha-1 antitrypsin deficiency. *N Engl J Med* 1980;302:272–275.

214. Putnam CW, Porter KA, Peters RL, et al. Liver replacement for alpha-1 antitrypsin deficiency. *Surgery* 1977;81:258–261.

215. Starzl TE, Van Thiel D, Tzakis AG, et al. Orthotopic liver transplantation for alcoholic cirrhosis. *JAMA* 1988;260:2542–2544.

216. Lucey MR, Merion RM, Henley KS, et al. Selection for and outcome of liver transplantation in alcoholic liver disease. *Gastroenterology* 1992;102:1736–1741.

217. Gish RG, Lee AH, Keeffe EB, et al. Liver transplantation for patients with alcoholism and end-stage liver disease. *Am J Gastroenterol* 1993;88:1337–1342.

218. Keeffe EB. Assessment of the alcoholic patient for liver transplantation: comorbidity, outcome and recidivism. *Liver Transpl Surg* 1996;2:12–20.

219. Osorio RW, Ascher NL, Avery M, et al. Predicting recidivism after orthotopic liver transplantation for alcoholic liver disease. *Hepatology* 1994;20:105–110.

220. Poynard T, Barthelemy P, Fratte S, et al. Evaluation of efficacy of liver transplantation in alcoholic cirrhosis by a case-control study and assimilated controls. *Lancet* 1994;344:502–507.

221. Todo S, Demetris AJ, Van Thiel D, et al. Orthotopic liver transplantation for patients with hepatitis B virus-related liver disease. *Hepatology* 1991;13:619–626.

222. Davies SE, Portmann BC, O'Grady JG, et al. Hepatic histological findings after transplantation for chronic hepatitis B virus infection, including a unique pattern of fibrosing cholestatic hepatitis. *Hepatology* 1991;13:150–157.

223. Benner KG, Lee RG, Keeffe EB, et al. Fibrosing cytolytic liver failure secondary to recurrent hepatitis B after liver transplantation. *Gastroenterology* 1992;103:1307–1312.

224. Luketic VA, Schiffman ML, McCall JB, et al. Primary hepatocellular carcinoma after orthotopic liver transplantation for chronic hepatitis B infection. *Ann Intern Med* 1991;114:212–213.

225. Mason AL, Wicke M, White HM, et al. Increased hepatocyte expression of hepatitis B virus transcription in patients with features of fibrosing cholestatic hepatitis. *Gastroenterology* 1993;105:237–244.

226. Fang J, Tung F, David G, et al. Fibrosing cholestatic hepatitis in a transplant recipient with hepatitis B virus pre-core mutant. *Gastroenterology* 1993;105:901–904.

227. Angus P, Locarnini S, McCaughan G, et al. Hepatitis B virus precore mutant infection is associated with severe recurrent disease after liver transplantation. *Hepatology* 1995;21:14–18.

228. Samuel D, Muller R, Alexander G, et al. Liver transplantation in European patients with hepatitis B surface antigen. *N Engl J Med* 1993;329:1842–1847.

229. Gish RG, Keeffe EB, Lim J, et al. Survival after liver transplantation for chronic hepatitis B using reduced immunosuppression. *J Hepatol* 1995;22:257–262.

230. Terrault NA, Zhou S, Combs C, et al. Prophylaxis in liver transplant recipients using a fixed dosing schedule of hepatitis B immunoglobulin. *Hepatology* 1996;24:1327–1333.

231. McGory RW, Ishitani MB, Oliveira WM, et al. Improved outcome of orthotopic liver transplantation for chronic hepatitis B cirrhosis with aggressive passive immunization. *Transplantation* 1996;61:1358–1364.

232. Jurim O, Martin P, Shaked A, et al. Liver transplantation for chronic hepatitis B in Asians. *Transplantation* 1994;57:1393–1411.

233. Ho BM, So SK, Esquivel CO, et al. Liver transplantation in Asian patients with chronic hepatitis B. *Hepatology* 1997;25:223–225.

234. Crippen J, Foster B, Carlen S, et al. Retransplantation in hepatitis B—a multicenter experience. *Transplantation* 1994;57:823–826.

235. Flowers M, Sherker A, Sinclair SB, et al. Prostaglandin E in the treatment of recurrent hepatitis B infection after orthotopic liver transplantation. *Transplantation* 1994;58:183–191.

236. Krüger M, Tillmann HL, Trautwein C, et al. Famciclovir treatment of hepatitis B virus recurrence after orthotopic liver transplantation—a pilot study. *Liver Transpl Surg* 1996;2:253–262.

237. Gish RG, Lau YNJ, Brooks L, et al. Ganciclovir treatment of hepatitis B virus infection in liver transplant recipients. *Hepatology* 1996;23:1–7.

238. Perrillo R, Rakela J, Dienstag J, et al. Multicenter study of lamivudine therapy for hepatitis B after liver transplantation. Lamivudine Transplant Group. *Hepatology* 1999;29:1581–1586.

239. O'Grady JG, Polson RJ, Rolles K, et al. Liver transplantation for malignant disease: results in 93 consecutive patients. *Ann Surg* 1988;207:373–379.

240. Penn I. Hepatic transplantation for primary and metastatic cancers of the liver. *Surgery* 1991;110:726–735.

241. Goldstein RM, Stone M, Tillery GW, et al. Is liver transplantation indicated for cholangiocarcinoma? *Am J Surg* 1993;166:768–771.

242. Iwatsuki S, Starzl TE, Sheahan DG, et al. Hepatic resection versus transplantation for hepatocellular carcinoma. *Ann Surg* 1991;214:221–228.

243. Haug CE, Jenkins RL, Rohrer RJ, et al. Liver transplantation for primary hepatic cancer. *Transplantation* 1992;53:376–382.

244. Berman MA, Burnham JA, Sheahan DG. Fibrolamellar carcinoma of the liver. An immunohistochemical study of 19 cases and a review of the literature. *Hum Pathol* 1988;19:785–794.

245. Tan CK, Gores GJ, Steers JL, et al. Orthotopic liver transplantation for preoperative early-stage hepatocellular carcinoma. *Mayo Clin Proc* 1994;69:509–514.

246. Rizzi PM, Kane PA, Ryder SD, et al. Accuracy of radiology in detection of hepatocellular carcinoma before liver transplantation. *Gastroenterology* 1994;107:1424–1429.

247. Dushieko GM, Hobbs KEF, Dick R, et al. Treatment of small hepatocellular carcinomas. *Lancet* 1992;340:285–288.

248. Stone MJ, Klintmalm GB, Polter D, et al. Neoadjuvant chemotherapy and liver transplantation for hepatocellular carcinoma: a pilot study in 20 patients. *Gastroenterology* 1993;104:196–202.

249. Venook AP, Ferrell LD, Roberts JP, et al. Liver transplantation for hepatocellular carcinoma: results with preoperative chemoembolization. *Liver Transpl Surg* 1995;1:242–248.

250. Mazzaferro V, Regalia E, Doci R, et al. Liver transplantation for the treatment of small hepatocellular carcinomas in patients with cirrhosis. *N Engl J Med* 1996;334:693–699.

251. Ojogho ON, So SKS, Keeffe EB, et al. Orthotopic liver transplantation for hepatocellular carcinoma: factors affecting long-term patient survival. *Arch Surg* 1996;131:935–941.

252. Reynolds TB. Budd-Chiari syndrome. In: Schiff L, Schiff ER, eds. *Diseases of the liver*, 6th ed. Philadelphia: JB Lippincott, 1987:1466–1472.

253. Bismuth H, Sherlock DJ. Portasystemic shunting versus liver transplantation for the Budd-Chiari syndrome. *Ann Surg* 1991;214:581–589.

254. Shaked A, Goldstein RM, Klintmalm GB, et al. Portosystemic shunt versus orthotopic liver transplantation for the Budd-Chiari syndrome. *Surg Gynecol Obstet* 1992;174:453–459.

255. Halff G, Todo S, Tzakis AG, et al. Liver transplantation for the Budd-Chiari syndrome. *Ann Surg* 1990;211:43–49.

256. Orloff MJ, Orloff MS, Daily PO. Long-term results of treatment of Budd-Chiari syndrome with portal decompression. *Arch Surg* 1992;127:1182–1188.

257. Campbell DA Jr, Rolles K, Jamieson N, et al. Hepatic transplantation with perioperative and long term anticoagulation as treatment for Budd-Chiari syndrome. *Surg Gynecol Obstet* 1988;166:511–518.

258. Oldhafer KJ, Ringe B, Wittekind C, et al. Budd-Chiari syndrome: portacaval shunt and subsequent liver transplantation. *Surgery* 1990;107:471–474.

259. Seltman HJ, Dekker A, Van Thiel DH, et al. Budd-Chiari syndrome recurring in a transplanted liver. *Gastroenterology* 1983;84:640–643.

260. Burdelski M, Rodeck B, Latta A, et al. Treatment of inherited metabolic disorders by liver transplantation. *J Inherit Metab Dis* 1991;14:604–618.

261. Alagille D, Estrada A, Hadchouel M, et al. Syndromic paucity of interlobular bile ducts (Alagille syndrome or arteriohepatic dysplasia): review of 80 cases. *J Pediatr* 1987;110:195–200.

262. Keeffe EB, Pinson CW, Ragsdale J, et al. Hepatocellular carcinoma in arteriohepatic dysplasia. *Am J Gastroenterol* 1993ˣ:1446–1449.

263. Tzakis AG, Reyes J, Tepetes K, et al. Liver transplantation for Alagille's syndrome. *Arch Surg* 1993;128:337–339.

264. Everson GT. Hepatic cysts in autosomal dominant polycystic kidney disease [Editorial]. *Mayo Clin Proc* 1990;65:1020–1025.

265. Gabow PA. Autosomal dominant polycystic kidney disease. *N Engl J Med* 1993;239:332–342.

266. Ringe B, Pichlmayr R, Ziegler H, et al. Management of severe hepatic trauma by two-stage total hepatectomy and subsequent liver transplantation. *Surgery* 1991;109:792–795.

267. Esquivel CO, Bernardos A, Makowka L, et al. Liver replacement after massive hepatic trauma. *J Trauma* 1987;27:800–802.

268. Angstadt J, Jarrell B, Moritz M, et al. Surgical management of severe liver trauma: a role of liver transplantation. *J Trauma* 1989;29:606–608.

269. Pepys MB. Amyloidosis. In: Samter M, Talmage DW, Frank MM, et al., eds. *Immunologic diseases,* 4th ed. Boston: Little, Brown and Company, 1988:631–674.

270. Holmgren G, Ericzon BG, Groth CG, et al. Clinical improvement in amyloid regression after liver transplantation in hereditary trans-thyretin amyloidosis. *Lancet* 1993;341:1113–1116.

271. Keeffe EB. Sarcoidosis in primary biliary cirrhosis: literature review and illustrative case. *Am J Med* 1987;83:977–980.

272. Casavilla FA, Gordon R, Wright HI, et al. Clinical course after liver transplantation in patients with sarcoidosis. *Ann Intern Med* 1993; 118:865–866.

Transplantation of the Liver, edited by Willis C. Maddrey, Eugene R. Schiff, and Michael F. Sorrell. Lippincott Williams & Wilkins, Philadelphia © 2001.

CHAPTER 3

Prognostic Models to Assist in Timing Liver Transplantation

W. Ray Kim and E. Rolland Dickson

At the dawn of the new millennium, the biggest challenge facing the field of liver transplantation is the critical shortage of donor organs, which has led to a dramatic increase in the number of patients on the waiting list as well as in their waiting time. Figure 3.1 illustrates the median waiting time by blood group reported by the United Network for Organ Sharing (UNOS). Although there is some variability by blood group, most transplant recipients wait well more than a year before finally receiving an organ.[1]

The increase in the waiting time presents a difficult dilemma for practicing transplant physicians and surgeons. Patients often experience severe complications of decompensated liver disease, partly because the organ distribution policy gives priority to the sickest patients. Most transplants are performed for patients with a high-priority status; thus, liver transplant candidates usually deteriorate substantially before they are given a high enough priority to receive an organ. To prevent patients from developing life-threatening complications, transplant physicians must therefore make timely decisions to enlist their patients for transplantation. Ideally, liver transplantation should be performed early enough so that the patient is able to tolerate the surgery, yet sufficiently late in the course of the disease so that prolonged survival is unlikely without a liver transplant.[2] In practice, however, determining such an optimal time for transplantation may not be that straightforward.

In today's health care environment, the decision regarding the optimal timing of liver transplantation involves consideration of posttransplantation morbidity and the resultant use of resources in addition to how to maximize the chance for posttransplantation survival.[3] Transplantation procedures in general and liver transplantation in particular have been criticized for being expensive.[4] Although most of the government and private insurance carriers cover liver transplantation, there is a pervasive trend for transplant centers to be held accountable for the financial consequences of their practice. For example, a typical contract with a managed care organization stipulates a certain payment level a priori, exposing transplant centers to a financial loss if expenditures for individual patients exceed the set limit.[5] Therefore, although the expectation continues for the transplant community to act as an advocate of society in the allocation of scarce resources, individual centers must also take into account their own financial interest to sustain their viability.

For transplant physicians to be able to make sound transplant decisions incorporating all these factors requires an ability to estimate not only the natural progression of liver diseases but also the outcome of liver transplantation. This

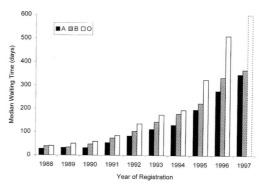

FIG. 3.1. Median waiting time of liver transplant recipients by blood group (year of registration from 1988–1997). For all blood groups, there was a dramatic increase in the waiting time. Most patients now wait more than 1 year on the waiting list.

W. R. Kim and E. R. Dickson: Department of Medicine, Mayo Medical School and Division of Gastroenterology and Hepatology, Mayo Clinic and Foundation, Rochester, Minnesota, 55905

chapter first reviews the prognostic indices that help determine the survival of patients without a transplant. These indices include non-disease-specific systems such as Child-Pugh score and disease-specific models such as the Mayo models for primary biliary cirrhosis and primary sclerosing cholangitis. Second, this chapter discusses how these systems may be useful in predicting the outcome of liver transplantation, including survival of patients, morbidity, complications, and resource utilization.

PROGNOSTIC INDICES FOR PATIENTS WITH CHRONIC LIVER DISEASE

Child-Pugh Classification

The Child-Pugh classification is a widely used disease severity index for patients with liver cirrhosis.[6] The origin of this system, the Child-Turcotte classification, is found in a monograph entitled *The Liver and Portal Hypertension,* published in 1964.[7] The purpose of this system was to assess the operative risk in patients undergoing surgical portosystemic shunt. The Child-Turcotte score is based on five variables (Table 3.1A): the three clinical factors of ascites, encephalopathy, and nutritional status, and the two laboratory parameters of the serum bilirubin and albumin concentrations. Upper gastrointestinal variceal hemorrhage, the most dramatic and life-threatening complication of liver cirrhosis and portal hypertension, is not included in the Child-Turcotte classification because the system was designed for patients who had already experienced gastrointestinal bleeding. The Child-Turcotte classification represented a collective wisdom accumulated over time by surgeons performing portosystemic shunts.[6] For example, the original description of the classification presented no data analysis to justify inclusion of the variables or their cut-off criteria, whereas Wantz and Payne used an almost identical system in their paper published in the *New England Journal of Medicine* in 1961, several years before the monograph by Child and Turcotte.[8]

In 1973, Pugh and colleagues used a modified version of the Child-Turcotte classification in describing the outcome of patients undergoing surgical ligation of esophageal varices.[9] They assigned a score ranging from 1 to 3 to each of the variables in the classification. Classes A, B, and C were designated by criteria applied to the sum of the individual scores (Table 3.1B). Nutritional status in the Child-Turcotte classification was also replaced with prothrombin time. Although the numerical scoring system imparts a scientific look to this version of the classification, little data were provided to support the rationale for the variable selection.

Although the Child-Pugh classification was not developed based on a strong statistical foundation, it has been repeatedly shown to be useful in the assessment of the prognosis of patients with liver cirrhosis. One such example is the work by Christensen et al. in which the Child-Pugh score was analyzed in a group of patients with liver cirrhosis from a variety of etiologies.[10] The investigators found that each of the five individual variables as well as the overall Child-Pugh class had prognostic significance. In another retrospective study of 620 patients with chronic liver disease of a variety of etiologies, the Child-Pugh classification was able to distinguish patients by their likelihood of survival.[11] A number of investigators have tried to improve the classification by either adding new variables or employing more sophisticated measures to produce a prognostic index.[12–14] In general, these efforts resulted in only a marginal improvement, while lacking the practicality or generalizability of the existing system.

Child-Pugh Classification as the Minimal Listing Criteria for Liver Transplantation

In February 1997, an expert panel organized by the American Society of Transplant Physicians and the American Association for the Study of Liver Diseases met at the National Institutes of Health to develop organ-specific criteria

TABLE 3.1. *Child-Turcotte-Pugh classification*

Variable	Points		
	1	2	3
A. The original Child-Turcotte classification			
Bilirubin level (mg/dL)	<2	2–3	>3
Albumin level (g/dL)	>3.5	3.0–3.5	<3.0
Encephalopathy grade	None	Minimal	Advanced, coma
Ascites	None	Easily controlled	Poorly controlled
Nutritional status	Excellent	Good	Poor, wasting
B. Pugh's modification of the Child-Turcotte classification[a]			
Encephalopathy grade	None	1–2	3–4
Ascites	Absent	Slight	Moderate
Albumin level (g/dL)	>3.5	2.8–3.5	<2.8
Prothrombin time (seconds prolonged)	<4	4–6	>6
Bilirubin level (mg/dL)	<2	2–3	>3
For cholestatic diseases)	(<4)	(4–10)	>10

[a]Child-Pugh class A, score = 5 or 6; class B = 7 to 9; class C = 10 to 15.

for entry into the UNOS waiting list for liver transplantation. These criteria were formulated as minimal listing criteria for potential liver transplant recipients.[15] The goal of this endeavor was to formulate criteria for registering patients on the waiting list that were simple, verifiable, and scientifically justifiable.

The participants of the panel agreed that, in general, a minimum criterion for a patient with chronic liver disease to qualify for the waiting list for liver transplantation should be a 90% chance or less of surviving 1 year. As a non-disease-specific criterion, the Child-Pugh score was deemed to best satisfy the stated objectives. It was recognized that once hepatic decompensation develops, survival of patients with liver cirrhosis sharply decreases. Events defining hepatic decompensation include ascites, hepatic encephalopathy, and variceal bleeding. Once these events occur, the estimated 1-year survival rate may range from 38% in patients with spontaneous bacterial peritonitis to 92% in patients with variceal hemorrhage successfully treated by endoscopic means.[16,17]

The panel concluded that a patient with cirrhosis and a Child-Pugh score of 7 or higher (Child-Pugh class B or C) would meet the requirement for a predicted 1-year survival rate of 90% or less. They also recognized the limitations of the Child-Pugh score with respect to important factors such as portal hypertensive gastrointestinal bleeding or spontaneous bacterial peritonitis. Since the criteria were officially adopted, the Child-Pugh classification has been widely used in consideration for liver transplant candidacy.

Disease-Specific Models

Natural History Models for Cholestatic Liver Disease

Cholestatic liver diseases, namely primary biliary cirrhosis (PBC) and primary sclerosing cholangitis (PSC), are characterized by the destruction of interlobular and septal bile ducts, leading to cholestasis, inflammation, fibrosis, and eventually cirrhosis.[18] These disorders contrast to parenchymal liver diseases such as viral, autoimmune, or alcoholic liver disease in which hepatocytes are the primary target of the disease process. Whereas the disease progression of these parenchymal liver diseases tends to be more erratic with a larger degree of variability among individual patients, both PBC and PSC

TABLE 3.2. *Prognostic variables in primary biliary cirrhosis*

European[19]	Yale[20]	Mayo[21]
Age	Age	Age
Bilirubin level	Bilirubin level	Bilirubin level
Albumin level	Hepatomegaly	Albumin level
Cirrhosis	Fibrosis/cirrhosis	Prothrombin time
Cholestasis		Edema

progress at a slower pace and with more consistency. The disease span (from the time of the very first sign of disease until hepatic failure) of PBC and PSC may be as long as 20 years. These characteristics of PBC and PSC lend themselves to mathematical modeling of disease progression and patient survival.

In the 1980s, advances in statistical methods for analyzing survival and the increased availability of computers facilitated the development of prognostic models for a variety of conditions. A number of investigators applied the Cox proportional hazards methodology in modeling the natural history of PBC and PSC. At least three models have been developed for PBC[19–21] and four or more for PSC.[22–25] Most of these models incorporate clinical and biochemical variables to compute a numerical index of disease severity that, in turn, may be used in an equation to arrive at the survival prediction. The clinical variables identified in these models as independent predictors of survival in patients with PBC are summarized in Table 3.2. Of these, the prognostic models developed by investigators at the Mayo Clinic have been the most extensively validated models[26] and, at least in North America, the most widely used.

Mayo Model for Primary Biliary Cirrhosis

The Mayo model for PBC was developed based on 312 patients who had been carefully diagnosed and enrolled in clinical trials for D-penicillamine.[21] Because this medication was found not to provide therapeutic benefits and the study protocol stipulated that patients should not take any other medications that might potentially influence the clinical course of the disease, the progression of disease in this group of patients was deemed appropriate to represent the natural history of PBC. Of the 312 patients, 125 died after

TABLE 3.3. *Mayo natural history model for primary biliary cirrhosis*

A. Computational formula for the risk score (R) for PBC

$$R = 0.04(\text{age [years]}) + 0.87 \log_e(\text{bilirubin [mg/dL]}) - 2.53 \log_e(\text{albumin [g/dL]}) + 2.38 \log_e(\text{prothrombin time [seconds]}) + 0.86(\text{edema}^a)$$

B. Underlying survival function for Mayo PBC model: $S(t) = S_0(t)^{\exp(R-5.1)}$

t (years)	0	1	2	3	4	5	6	7
$S_0(t)$	1	0.970	0.941	0.883	0.833	0.774	0.721	0.651

PBC, primary biliary cirrhosis.
^{a}0, no edema without diuretic therapy; 0.5, edema without diuretic therapy or edema resolved with diuretic therapy; 1, edema despite diuretic therapy.

a median follow-up period of 66 months. Nineteen underwent liver transplantation, and 160 were alive and being followed. From an array of demographic, clinical, biochemical, and histologic variables noted in these patients, five variables were identified as statistically and clinically significant predictors of survival. Based on these variables, a summary score, or risk score (R), is obtained, which in turn is used to calculate expected survival (Table 3.3).

This model has been validated using a number of different data sets. Initially, the model was applied to 106 patients with PBC at the Mayo Clinic who were not included in the treatment trial.[21] Subsequently, extramural validation was undertaken using data on 176 patients from two institutions outside the Mayo Clinic.[26] On both occasions, the model was able to predict the actual survival accurately. Although a few other models had been published previously, the Mayo model gained the most popularity for two reasons: It had the advantage of not requiring liver histology, and the model was subjected to rigorous validation.

Mayo Model for Primary Sclerosing Cholangitis

The first Mayo model to estimate the survival of patients with PSC was published in 1989.[22] This model was updated in 1992 to incorporate data from a number of other institutions.[24] These models included variables such as age, bilirubin level, hemoglobin level, splenomegaly, inflammatory bowel disease, and histologic stage on liver biopsy.[22–25]

Most recently, we reported a revised natural history model for PSC. This revision was undertaken to enhance the clinical utility of the model by excluding the histologic stage as a variable and thereby obviating the need for a liver biopsy.[27] Instead, more emphasis was placed on the reproducibility and generalizability of the variables. The revised model is based on five variables: the patient's age; serum levels of bilirubin, albumin, and aspartate aminotransferase; and a history of variceal bleeding (Table 3.4). This model has been validated using at least one independent data set.

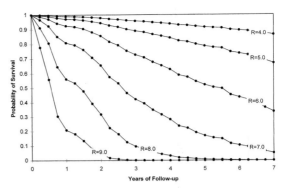

FIG. 3.2. Survival estimates as predicted by the Mayo model for primary biliary cirrhosis by risk score.

Numeric Examples of the Mayo Models

Although the derivation of the survival model and the inherent intricacies of survival analysis may be deemed complex to the uninitiated, the actual application of the model is relatively straightforward. The expected survival is obtained in two steps: First, a risk score is computed according to the formula for the respective disease. Then, by entering the risk score as the exponent in the equation $S(t) = S_0(t)^{\exp(R-R_0)}$, the survival probability may be computed. All these computations can be readily performed on a programmable hand-held calculator or a personal computer.*

Consider a hypothetical patient with PBC and the following variables: age, 48; serum total bilirubin level, 3.5 mg/dL; serum albumin level, 3.0 g/dL; prothrombin time, 12 seconds; and peripheral edema that was resolved with diuretic treatment. The risk score for this PBC patient is computed as follows:

$$R = 0.04 \, (\text{age}) + 0.87 \log (\text{bilirubin}) - 2.53 \log (\text{albumin}) + 2.38 \log (\text{prothrombin time}) + 0.86 \, (\text{edema})$$

$$= 0.04 \, (48) + 0.87 \log (3.5) - 2.53 \log (3.0) + 2.38 \log (12) + 0.86 \, (0.5)$$

$$= 6.5$$

The probability of survival at time t, $S(t)$, is a constant $S_0(t)$ raised to the power of $e^{(R-R_0)}$, where R_0 is a constant (5.1 for PBC). For example, to compute the estimated 1- and 5-year survival in this patient, $S_0(1) = 0.970$ and $S_0(5) = 0.774$ are taken from Table 3.3B. Inserting an R of 6.5 in the equation $S(t) = S_0(t)^{\exp(R-R_0)}$, we get $S(1) = 0.970^{\exp(6.5-5.1)} = 0.88$ and $S(5) = 0.774^{\exp(6.5-5.1)} = 0.33$. Thus, this patient, who has a risk score of 6.5, has an 88% chance of surviving the next year and a 33% chance of surviving the next 5 years (Fig. 3.2). The model for PSC is applied in an identical manner (Fig. 3.3).

TABLE 3.4. *Mayo natural history model for primary sclerosing cholangitis*

A. Computational formula for the risk score (R) for PSC

$R = 0.03$ (age [years]) $+ 0.54 \log_e$ (bilirubin [mg/dL]) $+ 0.54 \log_e$ (AST [IU/L]) $- 0.84$ (albumin [g/dL]) $+ 1.24$ (variceal bleeding[a])

B. Underlying survival function for Mayo PSC model: $S(t) = S_0(t)^{\exp(R-1.0)}$

t (year)	1	2	3	4
$S_0(t)$	0.963	0.919	0.873	0.833

PSC, primary sclerosing cholangitis; AST, aspartate aminotransferase.

[a]0, no variceal bleeding; 1, previous history of bleeding.

---

*The authors have created a user-friendly software program with which to apply the Mayo models. The software has been incorporated as an online worksheet on the Internet (http://www.mayo.edu/int-med/gi/model/mayomodl.htm).

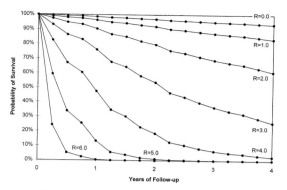

FIG. 3.3. Survival estimates as predicted by the Mayo model for primary sclerosing cholangitis by risk score.

Users of these models should be aware that these survival predictions only represent point estimates generated by the model.[21] There are always individual variations among patients that statistical models may or may not account for. Thus, it is useful practice to consider confidence bands around the estimates provided by the model. In addition, these models only attempt to reproduce observations in the data from which the models were generated. No matter how sophisticated a system may be designed to refine the predictability of these models, such a model will always require human interpretation to be informative and useful. The utility of these models is maximized when they are used as an aid in decision making based on sound clinical judgment.

Another minor point to be aware of when using the Mayo models is that the models were based on albumin levels measured by electrophoresis.[21] Most clinical laboratories employ colorimetric methods for measurement of serum albumin concentrations, which tend to overestimate the albumin level. Although the difference between the two techniques is usually small and its impact on the risk score minor, the user must be aware of such.

PROGNOSTIC MODELS TO PREDICT POSTTRANSPLANTATION OUTCOME

Pretransplantation Morbidity and Outcome of Liver Transplantation

In the early 1980s, Shaw championed the concept that pretransplantation morbidity level has a direct influence on the outcome of liver transplantation.[28] Based on data from 160 primary liver transplant recipients at the University of Pittsburgh, a scoring system was proposed to predict the outcome of liver transplantation. The variables used in the system included hepatic encephalopathy, age, bilirubin level, and prothrombin time, as well as intraoperative blood transfusion requirements (Table 3.5). Patients were classified into low risk (score 0–3), intermediate risk (score 4–6), and high risk (score 7 and above). The system was designed to correlate the scores with posttransplantation survival (Fig. 3.4).

More recently, investigators at the University of Michigan evaluated the relationship between pretransplantation risk factors and mortality during the initial hospitalization for liver transplantation.[29] In a retrospective fashion, they reviewed their experience with 229 consecutive adult liver transplant recipients. Of a number of preoperative risk factors considered in the analysis, Child-Pugh class C was associated with a higher in-hospital mortality rate (24%) than Child-Pugh class A (0%) or B (10%). Patients in Child-Pugh class C were more likely to need renal support in the perioperative period (30.4% for class C versus 12.5% for class B and 0% for class A). The Child-Pugh class was also associated with an increased occurrence of bacterial and fungal sepsis. Similarly, patients who were in the intensive care unit or had renal dysfunction preoperatively consistently had poorer outcome.

Application of Mayo Models for an Optimal Timing of Liver Transplantation

The Mayo natural history models have also been used as indices of pretransplantation morbidity in predicting the

TABLE 3.5. *Shaw's scoring system*

Variable	Points				
	−1	0	1	2	6
Coma	—	None	Grade 1–2	Grade 3	Grade 4
Malnutrition	—	None	Mild to moderate	Severe, generalized wasting	—
Ascites	—	None	Moderate, controlled	Massive, uncontrollable	—
Bilirubin level	<10 mg/dL	—	—	>30 mg/dL	—
Age	—	—	>40 yr	—	—
Operative blood loss	—	—	>35 units	—	—
Coagulopathy	<15 sec	—	—	—	—

Additional modification: If total score is greater than 5, subtract 2 points if age is less than 25 years, and subtract 1 point if red blood cell transfusion is less than 10 units.

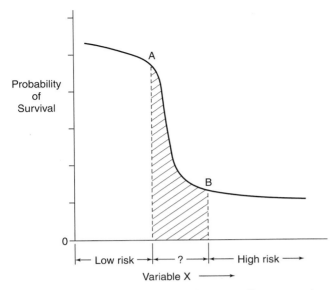

FIG. 3.4. Probability of survival following liver transplantation by preoperative risk as defined by Shaw et al. (From Shaw BW Jr, Wood RP, Gordon RD, et al. Influence of selected patient variables and operative blood loss on six-month survival following liver transplantation. *Semin Liver Dis* 1985;5:385–393, with permission.)

outcome of liver transplantation.[30,31] In these studies, actual patient survival following liver transplantation was compared with survival without transplantation as estimated by the models. Liver transplantation provides significantly higher survival than the model's prediction.

More significantly, preoperative risk scores have been shown to affect posttransplantation survival. Markus et al. applied the Mayo PBC model in 161 patients with PBC undergoing liver transplantation at the University of Pittsburgh and Baylor University Medical Center between 1980 and 1987.[30] Patients were divided according to their pretransplantation risk score into three groups (low, medium, and high risk). At each risk level, the actual survival beyond 3 months after transplantation was significantly better than the survival predicted by the Mayo model. Patients who had lower risk scores had significantly better posttransplantation survival than those with higher scores. Low-risk patients ($R < 8.6$) had a 4-month survival rate of 91%, compared with 78% in the intermediate-risk ($8.6 < R < 9.9$) and 57% in the high-risk ($R > 9.9$) groups. Thus, the difference in survival was mostly due to higher early postoperative mortality in the higher risk groups.

A similar study was conducted by Neuberger et al., who analyzed the outcome of liver transplantation in 70 patients with PBC.[32] Patients were divided into three groups according to their bilirubin level and the European prognostic index. The 1-year posttransplantation survival in patients in the low-risk group (median bilirubin con-

centration 4.9 mg/dL; expected survival without transplantation greater than 9 months) was 78%, whereas that of the high-risk group (median bilirubin concentration 27.3 mg/dL; expected survival less than 4 months) was only 50%.

We recently updated our report on the outcome of liver transplantation for PBC, based on data from 143 patients who underwent liver transplantation at Baylor University Medical Center and the Mayo Clinic between July 1987 and June 1994.[3] Patients were followed to December 1995, for a median follow-up of 35.8 months. Patient survival rates were 93% at 1 year, 90% at 2 years, and 88% at 5 years following transplantation. These rates were significantly higher than those in the report by Markus et al. a decade previously, in which the 1-, 2-, and 3-year survival rates were 76%, 75%, and 72%, respectively.

Figure 3.5 shows the relationship between the risk of death following transplantation and the pretransplantation risk score. The risk of death remains relatively constant until the risk score reaches 7.8, after which the risk starts to climb in an exponential fashion. Proportional hazards analysis indicates that an increase of 1 unit in the risk score beyond 7.8 is associated with an increase in the risk of death by 1.5 fold (95% confidence interval: 1.2–2.0). Figure 3.6 demonstrates the relationship between pretransplantation risk score and resource utilization. Resource utilization, as measured by days in the intensive care unit (ICU), hospital length of stay, and intraoperative blood transfusion requirements, was directly related to the pretransplantation risk score.

The Mayo model for PSC has been applied to patients undergoing liver transplantation. Two hundred sixteen patients with PSC received transplants at the University of Pittsburgh and the Mayo Clinic between 1981 and 1990.[31] Patients were divided into three groups according to their pretransplantation risk score. Similar to PBC, the risk score had a significant impact on short-term

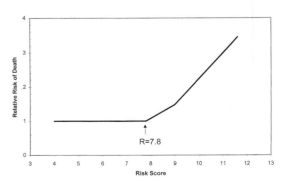

FIG. 3.5. Application of the Mayo model for primary biliary cirrhosis in the prediction of posttransplantation mortality. The risk of death following transplantation does not increase until a risk score of 7.8 is reached, at which point the risk starts to increase at an exponential rate.

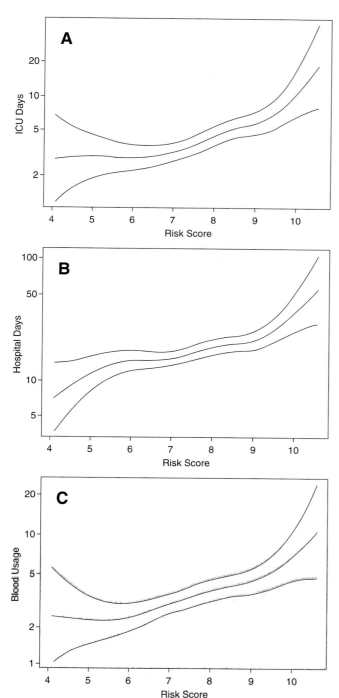

FIG. 3.6. Application of the Mayo model for primary biliary cirrhosis in the prediction of posttransplantation morbidity [**(A)** length of stay in intensive care unit, **(B)** length of stay in hospital, and **(C)** intraoperative requirement of red blood cell transfusion]. Main estimates and 95% confidence bands are shown. Posttransplantation morbidity and resource utilization increase in parallel to the pretransplantation risk score.

(first 3 months) survival ($p = 0.01$), although the overall long-term survival was similar in all three groups ($p = 0.26$).

More recent data on the impact of the pretransplantation severity of liver disease in PSC on posttransplantation morbidity and resource utilization have been reported.[33] As was the case with primary biliary cirrhosis, the Mayo model was found to be a useful predictor of various parameters of liver transplant outcome. As shown in Table 3.6, the pretransplantation Mayo risk score was able to effectively classify patients according to their posttransplantation outcome.

Other Models for Predicting Outcome of Liver Transplantation

Preoperative variables other than the severity of liver disease per se have been evaluated as predictors of the outcome of liver transplantation. As was suggested by Neuberger et al., to the extent that modern transplant technique can replace the diseased organ with a considerable consistency, the outcome of liver transplantation depends on the integrity of extrahepatic organ system function as well as the degree of pretransplantation hepatic dysfunction.[34]

Neuberger et al. analyzed the survival of 82 patients with PBC who underwent liver transplantation at the King's-Cambridge program.[34] Using the Cox regression analysis, the investigators found that after adjusting for the era in which the liver transplantation was performed, the variables that had a significant association with survival after liver transplantation were pretransplantation serum levels of bilirubin and urea and the presence of diuretic-responsive ascites. With use of these clinical variables, a prognostic index may be calculated for estimating survival for 6 months after liver transplantation (Fig. 3.7). As the prognostic index increases, the 6-month survival probability following liver transplantation decreases. The utility of this model is limited by the fact that the model was derived from data that showed a 6-month survival rate of 58%, which is substantially lower than what would be expected from current practice. Although it is possible that the predictor variables are still significant today, the survival estimates are clearly outdated. Therefore, caution is recommended in applying this model.

A similar analysis was recently performed for patients with PSC by Neuberger et al.[35] The analysis was based on 118 patients with PSC who underwent liver transplantation at the Queen Elizabeth Hospital in Birmingham, United Kingdom, between 1986 and 1997. The investigators' multivariate analysis identified five variables as having important prognostic significance. These included inflammatory bowel disease, previous abdominal surgery, ascites, cholangiocarcinoma, and the serum creatinine level. Based on these variables, survival probability for the first posttransplantation year may be estimated (Fig. 3.8).

TABLE 3.6. *Application of the Mayo model for primary sclerosing cholangitis to predict posttransplantation morbidity and resource utilization*

Variable	Risk score (R) <3.5	Risk score (R) ≥3.5	p
ICU stay (days)	3 (2–4)	5 (3–1)	<0.01
Hospitalization (days)	14 (10.5–19.0)	18 (12.5–65.0)	<0.01
RBC transfusion (L)	2.4 (1.2–4.6)	4.9 (2.3–12.2)	<0.01

Patients whose pretransplantation risk score was 3.5 or greater had significantly worse outcome. Median and interquartile ranges are compared. ICU, intensive care unit; RBC, red blood cell.

We completed a study in which we evaluated commonly available preoperative variables for their relationship with postoperative morbidities.[36] This study included 456 patients with PBC (n = 228) and PSC (n = 208) who underwent liver transplantation at the University of Pittsburgh, Baylor University, and the Mayo Clinic. The median posttransplantation follow-up was 2 years, with an overall 2-year patient survival of 90% and graft survival of 82%. The outcome parameters that were evaluated included intraoperative blood use, number of days in the ICU, and severe complications occurring within 30 days of liver transplantation. In the univariate analysis, most of the variables reflecting preoperative morbidity, such as the Mayo risk score, Karnofsky score, presence of ascites and encephalopathy, and serum albumin level, were associated with early postoperative morbidities. A multivariate analysis identified four variables of prognostic significance. These variables included age, renal insufficiency (as defined by a serum creatinine concentration greater than 2.0 mg/dL), Child's class, and UNOS status. Based on these variables a scoring system was devised whereby a quantitative assessment may be made for each outcome parameter, namely intraoperative blood use, length of stay in the ICU, and number of severe complications occurring in the first 30 days of transplantation.[36]

The predictors of postoperative morbidities identified in this study have been evaluated in other liver transplant recipient populations. The best-known example is the functional status as most often measured by the UNOS status. Until recently, patients were classified into four levels according to their urgency: homebound, hospitalized, in intensive care, and on life support. Critically ill patients dependent on life-support devices in an intensive care unit have a uniformly lower survival rate posttransplantation.[37,38] The most recent UNOS report demonstrates a difference in survival between the homebound and life-support groups of as much as 23% at 1 year and 18% at 2 years.[1] This difference is probably attributable to the poor outcome associated with postoperative multiorgan failure in patients with marked impaired functional status.[39] Similarly, Muto et al. concluded that preoperative recipient physiology is the most important determinant of survival in a study that evaluated pretransplantation variables such as the Acute Physiology and Chronic Health Evaluation (APACHE) II score, Blue Cross/Blue Shield risk stratification, and UNOS status.[40]

Serum creatinine concentrations have been found to be a significant predictor of patient survival,[41] graft failure,[42] intraoperative blood loss,[43] and early postoperative sepsis.[29] In a multivariate analysis, Ploeg et al. identified recipient renal failure as an independent risk factor for initial poor function

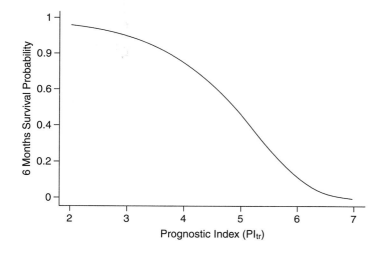

FIG. 3.7. The relationship between the prognostic index for survival after transplantation (PI) and the estimated probability of survival 6 months after transplantation in primary biliary cirrhosis. PI = 0.60 × log(serum bilirubin level in mg/dL) + 0.82 × log(serum urea level in mmol/L) + 1.14 × (transplantation before 1985) − 0.92 × (diuretic-responsive ascites) + 1.70. (From Neuberger J, Altman DG, Polson R, et al. Prognosis after liver transplantation for primary biliary cirrhosis. *Transplantation* 1989;48:444–447, with permission.)

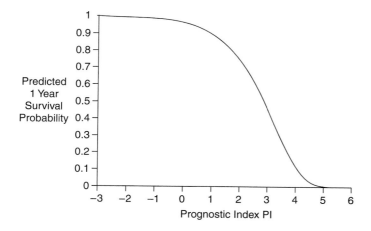

FIG. 3.8. The relationship between the prognostic index for survival after transplantation (PI) and the estimated probability of survival 6 months after transplantation in primary sclerosing cholangitis. PI = 0.534 × (inflammatory bowel disease*) + 1.393 × (previous upper abdominal surgery†) + 1.431 × (ascites†) + 1.111 (serum creatinine‡) − 1.191 × (cholangiocarcinoma†). *No inflammatory bowel disease = 0; ulcerative colitis = −1; Crohn's disease = 4. †Absent = 0, present = 1. ‡<100 umol/L = 0; ≥ 100 umol/L = 1. (From Neuberger J, Gunson B, Komolmit P, et al. Pretransplant prediction of prognosis after liver transplantation in primary sclerosing cholangitis using a Cox regression model. *Hepatology* 1999;29:1375–1379, with permission.)

of the graft.[44] In a series of 569 liver transplant recipients in whom pretransplantation renal function was measured by the glomerular filtration rate, those with hepatorenal syndrome had a significantly lower posttransplantation survival.[45] In patients without hepatorenal syndrome, postoperative mortality was not dependent on pretransplantation renal function, although postoperative morbidity was not considered in this analysis. Overall, we believe that increased creatinine concentration and renal insufficiency are independent risk factors for posttransplantation morbidities.

In summary, in contrast to the early years of liver transplantation, when patient survival was the sole outcome of interest, recent reports emphasize outcome measures such as posttransplantation morbidity, resource utilization, and quality of life. Pretransplantation recipient morbidity remains an important determinant of the outcome of liver transplantation, particularly during the first year after transplantation. Once the patient recovers from the initial insult of the transplant operation, his or her subsequent survival and functional recovery may not be affected by the degree of damage to the liver that has already been replaced.

As shown in the example of primary biliary cirrhosis, current standards of care in liver transplantation are able to achieve a robust posttransplantation outcome unless the recipient's physiology is deranged so severely that the extent or speed of recovery is reduced following the transplantation. Thus, to optimize outcomes, liver transplantation should be timed such that patients undergo transplantation while their physiology is reasonably maintained. The degree of hepatic dysfunction prior to transplantation may be measured by non-disease-specific indices such as the Child-Pugh classification or disease-specific indices such as the Mayo models. In addition, the functional integrity of the extrahepatic organ systems, such as the renal system, has become increasingly important as a determinant of posttransplantation outcome. A patient's overall functional status may be evaluated by measures such as the UNOS status or the Karnofsky score.

STRATEGY FOR THE OPTIMAL TIMING OF LIVER TRANSPLANTATION

In defining strategies for selecting candidates and the best timing for liver transplantation, the transplant community must act as an advocate for society in making the best use of the finite resources available, namely, donor organs and health care funds. The most rational strategy aims for a maximal benefit to society at the least possible human and material cost. In formulating such a strategy, several dimensions must be considered (Fig. 3.9).

The first set of variables to consider are the expected survival of patients with and without transplantation. Figure 3.10 illustrates a hypothetical patient being followed. At the beginning of the illness, the severity of disease is low and the chance for short-term survival is excellent. As time progresses, however, the severity of disease increases gradually, accompanied by a slow reduction in the probability of survival. These changes are gradual until a point is reached at which the progression of disease accelerates along with a reduction in the probability of survival.

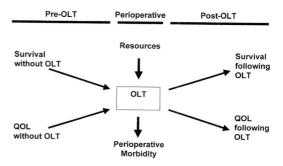

FIG. 3.9. Factors to be considered in the decision concerning patient selection and timing in liver transplantation. The benefit of transplantation is the difference between the quality of life and survival after transplantation minus the quality of life and survival without transplantation. Perioperative morbidities and resource utilization are the other dimensions to be considered.

If one considers liver transplantation at point A, the liver disease is not advanced and the patient is expected to have low postoperative mortality and morbidity. On the other hand, the patient has a good chance for a long-term survival without transplantation. In contrast, if liver transplantation is postponed until point C, the patient may be saved from the rapidly declining survival probability, but at the expense of higher posttransplantation mortality and morbidity. Thus, an optimal time for transplantation would be a point at which survival probability without a transplant is decreasing rapidly, whereas the severity of the liver disease and overall patient status is such that there is no great increase in postoperative mortality and morbidity (point B).

In patients with PBC and PSC, the Mayo models may be useful as markers of disease severity. Our data indicate that a PBC risk score of 7.8 and PSC risk score of 3.5 may be equivalent to point B in Fig. 3.10. From the standpoint of patient survival, these risk scores may be used to select the optimal timing of transplantation and avoid unnecessary mortality risk.

The second set of variables that are becoming increasingly important include short-term morbidity and resource utilization. As discussed in the previous sections, patients with impaired functional status and multiorgan system failure are at a much higher risk of developing postoperative complications that lead to higher resource utilization. This consideration is extremely relevant in this era of health care cost containment and managed competition.

The last variable whose importance is also increasingly recognized is the quality of life in patients before and after transplantation. However, our knowledge in this area is still incomplete. Ideally, we would like to be able to estimate how the quality of life changes over time in patients with end-stage liver disease without transplantation, how the quality of life changes following transplantation, and what variables influence the changes. For example, in a recent study in patients who had liver transplantation for PBC and PSC, although pretransplantation morbidity and quality of life were important determinants of the quality of life posttransplanta-tion, those variables only explained a fraction of the variability seen in the posttransplantation quality of life.[46]

In summary, the decision process for patient selection and timing for liver transplantation is complex and incorporates multiple factors: survival rates, morbidities, resource utilization, and quality of life. As the patient survival rate posttransplantation improves steadily, more emphasis is being given to the consideration of postoperative morbidities. Such a trend will also be significant from the perspective of the allocation of societal resources in support of transplant activities in the current health care environment. With the accumulation of the collective experience of the liver transplant community, an increasing body of data has become available to clinicians and has been incorporated into prognostic models, as reviewed in this chapter. Because the shortage of donor liver allografts is expected to increase, the utility of prognostic models to estimate patient outcome in longer terms will also increase. For clinicians who need to make critical decisions regarding the selection of candidates for and the timing of liver transplantation, prognostic models provide useful insight as aids for reaching the best-informed decisions.

REFERENCES

1. 1998 annual report of the U.S. Scientific Registry for Transplant Recipients and the Organ Procurement and Transplantation Network: transplant data: 1988–1997. Rockville, MD: U.S. Department of Health and Human Services, Health Resources and Services Administration, Office of Special Programs, Division of Transplantation; Richmond, VA: UNOS.
2. Starzl TE, Demetris AJ, Van Thiel D. Liver transplantation. *N Engl J Med* 1989;321:1014–1022.
3. Kim WR, Wiesner RH, Therneau TM, et al. Optimal timing of liver transplantation for primary biliary cirrhosis. *Hepatology* 1998;28:33–38.
4. Evans RW, Manninnen DL, Dong FB. An economic analysis of liver transplantation. Costs, insurance coverage, and reimbursement. *Gastroenterol Clin North Am* 1993;22:451–473.
5. Evans RW. Liver transplantation in a managed care environment. *Liver Transplant Surg* 1995;1:61–75.
6. Conn HO. A peek at the Child-Turcotte classification. *Hepatology* 1981;1:673–676.
7. Child CG, Turcotte JG. Surgery and portal hypertension. In: Child CG, ed. *The liver and portal hypertension.* Philadelphia: WB Saunders, 1964:50:1–85.
8. Wantz GE, Payne MA. Experience with portacaval shunt for portal hypertension. *N Engl J Med* 1961;265:721–728.
9. Pugh RN, Murray-Lyon IM, Dawson JL, et al. Transection of the oesophagus for bleeding oesophageal varices. *Br J Surg* 1973;60:646–649.
10. Christensen E, Schlichting P, Fauerholdt L, et al. Prognostic value of Child-Turcotte criteria in medically treated cirrhosis. *Hepatology* 1984;4:430–435.
11. Propst A, Propst T, Zangerl G, et al. Prognosis and life expectancy in chronic liver disease. *Dig Dis Sci* 1995;40:1805–1815.
12. Siegel JH, Williams JB. A computer based index for the prediction of operative survival in patients with cirrhosis and portal hypertension. *Ann Surg* 1969;169:191–201.
13. Milani A, Marra L, Siciliano M, et al. Prognostic significance of clinical and laboratory parameters in liver cirrhosis. A multivariate statistical approach. *Hepatogastroenterology* 1985;32:270–272.
14. Adler M, Verset D, Bouhdid H, et al. Prognostic evaluation of patients with parenchymal cirrhosis. Proposal of a new simple score. *J Hepatol* 1997;26:642–649.
15. Lucey MR, Brown KA, Everson GT, et al. Minimal criteria for placement of adults on the liver transplant waiting list: a report of a national conference organized by the American Society of Transplant Physi-

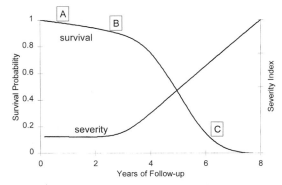

FIG. 3.10. Progression of liver disease and decrease in survival probability in a hypothetical patient.

cians and the American Association for the Study of Liver Diseases. *Liver Transplant Surg* 1997;3:628–637.

16. Andreu M, Sola R, Sitges-Serra A, et al. Risk factors for spontaneous bacterial peritonitis in cirrhotic patients with ascites. *Gastroenterology* 1993;104:1133–1138.

17. Rossle M, Haag K, Ochs A, et al. The transjugular intrahepatic portosystemic stent-shunt procedure for variceal bleeding. *N Engl J Med* 1994;330:165–171.

18. Ludwig J. New concepts in biliary cirrhosis. *Semin Liver Dis* 1987; 7:293–301.

19. Christensen E, Neuberger J, Crowe J, et al. Beneficial effect of azathioprine and prediction of prognosis in primary biliary cirrhosis: final result of an international trial. *Gastroenterology* 1985;89:1084–1091.

20. Roll J, Boyer JL, Barry D, et al. The prognostic importance of clinical and histologic features in asymptomatic and symptomatic primary biliary cirrhosis. *N Engl J Med* 1983;308:1–7.

21. Dickson ER, Grambsch PM, Fleming TR, et al. Prognosis in primary biliary cirrhosis: model for decision making. *Hepatology* 1989; 10:1–7.

22. Wiesner RH, Grambsch PM, Dickson ER, et al. Primary sclerosing cholangitis: natural history, prognostic factors and survival analysis. *Hepatology* 1989;10:430–436.

23. Farrant JM, Hayllar KM, Wilkinson M, et al. Natural history and prognostic variables in primary sclerosing cholangitis. *Gastroenterology* 1991;100:1710–1717.

24. Dickson ER, Murtaugh PA, Wiesner RH, et al. Primary sclerosing cholangitis: refinement and validation of survival models. *Gastroenterology* 1992;103:1893–1901.

25. Broome U, Olsson R, Loof L, et al. Natural history and prognostic factors in 305 Swedish patients with primary sclerosing cholangitis. *Gut* 1996;38:610–615.

26. Grambsch PM, Dickson ER, Kaplan M, et al. Extramural cross-validation of the Mayo primary biliary cirrhosis survival model establishes its generalizability. *Hepatology* 1989;10:846–850.

27. Kim WR, Therneau TM, Wiesner RH, Poterucha JJ, Benson JT, Malinchoc M, LaRusso NF, Lindor KD, Dickson ER. A revised natural history model for primary sclerosing cholangitis. *Mayo Clinic Proceedings* 2000;75;688–694.

28. Shaw BW Jr, Wood RP, Gordon RD, et al. Influence of selected patient variables and operative blood loss on six-month survival following liver transplantation. *Semin Liver Dis* 1985;5:385–393.

29. Baliga P, Merion RM, Turcotte JG, et al. Preoperative risk factor assessment in liver transplantation. *Surgery* 1992;112:704–710; discussion 710–711.

30. Markus BH, Dickson ER, Grambsch PM, et al. Efficacy of liver transplantation in patients with primary biliary cirrhosis. *N Engl J Med* 1989;320:1709–1713.

31. Abu-Elmagd KM, Malinchoc M, Dickson ER, et al. Efficacy of hepatic transplantation in patients with primary sclerosing cholangitis. *Surg Gynecol Obstet* 1993;177:335–344.

32. Neuberger JM, Gunson BK, Buckels JAC, et al. Referral of patients with primary biliary cirrhosis for liver transplantation. *Gut* 1990;31: 1069–1072.

33. Kim WR, Wiesner RH, Therneau TM, et al. Liver transplantation for primary sclerosing cholangitis in the 90's: patient survival and resource utilization [Abstract]. *Hepatology* 1998;28:389A.

34. Neuberger J, Altman DG, Polson R, et al. Prognosis after liver transplantation for primary biliary cirrhosis. *Transplantation* 1989; 48:444–447.

35. Neuberger J, Gunson B, Komolmit P, et al. Pretransplant prediction of prognosis after liver transplantation in primary sclerosing cholangitis using a Cox regression model. *Hepatology* 1999;29:1375–1379.

36. Ricci P, Therneau TM, Malinchoc M, et al. A prognostic model for the outcome of liver transplantation in patients with cholestatic liver disease. *Hepatology* 1997;25:672–677.

37. Delmonico FL, Jenkins RL, Freeman R, et al. The high-risk liver allograft recipient. Should allocation policy consider outcome? *Arch Surg* 1992;127:579–984.

38. Eghtesad B, Bronsther O, Irish W, et al. Disease gravity and urgency of need as guidelines for liver allocation. *Hepatology* 1994;20:56S–62S.

39. Spanier TB, Klein RD, Nasraway SA. Multiple organ failure after liver transplantation. *Crit Care Med* 1995;23:466–473.

40. Muto P, Freeman RB, Haug CE, et al. Liver transplant candidate stratification systems. Implications for third-party payers and organ allocation. *Transplantation* 1994;57:306–308.

41. Cuervas-Mons V, Millan I, Gavaler JS, et al. Prognostic value of preoperatively obtained clinical and laboratory data in predicting survival following orthotopic liver transplantation. *Hepatology* 1986;6:922–927.

42. Doyle HR, Marino IR, Jabbour N, et al. Early death or retransplantation in adults after orthotopic liver transplantation. Can outcome be predicted? *Transplantation* 1994;57:1028–1036.

43. Mor E, Jennings L, Gonwa TA, et al. The impact of operative bleeding on outcome in transplantation of the liver. *Surg Gynecol Obstet* 1993;176:219–227.

44. Ploeg RJ, D'Alessandro AM, Knechtle SJ, et al. Risk factors for primary dysfunction after liver transplantation—a multivariate analysis. *Transplantation* 1993;55:807–813.

45. Gonwa TA, Klintmalm GB, Levy M, et al. Impact of pretransplant renal function on survival after liver transplantation. *Transplantation* 1995;59:361–365.

46. Gross CR, Malinchoc M, Kim WR, et al. Quality of life before and after liver transplantation for cholestatic liver disease. *Hepatology* 1999;29:356–364.

Transplantation of the Liver, edited by Willis C. Maddrey, Eugene R. Schiff, and Michael F. Sorrell. Lippincott Williams & Wilkins, Philadelphia © 2001.

CHAPTER 4

Operative Procedures

Tomoaki Kato, David Levi, José R. Nery, Antonio D. Pinna, and Andreas G. Tzakis

STANDARD TECHNIQUE FOR DONOR HEPATECTOMY

Evaluation of the Liver Donor

Preoperative evaluation of the liver donor consists of two components: medical history and current condition. A precise medical history is essential for the evaluation and should include past medical history, particularly any history of liver disease, hypertension, diabetes mellitus, or malignancy; previous surgery; social history, particularly alcoholic intake; and history of high-risk behaviors, including intravenous drug use, multiple sexual partners, or incarceration. Important information regarding the donor's current condition includes etiology of brain death; hospital course; presence of cardiac or respiratory arrest, and the duration of cardiopulmonary resuscitation; blood loss and transfusion requirement; presence of abdominal trauma; ongoing infection; chest radiograph; physical examination; hemodynamic stability; urine output; inotropic requirement; and laboratory tests, including arterial blood gas, white blood cell count, plasma sodium concentration, liver function tests, serum bilirubin level, and viral serology.

Table 4.1 summarizes the general criteria for liver donors. Organ donors are frequently hypovolemic with electrolyte imbalances, particularly hypernatremia. This is usually due to diabetes insipidus or is the result of the medical treatment for brain edema.[1,2] Once the graft is accepted, the donor is medically managed according to an organ procurement protocol designed to control and stabilize these physiologic impairments.[3–13] If the plasma sodium level of the donor is greater than 160 mEq/L, it should be corrected before harvesting the organ because severe hypernatremia has been associated with early graft dysfunction.[14,15]

A final assessment of the quality of the graft is done at the time of surgery. Although there are no defined criteria for this assessment, a surgeon experienced in harvesting organs should be able to evaluate the graft by inspecting the color, texture, consistency, and shape of the liver and by observing the production of bile during organ retrieval. A frozen section biopsy of the graft helps to determine the degree of hepatic steatosis. Macrovesicular steatosis exceeding 30% is usually considered unacceptable because of the increased incidence of primary graft nonfunction.[16–19]

Donors who are positive for hepatitis B core antibodies can transmit the virus to recipients.[20–24] We are currently using livers from B core–positive donors for recipients who are also seropositive for B core antibody. When a B core–positive donor liver is transplanted into a B core–negative recipient in an emergency, a course of hepatitis B immune globulin (HBIG) and lamivudine immediately after the transplantation can help prevent transmission of the

Table 4.1. *General criteria for liver donors*

Consent for organ donation obtained
Age: no defined limit
No malignancy, except for nonmetastatic skin and brain cancer
No peritoneal contamination, no systemic sepsis
No transmissible disease
   HIV negative
   HTLV-1 negative
   Hepatitis B surface antigen negative
   Hepatitis B core antibody negative (see text)
   Hepatitis C antibody negative (see text)
Acceptable social history (low risk for transmissible disease)
Acceptable hemodynamics and oxygenation
Normalizing liver function tests
Normal or correctable prothrombin time
ABO identical or compatible

HIV, human immune deficiency virus; HTLV-1, human T-lymphotrophic virus 1.

T. Kato, D. Levi, J. R. Nery, A. D. Pinna, and A. G. Tzakis: Liver and Gastrointestinal Transplant Program, Division of Transplantation, University of Miami School of Medicine, Miami, Florida 33136

disease.[25] Livers from hepatitis C–positive donors are sometimes used in hepatitis C–positive recipients.[26,27] Liver biopsies should be performed in both B core–positive donors and hepatitis C–positive donors. These livers should only be used if there is no histologic evidence of hepatitis.

In recent years, liver grafts from older donors have been used in an effort to compensate for the shortage of hepatic grafts.[28–30] Although there is no clear age limit for the prospective liver donor, several reports suggest that the use of donors aged 60 years or older correlates with poor initial graft function, particularly when there is a prolonged cold ischemia time.[31–34] The precise cause of this phenomenon is unknown. One concern is the increased incidence of atherosclerotic disease among older donors. The hepatic artery is relatively well preserved from the effects of atherosclerosis, but it can be affected in advanced disease. Adequate attention should be directed to the quality of the hepatic artery in older donors.

Surgical Techniques

The classic technique for the donor hepatectomy described by Starzl et al. includes dissection of the hepatic hilum before cold perfusion.[35] If the donor is hemodynamically unstable, the technique is modified to minimize the period of time before cold perfusion. A method known as the rapid flush technique was developed to improve organ recovery in unstable donors.[36–39] We routinely use a modification of the rapid flush technique in most cases because it helps to reduce operative time. Our average time from the skin incision to aortic cross-clamp is about 30 minutes. If the heart and the pancreas are not removed, removal of the liver takes only 20 to 30 additional minutes. Shorter operative time minimizes the stress on the operating staff in the local hospital and decreases the cost of harvesting organs. Furthermore, it allows safe training of the inexperienced surgeon.

Our modification of the rapid flush technique begins with a midline skin incision made from the sternal notch to the symphysis pubis. A transverse extension is usually added bilaterally just below the umbilicus to maximize the exposure of the surgical field. The peritoneal cavity is thoroughly inspected for intraabdominal neoplasm or peritonitis.

The right colon and the duodenum are mobilized using Kocher's maneuver, continuing until the root of the superior mesenteric artery (SMA) is exposed. The anterior surface of the infrahepatic vena cava and the distal aorta are exposed. The aorta is encircled and taped just above the bifurcation of the iliac arteries. The inferior mesenteric artery is divided if necessary. The portal system is cannulated through either the superior mesenteric vein (SMV) or the inferior mesenteric vein. We prefer to use the SMV because it will accommodate a large cannula. The SMV can be found between the duodenum and the transverse mesentery or by dissecting the root of the mesentery. The gallbladder is opened and flushed. After systemic heparinization (20,000 units), the distal aorta is ligated and an aortic cannula is inserted. Another cannula is inserted in the SMV.

If the pancreas is to be harvested, the hepatic artery and the SMA must be dissected before cold perfusion. A detailed description of the technique for pancreas procurement is beyond the scope of this chapter. In brief, the common bile duct is ligated and transected just above the pancreas. The right gastric and the gastroduodenal arteries are divided between ties. The common hepatic artery is dissected toward the celiac axis. The root of the splenic artery is exposed and encircled. The portal vein is dissected to the level of splenic vein confluence. The coronary vein is usually divided during this dissection. The SMA is dissected at its root to explore for a possible aberrant right hepatic artery. For further details of pancreas procurement, readers should refer to the literature.[40–45]

After the aorta is cross-clamped, the viscera are perfused through both the aortic and portal vein cannulas with cold preservation solution (University of Wisconsin solution) and the viscera are packed in crushed ice (Fig. 4.1). If the heart is to be recovered simultaneously, the cardiac surgeon should vent the suprahepatic inferior vena cava. We usually delay placing a clamp at the thoracic aorta until after removal of the heart. Once the effluent fluid from the suprahepatic vena cava becomes clear (usually 4 L of cold solution from the aorta and 1 L from the portal vein are required), donor hepatectomy is performed.

After cold perfusion, dissection is done through planes away from important anatomic structures. The final dissec-

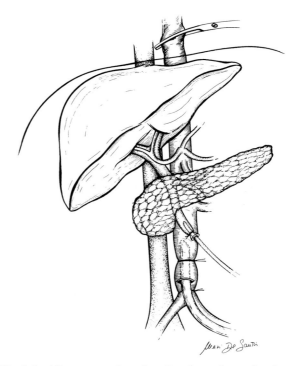

FIG. 4.1. After cross-clamping the thoracic aorta, the abdominal viscera are flushed with cold University of Wisconsin solution via cannulas in the infrarenal aorta and the superior mesenteric vein.

tion to clean the artery is done at the back table. The lesser curvature of the stomach is dissected. The branches of the left gastric artery are divided close to the serosa of the stomach to preserve an aberrant hepatic artery branch that may arise from the left gastric artery. This anomaly is encountered in approximately 10% of donors.[46,47] If the pancreas is not harvested, the splenic artery is divided along the body of the pancreas. The descending thoracic aorta is divided and dissected to the level of the diaphragm. The head of the pancreas is dissected. The gastroduodenal artery is identified and divided on the pancreas. The portal vein is identified and dissected toward the level of the splenic vein confluence. The splenic vein and the SMV are transected and the portal vein is freed from the posterior connective tissue. The pancreas head is further dissected, carefully preserving an aberrant right hepatic arterial branch from the SMA. Identification of this branch by palpation is sometimes unreliable, particularly without dissecting the hilum. The pancreatic tissue is usually divided to avoid endangering this branch. Final identification and dissection of the aberrant right hepatic artery branch should be done at the back table. The common bile duct is divided during dissection of the pancreas head. With the mesentery retracted upward, the SMA is identified from its inferior aspect and divided away from its origin to preserve a possible aberrant arterial branch going into the liver. This branch is usually found within 2 cm of the origin of the SMA in approximately 10% of donors.[46,47] The SMA is dissected toward its origin. When the pancreas is harvested simultaneously, the SMA should be divided just distal to the takeoff of the right replaced hepatic artery, thereby preserving a segment of the SMA for the liver.[44,45] The left side of the aorta is dissected at the level of the origin of the SMA, dividing the surrounding ganglion and lymphatics. Care should be taken to preserve the upper pole left renal artery if present. A small incision is made on the aorta, just below the origin of the SMA, and the left lateral wall of the aorta is divided obliquely to preserve any upper pole artery of the kidneys. After the origin of the right renal artery is identified from the inside of the aorta, the right wall of the aorta is divided. The infrahepatic vena cava is divided above the level of the left renal vein. It is also important to open the anterior wall of the infrahepatic vena cava and to identify the origin of the right renal vein from inside. The back wall of the infrahepatic vena cava is transected to leave a cuff for the right renal vein, thereby separating the liver from the kidneys.

To complete the removal of the liver, the diaphragm is divided; however, because the lower tip of the right triangular ligament is easily torn from the liver, it should be mobilized before the right diaphragm is divided. Once the liver and the kidneys are removed, the iliac vessels are harvested. If severe atherosclerotic disease is present, any well-preserved artery should be harvested for the vascular graft; the SMA is usually well preserved and may be useful.

Back-table Procedure

During the back-table procedure, the donor liver should be submerged in cold preservation solution to maintain a tissue temperature of 0°C to 4°C. First, the diaphragmatic tissue is removed from the suprahepatic vena cava, ligating the phrenic veins. The right adrenal vein is ligated at the infrahepatic vena cava, and the adrenal gland is removed. Connective tissue around the portal vein is dissected to the level of bifurcation. The artery is dissected from the aorta to the level of the common hepatic artery between the splenic artery and the gastroduodenal artery. We minimize dissection of the artery during the donor surgery, so this back-table procedure should be performed carefully to avoid injuring the artery. The SMA should be examined routinely to identify a right replaced hepatic artery that may have been overlooked during the donor surgery. An aberrant left hepatic artery arising from the left gastric artery is easily recognized before flushing during the donor surgery. The left gastric artery is dissected to the takeoff of the left hepatic branch when it is present. The gastroduodenal artery is ligated if it was not ligated during the donor surgery.

There are two major methods for reconstructing the right replaced artery from the SMA,[48-51] and both can be performed at the back table. One method is to place the SMA between the recipient hepatic artery and the donor celiac artery (Fig. 4.2A–B). Most commonly, the proximal SMA is anastomosed to the donor celiac artery (Fig. 4.2B). The other method involves connecting the right replaced artery to the splenic artery, creating a Carrel's patch from the SMA if necessary (Fig. 4.2C–D). If the splenic artery is not usable, the right replaced hepatic artery can be anastomosed to the gastroduodenal artery.

En Bloc Harvesting of Multiple Viscera

The multivisceral graft, including the stomach, pancreas, liver, and intestine, can be harvested en bloc[52-54] (see Transplantation of the Liver Together with Digestive Organs, later in this chapter). The graft includes all the abdominal organs perfused by the celiac artery and the SMA. The graft is flushed only via the aorta.

The right colon and the duodenum are mobilized before the cold perfusion to expose the root of the SMA. After cold perfusion, the spleen and the pancreas are mobilized from the retroperitoneum. If the kidneys are included in the multivisceral graft, both kidneys are mobilized from the retroperitoneum, and the ureters are transected distally. If the kidneys are to be used separately, the aorta is transected between the SMA and the renal arteries, and the vena cava is divided just above the renal veins. The esophagus is transected above the diaphragm, and the descending colon is transected. The aorta and the vena cava are mobilized from the vertebral bodies, and the organs are removed by dividing the diaphragm. The organs that are not to be used are removed at the back table. (The colon can be separated before the cold perfusion.)

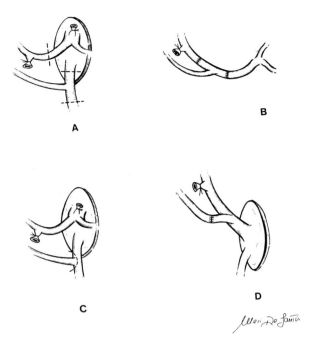

FIG. 4.2. Back-table reconstruction of the aberrant right hepatic artery from the superior mesenteric artery (SMA). (A–B) The SMA is placed in between the recipient hepatic artery and the donor celiac artery (SMA interposition). (C–D) The aberrant hepatic right artery is anastomosed to the splenic artery of the donor.

En bloc harvesting of the liver and the pancreas is useful when both are to be used at the same institution.[55,56] In addition to the usual liver harvesting, the spleen and the pancreas are mobilized from the retroperitoneum. The duodenum is transected at the pylorus proximally and at the ligament of Treitz distally. The liver and the pancreatico-duodenal complex are harvested en bloc. This technique is particularly useful in the unstable donor.

STANDARD TECHNIQUE FOR THE RECIPIENT PROCEDURE

Patient Position, Line Placement, and Skin Incision

The patient is placed in the supine position. We usually place an introducer for a Swan-Ganz catheter, a 12 French dialysis catheter for rapid blood product and fluid administration, a triple-lumen catheter for medications, and bilateral radial arterial lines. To monitor cardiac status during the procedure, we place a transesophageal echo probe in most adult recipients.

The skin is prepared from the upper chest to the upper thigh level, including both groins and axillae. A bilateral subcostal incision with upper midline extension (so-called Mercedez incision) is used. The right subcostal incision should be extended far laterally to provide adequate exposure of the right side of the liver, whereas the left side incision should be limited to the lateral border of the rectus muscle. The midline incision should be extended to the level of the xiphoid. The fal-

ciform ligament is divided and removed together with the fat tissue. The xiphoid is usually removed during this process. If venovenous bypass is indicated, the incisions for it should be made before the retractor is applied. Because proper exposure is crucial for the recipient surgery, the retractor should be sufficiently strong to lift the right rib cage cephalad and outward. We use a Rochard retractor (Aesculap, Burlingame, CA).

Recipient Hepatectomy

Standard, or conventional, hepatectomy includes removal of both the vena cava and the liver. Interrupting the inferior vena cava markedly decreases venous return to the heart, leading to hemodynamic instability. Pump-driven venovenous bypass maintains hemodynamic stability during the vena caval interruption by returning the inferior vena caval and the portal venous flow to the heart through the axillary vein (Fig. 4.3).[57–59] It also decompresses the splanchnic venous system, minimizing bowel edema.

Piggyback Method

Preservation of the retrohepatic vena cava during the recipient hepatectomy—the piggyback method—was first described by Calne et al.[60] Since 1989 Tzakis and colleagues have used it predominantly in pediatric patients.[61]

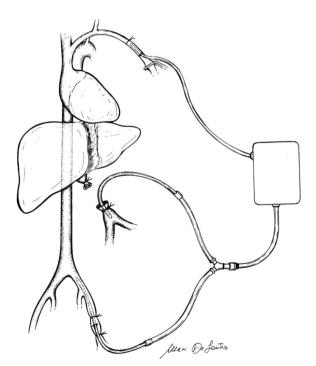

FIG. 4.3. Pump-driven venovenous bypass helps maintain hemodynamic stability during vena caval interruption by returning the inferior vena caval flow and the portal venous flow to the heart via the axillary vein. It also decompresses the splanchnic venous system, minimizing bowel edema.

More recently, this technique has been used in adult patients as well as children.[62-64] Initially applied for hemodynamically unstable pediatric recipients, the piggyback method has several advantages: It decreases warm ischemia time by eliminating the infrahepatic caval anastomosis, eliminates the need for venovenous bypass in most cases, and eases retransplantation.

We only use venovenous bypass with the piggyback method in the presence of few or no portal hypertensive collaterals (i.e., fulminant hepatic failure), a transjugular intrahepatic portosystemic shunt (TIPS), and hemodynamic instability in a recipient who is not expected to tolerate the portal vein clamp. As an alternative to the venovenous bypass, a temporary portacaval shunt (see page 60) can be used for portal decompression with the piggyback method.[65]

After the abdomen is entered and a retractor is placed, the abdominal cavity is inspected. The first step of the hepatectomy is mobilizing the left triangular ligament. The tip of the left lateral segment of the liver should be divided between ties. The remainder of this dissection is usually done with electrocautery. The lesser omentum is entered at its clear portion and divided. The hepatic hilum is approached by dissecting the hepatic artery and dividing it between ties. Although the hepatic artery is usually easily divided above the bifurcation, it can be divided at a lower level because it is usually reconstructed at the level of the common hepatic artery.

The common bile duct is isolated and divided. For duct-to-duct reconstruction, separately dividing the common hepatic duct and the cystic duct can help to obtain adequate length of the native bile duct. If a right replaced hepatic artery arising from the SMA is present, it is usually located behind the portal vein and should be recognized after the transection of the bile duct. This artery is sometimes large and can be used for arterial reconstruction.

The portal vein is dissected by dividing the overlying lymphatic structure circumferentially. A branch from the pancreas often drains into the anterior portion of the portal vein and requires ligatures. To minimize the time the portal vein is clamped, the portal vein flow should be maintained until the retrohepatic cava is dissected. Unless the operator chooses to use an end-to-side anastomosis at the level of the gastroduodenal confluence, the gastroduodenal artery is usually divided as the hepatic artery is dissected. The division of the gastroduodenal artery should be away from its origin because it can be used as a patch during the arterial reconstruction. The hepatic artery is dissected to the celiac axis to obtain enough length for arterial reconstruction. It is important to evaluate the hepatic artery for adequate arterial inflow. If the artery is too small or diseased, alternative sites should be considered. The presence of a large right replaced hepatic artery often indicates an inadequate common hepatic artery. The most common alternative site for arterial inflow is the infrarenal aorta, using an interposition graft of donor iliac artery. After the arterial dissection is completed, the portal vein is exposed to the superior border of the pancreas to create enough freedom for reconstruction.

The coronary vein is divided if necessary. The patient is placed on venovenous bypass at this point if indicated. If the operator chooses to use a temporary portacaval shunt, it is also performed now.

The right triangular ligament is then mobilized by opening the avascular plane between the liver and the diaphragm. Dissection is continued to the level of the vena cava, leaving the right adrenal gland in the retroperitoneum. The suprahepatic veins are dissected. Usually, the left and middle hepatic veins share a common trunk, and the right hepatic vein enters the cava separately.

The retrohepatic cava can be approached from several directions (Fig. 4.4). We present a commonly used method; nevertheless, to ensure a safe dissection, the operator must be flexible and able to change approach. The right side of the retrohepatic caval dissection includes division of the inferior vena cava ligament, a connective tissue bridge joining the left and right sides of the caudate lobe behind the vena cava. A right-angle clamp should be carefully inserted between the vena cava and the ligament. The ligament should be divided, placing the ligature between the ligament and the vena cava. The hepatic tissue of the caudate lobe sometimes extends far posteriorly, wrapping around the vena cava. In extreme cases, the vena cava can be totally surrounded by the liver parenchyma. Even in these cases, the tissue bridge can be cautiously divided. However, if the division proves difficult or dangerous, converting the procedure to a conventional method may be preferable.

After the right side of the vena cava ligament is freed, the retrohepatic veins (short hepatic veins) are carefully dissected with a right-angle clamp and are divided between ligatures. Any resistance to the clamp should not be forced because these small veins can be easily torn. A large hepatic vein draining the inferior-posterior part of the right lobe is often present. If the vein is too large to ligate, it should be oversewn. After the right side of the dissection is completed, the left lateral lobe is retracted to expose the left caudate lobe. The peritoneum between the vena cava and the left caudate lobe is incised and the left side of the caudate lobe is mobilized from the vena cava. The short hepatic veins are divided between ligatures. To minimize bowel edema, it is preferable to complete the retrohepatic caval dissection without dividing the portal vein. However, if necessary, the operator should divide the portal vein to improve exposure. The portal vein should be ligated and divided at the level of bifurcation. The retrohepatic cava is further dissected to the level of the major hepatic veins. We usually place two clamps on the suprahepatic veins: one on both the left and middle hepatic veins, and the other on the right. To preserve length, the veins are divided as they enter the liver parenchyma. If dissection of the right side of the vena cava is incomplete due to poor exposure, dividing the left and middle hepatic vein will facilitate the exposure. The right hepatic vein and other untied branches are easily identified after the left and middle hepatic veins are divided. The liver is now removed from the field.

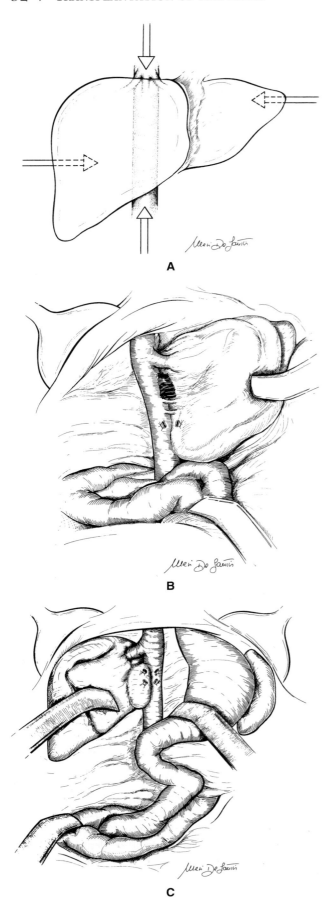

A

B

C

After the hepatectomy is completed, hemostasis is achieved in the retroperitoneum. The portal clamp often exacerbates oozing in the field. Unless the bleeding is excessive, the operator should not spend a great deal of time completing hemostasis because the oozing will decrease after the portal vein is unclamped and the liver is reperfused.

Conventional Method

The structures in the hepatoduodenal ligament are dissected as described in the previous section. The patient is usually placed on a venovenous bypass after the hilar dissection is completed. Cannulas are placed in the femoral vein, the portal vein, and the axillary vein. After the patient is placed on venovenous bypass, the right triangular ligament is mobilized. To accommodate a vascular clamp, the infrahepatic cava is dissected circumferentially. The right side of the vena cava is dissected off the retroperitoneum, and the adrenal vein is identified and divided between ties. The left lateral segment of the liver is then retracted to the right side, and the retroperitoneum is entered along the left side of the caudate lobe. An index finger is used to dissect both the left and right sides of the vena cava from the retroperitoneum. Any resistance encountered behind the vena cava may represent retroperitoneal venous collateral draining into the vena cava; it should be identified and ligated and divided. After the liver is completely liberated from the retroperitoneum, vascular clamps are placed on both the suprahepatic and infrahepatic vena cava. The infrahepatic vena cava is divided as high as possible, and the suprahepatic cava and suprahepatic veins are divided at the surface of the liver, leaving as much vena cava tissue as possible. After the liver is removed, the retroperitoneum is oversewn to cover the bare area.

Hepatectomy in the Patient with Previous Upper Abdominal Surgery

Hepatectomy in patients with previous surgery can be very difficult and can result in excessive blood loss due to the presence of venous collaterals and vascularized adhesions. The degree of these adhesions varies in each patient. In general, an open cholecystectomy does not promote significant adhesions. On the other hand, upper abdominal procedures such as gastric resection or devascularization often cause extensive adhesions.

The skin incision should be modified to include the previous incision when possible. The abdomen should be

FIG. 4.4. (A) The retrohepatic vena cava can be approached from several different directions. **(B)** The retrohepatic caval dissection from the right side. **(C)** The retrohepatic caval dissection from the left side. The left side of the caudate lobe is mobilized from the retroperitoneal reflection.

entered through an upper midline because this approach allows the surgeon to enter on the liver surface where few collaterals have developed. To avoid encountering adhesions, subcostal incisions should be placed higher than usual. After the abdomen is entered and the retractor is placed, dissection should begin at the inferior border of the liver. In principle, the plane between the liver capsule and the adhesion is avascular and can be entered with electrocautery. The surgeon should carefully enter this plane with an electrocautery on a low setting while an assistant surgeon applies gentle traction to the adhesed tissue. Once this dissection is completed and the hepatoduodenal ligament is exposed, the rest of the procedure can be done using either the conventional or piggyback method.

Liberating adhesed tissue at the right side of the hepatoduodenal ligament can be more difficult than liberating it from the left side. In an extreme case, once the left side of the hepatoduodenal ligament is exposed, the liver can be removed from above. An index finger should be inserted from the left side behind the hepatoduodenal ligament to locate the right border of the ligament. After the limit of the hilum of the liver is identified, a large vascular clamp is placed on the hilum en masse. Once the inflow to the liver is controlled with this maneuver, the suprahepatic veins can be approached. In the presence of little collaterals or vascularized adhesions on the surface of the liver, an appropriate plane should be entered, and the suprahepatic veins quickly explored with minimal blood loss. The suprahepatic veins are isolated, clamped, and divided, and the retrohepatic vena cava is dissected from above. Short hepatic veins are ligated and divided. After dissection is completed, the liver is mobilized anteriorly. The hepatic hilum is exposed from behind and divided, enabling the liberation of all adhesed tissue from the liver without difficulty.

Hepatic Outflow and Portal Vein Reconstruction

Piggyback Method

After the liver is removed, a large vascular clamp is placed to encompass all three hepatic veins. The bridge of tissue between the veins is divided to form a joined ostium for the suprahepatic caval anastomosis (Fig. 4.5). We routinely use all three major hepatic veins for upper caval anastomosis. The placement of the clamp at the base of hepatic veins occludes the inferior vena cava at least partially and can cause transient hypotension. After completing the upper vena caval anastomosis, the clamp can be replaced on the donor side of the anastomosis, thereby restoring the flow to the vena cava. This step takes 10 to 20 minutes; the anesthesiologist should be able to maintain blood pressure with fluid boluses.

After the hepatic veins are prepared, the donor liver is brought to the field. The anastomosis between the donor suprahepatic cava and the joined ostium is constructed in a running fashion with 3-0 or 4-0 Prolene. If the ostium of the

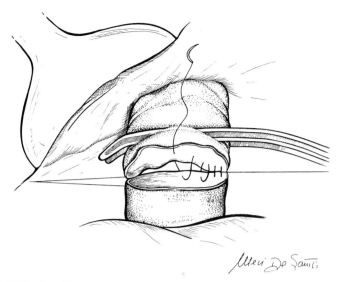

FIG. 4.5. The suprahepatic caval anastomosis. A cunning horizontal mattress stitch is used to compensate for size discrepancy between the ostium of the joined recipient hepatic veins and the donor vena cava.

recipient is larger than that of the donor, a few stitches should be placed horizontally on the recipient side to compensate for the size discrepancy (Fig. 4.5). When the recipient hepatic veins are not usable because they are short or a TIPS is present, the suprahepatic veins are oversewn and a venotomy is made longitudinally below the native hepatic veins (Fig. 4.6A). The posterior wall of the donor vena cava is opened and an end-to-side anastomosis is performed (Fig. 4.6B). If the suprahepatic cava of the donor is short, the infrahepatic vena cava can be used for anastomosis (Fig. 4.6C).

To construct the portal vein anastomosis, we use a "rollover sleeve" technique (Fig. 4.7).[66] This technique, which usually uses a 6-0 Prolene stitch, ensures approximation of the intima. The anastomosis is completed allowing for a growth factor of one-half to three-quarters of the diameter of the portal vein. After the anesthesiologist has been informed, the clamp on the native portal vein is released and the liver is flushed with blood through the infrahepatic vena cava of the donor. After 200 cc to 400 cc of blood has been flushed, the donor infrahepatic vena cava is clamped and the clamp on the suprahepatic vena cava is released. Reperfusion of the liver is now completed. After hemostasis is secured, the infrahepatic vena cava of the donor is ligated.

Conventional Method

After the liver is removed, the tissue bridges between hepatic veins and the cava are divided to form a single ostium. The suprahepatic caval anastomosis is constructed with 3-0 or 4-0 Prolene in a running fashion. The infrahepatic caval

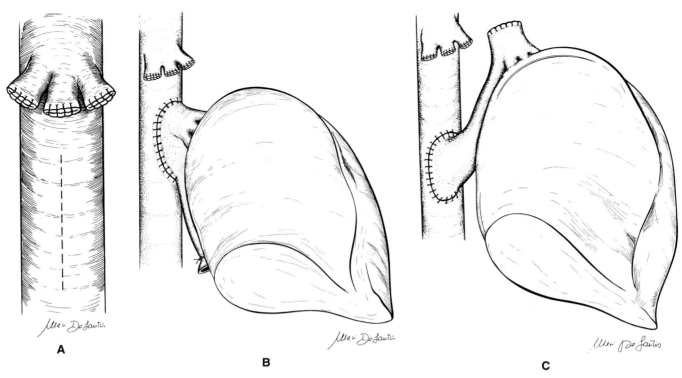

FIG. 4.6. A variation of the piggyback technique. **(A)** The suprahepatic veins are oversewn and a longitudinal venotomy is made below the native hepatic veins. **(B)** The posterior wall of the donor vena cava is opened and an end-to-side anastomosis is performed. **(C)** If the suprahepatic cava of the donor is short, the infrahepatic vena cava can be used for this anastomosis.

anastomosis is then performed with 4-0 Prolene in the same way. Care must be taken to ensure that the reconstructed vena cava is not too long. Redundant length can cause kinking or twisting of the cava, leading to vena caval stricture. While the infrahepatic caval anastomosis is being completed, cold lactated Ringer's solution is infused into the portal vein to flush the preservation solution from the liver. The cannula in the portal vein is removed and portal vein reconstruction is performed as described in the previous section. After completion of the portal vein anastomosis, the three clamps on the veins are released and the liver is reperfused.

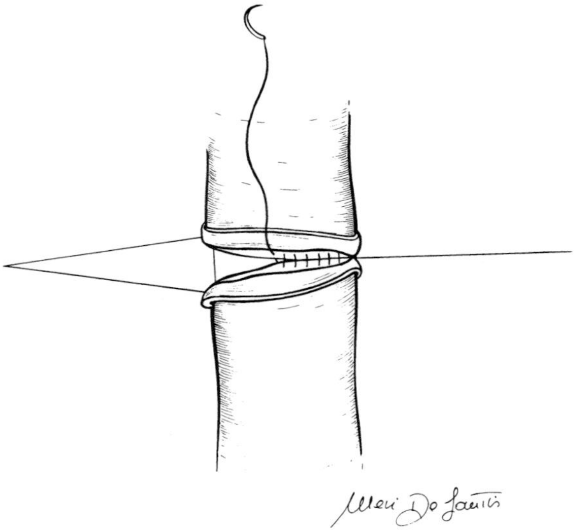

Arterial Reconstruction

Arterial reconstruction, essential for oxygenation of the liver and perfusion of the biliary tree, is usually performed soon after portal venous reperfusion. Sometimes the artery can be reconstructed prior to portal reperfusion, and the two are reperfused together. It is unclear whether simultaneous reperfusion of the artery and portal vein has any advantages other than facilitating the arterial anastomosis. (Arterial anastomosis after portal reperfusion is sometimes very difficult because the artery is usually posterior to the portal vein.) Simultaneous reperfusion may also be beneficial when bleeding, hypotension, or hepatic congestion may delay arterial reconstruction after portal vein reconstruction.

Early hepatic arterial thrombosis is a technical complication usually attributable to inadequate inflow, or a kink or twist at the anastomosis. The hepatic artery of the recipient should be carefully evaluated during hepatectomy. If it is

FIG. 4.7. The "rollover sleeve" technique. Both the donor and the recipient portal vein edges are everted to ensure intimal approximation.

inadequate, a jump graft should be placed before the graft liver is sewn in place.

End-to-end Anastomosis

The arterial reconstruction should be flexible and individualized for each recipient and donor liver. The goal is to join donor and recipient arteries of near-equal caliber without rotation, redundancy, or stenosis. The common hepatic artery at the gastroduodenal confluence of the recipient is most commonly used to provide inflow through an end-to-end anastomosis. The gastroduodenal artery is usually divided and its stump used for a patch (Fig. 4.8). An end-to-side anastomosis can be constructed at the origin of the splenic artery if the native common hepatic artery is deemed insufficient to handle the hepatic inflow (Fig. 4.9). The right replaced hepatic artery arising from the SMA of the recipient can be used if it is of adequate size for the arterial reconstruction. If this artery is used for reconstruction, extra caution must be taken when performing the biliary reconstruction because a duct-to-duct anastomosis may twist the artery and cause a kink. We prefer to perform a Roux-en-Y choledochojejunostomy for a bilary reconstruction in these cases. The donor hepatic artery is commonly anastomosed at the origin of the celiac artery with a

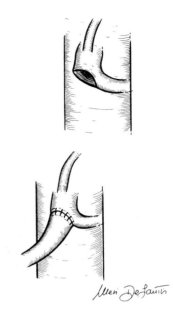

FIG. 4.9. An end-to-side anastomosis can be constructed at the origin of the splenic artery if the native common hepatic artery is deemed insufficient for hepatic inflow.

Carrel's patch (Fig. 4.10) or at the level of splenic artery confluence (Fig. 4.10).

The arterial reconstruction is usually performed in a running fashion with 6-0 or 7-0 Prolene. A small growth factor can be used to prevent "purse stringing" of the anastomosis when constructed without a patch.

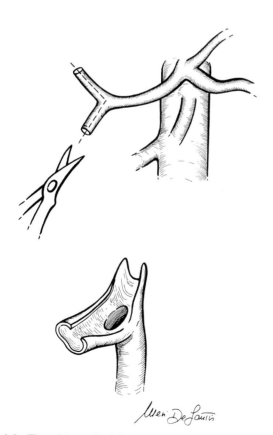

FIG. 4.8. The side wall of the hepatic artery and the gastroduodenal artery is incised to create a patch for the arterial anastomosis.

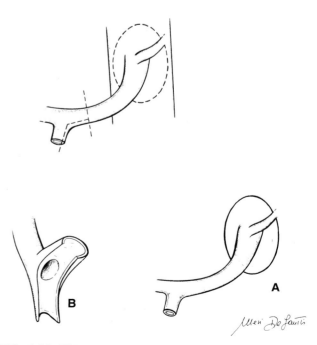

FIG. 4.10. The donor hepatic artery is commonly anastomosed at the origin of the celiac artery with a Carrel's patch **(A)** or at the level of splenic artery confluence **(B)**.

Use of a Jump Graft

When the native artery is not suitable for the arterial reconstruction, a donor iliac artery conduit can be used as a graft (jump graft), originating most commonly from the infrarenal aorta.[67] For this anastomosis, a partial occlusive vascular clamp is placed on the infrarenal aorta, and an end-to-side anastomosis is performed in a running fashion with 5-0 Prolene (Fig. 4.11). The iliac conduit is brought through the transverse mesocolon anterior to the pancreas.

Because the supraceliac aorta is usually well preserved, it can be used as the site for the jump graft if the infrarenal aorta is severely atherosclerotic. A graft from this site usually provides a short, straight route to the liver. However, placement of the graft at the supraceliac aorta is not easy. This anastomosis should be performed during the anhepatic phase before the liver is sewn in place because crossclamping of the supraceliac aorta decreases mesenteric arterial flow; consequently, portal flow decreases, causing marked ischemic damage to the liver.

Biliary Reconstruction

A duct-to-duct anastomosis is the preferred method of reconstruction at most transplantation centers. However, this reconstruction may compromise the vascular reconstruction.

If the donor and the recipient bile ducts are far apart after arterial reconstruction is completed, approximating the two ends may kink the arterial anastomosis. We prefer to create hepaticojejunostomy using a Roux-en-Y limb in the following situations: (a) patients with primary sclerosing cholangitis, (b) size mismatch between donor and recipient bile ducts, (c) large venous collaterals around the native bile duct, and (d) relatively redundant arterial reconstruction or reconstruction using a recipient right replaced hepatic artery from the SMA.

Duct-to-duct Reconstruction

Duct-to-duct reconstruction is the most commonly used method of biliary reconstruction. During the past, this anastomosis was performed routinely over a T tube, but several recent series have shown the T tube to be unnecessary.[68-70] In preparing a duct-to-duct anastomosis, the donor bile duct should be transected relatively high in the hilum to secure adequate blood supply. We often divide the donor bile duct above the cystic duct confluence. Care must be taken to avoid making the reconstructed duct too long because redundancy can lead to kinking. For this anastomosis, we

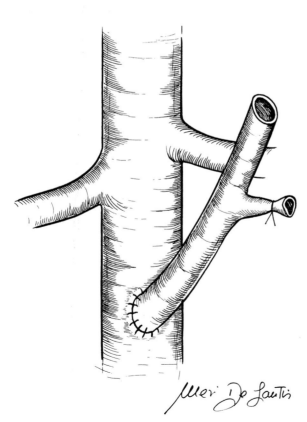

FIG. 4.11. The donor iliac artery is anastomosed to the recipient infrarenal aorta in an end-to-side fashion.

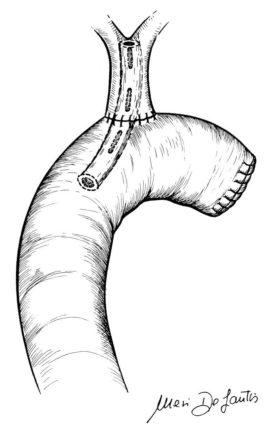

FIG. 4.12. An end-to-side hepaticojejunostomy. A multiperforated internal stent is placed.

usually use 5-0 or 6-0 absorbable monofilament suture in either interrupted or running fashion.

Roux-en-Y Choledochojejunostomy

A Roux-en-Y choledochojejunostomy is used when a duct-to-duct anastomosis is not suitable. To ensure a good blood supply, the donor bile duct should be transected high in the hilum, then anastomosed in an end-to-side fashion to the recipient Roux limb. The anastomosis is done with either running or interrupted stitches. An internal stent can be placed across the anastomosis if desired (Fig. 4.12).

Abdominal Closure

Closure of the abdomen can be difficult if the donor liver is large, or if there is considerable bowel or retroperitoneal edema. In these cases, we opt for a temporary mesh closure. Closing the abdomen too tightly may lead to pressure necrosis of the liver, abdominal compartment syndrome, or respiratory compromise. We prefer to use a Silastic or PTFE mesh for this purpose. In most cases, the edema improves after a few days of diuresis and the patient is taken back to the operating room for closure.

SPECIAL TECHNIQUES FOR RECIPIENT SURGERY

Technique for Patients with Portal Vein Thrombosis

In the past, a thrombosed portal vein was considered a relative contraindication for liver transplantation. Although liver transplantation in patients with portal vein thrombosis (PVT) is now routinely performed in most centers, the complexity of these cases should not be underestimated. Because the patient with PVT has extensive collaterals, the surgery can be complicated. When PVT is accompanied by a previous history of upper abdominal surgery, the surgeon should be prepared for excessive blood loss. Thorough planning is essential for a successful outcome.

Preoperative Evaluation

If a pretransplantation Doppler ultrasound study demonstrates an abnormality in the portal venous flow, a mesenteric angiogram and indirect portogram should be obtained to verify the presence and extent of a thrombus. Planning of portal reconstruction is dependent on the angiographic findings. Portal vein thrombectomy is usually possible when a thrombus is relatively fresh and both the SMV and the splenic vein are patent at the level of the confluence. When a thrombus is well organized and extends beyond the level of splenic vein confluence, a jump graft should be considered.[71] In such cases, the surgeon should carefully assess the angiogram to find the appropriate portion of the SMV for reconstruction of the portal vein. Although the thrombosis may be present in the proximal SMV, the branches of the distal SMV or large varices may be used for portal inflow.[72,73] If there is no sizable patent splanchnic vein, the patient should be considered for a portacaval hemitransposition.[74]

Portal Thrombectomy and Jump Graft

In cases of PVT, the hilar dissection can be extremely difficult because of extensive collateral formation and inflammatory changes around the portal vein. The portal vein should be explored proximally because the inflammatory changes are usually less prominent at this level. The portal vein is dissected to the level of splenic vein confluence. At this location, a clamp can be placed below the thrombus. Once the portal vein is transected, the thrombus is "peeled off" with scissors or a scalpel and removed with gentle traction (Fig. 4.13). Care must be taken not to tear the portal vein wall. If the usable portion of the portal vein above the splenic confluence is short, an elongation vein graft may be interposed (Fig. 4.14A).

In patients with PVT, dissection of the hepatic hilum can be very difficult and can cause massive blood loss. Mass clamping of the hilum can help reduce blood loss. Two

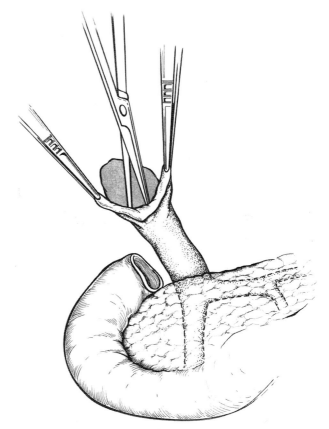

FIG. 4.13. Once the portal vein is transected, the thrombus is "peeled off" with scissors or a scalpel and removed with gentle traction.

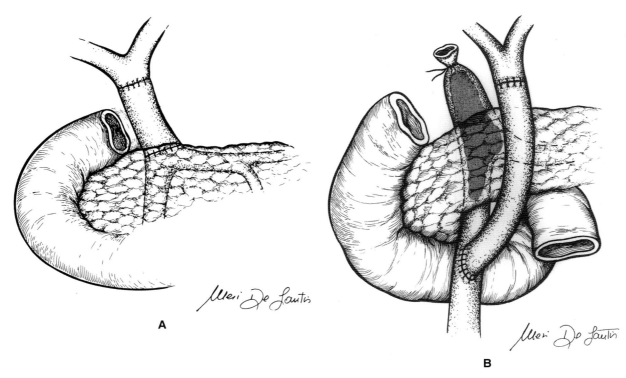

FIG. 4.14. (A) If the usable portion of the portal vein above the splenic confluence is short, an elongation vein graft may be interposed. **(B)** An end-to-side anastomosis is performed between the side of the superior mesenteric vein and the end of the donor iliac vein graft.

large vascular clamps are placed across the hepatoduodenal ligament, and the ligament is divided between clamps. The hepatic side of the ligament is oversewn with a running large (2-0 or 0) Prolene stitch. The hepatic artery and portal vein are identified in the proximal stump of the ligament, and vascular clamps are placed individually. The rest of the hilar strictures can be oversewn.

When a thrombus extends below the level of splenic vein confluence, a venous jump graft from the SMV is usually necessary. If this situation is recognized before transplantation, a graft can be placed early in the procedure before the hilar dissection. The root of the small bowel mesentery is dissected below the transverse mesocolon, and the anterior surface of the SMV is exposed. A partial occlusion vascular clamp should be placed on the SMV, and an end-to-side anastomosis performed between the side of the SMV and the end of the donor iliac vein graft (Fig. 4.14B). Dissection of the posterior wall of the SMV should be limited because it may cause injury to branches draining into the back wall. The iliac vein graft is tunneled through the transverse mesocolon. Once the jump graft is placed and the venous inflow to the graft is prepared, the entire hepatoduodenal ligament may be clamped en masse.

Portacaval Hemitransposition

Thrombosis of the entire splanchnic venous system was once an absolute contraindication for liver transplantation.

Multivisceral transplantation was an option, albeit an aggressive one. Portacaval hemitransposition is a more appealing alternative to ensure portal flow.[74] For this technique, the donor portal vein is anastomosed to the recipient inferior vena cava, thereby restoring hepatopetal blood flow in the portal vein (Fig. 4.15A–B). When the entire mesenteric venous system is thrombosed, blood return from the viscera travels through numerous unnamed collaterals into the systemic venous circulation.

Before this technique is used, the patient's abdomen should be extensively explored to search for a usable splanchnic vein. If no sizable splanchnic vein is found, the portal vein of the donor is anastomosed to the inferior vena cava either in an end-to-end or end-to-side fashion (Fig. 4.15). The patient considered for this procedure often has a history of splenectomy or gastric devascularization, or both. If the patient has not had splenectomy despite a history of variceal bleeding, a splenectomy and devascularization of the stomach may be added to the procedure because this technique does not alleviate portal hypertension. The patient may develop ascites after the procedure, but it usually disappears over time.

Technique for Patients with Prior Portosystemic Shunt

Prior Surgical Portosystemic Shunt

The technical aspects of liver transplantation for patients with prior portosystemic shunts have been described in several se-

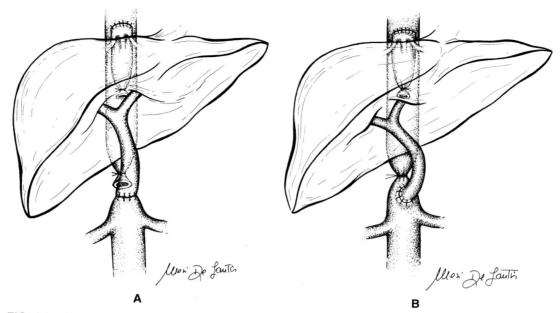

FIG. 4.15. The portacaval hemitransposition. The infrahepatic vena cava is anastomosed to the donor portal in an end-to-end fashion **(A)** or an end-to-side fashion **(B)**.

ries.[75–77] The complexity of the transplantation in patients with prior surgical shunts largely depends on the type of shunt. The central nonselective shunts, such as the end-to-side portacaval shunt or the side-to-side portacaval shunt, pose the greatest difficulty because the hilum has been violated. These shunts should be dismantled before portal vein reconstruction. More commonly performed selective shunt procedures, such as the distal splenorenal shunt or side-to-side mesocaval shunt (H graft), do not increase the complexity of the transplantation as much because the hepatic hilum is left untouched. In patients with mesocaval H grafts, the H graft should be kept intact during the anhepatic phase for portal decompression and simply ligated after the donor liver is reperfused.

Designed to maintain portal perfusion by separating the portomesenteric system from the gastrosplenic system, the distal splenorenal shunt (DSRS) is the most commonly performed selective shunt procedure.[78,79] Theoretically, if the selectivity of the shunt is maintained, dismantling the shunt is not necessary during liver transplantation. In our experience, however, most patients referred for liver transplantation have lost the selectivity of the shunt, and portal vein flow has been reversed or significantly reduced. This phenomenon of "centralization" of the DSRS is caused by the formation of collaterals between the portomesenteric system and the gastrosplenic system and often leads to a thrombosis of the portal vein.[80] If the shunt is already centralized, it should be dismantled during the transplant; otherwise, "stealing" by the shunt decreases portal perfusion and may lead to portal vein thrombosis. Direct ligation of the shunt is difficult, and splenectomy alone does not sufficiently substitute for shunt ligation because the collaterals that centralize the shunt lie in the peripancreatic area. Ligation of the left renal vein may be an alternative to direct ligation. To ad-

dress this problem, we have anastomosed the left renal vein to the donor portal vein in an end-to-end fashion in five patients with prior DSRS.[81] These cases included two patients with PVT, two with hepatofugal flow in the portal vein, and another with an extremely small phlebosclerotic portal vein. This method facilitates the procedure while securing adequate portal perfusion. Patients with prior DSRS should be carefully evaluated to check the patency of the shunt and the direction of the portal vein flow before the transplantation.

Prior Transjugular Intrahepatic Portosystemic Shunt

Transjugular intrahepatic portosystemic shunt has been gradually assuming the role of the surgical portosystemic shunt.[82,83] Used for variceal bleeding that is resistant to endoscopic therapy and for intractable ascites or hepatohydrothorax, TIPS has become a common intervention in the pretransplantation population.[82,83]

The TIPS prosthesis is placed within the liver parenchyma between the right hepatic vein and the right portal vein. Migration of the stent into the vena cava or the portal vein must be recognized before transplantation. A stent that has migrated into the main portal vein may cause inflammatory changes in the hepatic hilum and thrombosis of the portal vein.[84,85] The portal vein should be evaluated carefully before the transplantation. Migration of the TIPS into the vena cava is a greater problem.[86] Sometimes, opening the pericardium and clamping the vena cava above the diaphragm is the only way to retrieve the stent. The piggyback procedure can still be performed, but inflammatory change prohibits use of the right hepatic vein for the anastomosis. In such cases, the native suprahepatic veins are oversewn and the graft is anastomosed to the vena cava below the hepatic veins. Venovenous bypass is recommended for patients with TIPS because caval clamping may occur during the hepatectomy. In addition, collaterals are poorly developed in patients with TIPS, so portal clamping without venovenous bypass may result in severe bowel congestion.

Temporary Portacaval Shunt

Tzakis et al. first described the use of a temporary portacaval shunt during piggyback hepatectomy.[65] Designed to decompress the portal vein and to prevent bowel edema during the anhepatic phase, the shunt stabilizes the patient hemodynamically and positively influences posttransplantation renal function.[87] This shunt is used together with piggyback hepatectomy as an alternative to venovenous bypass in patients with relatively poor formation of portal hypertensive collaterals.

The shunt is placed after dissecting the hepatoduodenal ligament. A partial occlusion clamp is placed on the infrahepatic vena cava, and a venotomy is made. The portal vein is transected above the bifurcation and is anastomosed to the vena cava in an end-to-side fashion (Fig. 4.16A). This shunt should be kept in place until the suprahepatic caval anastomosis is completed. To perform portal vein anastomosis, the shunt is simply ligated and divided (Fig. 4.16B).

Transplantation of the Liver Together with Digestive Organs

Indication

Transplantation of the liver together with digestive organs has been performed for patients with both liver and intestinal failure.[88–91] Intestinal failure is defined as the inability of the intestine to maintain nutrition and/or positive fluid and electrolyte balance without parenteral support.[92] Most intestinal failure is secondary to the anatomic loss of the absorptive surface of the intestine, known as short gut syndrome. Intestinal failure also results from rare diseases or functional abnormalities of the intestine, such as pseudo-obstruction syndrome or microvillus inclusion disease. Liver and intestinal transplantation (LITx) is typically performed in patients with intestinal failure who develop liver failure secondary to the use of long-term total parenteral nutrition (TPN). Multivisceral transplantation, which includes the stomach and pancreaticoduodenal complex in addition to the liver and intestines, is indicated for patients with liver and intestinal failure whose stomach and pancreas must be removed because of their original disease or severe upper abdominal inflammation. Kidney(s) can be included with either graft. A more detailed description of the nonsurgical aspects of the intestinal transplantation is provided in Chapter 8.

Surgical Technique for Liver and Intestinal Transplantation

The graft for LITx is usually prepared at the back table from an en bloc multivisceral graft. The stomach and the pancreaticoduodenal complex are removed during this process by preserving the entire vascular pedicle to the liver, including the portal vein and the hepatic artery. The bile duct must be transected and reconstructed in the recipient (Fig. 4.17). To avoid this complex back-table procedure in

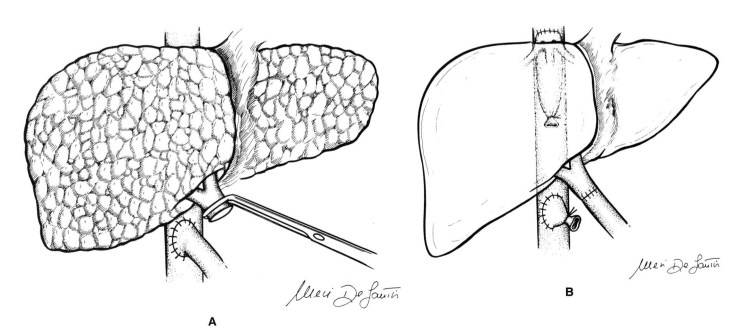

FIG. 4.16. The temporary portacaval shunt. **(A)** The portal vein is transected above the bifurcation and is anastomosed to the vena cava in an end-to-side fashion. **(B)** When performing the portal vein anastomosis, the shunt is simply ligated and divided.

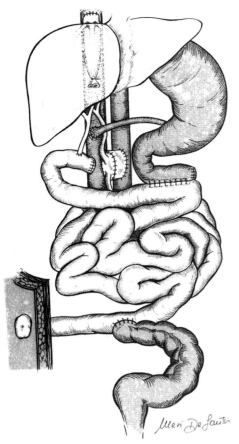

FIG. 4.17. Combined liver and intestinal transplantation. The donor bile duct is anastomosed to a Roux-en-Y limb. An interposition arterial graft is placed from the infrarenal aorta. A native portal vein to the vena caval shunt is created. The terminal end of the donor ileum is exteriorized as an ileostomy. The native rectum is anastomosed to the side of the donor ileum.

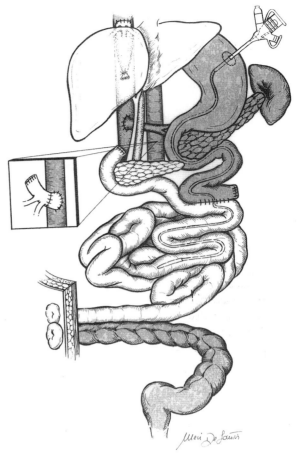

FIG. 4.18. Liver and intestinal transplantation with the entire donor pancreaticoduodenal complex. A biliary drainage procedure is unnecessary. An interposition arterial graft is placed from the infrarenal aorta. The terminal ileum of the donor and the native colon are exteriorized together (Mikulicz ileocolostomy). A double-lumen gastrojejunostomy tube is placed via gastrostomy.

small pediatric donors, the entire pancreas or the head of the pancreas together with the duodenum can be included in the graft (Fig. 4.18).[93,94]

Recipients of LITx usually have an extensive history of previous abdominal surgeries; therefore, entering the abdomen can be very difficult. Opening the peritoneum over the liver often facilitates the process. The operator should avoid entering the left upper abdomen of a patient with a preexisting gastrostomy. Upon entering the peritoneal cavity, the operator should carefully explore the remaining bowel. If the colon is not diseased, it should be carefully preserved. The hepatic hilum is dissected and the hepatic artery and the bile duct are divided. We usually create an end-to-side portacaval shunt to drain the native portal vein. The native portal vein can be drained into the donor portal system by anastomosis of the native portal vein to the donor splenic vein. We prefer removing the liver with the piggyback technique because the venovenous bypass is frequently unusable due to venous thrombosis secondary to long-term TPN use.

Arterial inflow is usually obtained from the infrarenal aorta. An interpositional arterial graft (the thoracic aorta

of the donor is most commonly used) is placed. The distal aorta of the donor, which is transected between the origin of the SMA and the renal arteries, is anastomosed to the interpositional graft (Fig. 4.18). The proximal aorta is ligated. A Carrel's patch including the origin of the celiac artery and the SMA can also be used for the anastomosis (Fig. 4.17). The suprahepatic vena cava of the donor is anastomosed to the joined ostium of the recipient suprahepatic veins using the piggyback technique.

The proximal intestinal anastomosis is made between the recipient jejunum (duodenum) and the donor jejunum in an end-to-side fashion. If the pancreas and the duodenum are not included in the graft, the proximal jejunum is anastomosed to the bile duct. The reconstruction of the distal gastrointestinal tract depends on the remaining distal bowel of the recipient. A terminal ileostomy is created for patients with minimal rectum. Either a Mikulicz double-barrel ostomy or the Bishop-Koup ileostomy is most commonly used for patients with a healthy large-bowel segment (Figs. 4.17,

4.18).[95,96] The Mikulicz ostomy is the safer technique because an anastomosis is avoided. A double-lumen gastrojejunostomy tube is usually placed via gastrostomy (Fig. 4.18).

Surgical Technique for Multivisceral Transplantation

Multivisceral transplantation is indicated for the patient whose stomach or pancreas, or both, must be removed. We consider multivisceral transplantation for the patient whose disease process involves the stomach, chronic pancreatitis, or severe adhesion or enterocutaneous fistula in the upper abdomen.

With the exception of the colon, all the abdominal organs supplied by the celiac artery and the SMA are included in a multivisceral graft. At the back table, the esophagus is again transected and oversewn at the gastroesophageal junction. A pyloroplasty is performed, and the colon is removed. It is preferable to preserve the omentum with the stomach.

The recipient total enterohepatectomy is performed in the following manner. For multivisceral transplantation, the stomach, pancreas, liver, and remaining small bowel are all removed en bloc. To minimize bleeding, the retroperitoneum behind the spleen and the pancreas is dissected, thereby exposing the roots of the celiac artery and the SMA. These arteries are clamped and transected. This maneuver markedly reduces oozing from the surgical field. The liver is removed using the piggyback technique.

Arterial inflow to the graft is usually obtained from the suprarenal aorta at the roots of the celiac artery and the SMA. A partial occlusive clamp is placed on the aorta, and both the roots of the celiac artery and the SMA are resected. The donor thoracic aorta is anastomosed to this ostium in an end-to-side fashion (Fig. 4.19). The distal aorta of the donor is closed with a piece of artery obtained from the proximal thoracic aorta of the donor as a "hatch" (Fig. 4.19).

The proximal anastomosis of the gastrointestinal tract is performed between the recipient esophagus and the donor stomach. This anastomosis is placed anterior to the closure of the donor esophagus. A gastrostomy to the donor stomach is difficult because it lies posterior in the abdominal cavity. As an alternative, a defunctionalized loop of jejunum is usually created for a feeding jejunostomy tube. The distal anastomosis of the gastrointestinal tract is performed in the same manner as described in the previous section.

Domino Liver Transplantation

Domino liver transplantation using a liver from a patient with familial amyloid polyneuropathy (FAP) is an interesting recent inovation.[97,98] This technique salvages livers that are essentially normal except for a single enzyme abnormality. The recipient of the amyloid liver can theoretically develop amyloidosis. However, it may take more than 20 years before the recipient develops symptoms related to amyloidosis; therefore, the liver can be suitable for elderly

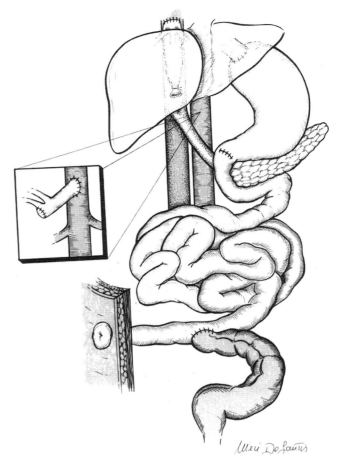

FIG. 4.19. Multivisceral transplantation. The donor thoracic aorta is anastomosed to the recipient suprarenal aorta. The distal stump of the donor aorta is closed with a piece of aortic wall.

patients. The recipient of the amyloid liver should be ABO identical and matched for size with the patient with FAP. We have been selecting elderly recipients (older than 60 years) as domino recipients. The patient with a relatively large malignant tumor may also be considered as a domino recipient.

The removal of the domino donor liver uses a conventional technique. The hepatic vasculature should be left intact until the liver is completely mobilized. The hepatic artery is usually transected directly above the level of the splenic artery takeoff, and the portal vein is transected directly above the pancreas. Anomalies in arterial anatomy must be identified and dissected to their origin to ensure adequate length for the liver graft. The transection of the vena cava is the most complicated aspect of the hepatectomy. The suprahepatic cava should be divided away from the liver. However, the suprahepatic vein in the domino donor liver is usually not long enough to use for anastomosis in the domino recipient. We usually oversew the suprahepatic cava and anastomose the infrahepatic vena cava in an end-to-side fashion to the domino recipient's retrohepatic vena cava.[99,100,101,102] The hepatectomy in the domino recipient should be performed using the piggyback technique; otherwise, no specific technical alternatives are required.

ACKNOWLEDGMENTS

The authors would like to thank Susan E. Siefert, ELS, CBC, for her helpful comments and suggestions in writing the manuscript. They also thank Roberto Verzaro, MD, for his help in preparation of the figures.

REFERENCES

1. Outwater KM, Rockoff MA. Diabetes insipidus accompanying brain death in children. *Neurology* 1984;34:1243–1246.
2. Marks JF, Arant BS Jr. Central diabetes insipidus. In: Levine DL, Morriss FC, eds. *Essentials of pediatric intensive care.* St Louis: Quality Medical Publishing, 1990:432–433.
3. Montefusco CM, Mollenkopf FP, Kamholz SL, et al. Maintenance of potential organ donors in multiple organ procurement. *Hosp Physician* 1984;20:9.
4. Robinette MA, Marshall WJS, Arbus GS, et al. The donation process. *Transplant Proc* 1985;17(suppl 3):45–65.
5. Squifflet JP, Carlier M, Gribomont B, et al. The preoperative management in multiple organ donors: a crucial phase in organ transplantation. *Acta Anaesthesiol Belg* 1986;37:71–76.
6. Novitzky D, Cooper DKC, Reicha B. Hemodynamics and metabolic responses to hormonal therapy in brain-dead potential organ donors. *Transplantation* 1987;43:853–854.
7. Klintmalm GB. The liver donor: special considerations. *Transplant Proc* 1988;20(suppl 7):9–11.
8. Darby JM, Stein K, Grenvik A, et al. Approach to management of the heartbeating "brain dead" organ donor. *JAMA* 1989;261:2222–2228.
9. Soifer B, Gelb AW. The multiple organ donor: identification and management. *Ann Intern Med* 1989;110:814–823.
10. Morris JA, Slaton J, Gibbs D. Vascular organ procurement in trauma population. *J Trauma* 1989;29:782–788.
11. Ashwal S, Schneider S. Brain death in the newborn. *Pediatrics* 1989;84:429–437.
12. Bodenham A, Park GR. Care of the multiple organ donor. *Intensive Care Med* 1989;15:340–348.
13. Ballew AB, Haid S. Identification and medical management of the pediatric organ donor. In: Levin DL, Morriss FC, eds. *Essentials of pediatric intensive care.* St Louis: Quality Medical Publishing, 1990:212–218.
14. Gonzalez FX, Rimola A, Grande L, et al. Predictive factors for primary dysfunction after liver transplantation. *Hepatology* 1994;20:565–573.
15. Figueras J, Busquets J, Grande L, et al. The deleterious effect of donor high plasma sodium and extended preservation in liver transplantation—a multivariate analysis. *Transplantation* 1996;61:410–413.
16. Todo S, Demetris AJ, Makowka L, et al. Primary nonfunction of hepatic allograft with preexisting fatty infiltration. *Transplantation* 1989;47:903–905.
17. Markin RS, Wood RP, Stratta RJ, et al. Predictive value of intraoperative liver biopsies of donor organs in patients undergoing orthotopic liver transplantation. *Transplant Proc* 1990;22:418–419.
18. Adams R, Reyenes M, Johann M, et al. The outcome of steatotic grafts in liver transplantation. *Transplant Proc* 1991;23(suppl 1, pt 2):1538–1540.
19. D'Alessandro AM, Kalayoglu M, Sollinger HW, et al. The predictive value of donor liver biopsies on the development of primary nonfunction (PNF) after orthotopic liver transplantation (OLT). *Transplantation* 1991;51:157–163.
20. Lowell JA, Howard TK, White HM, et al. Serological evidence of past hepatitis infection in liver donor and hepatitis B infection in liver allograft. *Lancet* 1995;345:1084–1085.
21. Wachs MF, Amend WJ, Ascher NL, et al. The risk of transmission of hepatitis B from HbsAg(−), HBcAb(+), HBIgM(−) organ donors. *Transplantation* 1995;59:230–234.
22. Dickson RC, Everhart JE, Lake JR, et al. Transmission of hepatitis B by transplantation of liver from donors positive for antibody to hepatitis B core antigen. The National Institute of Diabetes and Digestive and Kidney Diseases, Liver Transplantation Database. *Gastroenterology* 1997;113:1668–1674.
23. Dodson SF, Issa S, Araya V, et al. Infectivity of hepatic allograft with antibodies to hepatitis B virus. *Transplantation* 1997;64:1582–1584.
24. Uemoto S, Sugiyama K, Marusawa H, et al. Transmission of hepatitis B virus from hepatitis B core antibody-positive donors in living related transplants. *Transplantation* 1998;65:494–499.
25. Dodson RF, Bonham A, Geller DA, et al. Prevention of de novo hepatitis B infection in recipients of hepatic allograft from anti HBc positive donors. *Transplantation* 1999;68:1058–1061.
26. Sheiner PA, Mor E, Schwartz ME, et al. Use of hepatitis C positive donors in liver transplantation. *Transplant Proc* 1993;25:3071.
27. Wright TL, Donegan E, Hsu HH, et al. Recurrent and acquired hepatitis C viral infection in liver transplant recipients. *Gastroenterology* 1992;103:317–322.
28. Jimenez Romero C, Moreno Gonzalez E, Colina Ruiz F, et al. Use of octogenarian livers safely expands the donor pool. *Transplantation* 1999;68:572–574.
29. Mazziotti A, Cescon M, Grazi GL, et al. Successful liver transplantation using an 87 year-old donor. *Hepatogastroenterology* 1999;46:1819–1822.
30. Emre S, Schwartz ME, Altaca G, et al. Safe use of hepatic allografts from donors older than 70 years. *Transplantation* 1996;62:62–65.
31. Adams R, Sanchez I, Astarcioglu I, et al. Deleterious effect of extended cold ischemia time on the posttransplant outcome of aged livers. *Transplant Proc* 1995;27:1181–1183.
32. Marino IR, Doyle HR, Aldrighetti L, et al. Effect of donor age and sex on the outcome of liver transplantation. *Hepatology* 1995;22:1754–1762.
33. Yersiz H, Shaked A, Olthoff K, et al. Correlation between donor age and the pattern of liver graft recovery after transplantation. *Transplantation* 1995;60:790–794.
34. Washburn WK, Johnson LB, Lewis WD, et al. Graft function and outcome of older (≥60 years) donor livers. *Transplantation* 1996;61:1062–1066.
35. Starzl TE, Hakala TR, Shaw BW Jr, et al. A flexible procedure for multiple cadaveric organ procurement. *Surg Gynecol Obstet* 1984;158:223–230.
36. Starzl TE, Miller C, Broznick B, et al. An improved technique for multiple organ harvesting. *Surg Gynecol Obstet* 1987;165:343–348.
37. Nakazato PZ, Concepcion W, Bry W, et al. Total abdominal evisceration: an en bloc technique for abdominal organ harvesting. *Surgery* 1992;111:37–46.
38. Miller CM, Mazzaferro V, Makowka L, et al. Rapid flush technique for donor hepatectomy: safety and efficacy of an improved method of liver recovery for transplantation. *Transplant Proc* 1988;20:948–950.
39. Starzl TE, Iwatsuki S, Esquivel CO, et al. Refinements in the surgical technique of liver transplantation. *Semin Liver Dis* 1985;5:349–356.
40. Sollinger HW, Vernon WB, D'Alessandro AM, et al. Combined liver and pancreas procurement with Belzer-UW solution. *Surgery* 1989;106:685–691.
41. Delmonico FL, Jenkins RL, Auchincloss H Jr, et al. Procurement of a whole pancreas and liver from the same cadaver donor. *Surgery* 1989;105:718–723.
42. Marsh CL, Perkins JD, Sutherland DE, et al. Combined hepatic and pancreaticoduodenal procurement for transplantation. *Surg Gynecol Obstet* 1984;158:223–230.
43. Dunn DL, Morel P, Schlumpf R, et al. Evidence that combined procurement of pancreas and liver graft does not affect transplant outcome. *Transplantation* 1991;51:150–157.
44. Ames SA, Kisthard JK, Smith JL, et al. Successful combined allograft retrieval in donors with a replaced right hepatic artery. *Surg Gynecol Obstet* 1991;173:216–222.
45. Shaffer D, Lewis WD, Jenkins RL, et al. Combined liver and whole pancreas procurement in donors with a replaced right hepatic artery. *Surg Gynecol Obstet* 1992;175:204–207.
46. Todo S, Makowka S, Tzakis AG, et al. Hepatic artery in liver transplantation. *Transplant Proc* 1987;19(suppl 1, pt 3):2406–2411.
47. Hiatt JR, Gabbay J, Busuttil BW. Surgical anatomy of the hepatic artery in 1000 cases. *Ann Surg* 1994;220:50–52.
48. Brems JJ, Millis JM, Hiatt JR, et al. Hepatic artery reconstruction during liver transplantation. *Transplantation* 1989;47:403–406.

49. Colledan M, Ferla G, Rossi G, et al. Bench reconstruction of the graft arterial supply in liver transplantation. *Transplant Proc* 1990;22:408–409.

50. Gordon RD, Shaw BW Jr, Iwatsuki S, et al. A simplified technique for revascularization of homografts of the liver with a variant right hepatic artery from the superior mesenteric artery. *Surg Gynecol Obstet* 1985;160:474–476.

51. Quinones-Baldrick WJ, Memsic L, Ramming K, et al. Branch patch for arterialization of hepatic grafts. *Surg Gynecol Obstet* 1986;162:489–490.

52. Casavilla A, Selby R, Abu-Elmagd K, et al. Logistics and technique for combined hepatic-intestinal retrieval. *Ann Surg* 1992;216:605–609.

53. Starzl TE, Todo S, Tzakis AG, et al. The many faces of multivisceral transplantation. *Surg Gynecol Obstet* 1991;172:335–344.

54. Fragulidis G, Khan M, Nery J, et al. Intestinal and multiorgan transplantation. In: Mazziotti A, Cavallari A, eds. *Techniques in liver surgery.* London: Greenwich Medical Media, 1997:337–346.

55. Imagawa DK, Olthoff KM, Yersiz H, et al. Rapid en bloc technique for pancreas-liver procurement. Improved early liver function. *Transplantation* 1996;61:1605–1609.

56. Pinna AD, Dodson FS, Smith CV, et al. Rapid en bloc technique for liver and pancreas procurement. *Transplant Proc* 1997;29:647–648.

57. Shaw BW Jr, Martin DJ, Marquez JM, et al. Venous bypass in clinical liver transplantation. *Ann Surg* 1984;200:524–534.

58. Griffith BP, Shaw BW Jr, Hardesty RL, et al. Venovenous bypass without systemic anticoagulation for transplantation of the human liver. *Surg Gynecol Obstet* 1985;160:270–272.

59. Shaw BW Jr, Martin DJ, marquez JM, et al. Advantages of venous bypass during orthotopic transplantation of the liver. *Semin Liver Dis* 1985;5:344–348.

60. Calne RY, William R. Liver transplantation in man. I. Observations on technique and organization in five cases. *Br Med J* 1968;4:535–540.

61. Tzakis AG, Todo S, Starzl TE. Orthotopic liver transplantation with preservation of the inferior vena cava. *Ann Surg* 1989;210:649–652.

62. Fleitas MG, Casanova D, Martino E, et al. Could the piggyback operation in liver transplantation be routinely used? *Arch Surg* 1994;129:842–845.

63. Nery J, Jacque J, Weppler D, et al. Routine use of the piggyback technique in pediatric orthotopic liver transplantation. *J Pediatr Surg* 1996;31:1644–1647.

64. Busque S, Esquivel CO, Concepcion W, et al. Experience with the piggyback technique without caval occlusion in adult orthotopic liver transplantation. *Transplantation* 1998;65:77–82.

65. Tzakis AG, Reyes J, Nour B, et al. Temporary end to side portacaval shunt in orthotopic hepatic transplantation in humans. *Surg Gynecol Obstet* 1993;176:181–183.

66. Tzakis AG, Stieber AC. A simple and safe roll over sleeve technique for venous anastomosis. *Surg Gynecol Obstet* 1990;170:77.

67. Shaw BW Jr, Iwatsuki S, Starzl TE. Alternative methods of arterialization of the hepatic graft. *Surg Gynecol Obstet* 1984;159:490–493.

68. Rolles K, Dawson K, Novell R, et al. Biliary anastomosis after liver transplantation does not benefit from T tube splintage. *Transplantation* 1994;57:402–404.

69. Vougas V, Rela M, Gane E, et al. A prospective randomised trial of bile duct reconstruction at liver transplantation: T tube or no T tube? *Transpl Int* 1996;9:392–395.

70. Randall HB, Wachs ME, Somberg KA, et al. The use of the T tube after orthotopic liver transplantation. *Transplantation* 1996;61:258–261.

71. Tzakis A, Todo S, Stieber A, et al. Venous jump grafts for liver transplantation in patients with portal vein thrombosis. *Transplantation* 1989;48:530–531.

72. Shaw BW Jr, Iwatsuki S, Bron K, et al. Portal vein grafts in hepatic transplantation. *Surg Gynecol Obstet* 1985;161:66–68.

73. Pinna AD, Lim JW, Sugitani AD, et al. "Pants" vein jump graft for portal vein and superior mesenteric vein thrombosis in transplantation of the liver. *J Am Coll Surg* 1996;183:527–528.

74. Tzakis AG, Kirkegaard P, Pinna AD, et al. Liver transplantation with cavoportal hemitransposition in the presence of diffuse portal vein thrombosis. *Transplantation* 1998;65:619–624.

75. Esquivel CO, Klintmalm G, Iwatsuki S, et al. Liver transplantation in patients with patent splenorenal shunts. *Surgery* 1987;101:430–432.

76. Brems JJ, Hiatt JR, Klein AS, et al. Effect of prior portasystemic shunt on subsequent liver transplantation. *Ann Surg* 1989;209:51–56.

77. Lagnans AN, Marujo WC, Stratta RJ, et al. Influence of a prior portasystemic shunt on outcome after liver transplantation. *Am J Surg* 1992;87:714–718.

78. Warren WD, Zeppa R, Fomon JJ. Selective trans-splenic decompression of gastroesophageal varices by distal splenorenal shunt. *Ann Surg* 1967;166:437–455.

79. Henderson JM. The splenorenal shunt. *Surg Clin North Am* 1990;70:405–423.

80. Maillard J, Flamant YM, Hay JM, et al. Selectivity of the distal splenorenal shunt. *Surgery* 1979;86:663–671.

81. Kato T, Levi DM, DeFaria W, Nishida S, Tzakis AG. Liver transplantation with renoportal anastomosis after distal splenorenal shunt. *Arch Surg.* in press.

82. Kamath PS, McKusick MA. Transvenous intrahepatic portosystemic shunts. *Gastroenterology* 1996;111:1700–1705.

83. Brown RS Jr, Lake JR. Transjugular intrahepatic portosystemic shunt as a form of treatment for portal hypertension: indications and contraindications. *Adv Intern Med* 1997;42:485–504.

84. Clavien PA, Selzner M, Tuttle-Newhall JE, et al. Liver transplantation complicated by misplaced TIPS in the portal vein. *Ann Surg* 1998; 227:440–445.

85. Millis JM, Martin P, Gomes A, et al. Transjugular intrahepatic portosystemic shunts: impact on liver transplantation. *Liver Transpl Surg* 1995;1:229–233.

86. Wilson MW, Gordon RL, LaBerge JM, et al. Liver transplantation complicated by malpositioned transjugular intrahepatic portosystemic shunts. *J Vasc Interv Radiol* 1995;6:695–699.

87. Nery J, Kato T, Weppler D, et al. Temporary portal caval shunt in liver transplantation. In: Abe o, Inokuchi K, Takasaki K, eds. *XXX World Congress of the International College of Surgeons* [proceedings], vol 1. Bologna, Italy: Mouduzzi Editore, 1996: 791– 794.

88. Todo S, Reyes J, Furukawa H, et al. Outcome analysis of 71 clinical intestinal transplantations. *Ann Surg* 1995;222:270–282.

89. Lagnas AN, Shaw BW, Antonson DL, et al. Preliminary experience with intestinal transplantation in infants and children. *Pediatrics* 1996;97:443–448.

90. Asfer S, Zhong R, Grant D. Small bowel transplantation. *Surg Clin North Am* 1994;74:1197–1210.

91. Goulet O, Jan D, Brousse N, et al. Intestinal transplantation. *J Pediatr Gastroenterol Nutr* 1997;25:1–11.

92. Fleming CR, Remmington M. Intestinal failure. In: Hill GL, ed. *Clinical surgery international.* Edinburgh: Churchill Livingstone, 1981: 219–235.

93. Kato T, Romero R, Verzaro R, et al. Inclusion of entire pancreas in the composite liver and intestinal graft in pediatric intestinal transplantation. *Pediatr Transplantation* 1999;3:210–214.

94. Bueno J, Abu-Elmagd K, Mazariegos G, Madriaga J, Fung J, Reyes J. Composite liver-small bowel allografts with preservation of donor duodenum and hepatic biliary system in children. *J Pediatr Surg* 2000;35:291–295.

95. Roseman JE, Kosloske AM. A reappraisal of the Mikulicz enterostomy in infants and children. *Surgery* 1982;91:34–37.

96. Bishop HC, Koop CE. Management of meconium ileus: resection, Roux-en Y and ileostomy with pancreatic enzymes. *Ann Surg* 1957; 145:410–414.

97. Hesse U, Troisi R, Pattyn P, et al. Successful sequential orthotopic liver transplantation in the treatment of familial amyloidotic polyneuropathy. *Transpl Int* 1997;10:478–479.

98. Furtado A, Tome L, Oliveira FJ, et al. Sequential liver transplantation. *Transplant Proc* 1997;29:467–468.

99. Nishida S, Pinna A, Verzaro R, Levi D, Kazo T, Nery JR, Yamamoto S, Reddy RK, Ruiz P, Tzakis AG. Domino liver transplantation with end-to-side infrahepatic vena cavocavoscomy. *J Am Coll Surg.* in press.

100. Azowlay D, Samuel D, Castaing D, Adam R, Adams D, Said G, Bismuth H. Domino liver transplants for metabolic disorders: experience with familial amyloidotic polyneuropathy. *J. Am Coll Surg* 1999;189:584–593.

101. Sangou AJ, Heaton ND, Rela M, Pepys MB, Hawkins PN, Williams R. Domino hepatic transplantation using the liver for a patient with familial and amyloid polyneuropathy. *Transplantation* 1998;65:1496–1498.

102. Hemming AW, Carral MS, Chari KS, Gerg PD, Lilly LB, Ashby P, Lery GA. Domino liver transplantation for familial amyloid polyneuropathy *Liv Transpl Surg* 1998;4:236–238.

Transplantation of the Liver, edited by Willis C. Maddrey, Eugene R. Schiff, and Michael F. Sorrell. Lippincott Williams & Wilkins, Philadelphia © 2001.

CHAPTER 5

Current Status of Partial Liver Transplantation in Adults from Cadaveric and Living Donors

Debra L. Sudan

The tremendous success of liver transplantation as an effective treatment for patients with advanced liver failure has led to a dramatic increase in the number of individuals on the waiting list for liver transplantation in the United States. Over the last decade the number of people on the liver waiting list has increased approximately 25-fold; as of February 2000 it numbered 14,722 [based on data from the United Network for Organ Sharing (UNOS) Scientific Registry]. Unfortunately, the number of cadaveric donor livers available for transplantation has increased little from 1995 (3,879) to 1999 (4,406). The disparity between the number of potential recipients and the number of available cadaveric donors has led to an inevitable increase in the number of deaths of patients on the waiting list. In 1997 there were 1,130 waiting list deaths; this number rose to 1,319 in 1998, an increase of almost 20% (Fig. 5.1).

In response to the increasing risk of death for patients awaiting transplantation, alternatives to whole-organ cadaveric grafts have been sought. The most commonly used clinical alternative to whole cadaveric liver transplants has been partial liver transplantation (reduced-size, split-liver, and living-related transplantation). Reduced-size liver transplantation (RSLT) implies the use of a portion of the donor liver and was the first form of partial liver transplantation introduced. The technique of reduction of the liver allows livers from larger donors to be used in smaller recipients, who traditionally have had higher rates of mortality on the waiting list (25% to 50%).[1] With experience it became apparent that these reduced-size livers functioned as well as full-sized organs, with comparable rates of postoperative complications. The successful application of reduced-size liver transplantation led to efforts to divide the liver in such a way that

not only could a pediatric patient receive a transplant, but also a second (usually adult) patient could receive the larger right side of the liver. This technique has become known as split-liver transplantation.

As clinical experience with liver resections and partial liver grafts from cadaveric donors increased, it appeared feasible to safely use living donors for partial liver transplantation. In 1989 and 1990 the first reports of procurement of partial liver grafts for pediatric recipients from living donors emerged.[2,3] Nearly a decade later, living donor liver transplantation was introduced for adult recipients.[4–6] The current experience with partial human liver grafts from both cadaveric and living donors is the focus of this chapter.

ANATOMIC CONSIDERATIONS

There are several frequent anatomic variations that the surgeon must be aware of in the use of partial liver grafts. These anatomic variations apply generally to all types of partial grafts but are most important when a cadaveric liver is being split or the donor is living. In these cases it is crucial that both portions of the liver have perfect function, and therefore one cannot compromise hepatic artery or portal venous blood flow or biliary drainage to either segment. Variations in the normal arterial, venous, or biliary anatomy occur in as many as 10% to 40% of the population.[7–10] The normal variations of biliary anatomy are outlined in Fig. 5.2. In 41% of right lobe partial grafts there are two separate hepatic ducts that separately drain the anterior and posterior segments of the right lobe (i.e., all except variant A, Fig. 5.2). In the left lateral segment donor, care in division of the left hepatic duct distal to the aberrant right anterior or posterior hepatic duct must be made to avoid complications in the living donor or the recipient of the right split graft.

Figures 5.3 and 5.4 show hepatic angiograms in the arterial and portal venous phases with branches to segment 4

D. L. Sudan: Department of Surgery, University of Nebraska Medical Center, Organ Transplant Program, Omaha, Nebraska 68198

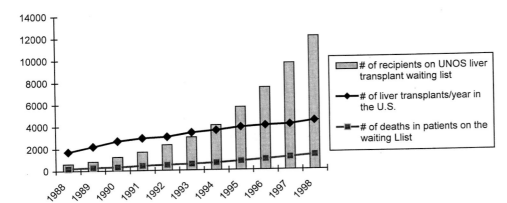

# of recipients on UNOS liver transplant waiting list

# of liver transplants/year in the U.S.

# of deaths in patients on the waiting Llist

FIG. 5.1. Trends in number of patients listed for liver transplantation with the United Network for Organ Sharing (UNOS), number of liver transplants performed, and number of patients who died while on the UNOS waiting list from 1988 to 1998 (based on UNOS Scientific Registry data, March 2000).

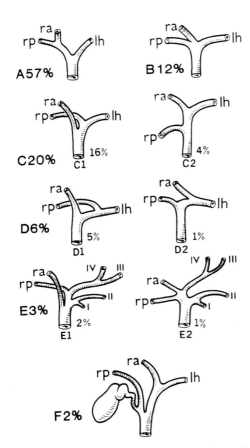

FIG. 5.2. Commonly encountered normal variations in human biliary anatomy. **(A)** Typical anatomy. **(B)** Trifurcation of hepatic ducts into right anterior (ra) and right posterior (rp) segmental ducts and left hepatic (lh) duct. **(C)** Aberrant origin of right segmental bile ducts (ra and rp) into common hepatic duct (**C1**, right anterior; **C2**, right posterior). **(D)** Aberrant drainage of right segmental ducts into left hepatic duct. **(E)** Absence of the hepatic duct confluence. **(F)** Absence of right hepatic duct, and ectopic drainage of right posterior duct into cystic duct. (From Bismuth H, Chiche L. The biliary tract and the anatomy of biliary exposure. In: Blumgart LH, ed. *Surgery of the liver and biliary tract,* 2nd ed. Vol. 1. New York: Churchill Livingstone, 1994:11–24, with permission.)

originating from the right hepatic artery and right portal vein, respectively. These figures emphasize the importance of preoperative studies and careful dissection of hilar structures in circumstances in which the liver is to be divided into two functional units.

REDUCED-SIZE LIVER TRANSPLANTATION

The technique of RSLT was introduced clinically in 1981, and Bismuth first reported the successful transplantation of a reduced-size liver graft in 1984.[11] In general, recipients of reduced-size liver transplants are the smallest children awaiting transplantation. Bilik et al. reported that pediatric RSLT recipients were approximately half the body size of recipients of full-size cadaveric organs (13.5 kg vs. 23.8 kg), and RSLT accounts for as many as 75% of transplants performed on children weighing less than 10 kg.[12] The major goal of RSLT has been met, with a decrease in pretransplantation mortality in this population from 25% in 1989 to less than 10% today.[13] Although this technique has increased the number of livers available for transplantation in children, it has had the undesired effect of reducing the pool of cadaveric organs available for adult recipients, who currently make up 94% of the patients on the waiting list (based on UNOS Scientific Registry data as of February 2000).

Technical Considerations

The preparation of a reduced-size liver for transplantation can be viewed as an *ex vivo* liver resection performed on a cadaveric donor. Reduced-size grafts consist most commonly of either the left lateral segment (Couinaud segments 2 and 3) or the full left lobe (Couinaud segments 2, 3, and 4) (Fig. 5.5). The techniques of *ex vivo* liver reduction can also be used to form a full right lobe graft for use in a small adult, although this application is far less common. In determining the specific segments to include, the transplant surgeon must examine the relationship of the body size of the donor and the body size of the recipient.[14] The full left lobe graft or full right lobe graft (Fig. 5.6 line B) is generally used in circum-

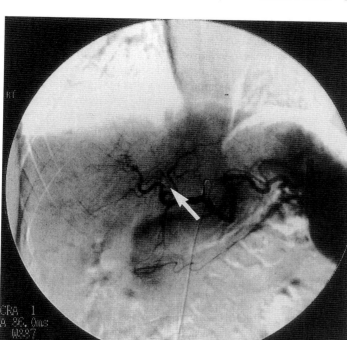

FIG. 5.3. Hepatic arterial branches supplying Couinaud segment 4 originate from the right hepatic artery in this living donor. (From Marcos A, et al. Right lobe living donor transplantation: a review. *Liver Transpl* 2000;6:3–20, with permission.)

stances in which the donor-to-recipient body weight ratio is from 1.5:1 to 3:1.[15] The left lateral segment or, in rare instances, a monosegment graft is preferred in circumstances of a greater donor-to-recipient size discrepancy.[15–17]

The two surgical techniques used for the implantation of reduced-size grafts differ primarily on the decision of whether to include the donor inferior vena cava. The initial description by Bismuth and Houssin included the donor inferior vena cava with segments 1, 2, and 3.[11] In the recipient, therefore, the graft was implanted similar to the standard method of orthotopic liver transplantation, with replacement of the native retrohepatic inferior vena cava (Fig. 5.7). The main drawback

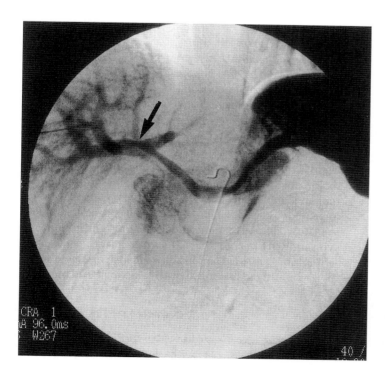

FIG. 5.4. Portal venous branches supplying Couinaud segment 4 arising from the right portal vein are evident in this portal phase image. (From Marcos A, et al. Right lobe living donor transplantation: a review. *Liver Transpl* 2000;6:3–20, with permission.)

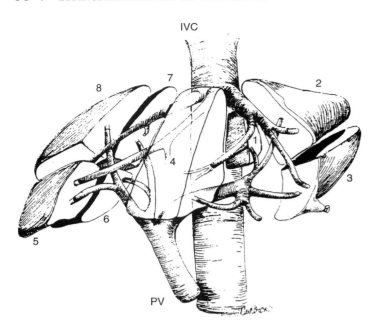

FIG. 5.5. Couinaud segmental anatomy of the liver. Segment 1: Caudate lobe. Segments 2 and 3: Left lateral segment. Segments 2, 3 and 4: Left lobe. Segments 5, 6, 7, and 8: Right lobe. Segments 4, 5, 6, 7, and 8: Extended right lobe. IVC, inferior vena cava; PV, portal vein. (From Busuttil RW, Goss JA. Split liver transplantation. *Ann Surg* 1999;229:313–321, with permission.)

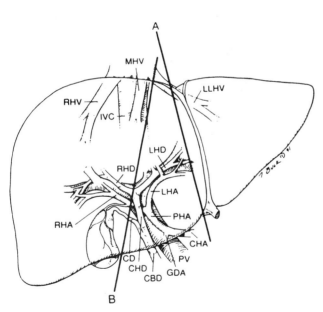

FIG. 5.6. Topical anatomy of the liver. Line A represents the plane for hepatic parenchymal transection for procurement of a left lateral segment graft (segments 2 and 3). Line B represents Cantle's line separating the left and right hepatic lobes. CBD, common bile duct; CD, cystic duct; CHA, common hepatic artery; CHD, common hepatic duct; GDA, gastroduodenal artery; IVC, inferior vena cava; LHA, left branch of the hepatic artery; LHD, left hepatic duct; LLHV, left lobe hepatic vein; MHV, middle hepatic vein; PHA, proper hepatic artery; PV, portal vein; RHA, right branch of the hepatic artery; RHV, right hepatic vein. (From Heffron TG. Living related liver transplantation. *Semin Liv Dis* 1995;15:165–172, with permission.)

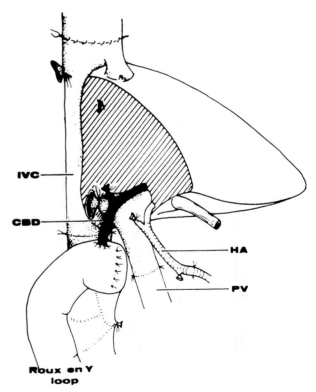

FIG. 5.7. Implantation of a reduced-size graft orthotopically. Here the native retrohepatic inferior vena cava (IVC) is replaced with the donor IVC. There are direct portal vein (PV) and hepatic artery (HA) anastomoses and biliary drainage by Roux-en-Y hepaticojejunostomy. CBD, common bile duct. (From Bismuth H, Houssin D. Reduced-size orthotopic liver graft in hepatic transplantation in children. *Surgery* 1984;95:367–370, with permission.)

of this technique is that there can be considerable size discrepancy between the donor and recipient inferior vena cava.

The method reported by Strong et al. excludes the donor inferior vena cava and retains the recipient inferior vena cava, forming an anastomosis between the donor left hepatic vein and an appropriately sized opening in the inferior vena cava at the level of the native hepatic veins (Fig. 5.8).[18] This technique has since become known as the piggyback technique.[19] In the smallest pediatric recipients (weighing less than 5 kg) the technique of RSLT has been expanded even further to form a functional liver graft from a single hepatic segment—either segment 2 or segment 3 (Fig. 5.9).[16,17]

Results

Patient survival after RSLT is equivalent to, and in some circumstances better than, survival after receiving full-size grafts.[11,20–24] One study reported worse patient and graft survival after reduced-size liver transplantation compared with whole-organ transplantation or transplantation using a living donor.[25] There were, however, significant differences in recipient parameters in this study; in particular, recipients of reduced-size cadaveric livers were far more likely to be younger than 1 year or critically ill in the intensive care unit, or both.[25]

Generally, pediatric recipients of whole cadaveric liver transplants have had higher rates of hepatic artery thrombosis than adult recipients. This is probably due at least in part to the small size of the donor hepatic artery (in many cases even less than 2 mm in diameter). The use of RSLT is associated with a decreased risk of hepatic artery thrombosis in pediatric recipients, probably because of the larger size of the donor vessels.[15,26] Biliary complications and bleeding appear to be more common, however, in comparison with

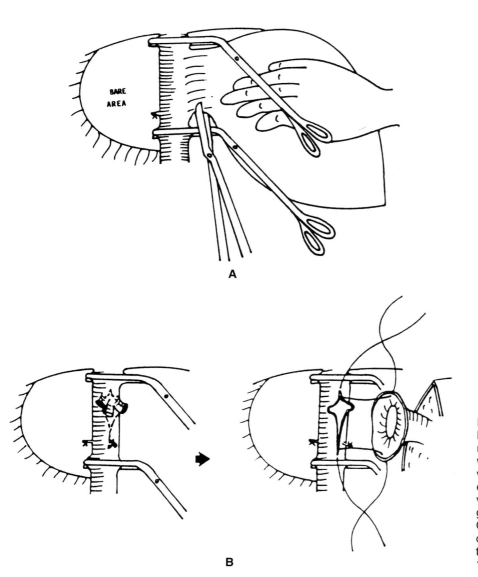

FIG. 5.8. Implantation of reduced-size liver graft by the native piggyback technique. **(A)** Removal of the native liver with preservation of the native inferior vena cava. **(B)** Opening of the confluence of the middle and left hepatic veins for anastomosis with the partial graft hepatic vein. (From Strong R, Ong TH, Pillay P, et al. A new method of segmental orthotopic liver transplantation in children. *Surgery* 1988;104: 104–107, with permission.)

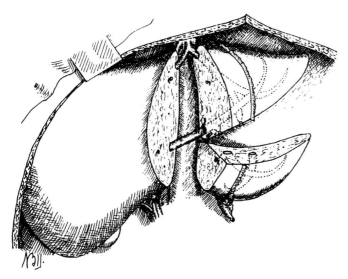

FIG. 5.9. *In situ* preparation of a segment 2 liver graft. (From de Santibanes E, McCormack L, Mattera J, et al. Partial left lateral segment transplant from a living donor. *Liver Transpl* 2000;6:108–112, with permission.)

whole-liver grafts. Because of the cut surface and the incomplete control of vasculature orifices on the back table, there is generally an increased need for blood transfusion intraoperatively, and in some cases early postoperatively, in comparison with whole-organ grafts.[12,26] In one series, bleeding from the cut surface of the liver required repeat laparotomy in nearly 20% of recipients of reduced-size liver grafts.[27]

Overall, it appears that the 1-year patient and graft survival rate is comparable between whole-liver transplantation and RSLT. The ultimate goal of RSLT was to reduce pretransplantation deaths in small children; this goal has been met. Demonstrating comparable results with reduced-size grafts was essential in the development of other sources for partial liver grafts, including split-liver transplantation and living-related liver transplantation.

Auxiliary Liver Transplantation

One additional application of the RSLT technique is reduced-size auxiliary liver grafts. Auxiliary partial orthotopic liver transplantation (APOLT) refers to a technique of partial native liver resection and orthotopic replacement with either a smaller full-sized or a partial liver graft. This technique has achieved good success in the treatment of patients with fulminant hepatic failure and metabolic liver diseases in which there is a defective enzyme but the native liver is not cirrhotic. In patients with fulminant hepatic failure, APOLT is used to bridge the patient to full recovery because of the potential for native liver regeneration.[28–30] In hepatic metabolic defects without cirrhosis, APOLT can replace the missing enzyme with the function of the partial hepatic graft and at

the same time reduce the risks associated with primary graft failure by preserving a portion of the native liver.[31–33] The Kyoto group has reported another application of this technique in the adult patient with cirrhosis for whom the living donor liver graft is "small for size."[34] In large part, however, APOLT for the adult patient with cirrhosis has been replaced by the use of right lobe grafts, which will be further discussed in the section on living donor transplantation.

SPLIT-LIVER TRANSPLANTATION

Split-liver transplantation refers to making use of a single cadaveric liver for two recipients. Typically, the left lateral segment is transplanted into a child and the right lobe into an adult (or large child). The first reported attempt at split-liver transplantation was by Pichlmayr et al. in 1988, who transplanted the right lobe into an adult with primary biliary cirrhosis and the left lateral segment into a child with biliary atresia.[35] Bismuth et al. then reported using the technique for transplantation in two patients with fulminant hepatic failure.[36]

The standard application of split-liver transplantation by transplant centers has been reported to increase the number of available liver grafts from cadaveric donor livers by as much as 26% to 28%.[37,38] Generally, only optimal cadaveric donors are considered candidates for splitting because of the potential for increased preservation injury, especially if the splitting occurs *ex vivo*. Estimates based on the usual donor characteristics in the United States reveal that between 15% and 25% of cadaveric donor livers may be suitable for splitting.[39]

Ex Vivo Technique

The technique of *ex vivo* splitting begins with a standard whole-organ procurement and preservation in University of Wisconsin solution. After the graft is transported to the recipient transplant center, the graft is divided on the back table. Some European centers recommend cholangiography and arteriography prior to division to delineate anatomy,[37,40] whereas others feel this is unnecessary.[38,41,42] Whether or not contrast studies are done, the hilar structures (hepatic artery, portal vein, and bile duct) are dissected and divided between the two hemilivers. There are varying opinions as to how the vessels should be divided. Some centers routinely retain the full length of the hepatic artery and portal vein with the left hemiliver, whereas other centers routinely retain the full length of the vessels with the right hemiliver (Fig. 5.10). Because the left biliary anatomy is more consistent, the left bile duct, which is generally a single duct, is divided above the hepatic bifurcation. The parenchymal transection is performed either with the mosquito fracture technique or by sharp dissection with a scalpel blade (or amputation knife). The line of transection extends from the confluence of the left and middle hepatic veins to the right side of the falciform ligament and umbilical fissure down to the hilar plate

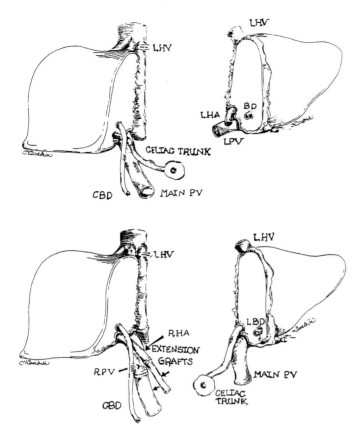

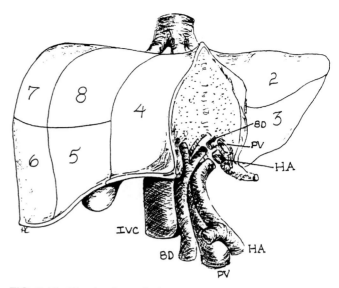

FIG. 5.11. The *in situ* technique of liver splitting is similar to the living donor technique for pediatric recipients. Segments 2 and 3 are separated from the remaining liver in the heart-beating cadaver. BD, biliary duct; HA, hepatic artery; IVC, inferior vena cava; PV, portal vein. (From Busuttil RW, Goss JA. Split liver transplantation. *Ann Surg* 1999;229:313–321, with permission.)

FIG. 5.10. *Ex vivo* split-liver technique. The left graft consists of Couinaud segments 2 and 3; the right graft consists of segments 5 to 8. **Top:** The full lengths of donor vessels are retained by the right graft. **Bottom:** The left lateral segment graft has retained the full length of the donor hepatic artery, and portal vein and extension grafts of donor iliac vessels are sewn to the right portal vein and right hepatic artery. BD, bile duct; CBD, common bile duct; LBD, left bile duct; LHA, left hepatic artery; LHV, left hepatic vein; PV, portal vein; RHA, right hepatic artery; RHV; right hepatic vein. (From Busuttil RW, Goss JA. Split liver transplantation. *Ann Surg* 1999;229:313–321, with permission.)

(Fig. 5.6 line A).[15,42] In most centers, segments 1 and 4 are resected and discarded to avoid acute necrosis or, less commonly, gradual atrophy.[42,43] Several vascular anomalies have been identified that preclude splitting of the liver, including absence of a portal vein bifurcation and right hepatic artery branches passing posterior to the main portal vein.[44]

In Situ Technique

The *in situ* split technique was developed as an application of the living liver donor technique discussed later in this chapter (Fig. 5.11). Rogiers et al. reported the first case using the *in situ* technique in 1995[45] and a series of 14 split grafts in 1996.[46] A left lateral segmentectomy was completed in the heart-beating cadaveric donor and flushed on the back table. Rogiers then proceeded with standard mul-

tiorgan procurement of the remainder of the intraabdominal organs with *in situ* flushing of University of Wisconsin solution. Hepatic segments 1 and 4 were evaluated prior to removal to assess viability and removed only if the appearance suggested that they were not well perfused.[46] Busuttil et al. likewise performed the hepatic transection without vascular interruption; however, Busuttil flushed both hepatic segments *in situ* prior to removal from the cadaveric donor.[39]

Implantation of the right and left split-liver grafts is similar to techniques described previously in the section on reduced-size liver grafts and is generally independent of the method of procurement (*ex vivo* or *in situ*). Generally, the right split graft retains the donor retrohepatic inferior vena cava and is therefore transplanted in the standard orthotopic technique described for whole-organ grafts (Fig. 5.12). The left split graft is generally implanted in the so-called piggyback technique to the confluence of the native middle and left hepatic veins. Extension grafts of donor iliac vessels may be used with either the left or right split graft for the hepatic artery or portal vein as needed (Fig. 5.10). Bile drainage is frequently performed by formation of a hepaticojejunostomy; however, choledochocholedochostomy has also been reported.[46]

Results

Until recently, patient and graft survival rates for recipients of split-liver grafts (50%–67% and 43%–50%, respectively)

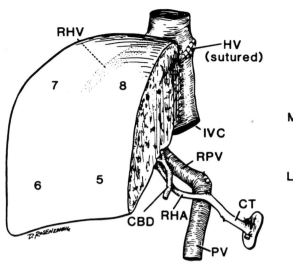
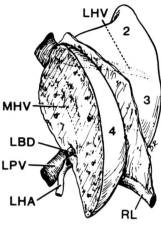

FIG. 5.12. Implantation of split-liver grafts. Right lobe split-liver grafts (segments 5–8) generally retain the donor inferior vena cava and are implanted in orthotopic fashion. Left lateral segment or left lobe split-liver grafts (segments 2 and 3, or 2, 3, and 4) are implanted using the piggyback technique. CBD, common bile duct; CT, celiac trunk; HV, hepatic vein; IVC, inferior vena cava; LBD, left bile duct; LHA, left branch of the hepatic artery; LHV, left hepatic vein; LPV, left portal vein; MHV, middle hepatic vein; PV, portal vein; RHA, right branch of hepatic artery; RHV, right hepatic vein; RL, right lobe. (From Emond JC, Whitington PF, Thistlethwaite JR, et al. Transplantation of two patients with one liver. *Ann Surg* 1990;212:14–22, with permission.)

were lower than these rates for whole-organ transplantation.[38,47,48] The decrease in patient and graft survival was most pronounced for recipients of the right lobe. The diminished survival was probably a result of poor recipient selection combined with prolonged cold ischemia and warming of the graft during the *ex vivo* preparation.[39] By limiting split-liver transplantation to elective situations, the results have improved and are now comparable with whole-organ grafts even for the right lobe graft.[37,41] Reports of *in situ* splitting revealed that this technique can be used even in urgent recipients without compromising patient and graft survival.[39]

Transplantation with a split graft was initially associated with increased bleeding. In early series as many as one-third of *ex vivo* split-liver graft recipients required reoperation or transfusion for early postoperative bleeding.[38] In contrast, bleeding after *in situ* split-liver grafting occurred in less than 3% of recipients.[39,46] *Ex vivo* splitting is also associated with a higher risk of biliary complications (22% to 27%) compared with whole-organ (4%) or *in situ* split grafts (0% to 3%).[37–39,46] Rates of arterial thrombosis and primary graft nonfunction in recent series are similar regardless of graft source.[39,44,46]

Split-liver grafts clearly are a more efficient use of cadaveric donors than RSLT because the total number of livers available for transplantation is doubled. Furthermore, with split-liver grafts the redistribution of adult cadaveric livers to pediatric recipients is avoided. Unfortunately, the most attractive potential application of the technique (i.e., splitting a liver for two adult recipients) is not possible for most adults in the United States. The left lateral segment and usually the full left lobe of the liver provide inadequate functional hepatic mass for most adult recipients in the United States. The acceptable range of hepatic mass re-

quired to achieve successful hepatic function is discussed further in the next section.

ADULT LIVING DONOR LIVER TRANSPLANTATION

Use of the live donor for transplantation has taken on a greater role as the number of patients listed for transplantation increases and the number of cadaveric donors remains unchanged. According to UNOS, in 1998 about one-third of all kidney transplants made use of a living donor. Living donor liver transplantation (LDLT) has become a routine alternative to cadaveric transplantation in pediatric recipients (see Chapter 7). This section focuses on a review of the current experience with living donor liver transplantation for adult recipients.

The major impediments to broader application of LDLT to adult recipients were twofold. First, surgeons were concerned about providing adequate hepatic mass for the recipient; second, they were concerned with donor safety after larger hepatic resections.

Two methods for determining if a graft will have adequate functional hepatic mass have been developed. One method is to calculate the graft-to-recipient-weight ratio (GRWR), which compares the mass of the graft with the overall body mass of the recipient.[49] The second method is to calculate the liver volume as a percentage of the standard liver volume (SLV) as determined by a mathematical formula based on measurements of the liver at autopsy.[50] Table 5.1 shows examples of both of these calculations. A recent review shows that there is nearly perfect (i.e., linear) correlation between these two estimates of liver volume; both methods can therefore be used interchangeably.[49]

TABLE 5.1. *Methods for determining the functional hepatic mass of grafts*

Graft-to-recipient-weight ratio (GRWR)
Optimal GRWR: 1% to 3%
Example
   Recipient body weight = 70 kg
   Graft weight = 700 g
   GRWR = 700 g / 70 kg = 0.01 (or 1%)

Calculation of standard liver volume (SLV)
Japanese formula:[49] SLV (mL) = 706.2 × [body surface area (m²)] + 2.4
Optimal SLV: 50% or greater
Example
   Body surface area (BSA)[a] = 1.88 m²
   SLV = 1.33 L (or approximately 1,330 g) using the Japanese formula
   Donor right lobe = 700 g (estimate based on computed tomography)
   SLV = 700 g / 1,330 g = 0.53 (or 53%)
Because North European and American white individuals are generally larger than Japanese individuals, the revised formula by Heinemann et al.[64] may be more accurate in these populations: SLV (mL) = 1072.8 × [body surface area (m²)] − 345.7

[a]Assuming a recipient who is 5'8" tall and weighs 75 kg.

The earliest experience with transplantation in adults using living donors merely extended the pediatric experience, using either the left lateral segment or full left lobe grafts (with or without the middle hepatic vein).[4,51,52] The size of partial left liver grafts, however, in most cases corresponds to only 20% to 35% of the recipient's expected SLV (Table 5.1). Although successful graft function has occurred with grafts as small as 0.6% GRWR (25% SLV),[53] others have reported an increased risk for postoperative morbidity and mortality with the use of grafts of less than 1.0% GRWR (50% SLV).[49,50,54] Grafts of less than 0.8% to 1.0% GRWR, or "small-for-size grafts," generally demonstrate poor graft function marked by pronounced cholestasis and prolonged coagulopathy.[54] The use of left lobe grafts in adult recipients is therefore limited to recipients with a body weight in the range of 45 to 55 kg. In the United States one would expect this weight restriction to represent only a minority of individuals on the waiting list. Indeed, at the University of Nebraska Medical Center this represents only 11% of the adult waiting list.

The right lobe of the liver, on the other hand, approximates 60% of the hepatic parenchyma and for most adults in the United States would provide at least 1% GRWR. The Kyoto group performed the first right lobe liver transplant in a child in 1994; however, because of concerns about donor safety, right lobe living donor liver transplants were not offered to adult recipients until 1998.[55,56] Since 1998, right lobe liver grafts from living donors have become the standard graft for adult recipients.[5,6]

Donor Selection

There are two key issues in donor selection. First, living liver donation should be voluntary, without coercion and without financial incentives. Second, the potential donor should have no medical conditions that would increase the risk of the donor operation. Most living donors have been immediate family members; rarely, a close friend is the donor.[5,6] Caution must be exercised, however, because family members may intentionally or unintentionally place pressure on relatives of appropriate age and blood type to donate. The evaluation process includes an interview with the potential donor in the absence of other family members. During this interview the potential donor can be provided with the option for the transplant team to provide a "medical excuse" at any time if he or she chooses not to donate. Furthermore, the individual must be able to give an informed consent; therefore, minors are excluded from living donation. In contrast to living donor transplantation in pediatric recipients, the adult recipient may have concerns about placing a loved one at risk or about potential complications he or she might suffer, and therefore the recipient's consent must also be obtained. There is some concern in the transplant community over the issue of informed consent given the limited experience that currently exists.[57] In a position paper presented at the May 2000 meeting, the American Society of Transplant Surgeons (ASTS) concurs that insufficient information currently exists "to accurately assign risk for the donor." The consent process must therefore clearly delineate the known experience and acknowledge that all potential risks are not yet known.

During the evaluation process the blood type of the potential donor should be determined and confirmed to be compatible with the recipient's blood type. Other commonly performed laboratory tests include liver and kidney function tests and viral serologies. The evaluation also includes a physical examination, performed when possible by a hepatologist familiar with liver diseases. Most donors in published series have been between 24 and 61 years old.[5,50] Age is not an absolute contraindication to living donation; however, older individuals have a higher likelihood of silent cardiac or cerebrovascular disease that may increase the perioperative risks.

After it has been determined that the potential donor is doing so without undue coercion and has no underlying medical conditions that would place him or her in jeopardy, the evaluation process continues with a determination of the size and shape of the donor liver. The donor liver will need to provide adequate functional mass for the potential recipient, and the remaining hepatic mass must be sufficient to minimize the risk of postoperative liver dysfunction in the donor. Traditionally, the estimation of liver volume has been accomplished by using computed tomography (CT) and, more recently, magnetic resonance imaging (MRI).[5,6,58] Both appear to provide relatively accurate assessments of liver volume, but experience increases accuracy. MRI has the potential advantage of assessment of arterial and biliary anatomy without further invasive testing.[5] Currently, however, hepatic arteriography is performed in addition to the CT or MRI scan in most centers to confirm hepatic arterial anatomy and to assess the portal venous anatomy, with specific attention to the blood supply to segment 4.[5] Perhaps in the future magnetic resonance hepatic angiography will replace the more invasive standard angiography.

Technique for Living Donor Right Lobe Graft

The procurement of the right lobe graft from the donor begins with a bilateral subcostal incision and division of the hepatic ligaments to the right hepatic lobe. The ligamentous attachments of the left lobe remain intact to prevent torsion of the remnant liver after right lobectomy. The liver is then mobilized off the retrohepatic vena cava, carefully ligating small accessory hepatic veins. Marcos et al. recommend preservation of any accessory hepatic vein greater than 5 mm in diameter for reimplantation.[5] Intraoperative ultrasound is then used to identify the intrahepatic course of the right and middle hepatic veins to determine the optimal line of transection. Hilar dissection is performed to identify the branches to the right lobe from the hepatic artery and portal vein. Minimal, if any, dissection is performed of the right hepatic duct(s) and left hilar structures. Cholecystectomy and cholangiography are then performed to assess biliary anatomy. Potential vascular and biliary anomalies were described in detail previously (Figs. 5.2 to 5.4). The right hepatic vein is also isolated prior to parenchymal transection and controlled with a vessel loop. In our center the Cavitron Ultrasonic Surgical Aspirator (CUSA) ultrasonic dissection is used to transect the hepatic parenchyma. Although this is a somewhat tedious process, it allows identification and ligation of large portal and hepatic venous branches that cross the plane of transection, thereby minimizing blood loss. No inflow or outflow vascular obstruction is performed during the process of hepatic parenchymal transection in order to minimize ischemic injury to either portion of the liver. Figure 5.13 depicts the right lobe graft after parenchymal transection and division of the hepatic artery, portal vein, right hepatic duct, and right hepatic vein.

Figure 5.14 demonstrates the method of implantation of this right hepatic lobe graft. This method differs from the technique used for reduced-size or split-liver right lobe grafts as demonstrated in Fig. 5.12 because of the absence of the donor inferior vena cava. In the recipient of the living donor right lobe graft, the native inferior vena cava is preserved and the donor right hepatic vein is anastomosed directly to the recipient right hepatic vein orifice in the so-called piggyback technique. Extension vascular grafts are rarely required with the right lobe graft. Biliary drainage is

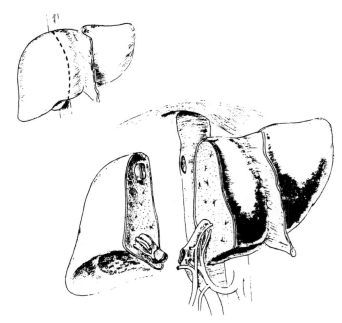

FIG. 5.13. Living donor right lobe graft procurement. The hepatic parenchyma is divided without inflow or outflow occlusion until the only remaining structural attachments are the right hepatic artery, portal vein, and hepatic vein. The vessels are sharply divided, and the graft removed to the back table to flush with University of Wisconsin solution. (From Wachs ME, Bak TE, Karrer FM, et al. Adult living donor liver transplantation using a right hepatic lobe. *Transplantation* 1998;66:1313–1316, with permission.)

most commonly performed by Roux-en-Y hepaticojejunostomy, although duct-to-duct anastomosis has also been reported.[56]

Donor Safety

A recent survey by Busuttil et al. reveals that between 150 and 200 right lobe transplants from living donors have been performed in the United States at 29 liver transplant centers (R.W. Busuttil, personal communication, 2000). An additional 165 right lobe transplants from living donors have been performed in other countries (K. Tanaka, personal communications, 2000; G. Testa, personal communications, 2000). Interestingly, many of the largest centers in the United States have been slow to adopt this technique primarily because of concerns over donor safety. The ASTS has proposed establishing a registry to track donor morbidity and mortality, which it is hoped will guide future application of this valuable technique.

Risk for Donor Mortality

Although the number of cases are few, the current experience appears to indicate that the risk of death from right hepatic lobectomy in the healthy donor is approximately 0.3%, which is similar to the reported rate of 0.1% to 0.2% for left

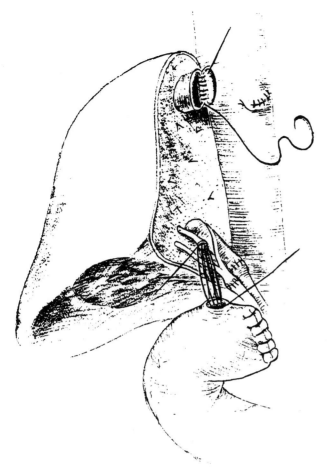

FIG. 5.14. Implantation technique for living donor right lobe graft. The technique differs from reduced-size liver transplantation and split-liver transplantation by the absence of a donor inferior vena cava. Therefore, implantation is by the piggyback technique, in which the donor right hepatic vein is anastomosed to the recipient right hepatic vein orifice. (From Wachs ME, Bak TE, Karrer FM, et al. Adult living donor liver transplantation using a right hepatic lobe. *Transplantation* 1998;66:1313–1316, with permission.)

lateral segment or left lobe living liver donors. There has been at least one donor death after right hepatic lobectomy (publicized in the news media).[59] Prior to beginning the adult LDLT program in our center, we reviewed all published series of major hepatic resection since 1993. Although the majority of these resections were for malignancy, we felt that examination of mortality rates would be helpful in estimating the risk for a healthy donor. Liver failure was the most common cause of death; however, this was not reported in the absence of underlying cirrhosis. We recognize nonetheless that with extensive hepatic resection, liver failure could be a risk even in the healthy liver donor. The remaining causes of death identified after major hepatic resection (excluding recurrent malignancy) include cardiac complications, bile leak and associated sepsis, pulmonary embolus, and operative complications, with an estimated overall incidence of 0.5% mortality for the 3,479 resections reported. This correlates closely with the early reported experience with right hepatectomy in living donors.

Donor Morbidity after Right Hepatectomy

Following right hepatectomy in the donor, the remaining liver has demonstrated mild dysfunction similar to that seen following right hepatectomy for cancer. However, comparisons of mean peak aspartate aminotransferase (AST) levels and total bilirubin levels would seem to indicate a higher level of dysfunction after donor right lobectomy than left lateral segmentectomy. Mean peak serum AST levels between 100 and 265 U/L have been reported after left lateral segmentectomy, compared with 205 to 379 U/L after right hepatectomy.[6,60] Transient hyperbilirubinemia with a peak of 4.4 mg/dL was reported after the first living donor right lobectomy.[61] In a series of 26 living right lobe donors for adult recipients, the Kyoto group reported a mean peak total bilirubin level of 3.2 mg/dL, which returned to normal within the first week.[6] In comparison, peak total bilirubin levels after left lateral segmentectomy remained within the normal range (less than 2.0 mg/dL) throughout follow-up.[6] Furthermore, coagulopathy with mean peak prothrombin time of 18.7 seconds has been reported in the first 7 days after extended right lobectomy in living donors.[62]

Other surgical complications reported after right hepatic lobectomy include the need for homologous blood transfusion, incisional hernia, bile leak, biliary stricture, sepsis, pancreatitis and sepsis, and patient death.[5,6,56,59] In addition, pulmonary embolus has been reported after left lobe and left lateral segment living donation.[52,63]

Recipient Results

At this time, most series of living-donor right lobe transplants are performed in the context of recipients who are UNOS status 2B or 3. The reason for limiting adult-to-adult LDLT to more elective patients is so that recipients will have the maximum chance for survival. This was also the approach early in the experience of living donor transplantation for pediatric recipients. Furthermore, the severely ill recipient may not tolerate a smaller volume of hepatic mass than is provided with a whole-organ cadaveric graft. Although overall experience with adult LDLT is still small, patient and graft survival rates are generally better with right lobe grafts than left. It also appears that right lobe grafts have comparable survival rates to those seen with whole cadaveric liver grafts. Current published results of right lobe LDLT in adults are summarized in Table 5.2.

Biliary complications, including anastomotic leak, anastomotic stricture, and biloma, are reported to occur in 15% to 40% of adult LDLT recipients,[5,6] which is more frequent than after whole-organ cadaveric liver transplantation. Other complications appear to occur with a similar frequency as in whole-organ cadaveric grafts and include

TABLE 5.2. *Current published experience with adult-to-adult living donor right lobe liver transplantation*

Ref.	Year	No. of recipients	Type of graft	Graft weight	Blood loss (donor)	Patient survival (%)	Graft survival (%)	Recipient complications (no. of cases)	Donor transfusion	Donor complications (no. of cases)
60	1997	7	Ext. right lobe	490–1140 g	900 mL	86	86	Biliary stricture (2) Biliary leakage (1) Abdominal abscess (1) Pancreatitis (1) Appendicitis (1) Postbiopsy hemorrhage (1) Abdominal candidiasis (1) Cerebrovascular accident (1) Necrosis of cut surface of the liver (4) Hepatic vein thrombosis (1)	No	Incisional hernia (1) Bile duct stricture (1)
56	1998	2	Right lobe	812 mL, 830 mL	1800 mL, 800 mL	100	100	Biliary stricture (1)	Yes	None
5	1999	25	Right lobe	884 + 162 g	665 + 607 mL	88	88	Biliary complications (24%) Biloma (5) Anastomotic leak (1) Anastomotic stricture (1) Sepsis (3) Gastrointestinal bleeding (2) Seizures (2)	No	Pressure sores(2) Atelectasis (1) Phlebitis (1) Prolonged ileus (1)
6	2000	26	Right lobe	465–900 g	338 + 175 mL	73	73	Hepatic venous outflow obstruction (1) Bile leak (4) Bile stricture (4) Postoperative bleeding (5) Intestinal perforation (2)	No	Bile leak (2)

sepsis, gastrointestinal bleeding, seizures, and acute rejection. With increased experience it will be possible to determine if the potential advantage of decreased pretransplantation mortality will outweigh the risks of perioperative complications in both donors and recipients.

SUMMARY

Reduced-size liver grafts were an important step in the development of partial liver grafts. In large part, however, RSLT has been abandoned in favor of techniques that increase the overall number of transplants that can be performed. Split-liver transplantation and adult LDLT using right lobe grafts are technically demanding procedures. Currently, only a few centers have gained experience with either technique. These methods of liver graft procurement differ from standard liver resection by the preservation of blood flow during hepatic parenchymal transection. Clearly, when either split-liver transplantation or adult-to-adult living donor liver transplantation is performed by surgeons experienced with these techniques, the procedures can be carried out safely with excellent graft function. As with any new procedure, over time more centers will begin to offer these options to patients on their waiting lists. The enthusiasm to decrease pretransplantation mortality, however, must be restrained by caution to do no harm to either the donor or recipient.

REFERENCES

1. Heffron TG. Living related liver transplantation. *Semin Liver Dis* 1995;15:165–172.
2. Raia S, Nery JR, Mies S. Liver transplantation from live donors [Letter]. *Lancet* 1989;2:497.
3. Strong RW, Lynch SV, Ong TH, et al. Successful liver transplantation from a living donor to her son. *N Engl J Med* 1990;322: 1505–1507.
4. Hashikura Y, Makuuchi M, Kawasaki S, et al. Successful living-related partial liver transplantation to an adult patient [Letter]. *Lancet* 1994;343:1233–1234.
5. Marcos A, Fisher RA, Ham JM, et al. Right lobe living donor liver transplantation. *Transplantation* 1999;68:798–803.
6. Inomata Y, Uemoto S, Asonuma K, et al. Right lobe graft in living donor liver transplantation. *Transplantation* 2000;69:258–264.
7. Chaib E, Bertevello P, Pinto FC, et al. Main variations of the extrahepatic biliary system and their application to the so-called "split-liver" transplantation technique [in Portuguese]. *Rev Hosp Clin Fac Med Sao Paulo* 1995;50:311–313.
8. Chaib E, Antonio LG, Ishida RY, et al. Hepatic venous system and its application in the so-called split-liver transplantation technique [in Portuguese]. *Rev Hosp Clin Fac Med Sao Paulo* 1995;50:49–51.
9. Asonuma K, Shapiro AM, Inomata Y, et al. Living related liver transplantation from donors with the left-sided gallbladder/portal vein anomaly. *Transplantation* 1999;68:1610–1612.
10. Couinaud C, Houssin D. Bisection of the liver for transplantation. Simplification of the method [in French]. *Chirurgie* 1992;118:217–222.
11. Bismuth H, Houssin D. Reduced-sized orthotopic liver graft in hepatic transplantation in children. *Surgery* 1984;95:367–370.
12. Bilik R, Greig P, Langer B, et al. Survival after reduced-size liver transplantation is dependent on pretransplant status. *J Pediatr Surg* 1993;28:1307–1311.
13. Malatack JJ, Schaid DJ, Urbach AH, et al. Choosing a pediatric recipient for orthotopic liver transplantation. *J Pediatr* 1987;111:479–489.
14. Boillot O. Graft reduction in pediatric hepatic transplantation: value, technique and results [in French]. *Pediatrie* 1991;46:351–356.
15. Langnas AN, Marujo WC, Inagaki M, et al. The results of reduced-size liver transplantation, including split livers, in patients with end-stage liver disease. *Transplantation* 1992;53:387–391.
16. Bonatti H, Muiesan P, Connelly S, et al. Hepatic transplantation in children under 3 months of age: a single centre's experience. *J Pediatr Surg* 1997;32:486–488.
17. de Santibanes E, McCormack L, Mattera J, et al. Partial left lateral segment transplant from a living donor. *Liver Transpl* 2000;6: 108–112.
18. Strong R, Ong TH, Pillay P, et al. A new method of segmental orthotopic liver transplantation in children. *Surgery* 1988;104:104–107.
19. Tzakis A, Todo S, Starzl TE. Orthotopic liver transplantation with preservation of the inferior vena cava. *Ann Surg* 1989;210:649–652.
20. Badger IL, Czerniak A, Beath S, et al. Hepatic transplantation in children using reduced size allografts. *Br J Surg* 1992;79:47–49.
21. Broelsch CE, Stevens LH, Whitington PF. The use of reduced-size liver transplants in children, including split livers and living related liver transplants. *Eur J Pediatr Surg* 1991;1:166–171.
22. Broelsch CE, Emond JC, Thistlethwaite JR, et al. Liver transplantation, including the concept of reduced-size liver transplants in children. *Ann Surg* 1988;208:410–420.
23. Broelsch CE, Emond JC, Thistlethwaite JR, et al. Liver transplantation with reduced-size donor organs. *Transplantation* 1988;45:519–524.
24. Alexander JW, First MR, Hariharan S, et al. Chapter 17, Recent contributions to transplantation at the University of Cincinnati. Alexander JW, First MR, Hariharan S, Penn I, Schroder T, Ryckman Munda R, Bhat G, Bolce R in Terasaki PI, editor. *Clinical Transplants* 1991. UCLA Tissue Typing Laboratory, Los Angeles CA, 159–178, 1991.
25. Sindhi R, Rosendale J, Mundy D, et al. Impact of segmental grafts on pediatric liver transplantation—a review of the United Network for Organ Sharing Scientific Registry data (1990–1996). *J Pediatr Surg* 1999;34:107–110; discussion 110–111.
26. Houssin D, Soubrane O, Boillot O, et al. Orthotopic liver transplantation with a reduced-size graft: an ideal compromise in pediatrics? *Surgery* 1992;111:532–542.
27. Bilik R, Yellen M, Superina RA. Surgical complications in children after liver transplantation. *J Pediatr Surg* 1992;27:1371–1375.
28. Sudan DL, Shaw BW Jr, Fox IJ, et al. Long-term follow-up of auxiliary orthotopic liver transplantation for the treatment of fulminant hepatic failure. *Surgery* 1997;122:771–777; discussion 777–778.
29. Boudjema K, Cherqui D, Jaeck D, et al. Auxiliary liver transplantation for fulminant and subfulminant hepatic failure. *Transplantation* 1995; 59:218–223.
30. Egawa H, Tanaka K, Inomata Y, et al. Auxiliary partial orthotopic liver transplantation from a living related donor: a report of two cases. *Transplant Proc* 1996;28:1071–1072.
31. Yazaki M, Ikeda S, Takei Y, et al. Complete neurological recovery of an adult patient with type II citrullinemia after living related partial liver transplantation. *Transplantation* 1996;62:1679–1684.
32. Uemoto S, Yabe S, Inomata Y, et al. Coexistence of a graft with the preserved native liver in auxiliary partial orthotopic liver transplantation from a living donor for ornithine transcarbamylase deficiency. *Transplantation* 1997;63:1026–1028.
33. Rela M, Muiesan P, Vilca-Melendez H, et al. Auxiliary partial orthotopic liver transplantation for Crigler-Najjar syndrome type I. *Ann Surg* 1999;229:565–569.
34. Inomata Y, Kiuchi T, Kim I, et al. Auxiliary partial orthotopic living donor liver transplantation as an aid for small-for-size grafts in larger recipients. *Transplantation* 1999;67:1314–1319.
35. Pichlmayr R, Ringe B, Gubernatis G, et al. Transplantation of a donor liver to 2 recipients (splitting transplantation)—a new method in the further development of segmental liver transplantation [in German]. *Langenbecks Arch Chir* 1988;373:127–130.
36. Bismuth H, Morino M, Castaing D, et al. Emergency orthotopic liver transplantation in two patients using one donor liver. *Br J Surg* 1989; 76:722–724.
37. Azoulay D, Astarcioglu I, Bismuth H, et al. Split-liver transplantation. The Paul Brousse policy. *Ann Surg* 1996;224:737–746; discussion 746–748.
38. Emond JC, Whitington PF, Thistlethwaite JR, et al. Transplantation of two patients with one liver. Analysis of a preliminary experience with 'split-liver' grafting. *Ann Surg* 1990;212:14–22.
39. Busuttil RW, Goss JA. Split liver transplantation. *Ann Surg* 1999;229: 313–321.

40. Otte JB, de Ville de Goyet J, Alberti D, et al. The concept and technique of the split liver in clinical transplantation. *Surgery* 1990;107:605–612.
41. Kalayoglu M, D'Alessandro AM, Knechtle SJ, et al. Preliminary experience with split liver transplantation. *J Am Coll Surg* 1996;182:381–387.
42. Rela M, Vougas V, Muiesan P, et al. Split liver transplantation: King's College Hospital experience. *Ann Surg* 1998;227:282–288.
43. Couinaud C. A "scandal": segment IV and liver transplantation [in French]. *J Chir* (Paris) 1993;130:443–446.
44. Rela M, McCall JL, Karani J, et al. Accessory right hepatic artery arising from the left: implications for split liver transplantation. *Transplantation* 1998;66:792–794.
45. Rogiers X, Malago M, Habib N, et al. *In situ* splitting of the liver in the heart-beating cadaveric organ donor for transplantation in two recipients. *Transplantation* 1995;59:1081–1083.
46. Rogiers X, Malago M, Gawad K, et al. *In situ* splitting of cadaveric livers. The ultimate expansion of a limited donor pool. *Ann Surg* 1996;224:331–339; discussion 339–341.
47. Shaw BW Jr, Wood RP, Stratta RJ, et al. Management of arterial anomalies encountered in split-liver transplantation. *Transplant Proc* 1990;22:420–422.
48. Broelsch CE, Emond JC, Whitington PF, et al. Application of reduced-size liver transplants as split grafts, auxiliary orthotopic grafts, and living related segmental transplants. *Ann Surg* 1990;212:368–375; discussion 375–377.
49. Kiuchi T, Kasahara M, Uryuhara K, et al. Impact of graft size mismatching on graft prognosis in liver transplantation from living donors. *Transplantation* 1999;67:321–327.
50. Kawasaki S, Makuuchi M, Matsunami H, et al. Living related liver transplantation in adults. *Ann Surg* 1998;227:269–274.
51. Lee SG, Hwang S, Lee YJ, et al. Regeneration of graft liver in adult-to-adult living donor liver transplantation using a left lobe graft. *J Korean Med Sci* 1998;13:350–354.
52. Ikai I, Morimoto T, Yamamoto Y, et al. Left lobectomy of the donor: operation for larger recipients in living related liver transplantation. *Transplant Proc* 1996;28:56–58.
53. Lo CM, Fan ST, Liu CL, et al. Minimum graft size for successful living donor liver transplantation. *Transplantation* 1999;68:1112–1116.
54. Emond JC, Renz JF, Ferrell LD, et al. Functional analysis of grafts from living donors. Implications for the treatment of older recipients. *Ann Surg* 1996;224:544–552; discussion 552–554.
55. Yamaoka Y, Washida M, Honda K, et al. Liver transplantation using a right lobe graft from a living related donor. *Transplantation* 1994;57:1127–1130.
56. Wachs ME, Bak TE, Karrer FM, et al. Adult living donor liver transplantation using a right hepatic lobe. *Transplantation* 1998;66:1313–1316.
57. Strong RW. Whither living donor liver transplantation? *Liver Transpl Surg* 1999;5:536–538.
58. Heymsfield SB, Fulenwider T, Nordlinger B, et al. Accurate measurement of liver, kidney, and spleen volume and mass by computerized axial tomography. *Ann Intern Med* 1979;90:185–187.
59. Liver donor's death sets transplant specialists abuzz. *The News and Observer* 1999 Oct 3:1A.
60. Lo CM, Fan ST, Liu CL, et al. Adult-to-adult living donor liver transplantation using extended right lobe grafts. *Ann Surg* 1997;226:261–269; discussion 269–270.
61. Tanaka K, Uemoto S, Tokunaga Y, et al. Surgical techniques and innovations in living related liver transplantation. *Ann Surg* 1993;217:82–91.
62. Lo CM, Fan ST, Liu CL, et al. Increased risk for living liver donors after extended right lobectomy. *Transplant Proc* 1999;31:533–534.
63. Sterneck MR, Fischer L, Nischwitz U, et al. Selection of the living liver donor. *Transplantation* 1995;60:667–671.
64. Heinemann A, Wischhusen F, Puschel K, et al. Standard liver volume in the Caucasian population. *Liver Transpl Surg* 1999;5:366–368.

Transplantation of the Liver, edited by Willis C.
Maddrey, Eugene R. Schiff, and Michael F.
Sorrell. Lippincott Williams & Wilkins,
Philadelphia © 2001.

CHAPTER 6

Pediatric Liver Transplantation

Rafik M. Ghobrial, Farin Amersi, Sue V. McDiarmid, and Ronald W. Busuttil

Orthotopic liver transplantation (OLT) has become a well-established modality for the treatment of previously fatal disease in children. Remarkable progress has been made since the first OLT was performed in a pediatric patient in 1963.[1] The number of OLTs dramatically increased after liver transplantation was given a therapeutic status by the National Institutes of Health.[2] The advent of new immunosuppressive agents and the refinement of surgical techniques have accounted for the remarkable improvement in 1-year patient survival from 20% to 30% in the 1970s to 80% to 90% in the 1990s. However, two important factors must be considered in the application of OLT for childhood diseases: the increasing gap between the donor supply and patients awaiting OLT, and the high financial costs incurred. This chapter highlights the aspects of liver transplantation that are pertinent to the pediatric patient, including childhood diseases, technical considerations, and complications.

INDICATIONS FOR TRANSPLANTATION

The diseases in pediatric patients treated with OLT are listed in Table 6.1. The end points that require transplantation include severe cholestasis, variceal bleeding, unmanageable ascites, intractable pruritus, failed synthetic function, encephalopathy, an unacceptable quality of life, and failure to thrive.[3]

Cholestatic Liver Disease

Obstructive Cholestatic Liver Disease

Biliary atresia is the most common indication for liver transplantation in children. It is defined as a partial or complete absence of patent bile ducts. The incidence varies from 1 in 8,000 to 1 in 10,000, with a 4- to 5-fold increase in Pacific and Indian Ocean areas.[4] In approximately 2% to 3% of cases of extrahepatic biliary atresia, surgical exploration reveals a dilated hilar structure that may communicate with intrahepatic bile ducts, the so-called correctable type of extrahepatic biliary atresia. Before 1959, the natural history of patients with "uncorrectable" biliary atresia was progressive liver failure and death before the age of 2 months. In 1959, Kasai and Suzuki devised the operation of portoenterostomy, which used a defunctionalized loop of jejunum to drain microscopic ducts within the porta hepatis.[5] Since then, numerous modifications of the procedure have occurred.[6] Successful bile flow is achieved in 40% to 60% of patients who are operated on early in life. However, even if the Kasai procedure is performed before the age of 3 months, 75% of children with biliary atresia will eventually require transplantation.[7,8] The most common clinically identifiable cause of failure of an initially successful portoenterostomy is cholangitis,[9] and many patients experience progressive cholestasis followed by cirrhosis, possibly due to intrahepatic causes.[10] Ninety percent of children in whom a portoenterostomy fails to provide adequate permanent bile drainage will die by the age of 5 years.[11] Reattempts at biliary drainage after an initially unsuccessful portoenterostomy are uniformly unsuccessful.[12,13]

In a 1984 report on a group of 31 patients who underwent transplantation for biliary atresia at Pittsburgh, early survival was 84% (follow-up of 2 to 36 months), and prior biliary surgery did not significantly affect survival after OLT.[12] In 1987, Starzl reported a 5-year survival rate of 64% in 137 patients with biliary atresia.[14] In the largest series, Goss et al. from the University of California at Los Angeles (UCLA) demonstrated 1-, 2-, and 5-year patient survival rates of 83%, 80%, and 78%, respectively, for 190 children who received transplants for biliary atresia.[8] In conclusion, children with biliary atresia should undergo early portoenterostomy, but should be referred for OLT evaluation at the first sign of failure.

R. M. Ghobrial and F. Amersi: Department of Surgery, Liver and Pancreas Transplantation, UCLA School of Medicine, Los Angeles, California 90095.

S. V. McDiarmid: Departments of Pediatrics and Surgery, UCLA School of Medicine, Los Angeles, California 90095.

R. W. Busuttil: Division of Liver and Transplantation, UCLA School of Medicine, Los Angeles, California 90095.

TABLE 6.1 *Indications for pediatric liver transplantation*

Cholestatic liver disease
Biliary atresia
Paucity of intrahepatic bile ducts
  Syndromic (Alagille syndrome)
  Nonsyndromic
Sclerosing cholangitis
Familial cholestasis syndromes
Fulminant liver failure
Viruses (hepatitis A, hepatitis B)
Toxins (drugs, mushrooms)
Metabolic (Wilson's disease)
Drugs (acetaminophen, isonicotinic acid hydrazide)
Metabolic disorders
α_1-Antitrypsin deficiency
Wilson's disease
Tyrosinemia
Urea cycle defects
Familial hypercholesterolemia
Selected lipid storage diseases
Glycogen storage diseases (IA and IV)
Neonatal iron storage disease
Crigler-Najjar syndrome
Disorders of bile acid metabolism
Hyperoxaluria type I
Hematologic disorders
  Hemophilia A or B
  Protein C deficiency, porphyria
Selected organic acidemias
Chronic active hepatitis or cirrhosis
Autoimmune
Neonatal hepatitis
Chronic hepatitis C or B
Cryptogenic cirrhosis
Neoplasia
Hepatoblastoma
Hemangioendothelioma
Sarcomas
Hepatocellular carcinoma or sarcoma
Miscellaneous
Budd-Chiari syndrome
Trauma
Cystic fibrosis
Caroli's disease
Cirrhosis secondary to parenteral nutrition

Sclerosing cholangitis is another form of obstructive cholestatic liver disease that may require transplantation.[15] OLT is indicated in this rare condition for increasing jaundice cholangitis and portal hypertension. Children with sclerosing cholangitis should be evaluated for underlying autoimmune or inflammatory bowel disease prior to transplantation.

Familial Cholestasis Syndromes

The term *idiopathic obstructive cholangiopathies* has been used to describe the poorly understood familial cholestasis syndromes. Following an initial inflammatory stage, some children develop paucity of the intrahepatic biliary system. In some, the disease is relatively benign, with mild cholestasis and pruritus that only require medical management.

In others, severe cholestasis and pruritus are pronounced, in addition to malabsorption and failure to thrive. Under such circumstances, transplantation is warranted.[15]

Paucity of Intrahepatic Bile Ducts

The syndromic form (Alagille syndrome[16]) of a paucity of intrahepatic bile ducts is characterized by extrahepatic anomalies, particularly involving the heart. The most common anomalies include pulmonary stenosis and tetralogy of Fallot. Both the syndromic and nonsyndromic forms require ongoing evaluation for OLT. Only a minority of children will present with marked hepatic dysfunction that requires transplantation; most experience symptomatic improvement with age and do not need OLT.[15]

Inborn Errors of Metabolism

OLT has been performed for a wide variety of metabolic disorders.[15] However, it is important to determine before transplantation whether liver replacement will improve or prevent further deterioration of accompanying extrahepatic manifestations. Thus, OLT should only be offered if (a) the metabolic defect is exclusively in the liver (e.g., Crigler-Najjar syndrome), (b) the clinical impact of an extrahepatic enzymatic defect will be overridden by a normal liver (e.g., tyrosinemia), and (c) the extrahepatic manifestations of the metabolic disorder do not preclude transplantation (e.g., Wilson's disease).

α_1-Antitrypsin Deficiency

α_1-Antitrypsin deficiency is the most common metabolic disorder for which OLT is performed. α_1-Antitrypsin (ATT) is one of several serine proteases that are synthesized by the liver to inhibit a wide variety of proteolytic enzymes, including trypsin.[17] The gene for the enzyme has 24 alleles that exhibit autosomal codominance. The normal phenotype of the ATT protease inhibitor (Pi) is designated MM. End-stage liver disease is associated with the PiZZ phenotype, in which only 10% to 15% of normal serum ATT levels (200–400 mg/dL) are detected. However, end-stage liver disease occurs only in a minority of children with the PiZZ phenotype.[17,18] PiZZ was detected in only 125 of 200,000 infants (0.06%) who were screened for the anomaly. Fourteen of these 125 infants (11%) exhibited neonatal jaundice, and at the age of 2 years, only 3 of the 14 (27%) had progressed to cirrhosis. Thus, the apparent overall incidence of cirrhosis in the PiZZ phenotype is 3 in 200,000.[18]

Hepatic injury may be caused by accumulation of ATT deposits within the hepatocytes or by hepatocyte damage due to uninhibited proteolysis, or both.[19] Although neonatal cholestasis may develop before 10 weeks of age, it usually abates until late childhood or early adolescence, when cirrhosis and portal hypertension become apparent. The diagnosis should be considered in any neonate with jaundice.

An absent α_1-globulin peak in serum electrophoresis increases suspicion, which can be confirmed by low serum ATT activity, quantitative measurements of serum ATT, and genetic Pi typing.[20] OLT is offered to patients with cirrhosis and evidence of progressive hepatic decompensation. Following successful OLT, recipients acquire the phenotype of the donor, and ATT levels normalize.[21] Progression of pulmonary disease, which accompanies α_1-antitrypsin deficiency, is presumably eliminated by OLT. The 5-year actuarial survival rate of children who receive transplants for α_1-Antitrypsin deficiency is greater than 80%.[22]

Tyrosinemia

The hereditary disorder tyrosinemia is characterized by a deficiency of *p*-hydroxyphenolpyruvate hydroxylase, an enzyme that degrades the metabolic products of tyrosine.[23,24] Tyrosinemia may present as acute liver failure in infancy or with a more insidious onset that slowly progresses to cirrhosis in childhood. The development of hepatocellular carcinoma in up to 37% of children older than 2 years[25,26] has made preemptive transplantation the treatment of choice even before end-stage liver disease supervenes.[27] The use of 2-(2-nitro-4-trifluromethylbenzoyl)-3-cyclohexanedione (NTBC), which prevents the accumulation of toxic metabolites, is under investigation.[28] However, it is not known whether NTBC therapy can reliably prevent or delay the onset of hepatocellular carcinoma.

Wilson's Disease

Wilson's disease is an autosomal recessive disorder characterized by copper accumulation in the liver, central nervous system, kidney, eyes, and other organs. The prevalence rate is 1 in 30,000 worldwide, with a carrier frequency of 1 in 90 individuals.[29] Lack of copper excretion from hepatocellular lysozymes leads to its accumulation, with subsequent hepatic damage. When hepatic capacity is exceeded, copper diffuses into the bloodstream and is deposited in other organs. Kayser-Fleischer rings, for example, are characteristic copper deposits in Descemet's membrane of the cornea.[29] Diagnosis is generally made by identifying low serum ceruloplasmin levels (<20 mg/dL) and the presence of Kayser-Fleischer rings. Liver biopsy with quantitative copper measurements and increased urinary copper excretion confirm the diagnosis.[30]

Hepatic manifestations may be either acute or exhibited by an insidious onset of progressive hepatic insufficiency accompanied by synthetic dysfunction and portal hypertension. Acute hepatic disease may be self-limiting or progress to fulminant failure, which is most commonly encountered in adolescent patients.[30] Wilson's disease, if diagnosed early before the onset of tissue damage, can often be managed medically with chelating agents such as D-penicillamine.[31]

However, such treatment is ineffective in fulminant or severe subacute hepatitis.

Patients should undergo OLT for Wilson's disease if they develop fulminant hepatitis or if they have cirrhosis with hepatic decompensation and fail adequate D-penicillamine therapy of 2 to 3 months.[30] Plasma levels of copper and ceruloplasmin are expected to normalize after OLT.[32]

Crigler-Najjar Syndrome

In 1952, Crigler and Najjar described a syndrome of "congenital familial nonhemolytic jaundice," which is now known by their names.[33] Currently, this syndrome is divided into type I and type II. Type I is characterized by undetectable bilirubin glucuronyl transferase activity in liver tissue and unresponsiveness to phenobarbital therapy. Such patients progress to death from kernicterus, usually before the age of 15 months,[34] and should be considered early for OLT. Type II disease, on the other hand, is less severe and often responds to phenobarbital therapy.

Hematologic Disorders

Porphyria is an autosomal dominant disease characterized by elevated levels of protoporphyrin in erythrocytes and plasma, caused by deficient heme synthetase activity.[34] Photosensitivity is the main clinical manifestation, but liver disease due to porphyrin deposition occasionally occurs and may progress to cirrhosis. Medical treatment of the disease is with cholestyramine;[35] OLT has successfully treated refractory cases.[32]

Life-threatening thromboses that occur in protein C deficiency can be averted by liver transplantation.[15] OLT may also be indicated in hemophilia A and B to increase the production of factors VIII and IX, respectively. However, OLT has only been performed in patients with hemophilia who have secondary liver disease caused by hepatitis B or C.[36]

Disorders of Lipid Metabolism

Lipid storage diseases (Gaucher's disease, Niemann-Pick disease, Wolman's disease, cholesterol ester storage disease) and other lysosomal storage diseases (mucopolysaccharidoses) are characterized by widespread extrahepatic enzyme deficiencies that result in progressive disease after liver transplantation, particularly involving the central nervous system.[37] Thus, OLT alone is not recommended because of the probability of progressive neurologic disease. Combined bone marrow transplantation and OLT may be considered in selected cases of mucopolysaccharidoses.[38] However, in familial hypercholesterolemia type 2A, early OLT alone may avoid the fatal consequences of cardiac atherosclerosis. Combined OLT and heart transplantation may reverse the metabolic defect and the life-threatening complications of an already established cardiac disease.[15]

Urea Cycle Defects

Among the disorders of amino acid metabolism, urea cycle defects may be cured by OLT[39] because the enzyme resides exclusively in the liver. Ornithine transcarbamylase deficiency is the most common defect, and profound neurologic damage is inevitable if OLT is not performed early in life.

Glycogen Storage Diseases

Disorders of carbohydrate metabolism for which OLT is indicated include galactosemia and the glycogen storage diseases. Liver disease due to galactosemia can be prevented by screening newborns and using dietary manipulation. OLT is reserved for children who develop cirrhosis or in whom hepatic adenomas develop.[40] Of the glycogen storage diseases, type IA can be controlled by dietary management alone, although there is a risk of development of hepatic adenomas.[41] Type IV is characterized by early cirrhosis. However, because the enzymatic defect is widespread, ongoing accumulation of amylopectin may still occur following transplantation,[42,43] albeit at a slower rate.

Other Metabolic Disorders

Neonatal iron storage disease is a poorly understood defect of iron metabolism that probably starts *in utero*. Some neonates present with advanced liver disease and succumb in the first few days of life. Others are less affected and thus enable transplantation to be performed in the first few weeks of life.[44] To date, no long-term sequelae of iron reaccumulation have been documented.

In primary oxalosis, the enzymatic defect is located in the liver. Although hyperoxaluria induces renal failure, only combined liver and kidney transplantation will allow the reversal of the metabolic defect.[45] Liver transplantation alone may be considered in selected patients, before the onset of renal failure.[46] OLT may be considered for disorders of bile acid synthesis in selected cases associated with end-stage liver disease. Similarly, OLT may be performed for selected cases of organic acidemias without central nervous system involvement.[15]

Acute Fulminant Liver Failure

Acute fulminant liver failure is defined as the development of liver necrosis and hepatic encephalopathy within 8 weeks of onset of symptoms in a patient without prior history of liver disease. The etiologies are diverse and include viral hepatitis (A, B, C, and non-A, non-B, non-C hepatitis), exposure to toxins (poisonous mushrooms), metabolic disorders (tyrosinemia and Wilson's disease), and drugs (acetaminophen and isonicotinic acid hydrazide). The clinical course is one of rapid deterioration of liver function and onset of neurologic failure, often progressing to coma and death. Mortality rates are excessively high (60% to 85%) despite maximal support-

ive medical therapy.[45–47] Liver transplantation for fulminant liver failure was first performed in 1968; since then, progressively more transplantations have been done, with a 5-year survival rate of greater than 75%.[48–50]

The most difficult aspect of evaluating fulminant patients for OLT is determining the timing of OLT weighed against the potential of spontaneous recovery. The evaluation attempts to determine when the liver failure becomes irreversible. OLT must be performed before the onset of fatal cerebral edema, however. Thorough neurologic evaluation is therefore essential to assess the reversibility of neurologic deficits. Monitoring for aggressive management of intracranial pressure and brain edema is increasingly recommended. However, the risks of intracranial bleeding must be considered. The best guide for timing of OLT still remains the poor prognostic indicators identified by O'Grady and co-workers: prothrombin time of more than 100 seconds, duration of jaundice more than 100 days, factor 5 levels of less than 20% to 30%, and age younger than 11 years or older than 40 years.[51]

Chronic Active Hepatitis and Cirrhosis

Chronic active hepatitis is a pathologic condition in which inflammatory and fibrotic hepatic lesions progress to cirrhosis and liver failure. This category is much less common in children than in adults. Etiologies are varied and include neonatal hepatitis, chronic viral hepatitis, autoimmune hepatitis, and cryptogenic cirrhosis (Table 6.1).

Neonatal hepatitis may result from an identified infectious agent (cytomegalovirus, toxoplasmosis, rubella) or may be used as a general term to describe the histologic appearance of hepatitis in infancy.[15] Most infants will resolve this early hepatitis-like illness, whereas some will proceed to develop liver failure and cirrhosis that requires OLT.[52] *De novo* hepatitis C in pediatric patients after liver transplantation exhibits an incidence of 4% to 6%. Affected children may exhibit a rapid progression to end-stage liver disease and a poor response to interferon therapy; death occurs in 23% of affected patients.[53] Retransplantation in such a population may be followed by graft reinfection, allograft failure, and death.

Autoimmune hepatitis, typically a disease of adolescent girls, may also occur in younger children of either sex. Steroid therapy may be beneficial in the early stages of the disease. However, steroids should be discontinued and OLT considered if unacceptable side effects or manifestations of advanced liver disease occur. Some children may present with rapidly decompensating liver disease and subfulminant failure that requires urgent transplantation.[54]

Neoplasia

Patients with tumors confined to the liver appear to be excellent candidates for OLT because of the absence of the disabling manifestations of chronic liver disease. Although short-term survival is excellent in these patients, approximately 50% eventually die from recurrent disease.[55]

Hepatoblastoma is the most common primary liver malignancy in childhood.[56] The tumor is usually locally invasive, and distant metastasis is late. If unresectable at diagnosis, chemotherapy may be used to allow resectability. OLT is indicated if the tumor is unresectable in the absence of distant spread.[57] Long-term survival of more than 50% has been achieved with OLT for hepatoblastoma.[58]

In contrast to hepatoblastoma, hepatocellular carcinoma in children is a highly malignant condition with a tendency for early metastasis. Most often it is associated with hepatitis B or long-standing cirrhotic liver disease.[59] OLT is indicated for unresectable tumors without metastasis. Other rare tumors for which OLT is performed include epithelial hemangioendotheliomas and sarcomas of the liver.

Miscellaneous

Budd-Chiari syndrome results from hepatic venous outflow obstruction. Etiologies in the United States include hypercoagulable states secondary to systemic lupus erythematosis, polycythemia, and oral contraceptive use. Mechanical causes include membranous obstruction or external compression from malignancy. A rapid onset of abdominal pain, ascites, and hepatomegaly that may be associated with liver failure is the usual presentation in a young patient. Diagnosis is confirmed via hepatic venous and inferior vena caval angiography, at which time venous pressures should be measured. If hepatic failure is absent, portosystemic shunting and anticoagulation are performed. A mesocaval H graft is recommended unless a gradient exists in the vena cava, in which case a mesoatrial shunt is indicated.[60] If hepatic failure is associated with the syndrome, OLT, which has an overall 3-year survival rate of 88%, should be performed. Posttransplantation anticoagulation is recommended if hypercoagulability is the underlying etiology.[61]

The severity of pulmonary disease and the risk of infections are serious considerations in evaluating patients with cystic fibrosis for OLT. In children with mild pulmonary disease, pulmonary function has improved after OLT, and infectious complications have not been life-threatening.[62,63] The role of combined liver and lung transplantation in the presence of severe pulmonary disease has not yet been assessed. Total parenteral nutrition with little or no enteral feeding is associated with progressive cirrhosis. Consideration should be given to combined liver and small bowel transplantation to prevent recurrence of cirrhosis in the transplanted liver.[64] Caroli's disease is a rare condition characterized by multiple focal dilatations of the biliary ducts that occur in the presence or absence of congenital fibrosis. Manifestations of the disease include jaundice and recurrent episodes of cholangitis. Antibiotics and local resection may control the disease if only a segment of the biliary tree is involved. OLT is indicated for intractable cholangitis caused by diffuse cystic dilatations. Congenital fibrosis alone, which results in presinusoidal por-

tal hypertension, is not an indication for liver transplantation but can be treated with portosystemic shunting.[15]

CONTRAINDICATIONS TO TRANSPLANTATION

Contraindications to OLT must be assessed not only at the time of initial evaluation but also at regular intervals during the waiting period for transplantation.

Absolute Contraindications

Absolute contraindications have become increasingly fewer with increasing experience and are currently summarized as follows:

1. Seropositivity for human immune deficiency virus (HIV)
2. Uncontrollable systemic sepsis of nonhepatic origin
3. Life-threatening disorder of extrahepatic origin that is not correctable by OLT
4. Extrahepatic malignancy

Relative Contraindications

Extrahepatic Disease

Children with poor neurologic function and no expected improvement after OLT should not undergo transplantation. Such a determination may be difficult in patients who suffer an acute insult after fulminant liver failure. Pulmonary complications that preclude OLT include severe pulmonary hypertension or ventilatory support with high oxygen and pressure requirements.[15] However, severe hypoxemia caused by the hepatopulmonary syndrome that is characterized by excessive pulmonary arteriovenous shunting should not be considered a contraindication for transplantation. Reversal of shunting and independence from oxygen can be achieved shortly after transplantation.[65] Children with cystic fibrosis that exhibit severely impaired pulmonary functions, active pulmonary infections, or colonization with *Pseudomonas cepacia* are poor candidates for transplantation.

Complex congenital heart disease, especially if accompanied with cyanosis and pulmonary hypertension not amenable to surgical correction, imposes an extremely high risk for OLT. Further, the overall poor condition of such children may preclude a combined heart-liver transplantation. Alagille syndrome and biliary atresia are both associated with an increased risk of congenital heart disease. Renal failure is seldom a contraindication for transplantation. Most commonly, renal failure is due to the hepatorenal syndrome, which resolves with a functioning liver graft. Acute tubular necrosis caused by multiorgan failure, on the other hand, carries a worse prognosis.[66]

Psychosocial and Financial Considerations

Psychosocial factors should never prevent children from receiving essential medical care. Aggressive steps that include counseling, foster care, or court orders may be necessary to allow life-saving therapy. Lack of financial means may limit access to OLT. However, this can almost always be solved by application to state or federally funded programs.

PATIENT EVALUATION AND SELECTION

The proper selection of patients for transplantation is crucial to a liver transplant program. A multidisciplinary approach is used. Evaluation is performed by a team that includes transplant surgeons, pediatric hepatologists, nephrologists, neurologists, psychiatrists, anesthesiologists, and infectious disease specialists. Routine blood chemistries and cultures are performed. Portal vein ultrasonography is used to assess patency. Computed tomography (CT) scanning is used to evaluate for the presence of extrahepatic malignancy when indicated. Donor-to-recipient matching is based on ABO status and size, and priority is given to urgent candidates.

Children are placed on the waiting list for transplantation and assigned points that are determined by urgency, waiting period, ABO compatibility, and size. This listing process is similar to that used for adults. However, in contradistinction to the adult system, the new UNOS regulations allow a different definition for status 1 in children. Status 1 includes all children (younger than 17 years) who require intensive care management and any hospitalized child with a metabolic disease that results in hyperammonemia or other toxic metabolites that affect the central nervous system.

TECHNICAL CONSIDERATIONS

Operative Procedure

The operative details of pediatric liver transplantation have been well described.[67,68] Recipient hepatectomy is the most challenging part of this complex procedure. Widespread portal hypertensive collaterals demand meticulous dissection to avoid relentless and, rarely, massive hemorrhage. Initially, diaphragmatic attachments of the left lobe are divided, followed by dissection of the hilar portal structures, including the hepatic artery, common bile duct, and portal vein. Prior operations, coagulopathies, episodes of spontaneous bacterial peritonitis, and vascularized adhesions all contribute to increased difficulties. Almost all children with biliary atresia have undergone a portoenterostomy prior to transplantation. Many have had multiple revision attempts with dense scarring. In such patients dissection of the hilum is initiated from the posterior aspect of the right lobe of the liver, in a previously unviolated plane. The duodenum and transverse colon are reflected away from the right hepatic lobe, and the Roux-en-Y limb is identified and traced to the hepatic hilum. Next, access to portal structures is gained by transecting the Roux-en-Y limb and reflecting it inferiorly.

After the portal structures and the diaphragmatic attachments of the right lobe are divided, the suprahepatic and infrahepatic vena cavae are isolated, clamped, and transected.

Division of the suprahepatic and infrahepatic vena cavae allows the implantation of a whole organ with the retrohepatic cava in position. In contrast to adults, in whom venovenous bypass is frequently used, infants and small children tolerate vena caval interruption well, and venovenous bypass is therefore seldom needed. After the native liver is removed, perfect hemostasis is achieved in the hepatic fossa by reapproximation of open peritoneal surfaces over the bare area and by triangular ligaments.

Allograft implantation in children is demanding because of the small caliber and delicate nature of their vessels. The anastomoses are performed in the following order: suprahepatic inferior vena cava, infrahepatic inferior vena cava, portal vein, hepatic artery, and biliary system. Vena caval anastomosis is performed with 4-0 or 5-0 polypropylene using interrupted anterior row and continuous posterior row sutures. Interrupted sutures facilitate the growth of the anastomosis. Portal vein anastomosis is performed with running or interrupted 6-0 or 7-0 polypropylene sutures. The new graft is then perfused with recipient portal blood during completion of the arterial anastomosis. We currently favor a microsurgical hepatic arterial reconstruction in which the aortic Carrell's patch of the donor is anatomosed to a branch patch constructed at the recipient gastroduodenal-hepatic or splenic–common hepatic artery confluence.[69] Fine interrupted suturing is performed with 8-0 polypropylene in conjunction with $3.5\times$ loupe magnification or with 9-0 nylon under the operating microscope. Conventional arterial reconstruction employs a running 7-0 polypropylene suture between donor and recipient vessels.[70] Interposition grafting with the same donor iliac, carotid, or innominate artery conduit, generally sited to the recipient supraceliac aorta, is used when the recipient's hepatic artery is judged to be inadequate. Biliary reconstruction in children is usually a Roux-en-Y choledochojejunostomy over an internal stent to a 40-cm defunctionalized limb of jejunum. If the duct is not diseased and is of sufficient caliber, an end-to-end choledochocholedochostomy with or without a T tube may be performed, but is rarely possible in the pediatric population. After the graft is implanted, three closed suction drains are placed before closure of the abdomen.

Currently, a vena cava–sparing procedure is increasingly performed in children. In such a modification, the vena cava is left in position and the recipient liver is resected off the retrohepatic cava after dividing the venous communications between the posterior surface of the liver and the anterior surface of the cava. The liver is thus left hanging by only the three hepatic veins. Transection of the hepatic veins allows removal of the liver. The vena cava–sparing technique allows piggyback implantation of the donor liver.[71] If a whole-organ graft is used, only a single venous anastomosis is performed between the donor suprahepatic vena cava and the common trunk of the recipient hepatic veins, while the donor infrahepatic cava is ligated. Left lateral segment allografts obtained from reduced-size grafts, living donors, or split livers are always implanted in a piggyback fashion because these grafts exhibit only a single venous outflow. The venous anastomosis is performed between the allograft left hepatic vein and the confluence of the recipient hepatic vein.

Liver Preservation

An exciting development in the history of liver transplantation was the extension of liver preservation using a solution developed by Belzer at the University of Wisconsin (UW solution). Initial studies demonstrated a mean preservation time of 12.7 (11–20) hours.[72] The solution evolved from Belzer's earlier work in which he showed the importance of phosphate and adenosine in kidney preservation.[73] In addition to such compounds, UW solution contains unique polymer sugars (hydroxyethyl starch, lactobionate) as nonionic osmotic agents, as well as glutathione and allopurinol as antioxidants and oxygen free radical scavengers. Since May 1988, UW solution has been routinely employed for liver preservation at UCLA. This has permitted significantly longer preservation times without compromise of graft function and allowed greater flexibility in the utilization of operating room time and resources.

Donor Organ Options

The severe shortage of whole-organ cadaveric grafts that are size matched for pediatric patients imposed an unacceptably high attrition rate for children awaiting transplantation. Because of this quantitative donor/recipient size disparity, pretransplantation mortality had been historically reported to be as high as 25% to 50% in children. To improve maximum donor organ utilization in children and small adults, three procedures have evolved from the fundamental principle that a component of the liver with a suitable vascular pedicle, bile duct, and venous drainage along with sufficient functional hepatocyte mass can sustain hepatic function in a patient as well as a whole organ can. Reduced-size liver transplantation was the wellspring for this effort, followed by living-related and cadaveric split-liver transplantation.

Reduced-Size Liver Transplantation

In reduced-size liver transplantation (RSLT), the liver graft can be tailored on the bench to a variety of functional lobes or segments. The most commonly employed parts of a graft used in children are segments 2 and 3 (left lateral segment) or segments 2, 3, and 4 (left lobe). Because of size discrepancy, the extended right lobe, segments 4 to 8, is rarely used in pediatric patients. In RSLT, when either a left lateral segment graft or a left lobe graft is used, the remaining right lobe is discarded.

Transplantation of part of a liver was initially performed in a heterotopic fashion, as first reported by Fortner.[74] Orthotopic transplantation of a reduced-size graft was first reported by Bismuth[75] in Europe, where organ shortage is even greater than in the United States. In 1988, Broelsch reported his experience with 14 children who received reduced liver grafts.[76] Thirteen of the 14 were urgent cases. Three right lobe grafts, nine left lobes, and two left lateral segments were utilized. The overall patient survival rate of 50% was similar to that of high-risk recipients of full-sized grafts. However, graft-related and extrahepatic complications were 71% and 93%, respectively. In a study by Otte et al. that included 54 patients, the overall 1-year patient survival was 82% for full grafts versus 68% for reduced-size grafts.[77] However, children who underwent elective transplantation exhibited a 1-year survival of 77%. In 1992, Langnas et al. demonstrated no significant difference in patient survival when comparing RSLT with whole-liver transplantation in the urgent recipient, but a diminished survival when compared with patients undergoing elective transplantation.[78] The results of this report demonstrated a 53% incidence of graft-related complications, as opposed to 75% as reported by Broelsch and co-workers.[79]

Thus, RSLT may represent a safe and effective therapy for critically ill children and significantly reduces the waiting periods for liver transplantation. However, although use of RSLT increases the number of pediatric donor organs, this technique does not increase the total number of organs available for transplantation, and it actually disadvantages the adult recipient pool, which has grown 12.1-fold over the past 8 years.

Living-Related Transplantation

Living-related liver transplantation (LRT) is a natural extension of reduced-size liver transplantation. Use of a portion of the liver from a living donor was attempted by Raia[80] in 1988 and was first successfully accomplished by Strong[81] in 1989. Over the past 10 years, approximately 1,000 LRTs have been performed throughout the world, achieving graft and patient survival rates equivalent or better than those observed with cadaveric whole organs or RSLT.[82–84]

The advantages offered by LRT include selection of an ideal donor in whom liver graft function is immediate and the ability to schedule the case electively, allowing maximal preparation of the recipient. The potential advantage of increased histocompatibility between donor and recipient favoring a lower incidence of rejection of living-related grafts has not been realized. Despite the success observed in pediatric LRT, there are still unresolved issues concerning the risks that are posed to donors, who are usually parents.

Split-Liver Transplantation

Split-liver transplantation (SLT) is the culmination of the stepwise progression from reduced-size liver transplantation and living-related transplantation. With this technique a whole adult cadaveric liver is divided into two functioning allografts: segments 2 and 3 for children (left lateral

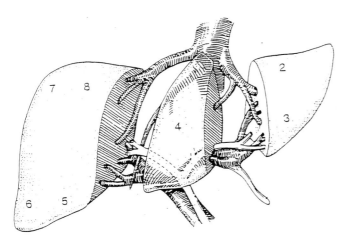

FIG 6.1. Segmental anatomy of the liver. Segment 1 (caudate lobe) is not shown. Segments 2 and 3 (left lateral segment) and segments 4 to 8 (extended right lobe) are used in split-liver transplantation.

segment), and segments 4 to 8 for adults (right trisegment) (Fig. 6.1). *Ex vivo* splitting of the liver is performed on the bench after removal from the cadaver, whereas the *in vivo* (*in situ*) technique accomplishes the division of the liver in the cadaver, in a similar fashion to the LRT procedure, prior to the procurement of the allograft. SLT not only overcomes the drawbacks of RSLT and LRT, but also increases the total number of donor organs. In fact, full development of split-liver transplantation may eliminate the need for RSLT and LRT procedures except in emergent circumstances.

Ex Vivo *Split-Liver Transplantation*

Pichlmayr and co-workers[85] in 1988 reported the first clinical attempt at SLT by placing a right graft into a 63-year-old woman with primary biliary cirrhosis and the left graft into a small child with biliary atresia. One year later Bismuth et al.[86] described two patients with fulminant hepatic failure who each received a split graft. Although both patients recovered from coma with improvement of liver function, death occurred from multiple organ failure on postoperative day 20 in one patient and from diffuse cytomegalovirus disease on postoperative day 45 in the other. The authors claimed that neither poor graft function nor technical problems contributed to the patients' demise. Broelsch et al.[87] reported the first series of 30 split-liver procedures in 21 children and 5 adults. In this early experience, patient survival was inferior to reported series of whole-organ cadaveric liver transplants, with only 67% of children and 20% of adults who received split grafts surviving.[88] Furthermore, technical problems were high, with a retransplantation rate and biliary complication rate of 35% and 27%, respectively.

Despite some skepticism of the lasting role of split-liver transplantation, several European centers—faced with increasing waiting list mortality because of donor scarcity—

cautiously pursued the split-liver option. A collective experience of 50 donor livers, providing 100 grafts over a 5-year period, was reported from the European Split Liver Registry by DeVille de Goyet.[89] In this series, graft and patient 6-month survival were stratified according to the elective or urgent status of the patient. In the elective situation, graft and patient survival rates were 80% and 88.9%, respectively, for children and 72.2% and 80% for adults. In the urgent setting, graft and patient survival rates were 61.3% and 61.3%, respectively, for children and 55.6% and 67.7% for adults. Twenty split grafts were lost because of complications related to the graft itself; other technical complications also occurred, including hepatic artery thrombosis (11.5%), portal vein thrombosis (4%), and biliary complications (18.7%). These results were compared with the European Liver Transplant Registry of conventional orthotopic liver transplantation performed during the same time period and did not show a significant difference. In fact, survival of elective adult patients receiving a split graft was higher than those who received a whole graft (88.9% versus 80.3%). Further, children who received an elective split graft experienced lower graft loss and retransplantation rates than those receiving whole grafts.

The results described from the European Split Liver Registry stimulated renewed interest in split-liver transplantation, as evidenced by more recent series reported by Azoulay et al.,[90] Kalayoglu et al.,[91] and Rela et al.[92] Despite marked improvement of outcome in these series, high-risk patients appeared to exhibit a worse outcome than nonurgent recipients. Further, this effect was more pronounced in adult patients who received right grafts. In addition, *ex vivo* SLT exhibits a high rate of biliary complications (in excess of 20%).

In Vivo *Split-Liver Transplantation*

A modification of the *ex vivo* splitting technique is *in vivo* splitting, which is an extension of the techniques established for living-related donor liver procurement but is completed in the heart-beating cadaver donor. At UCLA, we first attempted *in vivo* split-liver transplantation in 1992. Our first experience was not favorable, with only one of four grafts surviving. However, after establishing a living-related liver program and accruing an experience of 30 cases, we resumed the *in vivo* split-liver program in 1996. In that same year, Rogiers et al. reported their initial experience with 14 split grafts that resulted in 6-month patient and graft survival rates of 92.8% and 85.7%, respectively.[93] Furthermore, these authors described a lower rate of biliary complications, intraabdominal hemorrhage, and nonfunction of the right graft as compared with other series utilizing the *ex vivo* split-liver techniques.

There have been only a few published reports of *in vivo* split-liver transplants[93–95] because the procedure has only been performed regularly since 1996. Results from these series have shown improvement over the *ex vivo* experience, with higher patient and graft survival and lower incidence of technical complications associated with the hepatic artery, biliary anastomosis, and postoperative hemorrhage. The patients who received an *ex vivo* split liver at Kings College Hospital[92] have been the only patients who matched the results seen with *in vivo* split grafts. However, of these 41 patients who received *ex vivo* split livers, most were classified as elective cases except for 4 children and 1 adult (12%) who were classified as emergent. This contrasts with the *in vivo* experience, in which the number of emergent cases was substantially greater. In the Hamburg series[93] and the initial UCLA experience,[94] 21.4% and 38.5% of patients, respectively, were urgent recipients.

Our initial series at UCLA, which included 28 liver transplants generated from 15 *in vivo* splits, demonstrated overall 1-year patient and graft survival rates of 92.3% and 86%, respectively.[94] Urgent recipients exhibited 80% survival at 1 year. An expanded series of *in vivo* split-liver grafts performed since July 1, 1996, at UCLA confirmed these improved results in urgent patients when compared with *ex vivo* split grafts.[96] Of 92 patients who received a total of 100 *in vivo* split grafts, 47 (47%) were urgent recipients (UNOS status 1 and 2A), and 53 (53%) were nonurgent (UNOS status 2, 2B, and 3). Overall 1-year patient and graft survival rates were 80% and 77%, respectively. The type of graft used, whether a right trisegment or a lateral segment, did not significantly affect patient or graft survival. Although patient survival was significantly lower in urgent versus nonurgent recipients (71% versus 92%, $P < 0.002$), it was similar to survival rates achieved with whole-organ transplantation. Such encouraging results have allowed us to implement a policy to split every suitable liver. Since the implementation of *in vivo* SLT, we have decreased the waiting period for children younger than 1 year from 128 days to 24 days, and for children older than 1 year from 192 days to 30 days.

Thus, splitting of the cadaveric liver expands the donor pool of organs and may eliminate the need for living-related donation for children. Recent experience with the *ex vivo* technique, if applied to elective patients, results in patient and graft survival comparable with whole-organ transplantation, although postoperative complications are higher. *In vivo* splitting provides two grafts of optimal quality that can be applied to the entire spectrum of transplant recipients, and it may evolve into the method of choice for expanding the cadaveric liver donor pool.

IMMUNOSUPPRESSION

The recent explosive development of immunosuppressive agents that target characteristic enzyme pathways or distinctive receptors emanated from developments in immunology and pharmacology. During the first seven decades of research on immunosuppressive agents, radiation and chemical reagents were employed to nonselectively destroy rapidly dividing cells. In 1914 Murphy[97] documented the effects of the simple organic compounds benzene and toluene. In 1952

Baker et al.[98] noted that the combination of nitrogen mustards, corticosteroids, and splenectomy prolonged the survival of mongrel canine allografts. In 1959 Schwartz and Dameshek[99] demonstrated the antiproliferative effects of 6-mercaptopurine (6-MP), a competitive inhibitor of purine *de novo* synthesis and salvage pathways. The nitroimidazole derivative of 6-MP, azathioprine, was employed by Calne and co-workers[100] to prolong the survival of canine renal transplants. Corticosteroids were later added to the regimen in empiric fashion to improve immunosuppressive efficacy.

The second stage in the development of immunosuppression focused the attack upon T cells. Polyclonal antilymphocyte sera were investigated in rodent models by Russell and Monaco[101] and rapidly translated to the clinical arena by Starzl and colleagues.[102] Development of the hybridoma technology provided the basis for monoclonal antibody (MAb) therapy. Currently MAbs provide the clinician with a wide spectrum of selective reagents that eliminate cells bearing specific surface markers, including the T-cell receptor, accessory molecules, and other activation markers.

The third stage of pharmacologic immunosuppressive therapy sought to alter the alloreactivity of immune elements. The prototype of this family is cyclosporine (CsA). In 1976, Jean-Francois Borel[103] demonstrated the potent antilymphocytic effects of CsA. The clinical application of CsA ushered in a new era for transplantation and kindled the development of multiple new immunosuppressive agents. Tacrolimus[104] has evolved as the drug of choice in liver transplantation. Both CsA and tacrolimus inhibit cytokine synthesis. A second group of drugs, including rapamycin[105] and leflunomide,[106] block lymphokine signal transduction. A third group of drugs that inhibit nucleoside synthesis, including mizorbine, mycophenolate mofeteil,[107] and brequinar,[108] seek to replace the competitive inhibitor azathioprine.

The future rational use of immunosuppressive agents depends on elucidating their individual molecular targets and pharmacologic interactions. It is not unreasonable to expect that future use of synergistic immunosuppressive drug combinations will produce negative regulation of T cells with minimal toxic side effects. However, this impenetrable immunosuppressive shield inevitably predisposes transplant recipients to neoplastic and infectious complications. The following discussion seeks to highlight the important aspects of some clinically used immunosuppressive reagents.

Pharmacologic Agents

Inhibitors of Antigen Processing and Presentation

Corticosteroids are the prototypic agents for the inhibition of T-cell early activation events. Steroids impair interleukin (IL)-10[109] and IL-6[110] gene transcription, thereby inhibiting the generation of activation costimulatory signals. Moreover, steroids also inhibit gene expression of IL-2,[111] tumor necrosis factor (TNF),[112] and interferon gamma (IFN-γ). These compounds move across cell membranes where they bind a 97-kD intracytoplasmic and intranuclear receptor protein dimer. The activated complex reversibly binds and inhibits the transcription of DNA glucocorticoid response elements.[113] One of these sites is the AP-1 site present in the enhancer regions of multiple cytokine genes.

Steroids are universally employed in induction therapy in combination with other drugs. In addition, they are an essential component in the treatment of acute allograft rejection. Side effects are well known and include increased susceptibility to infection, growth retardation, gastrointestinal ulcers, fluid retention, truncal obesity, and osteoporosis. The dose of steroids is traditionally decreased with time to avoid such hazardous toxicities.

Lymphokine Synthesis Inhibitors

Cyclosporine

Cyclosporine is a cyclic oligopeptide extracted from *Tolypocladium inflatum Gams*. CsA inhibits processes dependent on an increased cytoplasmic calcium burst. Handschumacher demonstrated that CsA binds to a cytoplasmic protein, cyclophilin (CYP), which displays cis-trans peptidyl-prolylisomerase activity.[114] Such binding changes the substrate affinity of the isomerase such that it complexes with and inhibits calcineurins (CaN) A and B, serine-threonine phosphatases associated with Ca^{2+} and calmodulin (CaM).[115] The formation of the pentameric complex CaN-Ca^{2+}-CaM-CsA-CYP prevents enzymatic cleavage of the phosphate group necessary for nuclear translocation of nuclear factor of activated T cells, NF-AT, the first regulatory protein controlling the enhancer region of the IL-2 gene. CsA inhibits T-cell synthesis of not only IL-2, but also IL-3, IFN-γ, IL-6, and IL-7.[116] IL-1 synthesis and IL-2 receptor (IL-2R) generation appear to be calcium independent and therefore CsA resistant. T-helper and T-cytotoxic cells are the primary targets of CsA; T-suppressor cells are spared,[117] possibly due to a CsA-resistant activation cascade.

It is difficult to optimize CsA therapy because of the agent's marked interindividual variations.[118] Frequent measurement of the drug's level is required to maintain a therapeutic index. Although pharmacokinetic control of drug dosing may eliminate excessive immunodepression from CsA therapy, the apparent concentration-independent, drug-induced renal injury is still a problem. Utilization of CsA in liver transplant patients is further complicated by its dependency on bile for its absorption. Use of the new glycolfuran microemulsion formulation of CsA (Neoral), which appears to be absorbed independently of bile and food composition, may facilitate dose prediction and reduce some of the previously mentioned limitations.

Tacrolimus

Tacrolimus (FK506, Prograf) is a polycyclic macrolide produced by *Streptomyces tsukubaensis*[119] that inhibits T-cell production of IL-2, IL-3, and IFN-γ 10- to 100-fold more potently than CsA.[120] Tacrolimus, like CsA, inhibits Ca^{2+}-dependent intracellular pathways mediated by an interaction with an intracellular binding protein (FKBP), which, like CYP, is a member of the cis-trans prolyl isomerase "immunophilin" family.[121] Thus, the apparent antagonism between tacrolimus and CsA may be explained by the fact that they share a common intracellular pathway.

Both CsA and tacrolimus are metabolized by the cytochrome P-450 3A4 system and therefore display similar drug interactions.[122] Toxicity profiles for both agents are also similar. There was no difference in neurotoxicity, nephrotoxicity, or in the incidence of hypercholesterolemia, diabetes, or sepsis when both drugs were compared in the U.S. multicenter trial for primary immunosuppression in pediatric patients.[123] However, no hirsutism or gingival hypertrophy occurred in tacrolimus-treated children. The adult arm of the trial demonstrated similar findings, with a tendency to more neurotoxicity and hyperglycemia in the tacrolimus group.

Tacrolimus is metabolized in the liver and is excreted in the bile. Like CsA, tacrolimus displays variable absorption profiles and requires frequent level monitoring. However, its absorption is bile independent, a property that facilitates its use in liver recipients. The U.S. multicenter trial for primary immunosuppression[123] demonstrated no significant difference in patient and graft survival rates between tacrolimus and CsA. However, at 1 year, 48% of tacrolimus-treated children, compared with 21% of CsA-treated children, remained rejection free. With tacrolimus, only 21% of children required OKT3 treatment for rejection, whereas OKT3 was required in 32% of children receiving CsA therapy. Although the difference in the severity and incidence of rejection did not reach statistical significance in children, the incidence and severity of rejection was significantly lower with tacrolimus in the much larger adult arm of the trial. Further, the incidence of chronic rejection appears to be much decreased with tacrolimus.[122] In the U.S. multicenter trial,[124] rescue therapy with tacrolimus for chronic rejection in children was successful in 70.3% of converted children. A time interval of more than 90 days following transplantation and a bilirubin level of less than 10 mg/dL were significant prognostic indicators for the success of rescue.

Nucleoside Synthesis Inhibitors

Nucleoside synthesis inhibitors exploit the greater dependence of lymphocytes, compared with other rapidly dividing cell types, on *de novo* synthesis because of the low levels of nucleoside salvage pathways. The activity of antipurine agents is modest because of their nonselective actions on a variety of cells. This lack of selectivity suggests that therapeutic strategies with nucleoside synthesis inhibitors must depend on their synergistic potentiation of selective immunosuppressive agents.

Azathioprine

Azathioprine (AZA, Imuran), a nitroimidazole derivative, was the cornerstone of chemical immunosuppression in the 1960s. However, AZA exhibits multiple theoretical and practical limitations. Because AZA can be incorporated into DNA, it carries an increased proclivity to malignancy. It depresses bone marrow generation of rapidly dividing elements of the nonspecific immune response,[125] resulting in neutropenia, thrombocytopenia, and anemia. AZA also produces hepatotoxicity that potentiates CsA injury. Other toxicities include increased risk of infection and possibly pancreatitis. Although it still tends to be used as a third agent in CsA/steroid regimens, AZA has no demonstrable synergistic effects with CsA immunosuppression.[126] The limitations of AZA as an immunosuppressive drug led to an urgent need to identify new nucleoside synthesis inhibitors that (a) acted noncompetitively to inhibit synthesis of either purines (RS-61443, CellCept; Mizorbine) or pyrimidines (brequinar), (b) were not incorporated into DNA, and (c) showed reduced myelotoxicity.

Mycophenolate Mofetil

Mycophenolate mofetil (MMF) (RS-61443, CellCept) acts as a potent, noncompetitive, reversible inhibitor of inosine monophosphate dehydrogenase and guanylate synthetase of the de novo pathway, causing intracellular depletion of guanosine triphosphate and deoxyguanosine triphosphate rather than adenosine triphosphate and deoxyadenosine triphosphate. DNA synthesis is affected to a greater degree than RNA or protein synthesis, resulting in cell arrest at the S phase.[126] MMF selectively inhibits T- and B-cell lymphocytic function and spares other tissues from the detrimental effects of purine synthesis down-regulation. Side effects include gastritis, duodenitis, and esophagitis, but not hepatic or renal toxicities. The incidence of bone marrow suppression, manifested by leukopenia and thrombocytopenia, appears to be lower than with AZA. Currently, the role of MMF in hepatic transplantation is being defined. MMF alone or in combination with CsA may be an effective alternative therapy in patients failing CsA-based conventional therapy.[127] In addition, MMF may be of particular benefit in patients who do not tolerate CsA or tacrolimus.

Other Nucleoside Inhibitors

Mizorbine (MZB) is another purine synthesis inhibitor that noncompetitively inhibits inosine monophosphate dehydrogenase. As yet no clinical trials have been published outside Japan, and worldwide distribution of the drug is not anticipated. Brequinar noncompetitively and reversibly inhibits the de novo pyrimidine biosynthesis pathway. It exhibits a 100-fold greater potency than MMF or AZA. The potential for clinical application of brequinar is yet to be determined.[126]

Lymphokine Signal Transduction Inhibitors

Sirolimus

Sirolimus (rapamycin, RAPA, Rapamune), a macrolide antibiotic produced by the actinomycete *Streptomyces hygroscopicus,* is structurally related to tacrolimus.[128] Unlike CsA and tacrolimus, which influence the G_0-to-G_1 progression, sirolimus does not affect lymphokine synthesis, but rather inhibits lympokines' effects on the G_1 build-up phase necessary for lymphocyte activation and S-phase entry. Thus, RAPA inhibits a broad array of calcium-independent activation events mediated via CD-28,[129] protein kinase C, and lymphokine stimulation, possibly by blocking p70 S6 or the p34^{cdc2} kinases that are required for the proliferative responses induced by IL-2. Like tacrolimus, sirolimus binds FKBP to form RAPA-FKBP complex. However, unlike CsA and tacrolimus-immunophilin complexes that inhibit the Ca^{2+}-CAM-regulated serine-threonine phosphatase calcineurin, which plays an important role in lymphocyte activation, the RAPA-FKBP complex does not influence calcineurin activity. The actual mechanism of immuosuppressive effect is uncertain, but may involve the binding of the RAPA-FKBP complex with the mammalian homologues of the TOR1 and TOR2 yeast proteins.[130] Such mechanistic differences may also account for the different side effect profile of sirolimus, which includes thrombocytopenia, hyperlipidemia, and increased aminotransferase levels but not neurotoxicity, nephrotoxicity, or diabetogenesis.[131]

Sirolimus has been shown to be a powerful immunosuppressant both in vitro and in vivo.[126] The humoral arm of the immune response is also potently inhibited by sirolimus. Further, it inhibits transduction of all cytokine signals tested to date. It offers the promise of clinical usefulness because of its synergistic immunosuppressive effect with CsA.[132] Thus, the combination of RAPA and CsA may allow the use of both drugs at extremely low doses to produce a high immunosuppressive index with a low toxic profile. A pilot study that included 15 liver transplant recipients demonstrated the potent immunosuppressive effects of sirolimus alone or in combination with CsA.[133] Currently, sirolimus is undergoing phase III multicenter clinical trials in liver transplant patients in the United States.

Biologic Agents

Polyclonal Antibodies

Potent, nonspecific, immunosuppressive antibodies can be produced by immunizing a xenogeneic host with human lymphocytes. Such sera contain polyclonal antibodies that opsonize the corresponding peripheral blood cellular elements, including T cells, leading to their destruction. The resulting in vivo depletion or inactivation of T lymphocytes interferes with T-cell-mediated reactions, including allograft rejection, delayed hypersensitivity, and graft versus host reactions.

Antilymphocytic globulin or antithymocyte globulin has been used for prophylactic therapy during the first week after transplantation to reduce the frequency and severity of early rejection episodes. However, clinical studies have not yielded unequivocal evidence supporting the use of antilymphocytic globulin prophylactically.[126] Some centers demonstrated improved graft survival and fewer rejection episodes, with a relative paucity of the reported side effects of serum sickness, anaphylactoid reactions, vascular thrombosis, or cytomegalovirus infection. Recently, the use of polyclonal reagents in induction therapy with liver transplantation has fallen out of favor. However, polyclonal therapy may still be beneficial for the treatment of acute allograft rejection episodes.

Monoclonal Antibodies

The demonstration of clinical efficacy of OKT3, an anti-CD3 monoclonal antibody, has stimulated innovative development of MAbs that target cell surface epitopes involved in alloreactivity.[134] Hybridoma technology has yielded readily standardized, specific xenogeneic murine MAbs of greater purity and molecular specificity than the previously utilized polyclonal reagents. Currently, MAbs against T cell receptor (α/β-TcR), TcR-associated CD3 complex, CD4 and CD8 coreceptor molecules, adhesion molecules, and other markers of T-cell activation are readily available.[135] However, only MAbs directed against the CD3 complex or IL-2R promise wide use in liver transplantation.

Antibodies against TcR-Associated CD3 Complex. The murine IgG_{2a} monoclonal antibody OKT3 has become the agent of choice for treatment of steroid-resistant allograft rejection.[136] However, the development of anti-OKT3 antibody responses, including antiidiotypic and antiisotypic varieties, may preclude retreatment with mouse antibodies.[137] In addition, initial administration of OKT3 is associated with an acute clinical syndrome characterized by fever, chills, diarrhea, headache, and pulmonary edema. Such untoward side effects are due to cytokine release caused by a nonspecific *in vivo* T-cell activation caused by cross-linking of T cells to Fc receptor (FcR)–bearing antigen-presenting cells. In addition to the acute cytokine release reactions, excessive OKT3 therapy predisposes to cytomegalovirus infections and posttransplantation lymphoproliferative diseases.

Multiple experimental strategies have been employed to reduce such side effects. The first method was to coadminister soluble cytokine receptors during OKT3 therapy to mitigate cytokine activity. Another approach utilized the $F(ab')_2$ fragments of OKT3, which maintain antibody specificity but lack the ability to bind FcR+ cells.

Two innovations were adopted to avoid the production of idiotypic human antimouse antibodies following administration of mouse MAbs. Chimeric antibodies combine the variable regions of mouse antibodies with human antibody constant regions, and therefore present fewer foreign amino acid sequences to the host. However, one-third of the structure is still of mouse origin, which may stimulate the production of antiidiotypic antibodies. Humanized antibodies combine only the smallest part of a mouse antibody that is required for target recognition—the distinctive CDR regions—with human variable-region and constant-region frameworks.[138] Although extremely encouraging, the beneficial effects of humanized variants of mouse MAbs will only be clarified by undergoing randomized clinical trials.

Anti-IL-2R Antibody. The anti-IL-2R monoclonal antibody focuses the attack on expanding alloactivated T cells and spares T-cell progenitors from broad nonselective pan-T-cell suppression. It carries the potential advantage of reducing opportunistic infections and lymphomas.

IL-2 effects on target cells are mediated by its binding to IL-2R,[139] which comprises at least three distinct subunits: α chain (CD 25; IL-2Rα, Tac, p55), β chain (IL-2Rβ, p75), and γ chain (IL-2Rγ). Only the α and β chains bind IL-2. IL-2 binding to IL-2R may be blocked by MAbs directed against either the α or β chains, or more efficiently by targeting both subunits. IL-2R MAbs have been shown to be synergistic with CsA and to prolong allograft survival in mice, rats, and nonhuman primates.

In an initial randomized controlled trial, rat IL-2Rα MAb (33B3.1) was as effective as rabbit antithymocyte globulin (ATG) in prophylaxis of renal allograft rejection, with a significant reduction of infectious episodes seen in the MAb group.[140] In liver transplantation, the addition of either OKT3 or murine LO-Tact-1 anti-IL-2Rα MAb to conventional triple-drug immunosuppression therapy (CsA, AZA, and prednisone) significantly lowered rejection episodes over 2 years in the OKT3 and LO-Tact-1 groups. OKT3, but not LO-Tact-1, reduced the incidence of cytomegalovirus infections.[141] Compared with ATG, murine BT 563 MAb exhibited similar infectious complications but a lower incidence of rejection episodes in two separate prospective randomized trials.[142,143] Thus, the role of IL-2R MAbs in liver transplantation is currently under intense investigation.

Immunosuppression Protocol at UCLA

Induction and Maintenance Therapy

Before 1994, CsA-based triple-drug therapy was employed. CsA was administered intravenously or orally to maintain a whole blood trough level of 250 to 300 ng/mL. Methylprednisolone was started intravenously at the time of transplantation at 20 to 30 mg/kg and rapidly tapered to 0.3 to 0.5 mg/kg per day over the first week. When oral intake was resumed, oral prednisone was resumed at an equivalent dose. AZA was started at 1 to 2 mg/kg per day intravenously on the first day after transplantation and was later converted to the same oral dose. Severe sepsis, pancreatitis, or neutropenia (white blood cell count less than 4000/mL) were contraindications for AZA use.

In July 1994 we adopted our current dual tacrolimus-based immunosuppressive protocol. Tacrolimus is given orally at

0.1 to 0.2 mg/kg per day every 12 hours to maintain a whole blood trough level of 10 to 15 ng/mL during the first month, 10 ng/mL for the second month, and 5 to 10 ng/mL thereafter. Methylprednisolone is rapidly tapered from between 20 and 30 mg/kg to 0.3 mg/kg per day over 5 days, followed by oral prednisone at 0.3 mg/kg per day.

Steroid Withdrawal

Selected patients with at least 1 year survival after receiving an ABO-compatible graft and who are rejection free for 6 months are offered the option of steroid withdrawal.[50] Patients are excluded if there is a biopsy-proven rejection 6 months after transplantation, if there were two episodes of rejection posttransplantation, or if a previous graft was lost to acute or chronic rejection. Autoimmune hepatitis or a history of noncompliance are contraindications for steroid withdrawal. In eligible patients, prednisone is reduced by 0.5 mg bimonthly; after 1 week on 1 mg prednisone and 1 week on 0.5 mg, prednisone is discontinued. A diagnostic workup that includes a liver biopsy is performed on any patient who develops evidence of graft dysfunction. Acute rejection is treated with steroids, and the patient is maintained on prednisone thereafter.

Management of Rejection

Patients diagnosed with acute rejection are initially treated with intravenous methylprednisolone at 20 mg/kg, which is tapered over 5 days to the pretreatment dose. A second biopsy is performed on patients not responding to treatment, and a decision is made to either restart high-dose steroids or initiate treatment with muromonab (OKT3 MAb) at a dose of 2.5 mg per day for children weighing less than 30 kg and 5 mg per day for those weighing more than 30 kg. A typical course extends for 10 to 14 days. If CD3+ elements exceed 10%, OKT3 is administered at a higher dose. Prior to 1995 we utilized ATG for treatment of steroid-resistant rejection at a dose of 10 mg/kg administered for 10 days. In addition, after 1994, children with steroid-resistant rejection or evidence of chronic rejection were switched from CsA-based to tacrolimus-based regimens.

Risks of Immunosuppression

Allograft Rejection

Acute Cellular Rejection

Acute cellular rejection occurs in approximately one-third of patients following OLT. Symptoms are nonspecific and may include fever, abdominal pain, decreased bile production, elevated hepatic enzymes, and decreased synthetic function. If untreated, acute cellular rejection may progress to fulminant hepatic failure with neurologic and hemodynamic compromise. Tacrolimus therapy is associated with a slightly lower incidence of acute cellular rejection when compared with CsA therapy in children.[123]

Allograft biopsy is necessary to establish the diagnosis prior to treatment. Histologically, acute cellular rejection is defined by a triad of endothelialitis, portal triad lymphocytic infiltration with bile duct injury, and parenchymal cell damage.[144] Steroid bolus with a rapid taper is sufficient for the resolution of acute cellular rejection in 75% to 8-% of cases.[145] Steroid-resistant or recurrent rejection demands antilymphocyte OKT3 therapy, which is successful in 90% of cases.[146]

Chronic Rejection

Chronic rejection occurs in 5% to 10% of transplant recipients, with an equal frequency in adults and children. The syndrome can occur within weeks of transplantation or later in the clinical course. The usual presentation is progressive cholestasis with rising biliary ductal enzymes, including alkaline phosphatase and gamma glutamyl transferase. Alternatively the course may be asymptomatic or may follow an unsuccessful treatment of protracted rejection.[147]

The "vanishing bile duct syndrome" often characterizes the clinical course of chronic rejection. Injury is primarily to the biliary epithelium, where severe ductopenia is seen in at least 20 portal tracts.[148] The success of tacrolimus in the rescue therapy of at least 50% of children with chronic rejection[124] has led to the development of enhanced immunosuppressive protocols for this subgroup of patients.[149] Thus, retransplantation is occasionally necessary but is rarely emergent. Another subtype of chronic rejection is characterized by progressive injury to both the biliary epithelium and hepatic parenchyma, resulting in ductopenia in addition to ischemic necrosis and fibrosis. Such a clinical course is relentlessly progressive and often requires retransplantation.[148] Unfortunately, a high incidence of chronic rejection occurs in patients undergoing retransplantation for chronic rejection.

Infections

Infectious complications currently represent the most common cause of posttransplantation morbidity and mortality. Infection by multiple organisms and concurrent infections by different infectious agents are common.[150]

Bacterial infections in the immediate posttransplantation period are often caused by gram-negative organisms. All intraoperative lines should be removed as early as possible. Antibacterial prophylactic therapy should be discontinued within 24 to 48 hours after transplantation to minimize the risk of development of resistant organisms.

Candidiasis is the most common post-OLT fungal infection. However, aspergillosis and cryptococcosis are the most severe, and often fatal, infections. Severe fungal infections exhibit mortality rates that are greater than 80%.[147] Risk factors for the development of fungal infections include antilymphocyte preparations, retransplantation, previous bacterial infection, long-term antibiotic use, vascular complications, massive blood transfusions, and prolonged pretransplantation hospitalization. Some centers have advocated prophylactic antifungal therapy for such high-risk patients. Regimens using low-dose intravenous amphotericin or flucanazole have been administered as a means of preventing fungal infection. However, the efficacy of such measures remains to be determined.

The most common opportunistic infections following OLT are viral, which include cytomegalovirus (CMV), Epstein-Barr virus (EBV), and herpes simplex virus (HSV) infections. Despite recent advances in diagnosis and treatment, CMV continues to be a common cause of infection and disease in solid-organ transplant recipients. Risk factor analyses have provided important clues to identify those patients at high risk for symptomatic CMV infection. The major risk factors for the development of CMV infection and disease are seronegativity for CMV[151] (seronegative recipients receiving seropositive donor organs are at highest risk, followed by seropositive recipients receiving seropositive donor organs), treatment with OKT3 or other antilymphocyte preparations, hepatic artery thrombosis, and retransplantation. In addition to producing protean clinical manifestations, including fever, hepatitis, malaise, arthralgias, and pneumonitis in the first 6 months after transplantation, CMV infection appears to have an immunosuppressive effect and is a risk factor for superinfection with opportunistic pathogens. Prophylactic protocols such as (intravenous) IgG preparations, hyperimmune anti-CMV IgG, acyclovir, or ganciclovir have all achieved success in reducing the incidence of CMV and EBV infections.[152, 153]

EBV infection occurring in the postoperative period presents with a wide spectrum, including a mononucleosis-like syndrome, hepatitis, extranodal lymphoproliferative infiltration with bowel perforation, peritonsilar or lymph node enlargement, or encephalopathy.[147] EBV can manifest as a primary infection or as a reactivated past infection. Treatment consists of reduction of immunosuppressive therapy in combination with acyclovir or ganciclovir. Oral ganciclovir should be continued until resolution of lymphadenopathy.

Trimethoprim-sulfisoxazole prophylaxis for infection with *Pneumocystis carinii* has been extremely successful. However, allergic reactions and hepatic toxicity have been associated with long-term use of sulfa medications. In such patients pentamidine inhalation administered monthly for at least 1 year posttransplantation has been shown to provide adequate prophylaxis.

De Novo *Malignancy*

Lymphomas comprise by far the largest group of tumors (57%) that develop following liver transplantation. The shorter interval to the development of these tumors in liver transplant recipients may be a reflection of more intense immunosuppression, including the more frequent use of triple therapy and antilymphocyte preparations as compared with renal allograft recipients. In contrast to renal transplant recipients, a decreased incidence of skin cancers, carcinomas of the cervix, and carcinomas of the vulva and perineum is noted in liver transplant recipients and may reflect the relatively shorter follow-up period for liver patients.

EBV infection has been strongly implicated as a cause of a posttransplantation lymphoproliferative disease (PTLD) that ranges from a well-localized polyclonal proliferation with a good prognosis to a fully disseminated monoclonal malignant lymphoma with a high mortality. Hodgkin's disease and smooth muscle tumors have also been associated with EBV. The incidence of frank lymphomas in adult patients undergoing liver transplantation is 0.8% to 3%. In pediatric patients treated with CsA, the incidence of PTLD after OLT is 3% to 4% and increases to 6% to 13% under tacrolimus primary immunotherapy.[154] With OKT3 therapy the incidence of PTLD in children rises to 14% and is highest, up to 27%, in those who required tacrolimus conversion. Age (younger than 5 years), EBV seronegativity, and intense immunosuppression are all associated with increased PTLD.[155] At least in one series, PTLD was associated with a mortality rate of 60%. Of the patients who were rendered disease free with successful therapy, 38% developed ductopenic rejection.[155] Recently, mortality appears to have decreased to 10% to 20%, perhaps due to early diagnosis and treatment.

Patients with polyclonal B-cell proliferation frequently respond to a protocol of immediate decrease of immunosuppressive therapy and institution of anti-EBV treatment. However, patients with aggressive monoclonal malignancies have poor survival with such a protocol even with the addition of conventional chemotherapy and irradiation. Recent data suggest that preemptive therapy with ganciclovir in high-risk recipients, guided by the EBV polymerase chain reaction (PCR), successfully reduces the incidence of PTLD.[153,154]

POSTOPERATIVE COMPLICATIONS

Hepatic Complications

Hepatic Artery Thrombosis

Hepatic artery thrombosis (HAT), one of the most devastating complications following OLT, has been reported to occur in as many as 30% of pediatric OLT patients and is 3 to 4 times more frequent in this population than in adult transplant recipients.[156–158] Actuarial survival rates for patients with HAT are historically lower than for patients without HAT.[69] The presentation of HAT in the early postoperative period is generally categorized into three syndromes[158] that include (a) fulminant allograft failure with a rapid onset of hepatic decompensation, altered mental status, hypotension, and coagulopathy; (b) systemic sepsis and relapsing bacteremia; or (c) biliary complications, including bile leaks, cholangitis, biliary strictures, and obstruction.[159] Doppler studies are extremely valuable for the diagnosis of HAT.[160] However, false negative results do occur, and angiography may occasionally be required. Arterial thrombosis diagnosed in the perioperative period requires prompt reoperation. Thrombectomy and arterial reconstruction, if performed early, may salvage the graft.[161] Acute hepatic failure, diffuse biliary strictures, extensive hepatic necrosis, or focal abscesses demand immediate retransplantation. Biliary complications can be managed by stenting or percutaneous drainage to avoid infection until transplantation is undertaken.

Factors associated with an increased risk of HAT include small pediatric patients and recipients who require complex arterial reconstructions such as double donor arteries or iliac and aortic conduits. In one series of patients,[158] double donor arteries had a 24.1% incidence of arterial thrombosis, and iliac and aortic conduits exhibited thrombosis rates of 27.7% and 23.1%, respectively. Mazzaferro's analysis of 28 variables in 66 pediatric patients revealed 5 factors that significantly affected the development of HAT.[162] Such factors included an arterial diameter of less than 3 mm, the number of times the anastomosis was revised, use of iliac and aortic conduits, intraoperative administration of fresh frozen plasma, and postoperative anticoagulation. However, more recent studies demonstrated that aortohepatic interposition grafts exhibit a lower incidence of HAT compared with end-to-end anastomosis between donor and recipient hepatic arteries.[163] The largest series to date, which included 194 patients who underwent transplantation for biliary atresia, demonstrated that interrupted microsurgical anastomosis between the donor aortic Carrell's patch and the recipient branch patch constructed at the gastroduodenal-hepatic or splenic–common hepatic artery confluence virtually eliminated HAT.[69] Variables that influence HAT are summarized in Table 6.2.

Late HAT may be asymptomatic or present with slowly progressive biliary stenosis.[147,161] Collateral channels develop during the first postoperative months, rendering late thrombosis a silent event. Rarely, allograft necrosis occurs. If silent, late HAT can be carefully followed.

TABLE 6.2. *Factors associated with increased risk of hepatic artery thrombosis*

Donor or recipient size less than 10 kg
Allograft type
  Risk with living-related donor or split liver > with reduced-size liver > with whole liver
Anastomosis
  Primary hepatic artery > aortohepatic interposition
Allograft injury
  Prolonged cold ischemia
  Prolonged warm ischemia
  Acute cellular rejection
  Increased vascular resistance
Recipient hypotension
Hypercoagulability
  Administration of fresh frozen plasma
  Procoagulant factor deficiencies

Pseudoaneurysms and Rupture

Rupture of the hepatic artery from a pseudoaneurysm is an extremely rare complication following OLT. In a report of 11 pseudoaneurysms, 5 were nonanastomotic and were related to infection. Bacteria or fungi are often seen in the wall of the vessel on pathologic examination. Pseudoaneurysms are detected incidentally on imaging studies or may present with rupture, hemobilia, or an enteric fistula. Operative excision and revision of the anastomosis are necessary because of the high risk of significant complications.[164]

Portal Vein Complications

Complications related to the portal vein occur in 1% to 8.3% of transplant recipients.[161] Thrombosis may result from purse-stringing or stricturing of the anastomosis. Excessive length of the portal vein may lead to kinking and thrombosis of the vessel. Preexisting portal vein thrombosis, altered flow of the splanchnic bed caused by previous portosystemic shunting, reconstruction and vein grafting of the portal vein, allograft rejection, portal vein hypoplasia, and deficiencies of anticoagulant proteins have all been implicated in the pathogenesis of portal vein thrombosis.[147,161,165,166]

In the early postoperative course, portal vein thrombosis may present with severe allograft dysfunction, ascites, and variceal bleeding. Portal vein patency should be evaluated by duplex studies if the diagnosis is suspected. Immediate operative thrombectomy and revision of the portal anastomosis are required.[167] If unsuccessful, retransplantation is warranted.

With late thrombosis, liver function is usually well preserved because of the development of collateral vessels. Therapy is directed toward relieving the left-sided portal hypertension. Options for treatment include sclerotherapy, distal splenorenal shunting, or splenectomy with gastric and esophageal devascularization. Retransplantation is not required if the synthetic function is well maintained.

Hepatic Vein Complications

Thrombosis of the hepatic veins, although extremely rare (less than 1%), can be devastating and result in severe allograft dysfunction. Purse-stringing of the anastomosis or recurrence of Budd-Chiari syndrome are the major causes.[161] The risk of hepatic venous thrombosis is increased in patients who have received the left lateral segment of living-related, split, or reduced-size liver grafts. Because of mobility of the left lateral segment, twisting of the graft may lead to outflow venous obstruction. Duplex ultrasonography is sufficient to establish the diagnosis. Retransplantation may be necessary if liver dysfunction is severe. Deficiencies of anticoagulant proteins such as proteins C and S and antithrombin III must be excluded.[165] Anticoagulation is recommended in patients who underwent transplantation for Budd-Chiari syndrome.

Stenosis of the vena cava usually occurs at the level of the anastomosis. Suprahepatic vena caval stenosis presents with insidious onset of ascites, allograft dysfunction, and lower body edema. Infrahepatic vena caval stenosis does not cause graft dysfunction, but leads to ascites, lower extremity edema, and renal insufficiency. Duplex studies may be useful, but venography is essential to demonstrate the pressure gradient (greater than 8 cm H_2O) across the anastomosis. Balloon dilatation may be sufficient. Operative reconstruction is warranted if the stenosis is severe.

Bile Duct Complications

Biliary complications, once considered the Achilles' heel of liver transplantation, are less common today and often can be managed either radiologically or endoscopically without the need for surgical intervention or retransplantation. In the pediatric population the incidence of reported complications ranges from 7% to 20%.[168,169] The spectrum and treatment of bile duct complications are determined by the status of the hepatic artery and the type of allograft used. Some studies have demonstrated an increased risk of bile duct complications with reduced-size grafts compared with whole organs,[170] whereas others implied an equivalent rate of biliary complications.[78] Most series of *ex vivo,* but not *in vivo,* split-liver transplantations demonstrated a high incidence of bile duct complications.[171] This increased rate and the complexity of complications are the trade-offs for increased organ availability.

Bile duct complications represent a heterogeneous group of complications consisting of bile leaks, strictures, and obstruction due to stones or biliary sludge formation or both. The most common presentation is cholangitis. Transhepatic cholangiography is often required in children to establish the diagnosis,[172] and the integrity of the hepatic artery should be verified in all cases. One-third of biliary complications are diagnosed within 1 month of surgery, and 80% are diagnosed within 6 months, with leaks and strictures being the most common findings. After the first postoperative year, the incidence of bile duct complications drops significantly. Technical errors and graft ischemia are the major cause for early biliary leaks. Early biliary leaks in children with a Roux-en-Y choledochojejunostomy require surgical correction, which may vary from simple closure to revision of the anastomosis. Retransplantation may be warranted in the face of HAT. The most common cause of late biliary leaks in adults and older children is the T-tube site, following its removal in 10% to 15% of patients. Such leaks are managed endoscopically and rarely require laparotomy. Surgical correction is by Roux-en-Y choledochojejunostomy, which is the preferred reconstruction in most children and is required in all cases of biliary atresia.

Biliary strictures constitute the other major biliary complication. Presentation varies from acute cholangitis with recurrent mild fevers and elevated enzymes to progressive deterioration of allograft function. Anastomotic strictures are treated by balloon dilatation or surgical revision of the anastomosis. Retransplantation is required with severe allograft dysfunction.

The etiology of biliary strictures post-OLT is multifactorial. Numerous studies have suggested an association between the development of multiple or late intrahepatic nonanastomotic strictures in the absence of hepatic artery thrombosis with preservation injury (specifically, prolonged donor cold ischemia time of more than 12 hours), ABO incompatibility, chronic rejection, and CMV infection.[147,161,168] Often, such problems progress, and retransplantation may eventually be indicated because of graft failure. Moreover, biliary stricturing in patients with primary sclerosing cholangitis may represent recurrent disease or may be caused by the Roux-en-Y choledochojejunostomy. Nonanastomotic strictures generally appear 1 to 4 months after transplantation and are often treated with balloon dilatation or stenting using either a transhepatic or endoscopic approach. Although long-term patency of the biliary tree can be established in 80% of patients, approximately 20% will eventually develop secondary graft failure and will require retransplantation. The fact that recurrence of intrahepatic biliary strictures occurs following retransplantation further suggests that an autoimmune mechanism is important.

Primary Nonfunction

Primary nonfunction implies the absence of metabolic and synthetic hepatic allograft activity following transplantation. The reported incidence is 5% to 10%.[173,174] The result is a transplant patient who demonstrates frank hepatic failure with coma, acidosis, massive coagulopathy, renal failure, hypoglycemia, and shock. Patient survival depends on successful prompt retransplantation. Possible causes are outlined in Table 6.3.

Immediate posttransplantation immunologic events such as antibody-mediated hyperacute rejection have been implicated as a cause of immediate graft loss. Pretransplantation crossmatch is not clinically feasible, and potential liver donors are only matched for size and ABO compatibility.

TABLE 6.3. *Factors associated with increased risk of primary nonfunction*

Donor factors
Prolonged donor hospitalization
Severe biochemical abnormality
Hemodynamic instability
Prolonged cardiovascular compromise
Organ steatosis (>60% macrovesicular fat)
Recipient factors
Significant size disparity between donor and recipient
Prolonged cold ischemia time (>12–18 hr)
Prolonged warm ischemia time (>90 min)
Vascular thrombosis
Immunologic factors: ABO incompatibility, positive crossmatch

In pediatric patients, ABO compatibility is desirable, but not crucial, for the success of the transplant. Experience at Pittsburgh[175] demonstrated that results are significantly better in ABO-identical grafts than in ABO-nonidentical but compatible grafts, and are worst in ABO-incompatible grafts. In our pediatric experience, ABO-identical grafts yielded a survival rate of 96%, whereas 16 nonidentical but compatible grafts and 5 incompatible grafts yielded survival rates of 55% and 65%, respectively.[176] We reserve the use of nonidentical grafts for the most critical situations in which no other organs are available.

Nonhepatic Complications

Renal Complications

Varying degrees of renal impairment are common in liver transplant patients. Many exhibit renal insufficiency from the hepatorenal syndrome prior to transplantation. Postoperative oliguria may be caused by hypovolemia, intraoperative hypotension with acute tubular necrosis, sepsis, immunosuppressive therapy, or nephrotoxic drugs such as aminoglycosides or amphotericin. A study of renal function in our pediatric patients who have been on CsA for more than 1 year demonstrated that 85% of the patients exhibited true glomerular filtration rates that were less than the low normal rate for their age. CsA use was associated with progressive impairment of the renal function.[177] Adequate support of renal perfusion with volume replacement and close monitoring of immunosuppressive medications are critical. Volume overload is managed by diuretics. Ultrafiltration and hemodialysis may be required. The need for dialysis is associated with poor prognosis and high mortality rates in liver transplant recipients.[178]

Gastrointestinal Complications

Intraabdominal bleeding manifests with increasing abdominal girths and bloody drain outputs. Frequently no specific bleeding site is found at reoperation, and diffuse oozing is often secondary to coagulopathy.[161] Specific sites of bleeding may be located at the vascular anastomoses or the jejunojejunostomy. Other causes of bleeding include stress ulcers, gastritis, varices, herpes esophagitis, and CMV or candida colitis. Endoscopy and biopsies are usually needed for diagnosis. Portal vein thrombosis should be ruled out if variceal bleeding occurs after OLT.

Gastrointestinal perforation early after OLT is frequently caused by unrecognized intraoperative bowel injury or anastomotic leaks. The frequency is higher in patients with previous intraabdominal surgery and adhesions. Electrocautery burns to the duodenal serosa may progress to full-thickness perforation. Operative repair is necessary in patients presenting with intraabdominal sepsis or free intraabdominal air. Late perforation is less common and is usually secondary to PTLD or infectious ulcers. Bowel obstruction may result from postoperative adhesions. Other rare causes include herniation of the jejunojejunostomy or PTLD. Mild transient hyperamylasemia is common in OLT patients; usually no treatment is necessary. Significant pancreatitis is rare.[179]

Pulmonary Complications

Pulmonary morbidity occurs in almost all liver transplant recipients. Atelectasis, effusions, and infections are the most common complications. Atelectasis resolves with aggressive pulmonary toilet and ambulation. Right pleural effusions resolve over time. Thoracentesis or tube thoracostomy is necessary in only 15% to 20% of patients with large symptomatic effusions. Paralysis of the right hemidiaphragm after OLT may be caused by an intraoperative injury to the phrenic nerve during the application of vascular clamps on the suprahepatic vena cava.

Neurologic Complications

Seizures are common after OLT. Many are related to high CsA or tacrolimus levels accompanied by low magnesium levels. Patients respond well to lowering of immunosuppressive medications and magnesium infusions. Other complications include meningitis, extrapyramidal symptoms, and paresthesias. Positioning injuries that include the brachial plexus and the peroneal nerve are occasionally encountered. Intracranial hemorrhage occurs in patients with severe liver failure or fungal infections and is a frequent lethal event.

RESULTS

Although the potential for complications in pediatric liver transplantation is high, the rewards are tremendous. Recent analysis of long-term results demonstrated that children who underwent transplantation after 1993 exhibited significantly better survival than those who underwent transplantation earlier.[50] Overall patient survival in pediatric recipients is currently in excess of 89%.[50,181] Infants younger than 1 year or who weigh less than 10 kg now exhibit survival rates of 80% to 88%, versus previously reported rates of 50% to 60%.[50,147,181] Advancement in immunosuppressive therapy, refinement of operative techniques, improvements in postoperative management, aggressive preoperative nutritional intervention, and earlier referral and selection have all contributed to such progress.

Improvement in survival has also been accompanied by a decline in life-threatening and graft-threatening complications such as hepatic artery thrombosis and primary nonfunction in reduced-size and split-liver transplantation. The use of new immunosuppressive agents such as tacrolimus has decreased the incidence of acute and chronic allograft rejection.

In addition, transplant patients enjoy successful growth and development. In a study that included 19 patients who underwent transplantation at UCLA, 16 exhibited normal or accelerated growth after transplantation.[182] In the Pittsburgh pediatric series,[183] 50% of children who received transplants achieved accelerated growth, and 45 of 57 children were in an age appropriate school grade.

PROSPECTUS

Liver transplantation is a durable procedure that provides excellent long-term survival. Although there has been overall improvement in patient outcome with increased experience, such an effect is most pronounced in children younger than 1 year. Retransplantation, although meaningful in some patients, continues to carry a progressive decrement. The use of living-related and split-liver transplantation has dramatically reduced the waiting periods for children and improved survival. Continued development of future goals such as gene therapy for hereditary diseases, hepatocellular transplantation, improved immunosuppressive management, the development of clinically applicable tolerance protocols, and advances in xenogeneic transplantation should yield even greater future successes.

REFERENCES

1. Starzl TE, Marchiaro TL, Von Kaulla K, et al. Homotransplantation of the liver in humans. *Surg Gynecol Obstet* 1963;117:659–664.
2. NIH consensus development conference statement: liver transplantation. June 20–23. *Hepatology* 1984;4:107S.
3. McDiarmid SV, Millis MJ, Olthoff KM, So SK. Indications for pediatric liver transplantation. *Pediatr Transplantation* 1998;2:106–116.
4. Alagille D. Extrahepatic biliary atresia. *Hepatology* 1984;4:7S–10S.
5. Kasai M, Suzuki S. A new operation for "noncorrectable" biliary atresia: hepatic portoenterostomy. *Shujutsu* 1959;13:733–741.
6. Kasai M, Kimura S, Asakura Y, et al. Surgical treatment of biliary atresia. *J Pediatr Surg* 1968;3:665–672.
7. Otte JB, De Ville De Goyet J, Reding R, et al. Sequential treatment of biliary atresia with Kasai portoenterostomy and liver transplantation: a review. *Hepatology* 1994;20:41S–48S.
8. Goss JA, Shackleton CR, Swenson K, et al. Orthotopic liver transplantation for congenital biliary atresia. An 11-year, single-center experience. *Ann Surg* 1996;224:276–284.
9. Ohi R, Hanamatsu M, Mochizuki L, et al. Progress in the treatment of biliary atresia. *World J Surg* 1985;9:285–293.
10. Ito T, Horisawa M, Ando H. Intrahepatic bile ducts in biliary atresia: a possible factor in determining prognosis. *J Pediatr Surg* 1983;18:124–130.
11. Ascher NL, Najarian JS. Hepatic transplantation and biliary atresia: early experience in eight patients. *World J Surg* 1984;8:57–63.
12. Pettitt BJ, Zitelli BJ, Rowe ML. Analysis of patients with biliary atresia coming to liver transplantation. *J Pediatr Surg* 1984;19:77–85.
13. Altman RP. Results of reoperation for correction of extrahepatic biliary atresia. *J Pediatr Surg* 1979;14:305–309.
14. Starzl TE, Esquivel C, Gordon R, et al. Pediatric liver transplantation. *Transpl Proc* 1987;19:3230–3235.
15. McDiarmid SV, Mills MJ, Olthoff KM, et al. Indications for pediatric liver transplantation. *Pediatr Transplantation* 1998;2:106–116.
16. Alagille D, Estrada A., Hadchouel M, et al. Syndromic paucity of interlobular bile ducts (Alagille syndrome or arteriohepatic dysplasia): review of 80 cases. *J Pediatr* 1987;110:195–200.
17. Sharp HL. Alpha-1-antitrypsin: an ignored protein in understanding liver disease. *Semin Liver Dis* 1982;2:314–328.
18. Sveger T. Liver disease in alpha-1-antitrypsin deficiency detected by screening of 200,000 infants. *N Engl J Med* 1976;194:1316–1321.
19. Sveger T. The natural history of liver disease in alphalantrypsin deficiency in children. *Acta Paediatr Scand* 1988;77:847–851.
20. Alagille D. Alpha-1-antitrypsin deficiency. *Hepatology* 1984;4:llS–14S.
21. Hood JM, Koep LJ, Peters RL, et al. Liver transplantation for advanced liver disease with alpha-l-antitrypsin deficiency. *N Engl J Med* 1980;302:272–275.
22. Esquivel CO, Vincente E, Van Thiel R, et al. Orthotopic liver transplantation for alpha-l-antitrypsin deficiency: an experience in 29 children and 10 adults. *Transplant Proc* 1987;19(5):3798–3802
23. Carson NAJ, Biggart JD, Bitles AH, et al. Hereditary tyrosinemia: clinical, enzymatic, and pathological study of an infant with the acute form of the disease. *Arch Dis Child* 1976;51(2):106–113.
24. Kvittingen EA. Hereditary tyrosinemia type 1—an overview. *Scand J Clin and Lab. Invest* 1986;46:27–34.
25. Weinberg AG, Mize CE, Worthen HG. The occurrence of hepatoma in the chronic form of hereditary tyrosinemia. *J Pediatr* 1976;88:434.
26. Starzl TE, Zitelli BJ, Shaw BW Jr, et al. Changing concepts: liver replacement for hereditary tyrosinemia and hepatoma. *J Pediatr* 1985;106(4):604–606.
27. Sokal E, Bustos R, Van Hoof F, et al. Liver transplantation for hereditary tyrosinemia—early transplantation following patient stabilization. *Transplantation* 1992;54(5):937–939.
28. Lindstedt S, Holme E, Lock EA, et al. Treatment of hereditary tyrosinemia by inhibition of 4-hydroxyphenylpyruvate dioxygenase. *Lancet* 1992;340(8223):813–817.
29. Scheinberg IH, Sternlieb I. *Wilson's disease*. In Scheinberg IH ed. Wilson's disease. Philadelphia; WB Saunders 1984:9–16.
30. Sternlieb I. Wilson's disease: indications for liver transplants. *Hepatology* 1984;4:15S–17S.
31. Walshe JM. Copper chelation in patients with Wilson's disease. *Q J Med* 1973;42(167):441–452.
32. Esquivel CO, Iwatsuki S, Gordon RD, et al. Indications for pediatric liver transplantation. *J Pediatr* 1987;111:1039–1045.
33. Crigler JF, Najjar VA. Congenital familial nonhemolytic jaundice with kernicterus. *Pediatrics* 1952;10:169–173.
34. Bloomer JR, Sharp HL. The liver in Crigler-Najjar syndrome, protoporphyria, and other metabolic disorders. *Hepatology* 1984;4:18S–21S.
35. Bloomer JR. Protoporphyria. *Semin Liver Dis* 1982;2(2):143–153.
36. Bontempo FA., Lewis JH, Gorenc TJ, et al. Liver transplantation in hemophilia A. *Blood* 1987;69(6)1721–1724.
37. Carlson DE, Busuttil RW, Giudici TA, et al. Orthotopic liver transplantation in the treatment of complications of type I Gaucher disease. *Transplantation* 1990;49(6)1192–1194.
38. Krivit W, Pierpont ME, Ayaz K, et al. Bone marrow transplantation in Maroteaux-Lamy disease (mucopolysaccharoidosis IV): correction of the enzymatic defect. *N Engl J Med* 1984;311(25):1006–1011.
39. Todo S, Starzl TE, Tzakis A, et al. Orthotopic liver transplantation for urea cycle enzyme deficiency. *Hepatology* 1992;15(3):419–422.
40. Otto G, Herfarth C, Senninger N, et al. Hepatic transplantation in galactosemia. *Transplantation* 1989;47(5):902–903.
41. Malatack JJ, Iwatsuki S, Gartner JC, et al. Liver transplantation for type I glycogen storage disease. *Lancet* 1983;1(8333)1073–1075.
42. Selby R, Starzl TE, Yunis B, et al. Liver transplantation for type IV glycogen storage disease. *N Engl J Med* 1991;324(1):39–42.
43. Sokal EM, Van Hoof F, Alberti D, et al. Progressive cardiac failure following orthotopic liver transplantation for type IV glycogenosis. *Eur J Pediatr* 1992;151(3):200–203.
44. Esquivel CO, Marino IR, Fioravanti V, et al. Liver transplantation for metabolic diseases of the liver. *Gastroenterology* Clinics of N. America 1988;17(1):167–175.
45. European Association for the Study of the Liver. Randomized trial of steroid therapy in acute liver failure. *Gut* 1979;20(7):620–623.
46. Christensen E, Bremmelgoard A, Bannsen, M, et al. Prediction of fatality in fulminant hepatic failure. *Scand Gastroenterol* 1984;19:90–96.
47. Ring-Larsen H, Palazzo V. Renal failure in fulminant hepatic failure and terminal cirrhosis. *Gut* 1981;22(7):585–591.
48. Brems JJ, Hiatt JR, Ramming KP, et al. Fulminant hepatic failure: the role of liver transplantation as primary therapy. *Am J Surg* 1987;154(1):137–141.
49. Goss JA, Shackleton CR, Maggard M, et al. Liver transplantation for fulminant hepatic failure in the pediatric patient. *Arch Surg* 1998;133:839–846.
50. Goss JA, Shackleton CR, McDiarmid SV, et al. Long-term results of pediatric liver transplantation. An analysis of 569 transplants. *Ann Surg* 1998;3:411–420.
51. O'Grady JG, Alexander GJ, Hayllar KM, et al. Early indicators of prognosis in fulminant hepatic failure. *Gastroenterology* 1989;97(2):439–445.

52. Adrian-Casavilla F, Reyes J, Tzakis A, et al. Liver transplantation for neonatal hepatitis as compared to the two other leading indications for liver transplantation in children. *J Hepatol* 1994;21(6):1035–1039.
53. McDiarmid SV, Conrad A, Ament ME, et al. *De novo* hepatitis C in children after liver transplantation. *Transplantation* 1998;66(3):311–318.
54. Gregorio GV, Portmann B, Reid F, et al. Autoimmune hepatitis in childhood: a 20-year experience. *Hepatology* 1997;25(3):541–547.
55. Starzl TE, Iwatsuki S, Shaw BW Jr, et al. Treatment of fibrolamellar hepatoma with partial hepatectomy or with total hepatectomy and liver transplantation. *Surg Gynecol Obstet* 1986;162(2):145–148.
56. Newman KD. Hepatic tumors in children. *Semin Pediatr Surg* 1997;6(1):38–41.
57. Achilleos OA, Buist LJ, Kelly DA, et al. Unresectable hepatic tumors in childhood and the role of liver transplantation. *J Pediatr Surg* 1996;31(11):1563–1567.
58. Koneru B, Flye MW, Busuttil RW, et al. Liver transplantation for hepatoblastoma—the American experience. *Ann Surg* 1991;213(2):118–121.
59. Okuyama K. Primary liver cell carcinoma associated with biliary cirrhosis due to congenital bile duct atresia. *J Pediatr* 1965;67:89–93.
60. Ahn S, Yellin A, Sheng FC, et al. Selective surgical therapy of the Budd-Chiari syndrome provides superior survival rates than conservative management. *J Vasc Surg* 1987;5(1):28–37.
61. Campbell DA Jr, Rolles K, Jamieson N, et al. Hepatic transplantation with perioperative and long term anticoagulation as treatment for Budd-Chiari syndrome. *Surg Gynecol Obstet* 1988;166(6):511–518.
62. Cox KL, Ward RE, Furgiuele TL, et al. Orthotopic liver transplantation in patients with cystic fibrosis. *Pediatrics* 1987;80(4):571–574.
63. Revell SP, Noble-Jamieson G, Roberton NRC, et al. Liver transplantation in cystic fibrosis *J R Soc Med* 1993;86(2):111–112.
64. Todo S, Tzakis A, Abu-Elmagd K, et al. Cadaveric small bowel and small bowel-liver transplantation in humans. *Transplantation* 1992;53(2):369–376.
65. Hobeika J, Houssin D, Bernard O, et al. Orthotopic liver transplantation in children with chronic liver disease and severe hypoxemia. *Transplantation* 1994;57(2):224–228.
66. Ellis D, Avner ED, Starzl TE. Renal failure in children with hepatic failure undergoing liver transplantation. *J Pediatr* 1986;108(3):393–398.
67. Flye MW. *Atlas of organ transplantation.* Philadelphia: WB Saunders, 1995.
68. Warren KW, Jenkins RL, Steele GP. *Atlas of surgery of the liver, pancreas and biliary tract.* Norwalk, CT: Appleton & Lange, 1995.
69. Shackleton CR, Goss JA, Swenson K, et al. The impact of microsurgical hepatic arterial reconstruction on the outcome of liver transplantation for congenital biliary atresia. *Am J Surg* 1997;173:431–435.
70. Quinones-Baldrich WJ, Memsic L, Ramming K, et al. Branch patch for arterialization of hepatic grafts. *Surg Gynecol Obstet* 1986;162(5):488–490.
71. Tzakis A, Todo S, Starzl TE. Piggyback orthotopic liver transplantation with preservation of the inferior vena cava. *Ann Surg* 1989;210(5):649–652.
72. Kalayooglu M, Sollinger HW, Stratta RJ, et al. Extended preservation of the liver for clinical transplantation. *Lancet* 1988;1(8586):617–619.
73. Belzer FO, Sollinger HW, Glass NR, et al. Beneficial effects of adenosine and phosphate in kidney preservation. *Transplantation* 1983;36(6):633–635.
74. Fortner JG, Yeh SD, Kim DK, et al. The case for and technique of heterotopic liver grafting. *Transplant Proc* 1979;11(1):269–275.
75. Bismuth H, Houssin D. Reduced-sized orthotopic liver graft in hepatic transplantation in children. *Surgery* 1984;95(3):367–370.
76. Broelsch CE, Emond JC, Thistlethwaite JR, et al. Liver transplantation, including the concept of reduced-size liver transplants in children. *Ann Surg* 1988;208:410–420.
77. Otte JB, de Ville de Goyet J, Solak E, et al. Size reduction of the donor liver is a safe way to alleviate the shortage of size-matched organs in pediatric liver transplantation. *Ann Surg* 1990;211:146–157.
78. Langnas AN, Wagner CM, Inagaki M, et al. The results of reduced-size liver transplantation, including split livers, in patients with end-stage liver disease. *Transplantation* 1992;53:387–391.
79. Broelsch, CE, Emond JC, Whitington PF, et al. Application of reduced-size liver transplants as split grafts, auxiliary orthotopic grafts, and living related segmental transplants. *Annals of Surgery* 1990;(212)3:368–375.
80. Raia S, Nery JR, Mies S. Liver transplantation from live donors. *Lancet* 1998;2:497–503.
81. Strong RW, Lynch SV, Ong TN, et al. Successful liver transplantation from a living donor to her son. *N Engl J Med* 1990;322(21):1505–1507.
82. Jurim O, Shackleton CR, McDiarmid SV, et al. Living-donor liver transplantation at UCLA. *Am J Surg* 1995;169(5):529–532.
83. Millis JM, Alonso Em, Piper JB, et al. Liver transplantation at the University of Chicago. *Clinical Transplants* 1995;187–197.
84. Kiuchi T, Tanaka K. Living related donor liver transplantation: status quo in Kyoto, Japan. *Transplantation Proceedings* 1998;30(3):687–691.
85. Pichlmayr R, Ringe B, Gubernatis G, et al. Transplantation einer spenderbeber auf zwei empfanger (splitting–transplantation): eine neue methode in der weiterentwicklung der lebersegment transplantation. *Langenbecks Arch Chir* 1988;373:127–134.
86. Bismuth H, Marino M, Castaing D. Emergency orthotopic liver transplantation in two patients using one donor. *Br J Surg* 1989;76(7):722–724.
87. Broelsch CE, Emond JC, Whitington PF, et al. Application of reduced size liver transplants as split grafts, auxiliary orthotopic grafts and living related segmental transplants. *Ann Surg* 1990;(212)3:368–375.
88. Busuttil RW, Shaked A, Millis M, et al. One thousand liver transplants: the lessons learned. *Ann Surg* 1994;219(5):490–497.
89. De Ville de Goyet J. Split liver transplantation in Europe, 1988–1993. *Transplantation* 1995;59:1371–1376 vol(10).
90. Azoulay D, Astarcioglu I, Bismuth H, et al. Split liver transplantation: the Paul Brousse policy. *Ann Surg* 1996;224(6):737–746.
91. Kalayoglu M, D'Alessandro AM, Knechtle JS, et al. Preliminary experience with split liver transplantation. *J Am Coll Surg* 1996;182:381–387.
92. Rela M, Voregas V, Miniesan P, et al. Split liver transplantation: King's College Hospital experience. *Ann Surg* 1998;227:282–288 vol(2).
93. Rogiers X, Malago M, Gawad K, et al. *In situ* splitting of cadaveric livers: the ultimate expansion of the donor pool. *Ann Surg* 1996;224(3):331–339.
94. Goss JA, Yersiz H, Shackleton CR, et al. *In situ* splitting of the cadaveric liver for transplantation. *Transplantation* 1997;64(6):871–877.
95. Rogiers X, Malago M, Habib N, et al. *In situ* splitting of the liver in heart-beating cadaveric organ donor for transplantation in two recipients. *Transplantation* 1995;59(8):1081–1083.
96. Ghobrial RM, Farmer DG, Yersiz H, et al. Split liver transplantation for expansion of the donor pool. *Journal Transplantation* 1999;67:S548.
97. Murphy JB. Heteroplastic tissue grafting effected through roentgen ray lymphoid destruction. *JAMA* 1914;62:1459–1469.
98. Baker R, Gordon R, Huffer J, et al. Experimental renal transplantation: I. Effect of nitrogen mustard, cortisone and splenectomy. *Arch Surg* 1952;65:702–708.
99. Schwartz RS, Dameshek W. Drug-induced immunological tolerance. *Nature* 1959;183:1682–1689.
100. Calne RY, Alexandre GP, Murray JE. A study of the effects of drugs in prolonged survival of homologous renal transplants in dogs. *Ann N Y Acad Sci* 1962;99:743–753.
101. Russell PS, Monaco AP. Heterologous antilymphocyte sera and some of their effects. *Transplantation* 1967;5(4):1086–1099.
102. Starzl TE, Marchioro TL, Porter RA, et al. The use of heterologous antilymphoid agents in canine renal and liver homotransplantation and in human renal homotransplantation. *Surg Gynecol Obstet* 1967;124:301–309.
103. Borel JF, Feurer C, Gubler HU, et al. Biological effects of cyclosporin A: a new antilymphocytic agent. *Agents Actions* 1976;6(4):468–475.
104. Ochiai T, Nakajima K, Nagata M, et al. Studies of the induction and maintenance of long-term graft acceptance by treatment with FK506 in heterotopic cardiac allotransplantation in rats. *Transplantation* 1987;44:734–738 vol(6).
105. Calne RY, Collier DS, Lim S, et al. Rapamycin for immunosuppression in organ allografting. *Lancet* 1989;2(8656):227.
106. Bartlett RR, Dimitrijevic M, Mattar T, et al. Leflunomide (HWA 486), a novel immuno-modulating compound for the treatment of autoimmune disorders and reactions leading to transplantation rejection. *Agents Actions* 1991;32:10–21.
107. Sollinger SW, Deierhoi MH, Belzer FO, et al. RS-61443: a phase I clinical trial and pilot reserve study. *Transplantation* 1992;53:428–432 vol(2).
108. Kahan BD, Tejpal N, Gibbons S, et al. The synergistic interactions *in vitro* and *in vivo* of brequinar sodium with cyclosporine or rapamycin alone and in triple combination. *Transplantation* 1993;55:894–900 vol(4).

109. Synder DS, Unanue ER. Corticosteroids inhibit immune macrophages Ig expression and interleukin-1 production. *J Immunol* 1982;129(5):1803–1805.

110. Fowler B, Weltz G, Nieder RJ, et al. Evidence that glucocorticoids block expression of the human interleukin-6 gene by accessory cells. *Transplantation* 1990;49:183–189.

111. Bailey L, Lundry S, Razzouk A, Wang N. Pediatric Heart Manspianianos *Journal of Heart and Lung Transplantation* 1992;11(4PE): 5267–5271.

112. Waage A, Bajje O. Glucocorticoids suppress the production of tumor necrosis factor by lipopolysaccharide-stimulated human monocytes. *Immunology* 1988;63:299–302.

113. Tsai NY, Carlstedt-Duke J, Weigal NL. Molecular interactions of steroid hormone receptor with its enhancer element: evidence for receptor dimer function. *Cell* 1988;55:361–369.

114. Handschumacher RE, Harding MW, Rice J, et al. Cyclophillin-A: a specific cytosolic binding protein for cyclosporine A. *Science* 1984;26:544–547.

115. Liu J, Farmer JD, Lane WS, et al. Calcineurin is a common target of cyclophillin-cyclosporin A and FKBP-FK506 complexes. *Cell* 1991;66:807–815.

116. Kalman VK, Klimpel GR. Cyclosporine A inhibits the production of gamma interferon but does not inhibit production of virus induced IFN α/β. *Cell Immunol* 1983;78(1):22–29.

117. Kupiec-Weglinski JW, Filho MA, Strom TB, et al. Sparing of suppressor cells: a critical action of cyclosporine. *Transplantation* 1984;38(2):97–101.

118. Kahan BD. Overview: individualization of cyclosporine therapy using pharmacokinetic and pharmacodynamic parameters. *Transplantation* 1985;40(5):457–476.

119. Kino T, Hatanaka H, Hashimoto M, et al. FK 506, a novel immunosuppressant isolated from a streptomycetes. 1. Fermentation, isolation, and physiochemical and biological characteristics. *J Antibiot* 1988;41(8):999–1008.

120. Dumont FJ, Starvch MJ, Koprak SL, et al. Distinct mechanisms of suppression of murine T cell activation by the related macrolides FK506 and rapamycin. *J Immunol* 1990;144(1)251–258.

121. Liu J, Farmer JD, Lane WS, et al. Calcineurin is a common target of cyclophillin-cyclosporin A and FKBP-FK506 complexes. *Cell* 1991;66(4):807–815.

122. McDiarmid SV. The use of tacrolimus in pediatric liver transplantation. *J Pediatr Gastroenterol Nutr* 1998;26(1):90–102.

123. McDiarmid SV, Busuttil RW, Ascher NL, et al. FK(506) (tacrolimus) compared with cyclosporine for primary immunosuppression after pediatric liver transplantation. Results from the U.S. muticenter trial. *Transplantation* 1995;59(4):530–536.

124. Sher LA, Cosenza AA, Michel J, et al. Efficacy of tacrolimus as a rescue therapy for chronic rejection in orthotopic liver transplantation. *Transplantation* 1997;64(2):258–263.

125. Elion GB, Callahan S, Bieber S, et al. A summary of investigations with 2-amino-6-methy-4nitro-5-imidazolyothiopurine. *Cancer Chemother Rep* 1961;14:93–99.

126. Kahan BD, Ghobrial R. Immunosuppressive agents. *Surg Clin North Am* 1994;74(5):1029–1054.

127. Hebert FM, Ascher NL, Lake RJ, et al. Four year follow-up of mycophenolate mofetil for graft rescue in liver allograft recipients. *Transplantation* 1999;67(5):707–712.

128. Kahan BD, Chang JY, Seghal SN. Preclinical evaluation of a new potent immunosuppressive agent, rapamycin. *Transplantation* 1991; 52(2):185–191.

129. Pai SY, Calvo V, Wood M, et al. Cross-linking CD28 leads to activation of 70-kDa S6 kinase. *Eur J Immunol* 1994;24(10):2364–2368.

130. Brown EJ, Albers MW, Shin TB, et al. A mammalian protein targeted by G1-arresting rapamycin-receptor complex. *Nature* 1994;369:756–758.

131. Murgia M, Jordan S, Kahan BD. The side effect profile of sirolimus: a phase I study in quiescent cyclosporine-prednisolone-treated renal transplant patients. *Kidney Int* 1996;49(1):209–216.

132. Kimball PM, Kerman RH, Kahan BD. Production of synergistic but nonidentical mechanism of immunosuppression by rapamycin and cyclosporine. *Transplantation* 1991;51(2):486–490.

133. Watson CJE, Friend PJ, Jamieson NV, et al. Sirolimus: a potent new immunosuppressant for liver transplantation. *Transplantation* 1999;67(4):505–509.

134. Cosimi AB. Future of monoclonal antibodies in solid organ transplantation. *Dig Dis Sci* 1995;40(1):65–72.

135. Ghobrial R, Busuttil RW, Kupiec-Weglinski JW. Monoclonal antibodies. *Curr Opin Organ Transplant* 1997;2:82–93.

136. Colonna JO, Goldstein LI, Brems JJ, et al. A prospective study on the use of monoclonal anti-T3-cell antibody (OKT3) to treat steroid-resistant liver transplant rejection. *Arch Surg* 1987;122(10):1120–1123.

137. McIntyre JA, Kincade M, Higgins NG. Detection of IgA anti-OKT3-antibodies in OKT3-treated transplant recipients. *Transplantation* 1996;61(10):1465–1469.

138. Woodle SE, Thistlewaite JR, Jolliff LK, et al. Humanized OKT3 antibodies: successful transfer of immune modulating properties and idiotype expression. *J Immunol* 1992;148(9):2756–2763.

139. Theze J, Alzari PM, Bertoglio J. Interleukin-2 and its receptors: recent advances and new immunological functions. *Immunol Today* 1996;17(10):481–486.

140. Soulillou JP, Cantarovich D, Mauff B, et al. Randomized controlled trial of a monoclonal antibody against the interleukin-2 receptor (33B3.1) as compared with rabbit antithymocyte globulin for prophylaxis against rejection of renal allografts. *N Engl J Med* 1990;322(17):1175–1182.

141. Reding R, Feyaerts A, Vraux H, et al. Prophylactic immunosuppression with anti-interleukin-2 receptor monoclonal antibody LO-Tact-1 versus OKT3 in liver allografting. A two-year follow-up study. *Transplantation* 1996;61(9):1406–1409.

142. Nashan B, Schlitt HJ, Schwinzed R, et al. Immunoprophylaxis with a monoclonal anti-IL-2 receptor antibody in liver transplant patients. *Transplantation* 1996;61(4):546–554.

143. Lemmens HP, Langher JM, Bechstein WO, et al. Interleukin-2 receptor antibody vs ATG for induction immunosuppression after liver transplantation: initial results of a prospective randomized trial. *Transplant Proc* 1995;27(1):1140–1141.

144. Snover DC, Sibley RK, Freese DK, et al. Orthotopic liver transplantation: a pathological study of 63 serial liver biopsies from 17 patients with special reference to the features and natural history of rejection. *Hepatology* 1984;4(6):1212–1222.

145. Adams DH, Neuberger JM. Treatment of acute rejection. *Semin Liver Dis* 1992;12(1):80–88.

146. Ryckman FC, Schroeder TJ, Pedersen SH, et al. Use of monoclonal antibody immunosuppressive therapy in pediatric renal and liver transplantation. *Clin Transplant* 1991;5:186–193.

147. Alonso MH, Ryckman FC. Current concepts in pediatric transplant. *Semin Liver Dis* 1998;18(3):295–307.

148. Ludwig J, Wiesner RH, Batts KP, et al. The acute vanishing bile duct syndrome (acute irreversible rejection) after orthotopic liver transplantation. *Hepatology* 1987;7(3):476–483.

149. Freese DK, Snover DC, Sharp HL, et al. Chronic rejection after liver transplantation: a study of clinical, histopathological and immunological features. *Hepatology* 1991;13(5):882–891.

150. Kusne S, Dummer JS, Singh N, et al. Infections after liver transplantation. An analysis of 101 consecutive cases. *Medicine* 1988;67(2): 132–143.

151. Fox AL, Tolpin MD, Baker A, et al. Seropositivity in liver transplant recipients as a predictor of cytomegalovirus disease. *J Infect Dis* 1987;157(2):383–385.

152. Patel R, Snydman DR, Rubin RH, et al. Cytomegalovirus prophylaxis in solid organ transplantation. *Transplantation* 1996;61(9): 1279–1289.

153. Darenkov IA, Marcarelli MA, Basadonna GP, et al. Reduced incidence of Epstein-Barr virus-associated posttransplant lymphoproliferative disorder using preemptive antiviral therapy. *Transplantation* 1997;64(6):848–852.

154. McDiarmid SV, Jordan SJ, Lee GS, et al. Prevention and preemptive therapy of posttransplant lymphoproliferative disease in pediatric liver recipients. *Transplantation* 1998;66(12):1604–1611.

155. Newwell KA, Alonso EM, Whitington PF, et al. Posttransplant lymphoproliferative disease in pediatric liver transplantation: Interplay between primary Epstein-Barr virus in pechia and immunosuppression. *Transplantation* 1996;62(3):370–375.

156. Kalayoglu M, Stratta RJ, Sollinger HW, et al. Liver transplantation in infants and children. *J Pediatr Surg* 1989;24(1):70–76.

157. Hoffer FA, Teele RL, Lillehei CW, et al. Infected bilomas and hepatic artery thrombosis in infant recipients of liver transplants. *Radiology* 1988;169(2):435–438.

158. Tzakis AG, Gordon RD, Shaw BW, et al. Clinical presentation of hepatic artery thrombosis after liver transplantation in the cyclosporine era. *Transplantation* 1985;40(6):667–671.

159. Northover J, Terblanch J. Bile duct blood supply. Its importance in human liver transplantation. *Transplantation* 1978;26(1):67–69.

160. Penkrot RJ. Noninvasive evaluation of complications of orthotopic liver transplantation. *Semin Intervent Radiol* 1986;3:120–126.

161. Ozaki CF, Katz SM, Monsour H, et al. Surgical complications of liver transplantation. *Surg Clin North Am* 1994;74(5):1155–1167.

162. Mazzaferro V, Esquivel CO, Makowka L, et al. Hepatic artery thrombosis after pediatric liver transplantation—a medical or surgical event? *Transplantation* 1989;47(6):971–977.

163. Yandza T, Hamada F, Gauthier D, et al. Pediatric liver transplantation: effect of the site of arterial inflow on the incidence of hepatic artery thrombosis according to recipient weight. *Transplant Proc* 1994;26(1):169–170.

164. Tobben PJ, Zajko AB, Sumkin JH, et al. Pseudoaneurysms complicating organ transplantation: roles of CT, duplex sonography, and angiography. *Radiology* 1988;169(1):65–70.

165. Harper PL, Edgar PF, Liddington RJ, et al. Protein C deficiency and portal vein thrombosis in liver transplantation in children. *Lancet* 1988;2(8617):924–927.

166. Lerut J, Tzakis AG, Bron K, et al. Complications of venous reconstruction in human orthotopic liver transplantation. *Ann Surg* 1987;205(4):404–414.

167. De Goyet JD, Gibbs P, Clapuyt P, et al. Original extrahilar approach for hepatic portal revascularization and relief of extrahepatic portal hypertension related to late portal vein thrombosis after pediatric liver transplantation. Long term results. *Transplantation* 1996;62(1):71–75.

168. Peclet MH, Ryckman FC, Pedersen SH, et al. The spectrum of bile duct complications in pediatric liver transplantation. *J Pediatr Surg* 1994;29(2):214–219.

169. Stratta RJ, Wood P, Langnas AN, et al. Diagnosis and treatment of biliary tract complications after orthotopic transplantation. *Surgery* 1989;106(4):675–683.

170. Houssin D, Soubrane O, Boilot O, et al. Orthotopic liver transplantation with a reduced-size graft: an ideal compromise in pediatrics? *Surgery* 1992;111(5):532–542.

171. Busuttil RW, Goss JA. Split liver transplantation. *Ann Surg* 1999;229(3):313–321.

172. Zajko AB, Campbell WL, Bron KM, et al. Cholangiography and interventional biliary radiology in adult liver transplantation. *Am J Roentgenology* 1985;144(1):127–133.

173. Shaw BW Jr, Gordon RD, Iwatsuki S, Starzl, TE. Retransplantation of the liver. *Seminars in liver disease* 1985;5(4):394–401.

174. Miller C, Mazzaferro V, Makowka. L, et al. Rapid flush technique for donor hepatectomy: safety and efficacy of an improved method of liver recovery for transplantation. *Transplant Proc* 1988;20:948–949.

175. Gordon RD, Iwatsuki S, Esquivel CO, et al. Liver transplantation across ABO blood groups. *Surgery* 1986;100(2):342–348.

176. Busuttil RW, Seu P, Millis JM, et al. Liver transplantation in children. *Ann Surg* 1991;213(1):48–57.

177. McDiarmid S, Ettenger R, Hawkins R, et al. The impairment of true GFR in longterm CsA-treated pediatric allograft recipients. *Transplantation* 1990;49(1):81–85.

178. Wood RP, Shaw BW, Starzl TE, et al. Extrahepatic complications of liver transplantation. *Semin Liver Dis* 1985;5(4):377–384.

179. Alexander JA, Demetrius A, Gavaler JS, et al. Pancreatitis following liver transplantation. *Transplantation* 1988;45(6):1062–1065.

180. Otte JB, Yandza T, de Ville de Goyet J, et al. Pediatric liver transplantation: report on 52 patients with a 2-year survival of 86%. *J Pediatr Surg* 1988;23(3):250–253.

181. Beath S, Brook G, Kelly D, et al. Improving outcome of liver transplantation in babies less than one year of age. *Transplant Proc* 1994;26(1):180–182.

182. Spolidoro JV, Pehlivanoglu E, Berquist WE, et al. Growth acceleration in children after orthotopic liver transplantation (OLT). *Journal of Pediatrics* 1988;112(1):41–44.

183. Zitelli BJ, Gartner JC, Malatack JJ, et al. Pediatric liver transplantation. *Transplant Proc* 1987;19(4):3309–3316.

Transplantation of the Liver, edited by Willis C. Maddrey, Eugene R. Schiff, and Michael F. Sorrell. Lippincott Williams & Wilkins, Philadelphia © 2001.

CHAPTER 7

Living-Related Liver Transplantation for Children and Adults

Jean Emond

Extension of living-related liver transplantation (LRT) to adults has been one of the most dramatic clinical events in liver transplantation. It has been a challenging and controversial development, motivated by the inexorable entry of patients onto the waiting list, and has been the subject of intensive study and debate focusing on the perceived risk to the donor. The current state of the field is in marked contrast to that described in the second edition of this text, a time during which the transplant community was coming to terms with LRT as an acceptable alternative for the treatment of small children with liver disease. Our previous chapter, written in 1992, focused on the results of fewer than 100 LRTs in three international centers in Kyoto,[1] Chicago,[2] and Hamburg,[3] the only active centers offering this intervention systematically in that era. Based on personal communications and several informal registries, we estimate that nearly 1,000 children and over 200 adults have received the procedure since the first LRTs were performed in 1989.

The goal of this chapter is to review the evolution of LRT, to address physiologic and technical considerations as well as clinical outcomes, and finally, to speculate on the role of this innovation in the coming decade. The human drama of LRT is a fascinating tale that remains of great interest to the lay press as an account of heroism and advanced medical technology with serious ethical and public policy implications. The academic interest in LRT has also been enormous: A recent search of Index Medicus identified over 400 publications addressing LRT between 1989 and 1999, a rate of nearly one publication per two patients receiving the treatment during the decade. This attention is well deserved because the technical and physiologic considerations are complex; the innovation has also been a rich area for research in clinical medical ethics.

HISTORICAL OVERVIEW

The technical feasability of LRT was foreseen by Smith[4] nearly 30 years ago when he described the possibility of living donation of the left lateral segment for a child. Although a number of attempts at partial transplantation were described earlier in the oral lore of the transplant community, the first successful implantation of a partial liver, reduced *ex vivo* from a cadaveric donor liver, was described by Houssin and Bismuth in 1984.[5] The next intervening step was the introduction of split-liver transplantation in 1988,[6] in which a cadaveric liver was divided to treat two patients, essentially a procedure similar to living donation. The first successful LRT of an adult donating to a child was reported by Strong et al. in 1989,[7] followed shortly thereafter by the the first series of LRT in children, reported by Broelsch et al.[2] Improved results of the technique were reported in the ensuing years from Chicago[8] and Kyoto[9] after the introduction of the operating microscope.

After 1994, many pediatric centers accepted the feasability of LRT, and this option became available in many centers. Spurred by efforts in Hong Kong[9] and Tokyo,[10] efforts were made to initiate LRT in adults. Two general strategies were promoted: the use of auxiliary liver transplantation, in which the small graft obtained from the living donor was placed next to the recipient liver,[11] or increasing the extent of the donor hepatectomy, using the entire right lobe of the donor to obtain a graft of adequate size for the recipient. Wachs et al. reported the first cases of right lobe donor hepatectomy in North America.[12] In May 1999, Marcos et al. reported a large series of right lobe hepatectomies at the annual meeting of the

J. Emond: Department of Surgery, Columbia College of Physicians and Surgeons, and Center for Liver Disease and Transplantation, The New York Presbyterian Hospital, New York, New York 10032.

American Society of Transplant Surgeons.[13] This landmark paper coincided with acceptance of the need for LRT in adults as a response to the critical shortage of donor organs. At the same time, a widely publicized death in a donor alerted many to the escalation of donor risk posed by right hepatectomy in the healthy donor.[14]

ETHICAL CONSIDERATIONS

Although the introduction of LRT for the liver recipient has been considered radical, the fundamental ethical issues are not substantially different from those in kidney donation. These issues have been the subject of extensive review over several decades,[15–17] although the prominent attention given to liver donation by the media has drawn renewed attention to the ethical issues. One of the motivating forces for donation is altruism, which by custom and legal requirement in North America can be the only justification for donor participation in LRT. Paid donation is illegal, and the gravest concern faced in the evaluation of the donor is the detection and elimination of undue coercion extended by the recipient or extended family on the biologically suitable potential donor.

Prior to the initiation of the program in LRT at the University of Chicago, a clinical and ethical analysis was conducted to optimize the circumstances of the introduction of this radical innovative therapy.[18] In fact, LRT is a useful paradigm for a broader range of innovative therapies, in which defined end points and a strict process for protection of the rights of patient participants are crucial. Three general conditions should exist for the development of such new therapies:

1. A compelling need for the innovation that justifies the acceptance of some risk
2. An acceptable degree of risk and benefit to the participants
3. A structured process for informed consent and the protection of the rights of the participants

Need for the Innovation

We initially studied the problem of access to orthotopic liver transplantation (OLT) in children during our studies of the utility of partial or reduced-size liver transplantation in this population.[19] Prior to the widespread introduction of LRT, nearly 50% of the very small children eligible for liver transplantation died before receiving an organ. The great majority of the 500 children who receive liver transplants each year are younger than 5 years. According to data from the United Network for Organ Sharing (UNOS), about 300 organs from small children are available annually for these patients,[20] mandating redistribution of larger donor livers to the small children or, whenever possible, using LRT. The disparity between supply and demand varies even more dramatically for adults. Since 1994 the size of the waiting list has vastly surpassed the number of transplant procedures performed annually. Currently the number of patients on the waiting list is nearly 4 times the number of transplantations that can be performed annually (Fig. 7.1).[21] Because waiting times are elastic, the long waiting list has not yet translated into a dramatic increase in the waiting mortality.

Internationally, there has been substantial interest in LRT, particularly in Asia, where cultural objections to the concept of brain death have mandated the development of LRT. The earliest reports of adult LRT came from Asia in the early 1990s,[9,10] with the first use of a right lobe donation reported from Kyoto in 1992.[22] More troubling are reports of LRT being performed in countries in which the health care system is less advanced, with a remote likelihood of a successful outcome.[23]

Acceptable Risk and Benefits

The participant in an innovative therapy should face an acceptable risk and probability of benefit. Prior to our initial efforts in LRT, the risks of the donor hepatectomy were unknown and could only be estimated from the results of liver

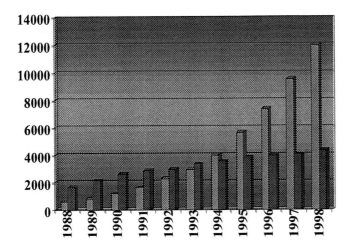

■ waiting list
■ transplant

FIG. 7.1. The growth in demand of liver transplantation in the last decade (United Network for Organ Sharing data).[21]

resection for benign disease in noncirrhotic patients.[18] It was our guess that a risk of 1% was acceptable, although the ethical parameters for deriving such a number are somewhat difficult to define. With a large body of data available for pediatric donation (usually a left lateral lobe donation), it appears that the mortality is similar to that faced by a kidney donor, 0.2%, based on nearly 1,000 LRTs performed in children and 2 documented donor deaths (Hamburg registry of LRT; X. Rogiers, personal communication, 1999). The risk from the more extensive resections needed for an adult recipient, either a full left or a full right lobe resection, is undoubtedly higher. A recent survey of U.S. centers suggests that between 150 and 200 LRTs have been performed for adult recipients (Renz J, personal communication, March 2000). Although no mortalities were reported in the survey, a donor death occurred recently that was publicized by the local print media.[14] This would indicate that the risk for adult donation would be at least 0.5%, although the experience of the centers performing LRT varies widely and undoubtedly affects local risk in each center.

The inevitable counterbalance to any risk taken by the donor is the probability of benefit to the recipient. Several factors can decrease this probability, including poor condition of the recipient or the use of LRT for advanced or hopeless disease. There is an emerging consensus that patients with decompensated cirrhosis should not be considered for LRT because the operation is more complex, takes longer, and introduces a graft that may not be of adequate size initially for the needs of the terribly ill patient. Others have been tempted to offer LRT to types of patients who have been shown to have unacceptably poor outcomes and who are not candidates for cadaveric transplants, such as patients with advanced hepatic malignancies or who are active alcoholics. We feel strongly that patients being considered for LRT should not be evaluated using broader selection criteria than those used for cadaveric transplantation. With respect to the added risk of LRT to the recipient when compared with standard orthotopic liver transplantation, the results of LRT for children are at least as good and possibly superior to those achieved with cadaveric livers. For adults, LRT has been associated with more complications[13] and is clearly a longer and more difficult procedure. The decreased size of the liver that is inevitable in LRT also leads to impairment in liver function.[24]

Informed Consent

We regard the process of informed consent as the most important element in the safe and optimal use of LRT. Coercion of the potential donor, either overt or concealed, is the greatest hazard in this process and has led some to argue that LRT is always coercive and therefore inherently unethical. A legitimate point can be made that, in a society that values altruism, living donation is always coercive. On the other hand, based on a doctrine of self-interest, restoration of health to a loved one can be justified as confer-

ring substantial benefit to the donor. We also think that the enhanced self-esteem brought on by the heroic act of the donor should not be underestimated as a benefit. In the aggregate we regard the balance of risk and benefit as being acceptable to justify the introduction of LRT for adults.

In our initial protocols for LRT, we went to great lengths to mitigate coercion.[18] We excluded emergencies to eliminate the pressure created by the urgent medical situation. In addition, the consent process required two separate steps separated in time to emphasize the need for the family to carefully consider the consequences of the decision to donate. Finally, the donor evaluation was conducted by a physician who was not a member of the transplant team in order to decrease the conflict of interest inherent when the recipient's physician makes medical decisions regarding the suitability of the donor. We have modified these rigorous conditions in recent years with the routine acceptance of LRT in pediatric patients for both elective and urgent transplantation. The rapid proliferation of LRT in adult transplant programs mandates that rigorous protocols be implemented to ensure donor safety and optimize informed consent.

TECHNICAL AND PHYSIOLOGIC CONSIDERATIONS

Functional Reserve and Regeneration

Several lines of investigation have documented the ability of the liver to regenerate when placed in a larger host.[25-28] The molecular events regulating the initiation of rejection seem to be the same in native and transplanted livers.[25] In addition to enlargment of the liver when it is too small, we have observed apoptosis in livers that are too large, which rapidly return to appropriate size for the host.[29] If the limits of graft size are exceeded (i.e., when the liver is too small), progressive damage to the graft may occur, leading to acute graft failure and the death of the recipient.[30] The lower limit of safe grafting has been studied empirically in a variety of centers; it appears that a minimum of 25% to 30% of the normal liver size is needed for a successful transplant. Urata et al.[31] developed an equation for accurately predicting the size of the "normal" liver that was needed for the recipient based on *in vivo* imaging. Developments in volumetric tomographic scanning permit the radiologist to accurately predict liver volume, a tool useful in planning LRT. Our studies suggest that grafts smaller than 50% of the recipient's needs will be associated with poor function and an increased risk of complications.[24]

Anatomic Considerations

The anatomic and technical studies that permitted the development of partial transplantation from cadavers provided the foundation for the introduction of LRT.[32] These clarified the requirements needed to obtain functional grafts of appropriate size for the recipients. The segmental anatomy of the liver, best described by Couinaud,[33] has been exploited for the creation of functionally intact grafts. Couinaud's nomenclature, in which the hepatic territories are divided into segments (eight portal segments are identified) and sectors derived from the portal venous inflow and hepatic vein outflows, provided a functional division of the liver that could be exploited in partial grafting.

The left lateral lobe, comprising portal segments 2 and 3, is used to create a liver comprising 15% to 20% of the adult liver mass and is optimal for transplanting into an infant. Addition of segment 4, the entire left hemiliver, creates a graft comprising 40% of the total liver and is satisfactory if the donor is larger than the recipient. The entire right lobe (segments 5 to 8), which typically comprises 60% of the mass of the liver, is used as the transplant for a recipient who is of comparable size or even larger than the donor. This is a substantial hepatectomy and is the mainstay of transplantation for adults from living donors.

Technical Considerations

The development and proliferation of LRT mandated the development of superior techniques for reconstruction of the vessels of the transplanted liver. Our efforts to use interposition grafts for this purpose were only partially successful, and the use of cryopreserved vessels was quite disappointing.[34] The routine application of microvascular reconstruction of the vessels by Tanaka and the Kyoto group was the most important technical advance in liver transplantation in the recent era.[35] The demonstration that vessels as small as 2 mm could be reconstructed with a 99% patency rate dispelled the persistent notion that arterial thrombosis is anything other than a technical failure.[36] Competence with microvascular technique has become an essential technical skill for LRT.

The original studies of positioning of the auxiliary liver transplant clarified the need for portal blood for the liver graft and the need for hepatic venous drainage near the chest.[37] Our clinical studies of partial liver transplantation drew attention to the importance of careful positioning of the liver in all types of partial transplantation.[38] The liver is exquisitely sensitive to obstruction of the hepatic vein outflow; thus, the anastomosis must be designed to accommodate the final resting position of the liver as the abdomen is closed. Failure to adhere to this principle led to lethal complications in our initial experiences with LRT. The other key element affecting the perfusion of the liver is the use of temporary prosthetic closure of the abdomen to create space if the liver is too big.[39] The freshly transplanted liver is exquisitely sensitive to abdominal compartment syndrome. Outflow problems when using the right lobe of the liver can be prevented by careful attention to the geometry of the partial graft and the creation of a generous anastomosis of the right hepatic vein to the recipient vena cava.

Finally, reconstruction of the biliary tree has posed exceptional challenges for the implantation of the graft from the living donor.[13,40,41] Many lessons were learned during the development and expansion of LRT for children, ultimately requiring renewed understanding of the intrahepatic anatomy of the left bile duct.[42] The more recent reports of right lobe LRT for adults suggest that the same efforts will be required for the perfection of techniques used with adult donation. Initial reports of right lobe donation suggest a biliary complication rate exceeding 50%, although this rate rapidly falls with increased experience with the technique.[13] At the minimum, transplantation of a segmental liver graft always requires hepaticojejunostomy for reconstruction of the biliary system.

Successful reconstruction requires detailed understanding of the intrahepatic biliary anatomy and careful preparation of the bile ducts during donor hepatectomy. The branching of the biliary tree occurs in three dimensions, with complex relationships between the territorial ducts and the vessels supplying these territories. Transplantation of a whole liver is akin to the insertion of a black box, in which the intrahepatic anatomy is of no significance. In contrast, for LRT, the biliary reconstruction requires anatomic precision, meticulous technique, and the creation of very fine anastomoses, ideally under high magnification to minimize technical flaws. Biliary complications in our own series include leaks from the cut surface, failure to recognize anatomic variants, technical flaws in the anastomoses, and finally, late strictures either at or above the anastomoses, likely caused by local impairment of the blood supply of the bile ducts.[43]

CURRENT RESULTS OF LIVING-RELATED LIVER TRANSPLANTATION

Pediatrics

LRT is routine in pediatrics and accounts for approximately 50% of children undergoing transplantation in our center. This is obviously an extreme example based on our long-standing interest and confidence in the technique. As expected, the proportion of LRT procedures performed varies from region to region based on the supply of livers and the preferences of the team. Nationally, fewer than 5% of patients have received LRT.[44] As noted earlier, recipient outcomes are comparable with (and may exceed) the results in those receiving standard liver transplants, and patient and graft survival should exceed 90% (Table 7.1). Technical

TABLE 7.1. *Results of living-related liver transplantation in pediatric and adult recipients*

Type	Patient survival (%)	Biliary leaks (%)	Peak bilirubin level (mg/dL)
Left lateral	95	5–10	<5
Left	90	5–10	5–15
Right	80–90	30–50	5–15

Percentages are estimated from personal experience and reported series.

TABLE 7.2. *Results of living-related liver transplantation for donors*

Type	Mortality (%)	OR time (h)	Hospital stay (d)	Reoperation rate (%)	Peak bilirubin level (mg/dL)
Left lateral	0.2	3–4.5	3–6	<1	2.5
Left	0.2	4–6	4–7	<1	2.5
Right	1.0	4.5–100	5–10	1–5	5–8

Percentages are estimated from personal experience and reported series.

complications differ somewhat; in general, biliary problems are more common after LRT, whereas nonfunction of a graft from a living donor is exceedingly rare.

The left lateral lobe donor operation has been refined substantially over the last decade, and in our center is accomplished with minimal blood loss in approximately 3 hours. The gall bladder is spared and there is a minimum of dissection of the structures supplying the right lobe (the donor's liver). Tanaka has poetically described the thick left liver often found in males as a "globefish" lobe, whereas other patients have a long thin left lobe akin to a "flatfish" (K. Tanaka, personal communication, 1998). Naturally, the time required to cut through the liver and the amount of blood loss seem to be related to the morphology and size of the lobe (unpublished data).

Because the extent of liver required for transplantation in an infant is modest (usually 15% to 20% of the liver), the effect on hepatic function of the donor is minimal, and donors generally leave the hospital after 3 to 5 days (Table 7.2). The need for reoperation is approximately 1%, although percutaneous treatment of biliary complications is slightly more frequent. A report of one donor death (from a pulmonary embolus) has been published,[45] and one other death has been described, for a total donor mortality of 2 in approximately 1,000 cases worldwide, a risk comparable with renal donation. Because the liver is able to regenerate, no long-term risk to the donor is anticipated; however, because the longest follow-up period has been 10 years as of this writing, this expectation has not yet been verified.

Adults

The earliest efforts to use LRT in adults were generally unsuccessful.[24] We had initially hoped to use the same hepatectomy as for pediatric cases, but it became apparent that grafts of this size were unable to provide satisfactory liver function in the adult recipient. Using more extensive resections and transplanting either the entire right or left lobe, several recent reports suggest that adult recipients of LRT have an outcome comparable with that of recipients of standard transplants (Table 7.1).[9,12,13,46] We recognize that this observation must be tempered to take into account the inevitable patient selection that occurs, which must influence results. Recipients of right lobes seem to have satisfactory liver function but appear to have a risk of biliary problems

substantially higher than that expected with standard OLT. Marcos' results indicate that the risk of biliary problems decreases with experience.[13]

Donors of the right lobe undergo a very significant reduction in hepatic parenchyma. The reduction in mass is even greater than that occurring in right hepatectomy for cancer, because in the latter case much of the volume of the resected lobe is tumor tissue, and the left lobe of the liver, which is left behind, has already regenerated.[47] In fact, in planning hepatic resection for cancer, the size of the remnant liver is considered prior to offering the procedure. Thus, right lobar donation for adult LRT is an unprecedented extent of hepatectomy in liver surgery. Operative time is much longer than for pediatric donation, up to 10 to 12 hours in Marcos' initial series.[13] Postoperatively, the patients are extremely fatigued and are at risk for narcotic overdose in the early postoperative period. Transient elevations of parameters of synthetic function, such as prothrombin time and bilirubin level, attest to the impact of these resections on hepatic function (Table 7.2; unpublished observations). Although little data are available, it is reasonable to suppose that, to some extent, the probability of complications will be related to the extent of resection.

SELECTION OF RECIPIENTS

We have had a long-standing interest in the structure of the donor evaluation, which has undergone substantial modifications over time. The tendency in pediatric LRT has been to simplify the donor evaluation as confidence with the procedure has increased and the operative risk decreased. Lest the source of the donor confuse the strategy, we insist that the first step in the evaluation of a potential transplant patient be the comprehensive assessment of the recipient. The indications for liver transplantation are well outlined elsewhere in this volume and, in our view, should not be modified in patients receiving LRT. Although families may be willing to donate in hopeless cases, we regard the safety of the donor to be a resource as precious as the scarce cadaveric liver: neither should be squandered.

In the first phase of the evaluation, the transplant team seeks to confirm the diagnosis of the prospective candidate's liver disease and determine the timing of transplantation. In fact, the principal benefit of LRT is the elective planning of transplantation, which is an enormous advantage that has been lost in cadaveric transplantation in the face of the scarcity of donor livers. LRT liberates the transplant from being confined to the sickest patients, a necessary triage that governs liver allocation for cadaveric recipients. LRT can be used to address quality-of-life indications such as non-life-threatening disability and can be adapted to the needs of the family, including such considerations as insurance and work-related disability, and even school holidays. In children with biliary atresia, it has long been accepted that the optimal time for transplantation is when growth failure occurs, but prior to frank hepatic decompensation or the development of complications of portal hypertension.[48] This optimal practice is only possible with LRT, because a baby who enters the waiting list for a cadaveric liver can face many months of decline prior to receiving a liver offer.

The use of LRT in fulminant hepatic failure has been accepted in pediatric practice.[49] The rapidly progressive nature of this disease, leading to brain edema within hours to days of admission, makes it uncertain whether a cadaveric donor will be located in time. Recent modifications in the allocation of cadaveric livers in North America have improved the chances of locating a donor in the time frame of this disease. In patients who are admitted in stage 3 or 4 hepatic coma, who may progress to herniation within 24 to 48 hours, we have compressed the donor evaluation to an overnight process and proceed with the transplantation within 24 to 36 hours of admission. We recognize the inherently coercive nature of the situation and offer the family the option of waiting for a cadaver donor, ultimately making a collaborative decision with the family to proceed with LRT if it seems unsafe to wait. The problem with this schedule is that families have difficulty truly accepting the enormity of the situation. In our experience, the donors tolerate the failure of a transplantation done in an urgent situation poorly from a psychological viewpoint, perhaps because there was insufficient time to truly embrace the risks and benefits.

The long waiting times faced by patients with primary hepatic malignancy have led to the use of LRT in this group. We know from older data that a high cure rate is possible for patients with hepatocellular carcinoma meeting strict criteria who receive OLT.[50,51] Unfortunately, patients with hepatocellular carcinoma who have stable liver function may wait several years on the waiting list, decreasing the probability of cure.[52] In addition, there are technical considerations to LRT in cancer patients. Ideally, the resection in the recipient must be radical to optimize the chance of a cure by resecting all the vessels and nodes of the portal hepatis. In children who have received LRT for hepatoblastoma, we have liberally used prosthetic vascular grafts to replace the vena cava, and saphenous vein to replace the portal vein and hepatic artery. It is not known whether the technical compromises necessary for LRT in cancer patients will result in the same cure rates that are achieved with cadaveric donors.

Because of the greater complexity of LRT in adults, and the fact that the graft will always be smaller than the ideal liver for the recipient, it has been recommended that LRT not be used in patients with advanced decompensation of chronic liver disease (currently listed as status 2A in the UNOS scheme).[13] Even standard OLT is more difficult in such patients; the operation is often prolonged, with increased blood loss, impaired renal and pulmonary function, and a decreased overall probability of a good outcome. In general, LRT should be done electively in ideal recipients to ensure optimal outcomes for both donors and recipients.

SELECTION OF DONORS

Based on our experience with pediatric OLT, we described a donor evaluation process that proceeds in phases and is coordinated with the evaluation of the recipient.[53] The process is summarized in Table 7.3 and represents an approach that changed little until the introduction of adult LRT, which has mandated a more rigorous anatomic evaluation of the donor than was necessary for pediatric donation. We have sought to simplify the evaluation. Three principal changes in our strategy include the acceptance of unrelated donors, early completion of serologic testing and blood typing to save time and stress for the family, and modification in the morphologic imaging of the donor.

In phase I, as the family is educated about the nature of the liver disease and the need for liver transplantation, the possibility of living donation is introduced systematically as part of the informational materials about transplantation.

TABLE 7.3. *Living donor evaluation criteria*

Phase I
Age: 18–60
Initial screening
    Emotionally related to recipient
    ABO compatible
    Negative serology for hepatitis viruses and HIV
Phase II
Psychosocial support
    Adequate psychosocial support systems as determined by transplant team, psychiatry, and social services
    Absence of coercion or financial benefit
Medical evaluation
    Comprehensive history and physical examination
    Exclusion of prospective donors with acute or chronic illness affecting operative risk
Laboratory evaluation
    Normal findings from hematologic, serum chemistry, and liver and kidney function tests
    Normal ECG and chest radiograph
    Negative serology for hepatitis viruses and HIV
Phase III
Graft assessment
    Volumetric MR scan excludes occult mass lesions, documents adequate liver volume, and defines hepatic vascular anatomy
    Graft represents ≥50% of expected recipient liver mass
    Arteriography (used selectively) documents arterial supply for the anticipated graft

ECG, electrocardiogram; HIV, human immunodeficiency virus; MR, magnetic resonance.

The goal of telling every family about LRT, particularly in the context of anonymous informational materials, is to allow them a chance to consider the possibility in a non-threatening way rather than to feel obligated to donate to please the transplant team. Although imperfect, this is an example of a measure to mitigate the detrimental effects of coercion. In our center, a formal curriculum is presented to candidates and their families that addresses, among other topics, the listing and selection process and the function of UNOS and the allocation of livers. All patients need to be placed on the cadaveric list even if a potential donor is available, so that the patient does not lose waiting time if subsequent events preclude use of the living donor. Furthermore, the outcomes of patients need to be tracked by the organ procurement and distribution system to properly document national transplant activities even if a donor is not obtained from the cadaveric waiting list.

It is often possible to exclude potential donors with very little investigation in phase I. It seems that the requirement for genetic relatedness is no longer mandatory because of the improved results of immunosuppression for nonrelated transplants; there is widespread acceptance of the appropriateness of emotionally related donors, most dramatically donation between spouses. Based on the initial encounter, if the donor is obviously healthy and desires to proceed, blood typing and serologic testing for human immunodeficiency virus (HIV) and hepatitis viruses are carried out promptly to decrease the time of uncertainty about whether LRT is possible. This initial phase identifies the majority of potential contraindications to donation; in fact, in our previous report, 98% of seemingly healthy donors were found to be suitable on subsequent detailed medical evaluation.[53]

In phase II, a comprehensive medical and psychosocial evaluation is conducted. The comprehensive psychosocial assessment by the transplant social worker and psychiatrist seeks to evaluate the donor and recipient as individuals as well as in the context of their relationship. We consider that this process serves both an educational and diagnostic function, familiarizing the family with the steps involved in the procedure and, once again, helping the family decide whether living donation is appropriate. We also seek to identify external social constraints that may place undue stress on either the donor or the recipient, or their dependents, who may be involuntary participants in the risks assumed by the donor. Such constraints may include a limited ability of the family to care for two patients, or significant financial hardship if the primary breadwinner becomes the donor. I am most concerned about the effects of donation on the children of the donor, particularly if the recipient is not a member of the immediate family. It is the responsibility of the transplant team to help the potential donor recognize and accept contraindications to donation. Next, a comprehensive medical assessment is conducted by a physician whose primary responsibility is the safety of the donor. In selecting the physician who will conduct the donor evaluation, the need for objectivity in this assessment must be balanced by the need for adequate experience with the medical issues surrounding transplantation, which will affect both donor and recipient.

The investigations of phase III concern the direct anatomic evaluation of the liver and the potential graft and are not perfomed until the candidacy of the donor has been fully established. Our approach has undergone some evolution since earlier descriptions of the process. For pediatric cases, we have decreased our reliance on volumetric scanning for determination of appropriate graft size. Because most infants with liver disease have enlarged livers, there is almost always room to accommodate the graft, even if it comes from very large donors. If needed, enlargement of the recipient abdominal cavity with a prosthetic closure can overcome even very great size disparities. In our current practice, we have adopted magnetic resonance imaging with vascular and biliary enhancement as the principal modality for the evaluation of the donor liver. This gives an ideal combination of arterial and venous anatomy for planning the procedure. If further information about the arteries is required, we selectively use arteriography. Although visualization of a nondilated biliary tree remains difficult with noninvasive imaging, we remain convinced that the benefits of preoperative cholangiography do not outweigh the risks of the procedure to the healthy living donor.

Volumetric imaging seems to offer some benefit for the assessment of the graft needed for the recipient.[54,55] If the recipient is a small child, the graft is limited to the left lateral lobe, whereas for adults either the full right or left lobe may be selected. The use of the left lobe graft for adult recipients has been championed by Miller et al.[46] and is an appealing alternative because the operation seems safer than the right lobe donation and has been used in larger children since the earliest days of LRT. The primary constraint is the size of the recipient, because the full left lobe is only about 40% of the total liver parenchyma. We currently use the left lobe if the donor is larger than the recipient (typically if a man is donating to a woman), whereas right lobe donation is necessary if the recipient is the same size or larger than the donor.

ROLE OF LIVING-RELATED TRANSPLANTATION

We are living in a paradoxical time in which the success of liver transplantation has created a crisis in the supply of a limited resource. Public debate about the allocation of cadaveric livers and the introduction of LRT has occurred in society at large, and the activities of our profession are under scrutiny as never before. As we promote living donation for our patients, we have a great responsibility to protect the safety of all participants and, most of all, to resist the natural tendency to pressure potential donors who are ambivalent.

An algorithm for the sequential strategy for the use of LRT is presented schematically in Fig. 7.2. In our center, we consider LRT for all potential recipients of liver transplantation,

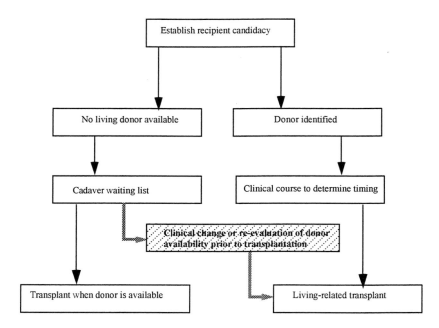

FIG. 7.2. Preoperative selection and candidacy.

children as well as adults. With this policy, approximately 50% of children and 25% of adults in our center have undergone transplantation using LRT in the past 2 years (unpublished data). Although it is clear that LRT can pose great hardship to the family, the worsening of the organ shortage forces us to face this risk. Elective LRT as an alternative to the progressive deterioration of the patient on the waiting list has sufficient merit to justify expanding its use on a scale comparable with that of renal donation. This statement is predicated on the assumption that the transplant team has adequate experience to perform LRT with acceptable risks and benefit.

In conclusion, we have demonstrated that LRT must meet three major ethical requirements: a convincing need for the innovation, an acceptable risk and benefit to the participants, and a satisfactory process for ensuring optimal informed consent and protecting the safety of the donor. The risk assessment is predicated on the ability of centers to offer adequate expertise in LRT, which requires a major committment and preparation on the part of the transplant team. As we witness the proliferation of right lobe donation, we run the risk of creating great harm if transplant surgeons do not approach LRT with the appropriate balance of humility and expertise.

REFERENCES

1. Tanaka K, Uemoto S, Tokunaga Y, et al. Surgical techniques and innovations in living related liver transplantation. *Ann Surg* 1993;217:82–91.
2. Broelsch CE, Whitington PF, Emond JC, et al. Liver transplantation in children from living related donors: surgical techniques and results. *Ann Surg* 1991;214:428–439.
3. Wadstrom J, Rogiers X, Malago M, et al. Experience from the first 30 living related liver transplants in Hamburg. *Transplant Proc* 1995; 27:1173.
4. Smith B. Segmental liver transplantation from a living donor. *J Pediatr Surg* 1969;4:126–132.
5. Bismuth H, Houssin C. Reduced size orthotopic liver graft in hepatic transplantation in children. *Surgery* 1984;95:367–370.
6. Emond JC, Whitington PF, Thistlethwaite JR, et al. Transplantation of two patients with one liver: analysis of preliminary experience with "split liver" grafting. *Ann Surg* 1990;212:14–22.
7. Strong RW, Lynch SV. Ethical issues in living related donor liver transplantation. *Transplant Proc* 1996;28:2366–2369.
8. Emond JC, Heffron TG, Kortz EO, et al. Improved results of living related liver transplantation (LRT) with routine application in a pediatric program. *Transplantation* 1993;55:835–840.
9. Fan ST, Lo CM, Liu CL. Technical refinement in adult-to-adult living donor liver transplantation using right lobe graft. *Ann Surg* 2000;231:126–131.
10. Hashikura Y, Makuuchi M, Kawasaki S, et al. Successful living-related partial liver transplantation to an adult patient [Letter]. *Lancet* 1994;343:1233.
11. Uryuhara K, Egawa H, Uemoto S, et al. Application of living related auxiliary partial liver transplantation in an adult recipient with biliary atresia. *J Am Coll Surg* 1998;187:562–564.
12. Wachs ME, Bak TE, Karrer FM, et al. Adult living donor liver transplantation using a right hepatic lobe. *Transplantation* 1998;66:1313–1316.
13. Marcos A, Fisher RA, Ham JM, et al. Right lobe living donor liver transplantation. *Transplantation* 1999;68:798–803.
14. Liver donor's death sets transplant specialists abuzz. *The News and Observer* 1999 Oct 3:1A.
15. DOT initiates study of factors influencing living related donors. *Transplant News* 1992;2:6.
16. Bay WH, Herbert LA. The living donor in kidney transplantation. *Ann Intern Med* 1987;106:719–727.
17. Najarian JS, Chavers BM, McHugh LE, et al. 20 years or more of follow-up of living kidney donors. *Lancet* 1992;340:807–810.
18. Singer PA, Siegler M, Lantos J, et al. Ethics of liver transplantation with living donors. *N Engl Med J* 1989;321:620–621.
19. Emond JC, Whitington PF, Thistlethwaite JR, et al. Reduced size liver orthotopic liver transplantation in children: use in the management of children with chronic liver disease. *Hepatology* 1989;10: 867–872.
20. Annual report of the US Scientific Registry of Transplant Recipients and the Organ Procurement and Transplantation Network, 1999. Bethesda, MD: Division of Organ Transplantation, Health Resources and Services Administration, 1999:36.
21. Annual report of the US Scientific Registry of Transplant Recipients and the Organ Procurement and Transplantation Network, 1999. Bethesda,

MD: Division of Organ Transplantation, Health Resources and Services Administration, 1999:216–217.

22. Ozawa K, Uemoto S, Tanaka K, et al. An appraisal of pediatric liver transplantation from living relatives. Initial clinical experiences in 20 pediatric liver transplantations from living relatives as donors. *Ann Surg* 1992;216:547.

23. Emond JC, Nelson RM, Blank EL, et al. Living related liver transplantation: request for an international ethics consultation from the Research Center for Surgery in Moscow. *Cambridge Q Healthcare Ethics* 1994;394:602–603.

24. Emond JC, Renz JF, Ferrell LD, et al. Functional analysis of grafts from living donor. Implication for the treatment of older recipients. *Ann Surg* 1996;224:544–554.

25. Emond JC, Xia RC. Reduced-size liver transplants (RLT) provide evidence of host regulation of hepatic regeneration [Abstract]. *Gastroenterology* 1991;100:A739.

26. Francavilla A, Zheng Q, Polimeno L, et al. Small-for-size liver transplanted into larger recipient: a model of hepatic regeneration. *Hepatology* 1994;19:210–217.

27. Van Thiel DH, Gavaler JS, Kam I, et al. Rapid growth of intact human liver transplanted into a recipient larger than the donor. *Gastroenterology* 1987;93:1414–1419.

28. Kam I, Lynch S, Svanas G, et al. Evidence that host size determines liver size: studies in dogs receiving orthotopic liver transplants. *Hepatology* 1987;7:362–366.

29. Bhagat G, Cataldeghirman G, Lefkwitch J, et al. Proliferation and apoptosis in living related liver allografts: correlation with graft size and rejection activity index. [Abstract] *Hepatology* 1999;30(suppl):303A.

30. Panis Y, McMullan DM, Emond JC. Progressive necrosis after hepatectomy and the pathophysiology of liver failure after major resection. *Surgery* 1997;1121:142–149.

31. Urata K, Kawasaki S, Matsunami H, et al. Calculation of child and adult standard liver volume for liver transplantation. *Hepatology* 1995;21:1317–1321.

32. Broelsch CE, Emond JC, Whitington PF, et al. Application of reduced size liver transplant as split grafts, auxiliary orthotopic grafts, and living related segmental transplants. *Ann Surg* 1990;212:368–375.

33. Couinaud C. *Le foie, etudes anatomiques et chirurgicales*. Paris: Masson, 1957.

34. Kuang AA, Renz JF, Ferrell LD, et al. Failure patterns of cryopreserved vein grafts in liver transplantation. *Transplantation* 1996;62:742–747.

35. Mori K, Nagata I, Yamagata S, et al. The introduction of microvascular surgery to hepatic artery reconstruction in living-donor liver transplantation—its surgical advantages compared with conventional procedures. *Transplantation* 1992;54:263–270.

36. Mazzaferro V, Esquivel CO, Makowka L, et al. Hepatic artery thrombosis after pediatric liver transplantation—a medical or surgical event? *Transplantation* 1989;47:971–977.

37. Then PK, Feldman L, Broelsch CE. Flow and vascular resistance measurements in auxiliary liver segments transplanted in orthotopic position. *Transplant Proc.* 1989 Feb;21(1 Pt 2):2378–2380.

38. Emond JC, Heffron TG, Whitington PF, et al. Reconstruction of the hepatic vein in reduced size hepatic transplantation. *Surg Gynecol Obstet* 1993;76:11–17.

39. Shun A, Thompson JF, Dorney SF, et al. Temporary wound closure with expanded polytetrafluoroethylene in pediatric liver transplantation. *Clin Transplant* 1992;6:315–317.

40. Heffron TG, Emond JC, Whitington PF, et al. Biliary complications in pediatric liver transplantation: comparison of reduced size and whole grafts. *Transplantation* 1992;53:391–395.

41. Egawa H, Uemoto S, Inomata Y, et al. Biliary complications in pediatric living related liver transplantation. *Surgery* 1998;124:901–910.

42. Reichart PR, Renz JF, D'Albuquerque LA, et al. Surgical anatomy of the left lateral segment as applied to living donor and split liver transplantation: a clinico-pathologic study *Ann Surg (in press)*.

43. Reichert PR, Renz JF, Bacchetti P, et al. Biliary complications of reduced-organ liver transplantation. *Liver Transplant Surg* 1998;4:343–349.

44. Annual report of the US Scientific Registry of Transplant Recipients and the Organ Procurement and Transplantation Network, 1999. Bethesda, MD: Division of Organ Transplantation, Health Resources and Services Administration, 1999:91.

45. Rogiers X, Malago M, Nollkemper D, et al. The Hamburg liver transplant program. *Clin Transplant* None listed in index med. 1997:183–190.

46. Miller CM, Emre S, Bem-Haim M, et al. Living transplantation using left lobe grafts from living adult donors in adult recipients: preliminary experience. [Abstract] *Transplantation* 1999:S548.

47. Emond JC, Renz JF. Surgical anatomy of the liver and its application to hepatobiliary surgery and transplantation. *Semin Liver Dis* 1994;14:158–168.

48. Whitington PF, Emond JC, Black DD, et al. Indications for liver transplantation in pediatrics. *Clin Transplant* 1991;5:155–160.

49. Hattori H, Higuchi Y, Tsuji M, et al. Living-related liver transplantation and neurological outcome in children with fulminant hepatic failure. *Transplantation* 1998;65:686–692.

50. Venook AP, Ferrell LD, Roberts JP, et al. Liver transplantation for hepatocellular carcinoma: results with preoperative chemoembolization. *Liver Transplant Surg* 1995;1:242–248.

51. Marsh JW, Dvorchik I, Subotin M, et al. The prediction of risk of recurrence and time to recurrence of hepatocellular carcinoma after orthotopic liver transplantation: a pilot study. *Hepatology* 1997;26:444–450.

52. Bruix J, Llovet JM, Aponte JJ, et al. Radical treatment of hepatocellular carcinoma during the waiting list for orthotopic liver transplantation: a cost-effectiveness analysis on an intention to treat basis. [Abstract] *Hepatology* 1999;30:233A.

53. Renz JF, Mudge CL, Heyman MB, et al. Donor selection limits use of living-related liver transplantation. *Hepatology* 1995;22:1122–1126.

54. Mittal R, Kowal C, Starzl T, et al. Accuracy of computerized tomography in determining hepatic tumor size in patients receiving liver transplantation or resection. *J Clin Oncol* 1984;2:637–642.

55. Lo CM, Fan ST, Liu CL, et al. Minimum graft size for successful living donor liver transplantation. *Transplantation* 1999;68:1112–1116.

Transplantation of the Liver, edited by Willis
C. Maddrey, Eugene R. Schiff, and Michael
F. Sorrell. Lippincott Williams & Wilkins,
Philadelphia © 2001.

CHAPTER 8

Liver and Small Bowel Transplantation

Alan Langnas and Kishore Iyer

Long-term total parenteral nutrition (TPN) has been the mainstay of therapy for patients with intestinal failure caused by the short bowel syndrome and other etiologies. Although TPN has significantly prolonged life in these patients, it is frequently complicated by central venous catheter infections, sepsis, and cholestatic liver disease with eventual cirrhosis. For these selected patients for whom TPN is not a viable option in the long term, intestinal transplantation has emerged as the standard of care. Although intestinal transplantation remains an evolving procedure, improvements in surgical technique, in the potency of immunosuppression, and in prophylactic regimens for infection and lymphoproliferative disease have led to improved results from different centers.

HISTORY

The long saga of the development of clinical intestinal transplantation must be viewed against the background of the enormous courage and fortitude displayed by the patients and their families in attempting to overcome near catastrophe. Alexis Carrel demonstrated the technical feasibility of intestinal transplantation in the early part of the twentieth century.[1] More than half a century later, Richard Lillehei began intestinal transplant studies in dogs while at the University of Minnesota.[2] Over the next 30 years, a succession of clinical trials of intestinal transplantation at different centers met with a singular lack of success.[3–5]

Limited clinical success from an intestinal graft was first achieved in 1987, when Starzl et al. reported survival for 192 days in one of two children who underwent multivisceral transplantation.[6] The child with short gut syndrome and liver failure secondary to TPN underwent excision of her stomach, duodenum, residual small intestine, and colon and received a vascularized composite graft of all the upper abdominal viscera up to the distal small bowel.[6] The immunosuppressive

regimen included cyclosporine, azathioprine, and prednisone. Death occurred from multifocal lymphoproliferative disease, uncontrolled sepsis, and multiorgan system failure. Williams et al. reported a similar course in one of two children, who died from extensive lymphoproliferative disease and sepsis 109 days after a multivisceral transplant.[7] Between 1987 and 1990 the Paris group of Goulet et al. performed nine small-intestinal transplants in seven children using cyclosporine-based immunosuppression.[8] One patient was alive, free of parenteral nutrition, and doing well at home 6 years after transplantation.[8]

In 1988, Grant et al. carried out what was to be the first successful small-bowel and liver transplantation;[9] the 41-year-old patient illustrates some of the problems encountered in this patient population prior to and after transplantation. The patient developed short bowel syndrome following thrombosis of the superior mesenteric artery, necessitating resection of her entire small bowel and colon. TPN was well tolerated, but the patient remained in the hospital for 18 months with intractable diarrhea, abdominal pain, recurrent pulmonary emboli, and repeated thrombosis of venous access sites.[9] She had low levels of antithrombin III, but the results of hematologic and liver function tests were otherwise normal. In the months leading up to the transplantation, central venous access was through a Hickman catheter placed in the superior vena cava at thoracotomy.

During her combined liver and small bowel transplantation, the donor and recipient inferior vena cavae were anastomosed end to end. The donor thoracic aorta was anastomosed to the side of the recipient's infrarenal aorta, and the stump of the donor aorta beyond the superior mesenteric artery was oversewn. The end of the recipient's portal vein was anastomosed to the side of the donor portal vein.[9] The recipient's distal large bowel was oversewn, and proximally the donor jejunum was anastomosed to the recipient duodenum. Immunosuppression was with cyclosporine, prednisone, and azathioprine, with a 2-week course of OKT3 for induction. Donor pretreatment was carried out with OKT3

A. Langnas and K. Iyer: Department of Surgery, University of Nebraska Medical Center, Omaha, Nebraska 68198.

and Minnesota antilymphocyte globulin.[9] Significant postoperative complications included an intraabdominal abscess drained percutaneously; Hickman catheter infection, requiring thoracotomy for removal; respiratory insufficiency necessitating tracheostomy and prolonged mechanical ventilation; phrenic nerve palsy; and disseminated *Candida* infection.[9] Despite the considerable morbidity, the patient was discharged 8 months after transplantation on an unrestricted oral diet, and continued to do well more than 4 years later.[4]

Since these landmark cases, a handful of centers have reported improved results.[10–15] Intestinal transplantation alone or as part of a composite graft with other organs has become the standard of care for the desperate patient with short bowel syndrome and TPN-related complications.

INDICATIONS AND PATIENT CHARACTERISTICS

The role for combined liver and small bowel (LSB) transplantation must be viewed within the context of the patient population in which it is indicated. In considering transplantation for the patient with intestinal failure, the widespread availability of highly effective and relatively safe long-term therapy in the form of TPN has to be clearly understood. Quigley's[16] 1996 observation that for the well-adapted patient who is doing well on home TPN, small intestinal transplantation cannot rival the established role of TPN is still valid. Therefore, intestinal transplantation is restricted at the present time to patients who develop life-threatening complications of TPN, such as advanced liver disease or loss of venous access due to repeated bouts of catheter sepsis and thrombosis.

The majority of candidates for combined LSB transplantation are in the pediatric age group. This is simply because of the preponderance of congenital causes of the short bowel syndrome and the very high incidence of TPN-associated liver disease in children, especially when TPN is started in the neonatal period. Of 51 LSB transplantations performed at the University of Nebraska Medical Center since 1992, there have been only 2 adult recipients (unpublished data). Both these adult patients had short bowel syndrome secondary to extensive resection with TPN-induced liver disease. Of the pediatric patients, 36 were younger than 5 years at the time of transplantation. The main diagnoses in the 51 patients who received liver–small bowel grafts are shown in Table 8.1.

The best results have been with isolated intestinal grafts.[11,12,14] This reflects the overall better health of the recipients at the time of transplantation, the shorter length of stay in intensive care and in the hospital,[17] and the earlier return to enteral feeding.[14] These results have persuaded us to pursue a more aggressive approach toward isolated intestinal transplants in patients with intestinal failure even in the presence of early TPN-induced liver disease. At the present time we do not view elevations in serum bilirubin or transaminase levels, or even mild degrees of fibrosis on liver biopsy, as contraindications to isolated intestinal transplantation. Our early experience with isolated intestinal transplants in 11 patients[18] is encouraging and differs from the experience of the Pittsburgh group.[19] The best guide for selecting which patients should be listed for combined LSB transplantation is based on establishing the diagnosis of end-stage liver disease.

RECIPIENT EVALUATION AND SELECTION

Evaluation of patients with intestinal failure for transplantation requires a multidisciplinary team of physicians (including pediatricians, gastroenterologists/hepatologists, transplant surgeons, and radiologists), dietitians, specialized nurses, social workers, and psychologists. The evaluation process is frequently complicated by ongoing problems with sepsis, coagulopathy, vascular access difficulties, and worsening liver failure. The goals of evaluation are listed in Table 8.2.

To this end, patients undergo a detailed history and physical examination with particular attention to nutritional history and episodes of catheter and other sepsis. Hematologic tests and biochemical tests of liver function are the same as those required for liver transplantation. Contrast studies of the small and large bowel are of particular value in developing an estimate of the enteral capabilities of potential candidates and are helpful in guiding the choice of allograft.

Supplementary information may be obtained by endoscopy, particularly if there is suspicion of portal hypertension and varices. A liver biopsy is essential to determine the

TABLE 8.1. *Causes of intestinal failure in recipients of liver–small bowel transplants at the University of Nebraska Medical Center*

Diagnosis	Number (N = 51)[a]
Midgut volvulus (malrotation)	13
Gastroschisis	12
Necrotizing enterocolitis	5
Pseudoobstruction	4
Atresias	4
Hirschsprung's disease	2
Other (massive resections, microvillus inclusion disease, intractable diarrheas of infancy, etc.)	11

[a]Includes 5 patients who received a combined liver, bowel, and pancreas transplant.

TABLE 8.2. *Goals of pretransplantation evaluation in intestinal failure*

Current status of venous access
Length of residual intestine
Functional status of intestine
Nutritional status of patient
Degree of liver dysfunction
Pertinent psychosocial issues
Overall appropriateness of intestinal transplantation
Type of allograft required (i.e., isolated or composite)

degree of liver damage; as indicated earlier, we do not consider early biopsy changes of TPN-induced cholestasis to be a contraindication for isolated intestinal transplantation. A baseline echocardiogram should be part of the evaluation in view of the association of hypertrophic cardiomyopathy with steroid and tacrolimus immunosuppression.[20]

The nutritional evaluation includes anthropometry, assessment of vitamin and mineral status, historical tolerance of enteral feedings, and reassessment of caloric requirements.

DONOR OPERATION

The donor operation is depicted in Fig. 8.1. Cadaveric donors should be less than 50% to 60% of recipient weight, ABO blood group compatible,[21] and hemodynamically stable. Larger donors can be used for the recipient who still has the majority or all of his or her native intestine intact (e.g., with pseudoobstruction) because the preservation of the peritoneal cavity and the availability of adequate room allow for the graft swelling that invariably follows reperfusion.

The principles and techniques of retrieval of the intestinal graft with or without the liver and other viscera have evolved over the last decade. The classic technique has been extensively described.[9,22–24] The complete multivisceral allograft specimen is conceptualized as a grape cluster with a double central stem consisting of the celiac axis and superior mesenteric artery (SMA).[24] The individual organs,

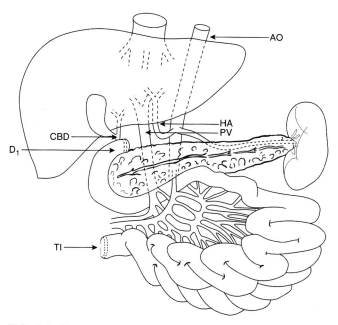

FIG. 8.1. Donor operation. Note that the liver, small bowel, pancreas, and spleen are procured en bloc. There is no hilar dissection, and the celiac trunk and superior mesenteric artery are included on a long segment of aorta. AO, thoracic aorta; HA, hepatic artery; PV, portal vein; CBD, common bile duct; D₁, first part of duodenum, stapled; TI, terminal ileum, stapled.

like grapes on a vine, can be removed or retained according to the surgical objectives, but both arterial structures are preserved except when only the intestine is to be transplanted. The venous outflow from the grape cluster is entirely toward the liver, and is kept intact up to or beyond the liver as required.[24] The bile duct is divided and the distal portion removed along with the donor duodenum and pancreas during back-table preparation to avoid any risk of donor pancreatitis or pancreatic duct fistula.[9]

Three technical problems were identified with the classic technique early in our experience at the University of Nebraska Medical Center:

1. Difficult back-table preparation, especially in infant donors. The major concerns were injury to the celiac trunk or SMA and the thin-walled portal vein during the extensive hilar dissection including pancreatoduodenectomy.
2. Bile leaks following biliary anastomosis between a Roux-en-Y loop of donor jejunum and liver allograft bile duct.
3. Torsion on the portal vein axis with venous congestion and risk of graft ischemia.

The new technique developed at the University of Nebraska Medical Center avoids hilar dissection, making graft preparation easier while virtually eliminating the risk of biliary complications and venous congestion or ischemia of the graft. The procedure for procurement of the liver–small bowel allograft has been previously reported[25] and is depicted in Fig. 8.1.

In brief, the hilar structures are left undisturbed. The stomach and colon are excluded from all grafts. Intravenous antithymocyte globulin (ATGAM, Upjohn, Kalamazoo, MI) and OKT3 (Ortho, Raritan, NJ) are administered to the donor immediately prior to commencement of the cold flush. Cold University of Wisconsin solution is administered through an infrarenal aortic cannula. An additional cannula is placed in the inferior mesenteric vein to assist with portal flushing, when size permits. The venous outflow is vented in the usual manner by transecting the cava above the diaphragm. The duodenum just beyond the pylorus and the distal ileum immediately proximal to the ileocecal valve are transected between double rows of staples. The inferior vena cava is divided at the level of the diaphragm and just cephalad to the renal veins. A long segment of thoracic aorta is procured in continuity with the celiac axis and the SMA. The distal aorta is divided a few millimeters below the SMA, leaving enough aortic length to be oversewn without compromising the flow into the SMA. The donor liver and the pancreas with attached spleen and intestines (stapled at both ends) are removed en bloc and placed in cold University of Wisconsin solution. No attempt is made at luminal decontamination of the donor. There is a frequent need for vascular conduits; to meet all exigencies, the donor team must retrieve good lengths of iliac artery and vein, and additional vessels in special cases.

On the back table, the celiac axis is dissected to the level of the splenic artery, which is ligated and divided. The SMA

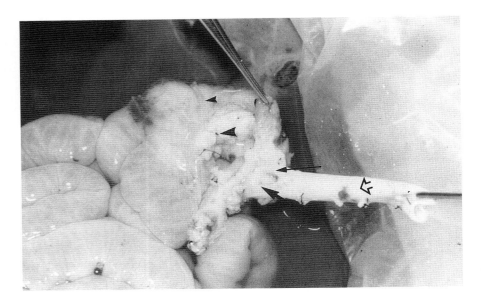

FIG. 8.2. Back-table preparation. The thoracic aorta is indicated by an open arrow, the celiac trunk by a thin arrow, and the superior mesenteric artery by a thick arrow. The larger arrowhead identifies the pancreas; the smaller arrowhead indicates the duodenum.

is dissected at its origin from the aorta up to the first jejunal branch, and the donor aorta inferior to the origin of the SMA is oversewn. The splenic vein is identified and dissected to its confluence with the superior mesenteric vein and portal vein. The pancreas is divided just to the right of the portal vein in order to leave a small remnant of pancreas and thereby preserve the continuity of the donor bile duct. The pancreatic duct is identified and ligated at the cut edge, and the pancreatic parenchyma is oversewn (Fig. 8.2).

RECIPIENT OPERATION

The recipient operation is depicted in Fig. 8.3. After removal of the native liver, the extent of remaining native gastrointestinal structures is delineated. Stomas are taken down, and any anastomosis between distal small bowel and colon is taken down and divided between double rows of staples. The suprahepatic and infrahepatic inferior vena caval anastomoses are performed end to end as in a standard liver transplantation. We prefer a supraceliac aortic anastomosis for the arterial inflow to the combined graft; further, we use a segment of donor thoracic aorta as an interposition graft (AO[I] in Fig. 8.3) to facilitate the supraceliac aortic anastomosis, without having the entire liver-bowel graft in the way. The aortic segment bearing the celiac trunk and SMA attached to the composite graft is then easily anastomosed to the free end of the conduit high up in the wound (AO[II] in Fig. 8.3). After completion of these anastomoses, clamps are released and the graft is revascularized.

To decompress the residual splanchnic viscera (native stomach, spleen, and pancreas), an end-to-side anastomosis between the native and donor portal veins is performed, as has been previously described.[7,24] An extension graft of donor iliac vein is interposed if required to avoid excessive tension. An alternative approach is to perform a native portacaval shunt to decompress the residual native viscera. Bowel continuity is established at the level of the remaining native bowel and proximal donor jejunum. An ileocolonic anastomosis is performed distally, and a diverting loop ileostomy is fashioned from the donor ileum approximately 10 cm proximal to the ileocolonic anastomosis to provide access for biopsies.

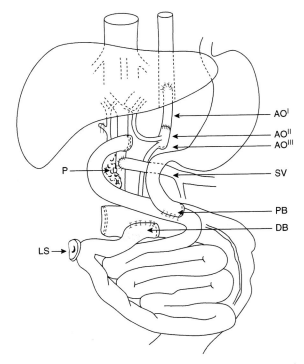

FIG. 8.3. Recipient operation. AO[I], interposition graft of aorta; AO[II], Carrel patch bearing celiac trunk and superior mesenteric artery; AO[III], aortic end oversewn, below superior mesenteric artery takeoff; SV, native splenic vein; P, pancreas, with duct and parenchymal edge oversewn; PB, proximal bowel anastomosis; DB, distal ileocolonic anastomosis; LS, diverting loop ileostomy.

POSTOPERATIVE MANAGEMENT

The high incidence of technical and infectious complications punctuated by numerous episodes of rejection following LSB transplantation[14,17,26–29] dictates meticulous attention to detail in the postoperative care of these sick patients. Infectious complications are common in the postoperative period. Bowel perforations, intestinal abscesses, and recurrent bouts of sepsis continue to be major postoperative problems. The patients are very susceptible to enteric viruses, enteritis caused by cytomegalovirus (CMV), and bacterial and fungal infections. Mortality is preeminently the result of infectious complications.[14]

Immunosuppression

At the current time, most, if not all, centers involved in intestinal transplantation use immunosuppression based on tacrolimus (FK506, Prograf) and steroids. The Pittsburgh group favors intravenous FK506, started intraoperatively at a dose of 0.15 mg/kg per day and converted to an oral dose when patients can tolerate oral intake.[17] The tacrolimus dose is adjusted to a target trough level of 15 to 30 ng/mL. Steroids (methylprednisolone) are started at a dose of 20 mg/kg and rapidly tapered over the next 5 to 7 days to a dose of 2 mg/kg per day. The patient is maintained on an oral prednisone dose of 0.3 mg/kg per day. The Pittsburgh group has also employed induction therapy with cyclophosphamide and subsequently switched to either mycophenolate mofetil or azathioprine.[17] We do not use any antilymphocyte induction therapy, and we administer tacrolimus intragastrically from the outset. With the introduction of IL-2 blocking agents, there may be a role for their use as part of initial immunosuppression, although the benefits of such an approach in intestinal transplantation remain to be documented.

Prostaglandin E_1 is started early at a dose of 0.02 to 0.03 μg/kg per minute and gradually increased up to a maximum dose of 0.09 μg/kg per minute through the first week. It is used both for its beneficial effects on fresh vascular anastomoses and for its prevention of microvascular thromboses, the damage-mediating event in acute cellular rejection and procurement injury.[17]

Rejection episodes are treated with intravenous bolus methylprednisolone at a dose of 10 mg/kg per day, and tacrolimus doses are increased by 20%. If patients fail to respond, they are treated with a further course of steroids or with an antilymphocyte preparation.

Diagnosis of Rejection

Diagnosing rejection accurately and in a timely fashion remains a problem even today. Despite numerous animal studies, a reliable marker for the diagnosis of rejection remains an elusive goal. Intestinal permeability, measured by chromium 51 ethylenediaminetetraacetic acid, may be one such marker.[9]

In recipients of liver–small bowel transplants, it is our practice to carry out protocol surveillance liver and intestinal biopsies at day 7, biweekly intestinal biopsies thereafter for 6 weeks and then as indicated. Indications for biopsies include unexplained fever, change in stoma output or appearance, gastrointestinal bleeding, and skin rash.[30]

Attempts to clarify the role of endoscopy in small intestinal transplantation[30,31] suggest that the gross appearance of the mucosa does not correlate with the histologic findings. Although there is a clear lack of endoscopic criteria for diagnosis of rejection, endoscopy with biopsy remains the gold standard for diagnosis of rejection in intestinal allografts.[30,32] The histopathologic changes of acute cellular rejection have been well described by Lee et al.[32,33] Rejection can be patchy in distribution, though it tends to be more pronounced at the ileal end. Acute rejection of an intestinal allograft is characterized by a varying combination of crypt injury, mononuclear mucosal infiltrate, and an increase in crypt cell apoptosis.[32]

Apoptosis is a morphologically distinct, gene-directed form of programmed cell death that contributes to both physiologic and pathologic processes.[32] The biological significance of apoptosis in intestinal rejection is not exactly clear. Apoptosis of gastrointestinal epithelium can be found occasionally in normal mucosa and in several other conditions, such as graft versus host disease, CMV infection, cytotoxic drug therapy or radiotherapy, idiopathic inflammatory bowel disease, drug-induced colitis, and immunodeficiency states.[32] Using a crude semiquantitative technique, increased apoptotic bodies were noted in 59% of acute rejection specimens but in only 8% of all other allograft specimens.[32] Thus, crypt cell apoptosis, although not a specific or absolute finding, is a distinctive feature of acute cellular rejection even when other changes are minimal.[33]

Chronic allograft rejection appears to be a very rare phenomenon and is hence less well understood. Obliterative arteriopathy was noted in 2 allografts resected at day 668 and 239 after transplantation from a total of 23 allografts;[32] no chronic changes were seen in 3,015 mucosal biopsy specimens in 62 recipients.[32] Mucosal biopsies from the 2 affected patients preceding graft removal showed a combination of nonspecific inflammation and acute rejection or a distinctive combination of reparative changes with apoptosis.[32]

Prevention of Infection

Our group does not practice intestinal decontamination of donor or recipient; however, Reyes et al. have reported allograft decontamination with polymyxin, tobramycin, and amphotericin B via the nasogastric tube for 2 weeks postoperatively, with quantitative stool cultures to assess overgrowth of resistant bacteria.[17] Broad-spectrum intravenous antibiotics are administered for 5 to 7 days; specific therapy is tailored to the infections that the patient may have had pretransplantation. In view of the concerns regarding lymphoproliferative disease driven by Epstein-Barr virus, all transplant recipients receive monthly intravenous immunoglobulin infusions and are treated prophylactically with acyclovir for the first postoperative year.[14] Prophylaxis against *Pneumocystis carinii* is employed using trimethoprim-sulfamethoxazole twice weekly. Antifungal therapy is used prophylactically.

Nutritional Management

Nutritional management of intestinal transplant recipients has been recently reviewed by Strohm et al.[34] TPN was initiated postoperatively in all patients. Caloric goals were based on patient status, taking into account such factors as endotracheal intubation, postsurgical complications, fever, rejection, and renal function.[34] Elemental jejunostomy feeds (commenced, on average, at 15 days) were advanced to peptide-based formula with medium chain triglyceride oil and subsequently to intact protein with fiber; a gradual transition was made in enteral feedings from continuous 24-hour infusion to cycled night-time feedings based on improvements in oral intake and absorption.[34]

Stoma losses of 40 to 50 mL/kg per day are deemed acceptable. Stool losses are often high in fluid and sodium content; thus these patients require very careful attention to intravenous replacement of ongoing losses. Most of these patients are very susceptible to osmotic diarrhea, and secretory diarrhea develops frequently in the presence of intercurrent infection or rejection.[14] Judicious use of antidiarrheal drugs such as loperamide hydrochloride (Imodium) may aid in slowing intestinal transit in selected patients. Pancreatic insufficiency or chylous ascites has not been a serious issue in the Omaha experience, but when it occurs it appears to respond to pancreatic enzyme supplements and conservative measures with full TPN and gradual reintroduction of elemental feeds.[34]

RESULTS

Intestinal transplantation remains a procedure in evolution. The gut's massive lymphocyte content and heavy bacterial load have provided formidable barriers to successful clinical transplantation for more than a quarter of a century.[11] Over the last 5 years, improved results have been reported from a few centers with improved surgical techniques, more potent immunosuppression, and standard prophylaxis for infections and lymphoproliferative disease.[10,14,15,17,35]

The 1997 report of the International Registry for Intestinal Transplantation provides useful information.[11] Since 1985, a total of 273 intestinal transplantations were performed in 260 patients by 33 transplant programs.[11] The types of transplants were as follows: only intestine in 113 patients (41%), intestine plus liver in 130 patients (48%), and multivisceral grafts that included the stomach, pancreas, intestine, and liver in 30 patients (11%). Nine grafts were obtained from living donors.

Patient and Graft Survival

The 1-year patient and graft survival rates continue to improve. The 1-year graft and patient survival figures since 1995 are 55% and 69%, respectively, for intestine alone; 63% and 66%, respectively, for small bowel–liver grafts; and 63% in both cases for multivisceral grafts.[11] Despite the apparent immunologic advantage conferred by simultaneous liver grafting with a small-bowel allograft, isolated intestinal allografts provided better patient survival and graft function at all follow-up times.[17] The preliminary experience from Omaha was similar, with reduced hospital and intensive care unit (ICU) stays for the recipients of isolated intestinal grafts compared with recipients of liver–small bowel grafts and a more rapid return to enteral feeding;[14] these observations have been sustained with accumulating experience.

As expected in such a complex undertaking, programs that had performed at least ten transplantations had better graft and patient survival rates than programs that had performed less than ten transplantations.[11] Patient survival was also better in cases of isolated intestinal transplantations. Of the nine patients receiving a graft from a living donor, six patients were alive, five with a functioning graft.[11] A total of 131 (50%) of the 260 recipients of intestinal transplants performed since 1985 have died.[11] Causes of death are listed in Table 8.3.

Retransplantation

The results of retransplantation have been disappointing, particularly for liver–small bowel recipients. Though experience is limited, all three liver–small bowel recipients who underwent retransplantation at Pittsburgh on the same day as primary graft removal died within 60 days of systemic bacterial infection, rejection, and lymphoproliferative disease, respectively.[17] Of the three patients, one received a liver-only retransplant following hepatic artery thrombosis, one patient received another LSB graft, and the third received a multivisceral retransplant. Our experience at the University of Nebraska has been similarly discouraging.

Nutritional Status

The nutritional status following transplantation is a major determinant of the quality of life in recipients of intestinal grafts. Of 126 patients who were alive, 95 (77%) were weaned from total parenteral nutrition, 17 (14%) required partial parenteral

TABLE 8.3. *Cause of death in 131 intestinal transplant recipients*

Cause of death	Number (Percentage) (n = 131 of 260 recipients)
Sepsis	59 (47%)
Multiorgan system failure	33 (26%)
Graft thrombosis	12 (10%)
Graft rejection	5 (4%)
Posttransplantation lymphoma	12 (10%)
Other causes	5 (4%)

[b]From registry data.

nutrition, 4 (3%) were receiving TPN with their graft intact, and 8 (6%) were receiving TPN after removal of their graft; this information was unavailable in 2 patients.[11] The median time to weaning from TPN in the Pittsburgh experience was 41 days (range 14 to 210).[17] Vitamins and trace elements, particularly zinc and selenium, frequently required supplementation. Weight decreased posttransplantation with loss of ascites and when TPN was discontinued.[34] Linear growth appears to be maintained, but was stunted by increased steroid doses for rejection episodes.[34]

COMPLICATIONS

Rejection

The incidence of acute graft rejection at 1 year remains high: 79% for intestine transplant alone, 71% for liver and intestine, and 56% for multivisceral transplants.[11] Immunosuppression was based on tacrolimus in 78%, cyclosporine in 19%, and other or no drugs in the remainder.[11]

Registry data for intestinal allograft rejection are in agreement with other observations that simultaneous liver grafting may reduce the risk of intestinal graft rejection.[9,36] However, as pointed out earlier, this immunologic advantage did not translate into better graft function or patient survival, with isolated intestinal grafts performing better at all follow-up times.[17] Reyes et al. reported the incidence of intestinal allograft rejection in the first 30 days after transplantation to be 88% for small-bowel grafts, 66% for liver–small bowel grafts, and 75% for multivisceral grafts.[17] This result was not affected by bone marrow augmentation. The need for OKT3 for the treatment of severe rejection was more common in recipients of small-bowel grafts (76%) versus recipients of liver–small bowel grafts (21%) or multivisceral (50%) grafts.

Infection

As discussed previously, infectious complications are frequent and include bacterial, fungal, and viral infections. Viral infections have been principally caused by cytomegalovirus and Epstein-Barr virus (EBV).

In the registry data summarized by Grant et al.,[11] the incidence of CMV disease was 24% for intestinal grafts, 18% for liver-intestinal grafts, and 40% for multivisceral grafts. In intestinal graft recipients, the median time to initial CMV infection was 54 days (range 21 to 274 days).[27,37] The intestinal graft itself is the commonest site of CMV infection. The risk factors for CMV infections in these patients include transplantation from CMV-seropositive donors to seronegative recipients, increased tacrolimus levels, and increased number of steroid boluses to treat rejection episodes.[27,37]

Post Transplantation Lympho Proliferative Disease

Registry figures for the incidence of posttransplantation lymphoproliferative disease (PTLD) are 7% for intestinal grafts, 11% for liver–small bowel grafts and 13% for multi-

visceral grafts.[11] Reyes et al. reported a much higher incidence, with PTLD occurring in 16 (29%) of 55 children.[17] Persistent intractable disease was seen in 7 patients, with death occurring in all of them.[17] The intestinal allograft was involved in 14 patients; in 3 patients, PTLD was discovered at routine endoscopy. Significant risk factors were noted to be the number of rejection episodes, the use of OKT3, splenectomy, and age.[17]

Use of a low-dose chemotherapy regimen may suffice to control resistant, disseminated PTLD without excessive side effects,[38] although rebound rejection is a significant contributor to morbidity and even mortality.[28,38] Initial data suggest that use of quantitative polymerase chain reaction (PCR) to detect elevations of EBV genome in peripheral blood lymphocytes may be predictive of progression to PTLD in some intestinal transplantation patients.[39] Even with early detection of EBV infection by quantitative PCR, the exact role for preemptive therapy with ganciclovir and high-titer CMV immune globulin (Cytogam) remains to be defined.

Graft versus Host Disease

The Pittsburgh group reported a 7% incidence of graft versus host disease,[17] an anticipated complication in view of the large lymphocyte mass in the allograft. Diagnosis is based on histopathologic criteria, which includes keratinocyte necrosis in biopsies of skin lesions, epithelial apoptosis of native gastrointestinal tract, or epithelial cell necrosis of oral mucosa.[17] Donor cell infiltration into the lesions, demonstrated immunohistochemically, is confirmatory.

Surgical Complications

Surgical complications, occurring in about 50% of recipients, are major contributors to morbidity and mortality. The most frequent of these are intraabdominal infections, which are usually consequent to other technical events such as anastomotic leaks and intestinal perforations precipitated by endoscopic biopsies.

QUALITY OF LIFE

Long-term parenteral nutrition is a safe, readily available, and highly effective therapy for the patient with short bowel syndrome and permits a reasonable quality of life for patients and their families.[40,41] The overall survival rate for patients receiving home parenteral nutrition is approximately 85% at 3 years.[42] The length of survival is related to the underlying diagnosis and indication for TPN. Because most adults and children do relatively well on home parenteral nutrition, the risks of intestinal transplantation are currently warranted only when standard therapies have failed. Thus, the current use of intestinal transplantation as salvage therapy for the selected group of patients who are doing badly on TPN or have life-threatening complications invalidates any comparison between the two modalities of treatment.

Even in this selected group of patients, overall cumulative patient survival is 72% at 1 year and 48% at 5 years, with graft survival of 64% and 40%, respectively.[43] The survival benefits are better in children than in adults, in whom the cumulative survival rate at 5 years is 68%.[43] In the Pittsburgh series, 51 (93%) of 55 current survivors are home, fully active, and completely weaned from TPN with full nutritional autonomy. Attempts to study quality of life in intestinal transplantation patients suggest a quality very similar to patients receiving long-term home TPN.[44] Interestingly, the quality of life in intestinal transplant recipients appears to improve over time as anxiety over functioning of the allograft decreases. These is an area that merits further long-term studies with larger sample sizes.

The average yearly cost of intestinal transplantation has significantly decreased in the last 4 years to an average of $132,285 for an isolated intestine, $214,716 for liver and intestine, and $219,098 for the multivisceral procedure.[43] The average yearly cost of TPN in 1992 was more than $150,000 per patient, excluding the cost of medical equipment and nursing care.[45] Based on these data, intestinal transplantation becomes cost effective by the second year after transplantation.

CURRENT CHALLENGES AND FUTURE PROSPECTS

Intestinal transplantation is an evolving procedure whose development has been seriously hindered by the twin specters of repeated severe rejection and life-threatening sepsis. At the present time the need for aggressive immunosuppression has to be fulfilled by relatively nonspecific agents. Although the development of tacrolimus has been a major advance, maintenance of adequate levels of this agent to control rejection of the intestinal allograft is associated with an unacceptably high incidence of sepsis and PTLD. Newer immunosuppressive agents with more specific cellular actions are urgently required.

In intestinal transplantation, the loss of mucosal integrity, such as that which occurs during severe rejection, leads to cytokine-mediated damage to the gut. Pharmacologic attempts to control cytokine release may be of value in protecting the graft from immune damage. This may also be critical in preventing bacterial translocation and systemic sepsis in the face of severe rejection.

The role of living-related transplantation needs further clarification. Although the procedure is clearly technically feasible and has been successful in some cases,[11,46,47] outcomes have to improve considerably before the procedure can be generally applied. Of even greater interest is the possibility of reduced-size and split orthotopic composite liver-intestinal allografts as described by Reyes et al.[48] The two initial recipients had poor graft outcomes, with death occurring for one recipient and a successful retransplantation for the other. Nevertheless, the technical feasibility of this procedure suggests a way to reduce the 50% to 60% mortality of children below 10 kg awaiting appropriate-sized liver–small bowel donors.

Isolated liver transplantation in infants with TPN-associated liver disease has been considered as an option in selected cases, but the fear of recurrent TPN-associated liver disease affecting the transplanted liver has inhibited enthusiasm for isolated liver transplantation. In Omaha, we have pursued an aggressive approach to the problem, and our preliminary experience is encouraging.[49] Six infants with short bowel syndrome and end-stage liver disease who were all TPN dependent but had a history of significant enteral tolerance underwent isolated liver transplantation. Four of the five surviving children are independent of parenteral feedings, and the fifth is receiving about 60% of food enterally. Of three additional children who underwent similar transplantations since that report, two are independent of TPN. The third developed recurrent cholestatic liver disease while receiving TPN, which was resolved by conservative measures; the child is now on full enteral intake. Clearly, isolated liver transplants can offer a long-term solution to end-stage TPN-associated liver disease in selected children with short bowel syndrome. Recurrent TPN-induced liver disease affecting the graft remains a possibility, and the care of these children requires a multidisciplinary team with experience in the management of intestinal failure.

REFERENCES

1. Carrel A. The transplantation of organs. A preliminary communication. *JAMA* 1905;45:1654.
2. Lillehei R, Goott B, Miller F. The physiologic response of the small bowel of the dog to ischemia including prolonged *in vitro* preservation of the bowel with successful replacement and survival. *Ann Surg* 1959;150:543–560.
3. Lillehei R, Idezuki Y, Feemster J, et al. Transplantation of stomach, intestine and pancreas: experimental and clinical observations. *Surgery* 1967;62:721–741.
4. McAlister V, Grant D. Clinical small bowel transplantation. In: Grant D, Wood R, eds. *Small bowel transplantation.* Boston: Edward Arnold, 1994:121–132.
5. Okumura M, Mester M. The coming of age of small bowel transplantation: a historical perspective. *Transplant Proc* 1992;24:1241–1242.
6. Starzl T, Rowe M, Todo S, et al. Transplantation of multiple abdominal viscera. *JAMA* 1989;261:1449–1457.
7. Williams J, Sankary H, Foster P, et al. Splanchnic transplantation—an approach to the infant dependent on parenteral nutrition who develops irreversible liver disease. *JAMA* 1989;261:1458–1462.
8. Goulet O, Jan D, Sarnacki S, et al. Isolated and combined liver-small bowel transplantation in Paris: 1987–1995. *Transplant Proc* 1996;28:2750.
9. Grant D, Wall W, Mimeault R, et al. Successful small-bowel/liver transplantation. *Lancet* 1990;335:181–184.
10. Abu-Elmagd K, Reyes J, Todo S, et al. Clinical intestinal transplantation: new perspectives and immunologic considerations. *J Am Coll Surg* 1998;186:512–527.
11. Grant D. Intestinal transplantation: 1997 report of the international registry. *Transplantation* 1999;67:1061–1064.
12. Reyes J, Todo S, Bueno J, et al. Intestinal transplantation in children: five year experience. *Transplant Proc* 1996;28:2755–2756.
13. Tzakis A, Webb M, Nery J, et al. Experience with intestinal transplantation at the University of Miami. *Transplant Proc* 1996;28:2748–2749.
14. Langnas A, Shaw B, Antonson D, et al. Preliminary experience with intestinal transplantation in infants and children. *Pediatrics* 1996;87:443–448.

15. Lacaille F, Jobert-Giraud A, Colomb V, et al. Preliminary experience with combined liver and small bowel transplantation in children. *Transplant Proc* 1998;30:2526–2527.
16. Quigley EMM. Small intestinal transplantation: reflections on an evolving approach to intestinal failure. *Gastroenterology* 1996;110: 2009–2011.
17. Reyes J, Bueno J, Kocoshis S, et al. Current status of intestinal transplantation in children. *J Pediatr Surg* 1998;33:243–254.
18. Sudan, D., Kaufman S, Shaw B, et al. Isolated intestinal transplantation for intestinal failure. *Am J Gastroenterol (in press)*.
19. Bueno J, Ohwada S, Kocoshis S, et al. Factors impacting the survival of children with intestinal failure referred for intestinal transplantation. *J Pediatr Surg* 1999;34:27–33.
20. Dhawan A, Mack D, Langnas A, et al. Immunosuppressive drugs and hypertrophic cardiomyopathy. *Lancet* 1995;345:1644–1645.
21. Sindhi R, Landmark J, Shaw B Jr, et al. Combined liver/small bowel transplantation using a blood group compatible but nonidentical donor. *Transplantation* 1996;61:1782–1783.
22. Todo S, Tzakis A, Abu-Elmagd K, et al. Intestinal transplantation in composite visceral grafts or alone. *Ann Surg* 1992;216:223–234.
23. Casavilla A, Selby R, Abu-Elmagd K, et al. Logistics and technique for combined hepatic-intestinal retrieval. *Ann Surg* 1992;216: 605–609.
24. Starzl T, Todo S, Tzakis A, et al. The many faces of multivisceral transplantation. *Surg Gynecol Obstet* 1991;172:335–344.
25. Sindhi R, Fox I, Heffron T, et al. Procurement and preparation of human isolated small intestinal grafts for transplantation. *Transplantation* 1995;60:771–773.
26. Tzakis A, Todo S, Reyes J, et al. Clinical intestinal transplantation: focus on complications. *Transplant Proc* 1992;24:1238–1240.
27. Foster P, Sankary H, McChesney L, et al. Cytomegalovirus infection in the composite liver/intestinal/pancreas allograft. *Transplant Proc* 1996;28:2742–2743.
28. Reyes J, Green M, Bueno J, et al. Epstein Barr virus associated post-transplant lymphoproliferative disease after intestinal transplantation. *Transplant Proc* 1996;28:2768–2769.
29. Reyes J, Abu-Elmagd K, Tzakis A, et al. Infectious complications after human small bowel transplantation. *Transplant Proc* 1992;24: 1249–1250.
30. Garau P, Orenstein S, Neigut D, et al. Role of endoscopy following small intestinal transplantation in children. *Transplant Proc* 1994; 26:136–137.
31. Tabasco-Minguillan J, Hutson W, Weber K, et al. Endoscopic features of acute cellular rejection. *Transplant Proc* 1996;28:2765–2766.
32. Lee R, Nakamura K, Tsamandas A, et al. Pathology of human intestinal transplantation. *Gastroenterology* 1996;110:1820–1834.
33. Lee R, Tsamandas A, Abu-Elmagd K, et al. Histologic spectrum of acute cellular rejection in human intestinal allografts. *Transplant Proc* 1996;28:2767.
34. Strohm SL, Koehler AN, Mazariegos GV, et al. Nutrition management in pediatric small bowel transplant. *Nutr Clin Pract* 1999; 14:58–63.
35. Goulet O, Michel J, Jobert A, et al. Small bowel transplantation alone or with the liver in children: changes by using FK 506. *Transplant Proc* 1998;30:1569–1570.
36. Calne R, Sells R, Pena J, et al. Induction of immunological tolerance by porcine liver allografts. *Nature* 1969;223:472–476.
37. Manez R, Kusne S, Green M, et al. Incidence and risk factors associated with the development of cytomegalovirus disease after intestinal transplantation. *Transplantation* 1995;59:1010–1014.
38. Gross T, Hinrichs S, Winner J, et al. Treatment of post-transplant lymphoproliferative disease (PTLD) following solid organ transplantation with low-dose chemotherapy. *Ann Oncol* 1998;9:339–340.
39. Green M, Reyes J, Jabbour N, et al. Use of quantitative PCR to predict onset of Epstein-Barr viral infection and post-transplant lymphoproliferative disease after intestinal transplantation in children. *Transplant Proc* 1996;28:2759–2760.
40. Stokes MA, Irving MH. Mortality in patients on home parenteral nutrition. *JPEN J Parenter Enteral Nutr* 1987;13:172–175.
41. Hall RCW, Beresford TP. Psychiatric factors in the management of long term hyperalimentation patients. *Psych Med* 1987;5:211–217.
42. Howard L, Malone M. Current status of home parenteral nutrition in the United States. *Transplant Proc* 1996;28:2691.
43. Abu-Elmagd KM, Reyes J, Fung J, et al. Evolution of clinical intestinal transplantation: improved outcome and cost effectiveness. *Transplant Proc* 1999;31:582–584.
44. Rovera G, DiMartini A, Schoen R, et al. Quality of life of patients after intestinal transplantation. *Transplantation* 1998;66:1141–1145.
45. Howard L, Ament M, Fleming CR, et al. Current use and clinical outcome of home parenteral and enteral nutrition therapies in the United States. *Gastroenterology* 1995;109:355–365.
46. Deltz E, Schroeder P, Gundlach M, et al. Successful clinical small bowel transplantation. *Transplant Proc* 1990;22:2501.
47. Pollard S, Lodge P, Selvakumar S, et al. Living related small bowel transplantation: the first United Kingdom case. *Transplant Proc* 1996; 28:2733.
48. Reyes J, Fishbein T, Bueno J, et al. Reduced-size orthotopic composite liver-intestinal allograft. *Transplantation* 1998;66:489–492.
49. Horslen S, Kaufman S, Sudan D, et al. Isolated liver transplantation in infants with TPN-associated end-stage liver disease. Presented at the annual meeting of the American Society of Transplant Surgeons, Chicago, May 1999.

Transplantation of the Liver, edited by Willis C.
Maddrey, Eugene R. Schiff, and Michael F.
Sorrell. Lippincott Williams & Wilkins,
Philadelphia © 2001.

CHAPTER 9

Auxiliary Liver Transplantation

Nigel D. Heaton and Mohamed Rela

The human liver is remarkable in many respects, not least in its ability to regenerate completely, even after severe acute liver failure. There is, however, a group of patients with acute liver failure who are unlikely to survive long enough for the injured liver to regenerate.[1] Orthotopic liver transplantation (OLT) has proved to be the most effective way of rapidly restoring liver function in these patients; however, this approach has some potential disadvantages. These include the risks of long-term immunosuppression, particularly nephropathy, malignancy, and graft failure. Finally, with the loss of the native liver there is no potential for liver regeneration. These facts have led to a reevaluation of a role for auxiliary liver transplantation (ALT).

The concept of ALT for acute liver failure is to transplant sufficient liver mass to support the patient for long enough to allow the native liver to recover. The first reported ALT was performed in dogs in 1955.[2] The extra liver was placed in a heterotopic position in the right paravertebral gutter, with portal venous inflow coming from the recipient iliac vein. The idea of heterotopic ALT was initially attractive because it avoided the need for native hepatectomy and an anhepatic phase, thus allowing for improved hemodynamic stability during transplantation. The first experience of auxiliary liver grafting in a patient was reported in 1965.[3] The early cases were performed in patients with chronic liver disease, and although a small number of successful transplantations were recorded,[4,5] the majority of patients died in the early postoperative period from graft failure, bleeding, and sepsis. In a review, Blankensteijn et al. reported survival of only 2 of 47 patients who underwent heterotopic auxiliary liver transplantations between 1964 and 1980.[6] The technique proved more difficult than that of OLT, technical complications were more common, and early graft function was less satisfactory. Finally, the development of hepatocellular carcinoma in the cirrhotic liver remnant of

one of the few long-term survivors[5] showed that hepatocellular carcinoma was a significant potential complication. Subsequent technical developments in OLT led to a loss of interest in the ALT technique.

More recently, interest has revived in ALT as a potential treatment for two groups of patients: those with reversible acute liver failure and those with noncirrhotic liver-based inborn errors of metabolism.[7–10] Examples of noncirrhotic inborn errors of metabolism that may be suitable for auxiliary transplantation include urea cycle defects, disorders of fatty acid metabolism, and Crigler-Najjar syndrome type 1.[11]

The use of auxiliary transplantation for chronic liver disease and the development of experimental models have enabled the key steps of the operation to be determined.[8] There is still some debate regarding the use of heterotopic versus orthotopic liver transplantation; however, the latter technique has gained favor in recent years. For successful ALT a number of problems need to be overcome. The lack of space available for the graft may result in compression of major venous vessels into and out of the graft. By resecting part of the native liver it is possible to create sufficient space for an appropriately shaped segmental graft, which will avoid the problems of graft and vessel compression. Using the orthotopic approach it is possible to place an appropriate reduced-size graft in this space and anastomose the graft venous outflow (left or right hepatic vein or suprahepatic inferior vena cava) to the native inferior vena cava as close to the right atrium as possible. This reduces the possibility of venous outflow hindrance by keeping the hepatic venous pressure low and avoiding a significant pressure gradient developing across the graft.[12] The pressure gradient between the liver sinusoids and the hepatic veins is approximately 2 mm Hg; in the upright position, the pressure in the inferior vena cava increases for every centimeter below the right atrium by 0.77 mm Hg. Thus a heterotopic graft below the liver will have a significantly higher pressure at the point of venous outflow when the patient is in the upright position.

N. D. Heaton and M. Rela: Institute of Liver Studies, King's
College Hospital, London SE5 9RS, United Kingdom.

The portal venous blood flow is maintained by an end-to-side anastomosis of the donor portal vein to the recipient portal vein. For ALT in acute liver failure, the native liver invariably has a higher resistance to venous inflow than the graft; this helps to divert blood to ensure that there is adequate portal venous inflow to the graft (Fig. 9.1). The situation is different in ALT for inborn errors of metabolism. In these cases the resistance to portal venous inflow in the native liver is less than that in the graft, and a ligature is usually required to narrow the recipient portal vein distal to the anastomosis with the graft portal vein to ensure that the graft receives a satisfactory portal blood supply. Graft atrophy has been noted when portal venous inflow has been unsatisfactory. Marchioro et al. concluded that graft atrophy occurred because of a lack of hepatotrophic growth factors rather than insufficient portal venous inflow.[13] In a series of experiments in the dog, Bengoechea-Gonzalez et al. showed that by ensuring satisfactory venous inflow to the graft by use of constricting tapes, it was possible to improve short-term survival and avoid sinusoidal venous congestion and necrosis.[14] However, the absolute need for portal venous inflow has not been established, at least in the dog.[15] Arterial integrity is essential for graft survival and long-term function and can be restored by constructing a suprarenal or infrarenal aortic conduit utilizing donor iliac artery (Fig. 9.2).

Anecdotal reports of successful ALT revived interest in this approach to patients with acute liver failure.[6,16] Currently there are no clear guidelines as to the type of graft that

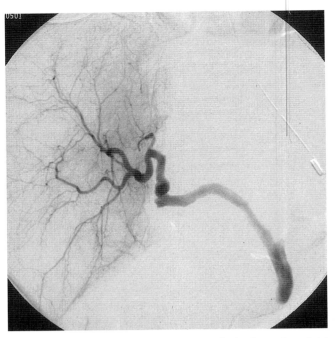

FIG. 9.2. Angiogram showing revascularization of a right auxiliary graft using the infrarenal donor iliac artery.

should be implanted. The auxiliary transplants have usually been based on segmental liver grafts and have included whole, right lobe, left lobe, or left lateral segments. Rough guidelines concerning the selection of a graft to be used depend on the quality of the donor liver, the size discrepancy between the donor and recipient livers, the severity of liver failure (degree of toxic liver syndrome), and the likelihood of recovery of the native liver. The selection of appropriate patients for this procedure remains a major difficulty.

At present, selection criteria for performing transplantation for acute liver failure identify patients with a predicted mortality of greater than 90% without transplantation.[1] The window available for transplantation in these patients before death from cerebral edema or sepsis is short, and a liver may not become available for transplantation. Patients with acute liver failure can be differentiated by their clinical course into two groups: those with hyperacute liver failure and those with subacute liver failure. Hyperacute liver failure (e.g., caused by acetaminophen toxicity) has a rapid onset and progression of liver failure. It is associated with a severe toxic liver syndrome with hemodynamic instability, cerebral edema, severe coagulopathy, and renal failure. However, if these patients should recover, regeneration occurs rapidly with restoration of the normal liver architecture. In contrast, subacute liver failure is associated with a more indolent course, with severe jaundice and moderate coagulopathy and usually with preservation of renal function. Even though these patients show evidence of regenerative nodules at the time of presentation (Fig. 9.3), the recovery and full regeneration of the liver is slow and the

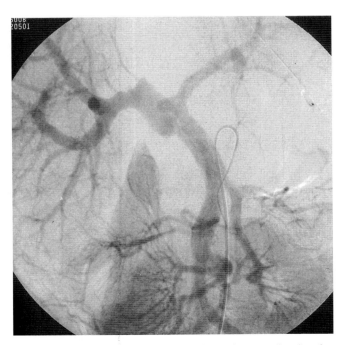

FIG. 9.1. Indirect portography to show the portal vein of a right auxiliary graft anastamosed close to the origin of the right branch of the recipient portal vein.

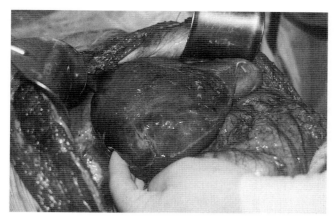

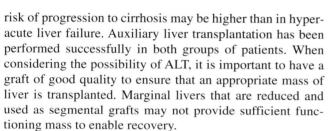

FIG. 9.3. Operative photograph of liver with regenerative nodules in a patient with subacute liver failure secondary to seronegative hepatitis.

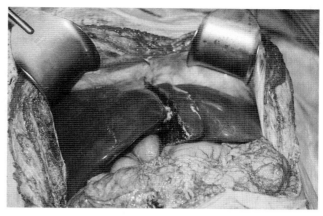

FIG. 9.4. Operative photograph of right auxiliary liver transplant for acute liver failure secondary to acetaminophen toxicity.

risk of progression to cirrhosis may be higher than in hyperacute liver failure. Auxiliary liver transplantation has been performed successfully in both groups of patients. When considering the possibility of ALT, it is important to have a graft of good quality to ensure that an appropriate mass of liver is transplanted. Marginal livers that are reduced and used as segmental grafts may not provide sufficient functioning mass to enable recovery.

Auxiliary liver transplantation is technically more demanding than whole-liver replacement, and careful consideration needs to be given to the condition of the recipient at the time of transplantation. Patients with severe intraoperative hemodynamic instability and raised intracranial pressure may not tolerate prolonged surgery, and whole-liver replacement may therefore be more appropriate. When considering patients with hyperacute liver failure, one must realize that ALT has some disadvantages compared with whole-liver replacement. These patients have severe toxic liver syndrome caused by liver necrosis and may be temporarily improved by total hepatectomy alone.[17] Therefore there is a need to resect the majority of the native liver in these patients to reduce the bulk of necrotic liver. If a significant volume of necrotic liver is left *in situ,* the patient may continue to experience cerebral edema and hemodynamic instability. In our experience an extended right hepatectomy should be performed to minimize the effects of toxic liver syndrome. Extended right hepatectomy has the additional advantage of creating space for a right lobe graft with a larger liver mass to be transplanted to ensure good early graft function (Fig. 9.4).

Small-for-size grafts should not be used in these circumstances because there is evidence from small-for-size living-donated grafts[18] to suggest that the graft-to-recipient-weight ratio should be greater than 1%. If a smaller graft is implanted, the risk of graft dysfunction and patient death from septic complications rises significantly. Patients with these grafts have prolonged cholestasis and gastrointestinal

hemorrhage with persistence of portal hypertension. In assessing small-for-size grafts, it is not enough to simply weigh the liver to determine graft volume. One must consider that marginal or fatty grafts may not have a functioning liver mass corresponding to their weight. We have observed this clinical scenario in adults given auxiliary grafts for acetaminophen-induced acute liver failure who received appropriately sized grafts that functioned suboptimally.[19] In these cases the surgeon should only use good-quality grafts to ensure that the graft size corresponds to its functional capacity. Marginal grafts are better transplanted as whole livers.

Patients with subacute liver failure usually show evidence of regeneration at the time of transplantation. Paradoxically, the selection of these patients is more difficult because some of them may not regenerate the liver, and the remnant of liver may progress to cirrhosis. In these patients, age older than 40 years and the presence of fibrosis on liver biopsy at the time of transplantation are associated with failure to regenerate. Fibrosis may also be observed in acute presentations of autoimmune hepatitis. From our experience of two such patients, whose livers failed to regenerate, we believe that these cases should not be considered for ALT. Conversely, children are more likely to experience liver regeneration regardless of the etiology of their liver disease.[20] Patients with subacute liver failure seldom have a severe toxic liver syndrome and it may be possible to leave a larger mass of native liver behind for regeneration. In addition, their clinical condition tends to be more stable; as a group, they will tolerate prolonged surgery. These patients therefore can be considered for either right or left lobe grafts. Even though the patient's recovery after a right lobe graft may be more rapid, liver regeneration occurs slowly and may be impaired by a large functioning graft. In these patients a smaller graft, such as a left lobe, to encourage liver regeneration may be more appropriate provided there is sufficient liver mass to avoid small-for-size syndrome.

There are further considerations for ALT in children. The possibility of obtaining a size-matched graft for children with acute liver failure is rare. A right auxiliary partial orthotopic liver transplantation (APOLT) can seldom be performed in children because of size discrepancy; however, the left lateral segment of an adult liver may provide sufficient liver mass to perform a successful ALT. All the smaller children in our pediatric series of 12 auxiliary transplants have received left lateral segment grafts.

SURGICAL TECHNIQUES

A number of different surgical techniques for ALT have been described (Figs. 9.5 and 9.6). These can be differentiated into heterotopic and orthotopic methods. Currently the majority of centers are performing orthotopic auxiliary transplantation because of the difficulties of creating sufficient space for the graft. After early experiences we would favor the orthotopic rather than heterotopic technique for ALT. It is possible to transplant a small whole liver in the space created by right hepatectomy. The most commonly used techniques, however, are right, left, or left lateral segment APOLT. Once the decision to perform APOLT has been made and the type of graft to be used is determined, the back-table reduction or split can be started. If the auxiliary graft is part of a split, the main vessels should preferably be retained with the auxiliary graft to ensure that surgical reconstruction is easier.

Left Auxiliary Partial Orthotopic Liver Transplantation

A left hepatectomy is performed for left APOLT (Fig. 9.5). The caudate lobe must be completely excised to adequately expose the retrohepatic inferior vena cava. This provides easy access to the vena cava for the suprahepatic caval anastomosis. We would recommend retaining the donor inferior vena cava with the graft for this procedure. The left hepatic artery is ligated and divided. It is important to confine the hilar dissection to the left side of the porta hepatis to expose the left branch of the portal vein. The donor portal vein is anastomosed in an end-to-end fashion to the left branch or in an end-to-side fashion to the main trunk of the recipient portal vein. The arterial revascularization is achieved using donor iliac artery conduit from the suprarenal or infrarenal aorta. The bile duct is drained by a Roux-en-Y hepaticojejunostomy. For left lateral segment auxiliary transplants, a cuff of left hepatic vein is anastomosed end to side to the recipient cava; otherwise, the operative technique is the same as for a left lobe graft.

Right Auxiliary Partial Orthotopic Liver Transplantation

In a right APOLT (Fig. 9.6), a recipient right hepatectomy is performed; the hilar dissection is confined to the right side, with minimal dissection of the bile duct. The right hepatic artery is ligated to the right of the common bile duct, and the right branch of the portal vein is exposed. The right side of the liver needs to be mobilized from the inferior vena cava sufficiently to expose the right hepatic vein and a satisfactory cuff of cava for subsequent anastomosis. The suprahepatic vena cava of the right lobe (or the right hepatic vein) is implanted using a piggyback technique to an extended right hepatic vein orifice as close to the diaphragm as possible. The donor portal vein is anastomosed in an end-to-end fashion to the right branch or in an end-to-side fashion to the main trunk of the recipient portal vein. The arterial revascu-

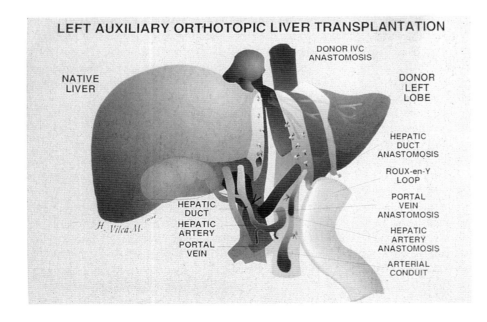

FIG. 9.5. Schematic representation of a left lobe auxiliary graft for acute liver failure. There is no ligature on the portal vein.

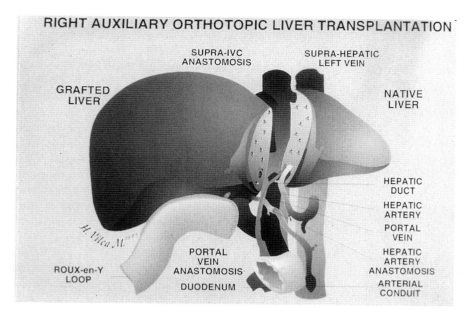

FIG. 9.6. Schematic representation of a right lobe auxiliary liver transplant for acute liver failure.

larization is achieved using donor iliac artery conduit from the suprarenal or infrarenal aorta. The bile duct is drained by a Roux-en-Y hepaticojejunostomy. We have not found it necessary to use a ligature to narrow the portal venous inflow to the native liver.

POSTOPERATIVE RESULTS

Auxiliary liver transplantation appears to have a higher risk of primary nonfunction and of vascular complications, particularly portal vein thrombosis, than orthotopic liver transplantation.[21] There is no doubt that the former operation is technically more demanding, and one would expect a higher incidence of technical complications. However, we believe that many of the previously observed poorly functioning grafts and vascular complications may have been the result of small-for-size grafts. This may offer an explanation for the persistent cholestasis and residual portal hypertension that is seen in some of these patients and that may predispose them to infection. These patients are also prone to infective complications because of the acute liver failure and the presence of two cut liver surfaces with a higher incidence of collections and bile leaks. It is not surprising, therefore, that the incidence of relaparotomy is higher to drain these collections or to manage cut surface bleeding. Secondary hemorrhage occurs more commonly because of associated renal failure and the continuing postoperative need for renal replacement therapy. The use of heparin and other anticoagulants should be considered carefully in this group of patients.

The postoperative recovery of liver function may differ from that observed after whole-liver transplantation. The coagulopathy may correct more slowly, particularly if the graft volume is small. The serum transaminase levels may not fall in the normal way because of a contribution from the native liver. This may pose problems in the diagnosis of early rejection. Protocol biopsies at 1 week are useful, but there is a risk of bleeding in patients with persistent coagulopathy or renal failure. Serial Doppler ultrasound is invaluable in assessing graft vasculature, particularly the portal venous inflow. One may observe reversal of flow within the segment of portal vein to the graft in severe rejection, with preferential flow to the native liver.

Computed tomographic (CT) or magnetic resonance (MR) imaging with guided biopsies of the graft and native livers in the early postoperative period provides a useful baseline to assess future regeneration (Fig. 9.7). Aortography may be indicated in severe graft dysfunction to exclude a technical complication, but otherwise has little role to play in the follow-up of these patients. We have found dimethyl iminodiacetic acid (HIDA) scintigraphy to be of value in assessing the differential function of the two livers and in following the recovery of the native liver (Fig. 9.8). Accurate assessment of native liver regeneration can only be made with a combination of investigations including serial CT volumetry, HIDA scintigraphy, and guided biopsies of the graft and native liver.[22] Currently we perform these investigations at 3, 6, and 12 months posttransplantation, and the decision to reduce immunosuppression is usually made after the investigations at 6 months.

Success in APOLT is defined as the long-term survival of the patient, with complete withdrawal of immunosuppression and recovery of native liver function. The majority of patients who survive long term can be withdrawn from their immunosuppressive therapy. However, this must be performed gradually; otherwise, an episode of severe acute rejection may be precipitated and may lead to premature graft loss before sufficient regeneration has occurred. The timing of immunosuppression reduction will depend on the rapidity of liver regeneration, which in turn is dependent on

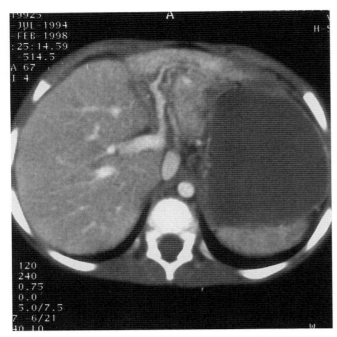

FIG. 9.7. Computed tomographic scan following right lobe auxiliary transplant for acute liver failure in a child. The native left lateral segment has not regenerated at this time.

the etiology of liver failure and the volume and function of graft transplanted. Patients with hyperacute liver failure will regenerate more rapidly. However, the larger volume of graft transplanted in this group (right lobe) will tend to inhibit native liver regeneration. Early immunosuppression reduction may encourage native liver regeneration, but this reduction needs to be done slowly and to be monitored carefully to control rejection. In the subacute group the regeneration is very slow, as observed by sequential imaging.

As a consequence, reduction and withdrawal of immunosuppression tends to be much later compared with the hyperacute group.

Immunosuppression withdrawal is associated with vascular complications, particularly in large grafts. Graft atrophy is usual with controlled immunosuppression withdrawal, and there is seldom a need to excise these grafts. However, if withdrawal is associated with vascular thrombosis resulting in graft necrosis or abscess formation, surgical excision may speed recovery (Fig. 9.9). Experience with immunosuppression withdrawal is limited; however, the collected European experience found that 65% of patients surviving more than 1 year with a successful ALT were free of immunosuppression.[21] In this series the overall 1-year patient survival rate of 62% in ALT was similar to that for OLT (61%).

Recurrence of the original disease may be a potential complication following ALT. Experience of ALT for acute hepatitis B has shown that there is clearance of hepatitis B surface antigen with the development of protective antibodies, as occurs after OLT, despite leaving behind part of the native liver. Our experience of two such cases has confirmed these case reports. These patients have been managed with a combination of lamivudine and hepatitis B immune globulin in the early postoperative period. There are no reports of disease recurrence, even though one patient received no prophylaxis.[23,24] Recurrent seronegative hepatitis has been described after OLT. Even though it is a potential risk, it has not been described thus far after ALT. Aplastic anemia may occur in up to one-third of children presenting with acute liver failure due to seronegative hepatitis. This represents a potential contraindication to ALT[25] because of susceptibility to infective complications. However, in our series of 12 children with acute liver failure, there are 10 long-term survivors, one of whom has successfully recovered from aplastic anemia.

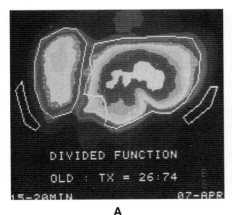
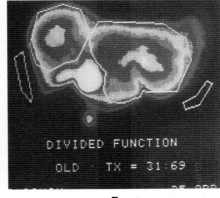
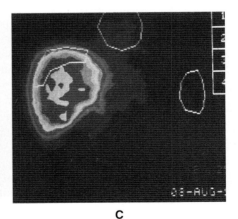

FIG. 9.8. A: A dimethyl iminodiacetic acid (HIDA) scintigraphy scan showing left lobe auxiliary liver graft at 2 months after transplantation. The native liver is contributing 26% of overall function. **B:** HIDA scan in same patient at 6 months after transplantation; the native liver is contributing 31% of overall function. **C:** HIDA scan in same patient at 1 year showing full regeneration of the native right liver. The left lobe auxiliary graft has atrophied.

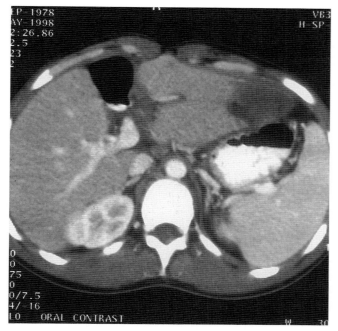

FIG. 9.9. Left lateral segment auxiliary graft with areas of necrosis following hepatic artery thrombosis 6 months post-transplantation after rapid immunosuppressant withdrawal.

With continuing refinement in surgical techniques and patient management, OLT is now the accepted treatment for severe acute liver failure. Although early survival rates are less satisfactory than for chronic liver disease, the majority of patients can look forward to long-term survival. The problems associated with long-term survival, particularly those related to immunosuppression, are more severe for this group of patients because they tend to be younger and to have significant renal injury at the time of transplantation. They are therefore more prone to renal failure long term. Auxiliary liver transplantation represents a way forward and is able to offer immunosuppression withdrawal in at least two-thirds of patients younger than 40 years. Improved understanding of patient and graft suitability and refinement of the surgical techniques have led many centers to reevaluate the potential of ALT.[26,27]

AUXILIARY LIVER TRANSPLANTATION FOR METABOLIC DISEASES

Orthotopic liver transplantation has been used successfully to treat liver-based metabolic disorders that produce structural and functional impairment of the liver. Liver replacement not only corrects the underlying metabolic defect but also resolves the problems posed by cirrhosis and portal hypertension. Some liver-based metabolic disorders do not cause cirrhosis but do cause severe or life-threatening extrahepatic complications. Orthotopic liver transplantation has been used to replace the defective enzyme or receptor site in

such disorders. Some of these conditions may be suitable for ALT; the rationale for this is that it is possible to provide sufficient liver mass to correct the underlying metabolic disorder while retaining the majority of the native liver. The advantage of this technique is that should the donor graft fail, it can be removed without necessarily endangering the life of the recipient. In addition, with retention of the native liver, gene therapy remains a possibility in the longer term. Gene therapy would avoid the need for life-long immunosuppression in these patients, who by the nature of the underlying disease tend to be very young children.

Auxiliary liver transplantation is not indicated for all non-cirrhotic inborn errors of metabolism. Conditions in which the liver is the site of production of an abnormal protein or enzyme that damages other target organs, such as familial amyloid polyneuropathy and primary hyperoxaluria type 1, require removal of the liver and orthotopic liver replacement.

Auxiliary liver transplantation has been used successfully to replace the defective enzyme in Crigler-Najjar syndrome type 1 (CNS1), which is characterized by an unconjugated hyperbilirubinemia due to complete lack of hepatic bilirubin UDP-glucuronyltransferase activity. The resulting high levels of serum bilirubin are not lowered by phenobarbitone, and patients are managed with daily phototherapy to maintain serum bilirubin levels between 200 and 400 μmol/L. Failure to control serum bilirubin levels can result in kernicterus and neurologic injury. For this reason OLT has been performed successfully for CNS1. There remains a significant morbidity and mortality following OLT, and the replacement of a structurally normal liver for a single enzymatic defect can be considered a drastic therapeutic measure. Experimental studies have shown that only 1% to 2% of the normal number of hepatocytes are needed for adequate bilirubin conjugation; thus, the idea that auxiliary partial orthotopic liver transplantation may provide an alternative treatment option for patients with CNS1 was put forward. APOLT has since been performed successfully for this condition. In this technique only a part of the patient's liver, usually the left lateral segment, is replaced with a size-matched donor graft that would allow conjugation of bilirubin.

Auxiliary transplantation for Crigler-Najjar syndrome was first reported from Chicago[28] in a 13-year-old girl who received a left lateral segment transplant from a living-related donor. The graft failed secondary to hepatic artery thrombosis, and she underwent retransplantation with a cadaveric donor left lateral segment. Recurrent rejection at 4 months was managed by conversion to tacrolimus, and 1 year later the serum bilirubin level was 70 μmol/L. Unfortunately, this patient later required orthotopic liver replacement; however, this report clearly indicated that ALT could successfully correct the underlying abnormality in CNS1. A second report described a patient who had the operation as part of an *in situ* split-liver procedure; unfortunately, graft function was poor because of early ischemic damage from insufficient portal venous inflow due to preferential flow to

TABLE 9.1. *Auxiliary partial orthotopic liver transplantation for Crigler-Najjar syndrome type 1*

Patient	Age (yr)	Bilirubin level at APOLT (μmol/L)	Phototherapy pre-APOLT (hr/d)	Neurology	Outcome	Follow-up period (months)	Follow-up bilirubin level (μmol/L)
1	10	418	16	Long tract signs	Died (LPD)	35	—
2	9	293	14	Normal	Alive	60	20
3	8	284	12	Normal	Alive	32	21
4	11	380	14	Normal	Alive	32	11
5	11	333	12	Normal	Alive	29	27
6	18	320	12	Normal	Alive	23	20

APOLT, auxiliary partial orthotopic liver transplantation; LPD, lymphoproliferative disease.

the native liver. This graft was removed and an orthotopic whole-liver transplantation performed.

The largest experience of ALT for this condition comes from our own unit, where we have performed seven APOLT procedures in six patients, with a median age at transplantation of 10.5 years (Table 9.1). All had received daily phototherapy from the first week of life with the objective of keeping the total serum bilirubin level below 300 μmol/L. Six of the seven transplantations were performed with left APOLT using segments 2 and 3 (Fig. 9.10); the seventh procedure was a right APOLT using a right lobe from a size-matched and ABO blood group–matched donor. Right APOLT was performed in this case because of prolonged waiting time for a size-matched organ and the opportunity to perform a split-liver transplant, resulting in two APOLTs in two patients.

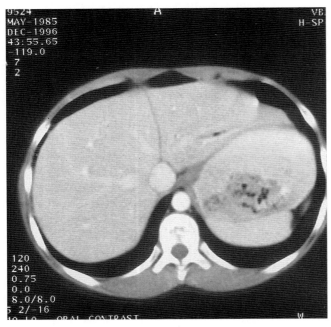

FIG. 9.10. Computed tomographic scan showing left lateral segment auxiliary graft for Crigler-Najjar syndrome type 1 at 1 year posttransplantation; the patient had a normal serum bilirubin level.

Postoperative immunosuppression was based on cyclosporin A, azathioprine, and prednisolone. The clinical course of all children except the first has been without major complications. In the first child, the Doppler study on day 1 showed no flow in the portal vein, but excellent arterial and left hepatic vein flow that was confirmed by arteriography. In view of satisfactory liver function, it was decided to continue observation; subsequent Doppler studies on day 3 showed satisfactory portal venous flow. However, the child developed episodes of intractable acute rejection resistant to pulse doses of steroids. Diagnosis of rejection was also delayed because no abnormalities in liver function tests were noted except for mild elevation of serum bilirubin that was initially interpreted as caused by poor graft function due to poor portal inflow. The diagnosis of rejection was only made on protocol biopsy. The patient's postoperative recovery was further complicated by glandular fever (IgM-positive Epstein-Barr virus) at 2 months that responded promptly to reduction of immunosuppression. He remained well, with a serum bilirubin level that fluctuated between 120 and 160 μmol/L for the next 12 months and then rose to 250 μmol/L, necessitating intermittent phototherapy. The patient underwent retransplantation with another left lateral segment APOLT 2.5 years after the first transplantation. The early postoperative recovery was uneventful; however, he was readmitted 6 months after retransplantation with diffuse lymphoma involving the central nervous system and died 2 weeks after admission.

The remaining five patients are alive, with serum bilirubin levels of less than 30 μmol/L (Fig. 9.11) at a median follow-up period of 32 months (range: 23–60 months) without phototherapy (Table 9.1). Three patients have experienced severe acute rejection that did not respond to pulse doses of steroids. They were converted to tacrolimus and are doing well, with good graft function. The child who received the right APOLT suffered a bile leak from the cut surface and required laparotomy and drainage; 3 months later the patient required revision of anastomotic biliary stricture. All surviving patients are well, and none has required phototherapy from the date of transplantation.

The problem of graft atrophy is significant in APOLT for metabolic liver disease and appears to be caused by poor portal venous inflow, impaired hepatic venous outflow, or pos-

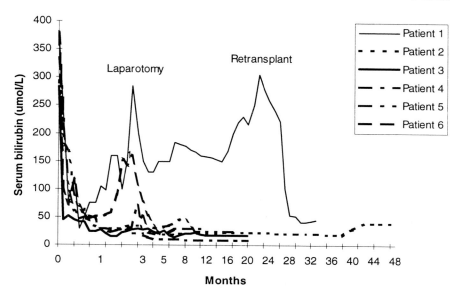

FIG. 9.11. Postoperative total serum bilirubin levels following auxiliary partial orthotopic liver transplantation.

sibly a lack of hepatotrophic substances, which may occur in the presence of a normal liver mass. In contrast to ALT for acute liver failure, in which narrowing of the native portal vein is not necessary, this step is an absolute necessity in APOLT for noncirrhotic metabolic liver disorders. In fulminant hepatic failure, the resistance to blood flow in the native liver is higher than in the graft, resulting in increased portal flow to the graft rather than the native liver. In contrast, the native liver in noncirrhotic metabolic disorders has a normal resistance to blood flow and the graft has a higher resistance, resulting in preferential portal flow to the native liver that renders the graft ischemic. This phenomenon was observed in the second reported case in the literature and in our first patient. It is accentuated by ongoing steroid-resistant rejection, resulting in a stiff graft. We try to narrow the portal vein to the native liver by up to 70% to encourage portal venous inflow to the graft. The experience reported from the Japanese literature is of disconnection of the portal vein to the native liver to completely divert the portal venous flow to the graft to prevent long-term graft atrophy.[29–31]

The diagnosis of acute rejection is difficult in these patients posttransplantation. There is minimal or no elevation in levels of hepatic enzymes such as aspartate aminotransferase and gammaglutamyl transferase in association with the rejection episodes. However, there is significant elevation in unconjugated serum bilirubin levels during such episodes, and rejection is always confirmed by biopsy before treatment. Diagnosis of rejection was delayed in our first patient because no abnormalities in liver function were noted other than an elevation of serum bilirubin level, which was thought to be due solely to poor portal venous inflow. The diagnosis was only made on liver biopsy. Our experience has shown that mild cases of unconjugated hyperbilirubinemia should be investigated with graft biopsy to exclude rejection.

APOLT has also been performed for other noncirrhotic liver-based inborn errors of metabolism such as propionic acidemia and urea cycle defects. We have performed a right APOLT for one child with propionic acidemia. The experience with orthotopic liver replacement for this condition is limited.[32] As with orthotopic replacement, ALT only partially corrects the underlying metabolic abnormality, and patients continue to have a high level of proprionyl-CoA metabolites in the plasma and urine that indicates the persistent metabolic abnormality in other organs. However, metabolic decompensation did not occur in our patient, and the child is leading a normal lifestyle with no dietary protein restriction. Tanaka and his colleagues have described APOLT for ornithine transcarbamoylase deficiency that relapsed following an episode of severe rejection and graft atrophy, but responded to the ligation of the portal venous supply to the liver.[31]

APOLT has potential in the management of other liver-based inborn errors of metabolism that do not structurally damage the liver, such as homozygous familial hypercholesterolemia, disorders of fatty acid metabolism, and hemophilia. It remains to be determined how much liver needs to be replaced for each of these conditions. Orthotopic ALT represents an alternative to liver replacement in the management of noncirrhotic inborn errors of metabolism. Long-term success will be defined as the ability to withdraw immunosuppression either following gene therapy or with the development of tolerance induction therapy. It is possible that advances in our understanding and our ability to induce tolerance to transplanted livers will make auxiliary grafting redundant. Until such time as these potential therapies are available, ALT is the only treatment that keeps all options open for the patient.

REFERENCES

1. O'Grady JG, Alexander GJM, Hallyar K, et al. Early indicators of prognosis in fulminant hepatic failure. *Gastroenterology* 1989;95:439–445.

2. Welch CS. A note on transplantation of the whole liver in dogs. *Transplant Bull* 1955;2:54–56.
3. Absolon KB, Hagihari PF, Griffen WO, et al. Experimental and clinical heterotopic liver transplantation. *Rev Intern Hepatology* 1965;15:1481–1487.
4. Fortner JG, Kinne DW, Shiu MH, et al. Clinical liver heterotopic (auxiliary) transplantation. *Surgery* 1973;74:739–751.
5. Houssin D, Berthelot P, Franco D, et al. Heterotopic liver transplantation in end-stage HBs Ag-positive cirrhosis. *Lancet* 1980;1:990–993.
6. Blankensteijn JD, Schalm SW, Terpstra OT. New aspects of heterotopic liver transplantation. *Transpl Int* 1992;5:43–50.
7. Fortner JG, Yeh SDJ, Kim DK, et al. The case for and technique of heterotopic liver grafting. *Transplant Proc* 1979;11:269–275.
8. Terpstra OT, Reuvers CB, Schalm SW. Auxiliary heterotopic liver transplantation. *Transplantation* 1988;45:1003–1007.
9. Gubernatis G, Pichlmayr R, Kemnitz J, et al. Auxiliary partial orthotopic liver transplantation (APOLT) for fulminant hepatic failure: first successful case report. *World J Surg* 1991;15:660–666.
10. Boudjema K, Jaeck D, Simeoni U, et al. Temporary auxiliary liver transplantation for subacute liver failure in a child. *Lancet* 1993;342:778–779.
11. Broelsch CE, Whitington PF, Emond JC. Evolution and future perspectives for reduced-size hepatic transplantation. *Surg Gynecol Obstet* 1990;171:353–360.
12. Jerusalem C, Heyde MN van der, Schmidt WJ, et al. Heterotopic liver transplantation. *Eur Surg Res* 1972;4:186–197.
13. Marchioro TL, Porter KA, Dickinson TC, et al. Physiologic requirements for auxiliary liver transplantation. *Surg Gynecol Obstet* 1985;121:17–31.
14. Bengoechea-Gonzalez E, Awane Y, Reetsma K. Experimental auxiliary liver homotransplantation. *Arch Surg* 1967;94:1–7.
15. Van der Hyde MN, Schalm L. Auxiliary liver-graft without portal blood: experimental autotransplantation of the left lobe. *Br J Surg* 1968;55:114–118.
16. Moritz MJ, Jarrell BE, Armenti V, et al. Heterotopic liver transplantation for fulminant hepatic failure—a bridge to recovery. *Transplantation* 1990;50:524–526.
17. Ringe B, Lubbe N, Kuse E, et al. Total hepatectomy and liver transplantation as a two-stage procedure. *Ann Surg* 1993;218:3–9.
18. Kiuchi T, Kasahara M, Uryuhara K, et al. Impact of graft size mismatching on graft prognosis in liver transplantation from living donors. *Transplantation* 1999;67:321–327.
19. Pereira SP, McCarthy M, Ellis AJ, et al. Auxiliary partial orthotopic liver transplantation for acute liver failure. *J Hepatol* 1997;26:1010–1017.
20. Chenard Neu MP, Boudjema K, Bernuau J, et al. Auxiliary liver transplantation: regeneration of the native liver and outcome in 30 patients with fulminant hepatic failure—a multicenter European study. *Hepatology* 1996;23:1119-1127.
21. van Hoek B, de Boer J, Boudjema K, et al. Auxiliary versus orthotopic liver transplantation for acute liver failure. EURALT Study Group. European Auxiliary Liver Transplant Registry. *J Hepatol* 1999;30:699–705.
22. Buyck D, Bonnin F, Bernuau J, et al. Auxiliary liver transplantation in patients with fulminant hepatic failure: hepatobiliary scintigraphic follow-up. *Eur J Nucl Med* 1997;24:138–142.
23. van Hoek B, Ringers J, Kroes AC, et al. Temporary heterotopic auxiliary liver transplantation for fulminant hepatitis B. *J Hepatol* 1995;23:109–118.
24. Bismuth H, Azoulay D, Samuel D, et al. Auxiliary partial orthotopic liver transplantation for fulminant hepatitis. The Paul Brousse experience. *Ann Surg* 1996;224:712–726.
25. Sudan DL, Langnas AN, Shaw BW Jr. Long-term follow-up of auxiliary liver transplantation for fulminant hepatic failure. *Transplant Proc* 1997;29:485–486.
26. Shaw BW Jr. Auxiliary liver transplantation for acute liver failure. *Liver Transpl Surg* 1995;1:194–200.
27. Neuhaus P, Bechstein WO. Split liver/auxiliary liver transplantation for fulminant hepatic failure. *Liver Transpl Surg* 1997;3:S55–S61.
28. Whittington PF, Edmond JC, Heffron TG, et al. Orthotopic auxiliary liver transplantation for Crigler Najjar syndrome type 1. *Lancet* 1993;342:779–780.
29. Kiuchi T, Edamoto Y, Kaibori M, et al. Auxiliary liver transplantation for urea-cycle enzyme deficiencies: lessons from three cases. *Transplant Proc* 1999;31:528–529.
30. Koebe HG, Schildberg FW, Yabe S, et al. Auxiliary partial orthotopic liver transplantation from living donors: significance of portal blood flow. *Transplantation* 1998;66:484–488.
31. Kaibori M, Uemoto S, Fujita S, et al. Native hepatectomy after auxiliary partial orthotopic liver transplantation. *Transpl Int* 1999;12:383–386.
32. Holmgren GH, Ericzon BG, Groth CG, et al. Clinical improvement and amyloid regression after liver transplantation in hereditary transthyretin amyloidosis. *Lanat* 1993;341:1113–1116.

Transplantation of the Liver, edited by Willis C. Maddrey, Eugene R. Schiff, and Michael F. Sorrell. Lippincott Williams & Wilkins, Philadelphia © 2001.

CHAPTER 10

Immediate Postoperative Care

Gregory T. Everson and Igal Kam

In 1999, there were 125 programs in liver transplantation in the United States, 14,517 patients were on the U.S. waiting list at the end of the year, and 4,487 transplantations were performed. The success of transplantation has increased steadily over the last two decades, with current 1-year patient and graft survival rates in the United States of 83.8% and 76.7%, respectively.[1] However, complications are common in the early postoperative period and contribute to significant morbidity and mortality.[2,3] Seventy-five percent to 85% of the deaths that occur in the first posttransplantation year happen within the first 3 months following the transplantation. Thus, knowledge of complications that emerge during the early postoperative period, early and accurate establishment of diagnosis, and prompt institution of appropriate interventions are essential for optimal patient and graft outcome. Uniform recommendations for postoperative care are often not possible because of the lack of standardization among transplant centers, the paucity of multicenter controlled trials, and the reliance on experience and observation.

DEFINITION

The immediate postoperative period begins with discharge from the operating room and includes the initial hospital stay, readmissions, and the clinical events and outpatient management that arise during the first 3 posttransplantation months. This period is characterized by wide interindividual variability in severity of illness, complications, need for acute care, lengths of stay, rates of readmission, and clinical outcomes. One patient may have an uncomplicated operation, undergo extubation in the operating room, transfer directly from the operating room to the transplant floor, and

G. T. Everson: Department of Medicine, University of Colorado School of Medicine, Denver, Colorado 80262.

I. Kam: Department of Surgery, University of Colorado School of Medicine, Denver, Colorado 80262.

be discharged from the hospital within 7 to 12 days of the transplant operation; such a patient may not require readmission and may undergo an uneventful postoperative recovery. In contrast, another patient may experience a difficult operation, require multiple transfusions of blood or blood products, transfer from the operating room to an intensive care unit (ICU), have a prolonged ICU course and hospitalization, transfer to a rehabilitation unit, and require close outpatient supervision and need repeated hospitalizations. The majority of patients experience a clinical course intermediate between these two extremes (Fig. 10.1).

DISPOSITION OF THE PATIENT AFTER SURGERY

Our center, and others, have used intraoperative assessment or evaluation in the recovery room to determine the feasibility of transferring the patient directly to the transplant floor, bypassing the surgical ICU. This practice is limited to the most stable liver recipients, that is, those with a functioning allograft who have been successfully extubated. Direct transfer to the transplant floor avoids unnecessary ICU days. Our criteria for early extubation and direct transfer to the floor are as follows:

1. Functioning allograft
2. Hemodynamic stability without active bleeding
3. Uncomplicated transplant operation
4. Rapid reversal of anesthetic effect with easy arousability and intact neurologic reflexes
5. Lack of active cardiopulmonary comorbidity

In contrast, other patients leave the operating room with a poorly functioning graft after a complicated operation, during which they received large volumes of blood products or manifested cardiovascular, respiratory, renal, or metabolic instability. These patients require life support; thus, they are transferred to the surgical ICU and monitored.

We have been able to directly transfer 40% of our patients to the floor. This group of patients was compared

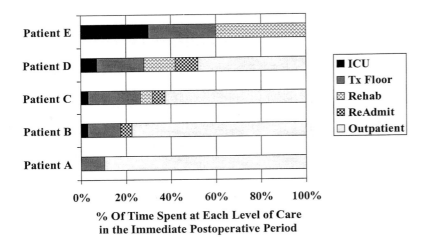

FIG. 10.1. Examples of the variability in immediate postoperative course. Patient A exhibited a benign course, was never admitted to the ICU, and was discharged from the hospital after 10 days and never readmitted. This course occurs in approximately 20% of cases. Patient E is representative of another 5% to 10% of patients, whose course is highly complicated by prolonged ICU and total hospital length of stay, with ongoing care required by transfer to a rehabilitation unit. The majority of patients (greater than 70%) exhibit an intermediate clinical course (patients B, C, and D).

with a cohort of patients who required immediate surgical ICU care (Table 10.1). The average total length of stay in the ICU was 1 day for the former group versus 7 days for the latter, the total hospital length of stay was 10 days versus 24 days, and the total charges were approximately $84,000 versus $163,000. Patients who were directly transferred to the ICU were more likely to have been in the ICU prior to transplantation (19% vs. 5%).

CLINICAL COURSE AND PREDICTORS OF OUTCOME

Intensive Care Unit

Four comorbidities extend the ICU stay: pulmonary hypertension, dialysis, infection, and cardiac disease. Pulmonary hypertension occurs in 2% to 4% of patients with chronic liver disease undergoing hepatic transplantation.[4–7] These patients are particularly demanding in terms of need for postoperative ICU care: they require Swan-Ganz monitoring, pressor support, volume management, and cardiac support.

Renal failure, defined as a creatinine level higher than 1.6 mg/dL, occurs in 40% of patients who undergo transplantation for fulminant hepatic failure and in 15% of those who undergo transplantation for cirrhosis.[8] The prevalence of renal failure is highest in Child's class C cirrhosis and in patients who were in the ICU prior to transplantation. Dialysis is required either prior to or after transplantation in 10% to 25% of patients with renal failure. The need for dialysis often correlates with the severity of liver disease and is associated with multisystem failure and a need for extended ICU care.

Underlying coronary artery disease is present in approximately 5% of patients undergoing liver transplantation.[9,10] One series reported a prevalence of 16.2% in recipients older than 50 years.[11] Manifestations of cardiac ischemia posttransplantation may include unexplained hypotension, pulmonary edema, or arrhythmia. Cardiac hemochromatosis, valvular heart disease, and idiopathic hypertrophic cardiomyopathy represent unique conditions that warrant special consideration.

Infection is present in many patients undergoing liver transplantation.[12,13] Active untreated infection, especially fungal infection, is associated with a greater likelihood of multisystem failure in the immediate postoperative period.

Donor characteristics predictive of poor graft function and reduced graft survival include female gender, age older than 60 years, macrosteatosis (more than 30%) on liver biopsy,

TABLE 10.1. *Positive impact of direct transfer to the transplant floor*

	Transfer to floor	Transfer to surgical ICU
Number of patients	57 (40%)	87 (60%)
Patient survival (%)	97	93
Retransplantations (%)	2	1
Length of ICU stay (d) (% of patients)		
Pretransplantation	0 ± 1 (5%)	2 ± 6 (19%)
Initial	0 ± 0	5 ± 12
Return to ICU	1 ± 7 (5%)	2 ± 7 (13%)
Length of hospital stay (d) (% of patients)		
Initial admittance	10 ± 12	24 ± 28
Readmittance, 90 d	9 ± 10 (78%)	7 ± 12 (73%)
Charges, initial stay ($)	84,060 ± 62,276	162,958 ± 161,514

ICU, intensive care unit.

serum [Na+] greater than 170 mEq/L, and cold ischemic time of more than 12 hours.[14,15] However, older grafts, even older than 70 years, may still offer excellent function if the procuring surgeon's assessment is that the donor liver is of good quality.[16,17]

Certain operative complications correlate with a need for prolonged monitoring in the ICU: intraabdominal bleeding requiring excessive transfusions, use of vascular grafts, poor intraoperative graft function, and total operative time.

Allograft function determines the stability of the patient in the postoperative period. Graft nonfunction or poor function is characterized by jaundice, aminotransferase elevation, hepatic dysfunction (elevated prothrombin time or international ratio) INR, hypoalbuminemia, ascites, encephalopathy), and electrolye and acid-base imbalance. Hemodynamic instability, susceptibility to infection, respiratory dysfunction, coagulopathy, and disordered metabolism of medications are consequences of poor graft function.

Inpatient Floor

Uncomplicated cases usually progress in three phases: patient recovery from the initial effects of the operation (control of pain, recovery of bowel function, removal of catheters and drains, resolution of diet and activity), stabilization of graft function and adjustment of immunosuppressive medications, and restoration of independence and development of understanding of transplant procedures, followup, and medications. A patient without complications may be discharged from the hospital between 7 and 12 days after liver transplantation.

Complications that delay discharge are allograft rejection, infection (bacterial, viral, or fungal), complications of immunosuppressive medications or inability to maintain satisfactory levels of immunosuppressive drugs, and neuropsychiatric instability. Excessive hospital length of stay is also related to deconditioning and need for physical rehabilitation, dietary therapy, nutritional support, physical therapy, and neuropsychiatric recovery.

Outpatient Clinic

Outpatients are monitored closely for signs of graft dysfunction. Graft dysfunction is usually asymptomatic, although severe injury may be heralded by jaundice or ascites. The primary marker of a problem emerging in the allograft is a rise in liver enzymes.

Figure 10.2 displays the means of posttransplantation liver tests for patients experiencing uncomplicated recovery. Aspartate aminotransferase (AST) generally is the first enzyme to return to a normal level and has very tight confidence limits. The other enzymes exhibit a similar pattern but do not return to normal levels in the first 2 weeks; the confidence limits about their means are much broader than for AST. For this reason, many programs monitor the AST level, since a sudden increase in AST may be the most sensitive early indicator of graft dysfunction.

An algorithm defining an approach to abnormal results from liver tests in the early posttransplantation period is shown in Fig. 10.3. Accurate diagnosis is dependent on demonstration of patency of vascular anastomoses, proper interpretation of liver biopsy, and performance of specific serologic tests or cultures. One of the more challenging diagnostic dilemmas is differentiating allograft rejection from recurrent hepatitis C.

Adequate plasma levels of immunosuppressive medication are required to prevent allograft rejection. Many of the drugs used as maintenance immunosuppression are dependent on bile for their intestinal absorption. In the

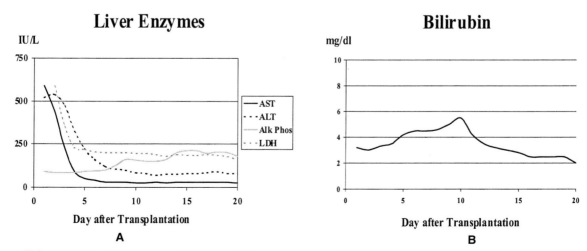

FIG. 10.2. The time course of changes in liver enzymes and bilirubin in 37 patients with uncomplicated recoveries. **A:** The pattern of change in liver enzymes. Aspartate aminotransferase (AST) is the first enzyme to return to normal and stabilize in the normal range. **B:** The change in total bilirubin level.

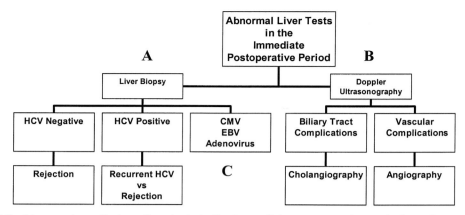

FIG. 10.3. Abnormal results from liver tests in the immediate postoperative period require prompt establishment of diagnosis. Liver biopsy **(A)** is essential for diagnosis of rejection and opportunistic viral infection; however, differentiation of rejection from hepatitis C may be difficult. Doppler ultrasonography **(B)** is used to evaluate patency of vessels. If vascular occlusion is suspected by ultrasonography, angiography may be required. Ultrasonography may also identify biliary complications and the need for cholangiography. Specific histologic stains, cultures, or serologic tests **(C)** are required to diagnose cytomegalovirus, Epstein-Barr virus, or adenovirus infections.

early posttransplantation period the liver is relatively cholestatic from ischemia-reperfusion injury, and bile secretion is impaired. Thus, absorption of orally administered medications may be erratic and unpredictable, contributing to fluctuating drug levels and periods of inadequate immunosuppression. An inadequate level of immunosuppressive medication is one cause of early allograft rejection.

Another major purpose of close outpatient monitoring is to detect and treat deficiencies in general health. Attention is paid to diet, nutrition, physical activity, and overall function, including neuropsychiatric recovery. Transplant coordinators educate the patient regarding side effects and toxicities of medications and emphasize compliance with treatment. The process of weaning the patient from the transplant center back to the referring physician is complex and dependent on the patient's sense of security, the resolution of all complications, the stabilization of graft function, and the establishment of the proper dose of maintenance immunosuppression. Most transplant centers have patient support groups to help guide not only patients but also families and loved ones through the healing process.

Experience of the Transplant Center

One of the key features defining a successful outcome from liver transplantation is the emphasis on a team approach to the care and management of these complicated patients. Surgical expertise is critical to the initial success of the transplant operation, and the level of competence and dedication of the surgical team will determine whether new surgical procedures, such as living donor liver transplantation, can be performed at a given center. Hepatologists evaluate candidates, guide pretransplantation care, aid in the post-

operative management of medical problems and immunosuppression, and work with transplant surgeons to direct the diagnostic approach and management of posttransplantation complications. The role of the transplant coordinator as a crucial liaison among patient, family, physicians, and surgeons cannot be overemphasized. Coordination of anesthesiology, nursing, pathology, radiology, and consult services is vital to optimal patient outcome.

Centers with large multidisciplinary teams are characterized by higher numbers of transplant procedures. A recent analysis by the United Network for Organ Sharing (UNOS) demonstrated that the patient survival rate in programs performing more than 20 transplantations per year is significantly better than that in programs performing fewer than 20 transplantations per year (Fig. 10.4).[18] The excess mortality in low-volume programs occurs primarily in the first 3 months after transplantation, further emphasizing the importance of an experienced team in managing complications occurring in the immediate postoperative period.

Recipient Age

The effect of recipient age at the time of transplantation on the postoperative course was examined in 735 adult patients who underwent transplantation at three U.S. medical centers between 1990 and 1994.[19] Patients were categorized into two groups: either younger than 60 or 60 years or older. The majority of elderly patients were women, white, and likely to have either cholestatic liver disease or cryptogenic cirrhosis. Disease severity, as assessed by Child-Turcotte-Pugh score, UNOS status, and Karnofsky score, was similar in the two groups. Elderly patients had extended ICU stays ($P < 0.01$) and prolongation of total hospitalization ($P < 0.03$). Graft survival was similar, but patient survival was

% of Patients who Died Posttransplantation

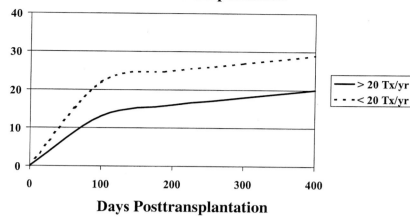

Days Posttransplantation

FIG. 10.4. Transplant programs performing more than 20 transplants per year are characterized by lower patient mortality. Nearly all the increase in patient mortality in low-volume programs occurs within the first 3 months after transplantation. (ret 18)

diminished in the elderly group (81% vs. 90%, $P < 0.004$). Excess mortality was due primarily to nonhepatic causes: infections, cardiac complications, and neurologic disease. Surviving elderly patients experienced the same improvement in quality of life as younger patients.

Early Allograft Dysfunction

Allograft dysfunction in the early postoperative period is predictive of subsequent patient outcome.[20–22] A study of 710 recipients defined early allograft dysfunction (EAD) as the early postoperative occurrence of a serum bilirubin level greater than 10 mg/dL, prothrombin time greater than or equal to 17 seconds, or hepatic encephalopathy.[20] Patients with EAD experienced prolonged lengths of stay in the ICU (4 vs. 3 days, $P < 0.0001$) and in the hospital (24 vs. 15 days, $P < 0.0001$) and had poorer graft and patient survival rates than patients without EAD (3-year patient survival was 68% vs. 83%, $P < 0.0001$; graft survival was 61% vs. 79%, $P < 0.0001$). Most of the excess mortality related to EAD had occurred by 3 months after transplantation.

Recipient factors associated with EAD include male gender, inpatient status at time of transplantation, and increased severity of pretransplantation liver disease. Donor characteristics associated with EAD are nonwhite race, donor age older than 50 years, cold ischemic time greater than 15 hours, fair or poor graft quality as assessed by the procurement surgeon, donor hospital stay greater than 3 days, donor acidosis, and ABO mismatch.

Marked elevation in aminotransferases also correlates with poor graft and patient outcome (Fig. 10.5).[21] The incidence of primary graft nonfunction increases and graft and patient survival rates decrease as the maximum concentration of posttransplantation AST increases (especially if AST is greater than 5000 IU/L). The increase in AST after transplantation correlates with a wide array of cytokines and markers of platelet and neutrophil aggregation and activation.[22] A summary of recipient, donor, and operative and perioperative factors predictive of graft loss or death is given in Table 10.2.

Patient survival after liver transplantation has improved steadily over the last decade. In the last UNOS review of

%

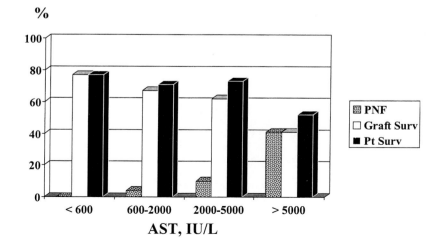

AST, IU/L

FIG. 10.5. Actuarial 1-year survival rates plotted against the maximum concentration of aspartate aminotransferase (AST) achieved in the immediate postoperative period. Patient and graft survival rates decrease as AST increases, particularly for AST higher than 5,000 IU/L. The decreased survival in all cases was related to an increased incidence of primary nonfunction (PNF). (ret 21)

TABLE 10.2. *Risk factors for graft loss or patient death within the first 6 months after liver transplantation*

Recipient factors	Donor factors	Operative and postoperative factors
Age >50 yr	Age > 50 yr	Excessive transfusion
Male gender	Female gender	Prolonged operative time
UNOS status 1	Nonidentical ABO match	Coagulopathy and hemodynamic instability
UNOS status 2A	DF/RM	Comorbidity (cardiopulmonary)
Fulminant hepatic failure	Macrosteatosis (>30%)	Prolonged cold ischemic time
Positive for HBsAg	Hypernatremia ([Na+] > 170 mEq/L)	AST > 2,500 IU/L
Creatinine level > 2 mg/dL		Bilirubin level > 10 mg/dL
Bilirubin level > 10 mg/dL		Prothrombin time > 17 sec
Albumin < 2.8 g/dL		Encephalopathy
Prothrombin time > 16 sec		

AST, aspartate aminotransferase; HBsAg, hepatitis B surface antigen; UNOS, United Network for Organ Sharing. Df/Rm, donor female/recipient male.

center-specific outcomes, several programs reported 1-year survival rates exceeding 85%.[23] The improvement in patient survival was paralleled by improvement in graft survival. Although advances in surgical technique are partly responsible for these improved outcomes, much of the enhanced survival is related to early diagnosis and appropriate therapy of complications occurring in the early posttransplantation period.

COMPLICATIONS

Major metabolic problems may be encountered in the first 48 to 72 hours of the initial ICU stay, including fluid and electrolyte imbalance, acid-base disturbance, and renal failure. Coagulopathy is common, and replacement with fresh frozen plasma, cryoprecipitate, specific factors, and platelets may be indicated. Persistent encephalopathy, underlying cardiopulmonary disease, and respiratory compromise may necessitate prolonged intubation. Cardiac arrhythmias may result from fluid and electrolyte imbalance, medications, use of vasopressors, or mechanical irritation from intracardiac catheters.

Allograft Dysfunction

Table 10.3 summarizes the complications that lead to allograft dysfunction.

Chronology

The timing of complications resulting in graft dysfunction is shown in Fig. 10.6. Graft injury within the first 3 days is most often caused by either primary nonfunction or hepatic artery thrombosis. Less common causes of graft dysfunction during this period include hyperacute rejection, portal vein thrombosis, and obstruction of the inferior vena cava. Between 3 and 14 days after transplantation, graft dysfunction is most commonly related to acute cellular rejection, recurrent hepatitis C virus (HCV), hepatic artery thrombosis, or biliary leak or cholangitis. Infrequent causes of dys-

function during this period are portal vein thrombosis, drug hepatotoxicity, and functional cholestasis. From 14 days to 3 months after transplantation, the most common causes of graft dysfunction include allograft rejection, recurrent HCV, biliary complications, cytomegalovirus (CMV) hepatitis, or drug hepatotoxicity. Vascular thromboses rarely present after the third week, and recurrence of hepatitis B virus (HBV) is typically delayed beyond 1 month.

Primary Nonfunction

Clinical Presentation

The most common cause of graft loss within the immediate postoperative period is primary nonfunction, or delayed ischemia-reperfusion injury.[24,25] Primary nonfunction (PNF) is characterized by acute liver failure (encephalopathy, asci-

TABLE 10.3. *Allograft dysfunction and surgical complications occurring in the immediate postoperative period*

Allograft dysfunction
  Primary nonfunction
  Primary poor function
  Acute cellular rejection
  Recurrent viral hepatitis
    Hepatitis B
    Hepatitis D
    Hepatitis C
  Drug and TPN hepatotoxicity
Surgical complications
Postoperative hemorrhage
Vascular complications
  Hepatic artery thrombosis
  Portal vein thrombosis
  Inferior vena caval or hepatic venous obstruction or thrombosis
  Other
Biliary tract complications
  Bile leak or fistula
  Biliary stricture

TPN, total parenteral nutrition.

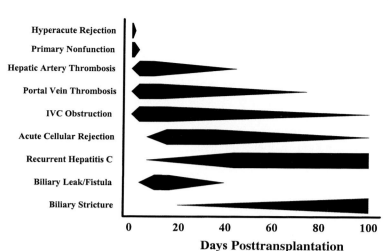

FIG. 10.6. The time course of development of various causes of graft dysfunction. Hyperacute rejection and primary nonfunction are restricted to the first few days after transplantation. Vascular complications tend to occur within the first few weeks but may present later. Acute cellular rejection emerges around postoperative day 7 and may occur at any time in the immediate postoperative period. Recurrent hepatitis C overlaps considerably with acute cellular rejection. Bile leaks tend to occur early, and strictures tend to occur later.

tes, coagulopathy, unstable hemodynamics), high levels of liver enzymes [AST and alanine aminotransferase (ALT) greater than 2,500 IU/L], and development of multiorgan failure (renal failure and pulmonary complications).[25] Reported rates of PNF, which requires retransplantation, range from 6.9% to 8.5%.[15,26–28]

Primary poor function (PPF) is a less severe form of PNF. Liver enzyme levels are usually lower (AST and ALT less than 2,500 IU/L), and synthetic function is partially preserved. Patients with PPF are typically not encephalopathic and have less severe coagulopathy, but they may have ascites. The treatment of PPF is supportive; most grafts eventually recover, but some continue to function poorly and require retransplantation.

Risk Factors

The cause of PNF is irreversible loss of hepatocyte function due primarily to ischemia-reperfusion injury. The risk of developing PNF is related to donor age older than 50 years, macrosteatosis (greater than 30%) on biopsy of donor liver, severe donor hypernatremia ([Na+] greater than 170 mEq/L), and prolonged cold ischemic time.[29–34]

Diagnostic Studies

PNF is established by the characteristic posttransplantation presentation of severe liver dysfunction with marked elevations in liver enzymes (AST greater than 2,500 IU/L). Arterial thrombosis is excluded by Doppler ultrasonographic evaluation, and PNF may be confirmed by liver biopsy. Histologic features include infiltration with mixed inflammatory cells, balloon degeneration of hepatocytes, and zonal necrosis.

Treatment

There is no effective therapy for PNF. Typically the damage in primary nonfunction is irreversible, and patient survival is dependent on early retransplantation. Because oxidant injury is thought to be a key factor in pathogenesis,[25] antioxidant and cytoprotective therapies have been investigated.[35–38] Prophylactic treatment of liver recipients with intravenous prostaglandin E$_1$ improved renal function and reduced the length of stay in the ICU, but did not reduce the incidence of PNF.[37,38]

Rejection

Hyperacute rejection is extremely rare in human liver transplantation, if it occurs at all, but is common in xenotransplantation.[39–42] This type of rejection occurs within minutes to hours of transplantation and is caused by preformed antibodies and complement-mediated destruction of endothelial cells with resultant thrombosis of the graft. The major risk factor for hyperacute rejection in allotransplantation is transplantation of an ABO-incompatible graft. Even so, successful transplantation across ABO barriers is possible. The most common form of rejection in human liver allotransplantation is acute cellular rejection.[43–48]

Clinical Presentation

Fifty percent of recipients of liver allografts will experience acute cellular rejection within the first 6 weeks after transplantation.[43] The median time to first rejection is 8 days. Twenty percent of recipients will experience two episodes of rejection, and 4% will have three episodes. Reported rates of rejection vary because of differences in methods used to detect rejection, such as protocol biopsy, and differences in immunosuppressive therapy. Acute cellular rejection is usually asymptomatic and heralded only by an increase in liver enzymes. Centers performing protocol biopsies may diagnose and treat rejection based solely on histology without requiring an abnormal liver test result.

Risk Factors

The risk of acute rejection is lowest in patients receiving the highest level of immunosuppression, for example, OKT3 induction or quadruple-drug immunosuppressive regimens. Rejection is also less likely in elderly patients and in those with significant pretransplantation comorbidity, including severe chronic liver disease, renal failure, and malnutrition. Conversely, young, relatively healthy recipients without renal failure are more likely to reject their grafts.[43,44,46] Other predictors of rejection include an increased number of HLA-DR mismatches, longer cold ischemic times, and older donor age.

Diagnosis

Liver biopsy is essential for diagnosis because changes in liver enzymes are nonspecific and simply reflect injury from any cause. Histologic examination reveals portal inflammation with a mixed cellular infiltrate with lymphocytes, polymorphonuclear leukocytes, plasma cells, mononuclear cells, and eosinophils. The biliary epithelium and vascular endothelium appear to be the targets of the inflammatory reaction.[45,47,49,50] Epithelial cells exhibit cellular unrest, reactive changes, apoptosis, and disruption of the epithelial lining of the duct. Endothelial cells swell, appear reactive, and are undermined by the inflammatory reaction. Focal thrombosis may be present in the region of vascular damage.

Treatment

Acute allograft rejection is nearly always reversible if diagnosed early and treated properly.[51-53] In some cases, mild rejection may resolve without treatment. Therapies include steroid pulse, steroid recycle, or antilymphocyte preparations [antilymphocyte globulin (ALG), antithymocyte globulin (ATG), or OKT3], and increasing the level of maintenance immunosuppression. Some studies suggest that adjuvant prophylaxis with ursodeoxycholic acid may lower the risk of rejection.[54,55]

Outcome

As opposed to other solid-organ transplants, the liver allograft may be relatively protected from both short- and long-term consequences of acute rejection. Rejection is readily reversible with current medical therapy, and immunologic graft loss is rare. Two-thirds or more of rejection episodes respond to steroid pulse therapy, and the minority require antilymphocyte therapy. The need for antilymphocyte therapy is directly related to the histologic severity of rejection. A single episode of rejection in a liver recipient is actually associated with improved graft and patient survival compared with recipients who have never experienced rejection.[43]

Recurrent Hepatitis B

Clinical Presentation

Recurrent HBV may be asymptomatic or present as an icteric illness with clinical features of acute viral hepatitis.[56,57] In nearly all cases, the acute hepatitis is followed by development of chronic hepatitis. Spontaneous virologic clearance does not occur in the setting of posttransplantation immunosuppression. An uncommon form of recurrence, fibrosing cholestatic hepatitis, is characterized by rapidly progressive jaundice that may lead to graft loss or death.[58,59] Recurrence of HBV is associated with reduced patient and graft survival rates.

Risk Factors

The major risk factor for allograft hepatitis B is a pretransplantation diagnosis of chronic hepatitis B; risk of recurrence is greatest in those who were positive for HBV DNA at the time of transplantation.[56,57] Prior to introduction of hyperimmune hepatitis B immune globulin (HBIG) or nucleoside analogue therapy, rates of recurrent HBV were approximately 75% at a mean ($\pm$ standard deviation) follow-up period of 3.2 ± 2.7 months. Current medical regimens using HBIG treatment are more than 80% effective in preventing reinfection.[60-62]

Another risk factor for allograft hepatitis B is receipt of an allograft from a donor positive for antibody to hepatitis B core antigen (anti-HBc).[63] Hepatitis B reactivates under immunosuppression in approximately 75% of these cases, causing allograft hepatitis, graft destruction, and reduced graft and patient survival. Currently, the use of donor livers positive for anti-HBc is commonly restricted to recipients who have hepatitis B and are already destined to receive posttransplantation HBIG or antiviral therapy. Some have suggested that anti-HBc–positive donor organs can be safely used in recipients who are negative for hepatitis B surface antigen (HbsAg) and antibody to HbsAg (anti-HBs) under cover of HBIG plus lamivudine.[64]

Diagnosis

The diagnosis of allograft hepatitis B is suspected when AST and ALT levels rise after the first posttransplantation month in a patient infected with HBV or in the recipient of a liver from an anti-HBc–positive donor. Serology results are positive for HBsAg, hepatitis B e antigen (HBeAg), and HBV DNA. Liver biopsy reveals features of acute hepatitis. Stains for surface antigen (HBsAg) or core antigen (HBsAg) are positive, and there is no evidence of rejection.

Prophylaxis against Allograft Hepatitis B

Current strategies use HBIG[60-62] to bind and clear HBsAg-positive viral particles or use nucleoside analogues[65-69] to inhibit hepatitis B viral replication. Although there is extreme variation in antiviral protocols among transplant centers, two regimens are often quoted: those from the University of Virginia (UVA) and the University of California at San Francisco (UCSF). The UVA protocol uses 10,000 IU HBIG given intravenously during the anhepatic phase and then daily for 6 days. Thereafter doses are given as needed to maintain the serum titer of anti-HBs at or above 500 IU/L. Although similar, the UCSF protocol involves 10,000 IU intravenous HBIG during the anhepatic phase daily for 7 days, and then monthly thereafter without adjustment for titer of anti-HBs. These HBIG strategies reduce the recurrence rate for allograft hepatitis B from over 75% for untreated patients to less than 20% for treated patients.* HBIG must be given according to schedule during the early postoperative period to avoid graft infection and to obtain the desired graft and patient survival rates.

Lamivudine is used with increasing frequency in transplant centers.[65–68] Often lamivudine is begun when the patient is on the waiting list, so that patients may undergo surgery with undetectable levels of circulating HBV DNA. Some centers continue to administer lamivudine as either monotherapy or in combination with HBIG beyond the day of transplantation.[68] One study of 12 patients after liver transplantation demonstrated prolonged effectiveness of lamivudine, without significant "breakthrough."† Lamivudine is relatively safe and appears to have little or no interaction with immunosuppressive drugs or other pharmaceuticals used in the posttransplantation period.

Pretransplantation famciclovir reduces viral DNA levels, but only 25% of treated patients are rendered HBV DNA negative prior to transplantation.[69] There is no information regarding the use of adefovir in prophylaxis against posttransplantation HBV. Prophylaxis with interferon is ineffective in reducing recurrent hepatitis B and is currently not recommended.

Treatment of Recurrent Hepatitis B

Treatment of allograft hepatitis B is usually an issue for later time points after transplantation, beyond 3 months. However, occasionally recurrence is early and aggressive, and treatment is initiated prior to 3 months. For this reason, a brief description of this issue is offered here.

Early experience with interferon in the treatment of recurrent hepatitis B was disappointing, and use of interferon had been discouraged. One recent series reported that 4 of 14 patients treated with interferon-alfa (3 MU three times a week for 23.5 weeks) cleared HBV DNA (28% response). One of the four cleared HBeAg and HBsAg, and another cleared HBeAg.[70] Others have suggested that long-term treatment (1 to 2 years) with modest doses (3 to 6 MU three times a week) may clear HBeAg and HBV DNA in some cases.[71,72]

Lamivudine is effective in suppression of HBV replication in the posttransplantation period.[65] However, clearance of HBeAg or HBsAg is rare. Relapse of hepatitis is the rule with discontinuation of treatment, and long-term therapy is associated with emergence of lamivudine-resistant strains of HBV, such as the YMDD mutation.[67] Lesser efficacy is achieved with famciclovir[73] or ganciclovir,[74] and nucleoside-resistant mutations may emerge with these agents.

Outcome

Recurrent or *de novo* hepatitis B in the liver allograft is becoming an increasingly rare event because of the effectiveness of current antiviral regimens. Successful antiviral therapy has translated into marked improvement in both patient and graft survival rates after liver transplantation. Graft survival rates now approach those achieved in transplantation for other nonmalignant hepatic diseases. The only drawback to this impressive positive turnaround is the need for lifelong HBIG, lamivudine, or combination therapy.

Recurrent Hepatitis C

Clinical Presentation

Allograft hepatitis C presents primarily as asymptomatic elevations in liver enzymes and is difficult to distinguish from rejection.[75] A minority of patients develop more severe evidence of hepatic dysfunction, and a rare patient may experience fibrosing cholestatic hepatitis. Although HCV RNA levels increase posttransplantation under the influence of immunosuppression, HCV RNA levels do not correlate well with the risk or severity of allograft hepatitis.

Risk Factors

A pretransplantation diagnosis of chronic HCV is the primary risk factor for allograft hepatitis C.[76,77] Recipient serology prior to transplantation predicts the likelihood of posttransplantation HCV infection: 86% if enzyme immunoassay is positive, 93% if recombinant immunoblot assay (RIBA) is positive, and 97% if HCV RNA is positive. HCV-negative recipients of a liver from a donor who is HCV RNA positive universally develop posttransplantation HCV.[78] HCV-negative recipients of a liver from a donor positive for HCV antibody but negative for HCV RNA may not develop posttransplantation HCV infection. Transplantation of HCV-infected livers into HCV-positive recipients does not appear to lead to a worse posttransplantation course.[79]

---

*At Colorado, we give HBIG 10,000 IU intravenously (40 mL) during the anhepatic phase, 5,000 IU (20 mL) intravenously daily for the first week posttransplantation, 2,500 IU (10 mL) intramuscularly every 2 weeks for 2 months, and then 2,500 IU (10 mL) intramuscularly monthly thereafter. In addition, we use no steroids for immunosuppression in our recipients with hepatitis B. Efficacy is similar to that reported with the higher-dose IV regimens.

†We give 100 mg to 150 mg lamivudine per day prior to transplantation, stop lamivudine the day after transplantation, and use the posttransplantation HBIG protocol mentioned in the previous footnote. No patient on this protocol has experienced recurrent HBV infection or disease.

Diagnosis

Allograft hepatitis C is suspected when an HCV-positive recipient develops asymptomatic elevations in AST and ALT. Liver biopsy demonstrates a predominantly portal inflammatory reaction. In general, there is a predominance of lymphocytes, but the reaction in early hepatitis is mixed, with all inflammatory cell types represented, making the distinction from allograft rejection difficult.[47,49,50] When present, lymphoid follicles and lobular hepatitis are features that tend to differentiate HCV from allograft rejection. Both HCV and allograft rejection can cause bile duct injury.

Treatment

There is currently no widely accepted successful intervention for prevention or treatment of HCV recurrence. Patients are monitored for evidence of recurrent hepatitis by liver function tests and liver biopsy. Antiviral interventions are typically used only after the patient has achieved a stable posttransplantation course and histologic changes of recurrent hepatitis C are documented. Unlike hepatitis B, there is no effective immunoglobulin prophylactic regimen for hepatitis C.

Treatment of patients with decompensated cirrhosis with interferon is complicated by underlying hypersplenism, neutropenia, and thrombocytopenia. Interferon causes neutropenia and thrombocytopenia, which can exacerbate these preexisting conditions. Ribavirin causes hemolytic anemia. Despite these concerns, some centers, including ours, have begun treating patients with decompensated cirrhosis with combination therapy and have observed an HCV RNA clearance rate on treatment of 20% to 30% (unpublished data). Several patients have required supplementation with either granulocyte colony-stimulating factor (G-CSF) or erythropoietin to maintain cell counts. Two of our patients rendered HCV RNA negative by combination therapy prior to transplantation have undergone transplantation and have normal ALT levels and are negative for HCV RNA 6 months posttransplantation.

Prophylaxis with interferon monotherapy may reduce the incidence and severity of recurrence of allograft hepatitis.[80] However, prophylaxis has not been shown to lower viral titer, reduce graft loss, or improve patient survival.

Posttransplantation treatment of established allograft hepatitis C with interferon monotherapy has been disappointing, with very few virologic responders.[81] Although responses may be better with combination therapy, this treatment is poorly tolerated. Anemia due to ribavirin may be more pronounced because of interference with renal excretion of ribavirin by cyclosporine or tacrolimus.

Outcome

Graft and patient survival rates during the immediate postoperative period in patients who undergo transplantation for HCV are similar to survival rates of non-HCV cohorts. In one analysis, 28% of all deaths in HCV-positive recipients were directly related to HCV recurrence.[76] Pretransplantation characteristics associated with mortality in HCV-infected recipients include HCV RNA level greater than or equal to 1×10^6 vEq/mL, Child-Pugh-Turcotte score of 10 or higher, nonwhite race, and advanced age.

Posttransplantation factors associated with increased mortality include treatment for acute cellular rejection, treatment for steroid-resistant rejection, and mean steroid dose greater than or equal to 100 mg per day in the first 42 days posttransplantation. Inappropriate use of steroids and other antirejection treatments in the early postoperative period in recipients infected with HCV might accelerate allograft hepatitis and result in poorer long-term outcomes.

Drug Hepatotoxicity

Drug toxicities may also emerge during the early postoperative period. Cyclosporine and tacrolimus typically cause cholestasis that is readily reversed by lowering the drug dosage. Azathioprine can cause a mixed hepatocellular injury with cholestasis, but this reaction is rare. Similarly, hepatic injury from mycophenolate mofetil, rapamycin (sirolimus), or steroids is distinctly uncommon.

This patient population may be uniquely predisposed to hepatotoxicity from total parenteral nutrition (TPN). Mechanisms of TPN-induced liver injury and cholestasis are poorly characterized but may involve abnormalities in metabolism of bile acids.[82] Posttransplantation impairment of synthesis of bile acids, reduced biliary secretion, and altered intestinal absorption may all predispose to TPN cholestasis. Treatment is reduction or removal of TPN. Additional interventions of unproven benefit include administration of ursodeoxycholic acid, vitamin E, glutamine, or *N*-acetylcysteine.

Surgical Complications

The surgical complications that occur in the immediate postoperative period are summarized in Table 10.3.

Postoperative Hemorrhage

Postoperative bleeding is the most common surgical complication occurring after liver transplantation. Published reports suggest that 10% to 15% of patients require reoperation for intraabdominal hemorrhage.[83] In our experience, 77 (12%) of 557 patients undergoing transplantation required reoperation for suspected surgical bleeding. Ten of the 77 had either primary nonfunction (n = 6), hepatic artery thrombosis (n = 3), or portal vein thrombosis (n = 1). Associated comorbidities in our 77 patients included blood transfusion (60%), thrombocytopenia requiring platelet transfusion (40%), perioperative renal dysfunction (44%), perioperative dialysis (29%), hyperglycemia requiring insulin (35%), and hypertension (14%).

Reports suggest that as many as two-thirds of patients undergoing reoperation for hemorrhage will die within 6 months of transplantation.[83] Our own experience contradicts this data; only 12 (15%) of our 77 patients died within 6 months of transplantation. Reoperation requires careful examination of all vascular anastomoses, but a point source of bleeding is found in only one-half of cases.

Bleeding related to coagulopathy is typically slower, and patients remain more stable, with less requirement for volume and blood replacement. Occasionally reoperation is required to be certain that there is no major vessel bleeding and to evacuate hematoma from the abdomen. The primary therapy is to identify and correct the coagulopathy, typically with fresh frozen plasma, cryoprecipitate, and platelets.[84] If liver allograft function recovers, the coagulopathy typically resolves quickly; if liver graft function is compromised, coagulopathy persists.

Hepatic Artery Thrombosis

Clinical Presentation

Hepatic artery thrombosis is the second leading cause of graft failure in the immediate postoperative period.[24] It complicates 2% to 8% of adult liver transplantations and accounts for 60% of all posttransplantation vascular complications.[85–89] Hepatic artery thrombosis has three main clinical syndromes: hepatic failure, delayed bile leak, and relapsing bacteremia. Hepatic failure is caused by complete thrombosis of the artery within the first few days to 2 weeks after the transplantation. AST and ALT rise precipitously and herald liver failure and multiorgan compromise. Emergent revascularization or retransplantation is required for survival. Delayed bile leak is caused by ischemic injury and necrosis of the donor bile duct and presents between 7 days to 2 months posttransplantation.[90] Bilomas commonly occur in this setting.[91] Occasionally, patients tolerate arterial thrombosis and do not experience significant graft dysfunction or major biliary injury. Patients in this group may experience relapsing bacteremia. Often the symptoms and bacteremia will respond to antibiotics, and the thrombosis may not be appreciated until a second or third episode triggers evaluation of the artery.

Hepatic artery stenosis without thrombosis may lead to insidious graft dysfunction, with a median time to diagnosis of 100 days.[92] Diagnosis of hepatic artery stenosis should trigger attempts at balloon angioplasty or surgery with revision of the anastomosis or implantation of vascular grafts (Fig. 10.7).

Risk Factors

The primary cause of hepatic artery thrombosis is technical difficulty with performance of the transplantation. Rates of hepatic artery thrombosis are increased in the pediatric population; thrombosis may occur in 10% to 25% of transplants in small-sized children (younger than 2 years). Allograft factors that may contribute to thrombosis include lack of arterial collaterals, prolonged cold ischemic time, rejection, variants in arterial anatomy, and need for vascular grafts. Grafts with hepatic arterial flows below 400 mL/min, or arterial flows below 7% of cardiac output, are 5 times more likely to develop thrombosis.[93] Recipient risk factors for thrombosis include ABO incompatibility, polycythemia, thrombocytosis, use of fresh frozen plasma, intrinsic or acquired hypercoagulable states, and comorbidity, such as CMV infection, sepsis, or postoperative pancreatitis.

Diagnosis

The preferred initial investigation of the hepatic artery is by Doppler ultrasonography, but its sensitivity and specificity for detection of thrombosis have yet to be defined. When hepatic artery thrombosis is detected by ultrasonography or highly suspected by clinical features, angiography is needed to establish the diagnosis and potentially to administer therapy (Fig. 10.7).[94–97] When angiography is contraindicated, one can attempt to assess arterial flow using magnetic resonance angiography or can urgently reoperate.

Treatment

Thrombosis complicated by infection requires antibiotic therapy directed against gram-positive bacteria, gram-negative bacteria, and enterococcus, and drainage of infected bilomas. Bile leaks and fistulas may require placement of internal stents [by endoscopic retrograde cholangiopancreatography (ERCP)] or external/internal biliary drains [by percutaneous transhepatic cholangiography (PTC)]. If arterial thrombosis is detected early, one may attempt to resolve the ischemic injury via angiographic means using dissolution agents, thrombectomy, or vascular stenting.[95,97] If radiologic intervention is contraindicated or unsuccessful, emergent reoperation and reconstruction of the arterial anastomosis may be required.[94,96] The reported success of attempts at early revascularization has varied widely, ranging from 20% to 75%.

Outcome

Mortality rates for patients whose transplantation is complicated by hepatic artery thrombosis range from 20% to 60%. We experienced 25 arterial thromboses in 577 transplants (4.3%). Nineteen (76%) were retransplanted, and 6 (24%) were not revascularized or retransplanted and the grafts are currently functional; there were only 4 deaths (16%).

The literature suggests that urgent revascularization may salvage 20% to 40% of grafts, but the majority of patients will require retransplantation. Salvage rates with urgent revascularization are best when patients are asymptomatic and the thrombosis is detected by routine screening Doppler ultrasonography (82% salvage rate).

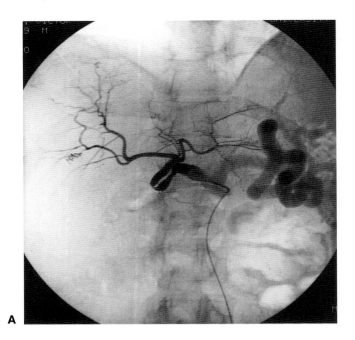
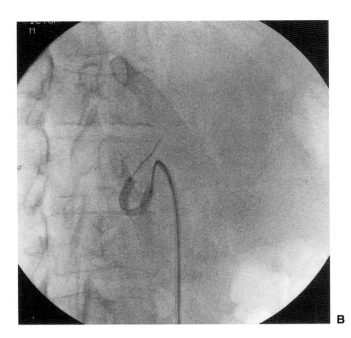
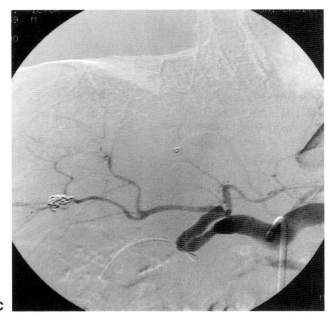

FIG. 10.7. Angiograms demonstrate **A:** stenosis of the hepatic artery, **B:** balloon dilation of stenosis, and **C:** the result of balloon angioplasty of the stenosis.

Once patients are symptomatic, only 15% of grafts are saved.[97]

Portal Vein Thrombosis

Clinical Presentation

Portal vein thrombosis is less common than hepatic artery thrombosis, occurring in only 1% to 3% of transplant re-

cipients.[98] Clinical manifestations include hepatic failure, complications of portal hypertension such as variceal hemorrhage or encephalopathy, and asymptomatic elevations seen in liver tests.[98–100] Hepatic failure is restricted to thromboses that occur within the first month. Associated manifestations may include edema, ascites, variceal hemorrhage, encephalopathy, and multiorgan failure. In contrast, presentation with complications of portal hypertension is more typical of thrombosis occurring after 1 month.

Cholangitis and biliary sepsis are not features of portal vein thrombosis.

Risk Factors

Technical factors associated with risk of portal vein thrombosis are misalignment or excessive vessel length, stenosis of anastomosis (Fig. 10.8), use of bypass catheters, retransplantation, and portosystemic shunt surgery. Other risk factors include allograft rejection, hypercoagulable states, and pretransplantation diagnosis of portal vein thrombosis or Budd-Chiari syndrome.

Diagnosis

The diagnosis is suspected when the patient experiences hepatic dysfunction or clinical manifestations of portal hypertension. Doppler ultrasonography or dual-phase computed tomographic (CT) scanning is used initially, but the diagnosis requires angiographic confirmation (Fig.).

Treatment

The choice of treatment will depend on the clinical presentation, residual amount of portal flow, and degree of liver injury. Patients with significant hepatic dysfunction should be considered for revascularization or retransplantation. In contrast, patients with established portal hypertension may be best served by radiologic thrombectomy, lytic therapy, stenting of underlying portal vein stenosis, or performance of decompressive shunt surgery.[101–105]

Outflow Obstruction (Inferior Vena Caval or Hepatic Venous Complications)

Clinical Presentation

The original surgical technique for liver transplantation described in 1963 by Starzl involved removal of the retrohepatic cava, use of venovenous bypass (femoral-portal-axillary), and performance of two end-to-end anastomoses of the donor inferior vena cava (IVC) with the recipient IVC. In 1968, Calne reported the first use of the piggyback technique, in which the donor hepatic veins are connected end to end to the recipient's hepatic veins, allowing preservation of IVC flow during the procedure and avoidance of venovenous bypass. Modifications of the latter technique have included use of patch grafts, performance of end-to-side anastomosis to the IVC, and inclusion of a portion of donor IVC with performance of side-to-side anastomosis.[106] Recent published series have indicated that as many as 80% of liver transplant procedures are currently performed using the piggyback technique or these modifications.[107]

The clinical presentation of outflow obstruction varies depending on the type of outflow anastomosis and the location

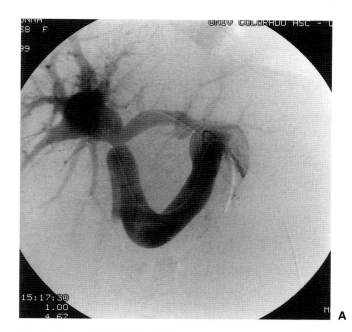

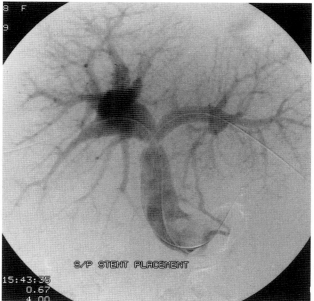

FIG. 10.8. A: Portal venography demonstrates stenosis at the portal venous anastomosis. **B:** Angioplasty and stenting of the stenosis corrected the portal hypertension and partially resolved the splenomegaly.

of the obstruction. A secondary consequence of venous obstruction and stagnation of blood flow is thrombosis. With the standard technique, IVC obstruction may occur at either the infrahepatic or suprahepatic caval anastomoses. Obstruction of the infrahepatic cava does not compromise graft function but impairs venous return from the lower extremities. The main clinical manifestations of infrahepatic caval obstruction are normal hepatic function, edema of the lower half of the body, and development of lumbar collaterals. Renal vein thrombosis may complicate caval obstruction.

Obstruction of the suprahepatic cava results in impairment of venous return from the lower half of the body and manifests the same clinical features noted for infrahepatic caval obstruction. In addition, the outflow from the graft is compromised and patients can manifest the entire spectrum of Budd-Chiari syndrome. With the piggyback technique, or its modifications, caval obstruction is rare; outflow obstruction is manifested as Budd-Chiari syndrome.

There are three main complications involving the venous outflow tract: hemorrhage, venous congestion, and Budd-Chiari syndrome. Hemorrhage (1% to 2% incidence) is related to either anastomotic leak or bleeding from collateral venous channels from the recipient IVC. It is usually recognized intraoperatively or within 24 hours of initial surgery.

Venous congestion, requiring repositioning of the graft or revision of the anastomosis, or Budd-Chiari syndrome occur in 1% to 3% of transplants. Signs and symptoms include hepatic dysfunction and portal hypertension with coagulopathy, jaundice, ascites, and gastrointestinal bleeding. Late presentation of hepatic outflow obstruction, more than 1 month posttransplantation, manifests primarily as hepatomegaly and ascites.

Risk Factors

Obstruction to outflow from the hepatic graft is primarily related to technical difficulties with performance of the vascular anastomoses. The risk of Budd-Chiari syndrome after the caval preservation operations may be reduced by use of a side-to-side caval patch. Recipient factors that increase the risk of outflow obstruction or Budd-Chiari syndrome include a hypercoagulable state, pretransplantation diagnosis of Budd-Chiari syndrome or portal vein thrombosis, pretransplantation diagnosis of hepatocellular carcinoma, and anatomic abnormalities of the IVC or hepatic veins (agenesis, fibrous stenosis).

Diagnosis

The results of liver blood tests may be normal or only mildly altered. Findings on biopsy that raise the possibility of outflow obstruction include central lobular congestion and necrosis, diapedesis of red blood cells into the space of Disse, and cholestasis in the absence of other features of rejection or hepatitis. Doppler ultrasonography reveals an enlarged liver with marked reduction of flow, stasis, or thrombosis in the hepatic venous outflow. Hepatic and IVC venography is the gold standard for diagnosis.

Treatment

Acute outflow obstruction presenting within the first few days after the transplantation is a graft- and life-threatening condition, usually necessitating emergent revision of the out-

flow anastomosis or retransplantation. Chronic outflow obstruction with preservation of graft function may be managed conservatively with diuretic therapy, radiologic evaluation of venous anastomoses, and angioplasty or stenting of outflow stenoses.[108] Transjugular intrahepatic portosystemic shunts may reverse Budd-Chiari syndrome, but they should be used selectively to avoid complications that would make performance of retransplantation more difficult.

Other Vascular Complications

Rare or unusual vascular complications include hepatic artery pseudoaneurysm, hepatic artery rupture, arteriovenous fistula, or arteriobiliary fistula.

Biliary Tract Complications

Biliary tract complications occur in approximately 10% to 20% of all liver transplant recipients.[109–124] Eighty percent of all biliary complications occur within the first 6 months after transplantation, and the vast majority of these within the first 3 months. In the early postoperative period (less than 3 months) two main types of biliary complications occur: bile leaks and strictures. These complications are caused by either technical complications at the anastomosis or ischemic injury related to compromised arterial blood supply. Preservation injury, immunologic factors (rejection of biliary epithelium), and ascending infection may contribute to destruction of the biliary system.[109]

Bile Leak

Clinical Presentation. Early bile leaks, occurring within the first few days after the transplantation, are usually caused by disruption of the surgical anastomosis. Late bile leaks are caused either by ischemic injury from hepatic artery thrombosis or by removal of T tubes.[109–113] Less common sites of bile leaks include the cut surface of reduced-size grafts, split livers, or partial grafts from living donors; the cystic duct remnant; unrecognized accessory ducts; or choledochoenteric anastomoses. Patients with bile leaks complain of pain in the right upper quadrant of the abdomen and may experience fever and leukocytosis. Fluid evacuated from abdominal drains may appear bilious.

Risk Factors. In general, early bile leak is from anastomotic sites and is related to technical complications with the surgical procedure or local ischemic injury to the donor duct. The surgical literature emphasizes the importance of adequate hepatic arterial flow, observation of bleeding at the cut ends of ducts prior to anastomosis, avoidance of excessive dissection of periductal tissue during organ procurement, prevention of excessive tension on the anastomosis, and avoidance of electrocautery.[114] Bile leak after T-tube removal is related to inadequate development of a fibrous fistulous tract along the course of the T tube, probably caused by impairment of fibrogenesis under immuno-

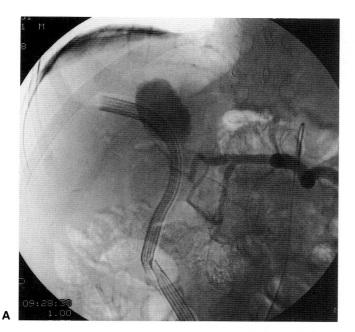 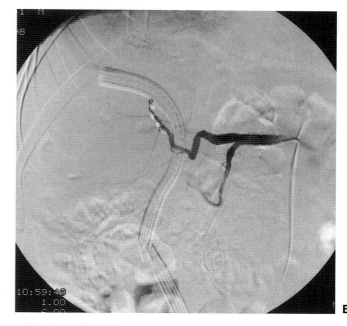

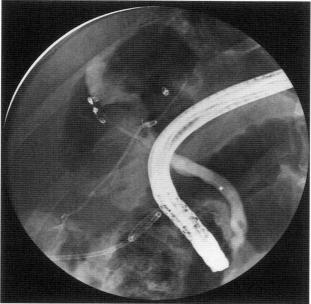

FIG. 10.9. Case of arteriobiliary fistula in patient with jaundice and upper gastrointestinal bleed. **A:** Arteriogram demonstrates arterial communication with amorphous space. **B:** Arteriographic coil enbolization of fistua. **C:** Cholangiogram obtained at endoscopic cholangiography (ERCP) demonstrates biliary leak/fistula.

suppression, especially with use of steroids.[120] Bile leak from T-tube removal is eliminated by the use of internal stents.[124]

Diagnosis. Liver test results may indicate hyperbilirubinemia without substantial increases in liver enzymes. Biliary scintigraphy is a noninvasive test that can be diagnostic with large bile leaks; it is less useful with small, contained leaks. Cholangiography (ERCP or PTC) is the gold stan-

dard for diagnosis (Fig. 10.9.c). Doppler ultrasonography for assessment of hepatic arterial flow is indicated in all patients sustaining a bile leak, except leaks directly related to T-tube removal.

Treatment. Early recognition of anastomotic bile leak is essential for achieving an optimal outcome.[119–124] In general, reoperation and surgical revision is required. Less invasive procedures, such as ERCP and stent placement, should be reserved for small, contained leaks. Management of late bile leaks related to hepatic artery thrombosis is focused on infectious complications and provision of biliary drainage (ERCP- or PTC-directed stenting) or drainage of infected bilomas. Ultimately, these patients may require retransplantation. Bile leak after T-tube removal has been effectively treated with endoscopic stenting and antibiotic therapy, avoiding the need for surgical intervention.

Biliary Strictures

There are two main types of strictures: anastomotic and ischemic. The mechanisms of injury that promote these types of biliary complications are similar to those noted previously for bile leaks.

Clinical Presentation. Anastomotic strictures typically evolve over an extended period of time and emerge clinically beyond the first month posttransplantation.[109–113] Patients may present with jaundice, cholangitis, or asymptomatic elevations seen in liver test results. Obstruction, uncomplicated by infection, typically causes a predominant increase in bilirubin, alkaline phosphatase, or γ-glutamyl transferase (GGT). Cases presenting with infection or cholangitis may be characterized by predominant elevations in AST and ALT. Choledocholithiasis does not complicate strictures presenting within the first 3 posttransplantation months, and the "biliary sludge syndrome" appears to be unique to biliary ischemia associated with hepatic artery thrombosis.[112]

Ischemic strictures typically are restricted to the donor side of the biliary anastomosis, are found in multiple locations, and are both intrahepatic and extrahepatic. Diffuse strictures in the setting of bile leaks and bilomas indicate hepatic artery thrombosis and the need for retransplantation. Focal intrahepatic strictures may occur in the setting of patency of the hepatic artery and may be managed conservatively without need for retransplantation.

Strictures caused by recurrent disease (primary sclerosing cholangitis) do not occur within the first 3 posttransplantation months.

Risk Factors. Some of the risk factors for development of biliary strictures were noted previously in the sections on bile leaks and hepatic artery thrombosis. Additional factors that may be particularly relevant to focal intrahepatic strictures include extended preservation times, ABO incompatibility, and ductopenic rejection. Conditions that impair the inflow of blood to the graft, in the absence of arterial thrombosis, may theoretically promote ischemic biliary injury. These include systemic hypotension, use of vasoconstrictive agents, and increased vascular resistance within the allograft (right heart failure, venous outflow obstruction, cellular rejection).[109]

Diagnosis. Cholangiography (ERCP or PTC) is the gold standard for the diagnosis and management of biliary strictures (Fig. 10.10). These procedures require antibiotic coverage to avoid or reduce the risk of septic complications.

Treatment. First-line therapy of anastomotic strictures is ERCP with balloon dilatation and stenting.[121,122] Surgical re-

vision is reserved for patients in whom ERCP (or PTC) is technically impossible or who have had prior unsuccessful attempts at endoscopic or radiologic management. Focal ischemic-type biliary strictures may also be managed with the same nonoperative interventions. However, the long-term patency rate is diminished compared with the results when similar methods are used for anastomotic strictures. Diffuse biliary strictures in the setting of hepatic artery thrombosis do not respond to either nonsurgical or surgical interventions and should trigger the need for retransplantation.

Outcome. The short- and long-term outcomes after treatment of anastomotic strictures are excellent. Late surgical revisions may be required in a minority of patients. Focal intrahepatic ischemic-type strictures typically require repeated dilatations and stent procedures. However, stents are prone to superimposed infectious complications, including fungal colonization. Some authors have advocated hepatic resection of the involved segment or lobe; however, data supporting this aggressive surgical approach are limited. Focal extrahepatic ischemic-type strictures are more amenable to endoscopic or radiologic management, but recurrence rates are high, necessitating repeated procedures. Surgical revision with fashioning of a Roux-en-Y anastomosis may ultimately be required. Diffuse intrahepatic and extrahepatic biliary strictures do not respond adequately to any of these interventions, and retransplantation is usually required. Late consequences of biliary strictures include choledocholithiasis, cholangitis, and pancreatitis.

Choledochocholedochostomy without T Tube

Duct-to-duct anastomoses in liver recipients are prone to edema and focal ischemia, narrowing, bile leaks, and strictures. For this reason, most surgical teams have used stenting or decompression to protect the anastomosis. The most common practice is to insert a T tube at the time of fashioning the anastomosis. T tubes allow external drainage of bile and maintenance of low pressure within the extrahepatic biliary tree. However, T-tube drainage interrupts the enterohepatic circulation of bile acids. Bile acids are responsible for micelle formation and are critical for adequate absorption of cyclosporine. Tacrolimus is less dependent on bile acids for its absorption.

External drainage of bile via T tubes may require use of intravenous forms of cyclosporine, which are more costly than oral preparations and are associated with an increased risk of adverse effects such as renal failure and neurotoxicity, including seizures. In addition, internal stents may be associated with a lower risk of stricture, and the risk of bile leak after T-tube removal is eliminated. Many programs have switched to internal stenting after choledochocholedochostomy.

Medical Complications

The medical complications that occur in the immediate posttransplantation period are summarized in Table 10.4.

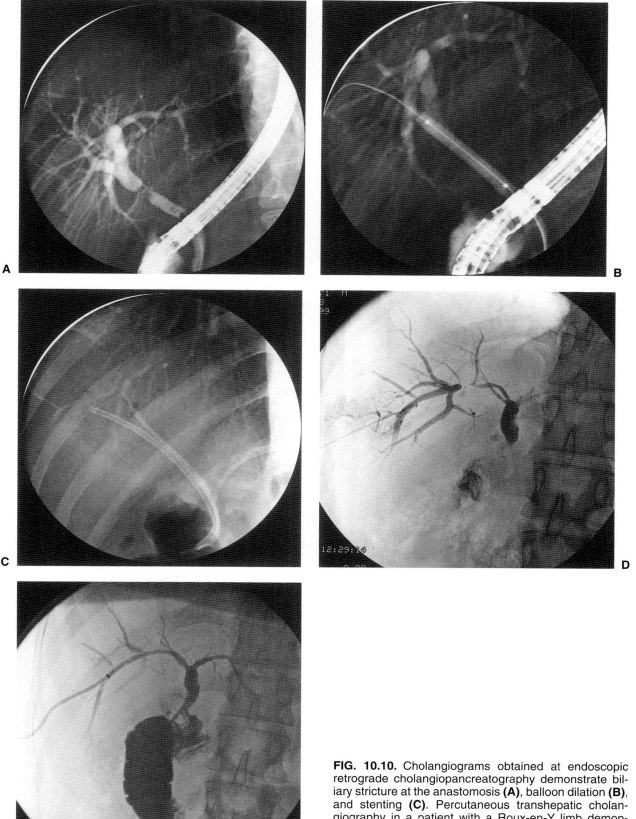

FIG. 10.10. Cholangiograms obtained at endoscopic retrograde cholangiopancreatography demonstrate biliary stricture at the anastomosis **(A)**, balloon dilation **(B)**, and stenting **(C)**. Percutaneous transhepatic cholangiography in a patient with a Roux-en-Y limb demonstrates a focal ischemic-type stricture of the right hepatic duct **(D)** and treatment by placement of external-internal biliary drain **(E)**.

TABLE 10.4. *Medical complications occurring in the immediate postoperative period*

Infections
  Bacterial
  Viral
    Cytomegalovirus
    Epstein-Barr virus
  Fungal
    Candidiasis, torulopsosis
    Pneumocystis carinii pneumonia
  Aspergillosis, mucormycosis
Respiratory complications
  Pneumonia
  Pulmonary edema
  Adult respiratory distress syndrome
  Portopulmonary hypertension
  Hepatopulmonary syndrome
Renal failure
Cardiovascular disease
  Hypertension
  Myocardial ischemia
  Valvular heart disease
  Cardiomyopathy
    Idiopathic hypertrophic subaortic stenosis
    Hemochromatosis
Neurologic complications
  Central pontine myelinolysis
  Seizures
  Central nervous system hemorrhage
  Ischemic events
Coagulopathy
  Thrombocytopenia
  Disseminated intravascular coagulation
Diabetes mellitus

Infections

The occurrence of infectious complications follows a predictable chronological sequence after transplantation (Fig. 10.11).[12,13] The majority of infectious complications occurring in the first week are bacterial, usually caused by indwelling catheters (~30%), pneumonia (~25%), abdominal or biliary infections (~15%), and wound infection (~10%). Gram-negative bacteremia should prompt investigation of the biliary tree. Bacteremia is more common in patients with underlying diabetes mellitus and poor nutritional state.[125] Fever and leukocytosis are often, but not invariably, associated with development of infection.[126,127] Mortality is higher in bacteremic patients and is primarily related to ICU stay, need for pressor support, and poor graft function. Prophylaxis with G-CSF is ineffective in preventing infectious complications.[128]

Opportunistic infections are rare within the first week, except for herpetic stomatitis or mucocutaneous candidiasis. Although graft injury from recurrent hepatitis C may occur within the first week, graft injury from hepatitis B is most often delayed beyond 1 month.

Tissue-invasive or systemic viral infections typically emerge after the first month and include infections from CMV, Epstein-Barr virus (EBV), varicella zoster virus (VZV), and adenovirus. Manifestations of CMV infections are hepatitis, gastritis, colitis, or CMV syndrome (flu-like symptoms with low-grade fever, leukopenia, and failure to thrive). EBV can emerge as hepatitis, mononucleosis-like syndrome, or posttransplantation lymphoproliferative disease (after 6 months). VZV emerges primarily as shingles and usually occurs later than 2 months posttransplantation. Adenovirus is rare but should be considered in the patient with unexplained severe hepatitis beyond the first month.

Other opportunistic infections that may emerge between months 1 and 3 include infections caused by *Nocardia asteroides*, *Listeria monocytogenes*, *Mycobacterium tuberculosis*, *Pneumocystis carinii*, *Aspergillus*, or *Mucor*, and tissue-invasive candidal infections.

Cytomegalovirus Infection

CMV infection is common; 60% to 90% of adults exhibit serologic evidence of prior exposure and infection. Eighty-one percent of our center's adult recipient population were seropositive for prior CMV infection. Immunosuppression activates CMV viral replication, leading to viremia and shedding of virus in urine and throat washings. The finding of CMV in low titer (100 to 1,000 vEq/mL) in blood or

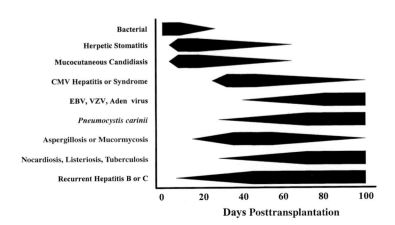

FIG. 10.11. The time course of occurrence of infectious complications. Bacterial infection predominates in the first week. Invasive opportunistic infections may appear in the first 2 to 3 weeks but more typically emerge after the first month. CMV, cytomegalovirus; EBV, Epstein-Barr virus; VZV, varicella zoster virus.

positive cultures of urine or throat washings are nonspecific and do not establish a diagnosis of CMV disease.

Clinical Presentation. CMV infection manifests as CMV hepatitis, CMV syndrome, and extrahepatic CMV.[129–134] CMV hepatitis is characterized by graft dysfunction and nonspecific constitutional complaints. There is a mild increase in aminotransferases, and leukopenia is common. Liver biopsy is required for diagnosis. It is extremely important to distinguish CMV hepatitis from rejection because treatment of CMV hepatitis involves reduction of immunosuppression. CMV syndrome is characterized by malaise, anorexia, arthralgia, myalgia, and headache, and is associated with low-grade fever and leukopenia. There is no evidence of graft dysfunction. Extrahepatic CMV typically manifests as colitis, gastritis, or enteritis, and rarely as pneumonitis, bone marrow infection, or chorioretinitis.

Risk Factors. The primary determinant of risk of CMV infection is the pretransplantation status of CMV serology in both donor and recipient (Table 10.5). Recipients naive to CMV have approximately a 50% chance of posttransplantation CMV disease if they receive a liver from a CMV-positive donor. Increased immunosuppression, especially OKT3, increases the risk of CMV disease. High levels of CMV DNA (using cutoffs between 2,000 and 7,000 vEq/mL) are independently predictive of CMV disease.[135,136]

Diagnosis. The diagnosis of CMV hepatitis is dependent on liver biopsy. Findings include microabscesses, lobular hepatitis, liver cell necrosis, and nuclear inclusions in hepatocytes (magenta-colored nuclear inclusion on hematoxylin and eosin stains, with a clear halo around the inclusion). Confirmatory tests include positive blood culture, positive blood CMV DNA, or positive culture of liver tissue. Diagnosis of CMV syndrome is supported by positive blood cultures for CMV or by positive CMV DNA with titer greater than 1,000 vEq/mL. Diagnosis of extrahepatic CMV is dependent on demonstration of CMV in biopsy specimens, resolution of signs and symptoms of disease with eradication of the virus, and recovery without recurrence of infection.

Prophylaxis. The CMV serologies of the donor and the recipient are reviewed by the blood bank at the time of transplantation. If both donor and recipient are CMV negative (~5% of cases), efforts are made to use only CMV-negative or leukocyte-poor blood products. This practice virtually eliminates the possibility of CMV disease in these recipients. Prophylaxis with ganciclovir, given either intravenously or orally for up to 3 months, is recommended for the specific situation in which the recipient is CMV negative and receives a graft from a CMV-positive donor (7 to 15% of cases). This prophylactic regimen reduces the risk of CMV disease in the recipient by 75%.[137–139] Similar prophylaxis is advised for patients treated with OKT3 or other antilymphocyte globulins, although efficacy is undefined. Prophylaxis with ganciclovir is superior to high-dose acyclovir (Fig. 10.12).

Treatment of Established Infection. There are three approaches to the treatment of established CMV infection: reduction in immunosuppression, antiviral therapy (ganciclovir, foscarnet), and use of immunoglobulin with high titers of CMV antibodies. The most experience has been gained with intravenous ganciclovir in doses of 5 mg/kg twice a day given initially and then followed by oral ganci-

TABLE 10.5. *Cytomegalovirus serology in liver recipients and risk of cytomegalovirus infection or disease*

	Percentage of recipients		Percentage risk of CMV disease or infection	
Serology	Study 1[a]	Study 2[b]	Study 1[c]	Study 2[d]
D+ / R+	50	56	18	40
D+ / R−	15	11	44	55
D− / R+	34	27	8	37
D− / R−	1	6	NE	25

CMV, cytomegalovirus; D+, donor positive for CMV antibody; D−, donor negative for CMV antibody; R+, recipient positive for CMV antibody; R−, recipient negative for CMV antibody; NE, not evaluated.

[a]Gane E, Saliba F, Valdecasas GJC, et al. Randomised trial of efficacy and safety of oral ganciclovir in the prevention of cytomegalovirus disease in liver transplant recipients. *Lancet* 1997;350:1729–1733.

[b]Winston DJ, Wirin D, Shaked A, et al. Randomized comparison of ganciclovir and high-dose acyclovir for long-term cytomegalovirus prophylaxis in liver transplant recipients. *Lancet* 1995;346:69–74.

[c]Rates reported are for CMV disease in untreated controls.

[d]Rates reported are for CMV infection in recipients treated intravenously and then orally with high-dose acyclovir for 100 days. The overall rate of CMV disease in this study was only 10% in the acyclovir arm and 0.8% in the intravenous ganciclovir arm (100 days).

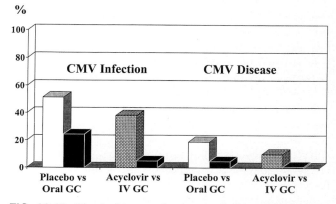

FIG. 10.12. The incidence of cytomegalovirus (CMV) infection and disease after liver transplantation from two separate studies.[138,139] Rates of CMV infection are approximately 50% for placebo (white bar), 38% for high-dose acyclovir given orally and intravenously, 25% for oral ganciclovir (GC), and 5% for intravenous ganciclovir. Rates of CMV disease are approximately 20% for placebo, 10% for high-dose acyclovir, 5% for oral ganciclovir, and 1% for intravenous ganciclovir. The duration of treatment was 98 days in one study and 100 days in the other.

clovir 1 gm three times a day for a total course of 6 weeks to 3 months. Complete or partial resolution of disease with CMV suppression occurs in over 90% of cases. Valganciclovir is currently being evaluated in clinical trials.[140] CMV antibody therapy may accelerate clearance of CMV, enhance the response to ganciclovir, and favor rapid resolution of disease. However, this treatment is expensive, has not been demonstrated to positively affect graft or patient outcome, and is not used routinely by most liver transplant centers. Recent analyses suggest that CMV disease occurring in the immediate postoperative period may increase hospital cost and length of stay, the risk of hepatic artery thrombosis, and the severity of HCV recurrence, and may reduce long-term patient survival.[131-134]

Epstein-Barr Virus Infection

Clinical Presentation. Manifestations of EBV infection that may occur in the early posttransplantation period include EBV viremia, EBV hepatitis, and EBV mononucleosis-like syndrome.[141] Patients experience constitutional, flu-like symptoms, and those with hepatitis exhibit nonspecific elevations in liver enzymes, with AST or ALT less than 200 IU/L. EBV-associated posttransplantation lymphoproliferative disease (PTLD) typically occurs later than the first 3 months after transplantation.[142]

Risk Factors. Ninety percent of recipients of adult liver transplants have serologic evidence of prior EBV infection. Seronegative recipients of a liver from a seropositive donor are at risk for acute EBV disease and hepatitis. EBV viremia, disease due to reactivation, acquired infection, and the likelihood of PTLD correlate with the level of immunosuppression.

Diagnosis. The clinical features of EBV mononucleosis-like syndrome and CMV syndrome are identical. Differentiation between these two diagnostic possibilities requires culture or quantitation of viral levels of both CMV and EBV. EBV disease is usually associated with viral loads of more than 1,000 vEq/10^5 lymphocytes; CMV disease is usually associated with viral loads of more than 7,000 vEq/mL. In the case of hepatitis, specific immunohistochemical stains of liver tissue or culture of liver tissue may establish the correct etiology.

Treatment and Outcome. Acute EBV disease may resolve after lowering immunosuppression. In some cases, resolution may be accelerated by use of antiviral therapy (ganciclovir or acyclovir) or immunoglobulin therapy. Relapse is the rule after antiviral therapy if immunosuppression cannot be lowered. The major risk of early EBV disease is the late development of PTLD.

Yeast Infections (Candidiasis, Torulopsis)

Clinical Presentation. The most common yeast infection is mucocutaneous candidiasis, primarily with oral or esophageal involvement.[12,13,143] Patients with a prior history of recurrent urinary tract infections or with indwelling catheters in the urinary bladder may also experience *Candida* cystitis or infection with *Torulopsis glabrata.* The major symptom of oral candidiasis is mouth soreness, especially after ingestion of hot liquids or of foods with high acidity. Esophageal involvement is signaled by development of dysphagia or odynophagia. Symptoms of fungal cystitis include urinary frequency, urinary urgency, dysuria, hematuria, persistent pyuria despite antibiotic therapy, and, rarely, unexplained fever. Colonization or superficial infections with yeast appear to predispose the patient to blood-borne dissemination of organisms and establishment of tissue invasion. Sites of dissemination include bone marrow, liver, spleen, kidney, heart (endocarditis), retina (chorioretinitis), and brain.[143-151]

Risk Factors. The risk of invasive fungal infection is directly related to the level of immunosuppression. Additional risk factors include long-term or repeated courses of antibiotics; chronic indwelling lines, catheters, or tubing; TPN; and extended length of ICU stay. Chronic internal/external biliary drainage catheters favor colonization of the biliary tract with yeast. Postsurgical complications may favor extension of infection from drain sites, biliary drains, or the biliary tract into the abdominal cavity and perihepatic space. Contamination of the operative field with yeast may result in infection of vascular anastomoses, mycotic aneurysm, and rupture of the hepatic artery.

Treatment and Outcome. Prophylaxis with fluconazole may lower the risk of both superficial and invasive infection with *Candida* species, excluding *Torulopsis glabrata.*[152] One recent randomized, double-blind, placebo-controlled trial demonstrated that fluconazole, 400 mg per day for 10 weeks posttransplantation, reduced the risk of superficial infection from 28% to 4% ($P < 0.001$) and the risk of invasive infection from 23% to 6% ($P < 0.001$).[152] No hepatotoxicity was reported, but drug interaction necessitated careful monitoring and adjustment of the cyclosporine dose. Despite the apparent microbiological benefit, neither patient nor graft survival were improved by fluconazole prophylaxis.

Treatment of established disease is more problematic. Mucocutaneous candidiasis is readily eradicated by fluconazole (200 to 400 mg per day) and lowering of immunosuppression. Resolution occurs in more than 90% of patients with a single course of therapy, but these patients may still be at risk for dissemination and tissue infection. Some authors have suggested that tissue-invasive infections with *Candida albicans* may also respond to long-term, high-dose fluconazole therapy, but most transplant centers recommend use of amphotericin B, preferably in liposomal or emulsified form.[153] Torulopsis is resistant to triazole therapy and requires use of amphotericin B. In contrast to mold infections (i.e., aspergillosis or mucormycosis), the majority of yeast infections respond to the combination of reduction in immunosuppression and institution of antifungal therapy.

Pneumocystis carinii *Infection*

Clinical Presentation. Pneumocystis carinii infection may present as early as 1 month posttransplantation, usually as pneumonia.[143–146] Clues to diagnosis of *Pneumocystis carinii* pneumonia (PCP) include fever, poorly productive cough, hypoxemia, and radiographic evidence of bilateral reticulonodular pulmonary infiltrates.

Treatment and Outcome. Prior to introduction of prophylactic regimens, the risk of PCP ranged from 10% to 12%.[12,13] Prophylaxis for 3 to 6 months with trimethoprim-sulfamethoxazole (TMP-SMX) (Bactrim DS, MWF), or with inhalation therapy with pentamidine for those with sulfa allergy, has virtually eliminated PCP. TMP-SMX prophylaxis is not only well tolerated but may also reduce the risk of other opportunistic infections such as listeriosis, nocardiosis, and toxoplasmosis.

The length of time of prophylaxis is dictated by the level of maintenance immunosuppression. Some centers continue prophylaxis indefinitely. We stop prophylaxis after 3 months because we taper our patients from steroids within 14 days of the transplant procedure and maintain our patients with relatively low-dose monotherapy (cyclosporine or tacrolimus). Readministration of prophylaxis is indicated whenever aggressive antirejection therapy is used.

Established PCP is diagnosed by bronchoscopically directed lavage, histochemical stains, antigen detection, and culture. Intravenous TMP-SMX is effective if administered early in the clinical course. Late recognition of PCP often results in progressive respiratory compromise, adult respiratory distress syndrome, respiratory failure, and death despite introduction of TMP-SMX therapy. High-dose, intravenous TMP-SMX may potentiate the nephrotoxicity of cyclosporine or tacrolimus. Creatinine concentration and renal function should be closely monitored under this treatment.

Mold Infections (Aspergillosis, Mucormycosis)

Clinical Presentation. Reported series suggest that invasive aspergillosis occurs in 1.5% to 10% of liver recipients.[144–150] A recent series, representing cases from the 1990s, reported a 1% incidence (n = 26) from 5 centers with 2,449 patients.[147] Mucormycosis is much less common, occurring in less than 0.1% of cases.

There are four main clinical presentations of *Aspergillus* infection: disseminated disease with involvement of two or more noncontiguous organs (~60%), pulmonary aspergillosis (~30%), fungal sinusitis (~1%), and wound infection (~10%). Disseminated aspergillosis is suspected in the patient who has unexplained fever that is unresponsive to antibiotics, who has had a complicated clinical course or prolonged ICU stay, or who has evidence of multiorgan failure. Seventy percent of current cases of invasive aspergillosis are diagnosed within the first 3 months posttransplantation.

Infection with *Aspergillus* or *Mucor* may present as fungal sinusitis.[151] This diagnosis is suspected when oral examination reveals a black, necrotic palatal ulcer or CT reveals sinusitis or sinus mass. These findings should prompt emergent otorhinolaryngologic evaluation and biopsy of the lesion with cultures and fungal stains, followed by prompt institution of liposomal amphotericin B treatment and reduction in immunosuppression. Untreated, *Mucor* invades by direct extension into the rhinencephalon and vascular bed, resulting in brain involvement and hematogenous dissemination that leads to death within a few days.

Risk Factors. Immunosuppression is the prerequisite for invasive mold infections. Older series, prior to 1990, indicated that approximately 70% to 80% of cases of invasive aspergillosis were associated with prior use of high-dose steroids or OKT3. Since 1990 only 8% of patients with invasive aspergillosis had received this augmentation of immunosuppression.[147] Thus, it is more likely that global immunosuppression, rather than specific immunosuppressive therapies, is the primary facilitating factor. Additional risk factors for invasive aspergillosis include a history of smoking, prior CMV infection, severe allograft dysfunction, retransplantation, renal failure, dialysis, and multiorgan failure.[143–151]

Treatment and Outcome. Invasive mold infection carries an ominous prognosis. Although anecdotal successes have been reported, in general the therapy of invasive mold infection has been ineffective. Reported series indicate mortality rates of 80% to 100% despite antifungal therapy with amphotericin B, liposomal amphotericin B, itraconazole, or combinations of amphotericin B preparations with either rifampin or flucytosine.[147–153]

Other Infections

Additional opportunistic infections that occur rarely in the setting of liver transplantation but may emerge within the first 3 months include listeriosis, nocardiosis, actinomycosis, histoplasmosis, cryptosporidiosis, and coccidioidomycosis. Certain preexisting parasitic infections, such as strongyloidiasis, toxoplasmosis, leishmaniasis, and trypanosomiasis, may be exacerbated within the first 3 months under immunosuppression.[12]

Mycobacterial infection represents a special condition in which suppression of host immunity may lead to exacerbation of infection. However, flare-up of tuberculosis is rare in liver recipients, with only 0.8% incidence in transplant patients worldwide, and rarer still in the early postoperative period.[12,13,154]

Respiratory Complications

Evaluation of Pulmonary Infiltrates

The risk of respiratory complications is related to hypoventilation and atelectasis caused by the pain and discomfort of major abdominal surgery and residual ascites, a large transfusion requirement, infusion of large volumes of intravenous fluids, preexistent or underlying cardiopulmonary disease, and immunosuppression. Published series suggest that approximately 50% of all liver recipients will have pulmonary infiltrates on radiologic evaluation during their initial recovery from transplantation in the ICU.[4,5,155,156] In approximately half of these patients, the infiltrate is due to intercurrent pulmonary infection.

A recent series (1995 to 1998) described a 44% incidence of pulmonary infiltrates in the ICU.[155] Etiologies included pneumonia (38%), pulmonary edema (40%), atelectasis (10%), adult respiratory distress syndrome (ARDS) (8%), contusion (3%), and unknown (3%). In this report, the most common causes of posttransplantation pneumonia were methicillin-resistant *Staphylococcus aureus* (MRSA) infection (27%), *Pseudomonas aeruginosa* infection (27%), and invasive aspergillosis (20%). Nearly all bacterial pneumonias, except for that caused by *Pseudomonas,* occurred within the first 30 days posttransplantation. Three separate series have suggested that the median time to diagnosis of pulmonary aspergillosis is 17 to 30 days.[147–150] *Pseudomonas* pneumonia emerges in the same time period, with most cases presenting after 30 days. Pulmonary embolus was not reported; in our experience, it is extremely rare posttransplantation.

Management of respiratory compromise is directed at reversing the underlying cause, but a key factor for recovery is restoration of allograft function. Nutritional support is essential; enteral formulas may be administered via a nasogastric or nasojejunal tube beginning the first or second postoperative day. Mechanical ventilation is maintained until ventilatory drive, oxygenation, and pulmonary function are restored. Culture of blood and pulmonary secretions is essential, and bronchoscopy may be required. Early institution of broad-spectrum antibiotics is essential (vancomycin plus levofloxacin or imipenem-cilastatin is our preference). Once specific infectious agents are identified, the antibiotic prescription is tailored to them.

Pulmonary edema is most often related to renal dysfunction and aggressive volume administration in the operative or perioperative period; it is not usually related to cardiac failure. For this reason, posttransplantation pulmonary edema usually resolves with restriction of fluids and administration of loop diuretics (furosemide, hydrochlorothiazide, or ethacrynic acid). Dialysis is used in the oliguric or anuric patient, and Swan-Ganz monitoring is required for patients with borderline cardiac function. Myocardial ischemia or infarction should be ruled out by serial electrocardiograms and cardiac enzyme tests if pulmonary edema fails to respond rapidly to volume removal.

Adult Respiratory Distress Syndrome

De novo ARDS after liver transplantation occurs in as many as 5% to 17% of liver recipients.[4,5,155,157] The major precipitating factor for ARDS is sepsis, occurring in 66% to 100% of cases. Additional risk factors for ARDS include UNOS status 1 or 2A, prolonged ICU stay, hemorrhage, large-volume transfusions, multiorgan failure, and use of OKT3. Nosocomial pneumonia (staphylococcal, gram-negative bacterial, or fungal) should be ruled out by appropriate cultures. Bronchoscopy is often required for rapid diagnosis and institution of appropriate antimicrobial therapy. Because pulmonary embolus is rare, performance of ventilation-perfusion scans or pulmonary angiography is rarely indicated.

Portopulmonary Hypertension

Pulmonary hypertension complicates cirrhosis in 2% to 4% of patients undergoing liver transplantation.[4–7,158] The main symptoms of pulmonary hypertension are fatigue, dyspnea on exertion, and peripheral edema. These symptoms are also highly prevalent in liver patients without pulmonary hypertension. Chest radiograph may demonstrate prominent pulmonary arteries and paucity of vascular markings in the periphery of lung fields. The diagnosis may be suspected by the finding of right bundle branch block, atrial premature contractions, right axis deviation, or right ventricular hypertrophy on electrocardiogram. Although these findings are clues to the diagnosis, echocardiography and confirmatory right heart catheterization are required. Currently, portopulmonary hypertension is defined by the presence of portalsystemic shunting, a mean pulmonary pressure above 25 mm Hg, a pulmonary vascular resistance of more than 120 dyne·s·cm^{-5}, and a pulmonary capillary wedge pressure below 15 mm Hg. Irreversible portopulmonary hypertension with mean pulmonary artery pressure (MPAP) above 45 mm Hg may be a contraindication to liver transplantation.

One recent series examined outcome based solely on MPAP.[159] The authors found that 8.5% of patients undergoing liver transplantation had a MPAP above 25 mm Hg. They defined mild pulmonary hypertension as MPAP between 25 and 44 mm Hg (6.7%), moderate pulmonary hypertension as MPAP between 45 and 59 mm Hg (1.2%), and severe pulmonary hypertension as MPAP of 60 mm Hg or above (0.6%). Patients with mild or moderate pulmonary hypertension had a survival rate equivalent to patients without pulmonary hypertension, but those with severe pulmonary hypertension had progressive pulmonary hypertension and a poor quality of life after transplantation. Mortality in the latter group was 42% at 9 months and 71% at 3 years.

The goals of therapy are improvement in cardiac output, decrease in pulmonary vascular resistance, and decrease in mean pulmonary artery pressure.[160–163] Standard vasodilators, such as oral or transdermal nitrates or calcium channel blockers, have not been effective. The two most promising agents are epoprostenol (2 to 10 ng/kg per minute), given either acutely or by continuous intravenous infusion for maintenance therapy, and nitrous oxide given by inhalation

(80 ppm). Epoprostenol has been evaluated in 15 patients with moderate to severe pulmonary hypertension: MPAP, 50 ± 14 mm Hg; pulmonary vascular resistance (PVR), 525 ± 286 dyne s cm^{-5}; and pulmonary capillary wedge pressure, 12 ± 5 mm Hg. Intravenous epoprostenol reduced the MPAP (-16%) and PVR (-34%) and increased cardiac output ($+21\%$); long-term maintenance infusions in responders further reduced the PVR (-47% from baseline).[160] The overall success of this therapy in management of the liver recipient with pulmonary hypertension is unknown.

Hepatopulmonary Syndrome

Hepatopulmonary syndrome (HPS) complicates cirrhosis in 1% to 2% of patients undergoing hepatic transplantation.[164–169] The diagnosis of HPS is dependent on advanced chronic liver disease, arterial hypoxemia (Pao$_2$ less than 70 mm Hg, or arterial-alveolar gradient greater than 20 mm Hg while breathing room air), and pulmonary vascular dilatations in the absence of intrinsic cardiopulmonary disease. Vascular dilatation is thought to be linked to nitric oxide metabolism. Others have suggested that anatomic microvascular shunts (analogous to spider telangiectasia) in the lung contribute to the ventilation-perfusion mismatch.

The diagnosis is confirmed by "bubble" echocardiography, and the severity of HPS can be assessed by simultaneously measuring the uptake in the lung and brain of intravenously administered macroaggregated albumin (MAA) labeled with technetium Tc 99m.[169] MAA shunt is calculated as the geometric mean of technetium counts (GMT) in brain relative to lung: $[GMT_{brain}/(GMT_{brain} + GMT_{lung})] \times 100\%$. Normoxemic cirrhotic patients without HPS and patients with intrinsic lung disease who lacked liver disease had MAA shunts of $2\% \pm 0.3\%$. In contrast, patients with HPS had markedly elevated MAA shunts, $30\% \pm 4\%$, and there was a highly significant inverse correlation of arterial Po$_2$ with MAA shunt.

The major manifestation of HPS is hypoxemia that responds variably to supplemental oxygen. The syndrome reverses in 60% to 90% of patients following liver transplantation, although prolonged treatment with supplemental oxygen may be necessary for several months following liver transplantation. Despite the apparent beneficial effects of transplantation, patient survival is reduced: 84% at 3 months and 62% at 1 year. Mortality is greatest in those with a pretransplantation Pao$_2$ below 50 mm Hg.

Renal Failure

Renal dysfunction is very common both prior to and after liver transplantation.[8,170,171] Typically, pretransplantation renal dysfunction is "prerenal" in nature and responds to volume replacement and successful transplantation. Hepatorenal syndrome, an ominous prognostic sign prior to transplantation, is a functional renal defect because it completely resolves after transplantation.

Seventy percent to 90% of all liver transplant patients experience an increase in serum creatinine level in the immediate postoperative period. Causes of renal dysfunction include a decrease in glomerular filtration rate from hypovolemia, renal vasoconstrictive effects of immunosuppressive drugs, acute tubular necrosis from intraoperative hypotension, transfusion of blood or blood products, infection, or tubular injury from drugs or medications. Prerenal causes of renal failure are characterized by urinary [Na$^+$] less than 20 mEq/L, fractional Na$^+$ excretion less than 1%, [creatinine]$_{urine}$ to [creatinine]$_{plasma}$ ratio greater than 40, and Osm$_{urine}$ to Osm$_{plasma}$ ratio greater than 1.5. Intrinsic renal disease causing oliguria is characterized by urinary [Na+] greater than 40 mEq/L, fractional Na$^+$ excretion greater than 1%, [creatinine]$_{urine}$ to [creatinine]$_{plasma}$ ratio less than 20, and Osm$_{urine}$ to Osm$_{plasma}$ ratio less than 1.1.[172]

Hypovolemia is corrected by the administration of fluids and colloid, primarily albumin. Renal vasoconstriction from cyclosporine and tacrolimus correlates with plasma levels of these drugs and is partially reversible by lowering the drug dosage. Acute tubular necrosis typically resolves with time; oliguric acute tubular necrosis may require temporary dialysis, but usually renal function resolves as allograft function improves. Dialysis in the setting of multiorgan failure is an ominous prognostic sign: Mortality approaches 50% to 60%.

The management of oliguria is controversial.[172–174] Our approach is stepwise. First, monitor the central venous pressure and restore the patient to a euvolemic state, primarily with albumin infusion. Second, if oliguria is not resolved, administer bolus diuretic therapy with either furosemide 200 mg IV or ethacrynic acid 50 to 100 mg IV. We have found ethacrynic acid superior to furosemide in converting the patient from oliguric to nonoliguric renal failure. High-dose therapy with either furosemide or ethacrynic acid is associated with hearing loss. Patients who fail these measures will likely require dialysis to maintain balance of fluids, electrolytes, and acid-base ratio.

The optimal frequency and duration of dialysis for treatment of acute renal failure is inadequately defined. Although randomized controlled trials are lacking, small series suggest that continuous hemofiltration (continuous arteriovenous hemodialysis or continuous venovenous hemodialysis) is preferable to intermittant hemodialysis in the management of acute renal failure. The primary reasons for preference of continuous hemofiltration are steady maintenance of volume, electrolyte, and acid-base status and avoidance of the volume shifts that commonly occur with intermittent hemodialysis. Use of biocompatible membranes rather than cellulose membranes in the performance of dialysis is associated with improved patient outcome.

Cardiovascular Disease

Hypertension

Hypertension occurs in 15% to 30% of patients recovering in the ICU after liver transplantation.[175–177] Treatment options depend on the volume status of the patient, the patient's cardiovascular and hemodynamic stability, and the availability of an oral versus intravenous route for administration of medications. Diuretics are indicated in the patient who is hypervolemic. Other antihypertensive agents used in this setting include beta-blockade with labetalol or esmolol; calcium channel blockade with nifedipine, amlodipine, or diltiazem; or vasodilation with nitroglycerin or hydralazine. Calcium channel blockers; particularly diltiazer, inhibit the metabolism of both cyclosporine and tacrolimus; levels of the latter drugs need to be carefully monitored, and doses lowered accordingly. We have preferred intravenous nitroglycerin over nitroprusside for management of hypertension that does not respond to more conservative measures.

Ischemia

Posttransplantation ischemic cardiac events are almost always restricted to recipients with two or more of the following characteristics: age older than 60 years, diabetes, obesity, hypertension, or positive family history of coronary disease. As the recipient waiting list continues to increase in the face of a fixed donor organ supply, patient selection committees will likely become increasingly restrictive in approving these high-risk patients.

The published prevalence of coronary artery disease in cirrhotic patients evaluated for liver transplantation is approximately 5%, but may be more than 15% in older recipients.[9–11] Myocardial infarction after liver transplantation is rare.[178]

Significant ischemia is detected during pretransplantation evaluation by stress evaluation of the heart, using dobutamine stress echocardiography. Positive stress evaluation is an indication for cardiac catheterization to define the nature of the coronary artery disease. Diffuse triple-vessel disease coupled with a positive stress evaluation is an absolute contraindication to liver transplantation. Focal coronary obstruction may be treated with angioplasty or stenting. Only those patients who achieve complete resolution of their previously abnormal stress evaluation should be considered for transplantation. The outcome after performing a transplantation in a patient with known symptomatic coronary artery disease has been poor, even if the patient was previously treated with coronary bypass. Perioperative mortality is approximately 20%, and 3-year mortality is estimated to be 50%.[9–11]

Hemochromatosis and the Heart

The overall outcome of patients who underwent transplantation for hemochromatosis is poor compared with other groups of transplant recipients.[179–181] Causes of increased mortality are infections and cardiac events such as heart block, arrhythmia, and congestive heart failure. The reasons for these cardiac events are not entirely clear but may relate to excessive cardiac accumulation of iron and development of fibrosis of the myocardium and conduction system. Patients with hemochromatosis may also suffer from complications of diabetes mellitus and have underlying ischemic coronary disease.

Idiopathic Hypertrophic Subaortic Stenosis

There has been little experience in liver transplantation of patients with the relatively rare condition of idiopathic hypertrophic subaortic stenosis. These patients are at risk for hypotension and central nervous system ischemic damage in the postoperative period. However, the most common problems are arrhythmia and heart block.[182,183] Sudden death has been described.

Valvular Heart Disease

Clinically important valvular disease is rare in patients undergoing hepatic transplantation. One series from Pittsburgh of 69 patients (a subset of 4,823 patients examined, 1% prevalence) indicated the following types of diseased valves: aortic valve (n = 44, 64%), mitral valve (n = 21, 30%), pulmonic valve (n = 2, 3%), and tricuspid valve (n = 2, 3%). The two most common diagnoses were aortic stenosis and postendocarditis valvular insufficiency.[184,185]

In the posttransplantation period, one is faced with either a patient who has previously undergone valve replacement or a patient who has untreated valvular heart disease. In the former case, valve replacement per se does not appear to adversely affect posttransplantation outcome if the valve is functioning properly. Antibiotic prophylaxis against endocarditis is warranted. In the latter case, one should monitor for signs of heart failure, support the patient medically, and avoid valve replacement surgery until the patient has fully recovered from the transplant procedure. Valve surgery, when performed late posttransplantation in a stable liver recipient, does not appear to adversely affect graft function or patient survival.

Neurologic Events

Alteration of mental status occurs in 10% to 30% of liver transplant recipients. In most cases this is related to pretransplantation encephalopathy, posttransplantation immunosuppressive medications (steroids, cyclosporine, tacrolimus), and the sleep deprivation and disorientation of ICU psychosis. The syndrome reverses with time, stabilization of immunosuppression, and transfer from ICU to the inpatient transplant floor.

Central pontine myelinolysis is a rare but potentially devastating neurologic complication.[186] Etiologic factors include prolonged ICU stay, severe hepatic dysfunction, and rapid fluctuations in fluid volume and concentration of electrolytes, particularly [Na+]. The neurologic deficits vary from isolated cranial neuropathy to "locked-in" syndrome. Magnetic resonance imaging (MRI) of the brain demonstrates evidence of demyelination in the central pons without evidence of hemorrhage or infarction.

Treatment is supportive, with a requirement for prolonged neurologic rehabilitation. Central pontine myelinolysis was once thought to be uniformly fatal; currently, however, most patients (more than 70%) recover significant neurologic function and ultimately return home. Nonetheless, residual neurologic dysfunction is the rule; most patients suffering this complication will be unable to return to gainful employment.

Seizures occurring posttransplantation are most often related to abnormalities in electrolytes, such as hypomagnesemia, or to intravenous infusion of cyclosporine or tacrolimus (especially in the setting of hypocholesterolemia). Occasionally seizures signal an intracranial event, such as hemorrhage, stroke, or cerebral edema. Brain imaging (CT or MRI) is indicated in any patient experiencing posttransplantation seizure activity.

Treatment of seizures is complicated by the fact that most antiseizure medications (such as phenobarbitol, dilantin, tegretol, and valproate) interfere with the metabolism of cyclosporine, tacrolimus, and rapamycin. Neurontin is the only antiseizure medication that lacks hepatic metabolism, is cleared by the kidney, and does not influence the plasma levels of immunosuppressive drugs.

Intracerebral hemorrhage, subdural hematoma, or epidural hematoma may occur spontaneously in the setting of severe coagulopathy, especially thrombocytopenia with a platelet count of less than 10,000. Other factors contributing to central nervous system hemorrhage include prior placement of intracranial pressure monitors, hypertension, prior head trauma, or underlying cardiovascular disease.

Ischemic cerebrovascular disease is rare and is caused either by thromboembolic events or by intrinsic atherosclerotic disease of the cerebral circulation. Risk factors for thromboembolic events include endocarditis, atrial fibrillation, valvular heart disease, and a hypercoagulable state. Risk factors for intrinsic cerebrovascular disease include cardiovascular or peripheral vascular disease, diabetes mellitus, and hypertension.

Cerebral edema is common in patients who have undergone hepatic transplantation for fulminant hepatic failure.[187–190] It may also complicate the course of patients with cirrhosis who have severe encephalopathy or of any patient undergoing liver transplantation whose operative course is complicated by marked shifts in fluids or electrolytes (particularly [Na$^+$]) and a need for massive volume replacement.[190]

One proposed mechanism of cerebral edema in liver patients involves the brain's utilization of ammonia to form glutamine. Ammonia accumulates in the brain, where it converts glutamate to glutamine. Glutamine accumulates in cerebral neurons and astrocytes, and the latter cells osmotically swell. Another hypothesis suggests that the necrotic liver releases inflammatory cytokines that affect movement of water into the brain. Still another hypothesis suggests that cerebral edema is a result of failure of appropriate autoregu-

lation of cerebral blood flow. All three of these mechanisms may interact in some way to produce cerebral edema.

A diagnosis of cerebral edema may be suspected when the patient exhibits worsening encephalopathy with increasing obtundation, stupor, or coma. CT imaging or MRI excludes hemorrhage, stroke, or subdural hematoma and may reveal brain edema. Intracranial pressure (ICP) monitoring confirms the raised pressure but should only be performed after correction of coagulopathy (platelets greater than 50,000; prothrombin time less than 1.7 international normalized ratio).

The goal of treatment is to keep ICP below 20 mm Hg, and cerebral perfusion pressure above 50 mm Hg. Mean arterial pressure should be maintained at or above 60 mm Hg by volume and pressors. CVVH is often required to maintain fluid balance. Additional measures include head-of-bed elevation, sedation with propofol or fentanyl to prevent agitation, and mild hyperventilation to maintain Pco_2 at 30 to 35 mm Hg and pH at 7.45 to 7.50. Mannitol is administered intravenously in doses of 0.5 to 1.0 mg/kg for ICP greater than 20 mm Hg that lasts longer than 5 minutes. Doses may be repeated every 2 to 4 hours as long as serum osmolarity does not exceed 320 mOsm/L and [Na$^+$] is less than 150 mEq/L. If intracranial pressure is unresponsive to these measures, it may be necessary to induce barbiturate coma by using a pentobarbital loading dose of 3 to 5 mg/kg over 15 minutes followed by continuous infusion of 0.5 to 2.0 mg/kg per hour.

Unproven therapies proposed for management of cerebral edema include N-acetylcysteine, prostacyclin, high-volume plasmapheresis, hypothermia, and indomethacin. Neither steroids nor benzodiazepine receptor blockade with flumazenil is of benefit in this setting. The key to recovery of the patient is recovery of liver function. Once allograft function improves, the cerebral edema resolves.

Coagulopathy

Prior to transplantation, nearly all patients with liver disease have multifactorial coagulopathy. Inadequate synthesis of humoral factors by the liver results in depression of most coagulation factors, particularly those that are dependent on the cofactor vitamin K (factors II, VII, IX, and X). Additional proteins made by the liver that may be deficient in the patient with advanced liver disease include fibrinogen, prothrombin, kininogen, factors V, VII, IX, X, XII, and XIII, plasminogen, α_2-antiplasmin, antithrombin III, protein C, and protein S.

Thrombocytopenia is common prior to transplantation and may worsen in the postoperative period. Hypersplenism, a common feature of portal hypertension, is the cause in most cases, but autoimmune thrombocytopenia may also occur.[191,192] Platelets and humoral factors may become critically depleted during transplantation because of consumption from bleeding and the need for multiple transfusions of blood and clotting factors. Surgery may also be complicated by disseminated intravascular coagulation. In general, treatment is directed at replacement of deficient factors by transfusion of fresh frozen plasma, cryoprecipitate (fibrinogen), and platelets.

Diabetes Mellitus

As many as 5% to 15% of patients undergoing liver transplantation have underlying diabetes mellitus.[193,194] Patients with long-standing diabetes mellitus are at risk for vascular and infectious complications posttransplantation. One recent analysis compared the outcome of 78 patients with diabetes mellitus, representing 7.8% of all transplant recipients, with a matched control population of nondiabetic patients (n = 78).[193] One-year and 5-year survival was significantly worse for patients with diabetes mellitus versus nondiabetic controls: 67.5% vs 90%, 61%, and 77%, respectively. Diabetic patients requiring either oral hypoglycemic agents or insulin had the worst prognosis. Causes of death in the diabetic population were often multifactorial and included sepsis, cardiac ischemic disease, and cerebrovascular complications.

LIVING DONOR LIVER TRANSPLANTATION IN ADULTS

Selection Process

The initial success of adult living donor liver transplantation (LDLT) in the United States has resulted in a growing interest in this procedure.[195–197] The impact of LDLT on liver transplantation will depend in part on the proportion of patients who are considered medically suitable for LDLT and the identification of suitable donors.

At Colorado, we consider LDLT for recipients who have first been approved for conventional liver transplantation by the institutional patient selection committee and who meet listing criteria for UNOS status 1, 2A, or 2B.[198] Of the first 100 evaluated recipients, 51 were rejected based on the following characteristics: imminent cadaveric transplant (n = 8), refusal of evaluation (n = 4), lack of financial approval (n = 6), and medical, psychosocial, or surgical problems (n = 33). Of the remaining 49 patients, who were considered to be ideal candidates for LDLT, 24 were unable to identify a suitable donor for evaluation. Twenty-six donors were evaluated for the remaining 25 potential recipients. Eleven donors were ruled out: Nine were rejected for medical reasons, and two refused donation after being medically approved. The remaining 15 donor-recipient pairs underwent LDLT.

Donor Surgery, Complications, and Recovery

At the time of this writing there have been over 100 living donor transplantations performed in adults, but few comprehensive reports on outcome.[195–197] In our experience (currently with 27 living donor transplants) we have not observed any donor deaths and little morbidity, outside that expected with major abdominal surgery. None of the donors required exogenous blood transfusion, and the mean time to discharge from the hospital was 6.5 days. One donor experienced an early bile leak, underwent reoperation and repair of the leak, and was discharged on postoperative day 7 relative to his initial operation. Another had a bile leak that corrected with prolonged drainage. Another donor required repair of an incisional hernia several months after the initial surgery. Outpatient recovery was rapid, and all have returned to their usual daily activities and occupations.

Recipient Outcome and Immediate Postoperative Period

The recipient outcome has been excellent. In our experience, only 2 of the 27 recipients have died (92% crude survival). One patient had severe end-stage HCV and hepatoma and died during the initial hospitalization. The other death occurred more than one year posttransplantation. Four patients underwent retransplantation for primary poor function (n = 1), hepatic artery or biliary complications (n = 2), or hepatic venous outflow obstruction (n = 1). Two differences between LDLT and standard orthotopic liver transplantation require emphasis: elevations in liver enzymes persist longer in LDLT, and the smaller vascular anastomoses increase the risk of vascular and biliary complications.

IMMUNOSUPPRESSION

The topic of immunosuppression is covered in detail in other chapters in this book; therefore, this section only comments on a few issues related to the immediate postoperative period. A wide array of immunosuppressive agents are currently in use in most transplant centers.[199–214] The goal of immunosuppression is prevention of both rejection and immunologic graft loss. A secondary objective is to avoid adverse consequences of the antirejection therapy.

It is common practice to use high-dose immunosuppression at the time of transplantation and then slowly taper the level of immunosuppression. The rate of reduction in immunosuppression varies widely among centers. One center may withdraw prednisone as early as 2 weeks posttransplantation or not use steroids at all. Another may never withdraw prednisone. Some centers use OKT3 for induction, whereas others restrict use of induction OKT3 to patients with renal failure or poor initial graft function. Still other programs use IL-2 receptor antibodies during the induction phase.

Given the wide array of immunosuppressive regimens, there is little uniformity among centers in tailoring and adjusting immunosuppression after liver transplantation. A list of the most commonly used immunosuppressive agents, how they are given, the principles of monitoring, and common adverse effects occurring in the immediate postoperative period is given in Table 10.6.

Many centers have adopted the practice of late steroid withdrawal in patients receiving chronic maintenance immunosuppression, and a few have begun to withdraw pred-

TABLE 10.6. *Immunosuppressants used in the immediate postoperative period: type, method of monitoring, and common adverse reactions*

Type	Monitoring	Adverse effects
Cyclosporine[a]	Blood level[b]	Nephrotoxicity,[c] neurotoxicity,[d] hypertension
Tacrolimus[e]	Blood level[f]	Nephrotoxicity, neurotoxicity, diabetes mellitus[g]
Prednisone	None	Hypertension, diabetes mellitus, neurotoxicity, fluid retention
Azathioprine	None (WBC count)	Neutropenia, thrombocytopenia, anemia
Mycophenolate mofetil[h]	None[i] (WBC count; ? blood level)	Neutropenia, dose-related increase in risk of HSV and CMV,[j] gastrointestinal symptoms
Sirolimus[k]	None[i] (Blood level)	Neutropenia, thrombocytopenia, hyperlipidemia[l]
OKT3[m]	CD3 count[n]	Pulmonary edema, cytokine release[o]
IL-2 receptor antibody[p]	None	None reported

CMV, cytomegalovirus; HSV, herpes simplex virus; IL, interleukin; WBC, white blood cell.

[a]Several different forms of cyclosporine are available. Additional adverse effects of cyclosporine that tend to occur beyond the immediate postoperative period include hirsutism, gingival hyperplasia, and hypercholesterolemia.

[b]Dosage of cyclosporine is adjusted primarily from trough plasma levels. Many different methods exist for measuring cyclosporine levels. The therapeutic range will differ depending on the method used and whether whole blood or plasma is assayed.

[c]Nephrotoxicity is defined by either a rise in serum creatinine concentration or a diminished glomerular filtration rate and is related to plasma concentrations of either cyclosporine or tacrolimus.

[d]Neurotoxicity includes paresthesias, neuropathy, and seizures. Neurotoxicity is more common with tacrolimus than cyclosporine.

[e]Tacrolimus was formerly known as FK506 and is available commercially as Prograf.

[f]Dosage of tacrolimus is adjusted primarily from trough levels. The plasma level of tacrolimus is currently measured by microparticle enzyme immunoassay (MEIA); the therapeutic range is 5 to 18 ng/mL.

[g]The incidence of diabetes mellitus is reduced by steroid withdrawal. Monotherapy with tacrolimus is more often associated with diabetes than is monotherapy with cyclosporine.

[h]Mycophenolate mofetil, Cellcept, is an inhibitor of inosine monophosphate dehydrogenase (IMPDH) and is used as a steroid-sparing or immunophilin-sparing agent.

[i]Currently there are no commercially available assays to measure drug levels for either mycophenolate mofetil or rapamycin (sirolimus).

[j]Risk of CMV infection during mycophenolate mofetil immunosuppression is dose related, with the greatest risk at doses of 3 g per day or more.

[k]Rapamycin is a newly described immunosuppressive agent that targets a protein involved in the initiation of the cell cycles.

[l]Hyperlipidemia is a major unique adverse effect of rapamycin.

[m]OKT3 is a mouse monoclonal antibody that binds to the CD3 determinant of the T-cell receptor. It is highly effective in aborting active rejection but is a potent immunosuppressant; repeated use may increase the risk of opportunistic infections and malignancy.

[n]CD3 count is the only way to determine whether OKT3 is inducing the desired immunosuppressive effect.

[o]OKT3 induces release of cytokines from T lymphocytes, resulting in "cytokine storm": headaches, fever, paresthesia, hypotension, hypoxemia, and abdominal and chest pain.

[p]IL-2 receptor antibodies are useful adjuncts to current immunosuppressive regimens.

nisone at 3 months posttransplantation.[215,216] Our center practices rapid, 14-day steroid withdrawal in the immediate postoperative period under monotherapy with either cyclosporine (Neoral) or tacrolimus (Prograf) with or without mycophenolate mofetil. This practice is not associated with increased risk of graft loss or patient mortality. On the contrary, we have observed marked reductions in the incidence of diabetes mellitus, hypertension, and hypercholesterolemia and in the risk of opportunistic infection in the immediate postoperative period (Table 10.7).

TABLE 10.7. *The effect of early steroid withdrawal, 14 days posttransplantation, on liver recipients*

Lack of consequences related to liver allograft
  No increase in risk or acute cellular rejection
  No immunologic graft loss
  No decrease in graft or patient survival
  Whether steroid withdrawal increases the risk of chronic rejection is unknown
Benefits to recipient
  Decrease in risk of developing and reduction in the severity of the following:
    Hypertension
    Diabetes mellitus
    Hypercholesterolemia
    Obesity
  Possible decrease in severity of recurrent HBV (and possibly HCV) infection
  Possible decreased risk of opportunistic infection

HBV, hepatitis B virus; HCV, hepatitis C virus.

SUMMARY

The immediate postoperative period, representing the first 3 months after liver transplantation, is one of the most critical periods in the clinical course of the liver transplant recipient. Interindividual variation in clinical course is extreme. Some recipients are fortunate to experience an uneventful course, with discharge from the hospital in 7 to 10 days. In contrast, others may have significant complications and experience extended ICU stay, prolonged hospitalization, and need for physical rehabilitation. Recipient, donor, and operative factors have been identified that increase the risk of a complicated postoperative course, graft loss, and patient death.

Complications arising during this period are classified as allograft dysfunction, surgical complications, and medical complications. The chronology and characteristics of each major complication were described in this chapter. Optimal outcome is dependent on early recognition of complications and prompt institution of appropriate therapy. An experienced team performing an adequate number of procedures (more than 20 transplants per year) is important for a positive outcome.

Despite the numerous potential complications that may arise in the immediate postoperative period, graft and patient survival rates after liver transplantation are excellent: 1-year patient survival rates now exceed 85% in most large-volume centers. Advances not only in surgical technique and immunosuppression but also in immediate postoperative management are responsible for the substantial improvements in outcome that have occurred over the last three decades.

REFERENCES

1. United Network for Organ Sharing OPTN and Scientific Registry data, 27 May 1999. From the Organ Procurement and Transplantation Network and the U.S. Scientific Registry of Transplant Recipients, http://www.unos.org, December 1999.
2. Cuervas-Mons V, Martinez AJ, Dekker A, et al. Adult liver transplantation: an analysis of the early causes of death in 40 consecutive cases. *Hepatology* 1986;6:495–501.
3. Gilbert JR, Pascual M, Schoenfeld DA, et al. Evolving trends in liver transplantation. *Transplantation* 1999;67:246–253.
4. Afessa B, Gay PC, Plevak DJ, et al. Pulmonary complications of orthotopic liver transplantation. *Mayo Clin Proc* 1993;68:427–434.
5. Jensen WA, Rose RM, Hammer SM, et al. Pulmonary complications of orthotopic liver transplantation. *Transplantation* 1986;42:484–490.
6. Kuo PC, Plotkin JS, Gaine S, et al. Portopulmonary hypertension and the liver transplant candidate. *Transplantation* 1999;67:1087–1093.
7. Castro M, Krowka M, Schroeder R, et al. Frequency and clinical implications of increased pulmonary artery pressures in liver transplant patients. *Mayo Clin Proc* 1996;71:543–551.
8. Brown RS Jr, Lombardero M, Lake JR. Outcome of patients with renal insufficiency undergoing liver or liver-kidney transplantation. *Transplantation* 1996;62:1788–1792.
9. Morris JJ, Hellman CL, Garvey BJ, et al. Three patients requiring both coronary artery bypass and orthotopic liver transplantation. *J Cardiothorac Vasc Anesth* 1995;9:322–332.
10. Plotkin JS, Benitez RM, Kuo PC, et al. Dobutamine stress echocardiography for preoperative cardiac risk stratification in patients undergoing orthotopic liver transplantation. *Liver Transplant Surg* 1998;4:253–257.
11. Carey WD, Dumot JA, Pimentel RR, et al. The prevalence of coronary artery disease in liver transplant candidates over age 50. *Transplantation* 1995;59:859–864.
12. Fishman JA, Rubin RH. Infection in organ-transplant recipients. *N Engl J Med* 1998;338:1741–1751.
13. Rubin RH. Prevention of infection in the liver transplant recipient. *Liver Transplant Surg* 1996;2:89–98.
14. Marino IR, Doyle HR, Aldrighetti L, et al. Effect of donor age and sex on the outcome of liver transplantation. *Hepatology* 1995;22:1754–1762.
15. Strasberg SM, Howard TK, Molmenti EP, et al. Selecting the donor liver: risk factors for poor function after orthotopic liver transplantation. *Hepatology* 1994;20:829–838.
16. Hoofnagle JH, Lombardero M, Zetterman RK, et al. Donor age and outcome of liver transplantation. *Hepatology* 1996;24:89–96.
17. Emre S, Schwartz ME, Altaca G, et al. Safe use of hepatic allografts from donors older than 70 years. *Transplantation* 1996;62:62–65.
18. Edwards EB, Roberts JP, McBride MA, et al. The effect of the volume of procedures at transplantation centers on mortality after liver transplantation. *N Engl J Med* 1999;341:2049–2053.
19. Zetterman RK, Belle SH, Hoofnagle JH, et al. Age and liver transplantation: a report of the liver transplantation database. *Transplantation* 1998;66:500–506.
20. Deschenes M, Belle SH, Krom RAF, et al., for the NIDDK Liver Transplantation Database. Early allograft dysfunction after liver transplantation: a definition and predictors of outcome. *Transplantation* 1998;66:302–310.
21. Rosen HR, Martin P, Goss J, et al. Significance of early aminotransferase elevation after liver transplantation. *Transplantation* 1998;65:68–72.
22. Kiuchi T, Oldhafer KJ, Schlitt HJ, et al. Background and prognostic implications of periperfusion tissue injuries in human liver transplants. *Transplantation* 1998;66:737–747.
23. 1998 annual report of the US Scientific Registry for Transplant Recipients and the Organ Procurement and Transplantation Network: transplant data: 1988–1997. Rockville, MD: U.S. Department of Health and Human Services, Health Resources and Services Administration, Office of Special Programs, Division of Transplantation; Richmond, VA: UNOS.
24. Quiroga J, Colina I, Demetris AJ, et al. Cause and timing of first allograft failure in orthotopic liver transplantation: a study of 177 consecutive patients. *Hepatology* 1991;14:1054–1062.
25. Bzeizi KI, Jalan R, Plevris JN, et al. Primary graft dysfunction after liver transplantation: from pathogenesis to prevention. *Liver Transplant Surg* 1997;3:137–148.
26. Mor E, Klintmalm GB, Gonwa TA, et al. The use of marginal donors for liver transplantation. *Transplant Proc* 1992;53:383–386.
27. Makowka L, Gordon RD, Todo S, et al. Analysis of donor criteria for the prediction of outcome in clinical liver transplantation. *Transplant Proc* 1987;19:2378–2382.
28. Ploeg RJ, D'Alessandro AM, Knechtle SJ, et al. Risk factors for primary dysfunction after liver transplantation: a multivariate analysis. *Transplantation* 1993;55:807–813.

29. Wall WJ. Predicting outcome after liver transplantation. *Liver Transplant Surg* 1999;5:458–459.
30. Seaberg EC, Belle SH, Beringer KC, et al. Long-term patient and retransplantation-free survival by selected recipient and donor characteristics: an update from the Pitt-UNOS liver transplant registry. In: Cecka JM and Terasaki PI, eds. *Clinical transplants 1997*. Los Angeles: UCLA Tissue Typing Laboratory, 1997:15–28.
31. Busuttil RW, Shaked A, Millis J, et al. One thousand liver transplants: the lessons learned. *Ann Surg* 1994;219:490–499.
32. Gayowski T, Marino IR, Singh N, et al. Orthotopic liver transplantation in high-risk patients: risk factors associated with mortality and infectious morbidity. *Transplantation* 1998;65:499–504.
33. Rufat P, Fourquet F, Conti F, et al., for the GRETHECO Study Group. Costs and outcomes of liver transplantation in adults. *Transplantation* 1999;68:76–83.
34. Marsman WA, Wiesner RH, Rodriquez L, et al. Use of fatty donor liver is associated with diminished early patient and graft survival. *Transplantation* 1996;62:1246–1251.
35. Lehr HA, Messmer K. Rationale for the use of antioxidant vitamins in clinical organ transplantation. *Transplantation* 1996;62:1197–1199.
36. Peltekian KM, Makowka L, Williams R, et al. Prostaglandins in liver failure and transplantation: regeneration, immunomodulation, and cytoprotection. *Liver Transplant Surg* 1996;2:171–184.
37. Klein AS, Cofer JB, Pruett TL, et al. Prostaglandin E1 administration following orthotopic liver transplantation: a randomized prospective multicenter trial. *Gastroenterology* 1996;111:710–715.
38. Schafer DF, Sorrell MF. Prostaglandins in liver transplantation: a promise unfulfilled. *Gastroenterology* 1996;111:819–820.
39. Ascher NL. Progress in transgenic pigs for xenotransplantation. *Liver Transplant Surg* 1998;4:180–181.
40. Flye MW, Pennington L, Kirkman R, et al. Spontaneous acceptance or rejection of orthotopic liver transplants in outbred and partially inbred miniature swine. *Transplantation* 1999;68:599–607.
41. Cozzi E, Tucker AW, Langford GA, et al. Characterization of pigs transgenic for human decay-accelerating factor. *Transplantation* 1997;64:1383–1392.
42. Weiss RA. Commentary: transgenic pigs and virus adaptation. *Nature* 1998;391:327–328.
43. Wiesner RH, Demetris AJ, Belle SH, et al. Acute hepatic allograft rejection: incidence, risk factors, and impact on outcome. *Hepatology* 1998;28:638–645.
44. Bathgate AJ, Hynd P, Sommerville D, et al. The prediction of acute cellular rejection in orthotopic liver transplantation. *Liver Transplant Surg* 1999;5:475–479.
45. Gaber LW, Moore LW, Gaber AO, et al. Utility of standardized histological classification in the management of acute rejection. *Transplantation* 1998;64:376–380.
46. Mor E, Solomon H, Gibbs JF, et al. Acute cellular rejection following liver transplantation: clinical pathologic features and effect on outcome. *Semin Liver Dis* 1992;12:28–40.
47. Ludwig J. Terminology of hepatic allograft rejection [Glossary]. *Semin Liver Dis* 1992;12:89–92.
48. Henley KS, Lucey MR, Appelman HD, et al. Biochemical and histopathological correlation in liver transplant: the first 180 days. *Hepatology* 1992;16:688–693.
49. Demetris AJ, Batts KP, Dhillon AP, et al. Banff schema for grading liver allograft rejection: an international consensus document. *Hepatology* 1997;25:658–663.
50. Ormonde DG, de Boer WB, Kierath A, et al. Banff schema for grading liver allograft rejection: utility in clinical practice. *Liver Transplant Surg* 1999;5:261–268.
51. Adams DH, Neuberger JM. Treatment of acute rejection. *Semin Liver Dis* 1992;12:80–88.
52. Dousset B, Hubscher SG, Padbury RTA, et al. Acute liver allograft rejection—is treatment always necessary? *Transplantation* 1993;55:529–534.
53. McVicar JP, Kowdley KV, Bacchi CE, et al. The natural history of untreated focal allograft rejection in liver transplant recipients. *Liver Transplant Surg* 1996;2:154–160.
54. Barnes D, Talenti D, Cammell G, et al. A randomized clinical trial of ursodeoxycholic acid as adjuvant treatment to prevent liver transplant rejection. *Hepatology* 1997;26:853–857.
55. Keiding S, Hockerstedt K, Bjoro K, et al. The Nordic multicenter double-blind randomized controlled trial of prophylactic ursodeoxycholic acid in liver transplant patients. *Transplantation* 1997;63:1591–1594.
56. Dickson RC. Management of posttransplantation viral hepatitis—hepatitis B. *Liver Transplant Surg* 1998;4(suppl 1):S73–S78.
57. Samuel D, Muller R, Alexander G, et al. Liver transplantation in European patients with the hepatitis B surface antigen. *N Engl J Med* 1993;329:1842–1847.
58. Davies SE, Portmann BC, O'Grady, et al. Hepatic histological findings after transplantation for chronic hepatitis B virus infection, including a unique pattern of fibrosing cholestatic hepatitis. *Hepatology* 1991;13:150–157.
59. Mason AL, Wick M, White HM, et al. Increased hepatocyte expression of hepatitis B virus transcription in patients with features of fibrosing cholestatic hepatitis. *Gastroenterology* 1993;105:237–244.
60. McGory RW, Ishitani MB, Oliviera WM, et al. Improved outcome of orthotopic liver transplantation for chronic hepatitis B cirrhosis with aggressive passive immunization. *Transplantation* 1996;61:1358–1364.
61. McGory R, Ishitani M, Oliviera W, et al. Hepatitis B immune globulin dose requirements following orthotopic liver transplantation for chronic hepatitis B cirrhosis. *Transplant Proc* 1996;28:1687–1688.
62. Terrault NA, Zhou S, Combs C, et al. Prophylaxis in liver transplant recipients using a fixed dosing schedule of hepatitis B immunoglobulin. *Hepatology* 1996;24:1327–1333.
63. Dickson RC, Everhart JE, Lake JR, et al. Transmission of hepatitis B by transplantation of livers from donors positive for antibody to hepatitis B core antigen. *Gastroenterology* 1997;113:1668–1674.
64. Dodson SF, Bonham CA, Geller DA, et al. Prevention of de novo hepatitis B infection in recipients of hepatic allografts from anti-HBc positive donors. *Transplantation* 1999;68:1058–1061.
65. Perillo R, Rakela J, Dienstag J, et al. Multicenter study of lamivudine therapy for hepatitis B after liver transplantation. *Hepatology* 1999;29:1581–1586.
66. Grellier L, Mutimer D, Ahmed M, et al. Lamivudine prophylaxis against reinfection in liver transplantation for hepatitis B cirrhosis. *Lancet* 1996;348:1212–1215.
67. Ling R, Mutimer D, Ahmed M, et al. Selection of mutations in the hepatitis B virus polymerase during therapy of transplant recipients with lamivudine. *Hepatology* 1996;24:711–713.
68. Markowitz JS, Martin P, Conrad AJ, et al. Prophylaxis against hepatitis B recurrence following liver transplantation using combination lamivudine and hepatitis B immune globulin. *Hepatology* 1998;28:585–589.
69. Singh N, Gayowski T, Wannstedt CF, et al. Pretransplant famciclovir as prophylaxis for hepatitis B virus recurrence after liver transplantation. 1997;63:1415–1419.
70. Terrault NA, Holland CC, Ferrell L, et al. Interferon alfa for recurrent hepatitis B infection after liver transplantation. *Liver Transplant Surg* 1996;2:132–138.
71. Janssen HLA, Gerken G, Carreno V, et al. Interferon alfa for chronic hepatitis B infection: increased efficacy of prolonged treatment. *Hepatology* 1999;30:238–243.
72. Ben-Ari Z, Shmueli D, Shapira Z, et al. Loss of serum HbsAg after interferon-alfa therapy in liver transplant patients with recurrent hepatitis B infection. *Liver Transplant Surg* 1997;3:394–397.
73. Kruger M, Tillman HL, Trautwein C, et al. Famciclovir treatment of hepatitis B virus recurrence after liver transplantation: a pilot study. *Liver Transplant Surg* 1996;2:253–262.
74. Gish RG, Lau JY, Brooks L, et al. Ganciclovir treatment of hepatitis B virus infection in liver transplant recipients. *Hepatology* 1996;23:1–7.
75. Everhart JE, Wei Y, Eng H, et al. Recurrent and new hepatitis C infection after liver transplantation. *Hepatology* 1999;29:1220–1226.
76. Charlton M, Seaberg E, Wiesner R, et al. Predictors of patient and graft survival following liver transplantation for hepatitis C. *Hepatology* 1998;28:823–830.
77. Feray C, Caccamo L, Alexander GJM, et al. European collaborative study on factors influencing outcome after liver transplantation for hepatitis C. *Gastroenterology* 1999;117:619–625.
78. Periera BJG, Milford EL, Kirkman RL, et al. Prevalence of hepatitis C virus RNA in organ donors positive for hepatitis C antibody and in the recipients of their organs. *N Engl J Med* 1992;327:910–915.
79. Vargas HE, Laskus T, Wang LF, et al. Outcome of liver transplantation in hepatitis C virus-infected patients who received hepatitis C virus-infected grafts. *Gastroenterology* 1999;117:149–153.
80. Sheiner PA, Boros P, Klion FM, et al. The efficacy of prophylactic interferon alfa-2b in preventing recurrent hepatitis C after liver transplantation. *Hepatology* 1998;28:831–838.
81. Wright TL, Combs C, Kim M, et al. Interferon-a therapy for hepatitis C virus infection after liver transplantation. *Hepatology* 1994;20:773–779.

82. Sandhu IS, Jarvis C, Everson GT. Total parenteral nutrition (TPN) and cholestasis. *Clinics Liver Dis* 1999;3:489–508.

83. Lebeau G, Yanaga K, Marsh JW, et al. Analysis of surgical complications after 397 hepatic transplantations. *Surg Gynecol Obstet* 1989; 170:123–147.

84. Everson GT. A hepatologist's perspective on the management of coagulation disorders prior to liver transplantation. *Liver Transplant Surg* 1997;3:646–652.

85. Lerut JP, Gordon RD, Iwatsuki S, et al. Human orthotopic liver transplantation: surgical aspects in 393 consecutive grafts. *Transplant Proc* 1988;20:603–606.

86. Langnas AN, Marujo W, Stratta RJ, et al. Vascular complications after liver transplantation. *Am J Surg* 1991;161:76–83.

87. Marujo WC, Langnas AN, Wood RP, et al. Vascular complications following liver transplantation: outcome and role of urgent revascularization. *Transplant Proc* 1991;23:1484–1486.

88. Wozney P, Zajko AB, Bron KM, et al. Vascular complications after liver transplantation: a 5-year experience. *AJR Am J Roentgenol* 1986; 147:657–663.

89. Tzakis AG, Gordon RD, Shaw BW, et al. Clinical presentation of hepatic artery thrombosis after liver transplantation in the cyclosporine era. *Transplantation* 1985;40:667–671.

90. Valente JF, Alonso MH, Weber FL, et al. Late hepatic artery thrombosis in liver allograft recipients is associated with intrahepatic biliary necrosis. *Transplantation* 1996;61:61–65.

91. Kaplan SB, Za, Ko AB, Koneru B. Hepatic bilomas in liver transplant. *Radiology* 1990;174:1031–1035.

92. Abbasoglu O, Levy MF, Vodapally MS, et al. Hepatic artery stenosis after liver transplantation—incidence, presentation, treatment, and long-term outcome. *Transplantation* 1997;63:250–255.

93. Abbasoglu O, Levy MF, Testa G, et al. Does intraoperative hepatic artery flow predict arterial complications after liver transplantation? *Transplantation* 1998;66:598–601.

94. Langnas AN, Marujo W, Stratta RJ, Wood RP, List Shaw BW Jr. Hepatic allograft rescue following arterial thrombosis. *Transplantation* 1991;51:86–90.

95. Hidalgo EG, Abad J, Canterro JM, et al. High-dose intra-arterial urokinase for the treatment of hepatic artery thrombosis in liver transplantation. *Hepatogastroenterology* 1989;36:529–532.

96. Pinna AD, Smith CV, Furukawa H, et al. Urgent revascularization of liver allografts after early hepatic artery thrombosis. *Transplantation* 1996;62:1584–1587.

97. Sheiner PA, Varma CVRR, Guarrera JV, et al. Selective revascularization of hepatic artery thromboses after liver transplantation improves patient and graft survival. *Transplantation* 1997;64:1295–1299.

98. Lerut J, Tzakis AG, Bron K, et al. Complications of venous reconstruction in human orthotopic liver transplantation. *Ann Surg* 1987; 205:404–414.

99. Helling TS. Thrombosis and recanalization of the portal vein in liver transplantation. *Transplantation* 1985;40:446–448.

100. Zajko AB, Bron KM. Hepatopedal collaterals after portal vein thrombosis following liver transplantation. *Cardiovasc Intervent Radiol* 1986;9:46–48.

101. Burke GW 3rd, Ascher NL, Hunter D, et al. Orthotopic liver transplantation: non-operative management of early, acute portal vein thrombosis. *Surgery* 1988; 104:924–928.

102. Rouch DA, Ring EJ, Roberts JP, et al. The successful management of portal vein thrombosis after liver transplantation with a splenorenal shunt. *Surg Gynecol Obstet* 1988;166:311–316.

103. Marino IR, Esquiveico, Zajko AB, et al. Distal splenorenal shunt for portal vein thrombosis after liver transplantation. *Am J Gastroenterol* 1989;84:67–70.

104. Scantelbury VP, Zajko AB, Esquivel CO, et al. Successful reconstruction of late portal vein stenosis after hepatic transplantation. *Arch Surg* 1989;124:503–505.

105. Olcott EW, Thistlewaite JR, Lichtosh, et al. Percutaneous transhepatic portal vein angioplasty and stent placement after liver transplantation: early experience. *J Vasc Interv Radiol* 1990;1:17–22.

106. Navarro F, Le Moine MC, Fabre JM, et al. Specific vascular complications of orthotopic liver transplantation with preservation of the retrohepatic vena cava: review of 1361 cases. *Transplantation* 1999; 68:646–650.

107. Parrilla P, Sanchez-Bueno F, Figueras J, et al. Analysis of the complications of the piggy-back technique in 1112 liver transplants. *Transplantation* 1999;67:1214–1217.

108. Orons PD, Hari AK, Zajko AB, et al. Thrombolysis and endovascular stent placement for inferior vena caval thrombosis in a liver transplant recipient. *Transplantation* 1997;64:1357–1359.

109. Porayko MK, Kondo M, Steers JL. Liver transplantation: late complications of the biliary tract and their management. *Semin Liver Dis* 1995;15:139–155.

110. Reichert PR, Renz JF, Rosenthal P, et al. Biliary complications of reduced-organ liver transplantation. *Liver Transplant Surg* 1998;4: 343–349.

111. Stratta RJ. Diagnosis and treatment of biliary tract complications after orthotopic liver transplantation. *Surgery* 1989;106:676–684.

112. Starzl TE. Biliary complications after liver transplantation: with special reference to the biliary cast syndrome and techniques of secondary duct repair. *Surgery* 1977;81:212–221.

113. Lerut J. Biliary tract complications in human orthotopic liver transplantation. *Transplantation* 1987;43:47–51.

114. Klein AS, Savader S, Burdick JF, et al. Reduction of morbidity and mortality from biliary complications after liver transplantation. *Hepatology* 1991;14:818–823.

115. Letourneau JG, Hunter DW, Ascher NL, et al. Biliary complications after liver transplantation in children. *Radiology* 1989;170:1095–1099.

116. Fisher A, Miller CM. Ischemic-type biliary strictures in liver allografts: the Achilles heel revisited? *Hepatology* 1995;21:589–591.

117. Sankary HN, McChesney L, Frye E, et al. A simple modification in operative technique can reduce the incidence of nonanastomotic biliary strictures after orthotopic liver transplantation. *Hepatology* 1995;21:63–69.

118. Sanchez-Urdazpal L, Gores GJ, Ward EM, et al. Ischemic-type biliary complications after orthotopic liver transplantation. *Hepatology* 1992;16:49–53.

119. Sanchez-Urdazpal L, Gores GJ, Ward EM, et al. Diagnostic features and clinical outcome of ischemic-type biliary complications after liver transplantation. *Hepatology* 1993;17:605–609.

120. Shuhart MC, Kowdley KV, McVicar JP, et al. Predictors of bile leaks after T-tube removal in orthotopic liver transplant recipients. *Liver Transplant Surg* 1998;4:62–70.

121. Osorio RW, Freise CE, Stock PG, et al. Nonoperative management of biliary leaks after orthotopic liver transplantation. *Transplantation* 1993;55:1074–1077.

122. Rizk RS, McVicar JP, Emond MJ, et al. Endoscopic management of biliary strictures in liver transplant recipients: effect on patient and graft survival. *Gastrointest Endosc* 1998;47:128–135.

123. Sawyer RG, Punch JD. Incidence and management of biliary complications after 291 liver transplants following the introduction of transcystic stenting. *Transplantation* 1998;66:1201–1207.

124. Rabkin JM, Orloff SL, Reed MH, et al. Biliary tract complications of side-to-side without T-tube versus end-to-end with or without T-tube choledochocholedochostomy in liver transplant recipients. *Transplantation* 1998;65:193–199.

125. Singh N, Paterson DL, Gayowski T, et al. Predicting bacteremia and bacteremic mortality in liver transplant recipients. *Liver Transplantation* 2000;6:54–61.

126. Pizzo PA. Fever in immunocompromised patients. *N Engl J Med* 1999;341:893–900.

127. Singh N, Gayowski T, Marino IR. Causes of leukocytosis in liver transplant recipients: relevance in clinical practice. *Transplantation* 1998;65:199–203.

128. Winston DJ, Foster PF, Somberg KA, et al. Randomized, placebo-controlled, double-blind, multicenter trial of efficacy and safety of granulocyte colony-stimulating factor in liver transplant recipients. *Transplantation* 1999;68:1298–1304.

129. Rubin RH. Importance of CMV in the transplant population. *Transpl Infect Dis Suppl* 1999;1:3–7.

130. Crumpacker CS. Ganciclovir. *N Engl J Med* 1996;335:721–729.

131. Falagas ME, Arbo M, Ruthazer R, et al. Cytomegalovirus disease is associated with increased cost and hospital length of stay among orthotopic liver transplant recipients. *Transplantation* 1997;63: 1595–1601.

132. Rosen HR, Chou S, Corless C, et al. Cytomegalovirus viremia: risk factor for allograft cirrhosis after liver transplantation for hepatitis C. *Transplantation* 1997;64:721–726.

133. Madalosso C, deSouza NF, Ilstrup DM, et al. Cytomegalovirus and its association with hepatic artery thrombosis after liver transplantation. *Transplantation* 1998;66:294–297.

134. Falagas ME, Paya C, Ruthazer R, et al. Significance of cyto-megalovirus for long-term survival after orthotopic liver transplantation: a prospective derivation and validation cohort analysis. *Transplantation* 1998;66:1020–1028.
135. Humar A, Gregson D, Caliendo AM, et al. Clinical utility of quantitative cytomegalovirus viral load determination for predicting cytomegalovirus disease in liver transplant recipients. *Transplantation* 1999;68:1305–1311.
136. Mendez J, Espy M, Smith TF, et al. Clinical significance of viral load in the diagnosis of cytomegalovirus disease after liver transplantation. *Transplantation* 1998;65:1477–1481.
137. Das A. Cost-effectiveness of different strategies of cytomegalovirus prophylaxis in orthotopic liver transplant recipients. *Hepatology* 2000;31:311–317.
138. Gane E, Saliba F, Valdecasas GJC, et al. Randomised trial of efficacy and safety of oral ganciclovir in the prevention of cytomegalovirus disease in liver transplant recipients. *Lancet* 1997;350:1729–1733.
139. Winston DJ, Wirin D, Shaked A, et al. Randomized comparison of ganciclovir and high-dose acyclovir for long-term cytomegalovirus prophylaxis in liver transplant recipients. *Lancet* 1995;346:69–74.
140. Pescovitz MD. Oral ganciclovir and pharmacokinetics of valganciclovir in liver transplant recipients. *Transpl Infect Dis Suppl* 1999;1:31–34.
141. Straus SE, Cohen JI, Tosato G, et al. Epstein-Barr virus infections: biology, pathogenesis, and management. *Ann Intern Med* 1993;118:45–58.
142. Paya CV, Fung JJ, Nalesnik MA, et al. Epstein-Barr virus-induced posttransplant lymphoproliferative disorders. *Transplantation* 1999;68:1517–1525.
143. Patterson JE. Epidemiology of fungal infections in solid organ transplant patients. *Transpl Infect Dis* 1999;1:229–236.
144. Paya CV. Fungal infections in solid organ transplantation. *Clin Infect Dis* 1993;16:677–682.
145. Walsh TJ, Groll AH. Emerging fungal pathogens: evolving challenges to immunocompromised patients for the twenty-first century. *Transpl Infect Dis* 1999;1:247–261.
146. Patterson TF. Approaches to fungal diagnosis in transplantation. *Transpl Infect Dis* 1999;1:262–272.
147. Singh N, Arnow PM, Bonham A, et al. Invasive aspergillosis in liver transplant recipients in the 1990s. *Transplantation* 1997;64:716–720.
148. Denning DW. Early diagnosis of invasive aspergillosis. *Lancet* 2000;355:423–424.
149. Collins LA, Samone MA, Roberts MS, et al. Risk factors for invasive fungal infections complicating orthotopic liver transplantation. *J Infect Dis* 1994;170:644–651.
150. Kusne S, Torre-Cisneros J, Manez R, et al. Factors associated with invasive lung aspergillosis and significance of positive culture after liver transplantation. *J Infect Dis* 1992;166:1379–1383.
151. DeShazo RD, Chapin K, Swain RE. Fungal sinusitis. *N Engl J Med* 1997;337:254–259.
152. Winston DJ, Pakrasi A, Busuttil RW. Prophylactic fluconazole in liver transplant recipients: a randomized, double-blind, placebo-controlled trial. *Ann Intern Med* 1999;131:729–737.
153. Tiphine M, Letscher-Bru V, Herbrecht R. Amphotericin B and its new formulations: pharmacologic characteristics, clinical efficacy, and tolerability. *Transpl Infect Dis* 1999;1:273–283.
154. Iseman MD. Treatment of multidrug-resistant tuberculosis. *N Engl J Med* 1993;329:784–791.
155. Singh N, Gayowski T, Wagener MM, et al. Pulmonary infiltrates in liver transplant recipients in the intensive care unit. *Transplantation* 1999;67:1138–1144.
156. Smetana GW. Preoperative pulmonary evaluation. *N Engl J Med* 1999;340:937–944.
157. Plevak DJ. Forum on critical care issues in sepsis, adult respiratory distress syndrome, and multiorgan system failure. *Liver Transplant Surg* 1997;3:58–87.
158. Fishman AP. Pulmonary hypertension: beyond vasodilator therapy. *N Engl J Med* 1998;338:321–322.
159. Ramsay MAE, Simpson BR, Nguyen AT, et al. Severe pulmonary hypertension in liver transplant candidates. *Liver Transplant Surg* 1997;3:494–500.
160. Krowka MJ, Frantz RP, McGoon MD, et al. Improvement in pulmonary hemodynamics during intravenous epoprostenol (prostacyclin): a study of 15 patients with moderate to severe portopulmonary hypertension. *Hepatology* 1999;30:641–648.
161. McLaughlin VV, Genthner DE, Panella MM, et al. Reduction in pulmonary vascular resistance with long-term epoprostenol (prostacyclin) therapy in primary pulmonary hypertension. *N Engl J Med* 1998;338:273–277.
162. McLaughlin VV, Genthner DE, Panella MM, et al. Compassionate use of continuous prostacyclin in the management of secondary pulmonary hypertension: a case series. *Ann Intern Med* 1999;130:740–743.
163. Kaspar MD, Ramsay MAE, Shuey CB Jr, et al. Severe pulmonary hypertension and amelioration of hepatopulmonary syndrome after liver transplantation. *Liver Transplant Surg* 1998;4:177–179.
164. Krowka MJ, Cortese DA. Hepatopulmonary syndrome: current concepts in diagnostic and therapeutic considerations. *Chest* 1994;105:1528–1537.
165. Krowka MJ, Wiseman GA, Steers JL, et al. Late recurrence and rapid evolution of severe hepatopulmonary syndrome after liver transplantation. *Liver Transplant Surg* 1999;5:451–453.
166. Rodriguez-Roisin R, Barbera JA. Hepatopulmonary syndrome: is *no* the right answer? *Gastroenterology* 1997;113:682–684.
167. Fallon MB, Abrams GA, Luo B, et al. The role of endothelial nitric oxide synthase in the pathogenesis of a rat model of hepatopulmonary syndrome. *Gastroenterology* 1997;113:606–615.
168. Rolla G, Brussino L, Colagrande P, et al. Exhaled nitric oxide and impaired oxygenation in cirrhotic patients before and after liver transplantation. *Ann Intern Med* 1998;129:375–378.
169. Abrams GA, Nanda NC, Dubovsky EV, et al. Use of macroaggregated albumin lung perfusion scan to diagnose hepatopulmonary syndrome: a new approach. *Gastroenterology* 1998;114:305–310.
170. Rimola A, Gavaler JS, Schade RR, et al. Effects of renal impairment on liver transplantation. *Gastroenterology* 1987;93:148–156.
171. Gonwa TA, Morris CA, Goldstein RM, et al. Long-term survival and renal function following liver transplantation in patients with and without hepatorenal syndrome—experience in 300 patients. *Transplantation* 1991;51:428–430.
172. Klahr S, Miller SB. Acute oliguria. *N Engl J Med* 1998;338:671–676.
173. Forni LG, Hilton PJ. Continuous hemofiltration in the treatment of acute renal failure. *N Engl J Med* 1997;336:1303–1309.
174. Adrogue HJ, Madias NE. Management of life-threatening acid-base disorders, parts I and II. *N Engl J Med* 1998;338:26–34; 107–111.
175. Taler SJ, Canzanello VJ, Schwartz L, et al. Role of steroid dose in hypertension early after liver transplantation with tacrolimus (FK506) and cyclosporine. *Transplantation* 1996;62:1588–1592.
176. Textor SC, Canzanello VJ, Taler SJ, et al. Cyclosporine-induced hypertension after transplantation. *Mayo Clin Proc* 1994;69:1182–1188.
177. Porayko MK, Textor SC, Krom RAF, et al. Nephrotoxic effects of primary immunosuppression with FK-506 and cyclosporine regimens after liver transplantation. *Mayo Clin Proc* 1994;69:105–109.
178. Sampathkumar P, Lerman A, Kim BY, et al. Post-liver transplantation myocardial dysfunction. *Liver Transplant Surg* 1998;4:399–403.
179. Brandhagen DJ, Alvarez W, Therneau TM, et al. Iron overload in cirrhosis—HFE genotypes and outcome after liver transplantation. *Hepatology* 2000;31:456–460.
180. Farrell FJ, Nguyen M, Woodley S, et al. Outcome of liver transplantation in patients with hemochromatosis. *Hepatology* 1994;20:404–410.
181. Fiel MI, Schiano TD, Bodenheimer HC, et al. Hereditary hemochromatosis in liver transplantation. *Liver Transplant Surg* 1999;5:50–56.
182. Maron BJ, Shen WK, Link MS, et al. Efficacy of implantable cardioverter-defibrillators for the prevention of sudden death in patients with hypertrophic cardiomyopathy. *N Engl J Med* 2000;342:365–373.
183. Watkins H. Sudden death in hypertrophic cardiomyopathy. *N Engl J Med* 2000;342:422–424.
184. Dec GW, Kondo N, Farrell ML, et al. Cardiovascular complications following liver transplantation. *Clin Transplantation* 1995;2:463–471.
185. Surindra NM, Griffith BP, Kormos RL, et al. Cardiac operations in solid-organ transplant recipients. *Ann Thorac Surg* 1997;64:1270–1278.
186. Fryer JP, Fortier MV, Metrakos P, et al. Central pontine myelinolysis and cyclosporine neurotoxicity following liver transplantation. *Transplantation* 1996;61:658–661.
187. Lopez OL, Estol C, Colina I, et al. Neurological complications after liver retransplantation. *Hepatology* 1992;16:162–166.
188. Martinez AJ, Estol C, Brenner RP, et al. Neurological complications after liver transplantation. *Neurol Clin* 1988;6:327–348.

189. Luerssen TG. Intracranial pressure: current status in monitoring and management. *Semin Pediatr Neurol* 1997;4:146–155.

190. Donovan JP, Schafer DF, Shaw BW Jr, et al. Cerebral oedema and increased intracranial pressure in chronic liver disease. *Lancet* 1998;351:719–721.

191. Chatzipetrou MA, Tsaroucha AK, Weppler D, et al. Thrombocytopenia after liver transplantation. *Transplantation* 1999;67:702–706.

192. West KA, Anderson DR, McAlister V, et al. Alloimmune thrombocytopenia after organ transplantation. *N Engl J Med* 1999;341:1504–1507.

193. Shields PL, Tang H, Neuberger JM, et al. Poor outcome in patients with diabetes mellitus undergoing liver transplantation. *Transplantation* 1999;68:530–535.

194. Merli M, Leonetti F, Riggio O, et al. Glucose intolerance and insulin resistance in cirrhosis are normalized after liver transplantation. *Hepatology* 1999;30:649–654.

195. Wachs ME, Bak TE, Karrer FM, et al. Adult living donor liver transplantation using a right hepatic lobe. *Transplantation* 1998;66:1313–1316.

196. Marcos A, Fisher RA, Ham JM, et al. Right lobe living donor liver transplantation. *Transplantation* 1999;68:798–803.

197. Inomata Y, Uemoto S, Asonuma K, et al. Right lobe graft in living donor liver transplantation. *Transplantation* 2000;69:258–264.

198. Trotter J, Wachs M, Trouillot T, et al. The evaluation of 100 recipients for living donor liver transplantation. *Liver Transplant Surg* 2000;6:290–295.

199. The US Multicenter FK506 Liver Study Group. A comparison of tacrolimus (FK506) and cyclosporine for immunosuppression in liver transplantation. *N Engl J Med* 1994;331:1110–1115.

200. European FK506 Multicenter Liver Study Group. Randomized trial comparing tacrolimus (FK506) and cyclosporin in prevention of liver allograft rejection. *Lancet* 1994;344:423–428.

201. Eckhoff DE, McGuire BM, Frenette LR, et al. Tacrolimus (FK506) and mycophenolate mofetil combination therapy versus tacrolimus in adult liver transplantation. *Transplantation* 1998;65:180–187.

202. Herrero JI, Quiroga J, Sangro B, et al. Conversion of liver transplant recipients on cyclosporine with renal impairment to mycophenolate mofetil. *Liver Transplant Surg* 1999;5:414–420.

203. Papatheodoridas GV, O'Beirne J, Mistry P, et al. Mycophenolate mofetil monotherapy in stable liver transplant patients with cyclosporine-induced renal impairment. *Transplantation* 1999;68:155–157.

204. Hebert MF, Ascher NL, Lake JR, et al. Four-year follow-up of mycophenolate mofetil for graft rescue in liver allograft recipients. *Transplantation* 1999;67:707–712.

205. Jain AB, Hamad I, Rakela J, et al. A prospective randomized trial of tacrolimus and prednisone versus tacrolimus, prednisone, and mycophenolate mofetil in primary adult liver transplant recipients. *Transplantation* 1998;66:1395–1398.

206. Paterson DL, Singh N, Panebianco A, et al. Infectious complications occurring in liver transplant recipients receiving mycophenolate mofetil. *Transplantation* 1998;66:593–598.

207. Watson CJE, Friend PJ, Jamieson NV, et al. Sirolimus: a potent new immunosuppressant for liver transplantation. *Transplantation* 1999;67:505–509.

208. Abraham RT, Wiederrecht GJ. Immunopharmacology of rapamycin. *Annu Rev Immunol* 1996;14:483–510.

209. Sehgal SN. Rapamune (RAPA, rapamycin, sirolimus): mechanism of action of immunosuppressive effect results from blockade of signal transduction and inhibition of cell cycle progression. *Clin Biochem* 1998;31:335–340.

210. Hirose R, Roberts JP, Quan D, et al. Experience with daclizumab in liver transplantation: renal transplant dosing without calcineurin inhibitors is insufficient to prevent acute rejection in liver transplantation. *Transplantation* 2000;69:307–311.

211. Mayforth RD, Quintans J. Designer and catalytic antibodies. *N Engl J Med* 1990;323:173–178.

212. Vincenti F, Kirkman R, Light S, et al. Interleukin-2-receptor blockade with daclizumab to prevent acute rejection in renal transplantation. *N Engl J Med* 1998;338:161–165.

213. Whiting JF, Fecteau A, Martin J, et al. Use of low-dose OKT3 as induction therapy in liver transplantation. *Transplantation* 1998;65:577–580.

214. Whiting JF, Rossi SJ, Hanto DW. Infectious complications after OKT3 induction in liver transplantation. *Liver Transplant Surg* 1997;3:563–570.

215. Belli L, DeCarlis L, Rondinara G, et al. Early cyclosporine monotherapy in liver transplantation: a 5-year follow-up of a prospective randomized trial. *Hepatology* 1998;27:1524–1529.

216. Everson GT, Trouillot T, Wachs M, et al. Early steroid withdrawal in liver transplantation is safe and beneficial. *Liver Transplant Surg* 1999;5:S48–S57.

Transplantation of the Liver, edited by Willis C. Maddrey, Eugene R. Schiff, and Michael F. Sorrell. Lippincott Williams & Wilkins, Philadelphia © 2001.

CHAPTER 11

Long-term Postoperative Care

Ashley St. J. M. Brown and Roger Williams

The postoperative recovery period following liver transplantation is highly variable. Some patients, such as those undergoing semielective transplantation, may be discharged from the hospital in under a week with few or even no postoperative complications. Others, such as those who have been extremely sick prior to transplantation (in particular, those requiring transplantation for acute liver failure), may have prolonged hospitalization with one setback after another.

In general, however, 3 months marks something of a milestone in the recovery of the majority of patients. By this stage, most patients will have recovered from the immediate effects of the surgery, the biliary t-tube (if used) will have been removed, and all wounds will have healed. In the majority of cases, graft function and immunosuppression requirements will have stabilized. Both physical and psychosocial rehabilitation should be well advanced. At this stage the frequency of follow-up and monitoring begins to be reduced, with the emphasis shifting from inpatient care to ambulatory and outpatient follow-up. This time marks the stage in many units where the continuing care of the patient reverts from the transplant team in the tertiary center to the referring physician in the home locality.

Many of the problems associated with the early stages of the posttransplantation period were addressed and to a large part overcome in the 1970s and 1980s; attention is now shifting to the problems of late posttransplantation morbidity and death. In a world where the demand for organs constantly exceeds the available supply, it is the duty of all parties to maximize graft survival. The supervising clinician in the long-term follow-up clinic must be constantly aware and vigilant of potential problems, and must address them at the earliest possible opportunity.

A. St. J. M. Brown and R. Williams: Institute of Hepatology, University College London, London WC1E 4HX, United Kingdom.

THE CLINIC VISIT

The frequency of follow-up visits is something for each unit to decide depending on local resources, the geographical location of patients, and the availability of support within the greater community. A framework is needed to guide new staff in the transplant clinic and thereby prevent unnecessary trips for the patient. As a general rule (assuming the patient has no obvious complications indicating the need for more frequent follow-up), we recommend monthly review for the first 6 months, bimonthly for the second 6 months, and review every 3 months thereafter for the next 2 years. After 2 years, the patient can be reviewed on a twice yearly or even yearly basis. It is essential that patients have access to transplant unit personnel at all times, and that a patient (or the patient's primary physician) should be able to arrange an unscheduled review appointment at extremely short notice.

At each clinic visit, a history should be taken and recorded. Enquiries should be made into the patient's general health, and the patient should be given the opportunity of responding to open questions before responding to directed questions concerning the possible long-term complications described in this chapter. Drug compliance should be checked, and a record made of all medications the patient is currently taking (including over-the-counter preparations). Some of the more common drug interactions are shown in Table 11.1. This list is not exhaustive, and the clinician has a duty to be aware of all possible interactions. By 3 months after transplantation, much of the antimicrobial prophylaxis can be safely discontinued; it is essential to check that patients are not taking any unnecessary medication. Attention should be directed toward potential underlying psychological and social issues.

The patient should be weighed, blood pressure should be measured, and the patient examined as appropriate. In particular, the abdomen should be palpated to assess graft size,

TABLE 11.1. *Common drug interactions of immunosuppressant drugs*

Drug	Interactions	Drugs implicated
Cyclosporine	Increases plasma concentration (risk of toxicity)	Grapefruit juice, erythromycin, ketoconazole, fluconazole, chloroquine, diltiazem, nicardipine, verapamil, high-dose methylprednisolone, progestogens, tacrolimus, cimetidine
	Reduces plasma concentration (risk of rejection)	Rifampin, trimethoprim (IV), carbamazapine, phenobarbitone, phenytoin
	Increases risk of nephrotoxicity	NSAIDs, aminoglycosides, co-trimoxazole, amphotericin, colchicine
	Increases risk of hyperkalemia	ACE inhibitors, spironolactone
	Other	Possible increased risk of myopathy with HMG-CoA reductase inhibitors
Tacrolimus	Increases plasma concentration (risk of toxicity)	Clarithromycin, erythromycin, clotrimazole, fluconazole, ketoconazole, cyclosporine, omeprazole
	Reduces plasma concentration (risk of rejection)	Rifampin
	Increases risk of nephrotoxocity	Ibuprofen, amphotericin
	Other	Possible reduced effectiveness of OCP
Azathioprine	Reduces plasma concentration (risk of rejection)	Rifampin
	Other	Allopurinol enhances effect with subsequent increased toxicity
Mycophenolate mofetil	Increases plasma concentration (risk of toxicity)	Acyclovir
	Reduces plasma concentration (risk of rejection)	Antacids, cholestyramine
Prednisolone	Reduces plasma concentration (risk of rejection)	Rifampin, carbamazepine, phenytoin, phenobarbitone
	Increases risk of hypokalemia	Amphotericin, loop diuretics, thiazides, salbutamol, terbutaline, carbenoxolone

ACE, angiotensin-converting enzyme; HMG-CoA, 3-hydroxy-3-methylglutaryl coenzyme A; NSAID, nonsteroidal antiinflammatory drug; OCP, oral contraceptive pill.

exclude the reaccumulation of ascites, and exclude the development of incisional hernias.

A battery of blood tests should be performed, including urea and electrolyte estimations, liver function tests (LFTs), full blood count, and measurement of blood levels of immunosuppressive drugs. Additional tests will need to be performed as symptoms or clinical signs dictate. Liaisons with pathology laboratories should result in tests that are reliable, cheap, and fast.[1] Prioritization by the laboratories should enable LFT results to be available the same day so that any abnormalities can be acted upon. Immunosuppressant levels should be available by the following day, and a system must exist whereby these results are reviewed and patients are contacted immediately when dosage adjustment is required. Some argue that the low specificity and sensitivity of standard LFTs mean that they should be supplemented with periodic histologic information in the form of yearly protocol biopsies.[2] However, the majority of transplant units argue that the role of liver biopsy is for the further investigation of biochemical abnormalities or clinical evidence of hepatic dysfunction.

The problems encountered at this stage of recovery are best divided into those relating to the transplantation surgery and the graft itself, those complications arising from long-term immunosuppressant medication, and those related to the recurrence of disease. In addition, a number of general features need to be considered.

COMPLICATIONS DIRECTLY RELATED TO SURGERY AND THE GRAFT

Stricture Formation

The most common cause of abnormal findings on LFTs more than 3 months posttransplantation remains biliary tract complications. These have been reported as occurring in up to 15% of cases.[3]

In the early era of hepatic transplantation, the surgical complications of the biliary anastomosis were termed the Achilles heel of the procedure.[4] Anastomotic strictures are more common after choledochojejunostomy than after direct choledochocholedochostomy.[5] Thankfully, refinement of surgical techniques has significantly improved the complication rate in this area.

With the reduction in surgical strictures, however, the number of ischemic strictures has become more apparent. Ischemic strictures usually occur as a late complication of hepatic artery thrombosis because, unlike the hepatic parenchyma, which enjoys a dual blood supply, the biliary epithelium relies on its arterial supply. These ischemic strictures occur both at the hilum of the liver and in the intrahepatic biliary tree. A diffuse series of strictures and cholangiectases may develop as a result of serial segmental arteriolar thrombosis, which results in disruption of bile flow. Although warm ischemic injury was previously implicated as the cause, the widespread use of University of Wisconsin preservation solution did not reduce the incidence of ischemic strictures. It is now generally held that the incidence of stricturing increases as a result of prolonged cold ischemic time (in excess of 12 hours).[5,6] Multiple ischemic strictures developing as a result of obliterative arteriopathy may also be a manifestation of chronic rejection.

Regardless of the nature of the stricture, the patient will present with cholestatic findings on LFTs and a rising serum bilirubin level. Depending on the level of the jaundice, the patient may complain of general malaise and anorexia. Where bile stasis occurs, ascending cholangitis remains a real threat. As with other posttransplantation infections, fever may be suppressed by the immunosuppressive treatment.

Investigation of the patient requires urgent ultrasonography and, once biliary dilation has been confirmed, early progression to visualization of the biliary tree either by endoscopic retrograde cholangiopancreatography (ERCP) or magnetic resonance cholangiography (MRC). Infection must be treated early and aggressively if further stricturing is to be avoided. In situations where sepsis has not already occurred, antibiotic prophylaxis at the time of biliary intervention should be considered mandatory.

Simple strictures are frequently amenable to percutaneous or endoscopic dilatation or stenting, or both. Occasionally, biliary casts that are not amenable to endoscopic intervention may develop as a result of biliary stasis. Other complications of biliary stasis include early formation of gallstones in the biliary tract (despite routine cholecystectomy of the donor graft), with an increased risk of ascending cholangitis. Reduced bile flow will affect the absorption of the oil-based formulations of cyclosporine, resulting in subtherapeutic levels, though this no longer appears to be a problem with microemulsion formulations of cyclosporine. Many centers advocate the use of ursodeoxycholic acid as a choleretic in an attempt to prevent biliary sludge formation, though there is little published evidence to support this. Occasionally, strictures require surgical biliary reconstruction with the formation of choledochojejunostomy or even hepaticojejunostomy. Early retransplantation needs to be considered in individuals with chronic rejection, hepatic artery thrombosis, or multiple established strictures that are not amenable to endoscopic intervention.

Acute Rejection

Although most acute rejection occurs during the first 3 posttransplantation months, episodes of acute rejection are by no means rare after this period and may occur for several years after orthotopic liver transplantation (OLT). The diagnosis must not be missed at this stage, because late acute rejection has a significantly worse prognosis than that occurring in the first 3 months. A significant proportion of cases of late acute rejection can be attributed to underimmunosuppression. This may occur because of noncompliance (often at this stage the patient will feel well and may inadvertently

omit medication) or as a result of the physician reducing the dose of medication in an attempt to minimize side effects. Alternatively the trough level of cyclosporine or tacrolimus (FK506) may fall as a result of reduced drug absorption, increased drug metabolism, or altered bioavailability. Nifedipine is known to reduce blood levels of tacrolimus, and rifampin, erythromycin, ketoconazole, and losartan can all affect blood levels of cyclosporine.

Patients may be asymptomatic during episodes of acute rejection, although many will describe general malaise or discomfort in the right upper quadrant, and the liver may be tender on palpation. The diagnosis must therefore be actively considered in any patient with a rising serum transaminase level, particularly if this is accompanied by subtherapeutic blood levels of immunosuppressant drugs.

Treatment should be aggressive. Liver biopsy is essential to confirm the diagnosis, though this should not delay institution of augmented immunosuppressive therapy. Although this therapy previously involved the use of intravenous corticosteroids, many units are now moving toward the outpatient management of acute rejection with high-dose oral corticosteroids. Repeated episodes of acute rejection may indicate the need for introduction of a second-line immunosuppressive agent. In those patients who underwent transplantation for viral hepatitis, there is evidence to suggest that a switch from cyclosporine to tacrolimus and the introduction of mycophenolate mofetil may be advantageous even after a single episode of acute rejection.[7]

One study by Cakaloglu et al. showed that a significant proportion of patients experiencing late acute rejection were suffering from concomitant viral infections (cytomegalovirus, 30%; herpes simplex virus, 5%; Epstein-Barr virus, 3%; and varicella zoster virus, 3%).[8] Because refractory rejection is more common in late episodes than in early episodes of acute rejection, it is essential that such viral infections are sought out and that appropriate antiviral agents, such as acyclovir and ganciclovir, are used in conjunction with augmented immunosuppression.

Chronic Rejection

Chronic rejection rarely occurs within the first 3 months after transplantation, and is usually not evident until at least 6 months after OLT. Nevertheless, in one of the earlier published series, chronic rejection accounted for 11.3% of graft losses at a mean of 496 days posttransplantation.[9] Figures have improved over time, and a more recent series records the rate of chronic rejection at approximately 1.3% in a pooled historical series of 1,174 primary grafts.[10] It is confidently predicted that these figures will continue to drop both as a result of improved immunosuppressive drugs (following the introduction of tacrolimus, Neoral, and mycophenolate) and improved extracorporeal graft preservation.[11]

Until such a time as the patient becomes cholestatic, chronic rejection is usually asymptomatic. The reviewing physician should be alerted to the possibility by gradual deterioration in liver function tests. Results of LFTs classically demonstrate an elevation of alkaline phosphatase and a proportionally lesser elevation of serum transaminases. Differential diagnoses at this stage will depend on the length of time since transplantation. Strictures with or without cholangitis (which usually has a more rapid onset and is accompanied by general malaise and fever) can occur many months or even years posttransplantation. The possibility of recurrence of underlying disease presenting as gradual progressive cholestasis must also be considered, and will be discussed later in this chapter.

Confirmation of chronic rejection requires liver biopsy. Chronic rejection is characterized by two distinct histologic entities: loss of small bile ducts and an obliterative angiopathy. Although the classic picture of chronic rejection is ductopenia with at least 50% of the portal tracts demonstrating absent bile ducts, these criteria may not be fulfilled in the early stages of development of the condition. In the early stages, chronic rejection may mimic acute rejection, with a dense portal tract infiltration and bile duct endotheliitis (hence the use of the all-encompassing term *cellular rejection*). The presence of foamy macrophage infiltration of arterial branches supports the diagnosis of early chronic rejection.

Because of the angiopathic changes, hepatic angiography has been used to support the diagnosis of chronic rejection. Angiography can demonstrate a number of changes in the graft vasculature, ranging from peripheral pruning to marked diffuse vascular sclerosis. It has been suggested that the presence of arteriographic changes positively predicts the chances of graft loss.[12]

Several studies have shown an association between the persistence of the cytomegalovirus (CMV) viral genome and progression to chronic rejection.[13,14] The association between HLA-DR matching and the vanishing bile duct syndrome has also been noted.[13] Other suggested associations with chronic rejection include chronic hepatitis C and positive cytotoxic T-cell crossmatching.[15]

Chronic (as opposed to acute) graft versus host disease (GVHD) usually develops at least 3 months posttransplantation and will affect up to one-third of long-term survivors.[16] Histologically, the bile duct changes associated with chronic GVHD may be indistinguishable from chronic rejection. However, angiopathic changes are not a feature of chronic GVHD. Early detection may prevent long-term damage.

COMPLICATIONS OF IMMUNOSUPPRESSIVE THERAPY

With respect to immunosuppression, the follow-up clinician has two roles: to optimize the dose of drugs by appropriate monitoring of drug levels and adjustment of dosages as indicated, and to be constantly vigilant for the signs and symptoms associated with immunosuppressant drug toxicity. As such, the clinician walks a tightrope, attempting to balance the known short- and long-term side effects of the immunosuppressant drugs with the knowledge that insufficient immunosuppression can seriously affect morbidity and graft survival. Individual immunosuppressant drugs will be covered in more detail in the relevant chapters. This chapter discusses the management of immunosuppression in the context of the transplant follow-up clinic.

Drug Monitoring

Monitoring of blood levels should take place at each clinic visit. More frequent monitoring may be required in particular cases both to avoid toxicity and to ensure adequate levels of immunosuppression. The assistance of primary physicians (family or general practitioners) can often be enlisted in this task, though it is essential that they understand the conditions and timing of sampling.

Monitoring of cyclosporine and tacrolimus has traditionally been based on trough level estimations (C_{min}). Data from renal transplant recipients suggest that freedom from rejection episodes has more to do with area under the (drug/time) curve (AUC) than with trough levels.[17] It has also been demonstrated that peak levels (C_{max}) determine the degree of calcineurin inhibition,[18] a factor known to predict the efficacy of immunosuppression. It is therefore possible that under current monitoring regimens, some patients are failing to obtain immunosuppressive protection because of a suboptimal C_{max} whereas others are experiencing toxicity because of a high AUC despite trough levels within the accepted range. It may well be that we need to look at improved methods of monitoring if the occurrence of both acute rejection and side effects from long-term drug use are to be avoided. Evidence from cardiac transplant recipients suggests that blood levels sampled 2 hours after a dose correlate with AUC and may be preferable to trough levels for monitoring purposes;[19] as yet, however, there are no published data on the use of this form of monitoring in liver transplant recipients.

Drug Regimens

Although unit-based immunosuppression policies, based on the latest findings in controlled clinical trials, are to be encouraged, ultimately each patient will require an individual regimen tailored according to his or her underlying disease, rejection episode history, experienced side effects, and comorbidity. The recent development of drugs such as tacrolimus, mycophenolate, and rapamycin has added to the clinician's armamentarium.

Because many of the adverse side effects experienced by the patient can be directly attributed to the use of corticosteroids, early tapering and, where possible, withdrawal of corticosteroids is to be encouraged. With increasing experience it is becoming apparent that lower doses, earlier withdrawal, and even complete avoidance of corticosteroids is possible if mycophenolate is used in the immunosuppressive regimen.[20] Whether this will translate into a reduction of the metabolic complications associated with corticosteroids has yet to be seen. Patients who underwent transplantation for chronic viral hepatitis should, when possible, be withdrawn from corticosteroids early. In contrast, some patients who underwent transplantation for autoimmune liver disease may require long-term low-dose corticosteroids.

A number of U.S. and European multicenter studies have attempted to compare the long-term benefits of tacrolimus and cyclosporine.[21-23] The 3-year follow-up data of the European Multicentre Tacrolimus Liver Study showed similar safety profiles for both drugs but a significant reduction in the incidence of acute, refractory acute, and chronic rejection and higher patient and graft survival rates in those patients receiving tacrolimus.[23] This study, however, compared tacrolimus with Sandimmune rather than Neoral. Other studies show no difference between the two treatment regimens in terms of improved 5-year graft and patient survival rates, patient tolerability, and side effect profiles.[24,25]

The conversion of patients from oil-based preparations of cyclosporine (Sandimmune) to a microemulsion-based formulation (Neoral) in the majority of centers has undoubtedly led to a 10% to 15% reduction in maintenance dosage requirements.[26] Because it is far less dependent on bile flow for absorption than Sandimmune, Neoral has also eliminated the need for intravenous cyclosporine during the immediate postoperative period[27]—a time when much of the damage to the kidney is done that may only become apparent many months or years later. It is hoped that this change will translate into a reduction in complications of cyclosporine toxicity in both the short term and the long term.

As the years posttransplantation progress, the balancing act becomes progressively easier. It is generally agreed that target blood levels of immunosuppressive therapy should be reduced as the time since operation progresses. It may therefore be necessary to reduce the maintenance dose at intervals. It is also becoming clear that a subgroup of patients may eventually be able to be withdrawn from immunosuppression completely in the long term, though further work is required to determine in which patients this can safely be carried out.[28,29]

Specific Problems

Renal Impairment

The nephrotoxicity of the mainstay immunosuppressive agents tacrolimus and Neoral is a significant cause for concern among those working in transplant follow-up clinics because it remains one of the major causes of patient morbidity and mortality after the first year of transplantation. Early studies indicated a reduction in glomerular filtration rate and effective renal plasma flow to between 45% and 60% of normal on standard cyclosporine regimens,[30] with cyclosporine causing acute and chronic renal dysfunction in 16% and 80% of patients, respectively.[31] The introduction

of tacrolimus has brought about a reduction in the incidence of renal problems.[32] These advantages appear to have been matched by the introduction of Neoral.[33] In addition to too high levels of immunosuppressant drugs, renal disease may predate the transplant or may have occurred as a result of early preoperative or postoperative hypotension or sepsis, or both. Diabetes (discussed later), which is common preoperatively and even more so postoperatively, contributes to diminished renal function.

Renal function should be measured at each clinic visit, because there is evidence that creatinine levels at 1 and 3 months posttransplantation are important predictors of long-term renal outcome.[34] Serious consideration must be given to the possibility of drug interactions, in particular the possible interaction with apparently innocuous drugs such as nonsteroidal antiinflammatory drugs (NSAIDs), which in many countries are available without prescription. Renal impairment can also be exacerbated by poor fluid intake, particularly in hot climates; patients thus need to be encouraged to keep up fluid intake.

Chronic renal failure necessitating long-term dialysis or transplantation as a result of immunosuppressive therapy has been well documented. Improved monitoring of blood levels of immunosuppressants, new formulations of cyclosporine, and the knowledge that patients can be maintained at a lower level of immunosuppression should all help to reduce the incidence of renal impairment in patients posttransplantation.

It has been suggested that a lower dose of tacrolimus supplemented with mycophenolate for the first 3 months results in a lower incidence of renal impairment than with standard tacrolimus-based regimens.[35] Many would also feel that at the first evidence of renal impairment, patients should be switched to tacrolimus and mycophenolate for the first 6 months, with withdrawal of the latter agent at 6 months.

Neither rapamycin nor FTY720 (a unique immunosuppressive drug produced by modification of a metabolite from *Isaria sinclairii*) have been found to have significant nephrotoxicity. The efficacy of these drugs has yet to be fully evaluated by the transplant community in controlled clinical trials, but they offer potential benefits both in patients who have preexisting renal impairment as well as those experiencing posttransplantation nephrotoxicity.

Cardiovascular and Metabolic Complications

A new emphasis for the reviewing clinician in the oupatient transplant follow-up clinic is the monitoring of, and where possible the treatment of, the known cardiovascular and metabolic complications that occur posttransplantation. The four major complications in this category—hypertension, hyperlipidemia, diabetes mellitus, and obesity—are inextricably linked. The contribution of these four conditions to the mortality and morbidity of the transplant population cannot be underestimated. Much work needs to be done on studying the underlying causes and optimal management of these conditions. Although we will attempt to discuss each of them individually, their interrelationship should be self-evident.

As long-term transplantation survival improves, cardiovascular complications are emerging as a major cause of both morbidity and mortality. In patients surviving more than 1 year after transplantation, the third most common cause of death (22.9%) is complications from cardiovascular disease.[36] The incidence of hypertension increases with the length of time from transplantation; various studies have reported incidences ranging from 15% at 3 months to 87% at 3 years posttransplantation.[37,38] These studies, however, were based on observations in patients treated with oil-based preparations of cyclosporine and with higher doses of corticosteroids than are generally used in clinical practice today. It is generally anticipated that the lower dose requirements of Neoral as well as the more widespread use of tacrolimus will reduce the incidence of hypertension in the future.

If left untreated, hypertension can have significant implications both for the graft and for the patient's general health. Therefore blood pressure must be monitored at every clinic visit, and hypertension treated early and aggressively. Although lifestyle factors should be addressed initially, and although occasionally hypertension can be improved by a reduction in the patient's immunosuppression dose (with close monitoring of LFTs) or even a switch to an alternative drug, in the majority of cases antihypertensive medication is required. Calcium channel blocking agents have proved to be the most effective drugs in this situation, with the angiotensin-converting enzyme inhibitors proving relatively ineffective. In certain situations multiple antihypertensive agents may be required.

Compounding the high incidence of hypertension is the fact that elevated lipid levels have been recorded in up to 30% of liver transplant recipients.[39] Evidence now links elevated lipid levels with allograft vasculopathy, an accelerated form of atherosclerosis,[40] and possibly even vanishing bile duct syndrome. Factors contributing to hyperlipidemia in the posttransplantation patient include obesity, corticosteroids, and cyclosporine. Cyclosporine is thought to inhibit the enzyme 26-hydroxylase (which is important in bile acid synthesis), resulting in reduced transport of cholesterol to the intestines. It is also thought to bind to low density lipoprotein (LDL) receptors.[41] Corticosteroids result in elevated levels of very low density lipoproteins, total cholesterol, and triglycerides, and in a reduction in high density lipoproteins. A number of studies have suggested that lipid levels are lower in patients receiving tacrolimus than in those receiving cyclosporine.[42,43] In the largest and most recent series,[43] mean cholesterol levels were consistently higher in those patients receiving cyclosporine and prednisolone compared with patients administered tacrolimus and prednisolone (Table 11.2). However, the greatest difference was noted when comparing patients given monotherapy with those still receiving prednisolone. In all patients in whom corticosteroid use was discontinued, mean cholesterol levels fell from 224 ± 70 mg/dL to 191 ± 48 mg/dL ($p < 0.001$). This drop was much more marked in the cyclosporine group. Hypercholesterolemia existed in 22% of the patients receiving cyclosporine monotherapy compared with 15% of those receiving tacrolimus ($p < 0.5$). This would seem to suggest that irrespective of the first-line agent, it is the early withdrawal of corticosteroids that has the most significant impact on lowering posttransplantation cholesterol levels.

Lipid levels should be checked in transplant recipients on a regular basis. Management should be based on diet and weight control and the tapering (and where possible, withdrawal) of corticosteroids. Although the use of HMG-CoA reductase inhibitors has been shown in a number of papers to have been beneficial for cardiac and renal transplant recipients in terms of reduced morbidity and mortality,[44] no data have yet been published concerning the inhibitors' effects in liver transplant recipients.

Patients with end-stage liver disease frequently exhibit glucose intolerance, and a proportion of them will require insulin treatment preoperatively. One series reports that 4.5% of patients are taking insulin or hypoglycemic agents prior to transplantation.[45] Although hyperglycemia is understandably common in the immediate postoperative period (reflecting the use of high-dose corticosteroids, reduced graft function, infection, and the use of parenteral nutrition), impaired glucose tolerance and the requirement for hypoglycemic medication will persist beyond the first 3 months in 4% to 17% of patients.[45,46]

TABLE 11.2. *Posttransplantation hypercholesterolemia*

	Mean serum cholesterol (mg/dL)[a]			
	Cyclosporine A + prednisolone	Cyclosporine monotherapy	Tacrolimus + prednisolone	Tacrolimus monotherapy
Pretransplantation	156 ± 31		160 ± 23	
1 yr posttransplantation	218.6 ± 53.8	183.3 ± 54.2	208.8 ± 58.1	223.8 ± 55.0
2 yr posttransplantation	223.3 ± 58.0	197.0 ± 63.8	183.0 ± 49.1	178.4 ± 53.5
3 yr posttransplantation	215.6 ± 53.7	199.8 ± 55.9	169.1 ± 59.4	168.7 ± 55.5

[a]normal < 220 mg/dL.
From Charco R, Canterell C, Vargas V, et al. Serum cholesterol changes in long-term survivors of liver transplantation: a comparison between cyclosporine and tacrolimus therapy. *Liver Transplant Surg* 1999;5(3):204–208, with permission.

Some of these patients will require insulin after discharge from the hospital; therefore, they should be educated to understand the relationship between blood glucose monitoring and insulin requirements and should be given the equipment and support to adjust their treatment accordingly. In these patients, home monitoring of blood sugar levels is important, supplemented by three monthly estimations of glycosylated hemoglobin levels. The assistance of the diabetic liaison team in the optimization of glycemic control can be valuable. The relationship between posttransplantation obesity and glucose intolerance cannot be underestimated, and weight control, as well as the adjustment of immunosuppressant drugs and good diabetic control, is an essential part of the management of patients with posttransplantation hyperglycemia.

Although initial reports suggested that the drug tacrolimus was potentially intrinsically diabetogenic, subsequent studies would appear to refute this. The use of mycophenolate to reduce steroid requirements may also reduce the incidence of posttransplantation diabetes.[47]

Obesity has effects on morbidity over and above its effects on diabetes and hypertension. Many patients who have had end-stage liver disease that led to transplantation will have suffered many years of anorexia and suboptimal nutritional status. Recovery of normal liver function commonly results in a rediscovery of appetite. Coupled with the weight-gaining effects of immunosuppressant medication, in particular corticosteroids, this can lead to rapid weight gain postoperatively, with the result that a significant proportion of transplant recipients become clinically obese.

In one study, 64.3% of patients became overweight posttransplantation.[48] A strong association was noted between obesity, hyperlipidemia, and diabetes. In the early posttransplantation period, weight gain was running at 1.5 kg per month, though the rate slowed in the second posttransplantation year. Obesity pretransplantation predicted posttransplantation weight gain. A second, larger study of 123 consecutive transplant recipients reported the incidence of obesity at 1 year posttransplantation as 41.9% in women and 39.3% in men.[49] This paper noted a significant reduction in each of the late metabolic complications posttransplantation (hypertension, hyperlipidemia, diabetes, and obesity) with the tapering of corticosteroid doses. A more recent long-term follow-up study of 774 patients found that 21.6% who were not obese prior to transplantation developed obesity within 1 year of transplantation.[50] This group reported pretransplantation predictors of obesity that included greater donor and recipient body mass index and being married, whereas posttransplantation predictors of obesity included absence of acute rejection episodes and the cumulative prednisone dose in the second postoperative year. Despite this, the incidence of obesity in the transplant population was only slightly greater than that of the U.S. population as a whole (though this is higher than in other western centers). Patients should be given advice on healthy eating, and the assistance of a dietician is invaluable in obtaining calorie

counts and in identifying unrecognized calorie sources in those not losing weight.

Two separate studies, one from the United States and the other from Germany, both reported a lower incidence of cardiovascular complications in patients receiving tacrolimus-based immunosuppression compared with those on more traditional cyclosporine-based regimens.[51,52] Only in the U.S. study did this apparent advantage reach levels of statistical significance, however. Follow-up in this study was for just 1 year, and whether the advantage was maintained has yet to be reported.

Osteoporosis

Many patients with chronic liver disease are severely osteopenic as a result of long-term reduced mobility and reduced absorption of fat-soluble vitamins. This is especially marked in patients with the chronic cholestatic syndromes, in particular primary biliary cirrhosis (PBC). In women undergoing transplantation for PBC, bone mineral density drops by 18% in the first 3 months posttransplantation and is severely aggravated by immobility and high-dose corticosteroids; it may take up to 1 year to regain the (suboptimal) preoperative levels. By 2 years, mineralization had only increased 5% above (a suboptimal) baseline (Fig. 11.1).[53]

Osteoporotic fractures can be one of the most difficult problems to manage postoperatively. Fractures can not only be disabling, but can also be life-threatening; there have been reports of cord transection occurring as a result of vertebral collapse. Nothing is more upsetting than to see a patient with PBC going through transplantation, losing the characteristic itch and pigmentation of that condition and as a result looking years younger, only to see the patient severely handicapped by fractures resulting from minimal trauma. The spontaneous fracture rate during the postoperative period was 65% for patients with PBC and between 17% and 38% for those patients with mixed etiologies.[53–55] The possibility of fracture must therefore be considered whenever patients report bone or back pain. The differential diagnosis of bone pain and pathologic fractures must include metastatic hepatoma in those patients with preoperative cirrhosis. Further investigations may therefore include radionucleotide bone scans and magnetic resonance imaging as well as plain radiographs.

Management of osteoporotic fractures is conservative. NSAIDs should be avoided because of the risk of exacerbating renal impairment. Pain control can therefore be difficult, and nerve blocks and transcutaneous electrical nerve stimulation (TENS) may be beneficial. Preoperative treatment with intravenous bisphosphonates can dramatically reduce the incidence of postoperative fractures.[56] The use of antiresorptive drugs such as etidronate may be beneficial in terms of improving vertebral bone mineral density in postoperative patients.[57] It has also been suggested that when managing certain subgroups of transplantation patients, such as those older than 60 years, immunosuppression regimens

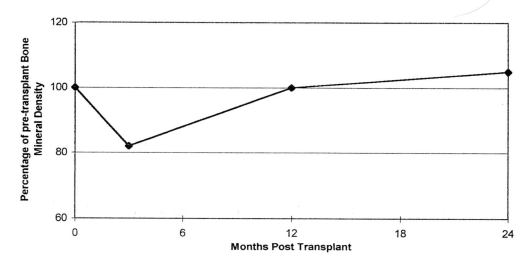

FIG. 11.1. Loss of bone mineral density in the perioperative period.

avoiding corticosteroids (i.e., cyclosporine/tacrolimus plus azathioprine or mycophenolate) can be utilized with no extra episodes of acute rejection and with possible benefits in terms of reduced orthopedic complications.[58]

Neurologic Complications

Many of the complaints mentioned by the patient in the transplant follow-up clinic will relate to the neurologic side effects of the immunosuppressant medication. Headaches are common and may at times be sufficiently severe so as to affect the patient's quality of life or result in clinical depression; on occasion, they have led to serious opiate addiction. Dose reduction may be of benefit in some patients. Although all the first-line immunosuppressant drugs have similar side effect profiles with respect to this complaint, sometimes a change of immunosuppressant drug may benefit the patient. The differential diagnosis is extensive, and the patient's complaints must be taken seriously and fully investigated, including performing computed tomographic (CT) scans of the head. Neurologic referral may be warranted in cases that are resistant to treatment.

Tremor is a well-recognized side effect of cyclosporine in a large number of patients. The symptoms can be distressing and even significantly disabling to the patient.[59] Reassurance is required, because often this symptom will improve with time or a reduction in drug dosage.

Some patients complain of memory loss and poor concentration postoperatively. Occasionally this may be as a result of cerebral hypotension at the time of surgery. Immunosuppressants have also been implicated.

Neurotoxicity of cyclosporine as a result of supratherapeutic blood levels can present in a number of ways, including tremulousness, restlessness, acute confusional state, psychosis, seizures, speech apraxia, and even cortical blindness.[60] Frequently the neurological presentation can be subtle; therefore, the reviewing physician needs to be constantly aware of the possibility of cyclosporine neurotoxicity, and receptive to any clues the patient may give him or her in the history.

Although seizures are not an uncommon occurrence in the immediate postoperative period (and frequently predict an unfavorable outcome), they usually have an underlying metabolic or infective cause. In a number of situations, seizures can be attributed to toxic blood levels of immunosuppressant medication. Whatever the cause, in those patients who survive, seizures do not tend to persist into the follow-up period and anticonvulsants are not generally required.[61]

Myeloproliferative Disorders

Based on currently available statistics, patients who underwent transplantation for conditions other than malignancy or viral hepatitis and who survive 12 months posttransplantation have a near normal life expectancy. One factor that reduces life expectancy, however, is the increased incidence of myeloproliferative disorders directly related to the duration and intensity of immunosuppression. The incidence is greatest in the pediatric population. Unpublished data from Kings College Hospital regarding 385 consecutive liver transplant recipients over a 20-year period show an incidence of 1% and the risk of lymphoproliferative syndromes as being 0.47% per year. In a series of 1,276 patients over a similar time period, Starzl's group reported the incidence as 3.6%.[62] The risk in pediatric patients would appear to be significantly higher.[63] Although studies of the use of tacrolimus have suggested a lower incidence of lymphoma with this drug,[64] it must be noted that the follow-up period for these studies has been short. An even greater association between OKT3 usage and the development of lymphoproliferative disorder has been demonstrated in pediatric[65] and cardiac transplant recipients.[66]

Cosmetic Considerations

Many patients will become concerned and distressed over the cosmetic side effects of the immunosuppressive therapy they are receiving. Cyclosporine is associated with hirsutism and gum hypertrophy. Corticosteroids can cause acne. Patients, in particular younger female patients, will need reassurance that these symptoms will frequently lessen with time, although a change of immunosuppressant may occasionally be indicated. Gynecomastia may be slow to resolve or may continue to develop if the patient is receiving postoperative spironolactone. Surgical referral for mastectomy may be required. Incisional hernias and scar tissue may cause physical or cosmetic concern to the patient and warrant surgical revision.

DISEASE RECURRENCE

The ongoing assessment of disease recurrence plays an integral part of the transplant follow-up clinic. The clinician must never lose sight of the initial indication for transplantation. In this way he or she can be alert to evidence of disease recurrence and thereby plan diagnostic investigation and treatment as appropriate.

The majority of conditions for which individuals undergo transplantation will recur at some point in time; these are discussed in more detail in the relevant chapters. The timing of disease recurrence is highly variable. Recurrence of viral hepatitis is early and universal, and efforts are directed at minimizing viral damage to the graft. Features of many of the autoimmune chronic cholestatic liver diseases will reappear over time. Recurrence of tumor in those patients undergoing transplantation for malignancy is often rapid and aggressive. Alcoholic liver disease will only recur if the patient decides to resume ethanol consumption. Only those undergoing OLT for inherited metabolic diseases in which the deficient enzyme is restricted to the liver can be said to be truly cured.

Viral Hepatitis

Because chronic viral hepatitis is now the primary indication for transplantation worldwide, a significant proportion of patients seen in the follow-up clinic will be affected. The use of human hepatitis B immune globulin (HBIG) has significantly improved the 5-year survival rates in patients undergoing transplantation for chronic hepatitis B virus (HBV) infection. The use of lamivudine, both to supress viral replication in the pretransplantation period and to maintain viral suppression posttransplantation, has further improved graft survival. Those patients in the clinic taking lamivudine will need to be monitored for potential side effects, in particular pancreatitis, as well as for evidence of viral breakthrough due to mutation as evidenced by a rising alanine aminotransferase (ALT) level and positive HBV DNA titer. More recently the use of high-dose HBIG infusions has improved the prognosis further,[67] although raising issues of cost and availability. Within the follow-up clinic, arrangements will need to be made for these regular infusions to be administered, and levels of antibodies to hepatitis B surface antigen (anti-HBs)

will need to be monitored regularly. Recurrent hepatitis B can bring about graft destruction either as a result of the chronic hepatitis leading to cirrhosis or as a result of fibrosing cholestatic hepatitis, a unique syndrome with characteristic histologic appearance.

The majority of patients who undergo transplantation for chronic hepatitis C will experience a mild chronic hepatitis following transplantation. A minority, however, will experience an aggressive recurrence that can lead rapidly to cirrhosis and may well require regrafting. In these patients it can be difficult to determine whether a rise in transaminases reflects viral recurrence or acute rejection; clearly, the treatments for each of these two options are antagonistic. Liver biopsy is mandatory, although histologic differentiation can be difficult. In patients with confirmed recurrence of hepatitis C, treatment with interferon and ribavirin must be considered. These patients will need to be reviewed on a frequent basis, not only to monitor the hepatitis but also to monitor the side effects of treatment (including hemolytic anemia and neutropenia), which can have more serious implications in the immunosuppressed patient. The management of viral recurrence is discussed in more detail in other chapters of this book.

Primary Sclerosing Cholangitis

Recurrence of primary sclerosing cholangitis (PSC) tends to occur late. Presentation is usually as a gradual rise of alkaline phosphatase with or without episodes of jaundice and cholangitis. Management consists of confirmation of diagnosis with ERCP. The differential diagnosis includes chronic ductopenic rejection. Anastomotic strictures are more common in patients who underwent transplantation for PSC. Single, dominant strictures are frequently amenable to dilatation. More extensive stricturing may require extensive surgical biliary reconstruction. Retransplantation may need to be considered. *De novo* autoimmune hepatitis has been described in patients who underwent transplantation for other indications.[68]

Malignancy

Patients who undergo transplantation for hepatocellular carcinoma or in whom hepatoma is found incidentally at the time of transplantation will require screening. α-Fetoprotein should be checked at each clinic visit and at other times if there is evidence of clinical deterioration. Recurrence is usually as a result of metastases, either occurring in the graft or distally. Therefore, ultrasound of the liver needs to be supplemented with other imaging modalities, including chest radiography and CT of those regions suspected of involvement.

Regression of Symptoms and Signs of Chronic Liver Disease

Although many of the signs and symptoms of chronic liver disease will regress rapidly following transplantation, others may persist well into the long-term follow-up period. It may take up to 12 months for hepatic hemodynamics to return to normal. As a consequence, patients may still have significant flow through portosystemic anastamoses for some time after transplantation. Cutaneous manifestations of liver disease regress differentially. Spider nevi, for example, should disappear rapidly, whereas the xanthomas associated with primary biliary cirrhosis may take months or years to regress and may never disappear completely. The rapidity with which the neurologic manifestations of Wilson's disease reverse after transplantation is highly variable. If symptoms do not appear to be regressing as rapidly as anticipated, the possibility of graft dysfunction or disease recurrence, or both, needs to be considered.

GENERAL ISSUES

Cancer Screening

Patients need to be reminded of the increased incidence of a number of malignancies while on long-term immunosuppression. One Birmingham series of 904 patients reported malignancy rates of 0.6%, 5.7%, and 10.2% at 1, 5, and 10 years posttransplantation.[69]

The incidence of skin malignancies can be significantly reduced by simple measures such as the use of high protection factor sunscreen and the wearing of a hat when outdoors. Patients who underwent transplantation for primary sclerosing cholangitis (PSC) who retain an intact colon should be enrolled into a colonoscopic surveillance program because the incidence of colon cancer is higher in immunosuppressed patients than in the healthy population. One study from the Mayo clinic reports a 4-fold increased risk of posttransplantation malignancy in patients with ulcerative colitis and PSC compared with the pretransplantation period. The cumulative incidence of dysplasia was 15% at 5 years and 21% at 8 years.[70] Although no guidelines exist on the frequency of surveillance, annual colonoscopy with multiple mucosal samplings would appear prudent. Female patients should be reminded of the need for regular cervical cytology screening and breast self-examination.

Psychosocial Issues

Many reviews attest to the improved quality of life experienced by the majority of patients undergoing transplantation for chronic liver disease.[71,72] Quality of life, however, relies not only on physical but also on mental well-being. The interpersonal dynamics of the chronically sick patient can be complex. Return to good health after transplantation can have profound effects on these relationships. In some cases the patient may persist in the sick role. In other situations family members who have adopted the role of caregiver over many months or years may suddenly find themselves redundant. Patients may not consider these problems of sufficient importance to concern their physician. However, these issues

are pivotal to the patient's full recovery and rehabilitation and can therefore not be dismissed. The assistance of social workers and outside agencies may need to be enlisted.

Alcohol and the Transplant Recipient

Much is written about the risks of alcoholic recidivism after transplantation for end-stage alcoholic liver disease. It is generally accepted that the incidence is underreported by patients, and therefore true figures are hard to obtain. Published statistics quote overall recidivism rates between 10%[73] and 18%,[74] though it is generally accepted that rates are higher in certain subgroups. Returning to alcohol consumption is frequently associated with rapid development of histologic changes of alcoholic liver disease.[75]

One factor that needs to be taken into account when assessing these studies is the definition of recidivism. In some studies, any alcohol consumption, even within the accepted "safe" limits, constitutes recidivism. It is generally believed that public knowledge of alcohol consumption by individuals who have received a transplant for end-stage alcoholic liver disease could adversely affect donation rates and the transplant program as a whole. Heavy drinking also raises issues of compliance with medication and alteration in pharmacokinetics. However, there is less evidence to suggest that occasional alcohol consumption has adverse effects on the health of the individual, and therefore many clinicians will tolerate occasional, moderate alcohol consumption in their patients.

This having been said, there is a significant proportion of patients who will resume heavy alcohol consumption. Because patient recall of abstinence advice is unreliable, and those who return to moderate or heavy drinking usually do so within the first year posttransplantation,[75] it is important that these patients be identified early and that appropriate counseling and support structures be put in place as early as possible. Some physicians advocate random testing for blood alcohol levels or monitoring of γ-glutamyltransferase levels at routine outpatient clinic visits. However, these methods are notoriously unreliable; it is preferable to rely on the doctor-patient relationship built on mutual trust and nonjudgmental understanding in order to detect and cope with this particular problem.

A more difficult problem is that of whether patients who undergo transplantation for nonalcoholic indications should be allowed to drink. It seems unnecessarily draconian to deny patients who have never previously shown an inability to control alcohol consumption a social pleasure enjoyed by the rest of the population. What is important, however, is consistency on the part of the whole team, since conflicting information given to the patient can be confusing and divisive.

Employment

Considering that the aim of transplantation is to return patients to a full and normal life, a disappointingly high percentage of patients do not return to full-time occupation. A number of reasons exist for this phenomenon. In a minority of cases, continuing ill health may prevent the patient from seeking full-time employment. In others, chronic ill health through adolescence and early life may have led to a lack of educational and training opportunities. Some employers have concerns about hiring workers posttransplantation, whether because of fear of underlying illness or a concern over future absenteeism. Often, all that is required is reassurance from the physician in charge. Wherever possible, the physician should be flexible in the timing of review of the patient to fit in with the patient's work schedule. In a certain number of cases, however, the patient may have fully assumed the sick role and never have considered the need to return to work. In these cases specialized counseling involving the services of social workers and occupational therapists as well as remedial training may be of benefit.

Fertility and Contraception

Although patients may (erroneously) feel that the transplant outpatient clinic is not the forum for the discussion of issues relating to sexual activity, these issues contribute significantly to quality-of-life values. Patients should be encouraged to discuss their concerns in order that advice or treatment can be given, or appropriate referrals made.

Increasing numbers of women of child-bearing age are undergoing transplantation for a range of diseases, in particular autoimmune hepatitis. Women with chronic liver disease demonstrate a high incidence of amenorrhea and secondary infertility. Forty-eight percent of women undergoing transplantation for chronic liver disease reported secondary amenorrhea of greater than 12 months' duration.[76] Lack of libido as a result of chronic disease is also well recognized. Similarly, men with chronic liver disease may experience a degree of hypogonadism resulting in erectile dysfunction and loss of libido. As a consequence of these factors, the need for contraception may have been absent in many relationships. Resumption of an active sex life postoperatively together with refound fertility may result in unwanted pregnancies unless patients are appropriately counseled at the time of operation. Conception before the resumption of menstruation has been reported.

With long-term survival rates greater than 80%, increasing numbers of women wish to pursue pregnancy. Pregnancy posttransplantation carries a slightly increased risk of obstetric complications and graft dysfunction. In a series reported by Patapis et al., 17 women underwent 27 pregnancies.[77] Seven pregnancies were terminated; of the remainder, 15 resulted in live births (3 by elective caesarean section) and 5 were miscarriages. In the mothers, there were two episodes of rejection, one responding to pulsed steroids, the other requiring retransplantation. Other centers confirm a higher risk of obsteric complications, including anemia, preterm delivery, eclampsia, and caesarean section.[78] In one study, 7 of 13 women who be-

came pregnant after transplantation had evidence of renal dysfunction at the time of the first prenatal visit. Renal dysfunction was found to be the primary determinant of adverse pregnancy outcome.[79]

Many successful pregnancies have been completed in women following liver transplantation, however, and in the majority of women, a planned pregnancy with successful outcome should be considered to be a natural expectation following OLT. It would seem sensible, though, to advise patients to use reliable contraception for the first year after transplantation, when the risks, both obstetric and hepatic, would appear to be greatest. After this stage, pregnancy should ideally be discussed and planned in conjunction with the patient's obstetrician and hepatologist.

There has been no evidence to date that cyclosporine or tacrolimus has teratogenic effects, though blood levels of immunosuppressants[80] and placental blood flow should be monitored carefully throughout pregnancy. Azathioprine has been linked with growth retardation and fetal immunosuppression[81] and should therefore be discontinued at least 3 months before conception is planned.

REFERENCES

1. Hickman PE, Potter JM, Pesce AJ. Clinical chemistry and post-liver-transplant monitoring. *Clin Chem* 1997;43:1546–1554.
2. Neuberger J, Wilson P, Adams D. Protocol liver biopsies: the case in favour. *Transplant Proc* 1998;30:1497–1499.
3. Lopez RR, Benner KG, Ivancev K, et al. Management of biliary complications after liver transplantation. *Am J Surg* 1992;163:519–524.
4. Calne RY. A new technique for biliary drainage in orthotopic liver transplantation utilising the gall bladder as a pedicle graft conduit between the donor and recipient bile ducts. *Ann Surg* 1976;184:605–609.
5. Colonna JO, Shaked A, Gomes AS, et al. Biliary strictures complicating liver transplantation: incidence, pathogenesis, management and outcome. *Ann Surg* 1992;163:519–524.
6. Sanchez-Urdazpal L, Gores GJ, Ward EM, et al. Ischaemic-type biliary complications after orthotopic liver transplantation. *Hepatology* 1992;16:49–53.
7. Platz KP, Mueller AR, Berg T, et al. Searching for the optimal management of hepatitis C patients after liver transplantation. *Transpl Int* 1998,11:S209–S211.
8. Cakaloglu Y, Devlin J, O'Grady J, et al. Importance of concomitant viral infection during late, acute, liver allograft rejection. *Transplantation* 1995;59:40–85.
9. Quiroga J, Colina I, Demetris AJ, et al. Cause and timing of first allograft rejection in orthotopic liver transplantation—associated risk factors and outcome. *Transplantation* 1991;14:1054–1062.
10. Abbasoglu O, Levy MF, Brkic BB, et al. Ten years of liver transplantation: an evolving understanding of late graft loss. *Transplantation* 1997;64:1801–1807.
11. Pirsch JD, Kalayoglu M, Hafez GR, et al. Evidence that the vanishing bile duct syndrome is vanishing. *Transplantation* 1990;49:1015–1018.
12. Devlin J, Page AC, O'Grady J, et al. Angiographically determined arteriopathy in liver graft dysfunction and survival. *J Hepatol* 1993;18:68–73.
13. Arnold JC, Portmann B, O'Grady J, et al. Cytomegalovirus infection persists in the liver graft in the vanishing bile duct syndrome. *Hepatology* 1992;16:285–292.
14. Manez R, White LT, Linden P, et al. The influence of HLA matching of cytomegalovirus hepatitis and chronic rejection after liver transplantation. *Transplantation* 1993;55:1067–1071.
15. Wong T, Donaldson P, Devlin J, et al. Repeat HLA-B and -DR loci mismatching at second liver transplantation improves patient survival. *Transplantation* 1996;61:440–444.
16. Demetris AJ. Immune cholangitis: liver allograft rejection and graft-versus-host-disease. *Mayo Clin Proc* 1998;73:367–379.

17. Lindholm A, Kahan BD. Influence of cyclosporine pharmacokinetics, trough concentrations, and AUC monitoring on outcome after kidney transplantation. *Clin Pharmacol Ther* 1993;54:205–218.
18. Batiuk TD, Pazderka F, Enns J, et al. Cyclosporine inhibition of leukocyte calcineurin is much less in whole blood than in culture medium. *Transplantation* 1996;61:158–161.
19. Cantarovich M, Barkun JS, Tchervenkov JI, et al. Comparison of Neoral dose monitoring with cyclosporine trough levels versus 2-hr postdose levels in stable liver transplant patients. *Transplantation* 1998;66:1621–1627.
20. McDiarmid S. The necessity for steroid induction or long-term maintenance after liver transplantation: the argument against. *Transplant Proc* 1998;30:1449–1451.
21. Wiesner RH. A long-term comparison of tacrolimus (FK506) versus cyclosporine in liver transplantation: a report of the United States FK506 study group. *Transplantation* 1998;66:493–499.
22. Jonas S, Guckelberger O, Bechstein WO, et al. Five year follow-up of tacrolimus as primary immunosuppressant after liver transplantation. *Transplant Proc* 1998;30:2179–2181.
23. Pichlmayr R, Winkler M, Neuhaus P, et al. Three year follow-up of the European multicentre tacrolimus (FK506) liver study. *Transplant Proc* 1997;29:2499–2502.
24. Busuttil RW, Holt CD. Tacrolimus is superior to cyclosporine in liver transplantation. *Transplant Proc* 1998;30:2174–2178.
25. Levy GA. Neoral is superior to FK506 in liver transplantation. *Transplant Proc* 1998;30:1812–1815.
26. Chueh SC, Tian L, Wang M, et al. Induction of tolerance toward rat cardiac allografts by treatment with allochimeric class I MHC antigen and FTY720. *Transplantation* 1997;64:1407–1414.
27. Hemming AW, Greig PD, Cattral MS, et al. A microemulsion of cyclosporine without intravenous cyclosporine in liver transplantation. *Transplantation* 1996;62:1798–1802.
28. Mazariegos GV, Reyes J, Marino IR, et al. Weaning of immunosuppression in liver transplant recipients. *Transplantation* 1997;63:243–249.
29. Devlin J, Doherty D, Thomson L, et al. Defining the outcome of immunosuppression withdrawal after liver transplantation. *Hepatology* 1998;27:926–933.
30. Wheatley HC, Datzman M, Williams JW, et al. Long-term effects of cyclosporine on renal function in liver transplant recipients. *Transplantation* 1987;43:641–647.
31. McCauley J. The nephrotoxicity of FK506 as compared with cyclosporine. *Curr Opin Nephrol Hypertens* 1993;2:662–669.
32. Tauxe WN, Mochizuki T, McCauley J, et al. A comparison of the renal effects (ERPF, GFR, and FF) of FK 506 and cyclosporine in patients with liver transplantation. *Transplant Proc* 1991;23:3146–3147.
33. Van Buren D, Payne J, Geevarghese S, et al. Impact of Sandimmune, Neoral, and Prograf on rejection incidence and renal function in primary liver transplant recipients. *Transplant Proc* 1998;30:1830–1832.
34. Fisher NC, Nightingale PG, Gunson BK, et al. Chronic renal failure following liver transplantation: a retrospective analysis. *Transplantation* 1998;66:59–66.
35. Eckhoff DE, McGuire BM, Frenette LR, et al. Tacrolimus (FK506) and mycophenolate mofetil combination therapy versus tacrolimus in adult liver transplantation. *Transplantation* 1998;65:180–187.
36. Asfar S, Metrakos P, Fryer J, et al. An analysis of late deaths after liver transplantation. *Transplantation* 1996;61:1377–1381.
37. O'Grady JG, Forbes A, Rolles K, et al. An analysis of cyclosporin efficacy and toxicity after liver transplantation. *Transplantation* 1988;45:575–578.
38. Hauters P, de Hemptinne B, Carlier M, et al. Long term analysis of glomerular filtration rate and hypertension in adult liver transplant recipients treated with cyclosporine A. *Transplant Proc* 1991;23:1458–1459.
39. Mathe D, Adam R, Malmendier C, et al. Prevalence of dyslipidemia in liver transplant recipients. *Transplantation* 1992;54:167–170.
40. Pirsch JD, D'Alessandro AM, Sollinger HW, et al. Hyperlipidemia and transplantation: etiologic factors and therapy. *J Am Soc Nephrol* 1992;2:S238–S242.
41. deGroen PC. Cyclosporine, low-density lipoprotein, and cholesterol. *Mayo Clin Proc* 1988;63:1012–1021.
42. Jindal RM, Popescu I, Emre S, et al. Serum lipid changes in liver transplant recipients in a prospective trial of cyclosporine versus FK506. *Transplantation* 1994;57:1395–1398.
43. Charco R, Canterell C, Vargas V, et al. Serum cholesterol changes in long-term survivors of liver transplantation: a comparison between cyclosporine and tacrolimus therapy. *Liver Transplant Surg* 1999;204–208.
44. Castelao AM, Grino JM, Andres E, et al. HMGCoA reductase inhibitors lovastatin and simvastatin in the treatment of hypercholesterolaemia after renal transplantation. *Transplant Proc* 1993;25:1043–1046.
45. Wahlstrom HE, Cooper J, Gores G, et al. Survival after liver transplantation in diabetics. *Transplant Proc* 1991;23:1565–1566.
46. Fung J, Abu-Elmagd K, Jain A, et al. A randomised trial of primary liver transplantation under immunosuppression with FK506 vs cyclosporine. *Transplant Proc* 1991;23:2977–2983.
47. Stegall MD, Wachs ME, Everson G, et al. Prednisone withdrawal 14 days after liver transplantation with mycophenolate: a prospective trial of cyclosporine and tacrolimus. *Transplantation* 1997;64:1755–1760.
48. Palmer M, Schaffner F, Thung SN. Excessive weight gain after liver transplantation. *Transplantation* 1991;51:797–800.
49. Stegall MD, Everson G, Schroter G, et al. Metabolic complications after liver transplantation. Diabetes, hypercholesterolaemia, hypertension and obesity. *Transplantation* 1995;60:1057–1060.
50. Everhart JE, Lombardero M, Lake JJR, et al. Weight gain and obesity after liver transplantation: incidence and risk factors. *Liver Transplant Surg* 1998;4:285–296.
51. Canzanello VJ, Schwartz L, Taler SJ, et al. Evolution of cardiovascular risk after liver transplantation: a comparison of cyclosporin A and tacrolimus (FK506). *Liver Transplant Surg* 1997;3:1–9.
52. Guckelberger O, Bechstein WO, Neuhaus R, et al. Cardiovascular risk factors in long-term follow-up after orthotopic liver transplantation. *Clin Transplant* 1997;11:60–65.
53. Eastell R, Dickson ER, Hodgson SF, et al. Rates of vertebral bone loss before and after liver transplantation in women with primary biliary cirrhosis. *Hepatology* 1991;14:296–300.
54. McDonald JA, Dunstan CR, Dilworth P, et al. Bone loss after liver transplantation. *Hepatology* 1991;14:613–619.
55. Haagsma EB, Thijn CJP, Post JG, et al. Bone disease after orthotopic transplantation. *J Hepatol* 1988;6:94–100.
56. Reeves HL, Francis RM, Manas DM, et al. Intravenous bisphosphonate prevents symptomatic osteoporotic vertebral collapse in patients after liver transplantation. *Liver Transplant Surg* 1998;4:404–409.
57. Valero MA, Loinaz C, Larrodera L, et al. Calcitonin and bisphosphonates treatment in bone loss after liver transplantation. *Calcif Tissue Int* 1995;57:15–19.
58. Tisone G, Angelico M, Vennarecci G, et al. Metabolic findings after liver transplantation within a randomised trial with or without steroids. *Transplant Proc* 1998;30:1447–1448.
59. LeDoux MS, McGill LJ, Pulsinelli WA, et al. Severe bilateral tremor in a liver transplant recipient taking cyclosporine. *Mov Disord* 1998;13:589–596.
60. Wijdicks EF, Wiesner RH, Krom RA. Neurotoxicity in liver transplant recipients with cyclosporine immunosuppression. *Neurology* 1995;45:1962–1964.
61. Wijdicks EF, Plevak DJ, Wiesner RH, et al. Causes and outcomes of seizures in liver transplant recipients. *Neurology* 1996;47:1523–1525.
62. Stieber AC, Boillot O, Scotti-Foglieni C, et al. The surgical implications of posttransplant lymphoproliferative disorders. *Transplant Proc* 1991;23:1477–1479.
63. Malatack JJ, Gartner JC, Urbach AH, et al. Orthotopic liver transplantation, Epstein Barr virus, cyclosporine, and lymphoproliferative disease: a growing concern. *J Pediatr* 1991;118:667–675.
64. Reyes J, Tzakis A, Green M, et al. Posttransplant lymphoproliferative disorders occuring under FK506 immunosuppression. *Transplant Proc* 1991;23:3044–3046.
65. Renard TH, Andrews WS, Foster ME. Relationship between OKT3 administration, EBV seroconversion, and lymphoproliferative syndrome in pediatric liver transplant recipients. *Transplant Proc* 1991;23:1473–1476.
66. Swinnen JL, Costanzo-Nordin MR, Fisher SG, et al. Increased incidence of lymphoproliferative disorder after immunosuppression with the monoclonal antibody OKT3 in cardiac transplant recipients. *N Engl J Med* 1990;323:1723–1728.
67. Nymann T, Shokouh-Amiri MH, Vera SR, et al. Prevention of hepatitis B recurrence with indefinite hepatitis B immune globulin (HBIG) prophylaxis after liver transplantation. *Clin Transplant* 1996;10:663–667.
68. Kerkar N, Hadzic N, Davies ET, et al. De novo autoimmune hepatitis after liver transplantation. *Lancet* 1998;351:409–413.
69. McMaster P, Gunson B, Min X, et al. Liver transplantation: changing goals in immunosuppression. *Transplant Proc* 1998;30:1819–1821.

70. Loftus EV Jr, Aguilar HI, Sandborn WJ, et al. Risk of colorectal neoplasia in patients with primary sclerosing cholangitis following orthotopic liver transplantation. *Hepatology* 1998;27:685–690.
71. Gross CR, Malinchoc M, Kim Wr, et al. Quality of life before and after liver transplantation for cholestatic liver disease. *Hepatology* 1999;29:356–364.
72. Seiler CA, Muller M, Fisch HU, et al. Quality of life after liver transplantation. *Transplant Proc* 1998;30:4330–4333.
73. Lucey MR. Liver transplantation for alcoholic liver disease. *Ballieres Clin Gastroenterol* 1993;7:717–727.
74. Fabrega E, Crespo J, Casafont F, et al. Alcoholic recidivism after liver transplantation for alcoholic cirrhosis. *J Clin Gastroenterol* 1998;11:204–206.
75. Tang H, Boulton R, Gunson B, et al. Patterns of alcohol consumption after liver transplantation. *Gut* 1998;43:140–145.
76. Cundy TF, O'Grady JG, Williams R. Recovery of menstruation and pregnancy after liver transplantation. *Gut* 1990;31:337–338.
77. Patapis P, Irani S, Mirza DF, et al. Outcome of graft function and pregnancy following liver transplantation. *Transplant Proc* 1997;29:1565–1566.
78. Casele HL, Laifer SA. Pregnancy after liver transplantation. *Semin Perinatol* 1998;18:149–155.
79. Casele HL, Laifer SA. Association of pregnancy complications and choice of immunosuppressant in liver transplant patients. *Transplantation* 1998;65:581–583.
80. Roberts M, Brown AS, James OF, et al. Interpretation of cyclosporin A levels in pregnancy following orthotopic liver transplantation. *Br J Obstet Gynaecol* 1995;102:570–572.
81. Laifer SA, Darby MJ, Scantlebury VP, et al. Pregnancy and liver transplantation. *Obstet Gynecol* 1990;76:1083–1088.

Transplantation of the Liver, edited by Willis C. Maddrey, Eugene R. Schiff, and Michael F. Sorrell. Lippincott Williams & Wilkins, Philadelphia © 2001.

CHAPTER 12

Metabolism of Drugs before and after Liver Transplantation

K. Vincent Speeg, Jr., Glenn A. Halff, and Steven Schenker

This chapter addresses the effects of severe pretransplantation liver disease on the disposition and elimination of therapeutic agents, as well as the changes in drug handling that occur during surgery, in the immediate (perioperative) period after liver transplantation, and during the postoperative stage. The liver is a key organ for the elimination of many drugs because of (a) its position astride the portal axis with direct contact with drugs taken orally and (b) its large complement of biotransforming enzymes, which render many drugs water soluble and thus more readily excreted by the liver or kidneys. Any significant insult to the liver may have an important impact on drug pharmacokinetics and, therefore, on drug use.

PRETRANSPLANTATION STAGE

Prior to a detailed discussion of the disposition of specific drugs in patients waiting for liver transplantation, some general comments are needed.

General Considerations

Type of Liver Disease

Patients qualifying for liver transplantation by definition have severe irreversible hepatic dysfunction. However, the nature and type of the liver disease varies. There are three major categories of patients:

1. Those with acute and subacute fulminant liver failure from viral or drug-induced hepatitis
2. Those with chronic parenchymal (primarily hepatocellular) liver disease (e.g., cirrhosis resulting from alcohol abuse or chronic hepatitis)
3. Those with chronic cholestatic hepatic dysfunction (e.g., primary biliary cirrhosis or primary sclerosing cholangitis)

In the first and second groups with parenchymal dysfunction, drug elimination, in general, is more affected than in biliary obstructive disease. Moreover, in acute or subacute disease, liver cell necrosis contributes more to impaired drug handling, whereas with cirrhosis the shunting of blood around viable hepatocytes is an important culprit.[1,2] In both instances, however, it is hepatic metabolism (i.e., intrinsic clearance) that appears to be primarily affected rather than blood flow and delivery of the drugs to the liver (even for those drugs with a high extraction normally).[3–5] In this context, intrinsic clearance refers to hepatic drug removal (capillarization, shunting, biotransforming enzyme content) independent of blood flow.[5]

Pharmacokinetic Considerations

Drug disposition and elimination by the liver depends on a variety of pharmacokinetic factors. The effects of severe pretransplantation liver disease on these dispositional factors are considered briefly next.

First-pass Effect

Drugs taken orally that are well absorbed pass first to the liver. With drugs that are extensively metabolized by the normal liver, less parent drug normally enters the systemic circulation than after intravenous administration (high first-pass effect; that is, low bioavailability). With liver disease,

K. V. Speeg Jr. and S. Schenker: Department of Medicine, Division of Gastroenterology and Nutrition, The University of Texas Health Science Center at San Antonio, San Antonio, Texas 78284.

G. A. Halff: Department of Surgery, Organ Transplantation Progam, The University of Texas Health Science Center at San Antonio, San Antonio, Texas 78284.

metabolism decreases and extraction is compromised, resulting in more drug entering the systemic circulation. In this fashion, orally ingested agents may accumulate in the plasma of patients with liver disease.[6,7]

Drug Binding

Some drugs are highly bound to plasma proteins. In severe liver disease, the serum albumin level often decreases, resulting in lower binding for some (mainly acidic and neutral) drugs.[8] There may also be a decrease in binding affinity for the albumin. The net effects for highly bound drugs may be increased availability of the drug to its sites of action and increased penetration of the unbound drug into various tissues, with a higher drug volume of distribution (drug sequestration at these sites). On the other hand, α_1-glycoprotein may be increased (as an acute phase reactant) in some of these patients and may enhance the binding of mainly basic drugs.

Drug Volume of Distribution

Many patients with severe liver disease have ascites and volume overload due to fluid retention. This promotes greater drug sequestration and often a greater drug volume of distribution (Vd, the space in which the drug distributes).[6] This process may be enhanced by lower drug binding (see previous section). It should be appreciated that Vd refers to drug concentration in a mathematical sense and that this does not correspond to any specific anatomic space, although it may correlate with a space, as with ascites.

Drug Elimination

Normally, high-extraction drugs depend on hepatic blood flow for elimination, whereas low-extraction drugs are flow independent and their removal by the liver is governed by hepatic metabolizing capacity (intrinsic clearance). With severe liver disease, both damage to the liver and portosystemic shunting decrease intrinsic clearance.[3-5] The clearance of such drugs is therefore decreased, primarily due to compromised hepatic function. Moreover, the elimination of high-clearance drugs becomes dependent on hepatic extraction.[3,4] In other words, even high-clearance drugs behave as if they were low-extraction agents. The hepatic factors that contribute to decreased hepatic clearance of drugs include sinusoidal capillarization with decreased hepatic drug uptake, cell damage with impaired drug metabolism, portosystemic shunting of drug in and around the liver, and, at times, impaired drug excretion into bile. To the extent that these various factors contribute to decreased drug removal, the concepts of sick hepatocytes or intact (shunted) hepatocytes have been promoted.[6,9]

Because clearance (the volume of blood from which drug is removed per unit time) controls drug dosage over a period of time, in the presence of severe liver disease the dosage of many drugs eliminated by the liver must be lowered to reduce drug accumulation and possible toxicity. The toxicity of any given drug, of course, will depend on its therapeutic index, that is, the difference between therapeutic and toxic concentrations and the duration of drug use. These concepts apply to agents that are metabolized in the liver to more polar substances prior to elimination. Some drugs are removed via the bile without prior biotransformation. For these, excretion is governed by the degree of intrahepatic obstruction, that is, cholestasis. The kidneys also contribute to drug removal, with or without prior hepatic biotransformation, and thus, when functioning normally, may serve as a safety valve when hepatic function is compromised. Total (systemic) clearance thus may be totally hepatic, totally renal, or a combination of both.[6] Because total and renal clearances are relatively easy to measure but hepatic clearance requires more invasive procedures, hepatic clearance is often assessed indirectly as the difference between total and renal clearance.

Another measurement of drug removal is the elimination half-life ($t_{1/2}$), which is the time needed for half of the drug to be removed from the circulation. Although often used, this is a hybrid parameter that correlates directly with the volume of distribution (Vd) and inversely with clearance (Cl) in the following manner:

$$t_{1/2} = (0.693 \times Vd) / Cl$$

Hence, any increase in Vd or fall in Cl will prolong the $t_{1/2}$, but offsetting changes in Vd and Cl may leave an unchanged $t_{1/2}$ value.[6,9] Clearance is thus a useful measure of drug elimination by the liver. In patients with severe liver disease, in whom there is an increase in Vd and a fall in Cl, there may be a substantial prolongation of $t_{1/2}$. In general, such prolongation provides a guide to frequency of dosing, with the time intervals increasing with longer $t_{1/2}$.

Drug Metabolism

What is the effect of liver disease on various metabolic pathways? There are two main types of drug biotransformations in the liver: oxidation and conjugation. Oxidation of drugs is more impaired with liver disease than is glucuronidation, the best studied conjugation reaction. The relative sparing of glucuronidation probably derives from the availability of extrahepatic glucuronidation and the presence of substantial glucuronidating reserves, which are less susceptible to injury than oxidation mechanisms, in the damaged liver. Upregulation of various isoforms of glucuronyltransferase also seems to take place.[10] With very severe hepatic dysfunction, however, all detoxifying mechanisms are impaired.[11] Nevertheless, the lesser effect of liver disease on glucuronidation and the absence of pharmacologic activity of most glucuronides (thus shortening the pharmacologic effects) makes these agents favorites for the treatment of patients with liver disease.

Pharmacodynamics

In addition to dispositional (pharmacokinetic) considerations, patients with severe liver disease may manifest end-organ sensitivity to some drugs (altered pharmacodynamics). A well-known example of this is the sensitivity of some of these patients to sedatives and analgesics, with precipitation of encephalopathy.[12] The mechanism of this, at least in part, has been attributed to sensitization of the γ-aminobutyric acid (GABA) supramolecular complex to endogenous benzodiazepine-like compounds.[13] Another explanation may simply be a summation of subliminal sedative influences. Another example of the sensitivity of these patients to certain drugs may be the untoward response of the kidneys to nonsteroidal analgesics (presumably due to inhibition of permissive prostaglandin-dependent renal function) as well as the greater toxicity in these patients of aminoglycosides. Patients with severe liver disease may thus exhibit greater target-organ sensitivity to various drugs independent of altered drug disposition. This consideration affects drug use in these patients.

Predictive Tests

Inasmuch as the elimination of many drugs may be impaired with liver disease, and conventional liver tests provide only a rough index of hepatic function, there has been a search for a liver function test that has predictive value. A variety of marker compounds (such as indocyanine green (ICG), which is normally flow dependent, and antipyrine, caffeine, or aminopyrine, which have a low extraction) have been used as predictive tests for other drugs. In general, however, the coefficient of correlation has ranged from 0.6 to 0.8, not considered to be of value in the individual patient.[14] Some have championed the use of lidocaine metabolism as a simple functional test, especially for the timing of liver transplantation and to assess the viability of the donor organ.[15,16] It is reasonable to state, however, that no test has substantially improved on the Child classification of severity of liver disease and that there is no predictive test available for hepatic drug elimination similar to renal creatinine clearance.

Accordingly, drug usage in these patients is based on knowledge of each agent's metabolism and route of elimination, its therapeutic index, titration of dose to individual patient response, and in many instances, decrease of drug dosage by 50% (a somewhat arbitrary figure) with anticipated prolonged drug usage.[6] In some instances, plasma drug assays may be helpful. It is hoped that with greater knowledge of the mechanisms of drug disposition, an agent may emerge as a sensitive and specific index of hepatic function.

Specific Drugs

This section considers the disposition and elimination of individual drugs commonly used in patients with severe liver disease. The information here is applicable both to patients in the pretransplantation stage and to those in whom the transplanted liver is failing (Table 12.1).

Agents Used for General Treatment of Liver Disease

Corticosteroids

Corticosteroid agents, such as prednisone or prednisolone, are commonly used for the treatment of autoimmune hepatitis and possibly for some types of drug-induced hypersensitivity reactions. They are also, of course, employed to prevent organ rejection after transplantation. For pharmacologic effect, prednisone has to be hydroxylated to prednisolone in the liver, raising the issue of optimal drug form. The available data indicate, however, that any decrease in hydroxylation of prednisone by the diseased liver is small and that there is interconversion of these two compounds. Either substance may thus be used effectively, although prednisolone administration may give more predictable steady-state levels. No dosage adjustment of this drug is needed with liver failure.[17–20]

TABLE 12.1. *Effects of severe liver disease on drug elimination*

Drug	Elimination
Corticosteroids	No significant change
Azathioprine	No significant change
Methotrexate	No significant change
Colchicine	Decreased
Ursodeoxycholic acid	Decreased
Interferon	Drug-drug interaction
Penicillins	No significant change[a]
Cephalosporins	No significant change
Metronidazole	Decreased
Quinolones	Drug-drug interaction
Isoniazid	No significant change
Ketoconazole	Decreased and drug-drug interaction
Diuretics	No significant change[b]
Beta-blockers	Decreased
Calcium channel blockers	Decreased
ACE inhibitors	No significant change[c]
Sedatives	Decreased[d]
Analgesics	
Narcotics	Decreased[e]
NSAIDs	Variable
Gastric acid suppressants	
H₂-receptor antagonists	Decreased
Omeprazole	Decreased

ACE, angiotensin-converting enzyme; NSAID, nonsteroidal antiinflammatory drug.
[a]Agents excreted in bile (e.g., nafcillin) may have decreased clearance.
[b]Triamterene clearance is decreased.
[c]Only one drug was studied.
[d]Oxidized drugs are decreased more than glucuronidated agents.
[e]Drugs with significant first-pass effect given orally require special caution.

Immunosuppressive Agents

Azathioprine (Imuran) and methotrexate have been used for the treatment of autoimmune liver disease and primary biliary cirrhosis, respectively. There are no specific studies on the pharmacokinetics of these agents in patients with severe liver disease, but in both instances renal excretion appears to be important. Methotrexate elimination is unaltered in hepatic fibrosis.[21] Accumulation of azathioprine or methotrexate to toxic levels as a result of hepatic dysfunction has not been reported as a clinical problem. Metabolism of methotrexate does not constitute an important part of its disposition. Mercaptopurine (the active moiety of Imuran) undergoes methylation and then oxidation of its sulfhydryl groups.

Colchicine

Colchicine has been used in alcoholic cirrhosis and primary biliary cirrhosis. Clearance of colchicine is impaired in cirrhosis, with a 50% fall on the average, and the half-life is equally prolonged.[22] One may estimate that steady-state levels of colchicine in cirrhotic patients given a dose of 0.6 mg every 12 hours would increase to 2.82 ng/mL, as compared with normal values of 1.12 ng/mL. The liver is an important route of colchicine elimination, with biliary secretion and, to a lesser extent, oxidation as the major excretory pathways.

Ursodeoxycholic Acid

Ursodeoxycholic acid is a bile acid that has been used primarily in cholestatic disorders. It is excreted unmetabolized via bile. The normal extraction ratio of this agent by the liver is 0.53; the ratio falls progressively with increasing severity of hepatic dysfunction. With severe liver disease,[23] it is only 0.07. Thus, the drug will accumulate in plasma with prolonged use in these patients. No untoward effects of the agent have been reported in this setting, however.

α-Interferon

It is unlikely that any patient with disease sufficiently severe to warrant liver transplantation will be on interferon therapy, but the drug is in sufficiently common use to warrant comment. The main concern with this agent as regards drug disposition is that it may interact with and affect the elimination of other agents metabolized via cytochrome P-450 3A.[24] Thus, during α-interferon therapy the elimination of erythromycin, nifedipine, quinidine, lidocaine, diltiazem, and theophylline may be decreased; discontinuation of interferon would theoretically enhance their degradation.[24–26] Consideration must be given to such drug-drug interactions, especially with low therapeutic index agents (e.g., cyclosporine after transplantation).

Antimicrobial Agents

Most of the antibiotics are eliminated by renal excretion, and for many others the therapeutic index is high; hence, no dosage restriction is needed in patients with severe liver disease, even though hepatic clearance may be depressed.[6] Some agents, however, do not fit this description and require more consideration. For instance, some semisynthetic penicillins (e.g., nafcillin) are primarily excreted in bile, and their dose should be reduced with cholestasis.[27] Others (e.g., mezlocillin) are eliminated by the kidneys and, to a lesser extent, in bile. In the presence of concomitant hepatic and renal disease, the drug dosage should be adjusted downward because side effects (e.g., central nervous system irritability) may ensue with drug accumulation.[28]

First- and second-generation cephalosporins (cephalothin, cefoxitin, cefamandole) are excreted primarily by the kidneys, and no dose adjustment is needed with liver disease alone. However, these agents apparently can interact with aminoglycosides to induce renal dysfunction selectively in cirrhotic patients.[29] Third-generation cephalosporins (cefoperazone, cefotaxime) depend on hepatic elimination, but no dose reduction is necessary. In fact, cefotaxime in customary doses is the antibiotic of choice for spontaneous bacterial peritonitis.[30] Metronidazole undergoes extensive hepatic metabolism by oxidation and conjugation. Although the data are somewhat conflicting, it would appear prudent to decrease drug dosage by 50% in the presence of severe liver dysfunction because this agent may cause peripheral neuropathy (the mechanism or mechanisms of this are uncertain).[31]

The quinolone derivatives (e.g., ciprofloxacin) are mainly removed by the kidneys. However, perfloxacin clearance is depressed in cirrhosis,[32] and norfloxacin is metabolized in the liver.[33] Both agents may interfere with the elimination of theophylline, caffeine, warfarin, and cyclosporine.[34] Because patients with liver disease a priori exhibit decreased demethylation of theophylline and because this agent has a low toxic and therapeutic threshold, caution in the use of the quinolone derivatives is recommended.

Antituberculous drugs are generally excreted by the kidneys. Pyrizinamide may be an exception, and toxicity may be dose dependent. Isoniazid is acetylated in the liver cytosol; this process may be somewhat decreased in cirrhosis. However, such an impairment is minor compared with genetically determined slow acetylation.[35] Moreover, isoniazid toxicity to the liver is idiosyncratic, that is, not dose dependent. Isoniazid use, however, can potentiate acetaminophen toxicity by induction of the shared cytochrome P-450 2EI isozyme.[36]

Antifungal agents deserve special mention. Ketoconazole and its surrogates undergo hepatic oxidative metabolism[6] and hence may accumulate in patients with severe hepatic dysfunction. Their metabolism via the cytochrome P-450 3A isozyme may interact with the elimination of nifedipine, erythromycin, and other agents, such as various antihistamines, with potentially serious cardiotoxicity.[37] As is discussed later, this isozyme also metabolizes cyclosporine, with possible toxic interaction.

Diuretics and β-Blockers

Furosemide half-life is increased in cirrhosis, but the clearance is largely unaltered. The data on spironolactone elimination are few and incomplete, but no reduction in dosage is required on pharmacokinetic grounds. Triamterene disposition, by contrast, is depressed more extensively.[38]

β-Blockers are used primarily to decrease portal pressure and forestall gastroesophageal bleeding. For propranolol, metoprolol, and labetalol, clearance is significantly depressed in patients with severe liver dysfunction, and lower doses are needed to reduce portal pressure without significant toxicity.[39–41]

Treatment of Hepatic Encephalopathy

The principal drug therapy of hepatic encephalopathy consists of lactulose or an antibiotic such as metronidazole. On occasion neomycin, orally or by enema, is employed. More recently sodium benzoate has been tried in efforts to remove ammonia as hippurate. The dose of metronidazole in severe liver disease may need to be decreased, as discussed earlier, and prolonged neomycin rarely may be absorbed sufficiently to become ototoxic and nephrotoxic if given to patients with underlying renal disease. Sodium benzoate in the doses recommended seems to be tolerated well in the few recent trials reported.[42]

Sedatives and Analgesics

Sedative agents have the propensity of precipitating hepatic encephalopathy, regardless of their pharmacokinetic profile, because of a pharmacodynamic effect on the brain of patients with cirrhosis (see earlier discussion). Moreover, benzodiazepines that are metabolized by oxidation (diazepam, chlordiazepoxide, alprazolam, clorazepate, flurazepam) are known to have a depressed clearance in patients with severe liver disease.[6,9] With prolonged therapy these drugs are likely to accumulate and induce unwanted sedation. By contrast, benzodiazepines that are glucuronidated to pharmacologically inactive derivatives (lorazepam, temazepam) seem to be metabolized better in such patients, except in the very decompensated disease state.[11]

Diphenhydramine (Benadryl) is often used as a sedative in children. In stable cirrhotic patients, there was a mild prolongation of drug half-life; hence, in severe cirrhosis with prolonged use, drug dosage should probably be reduced.[42] Less is known about the tricyclic antidepressants,

which generally are metabolized by oxidation in the liver and thus would be expected to accumulate. Thus, lower doses with prolonged therapy are suggested.[6] Chlorpromazine is extensively metabolized in the liver but seems to cause encephalopathy in these patients mainly on a pharmacodynamic basis.[43] All these agents require low doses and individual patient titration.

Analgesics are all metabolized by the liver, and those with narcotic effects can precipitate hepatic encephalopathy independent of their dispositional characteristics. Thus, a reduction in dose is needed for meperidine, pentazocine, morphine, and methadone when these are taken orally and first-pass effect (i.e., bioavailability) becomes an important consideration.[6,9] The degree of reduction with oral intake will vary from about 50% for meperidine to substantially less (~25%) for the other agents. With parenteral administration, a major decrease in clearance is seen with meperidine, and lesser changes with the other three drugs. Codeine has the advantage of a lesser first-pass effect and minimal protein binding. However, it too undergoes extensive hepatic metabolism, and its constipating characteristics may contribute to the development of hepatic encephalopathy in these patients. Thus, a significant reduction in long-term dosing is indicated. Other opioids (e.g., Lomotil, Imodium) have a substantial first-pass metabolism in liver that must be considered when calculating dosages for patients with severe liver disease.[44]

The nonsteroidal antiinflammatory analgesics pose a serious problem in patients with chronic severe liver disease. First, some are a frequent cause of hepatic toxicity. Second, they may precipitate renal dysfunction, presumably by inhibiting prostaglandin-mediated renal blood flow. This fact has limited pharmacokinetic studies of these agents in patients with severe liver disease. Third, they promote gastrointestinal bleeding in patients with underlying portal hypertension. Added to these concerns is evidence that many of these agents (e.g., ibuprofen, sulindac) undergo extensive hepatic metabolism. Although there are few data, some of these agents (e.g., ibuprofen) do not exhibit decreased removal in patients with liver disease.[45] On the other hand, sulindac elimination is decreased in these patients.[45] Some drugs in this group that are highly bound to albumin in plasma (e.g., salicylates, naproxen) may present with more unbound drug in these patients and greater access of the agent to target organs. Clearly, these agents must be used with extreme caution in patients with severe liver disease.

For the above reasons, acetaminophen is often recommended in this patient group. The drug is metabolized extensively by conjugation with glucuronide and sulfate, with only very minor oxidation. In mild or moderate liver disease, acetaminophen clearance is not affected,[46] but with severe dysfunction even conjugation is depressed.[47] The therapeutic index for the drug in these patients is relatively high, unless there has been prior chronic ethanol (or isoniazid) intake, which can induce the formation of the toxic metabolite. Theoretically, severe malnutrition with a major decrease in hepatic glutathione, to detoxify the oxidative metabolite, could be a risk factor. With these caveats, however, acetaminophen is a reasonable mild analgesic in patients with severe liver disease.

Gastric Acid Suppressants

H_2-receptor antagonists are often used in patients with decompensated cirrhosis who are prone to ulcer-induced gastroesophageal bleeding. These agents are primarily eliminated by the kidneys, and in well-compensated cirrhosis there is no decrease in their elimination. With decompensated cirrhosis, however, there is evidence for a decrease in overall clearance of cimetidine.[48] This is primarily caused by an impaired renal clearance of the drug, although in one report there was also a lower production of the sulfoxide metabolite. There are also single reports of decreased ranitidine and famotidine elimination in decompensated cirrhosis.[49] Presumably this is mainly due to subtle renal injury accompanying the severe liver disease. More studies in this area are warranted. Although accumulation of these agents is usually well tolerated, there are reports of occasional central nervous system irritability, and this may be seen in patients with severe liver disease. It appears, therefore, that in severe liver disease some modest decrease in H_2-antagonist dosage is warranted.

Elimination of the proton pump inhibitors omeprazole, lansoprazole, and rebeprazole has not been studied extensively in this patient population, but package insert information indicates that metabolism occurs, at least in part, through cytochrome P-450 3A and that removal of these drugs is significantly decreased with hepatic dysfunction. Few drug interactions have been reported, and the therapeutic indices of the drugs are high. Profound inhibition of gastic acid occurs; this may decrease absorption for organic cations.[34]

Antihypertensive Agents

Diuretics and β-blockers have been discussed earlier, and the subject is presented more extensively elsewhere.[9] Few studies are available with calcium channel blockers, but the clearance of both nifedipine and verapamil is decreased by about 50% in patients with cirrhosis.[50,51] On theoretical grounds, reduced dosage is probably also applicable to other drugs in this group.[6] Among angiotensin-converting enzyme (ACE) inhibitors, perindopril kinetics were not altered in these patients.[52]

PERIOPERATIVE DRUG METABOLISM

The perioperative period can be divided into an intraoperative and a postoperative period. The intraoperative period can in turn be divided into three surgical phases: pre-anhepatic, anhepatic, and postanhepatic, or postreper-

fusion. Hepatic drug metabolism in the perioperative period is influenced by a large number of variables, including preoperative and postoperative liver function, the difficulty of the operation and the amount of blood loss, hemodynamic stability, and the anesthetic agents that are used.

Pre-anhepatic Phase

Drug metabolism in the pre-anhepatic phase (prior to recipient liver removal) is affected by the preexisting degree of liver dysfunction and the effects of anesthesia. Parenchymal liver diseases tend to affect hepatic metabolic function more than either cholestatic diseases or tumor involvement of the liver. The degree of metabolic (synthetic and detoxifying) reserve remaining varies considerably among patients with parenchymal liver disease, depending on how early in the disease process the patients undergo transplantation and whether they undergo transplantation for chronic liver disease or fulminant hepatic failure. Because of this large variability, most medications need to be titrated on an individual basis to achieve the desired effect.[53]

Anesthesia may affect hepatic function and drug elimination directly, by an interaction of the anesthetic and the drug, or indirectly, by lowering hepatic blood flow and/or causing liver hypoxia. An instance of the former is the decreased intrinsic clearance of propranolol caused by halothane.[54] Halothane also is an example of the latter mechanism in that it may cause a selective increase in hepatic artery resistance, resulting in decreased hepatic blood flow and oxygenation.[55,56] Halothane is not recommended for use in liver transplant operations because it seems to impair hepatic function, blood flow, and oxygen supply more than other inhalational anesthetics such as isoflurane.[56]

Decreased hepatic perfusion may also be caused by the surgery itself.[57] Surgery in the upper abdomen may compromise hepatic blood flow secondary to decreased mesenteric venous flow resulting from bowel manipulation or from manipulation of the liver itself. Splanchnic vasoconstriction caused by endogenous vasopressor release may also play a role. If hemodynamic problems arise, the decrease in liver blood flow will readily compromise hepatic clearance of high-extraction drugs, an effect best documented for lidocaine.[58] A concomitant decrease in renal perfusion may accentuate this problem.

Because decreased blood flow to the liver may be severe enough to induce hepatic hypoxia, the elimination of drugs that depend on cellular oxidative metabolism may also be affected. This has been well documented for low-extraction, intrinsic-clearance-dependent drugs such as antipyrine and theophylline.[59] Thus, both high- and low-extraction drugs may be affected. Isoflurane and fentanyl citrate seem to minimize hepatic ischemic injury and optimize hepatic oxygen supply-and-demand requirements experimentally compared with several other anesthetics[60,61]; the two are used together clinically for liver transplantation on a routine basis. A large volume of blood loss may make drug dosing very difficult because the decrease in hepatic perfusion and oxygenation and the amount of drug lost with the blood is hard to quantitate.

General Anesthetic Drug Considerations

The pre-anhepatic period is relatively short, usually lasting only 1 to 2 hours, so some of the above considerations, such as decreased hepatic oxidative metabolism, are of more theoretical than clinical importance, especially since they are difficult to quantitate and there is so much interpatient variability. A higher initial dose of some medications will need to be given if the Vd is increased due to ascites. A lower initial dose may need to be given if significantly decreased albumin binding is present, resulting in an increased unbound drug fraction. Lengthened elimination half-lives caused primarily by decreased clearance are treated clinically by titrating the dose of anesthetic based on hemodynamic and other clinical parameters. Most of the anesthetics used are relatively nontoxic in somewhat elevated doses; because the patients are usually kept intubated for up to 12 hours postoperatively, the effect of an increased drug duration of action during the operation is not generally felt to be clinically significant.

Preoperative renal compromise may necessitate dosage adjustment of drugs eliminated by the kidneys, such as the muscle relaxant pancuronium. The usual amount of drug is required for the initial effect; however, it may be longer acting. Thus, overall dosage requirement over time may be reduced. Renal insufficiency related to the hepatorenal syndrome is seen in about 8% of liver transplant candidates.[62]

Specific Anesthetic Drug Use

Anesthesia typically consists of sedation with midazolam, induction with fentanyl followed by thiopental sodium and a muscle relaxant such as succinylcholine or vecuronium, and then maintenance with isoflurane, fentanyl, and a long-acting nondepolarizing muscle relaxant such as pancuronium[53] or doxacurium. A shorter-acting muscle relaxant, such as atracurium or vecuronium, may be used if the transplant procedure is likely to be relatively fast (3 to 4 hours).

Midazolam

Midazolam is typically given in a normal to low dose during anesthesia for anxiolysis, hypnosis, and amnesia. If it is given prior to entering the operating room, a low dose should be used because decreased protein binding may cause an increased free drug fraction and an increased cerebral effect.[63] The metabolism of midazolam is by phase I (oxidation) and then phase II (conjugation) routes, which would seem to account for the decreased clearance, based on decreased oxidative metabolism, in cirrhotic patients and to result in prolonged drug elimination. Although a decreased clearance, a normal Vd, and an increased elimination half-life have been

documented for midazolam, the mechanism is complex because decreased clearance did not correlate with the albumin level or ICG or antipyrine clearance.[64]

Thiopental Sodium

Thiopental has been reported to have a synergistic effect with midazolam. Thiopental is usually given in a normal to slightly low dose. It is normally highly bound to albumin, and a decrease in drug binding in cirrhotic patients may cause the active unbound fraction of the drug to be elevated and cause hypotension during induction. An increased, but not statistically significant, Vd and elimination half-life with a normal clearance have been seen in patients with moderate cirrhosis.[65]

Fentanyl Citrate

Fentanyl citrate may be given during the induction sequence and also for maintenance of anesthesia. It has the advantages of causing relatively little hemodynamic instability and of optimizing, experimentally, hepatic blood flow and oxygenation and minimizing hepatic ischemic injury.[60,61] Fentanyl is highly lipid soluble, highly protein bound (79% to 87%), and primarily metabolized by the liver.[66] Although the plasma clearance, Vd, and elimination half-life of fentanyl[67,68] and sufentanil[69] are not changed with mild to moderate cirrhosis, there is wide variation in the clearance and $t_{1/2}$ of fentanyl in patients with end-stage cholestatic liver disease. Clearance was very decreased, and $t_{1/2}$ much increased, in half the patients in one study, with a fairly normal Vd in all.[67] This may be explained by the variable loss of synthetic and detoxifying function in patients with cholestatic liver disease. Clinically, fentanyl is given in a normal dose with liver transplantation and then titrated appropriately. Some anesthesiologists prefer sufentanil as an alternative opioid to fentanyl. The pharmacokinetic and pharmacodynamic changes with this drug in patients with liver disease are similar to those with fentanyl.

Muscle Relaxants

The duration of action of succinylcholine may be increased due to decreased pseudocholinesterase levels,[70] but this is not clinically significant because the patients are kept intubated routinely for up to 12 hours postoperatively to ascertain good allograft function. The pseudocholinesterase levels return to normal with adequate allograft function.

Nondepolarizing muscle relaxants tend to require an increased initial dose in liver failure patients because of an increased Vd. They often have a decreased clearance and lengthened elimination half-life. The clearance of vecuronium is decreased and the elimination half-life lengthened in patients with severe liver disease.[71] This may be at least partly explained by the significant biliary excretion (25% to 50%) of the drug, since this function may be depressed in these patients. Several studies have shown that the pharmacokinetics in cirrhotic patients are affected by the dose of vecuronium that was given, with a 0.1 to 0.15 mg/kg dose (recommended initial dose 0.80–1.0 mg/kg) showing no change in clearance, Vd, or $t_{1/2}$, and a dose of 0.2 mg/kg having a decreased clearance and increased elimination half-life.[72–74] The interpretation of these studies is limited by inadequate quantification of liver failure and study of patients with only mild to moderate liver failure.

Pancuronium has an increased Vd (50%) and $t_{1/2}$ (doubled) and a decreased clearance (22%) in cirrhotic patients.[75] The initial dose is usually increased in patients with liver failure because of the increased Vd. Appropriate dosing is usually titrated by using a peripheral nerve stimulator.

Isoflurane

Isoflurane may be added for maintenance of anesthesia. It undergoes minimal biotransformation.[76] Like fentanyl, experimental evidence indicates that isoflurane is associated with less hepatic ischemic injury than halothane or enflurane.[60,61]

Anhepatic Phase

The anhepatic phase by definition implies no hepatic drug metabolism. Total oxygen consumption decreases by 25% during this period, with a marked increase in oxygen consumption after reperfusion.[77] With poor hepatic reperfusion, the increase in oxygen consumption is incomplete.[77] Although no hepatic metabolism is occurring during the anhepatic phase, several studies have shown that some metabolism occurs in extrahepatic sites during this period. This may be both phase I (oxidation) and phase II (glucuronidation) metabolism. Small amounts of midazolam, a benzodiazepine, are metabolized during the anhepatic period.[78] Measurable, but very low, levels of the morphine metabolites morphine-3-glucuronide and morphine-6-glucuronide, and the glucuronide metabolite of propofol, a short-acting anesthetic, have been found during the anhepatic phase.[79,80] The amount of extrahepatic metabolism is so small, however, and the anhepatic period so short that extrahepatic metabolism has little clinical significance.

No hepatic metabolism occurs during the anhepatic period, but the duration is usually so brief, usually less than 1 hour, that drug dosing is not usually affected. Because the liver contains 15% of the normal total blood volume,[81] the initial dose of some drugs may need to be adjusted if they are administered during this period because of a decreased volume of distribution. For example, flumazenil concentrations after a bolus injection were found to be much higher (4-fold) during the anhepatic period than in cirrhotic patients or normal subjects.[82]

Postanhepatic Phase

The postreperfusion phase is the initial part of a continuum leading into the postoperative period. The most important variable affecting hepatic metabolism during this time is the function of the new liver. Primary nonfunction occurs in 5% of liver transplants, and in this group drug metabolism will be especially poor because overall liver function is marginal. Lesser degrees of ischemic injury may occur with gradual recovery of hepatic function. Hypoxic injury to the transplanted liver can develop during the donor or recipient operative process and will depend on the degree of donor hemodynamic stability prior to the donor operation, the quality and length of organ preservation, and the recipient and donor surgery itself. Excessive bleeding during the postreperfusion phase will necessitate manipulation of the liver to expose potential bleeding sites; this may significantly affect hepatic blood flow and oxygenation.

Metabolism of drugs is very sensitive to hypoxia. This is especially true of the oxidative reactions. The sensitivity of individual enzymatic oxidative reactions to low oxygen varies. The Km_{O_2} is the oxygen concentration at which the activity of the enzyme is half maximal; the normal hepatic oxygen level is only 2- to 3-fold higher than the Km_{O_2} for many enzymes, so even moderate hypoxia is likely to affect them.[83] Conjugation reactions appear to be less susceptible to hypoxia than oxidation, and sulfation is probably more resistant than glucuronidation.[83] This may be due to the periportal location of sulfation for some drugs since the pericentral areas (zone 3) tend to be more hypoxic, as well as being the site where most oxidation reactions occur.

Indicators of Allograft Function

One of the earliest and most significant gross indicators that early liver function will be adequate is the production of bile of normal color, which often is seen immediately after reperfusion and before the bile duct is anastomosed. A steady decline in the lactate level, from a peak after the anhepatic phase, and gradual normalization of the prothrombin time over several days are also important measures of liver function. Continued good urine output and an alert mental status within 12 to 24 hours suggest that the liver is functioning properly. The early postoperative period is characterized by the gradual return of normal liver function over the first few hours to days or weeks, depending on the specific function examined. Oxidative metabolism of enflurane was demonstrated to be near normal in the first several hours after reperfusion in a patient with a significant ischemic insult to the liver.[84] Bile salt concentration returns to normal by day 5, but bile flow and bile salt output are not normalized until between postoperative days 10 and 12.[85]

The arterial ketone blood ratio of acetoacetate to β-hydroxybutyrate reflects the hepatic mitochondrial oxidation/reduction state. Arterial ketone body ratios of less than 0.7 were associated with primary nonfunction of hepatic grafts. The arterial ketone body ratio was above 1 by 16 hours postreperfusion in most of the grafts in the group that functioned well and above 1 in all of this group by 3 days postoperatively.[86]

Effect of Bile Duct Reconstruction

The majority of bile duct reconstructions in adults are done in a duct-to-duct fashion with or without a T tube stenting the anastomosis and decompressing and draining the common bile duct. The alternative is a donor bile duct to recipient jejunal limb (Roux-en-Y choledochojejunal) anastomosis that is not decompressed with an external T tube or drain. The T tube in a duct-to-duct anastomosis drains externally for an average of 1 week; during this time a significant proportion of the bile is diverted from the bowel, resulting in poor absorption of lipid-soluble drugs. After clamping the T tube, the absorption of fat-soluble compounds increases dramatically. A common example is oral cyclosporine, in which the dose-normalized area under the plasma concentration/time curve has been reported to increase about 3-fold[87] and the bioavailability to increase from 10.6% to 28.1% upon clamping the T tube.[88] The dose of cyclosporine is typically decreased at the same time as the T tube is clamped. The dosage of cyclosporine is usually adjusted based on a trough level.

Specific Drugs

Cyclosporine and Tacrolimus

Cyclosporine was previously given intravenously until the postoperative ileus resolved, and then a combination of oral and IV cyclosporine was given until an adequate drug level was achieved by the oral route. The oral dose was usually about two to three times the intravenous dose.[89] This sometimes required clamping of the T tube to increase the amount of bile in the bowel and, therefore, absorption. Occasionally drugs that decrease the metabolism of cyclosporine, such as diltiazem, were given to help wean patients from IV cyclosporine. The many interactions of cyclosporine with other drugs are discussed later in this chapter. Oral microemulsified cyclosporine (Neoral) is better absorbed and less dependent on bile flow than standard cyclosporine and has decreased the need for IV cyclosporine.

Tacrolimus (FK506), if used instead of cyclosporine, is well absorbed in oral form (or via nasogastric tube) beginning immediately posttransplantation. Use of IV tacrolimus is not necessary and may lead to significant nephrotoxicity.

Cyclosporine and tacrolimus are primarily metabolized by the liver via phase I (oxidative) metabolism, and the metabolites are excreted in the bile.[90,91] Therefore, patients with poor allograft liver function frequently need to have a reduction in cyclosporine or tacrolimus dosage.[92] This situation is exaggerated in the case of tacrolimus, where poor allograft function can lead to very toxic levels of tacrolimus.[93] A choledochojejunostomy causes bile to enter the mid- to distal jejunum; therefore, fat-soluble drugs that are absorbed in the proximal jejunum, such as cyclosporine, may have permanent decreased absorption.[94] Decreased cyclosporine absorption has also been noted in patients with a total bilirubin level greater than 10 mg/dL.[95]

Sedatives and Analgesics

The metabolism of intravenous midazolam, which undergoes oxidative and then glucuronidative metabolism, was studied in four patients immediately after liver transplantation. Central Vd and total plasma clearance appeared to be similar to that of healthy volunteers. Total Vd could not be calculated. The levels of the primary metabolite, alpha-midazolam, were higher in the liver transplant recipients than in the healthy volunteers, possibly indicating that subsequent glucuronidation of this metabolite was delayed. All patients required further sedation between 0.5 and 5 hours after the initial dose, which suggested that the duration of action of the active drug was not prolonged.[96]

The metabolism of morphine, which is by hepatic glucuronidation, was studied in seven patients by Shelly et al.[97] immediately after liver transplantation. The plasma clearance and Vd were both increased, with an elimination half-life of 2.4 hours, slightly longer than patients with normal liver function. Most of the drug was metabolized to morphine-3-glucuronide (85%), with 3.6% found as morphine-6-glucuronide and only 4.5% recovered as unchanged morphine over 24 hours.[97] Despite the relatively normal elimination half-life of morphine postoperatively, it is important not to give narcotics to these patients until they are awake and it is clear that the allograft is functioning well. Otherwise, the narcotics may confuse the clinical picture, in which mental status is an important variable. Also, since renal insufficiency may accompany poor graft function, active metabolites of some drugs may accumulate.

Of further interest, a study comparing postoperative analgesic use of morphine in liver transplant recipients and postcholecystectomy patients found that liver transplant recipients used less morphine, had lower plasma levels of morphine, and subjectively had better pain relief than the cholecystectomy patients ($p < 0.05$).[98] The mechanism is obscure, but this is probably not caused by lower protein binding because morphine is not highly bound (30%), and probably not caused by decreased metabolite excretion since the majority of morphine metabolites are inactive. Morphine-6-glucuronide, however, has been shown to be pharmacologically active.[99]

Antibiotics

The metabolism of ceftriaxone, a third-generation cephalosporin, has been studied in seven liver transplant recipients between postoperative days 3 and 5. The plasma drug clearance was decreased and the Vd was increased. The larger Vd was caused by decreased protein binding. The half-life of the drug was much longer in the transplant recipients than in normal subjects, 13.1 hours versus 5.8 hours, and the drug concentration at 12 and 24 hours was much higher. The decreased clearance may be explained by the fact that normally a significant percentage (40%) of ceftriaxone is eliminated in the bile, and in these patients the amount of drug excreted in bile was greatly decreased (1.5%).[100] This is not surprising because recovery of normal bile secretion after liver transplantation takes about 10 to 12 days.[85]

Cefotaxime, another cephalosporin, is metabolized by the liver to desacetylcefotaxime, which is active, and both the metabolite and the parent drug are excreted by the kidneys. A group of four patients in the postoperative recovery phase of liver transplantation and four patients with allograft nonfunction were given 1 gram of cefotaxime, and the drug and metabolite were measured over time. The terminal half-lives in the recovery phase were prolonged, ranging from 1.60 to 5.07 hours, compared with 3.54 to 11.34 hours in the group with graft nonfunction and 0.6 to 1.4 hours in healthy subjects from other studies. Plasma clearance was decreased in the recovery period (74–150 mL/min) compared with normal controls (250–350 mL/min), and severely altered (22–80 mL/min) in the hepatic nonfunction group.[101] The investigators recommended decreasing the dose to half in patients with poor graft function. Others have not advised a dose reduction with liver dysfunction because the agent has a high therapeutic index.[102]

The most critical issue relative to drug metabolism in patients with liver transplants is how rapidly and to what degree a transplanted liver is capable of recovering hepatic function. Both oxidative and conjugative drug-metabolizing abilities are similar to normal controls in stable liver transplant patients as measured by antipyrine and acetaminophen metabolism.[103,104] Drugs that are highly protein bound may have altered free (unbound) clearances because of the decreased albumin and increased α_1-acid glycoprotein concentrations posttransplantation.[94] Steroid metabolism is decreased compared with normal controls in these patients. However, this may be due to interaction with cyclosporine,[105] because other studies in the absence of cyclosporine do not show this. There is a wide variation in function due to the variability of individual allograft injury, but for the majority of liver transplants, in which recovery is relatively good, liver function and drug metabolism and elimination eventually approximate that of a normal liver.

POSTTRANSPLANTATION PERIOD

The metabolism of drugs following recovery from the transplantation surgery itself is influenced primarily by the degree to which the new liver functions normally and by the drugs being used in addition to cyclosporine or tacrolimus. The simplest case is that in which the new liver is normal and the primary influence on drug elimination will be that of the drug on either cyclosporine or tacrolimus. (That is, does the added drug inhibit cyclosporine or tacrolimus metabolism, does the drug induce the metabolism of cyclosporine or tacrolimus, or does cyclosporine or tacrolimus inhibit the metabolism or excretion of the added drug?) The most complicated case is that in which the new liver is significantly compromised by ongoing damage from ischemia, infection,

recurrent disease, or rejection. In this case, drug metabolism may be impaired as before transplantation (see previous discussion), with the possible added effects of cyclosporine or tacrolimus. Cyclosporine or tacrolimus metabolism may be decreased by the impaired liver per se. Added drugs may modulate cyclosporine or tacrolimus elimination by the damaged liver, or cyclosporine or tacrolimus may modulate the elimination of the added drug by the compromised liver. If there is significant cholestasis, drugs that are normally eliminated in bile will be affected.

Many drugs that might be used, however, have no interaction with cyclosporine or tacrolimus (i.e., cyclosporine or tacrolimus does not inhibit the metabolism or excretion of the drug, nor does the drug inhibit or induce the metabolism of cyclosporine or tacrolimus). Therefore, elimination of these drugs depends solely on the degree to which the transplanted liver and the kidneys function normally. Because this aspect has been discussed earlier for the abnormal (pretransplantation) liver, it will not be reiterated here. Rather, the emphasis will be on cyclosporine and tacrolimus handling and their interaction with other drugs, especially those metabolized by cytochrome P-450 3A.

Cyclosporine

Because cyclosporine was available before tacrolimus, there is more information available concerning drug-drug interactions involving cyclosporine. However, because tacrolimus and cyclosporine are both metabolized by cytochrome P-450 3A, similar drug-drug interactions can be anticipated. Many drugs interact with cyclosporine; an understanding of which drugs cause which effects is of critical clinical importance. Several reviews of cyclosporine-drug interactions or tacrolimus-drug interactions have been published.[106–110]

Drugs that increase cyclosporine levels have the potential for causing nephrotoxicity, which is characterized acutely by a rapid fall in urine output and creatinine clearance[111–113] or a rapidly progressive vasculopathy;[114] chronic cyclosporine nephrotoxicity is characterized by interstitial fibrosis and tubular atrophy.[115,116] Some drugs that have intrinsic nephrotoxicity may have an additive pharmacodynamic effect with cyclosporine (i.e., increased nephrotoxicity). Examples are acyclovir,[117] aminoglycosides,[118,119] amphotericin B,[120] and nonsteroidal antiinflammatory agents.[121,122]

Drugs that decrease cyclosporine levels have the potential of reducing immunosuppression and increasing the risk of organ rejection. Conversely, cyclosporine, because it is a substrate for cytochrome P-450 3A[123–125] and inhibits ATP-driven transport processes at the bile canaliculus,[126–130] has the potential to impair the elimination of some drugs and lead to untoward effects. When adding a new drug to an existing regimen, unless the new drug has been well studied it is generally a good practice to anticipate that an interaction with cyclosporine will occur and to monitor cyclosporine blood drug levels closely.

General Pharmacokinetic Principles

Drug Absorption

The bioavailability of oral cyclosporine is variable and incomplete, ranging from 1% to 67% with an average of 27% to 34%.[131,132] Bioavailability is influenced by gastrointestinal function (for example, cyclosporine absorption is impaired with diarrhea or gastroparesis and increased with prokinetics such as metoclopramide[133] or cisapride[34]), bile flow, and bile acids in the intestine (for example, chenodeoxycholic acid[94] or ursodeoxycholic acid[134,135] may increase absorption). Intestinal metabolism may also influence bioavailability. Intestinal mucosa contains the P-450 3A isozyme responsible for cyclosporine oxidation and likely contributes to low cyclosporine bioavailability following oral administration.[136–140] Other drugs that are metabolized by the same P-450 may also influence cyclosporine absorption. Modulation of intestinal cyclosporine metabolism may explain the effect of phenytoin[141] and erythromycin[142] on cyclosporine bioavailability. Preliminary data suggest that intestinal and liver cyclosporine oxidase may behave differently in response to inducers.[143]

Drug Distribution

Cyclosporine has a large volume of distribution (3.5–8.7 L/kg body weight). In blood, approximately half of cyclosporine is found in erythrocytes, and approximately 90% of that in plasma binds to lipoproteins. There would appear to be few if any examples where addition of a second drug displaces cyclosporine from its binding sites. There are also no examples of cyclosporine displacing other highly bound

drugs from their binding sites, although liver transplant patients also have lower albumin levels.[95] It would appear that changes in hematocrit or lipoprotein levels might be most likely to influence cyclosporine distribution.[144,145]

Drug Metabolism

Cyclosporine that reaches the systemic circulation is extensively metabolized in the liver, with subsequent elimination of metabolites in the bile.[146] The cytochrome P-450 3A isozyme apparently does not demonstrate genetic polymorphism.[109] A damaged liver would be expected to eliminate cyclosporine less well than a normal liver,[146] but clinically there is a large interindividual variation in the clearance of cyclosporine. A low dosage requirement to maintain therapeutic blood levels does not usually imply liver damage unless the requirement has changed recently (exclude the effects of other drugs).

Drugs That Decrease Cyclosporine Levels

Several drugs have been found to decrease cyclosporine levels and can be considered inducers of P-450 3A (cyclosporine oxidase) (Table 12.2). Pichard et al. have demonstrated both an increased enzyme activity and an increased P-450 3A level in human hepatocytes and microsomes following exposure to these agents.[147] Induction of this cytochrome (P-450 3A) is not specific for these drugs, however, and the inducers themselves may be metabolized by P-450 isozymes other than P-450 3A. The time course of induction and deinduction is generally not known but is likely dependent on the chemical characteristics (lipid solubility)

TABLE 12.2. *Drugs that decrease cyclosporine blood levels (inducers of cyclosporine oxidase)*

Drug	Change in CsA oxidase *in vitro*[a]	Change in P-450 3A level *in vitro*[a]	Substantiated interaction[b]	Reference for interaction
Anticonvulsant				
Carbamazepine	Decrease	Increase	Yes	148, 221
Phenobarbital	Increase	Increase	Yes	222, 223
Phenytoin	Increase	Increase	Yes	141, 224–227
Primidone	Not tested	Not tested	—	223, 228
Antiinflammatory				
Phenylbutazone	Increase	Increase	No	—
Antiinfective				
Nafcillin	Not tested	Not tested	—	229, 230
Isoniazid	No effect	No effect	Yes	149
Rifampicin	Increase	Increase	Yes	228, 231–239
Sulfadimidine	Increase	Increase	No	228, 240–242
Corticosteroid				
Dexamethasone	Increase	Increase	No	—
Uricosuric				
Sulfinpyrazone	Increase	Increase	No	243

CsA, cyclosporine.
[a]Studies used human hepatocytes or microsomes *in vitro;* P-450 3A was quantitated by Western blot using anti–P-450 3A7 antibody.[147]
[b]Validated by the weight of clinical experience, corroboratory evidence, or clear underlying mechanism.[191]

and pharmacokinetics of the inducer. Clinical experience would suggest that several days of exposure are required (2–10 days) for full induction and that deinduction is a slower process (days to weeks) once the inducer has been withdrawn.

As seen in Table 12.2, some of the interactions may be complex. For example, with the *in vitro* assessment, carbamazepine decreased cyclosporine oxidase activity yet increased P-450 3A enzyme content.[147] The overall clinical effect would appear to be induction of cyclosporine oxidase activity rather than inhibition.[148] The effects of prednisone and prednisolone *in vitro* were variable, whereas dexamethasone increased both cyclosporine oxidase activity and P-450 3A content.[147] Thus, because corticosteroids are both inducers of P-450 3A and substrates, the direction of an interaction is difficult to predict. Isoniazid did not appear to be an inducer of P-450 3A since it had no effect on either cyclosporine oxidase activity or P-450 3A content in the *in vitro* test systems.[147] Isoniazid is known, however, to be a potent inducer of P-450 2E1.[36] Although an effect on blood cyclosporine consistent with induction of metabolism has been reported,[149] the precise basis is not clear.

Tobacco smoking has not been demonstrated to have an effect on P-450 3A to our knowledge, although it is an inducer of P-450 1A2[150] and there are data from *in vitro* experiments that suggest that cyclosporine interacts with P-450 1A2[151] and that smoking induces a form of benzyloxyresorufin oxidase that is inhibitable by cyclosporine.[152]

Drugs That Increase Cyclosporine Levels

Numerous drugs have been reported to increase cyclosporine levels (Table 12.3). Although not certain in all cases, it would appear that the increase in cyclosporine level following addition of a second drug is a consequence of inhibition of cyclosporine oxidase in either the liver, the intestine, or both. Indeed, many of these added drugs would also appear to be substrates for P-450 3A, the enzyme family that oxidizes cyclosporine (Table 12.4). Generally, inhibition of drug metabolism is a rapid process and might be expected to be apparent within the first few days after addition of a second drug; similarly, reversal of inhibition can be expected to begin immediately upon removal of the inhibitor.

There are several broad categories of inhibitory drugs, including antifungal agents, calcium channel antagonists, and macrolide antibiotics. The azole antifungal agents include ketoconazole, itraconazole, and fluconazole. The inhibitory potential of these agents differs greatly, with keto-

TABLE 12.3. *Drugs that increase or might increase cyclosporine blood levels (inhibitors of cyclosporine oxidase)*

Drug	Change in CsA oxidase *in vitro*[a]	Change in P-450 3A level *in vitro*[a]	Substantiated interaction[b]	Reference for interaction
Azole antifungal agents				
Josamycin	None	None	Yes	244
Ketoconazole	Decrease	Increase	Yes	153, 154, 245–250
Miconazole	Decrease	None	No	—
Calcium channel blockers				
Diltiazem	None	None	Yes	251–256
Nicardipine	Decrease	None	Yes	257–259
Nifedipine	Increase	None	No	—
Verapamil	Not tested	Not tested	Yes	260–264
Macrolide antibiotics				
Triacetyloleandromycin	Decrease	Increase	No	—
Erythromycin	Decrease	Increase	Yes	142, 265–271
Midecamycin	None	None	No	—
Miocamycin	Not tested	Not tested	Yes	272
Steroids				
Ethinyl estradiol	None	None	No	—
Danazol	Not tested	Not tested	Yes	273
Norethisterone	Not tested	Not tested	Yes	273
Methyltestosterone	Not tested	Not tested	Yes	274
Progesterone	None	None	No	—
Oral contraceptives	Not tested	Not tested	No	275
Miscellaneous				
Bromocriptine	Decrease	None	No	—
Dihydroergotamine	Decrease	None	No	—
Ergotamine	Decrease	None	No	—

CsA, cyclosporine.
[a]Studies used human hepatocytes or microsomes *in vitro;* P-450 3A was quantitated by Western blot using anti-P-450 3A7 antibody.[147]
[b]Validated by the weight of clinical experience, corroboratory evidence, or clear underlying mechanism.[191]

TABLE 12.4. *Cyclosporine interactions with substrates for P-450 3A*

Known substrates	Interaction result	Reference
Cortisol	—	276
Dapsone	—	—
Diltiazem	Increased CsA level	251–256, 277, 278
Erythromycin	Increased CsA level	125, 142, 265–271
Ethinyl estradiol	Increased CsA level	279
FK506 (tacrolimus)	Increased CsA level	280
Ketoconazole	Increased CsA level	153, 154, 245–250
Lidocaine	—	281
Lovastatin	Increased lovastatin level	165, 166
Midazolam	—	282
Nicardipine	Increased CsA level	257–259
Nifedipine	No change in CsA level	124, 125, 256, 264, 283–285
Progesterone	—	286, 273
Quinidine	—	—
R-Warfarin	—	287
Testosterone	Increased CsA level	274
Triacetyloleandomycin	—	288
Triazolam	—	—
Suspected substrates		
Astemizole[a]	—	34
Bromocriptine[*,b]	—	289
Clarithromycin[c]	—	—
Danazol	Increased CsA level	273, 279
Dihydroergotamine[b]	—	290
Ergotamine[b]	—	291
Flurithromycin[c]	—	—
Itraconazole	Increased CsA level	290, 292, 293
Josamycin[c]	Increased CsA level	244
Methylprednisolone[b]	Variable effect on CsA level	294, 295
Miconazole[b]	—	—
Midecamycin[c]	—	—
Miocamycin[c]	Increased CsA level	272
Prednisolone[b]	Increased prednisolone level	162–164, 296
Prednisone[b]	—	—
Roxithromycin[c]	—	—
Terfenadine[a]	—	297, 298

CsA, cylcosporine.
[a]Based on interaction (decreased metabolism) with erythromycin and ketoconazole.
[b]Based on competitive inhibition of cyclosporine oxidase *in vitro*.[147]
[c]Based on similar interaction with P-450 as other macrolides.[158]

conazole having approximately 10-fold greater inhibitory potency than itraconazole.[153] Because of this potency, ketoconazole has been used to spare the cost of cyclosporine, as reviewed by Albengres and Tillement.[154] Fluconazole apparently has less inhibitory potency.[153] Fluconazole is frequently used, and an increase in either cyclosporine or tacrolimus levels can be seen clinically. There generally is decreased renal function, leading to an accumulation of fluconazole (80% eliminated as unchanged drug in urine) and eventually to inhibition of cytochrome P-450 3A. If cyclosporine or tacrolimus levels rise enough there may be further nephrotoxicity[155] and further increases in fluconazole and immunosuppressant levels. There are many other members of this class of drugs, but most are applied topically or intravaginally. An interaction has been reported for clotrimazole.[156]

The calcium channel antagonists diltiazem, nifedipine, and nicardipine are substrates for P-450 3A. Diltiazem and nicardipine can increase cyclosporine or tacrolimus levels, whereas nifedipine clinically does not, which seems at odds with theory. A recent report, however, indicates that a small interaction does occur.[155] Nitrendipine also did not increase cyclosporine levels when tested in renal transplant recipients.[157]

Macrolide antibiotics such as erythromycin and triacetyloleandomycin are substrates for P-450 3A and potent inhibitors of metabolism of various other substrates. These drugs form nitrosoalkanes and inactivate P-450. Other macrolides, such as josamycin, midecamycin, miocamycin, roxithromycin, clarithromycin, and flurithromycin, form complexes to a lesser extent and are less likely to inhibit P-450. Macrolides such as spiramycin, rokitamycin, dirithromycin, and azithromycin do not inactivate cytochrome P-450.[158] Numerous reports have documented an inhibitory effect of erythromycin and triacetyloleandomycin on the pharmacokinetics of theophylline, which is generally considered a substrate for P-450 1A2.

Alcohol is well known to affect the pharmacokinetics of many drugs[159] and has been characterized chronically as an inducer and acutely as an inhibitor of P-450 2E1. It is not certain that there is an effect on cyclosporine metabolism, although one report has suggested increased cyclosporine levels after heavy alcohol consumption.[160] Although abstinence does not appear to be required, moderate to heavy alcohol consumption may have a deleterious effect on the liver per se as well as on the metabolism of required drugs, and should be discouraged.

Drugs Whose Levels Are Increased by Cyclosporine

There are few documented instances of cyclosporine increasing the levels of other drugs. One example is the decreased ketoconazole clearance seen as a consequence of cyclosporine.[161] Metabolism of any drug metabolized by cytochrome P-450 3A might be inhibited by cyclosporine (Table 12.3); this would depend on the relative affinity of the drug and cyclosporine for P-450 3A. Whether inhibition would have a deleterious effect would depend on the particular drug (i.e., its therapeutic index) and its usage (i.e., dose and duration of therapy). Another example is the apparent inhibition of prednisolone metabolism by cyclosporine.[162-164] Lovastatin is a P-450 3A substrate whose metabolism could potentially be impaired by cyclosporine, leading to an increased incidence of side effects.[165,166]

Variability and Drug Interactions

There is significant variability in the bioavailability of oral cyclosporine and in the rate at which cyclosporine is oxidized, as demonstrated by a dosing range of 6 to 57 mg/kg per day to achieve therapeutic levels.[94] Through monitoring of cyclosporine blood levels, the oral dose is varied and the dosing interval is maintained at twice daily. Bioavailability, as mentioned earlier, is determined in part by intestinal P-450 3A enzyme activity, and elimination is primarily a consequence of hepatic P-450 3A enzyme activity. A transplant patient whose cyclosporine blood level can be maintained at a therapeutic level while on a small daily dose would have either better than average bioavailability (perhaps less than average cyclosporine metabolism by the gut) or a lower than average rate of hepatic oxidation, or both. Conversely, a person requiring a large daily dose of cyclosporine to maintain a therapeutic level might have lower than average bioavailability (perhaps increased gut metabolism of cyclosporine) or higher than average hepatic oxidation of cyclosporine, or both. Variable oxidation of cy-

closporine likely is genetically determined and thus may be susceptible to early testing in the future by using other substrates of this P-450 isozyme (e.g., the erythromycin breath test).[167]

As illustrated for a number of drugs, it appears that individuals with higher rates of drug clearance are more susceptible to inhibition by an added drug than are those with lower clearance. This phenomenon was demonstrated in individuals whose chlordiazepoxide pharmacokinetics were studied before and after the addition of ketoconazole.[168] The higher the basal chlordiazepoxide clearance, the greater the inhibition by ketoconazole. The phenomenon was also demonstrated for theophylline clearance before and after the addition of cimetidine; that is, the higher the basal theophylline clearance, the greater the decrease in clearance by cimetidine.[169] In this study, there was a correlation between basal clearance and percentage of inhibition of theophylline clearance following cimetidine use that cannot easily be explained by competitive inhibition. A similar effect of cimetidine on theophylline metabolism has also been reported in smokers[170,171] and in patients taking rifampin,[172] both of which are considered inducers of theophylline metabolism. The phenomenon was also found in a study of chlordiazepoxide clearance in cirrhotic and normal individuals before and after cimetidine use. The higher the basal clearance, the greater the degree of inhibition following addition of cimetidine in both the cirrhotic and normal individuals.[173] Thus, cimetidine resulted in a smaller decrease in clearance in cirrhotic patients than in normal subjects. This observation was also made with regard to organic cation secretion into urine.[174]

Conversely, it appears that those with the slowest drug clearance will have the greatest increase in clearance following the introduction of a drug that induces P-450. Thus, individuals who were slow initial metabolizers of antipyrine had the shortest antipyrine half-life following the introduction of phenobarbital.[175]

It could be speculated that decreases in cyclosporine levels are most commonly secondary to addition of P-450 inducers and that perhaps individuals on small doses of cyclosporine are at greatest risk of this interaction. Increases in cyclosporine levels are most commonly secondary to addition of P-450 3A inhibitors, and perhaps those at greatest risk are those requiring a large dose of cyclosporine to maintain blood levels.

Effect of Cyclosporine on P-Glycoprotein

Some drugs require active secretion into bile or urine for optimal elimination. Recently, ATP-dependent transport processes have been described in the biliary canaliculus that appear important for this function. These transporters may all be members of a superfamily[176] and include P-glycoprotein (also called multidrug resistance transporter or gp-170), an ATP-dependent bile acid transporter,[177] and an ATP-dependent organic anion transporter that would appear to recognize glutathione and glucuronide conjugates.[178–180] P-glycoprotein likely is responsible for secretion of colchicine, doxorubicin, erythromycin, vecuronium, and many other drugs.[181]

Cyclosporine inhibits P-glycoprotein in vitro[182,183] and also inhibits the biliary canalicular P-glycoprotein in vivo.[126,184] Cyclosporine has been reported to be a substrate for P-glycoprotein in some cell systems expressing high levels of P-glycoprotein,[185] but was not secreted into bile when assessed in vivo.[126] This is consistent with data suggesting that cyclosporine is extensively metabolized by P-450 3A in vivo[92,123,125] with little parent cyclosporine appearing in bile.[186] Cyclosporine inhibits the biliary secretion of bilirubin,[128,129] bromosulfophthalein,[128] and bile acids,[127,130,187] suggesting that it may inhibit ATP transporters other than P-glycoprotein. It seems probable that inhibition of P-glycoprotein by cyclosporine may explain, at least in part, interactions between cyclosporine and P-glycoprotein substrates such as doxorubicin,[188] colchicine,[189] etoposide,[188] atracurium,[190] vecuronium,[190] and pentazocine.[191] Many agents have been reported to interact with P-glycoprotein in vitro,[192,193] but it is uncertain whether these effects also occur in vivo. A better understanding of the drugs utilizing one of these canalicular transporters is required before predictions of interactions with cyclosporine can be made.

Cyclosporine also inhibits P-glycoprotein in the renal tubule but would appear not to have an effect on the organic anion and organic cation transporters also known to be present.[194] P-glycoprotein is distributed throughout the mucosal surface of the gastrointestinal tract and, although its function is unknown, this too is a potential site for inhibition by cyclosporine.

Tacrolimus

Tacrolimus (FK506) is a macrocyclic lactone that has shown efficacy as an immunosuppressive agent following liver transplantation. At least two features distinguish tacrolimus from cyclosporine: tacrolimus is much more potent than cyclosporine (the therapeutic level is 0.5–2.0 ng/mL for tacrolimus and 100–200 ng/mL for cyclosporine),[195] and tacrolimus is much less dependent on the presence of bile for absorption from the gastrointestinal tract.[196] Other comparisons have also been made.[195] Liver function is an important determinant of tacrolimus clearance, as with cyclosporine.[93,197] Tacrolimus is oxidized primarily to 13-desmethyl tacrolimus by the cytochrome P-450 isozymes of the P-450 3A subfamily, as is cyclosporine.[90,91] Like cyclosporine, tacrolimus is an inhibitor of P-450 3A activity and to a lesser extent of P-450 1A activity in vitro.[51,198]

In vitro, tacrolimus inhibits cyclosporine metabolism.[199–201] Ketoconazole is a far more potent inhibitor of cyclosporine metabolism than is tacrolimus, however.[199] In a study by Christians et al., cyclosporine failed to inhibit tacrolimus metabolism.[201] In an in vivo study in dogs, tacrolimus had no effect on the pharmacokinetics of cyclosporine given intravenously. The basis for these observations was thought to be inhibition of cyclosporine intestinal first-pass metabolism,[137–139,202] presumably by inhibition of intestinal P-450 3A, as has been suggested for erythromycin.[142]

Less is known about the effect of drugs on the metabolism of the immunosuppressant tacrolimus or the effect of tacrolimus on the disposition of other drugs. However, interactions have been described (but the mechanism not necessarily elucidated) for the antibiotics erythromycin,[195,203] clarithromycin,[204] chloramphenicol,[205] and metronidazole;[206] the antifungals ketoconazole,[155] itraconazole,[207] and clotrimazole;[156,195] danazol;[208] the HIV protease inhibitors saquinavir, ritonavir, nelfinavir, and indinavir;[209] the Serotonin Antagonist Reuptake Inhibitor (SARI) nefazodone;[210,211] and the calcium channel blocker mibefradil.[212] Several HMG-CoA reductase inhibitors (atorvastatin, cerivastatin, lovastatin, and simvastatin) are substrates for cytochrome P-450 3A and potentially can alter tacrolimus levels.[213] ACE inhibitors and the nucleoside analogue lamivudine have not been reported to change tacrolimus levels. Tacrolimus did not impair bromosulfophthalein biliary excretion in rats studied in vivo,[214] although impairment of bromosulfophthalein excretion does occur with cyclosporine.[128] Tacrolimus has been reported to be able to reverse multidrug resistance, presumably by inhibiting the multidrug transporter.[215] Drugs that are eliminated to a significant degree into bile by this mechanism could potentially be affected.

It can be anticipated that drugs that are inducers of P-450 3A (see Table 12.2) may result in increased tacrolimus metabolism and therefore a decrease in its blood level. Similarly, drugs that are competitive inhibitors of P-450 3A (see Table 12.3) might be expected to decrease tacrolimus metabolism and increase blood levels. However, due to the greater potency of tacrolimus and thus the smaller dosage required compared with cyclosporine, tacrolimus is unlikely to cause inhibition of P-450 3A–mediated metabolism of other drugs. Experience is limited, however, and clinical vigilance is required.

Mycophenolate Mofetil

Mycophenolate mofetil is a prodrug that is rapidly and completely absorbed and undergoes presystemic deesterification to the active immunosuppressant, mycophenolic acid. Mycophenolic acid inhibits inosine monophosphate dehydrogenase, an important enzyme in the de novo synthesis of guanosine nucleotides. Mycophenolic acid is glucuronidated in the liver to an inactive, stable phenolic glucuronide that is primarily excreted in the urine. There is some active tubular secretion of the glucuronide and potential for competition with other secreted organic anions. Some mycophenolic acid glucuronide is also excreted in bile and undergoes enterohepatic cycling. Mycophenolic acid is absorbed following deconjugation of mycophenolic acid glucuronide by colonic bacteria. No drug interactions have been described with mycophenolic acid, but antacids and cholestyramine can decrease the AUC.[216]

Sirolimus

Sirolimus is a macrolide that is structurally related to tacrolimus and binds to tacrolimus-binding immunophilin. It would appear to have much less potential for nephrotoxicity than cyclosporine or tacrolimus, perhaps because it does not inhibit the renal protease, calineurin.[217] Sirolimus is metabolized by cytochrome P-450 3A, as are cyclosporine and tacrolimus.[218,219] Coadministration of drugs metabolized by cytochrome P-450 3A might be expected to result in mutual inhibition of metabolism depending on concentration and affinity. Oral coadministration of cyclosporine and sirolimus in a rat model resulted in an increased AUC of both cyclosporine and sirolimus, whereas intravenous coadministration did not, suggesting that the intestinal P-450 3A activity may have been more affected than liver P-450 3A activity.[220] Because sirolimus will likely be administered with either cyclosporine or tacrolimus, renal function should be monitored closely. Further experience with sirolimus and other P-450 3A substrates such as cisapride is needed.

In the posttransplantation patient, the well-functioning liver may have essentially normal ability to metabolize drugs. Virtually all patients will be medicated with cyclosporine or tacrolimus, and both of these immunosuppressants are oxidized primarily by the liver cytochrome P-450 3A. Cyclosporine or tacrolimus may have an effect on the disposition of some drugs. Of more importance, many agents may either induce or inhibit P-450 3A and modulate the elimination of cyclosporine or tacrolimus, leading to deleterious clinical consequences. Experience with some drugs suggests no interaction occurs; however, it is important to note that most drugs have not been specifically tested. Therefore, it is prudent to assume that an interaction is possible with any drug taken in this setting.

REFERENCES

1. Preisig R, Rankin JG, Sweeting J, et al. Hepatic hemodynamics during viral hepatitis in man. *Circulation* 1966;34:188–197.
2. Branch RA. Drugs as indicators of hepatic function. *Hepatology* 1982; 2:97–105.
3. Pessayre D, Lebrec D, Descatoire V, et al. Mechanisms for reduced drug clearance in patients with cirrhosis. *Gastroenterology* 1978;74: 566–571.
4. Huet P-M, Villeneuve JP. Determinants of drug disposition in patients with cirrhosis. *Hepatology* 1983;3:913–918.
5. Roberts RK, Schenker S. Clearly there is intrinsic value in intrinsic clearance. *Hepatology* 1983;3:1036–1038.
6. Secor JW, Schenker S. Drug metabolism in patients with liver disease. *Adv Med* 1987;32:379–406.
7. Wilkinson GR, Shand DC. A physiological approach to hepatic drug clearance. *Clin Pharmacol Ther* 1975;18:377–390.
8. Blaschke TF. Protein binding and kinetics of drugs in liver diseases. *Clin Pharmacokinet* 1977;2:32–44.
9. Hoyumpa AM, Schenker S. Influence of liver disease on the disposition and elimination of drugs. In: Schiff L, Schiff E, eds. *Diseases of the liver,* 7th ed. Philadelphia: JB Lippincott, 1993;784–824.
10. Howard ML, Li Y, Mashford ML, et al. The effect of fibrosis and inflammation on the mRNA expression of UDP-glucuronyltransferase 1A1, 1A6, 2B7 and 2B15 [Abstract]. *Hepatology* 1999;30:322A.
11. Hoyumpa AM, Schenker S. Is glucuronidation truly preserved in patients with liver disease? *Hepatology* 1991;13:786–795.
12. Bakti G, Fisch HU, Kazlaganis G, et al. Mechanisms of the excessive sedative response of cirrhotics to benzodiazepines: model experiments with triazolam. *Hepatology* 1987;7:629–638.
13. Tallman JF, Paul SM, Skolnick P, et al. Receptors for the age of anxiety: pharmacology of the benzodiazepines. *Science* 1980;207:274–278.
14. Hepner GW, Vesell EF, Lipton A, et al. Disposition of aminopyrine, antipyrine, diazepam and ICG in patients with liver disease. *J Lab Clin Med* 1977;90:440–456.
15. Oellerich M, Raude E, Burdelski M, et al. Monoethylglycinexylidide formation kinetics: a novel approach to assessment of liver function. *J Clin Chem Clin Biochem* 1987;25:845–853.
16. Oellerich M, Ringe B, Gubernatis G, et al. Lignocaine metabolite formation as a measure of pre-transplant liver function. *Lancet* 1989;25: 640–642.
17. Schalm SW, Summerskill WHJ, Go VLW. Prednisone for chronic active liver disease: pharmacokinetics, including conversion to prednisolone. *Gastroenterology* 1977;72:910–913.
18. Uribe M, Summerskill WHJ, Go VLW. Comparative screen prednisone and prednisolone concentrations following administration to patients with chronic active liver disease. *Clin Pharmacokinet* 1982; 7:452–459.
19. Bergrem H, Ritland S, Opedal I, et al. Prednisolone pharmacokinetics and protein binding in patients with portasystemic shunts. *Scand J Gastroenterol* 1983;18:273–276.
20. Uribe M, Go VLW, Kluge D. Prednisone for chronic active hepatitis: pharmacokinetics and screen binding in patients with chronic active hepatitis and steroid major side effects. *J Clin Gastroenterol* 1984;6: 331–335.
21. Jones SK, Aherne GW, Campbell MJ, et al. Methotrexate pharmacokinetics in psoriatic patients developing hepatic fibrosis. *Arch Dermatol* 1986;122:666–669.
22. Leighton JA, Bay MK, Maldonado AL, et al. Colchicine clearance is impaired in alcoholic cirrhosis. *Hepatology* 1991;14:1013–1015.
23. Marigold JH, Bull HJ, Gilmore IT, et al. Direct measurement of hepatic extraction of chenodeoxycholic acid and ursodeoxycholic acid in man. *Clin Sci* 1982;63:197–203.
24. Craig PI, Topner M, Farrell GC. Interferon suppresses erythromycin metabolism in rats and human subjects. *Hepatology* 1993;17:230–235.
25. Williams SJ, Baird-Lambert JA, Farrell GC. Inhibition of theophylline metabolism by interferon. *Lancet* 1987;2:939–941.
26. Meredith C, Christian D, Johnson RF, et al. Effects of influenza virus vaccine on hepatic drug metabolism. *Clin Pharmacol Ther* 1985;37: 396–401.
27. Marshall JP, Salt WB, Elam RO, et al. Disposition of nafcillin in patients with cirrhosis and extrahepatic biliary obstruction. *Gastroenterology* 1977;73:1388–1392.
28. Bunke CM, Aronoff GR, Brier ME, et al. Mezlocillin kinetics in hepatic insufficiency. *Clin Pharmacol Ther* 1983;33:73–76.
29. Cabera J, Arroyo V, Ballesta AM, et al. Aminoglycoside nephrotoxicity in cirrhosis. *Gastroenterology* 1982;82:97–105.
30. Felisart J, Rimola A, Arroyo V, et al. Cefotaxime is more effective than is ampicillin-tobramycin in cirrhotics with severe infections. *Hepatology* 1985;5:457–462.
31. Farrell G, Baird-Lambert J, Cvejic M, et al. Disposition and metabolism of metroidazole in patients with liver failure. *Hepatology* 1984; 4:722–726.
32. Danan G, Montay G, Cunci R, et al. Perfloxacin kinetics in cirrhosis. *Clin Pharmacol Ther* 1985;38:439–442.
33. Eandi M, Viano I, DiNola F, et al. Pharmacokinetics of norfloxacin in healthy volunteers and patients with renal and hepatic damage. *Eur J Clin Microbiol* 1983;2:253–259.
34. *Physicians' Desk Reference,* 53rd ed. Montvale, NJ: Medical Economics, 1999.
35. Levi AJ, Sherlock S, Walker D. Phenylbutazone and isoniazid metabolism in patients with liver disease in relation to previous drug therapy. *Lancet* 1968;1:1275–1279.
36. Burk RF, Hill KE, Hunt RW Jr, et al. Isoniazid potentiation of acetaminophen hepatotoxicity in the rat and 4-methylpyrazole inhibition of it. *Res Commun Chem Pathol Pharmacol* 1990;69:115–118.

37. Watkins PB. Role of cytochromes P450 in drug metabolism and hepatotoxicity. *Semin Liver Dis* 1990;10:235–250.
38. Villeneuve JP, Rocheleau F, Raymond G. Triamterene kinetics and dynamics in cirrhosis. *Clin Pharmacol Ther* 1984;35:831–837.
39. Wood AJJ, Kornhauser DM, Wilkinson GR, et al. The influence of cirrhosis on steady-state blood concentrations of unbound propranolol after oral administration. *Clin Pharmacokinet* 1978;3:478–487.
40. Homeida M, Jackson L, Roberts CJC. Decreased first pass metabolism of labetalol in chronic liver disease. *Br J Med* 1978;2:1048–1050.
41. Sushma S, Dasarathy S, Tandon RK, et al. Sodium benzoate in the treatment of acute hepatic encephalopathy: a double-blind randomized trial. *Hepatology* 1992;16:138–144.
42. Meredith C, Christian D, Johnson RF, et al. Diphenylhydramine disposition in chronic liver disease. *Clin Pharmacol Ther* 1984;35:474–479.
43. Maxwell JD, Carrella M, Parker JD, et al. Plasma disappearance and cerebral effects of chlorpromazine in cirrhosis. *Clin Sci* 1972;43:143–151.
44. Karim A, Ranney RE, Evensen KL, et al. Pharmacokinetics and metabolism of diphenoxylate in man. *Clin Pharmacol Ther* 1972;13:407–419.
45. Juhl RP, Van Thiel DH, Dittert LW, et al. Ibuprofen and sulindac kinetics in alcoholic liver disease. *Clin Pharmacol Ther* 1983;34:104–109.
46. Benson GD. Acetaminophen in chronic liver disease. *Clin Pharmacol Ther* 1983;33:95–101.
47. Forrest JAM, Adriaenssens P, Finlayson NDC, et al. Paracetamol metabolism in chronic liver disease. *Eur J Clin Pharmacol* 1979;15:427–431.
48. Villeneuve JP, Fortunet-Fouin H, Arsene D. Cimetidine kinetics in patients with severe liver disease. *Hepatology* 1983;3:923–927.
49. Young CJ, Daneshmend TK, Roberts CJC. Effects of cirrhosis and aging on the elimination and bioavailability of ranitidine. *Gut* 1982;23:819–823.
50. Kleinbloesem CH, Van Harlan J, Wilson JPH, et al. Nifedipine: kinetics and hemodynamic effects in patients with liver cirrhosis after intravenous and oral administration. *Clin Pharmacol Ther* 1986;40:21–28.
51. Somogyi A, Albrecht M, Kliems G, et al. Pharmacokinetics, bioavailability and ECG response of verapamil in patients with liver cirrhosis. *Br J Clin Pharmacol* 1981;12:51–60.
52. Tsai HH, Lees KR, Howden CW, et al. The pharmacokinetics and pharmacodynamics of perindopril in patients with hepatic cirrhosis. *Br J Clin Pharmacol* 1989;28:53–59.
53. Gelman S, Kang Y, Pearson J. Anesthetic considerations in liver transplantation. In: Fabian J, ed. *Anesthesia for organ transplantation.* Philadelphia: JB Lippincott, 1992:115–139.
54. Reilly C, Wood A, Koshakji R, et al. The effect of halothane on drug disposition: contribution in changes in intrinsic drug metabolizing capacity and hepatic blood flow. *Anesthesiology* 1985;63:70–76.
55. Chapin J, Newland M, Hurlbert B. Anesthesia for liver transplantation. *Semin Liver Dis* 1989;9:195–201.
56. Gelman S, Fowler K, Smith L. Liver circulation and function during isoflurane and halothane anesthesia. *Anesthesiology* 1984;61:726–730.
57. Gelman S. Disturbances in hepatic blood flow during anesthesia and surgery. *Arch Surg* 1976;111:881–883.
58. Thomson P, Melmon K, Richardson J, et al. Lidocaine pharmacokinetics in advanced heart failure, liver disease, and renal failure in humans. *Ann Intern Med* 1973;78:499–508.
59. Vesell E. The antipyrine test in clinical pharmacology: conceptions and misconceptions. *Clin Pharmacol Ther* 1979;26:275–286.
60. Nagano K, Gelman S, Parks D, et al. Hepatic circulation and oxygen supply-uptake relationships after hepatic ischemic insult during anesthesia with volatile anesthetics and fentanyl in miniature pigs. *Anesth Analg* 1990;70:53–62.
61. Gelman S, Dillard E, Bradley E. Hepatic circulation during surgical stress and anesthesia with halothane, isoflurane, or fentanyl. *Anesth Analg* 1987;66:936–943.
62. Goldstine R, Soloman H, Holman M, et al. Liver transplantation 1990. A Dallas perspective. In: Terasaki P, ed. *Clinical transplants 1990.* Los Angeles: UCLA Tissue Typing Laboratory, 1990:127–128.
63. Trouvin J, Farinotti R, Haberer JP, et al. Pharmacokinetics of midazolam in anaesthetized cirrhotic patients. *Br J Anaesth* 1988;60:762–767.
64. MacGilchrist A, Birnie G, Cook A, et al. Pharmacokinetics and pharmacodynamics of intravenous midazolam in patients with severe alcoholic cirrhosis. *Gut* 1986;27:190–195.
65. Pandele G, Chaux F, Salvadori C, et al. Thiopental pharmacokinetics in patients with cirrhosis. *Anesthesiology* 1983;59:123–126.
66. Murphy M. Opioids. In: Barash P, Cullen B, Stoelting R, eds. *Clinical anesthesia.* Philadelphia: JB Lippincott, 1992:424–427.
67. Kang Y, Uram M, Shiu G, et al. Pharmacokinetics of fentanyl in end-stage liver disease [Abstract]. *Anesthesiology* 1984;61:A380.
68. Haberer J, Schoeffler P, Couderc E, et al. Fentanyl pharmacokinetics in anaesthetized patients with cirrhosis. *Br J Anaesth* 1982;54:1267–1270.
69. Chauvin M, Ferrier C, Haberer J, et al. Sufentanil pharmacokinetics in patients with cirrhosis. *Anesth Analg* 1989;58:1–4.
70. Aldrete J, O'Higgins J, Holmes J. Changes of plasma cholinesterase activity during orthotopic liver transplantation in man. *Transplantation* 1977;23:404–406.
71. Gelman S. Anesthesia and the liver. In: Barash P, Cullen B, Stoelting R, eds. *Clinical anesthesia.* Philadelphia: JB Lippincott, 1992:1185–1213.
72. Arden J, Cannon J, Lynam D, et al. Vecuronium pharmacokinetics and pharmacodynamics in hepatocellular disease [Abstract]. *Anesth Analg* 1987;66:S3.
73. Lebrault C, Berger J, D'Hollander A, et al. Pharmacokinetics and pharmacodynamics of vecuronium in patients with cirrhosis. *Anesthesiology* 1985;62:601–605.
74. Hunter J, Parker C, Bell C, et al. The use of different doses of vecuronium in patients with liver dysfunction. *Br J Anaesth* 1985;57:758–764.
75. Duvaldestin P, Agoston S, Henzel D, et al. Pancuronium pharmacokinetics in patients with liver cirrhosis. *Br J Anaesth* 1978;50:1131–1136.
76. Holaday D, Fiserova-Bergerova V, Latto I, et al. Resistance of isoflurane to biotransformation in man. *Anesthesiology* 1975;43:325–332.
77. Svensson K, Persson H, Henriksson B, et al. Whole body gas exchange: amino acid and lactate clearance as indicators of initial and early allograft viability in liver transplantation. *Surgery* 1989;105:472–480.
78. Park G, Manara A, Dawling S. Extra-hepatic metabolism of midazolam. *Br J Clin Pharmacol* 1989;27:634–637.
79. Bodenham A, Quinn K, Park G. Extrahepatic morphine metabolism in man during the anhepatic phase of orthotopic liver transplantation. *Br J Anaesth* 1989;63:380–384.
80. Veroli P, O'Kelly B, Bertrand F, et al. Extrahepatic metabolism of propofol in man during the anhepatic phase of orthotopic liver transplantation. *Br J Anaesth* 1992;68:183–186.
81. Kang Y, Gelman S. Liver transplantation. In: Gelman S, ed. *Anesthesia and organ transplantation.* Philadelphia: WB Saunders, 1987:139–185.
82. Park G, Podkowik B. Plasma concentrations of flumazenil during liver transplantation. *Anesthesia* 1992;47:887–889.
83. Angus PW, Morgan DJ, Smallwood RA. Review article: hypoxia and hepatic drug metabolism—clinical implications. *Aliment Pharmacol Ther* 1990;4:213–225.
84. Rosenberg P, Oikkonen M, Orko R, et al. A transplanted liver rapidly begins to metabolize enflurane in humans. *Anesth Analg* 1984;63:1131–1132.
85. Shiffman M, Carithers R, Posner M, et al. Recovery of bile secretion following orthotopic liver transplantation. *J Hepatology* 1991;12:351–361.
86. Konishi Y, Shaked A, Egawa H, et al. Correlation of hepatic injury, synthetic function, and mitochondria energy level in orthotopic liver transplantation. *J Surg Res* 1992;52:466–471.
87. Mehta M, Venkataramanan R, Burchart G, et al. Effect of bile on cyclosporin absorption in liver transplant patients. *Br J Clin Pharmacol* 1988;25:579–584.
88. Tredger J, Naoumov N, Steward C, et al. Influence of biliary T tube clamping on cyclosporine pharmacokinetics in liver transplant recipients. *Transplant Proc* 1988;20:512–515.
89. Groen P. Cyclosporine and the liver: how one affects the other. *Transplant Proc* 1990;22:1197–1202.
90. Vincent SH, Karanam BV, Painter SK, et al. *In vitro* metabolism of FK-506 in rat, rabbit, and human liver microsomes: identification of a major metabolite and of cytochrome P4503A as the major enzymes responsible for its metabolism. *Arch Biochem Biophys* 1992;294:454–460.
91. Sattler M, Guengerich FP, Yun CH, et al. Cytochrome P-450 3A enzymes are responsible for biotransformation of FK506 and rapamycin in man and rat. *Drug Metab Dispos* 1992;20:753–761.
92. Maurer G, Loosli HR, Schreier E, et al. Disposition of cyclosporine in several animal species and man. *Drug Metab Dispos* 1984;12:120–126.
93. Abu-Elmagd K, Fung JJ, Alessiani M, et al. The effect of graft function on FK-506 plasma levels, dosages, and renal function, with particular reference to the liver. *Transplantation* 1991;52:71–77.

94. Venkataramanan R, Habucky K, Burckart GJ, et al. Clinical pharmacokinetics in organ transplant patients. *Clin Pharmacokinet* 1989;16:134–161.

95. Huang ML, Venkataramanan R, Burckart GJ, et al. Drug binding proteins in liver transplant patients. *J Clin Pharmacol* 1988;28:505–506.

96. Shelly M, Dixon J, Park G. The pharmacokinetics of midazolam following orthotopic liver transplantation. *Br J Clin Pharmacol* 1989;27:629–633.

97. Shelly M, Quinn K, Park G. Pharmacokinetics of morphine in patients following orthotopic liver transplantation. *Br J Anaesth* 1989;63: 375–379.

98. Eisenach J, Plevak D, Van Dyke R, et al. Comparison of analgesic requirements after liver transplantation and cholecystectomy. *Mayo Clin Proc* 1989;64:356–359.

99. Osborne R, Joel S, Slevin M. Morphine intoxication in renal failure: the role of morphine-6-glucuronide. *Br Med J* 1986;292:1548–1549.

100. Toth A, Abdallah H, Vankataramanan R, et al. Pharmacokinetics of ceftriaxone in liver-transplant recipients. *J Clin Pharmacol* 1991;31:722–728.

101. Kuse E, Vogt P, Rosenkranz B. Pharmacokinetics of cefotaxime in patients after liver transplantation. *Infection* 1990;18:268–272.

102. Balant L, Dayer P, Auckenthaler R. Clinical pharmacokinetics of the third generation cephalosporins. *Clin Pharmacokinet* 1985;10:101–143.

103. Venkataramanan R, Kalp K, Rabinovitch M, et al. Conjugative drug metabolism in liver transplant patients. *Transplant Proc* 1989;21:2455.

104. Mehta M, Venkataramanan R, Burckart G, et al. Antipyrine kinetics in liver disease and liver transplantation. *Clin Pharmacol Ther* 1986;39:372–377.

105. Venkataramana R, Huang M, Delamos B, et al. Steroid metabolism in liver transplant patients. *Transplant Proc* 1989;21:2452.

106. Yee GC, McGuire TR. Pharmacokinetic drug interactions with cyclosporin (Part I). *Clin Pharmacokinet* 1990;19:319–332.

107. Yee GC, McGuire TR. Pharmacokinetic drug interactions with cyclosporin (Part II). *Clin Pharmacokinet* 1990;19:400–415.

108. Lake KD. Management of drug interactions with cyclosporine. *Pharmacotherapy* 1991;11:110S–118S.

109. Lake KD, Canafax DM. Important interactions of drugs with immunosuppressive agents used in transplant recipients. *J Antimicrobial Chemother* 1995;36(suppl B):11–22.

110. Paterson DL, Singh N. Interactions between tacrolimus and antimicrobial agents. *Clin Infect Dis* 1997;25:1430–1440.

111. Myers BD. Cyclosporine nephrotoxicity. *Kidney Int* 1986;30:964–974.

112. Shulman H, Striker G, Deeg HJ, et al. Nephrotoxicity of cyclosporin A after allogeneic marrow transplantation: glomerular thromboses and tubular injury. *N Engl J Med* 1981;305:1392–1395.

113. Basarab A, Jarrell BE, Hirsch S, et al. Use of the isolated perfused kidney model to assess acute pharmacologic effects of cyclosporine and its vehicle, cremophor EL. *Transplantation* 1987;44:199–201.

114. Wolfe JA, McCann RL, Sanfilippo F. Cyclosporine-associated microangiopathy in renal transplantation: a severe but potentially reversible form of early graft injury. *Transplantation* 1986;41:541–544.

115. Myers BD, Ross J, Newton L, et al. Cyclosporine-associated chronic nephropathy. *N Engl J Med* 1984;311:699–705.

116. Mihatsch MJ, Thiel G, Basler V, et al. Morphological patterns in cyclosporine-treated renal transplant recipients. *Transplant Proc* 1985;17:101–116.

117. Bennett WM, Pulliam JP. Cyclosporine nephrotoxicity. *Ann Intern Med* 1983;99:851–854.

118. Hows JM, Chipping PM, Fairhead S, et al. Nephrotoxicity in bone marrow transplant recipients treated with cyclosporin A. *Br J Haematol* 1983;54:69–78.

119. Whiting PH, Simpson JG, Davidson RJ, et al. The toxic effects of combined administration of cyclosporine A and gentamycin. *Br J Exp Pathol* 1982;63:554–561.

120. Kennedy MS, Deeg MJ, Siegel M, et al. Acute renal toxicity with combined use of amphotericin B and cyclosporine after marrow transplantation. *Transplantation* 1983;35:211–215.

121. Deray G, LeHoang P, Aupetit B, et al. Enhancement of cyclosporine A nephrotoxicity by diclofenac. *Clin Nephrol* 1987;27:213–214.

122. Whiting PH, Burke MD, Thomson AW. Drug interactions with cyclosporine: implications from animal studies. *Transplant Proc* 1986;18:56–70.

123. Kronbach T, Fischer V, Meyer UA. Cyclosporine metabolism in human liver: identification of a cytochrome P-450III gene family as the major cyclosporine-metabolizing enzyme explains interactions of cyclosporine with other drugs. *Clin Pharmacol Ther* 1988;43:630–635.

124. Aoyama T, Yamano S, Waxman DJ, et al. Cytochrome P-450 hPCN3, a novel cytochrome P-450 IIIA gene product that is differentially expressed in adult human liver. cDNA and deduced amino acid sequence and distinct specificities of cDNA-expressed hPCN1 and hPCN3 for the metabolism of steroid hormones and cyclosporine. *J Biol Chem* 1989;264:10388–10395.

125. Combalbert J, Fabre I, Fabre G, et al. Metabolism of cyclosporin A. IV. Purification and identification of the rifampicin-inducible human liver cytochrome P-450 (cyclosporin A oxidase) as a product of P450IIIA gene subfamily. *Drug Metab Dispos* 1989;17:197–207.

126. Speeg KV, Maldonado AL, Liaci J, et al. Effect of cyclosporine on colchicine secretion by a liver canalicular transporter studied *in vivo*. *Hepatology* 1992;15:899–903.

127. Thai BL, Dumont M, Michel A, et al. Cholestatic effect of cyclosporine in the rat: an inhibition of bile acid secretion. *Transplantation* 1988;46:510–512.

128. Cadranel JF, Dumont M, Mesa VA, et al. Effect of chronic administration of cyclosporin A on hepatic uptake and biliary secretion of bromosulfophthalein in rat. *Dig Dis Sci* 1991;36:221–224.

129. Roman ID, Monte MJ, Esteller A, et al. Cholestasis in the rat by means of intravenous administration of cyclosporine vehicle, cremophor EL. *Transplantation* 1989;48:554–558.

130. Moseley RH, Johnson TR, Morrissette JM. Inhibition of bile acid transport by cyclosporine A in rat liver plasma membrane vesicles. *J Pharmacol Exp Ther* 1990;253:974–980.

131. Kahan BD. Individualization of cyclosporine therapy using pharmacokinetic and pharmacodynamic parameters. *Transplantation* 1985;40:457–476.

132. Venkataramanan R, Burckardt GJ, Ptachcinski R. Pharmacokinetics and monitoring of cyclosporine following orthotopic liver transplantation. *Semin Liver Dis* 1985;5:357–368.

133. Wadhwa NK, Schroeder TJ, O'Flaherty E, et al. The effect of oral metoclopramide on the absorption of cyclosporine. *Transplant Proc* 1987;19:1730–1733.

134. Kallinowski B, Theilmann L, Zimmerman R, et al. Effective treatment of cyclosporine-induced cholestasis in heart-transplanted patients treated with urosodeoxycholic acid. *Transplantation* 1991;51:1128–1129.

135. Gutzler F, Zimmerman R, Ring GH, et al. Ursodeoxycholic acid enhances the absorption of cyclosporine in a heart transplant patient with short bowel syndrome. *Transplant Proc* 1992;24:2620–2621.

136. Watkins PB, Wrighton SA, Schuetz EG, et al. Identification of glucocorticoid-inducible cytochromes P-450 in the intestinal mucosa of rats and man. *J Clin Invest* 1987;80:1029–1036.

137. Kolars JC, Awni WM, Merion RM, et al. First-pass metabolism of cyclosporin by the gut. *Lancet* 1991;338:1488–1490.

138. Schwinghammer TL, Przepiorka D, Vendataramanan R, et al. The kinetics of cyclosporine and its metabolites in bone marrow transplant patients. *Br J Clin Pharmacol* 1991;32:323–328.

139. Kolars JC, Stetson PL, Rush BD, et al. Cyclosporine metabolism by P450IIIA in rat enterocytes—another determinant of oral bioavailability. *Transplantation* 1992;53:596–602.

140. Kolars JC, Schmiedlin-Ren P, Schuetz JD, et al. Identification of rifampin-inducible P450IIIA4 (CYP3A4) in human small bowel enterocytes. *J Clin Invest* 1992;90:1871–1878.

141. Rowland M, Gupta SK. Cyclosporin-phenytoin interaction: reevaluation using metabolite data. *Br J Clin Pharmacol* 1987;24:329–334.

142. Gupta SK, Bakran A, Johnson RWG, et al. Cyclosporin-erythromycin interaction in renal transplant patients. *Br J Clin Pharmacol* 1989;27:475–481.

143. Hebert MF, Roberts JP, Prueksaritanont T, et al. Clinical evidence of metabolic differences between intestinal and hepatic cytochrome P450 [Abstract]. *Clin Pharmacol Ther* 1993;53:190.

144. Niederberger W, Lemaire M, Maurer G, et al. Distribution and binding of cyclosporine in blood and tissues. *Transplant Proc* 1983;15:2419–2421.

145. Rosano TG. Effect of hematocrit on cyclosporine (cyclosporin A) in whole blood and plasma of renal transplant patients. *Clin Chem* 1985;31:410–412.

146. Ptachcinski RJ, Vendataramanan R, Burckart GJ. Clinical pharmacokinetics of cyclosporin. *Clin Pharmacokinet* 1986;11:107–132.

147. Pichard L, Fabre I, Fabre G, et al. Screening for inducers and inhibitors of cytochrome P-450 (cyclosporin A oxidase) in primary cultures of human hepatocytes and in liver microsomes. *Drug Metab Dispos* 1990;18:595–606.

148. Lele P, Peterson P, Yang S, et al. Cyclosporine and tegretol—another drug interaction [Abstract]. *Kidney Int* 1985;27:344.

149. Coward RA, Raftery AT, Brown CB. Cyclosporine and antituberculous therapy (Letter). *Lancet* 1985;1:1342–1343.

150. Sesardic D, Boobis AR, Edwards RJ, et al. A form of cytochrome P450 in man, orthologous to form d in the rat, catalyses the O-deethylation of phenacetin and is inducible by cigarette smoking. *Br J Clin Pharmacol* 1988;26:363–372.

151. Moochhala SM, Lee EJD, Earnest LL, et al. Inhibition of drug metabolism in rat and human liver microsomes by FK-506 and cyclosporine. *Transplant Proc* 1991;23:2786–2788.

152. Lee EJD, Moochhala SM. Selective inhibition of drug metabolism by cyclosporin A [Abstract]. *Eur J Clin Pharmacol* 1989;36: A268.

153. Back DJ, Tjia JF. Comparative effects of the antimycotic drugs ketoconazole, fluconazole, itraconazole and terbinafine on the metabolism of cyclosporin by human liver microsomes. *Br J Clin Pharmacol* 1991;32:624–626.

154. Albengres E, Tillement JP. Cyclosporin and ketoconazole, drug interaction or therapeutic association? *Int J Clin Pharmacol Ther Toxicol* 1992;30:555–570.

155. Assan R, Fredj G, Larger E, et al. FK506/fluconazole interaction enhances FK506 nephrotoxicity. *Diabetes Metab* 1994;20:49–52.

156. Mieles L, Venkataramanan R, Yokoyama I, et al. Interaction between FK506 and clotrimazole in a liver transplant recipient. *Transplantation* 1991;52:1086–1087.

157. Copur MS, Tasdemir I, Turgan C, et al. Effects of nitrendipine on blood pressure and blood cyclosporin A level in patients with posttransplant hypertension. *Nephron* 1989;52:227–230.

158. Periti P, Mazzei T, Mini E, et al. Pharmacokinetic drug interactions of macrolides. *Clin Pharmacokinet* 1992;23:106–131.

159. Lane EA, Guthrie S, Linnoila M. Effects of ethanol on drug and metabolite pharmacokinetics. *Clin Pharmacokinet* 1985;10:228–247.

160. Paul MD, Parfrey PS, Smart M, et al. The effect of ethanol on serum cyclosporine A levels in renal transplant recipients. *Am J Kidney Dis* 1987;10:133–135.

161. Myre SA, Schroeder TJ, Pesce AJ, et al. Influence of cyclosporine on ketoconazole relative oral bioavailability and clearance in the dog [Abstract]. *Clin Pharmacol Ther* 1993;53:164.

162. Ost L. Effects of cyclosporine on prednisolone metabolism (Letter). *Lancet* 1984;1:451.

163. Ost L, Klintmalm G, Ringden O. Mutual interaction between prednisolone and cyclosporine in renal transplant patients. *Transplant Proc* 1985;17:1252–1255.

164. Langhoff E, Madsen S, Flachs H, et al. Inhibition of prednisolone metabolism by cyclosporine in kidney transplanted patients. *Transplantation* 1985;39:107–109.

165. Norman DJ, Illingworth DR, Munson J, et al. Myolysis and acute renal failure in a heart-transplant recipient receiving lovastatin. *N Engl J Med* 1988;318:46–47.

166. East C, Alivizatos PA, Grundy SM, et al. Rhabdomyolysis in patients receiving lovastatin after cardiac transplantation. *N Engl J Med* 1988;318:47–48.

167. Watkins PB, Hamilton TA, Annesley TM, et al. The erythromycin breath test as a predictor of cyclosporine blood levels. *Clin Pharmacol Ther* 1990;48:120–129.

168. Brown MW, Maldonado AL, Meredith CG, et al. Effect of ketoconazole on hepatic oxidative drug metabolism. *Clin Pharmacol Ther* 1985;37:290–297.

169. Cremer KF, Secor J, Speeg KV. The effect of route of administration on the cimetidine-theophylline drug interaction. *J Clin Pharmacol* 1989;29:451–456.

170. Grygiel JJ, Miners JO, Drew R, et al. Differential effects of cimetidine on theophylline metabolic pathways. *Eur J Clin Pharmacol* 1984;26:336–340.

171. Cusack BJ, Dawson GW, Mercer GD, et al. Cigarette smoking and theophylline metabolism: effect of cimetidine. *Clin Pharmacol Ther* 1985;37:330–336.

172. Feely J, Pereira L, Guy E, et al. Factors affecting the response to inhibition of drug metabolism by cimetidine-dose response and sensitivity of elderly and induced subjects. *Br J Clin Pharmacol* 1984; 17:77–81.

173. Nelson DC, Avant GR, Speeg KV, et al. The effect of cimetidine on hepatic drug elimination in cirrhosis. *Hepatology* 1985;5:305–309.

174. Kosoglou T, Rocci ML Jr, Vlases PH. Trimethoprim alters the disposition of procainamide and N-acetylprocainamide. *Clin Pharmacol Ther* 1988;44:467–477.

175. Vesell ES, Page JG. Genetic control of the phenobarbital-induced shortening of plasma antipyrine half-lives in man. *J Clin Invest* 1969;48: 2202–2209.

176. Juranka PF, Zastawny RL, Ling V. P-glycoprotein: multidrug resistance and a superfamily of membrane-associated transport proteins. *Fed Am Soc Exp Biol J* 1989;3:2583–2592.

177. Nishida T, Gatmaitan Z, Che M, et al. Rat liver canalicular membrane vesicles contain an ATP-dependent bile acid transport system. *Proc Natl Acad Sci U S A* 1991;88:6590–6594.

178. Kobayashi K, Sogame Y, Hara H, et al. Mechanism of glutathione S-conjugate transport in canalicular and basolateral rat liver plasma membranes. *J Biol Chem* 1990;265:7737–7741.

179. Ishikawa T, Muller M, Klunemann C, et al. ATP-dependent primary active transport of cysteinyl leukotrienes across liver canalicular membrane. *J Biol Chem* 1990;265:19279–19286.

180. Oude Elferink RPJ, Bakker CTM, Roelofsen H, et al. Accumulation of organic anion in intracellular vesicles of cultured rat hepatocytes is mediated by the canalicular multispecific organic anion transporter. *Hepatology* 1993;17:434–444.

181. Kamimoto Y, Gatmaitan Z, Hsu J, et al. The function of GP170, the multidrug resistance gene product, in rat liver canalicular membrane vesicles. *J Biol Chem* 1989;264:11693–11698.

182. Slater LM, Sweet P, Stupeky M, et al. Cyclosporine A reverses vincristine and daunorubicin resistance in acute lymphatic leukemia in vitro. *J Clin Invest* 1986;77:1405–1408.

183. Twentyman PR. Modification of cytotoxic drug resistance by non-immunosuppressive cyclosporin. *Br J Cancer* 1988;57:254–258.

184. Speeg KV, Maldonado AL. Effect of cyclosporine on colchicine partitioning in the rat liver. *Cancer Chemother Pharmacol* 1993;32: 434–436.

185. Goldberg H, Ling V, Wong PY, et al. Reduced cyclosporin accumulation in multidrug-resistant cells. *Biochem Biophys Res Commun* 1988;152:552–558.

186. Burckart GJ, Starzl TE, Venkataramanan R, et al. Excretion of cyclosporine and its metabolites in human bile. *Transplant Proc* 1986; 18:46–49.

187. Stacey N, Kotecka B. Inhibition of taurocholate and ouabain transport in isolated rat hepatocytes by cyclosporin A. *Gastroenterology* 1988;95:780–786.

188. Kloke O, Osieka R. Interaction of cyclosporine A with antineoplastic agents. *Klin Wochenschr* 1985;63:1081–1082.

189. Menta R, Rossi E, Guariglia A, et al. Reversible acute cyclosporine nephrotoxicity induced by colchicine administration. *Nephrol Dial Transplant* 1987;2:380–381.

190. Gramstad L, Gjerlow JA, Hysing ES, et al. Interaction of cyclosporine and its solvent, cremophor, with atracurium and vecuronium. Studies in the cat. *Br J Anaesth* 1986;58:1149–1155.

191. Cockburn ITR, Krupp P. An appraisal of drug interactions with Sandimmune. *Transplant Proc* 1989;21:3845–3850.

192. Hofsli E, Nissen-Meyer J. Reversal of multidrug resistance by lipophilic drugs. *Cancer Res* 1990;50:3997–4002.

193. Dellinger M, Pressman BC, Calderon-Higginson C, et al. Structural requirements of simple organic cations for recognition by multidrug-resistant cells. *Cancer Res* 1992;52:6385–6389.

194. Speeg KV, Maldonado AL, Liaci J, et al. Effect of cyclosporine on colchicine secretion by the kidney multidrug transporter studied in vivo. *J Pharmacol Exp Ther* 1992;261:50–55.

195. Venkataramanan R, Jain A, Warty VS, et al. Pharmacokinetics of FK-506 in transplant patients. *Transplant Proc* 1991;23:2736–2740.

196. Furukawa H, Imventarza O, Venkataramanan R, et al. The effect of bile duct ligation and bile diversion of FK-506 pharmacokinetics in dogs. *Transplantation* 1992;53:722–725.

197. Jain AB, Venkataramanan R, Cadoff E, et al. Effect of hepatic dysfunction and T-tube clamping on FK-506 pharmacokinetics and trough concentrations. *Transplant Proc* 1990;22:57–59.

198. Shah IA, Whiting PH, Omar G, et al. Effects of FK-506 on human hepatic microsomal cytochrome P-450-dependent drug metabolism in vitro. *Transplant Proc* 1991;23:2783–2785.

199. Omar G, Shah IA, Thomson AW, et al. FK-506 inhibition of cyclosporine metabolism by human liver microsomes. *Transplant Proc* 1991;23:934–935.

200. Pichard L, Fabre I, Domergue J, et al. Effect of FK-506 on human hepatic cytochromes P-450: interaction with CyA. *Transplant Proc* 1991;23:2791–2793.

201. Christians U, Braun F, Sattler M, et al. Interactions of FK-506 and cyclosporine metabolism. *Transplant Proc* 1991;23:2794–2796.

202. Lampen A, Christians U, Guengerich FP, et al. Metabolism of the immunosuppressant tacrolimus in the small intestine: cytochrome P450, drug interactions, and interindividual variability. *Drug Metab Dispos* 1995;23:1315–1324.

203. Shaeffer MS, Collier D, Sorrell MF. Interaction between FK506 and erythromycin. *Ann Pharmacother* 1994;28:280–281.

204. Wolter K, Wagner K, Philipp T, et al. Interaction between FK506 and clarithromycin in a renal transplant patient. *Eur J Clin Pharmacol* 1994;47:207–208.

205. Schulman S, Shaw I, Jabs K, et al. Interaction between tacrolimus and chloramphenicol in a renal transplant recipient. *Transplantation* 1998;65:1397–1398.

206. Herzig K, Johnson DW. Marked elevation of blood cyclosporin and tacrolimus levels due to concurrent metronidazole therapy. *Nephrol Dial Transplant* 1999;14:521–523.

207. Furlan V, Parquin F, Penaud JF, et al. Interaction between tacrolimus and itraconazole in a heart-lung transplant recipient. *Transplant Proc* 1998;30:187–188.

208. Shapiro R, Venkataramanan R, Warty VS, et al. FK 506 interaction with danazol. *Lancet* 1993;341:1344–1345.

209. Sheikh AM, Wolf DC, Lebovics E, et al. Concomitant human immunodeficiency virus protease inhibitor therapy markedly reduces tacrolimus metabolism and increases blood levels. *Transplantation* 1999;68:307–309.

210. Olyaei AL, deMattos AM, Norman DJ, et al. Interaction between tacrolimus and nefazodone in a stable renal transplant recipient. *Pharmacotherapy* 1998;18:1356–1359.

211. Campo JV, Smith C, Perel JM. Tacrolimus toxic reaction associated with the use of nefazodone: paroxetine as an alternative agent. *Arch Gen Psychiatry* 1998;55:1050–1052.

212. Krahenbuhl S, Menafoglio A, Giostra E, et al. Serious interaction between mibefradil and tacrolimus. *Transplantation* 1998;66:1113–1115.

213. White MC, Chow MSS. A preview of the HMG-CoA reductase inhibitors. *US Pharm* 1998;HS19–HS29.

214. Farghali H, Sakr M, Gasbarrini A, et al. Effect of FK-506 chronic administration on bromosulfophthalein hepatic excretion in rats. *Transplant Proc* 1991;23:2802–2804.

215. Naito M, Oh-hara T, Yamazaki A, et al. Reversal of multidrug resistance by an immunosuppressive agent FK-506. *Cancer Chemother Pharmacol* 1992;29:195–200.

216. Bullingham RES, Nicholls AJ, Kamm BR. Clinical pharmacokinetics of mycophenolate mofetil. *Drug Dispos* 1998;34:429–455.

217. Andoh TF, Burdmann EA, Fransechini N, et al. Comparison of acute rapamycin nephrotoxicity with cyclosporine and FK506. *Kidney Int* 1996;50:1110–1117.

218. Streit F, Christians U, Schiebel HM, et al. Structural identification of three metabolites and a degradation product of the macrolide immunosuppressant sirolimus (rapamycin) by electrospray-MS/MS after incubation with human liver microsomes. *Drug Metab Dispos* 1996;24:1272–1278.

219. Sattler M, Guengerich FP, Yun CH, et al. Cytochrome P450 3A enzymes are responsible for biotransformation of FK506 and rapamycin in man and rat. *Drug Metab Dispos* 1992;20:753–761.

220. Stepkowski SM, Napoli KL, Wang M-E, et al. Effects of the pharmacokinetic interaction between orally administered sirolimus and cyclosporine on the synergistic prolongation of heart allograft survival in rats. *Transplantation* 1996;62:986–994.

221. Hillebrand G, Castro LA, van Scheidt W, et al. Valproate for epilepsy in renal transplant recipients receiving cyclosporine. *Transplantation* 1987;43:915–916.

222. Carstensen H, Jacobsen N, Dieperink H. Interaction between cyclosporine A and phenobarbitone. *Br J Clin Pharmacol* 1986;21:550–551.

223. Wideman CA. Pharmacokinetic monitoring of cyclosporine. *Transplant Proc* 1983;15:3168–3175.

224. Keown P, Stiller CR, Laupacis AL, et al. The effects and side effects of cyclosporine A: relationship to drug pharmacokinetics. *Transplant Proc* 1982;14:659–661.

225. Keown PA, Laupacis A, Carruthers G, et al. Interaction between phenytoin and cyclosporine following organ transplantation. *Transplantation* 1984;38:304–306.

226. Freeman DJ, Laupacis A, Keown PA, et al. Evaluation of cyclosporine-phenytoin interaction with observations on cyclosporine metabolites. *Br J Clin Pharmacol* 1984;18:887–893.

227. D'Souza MJ, Pollock SH, Solomon HM. Cyclosporine-phenytoin interaction. *Drug Metab Dispos* 1988;16:256–258.

228. Klintmalm G, Sawe J, Ringden O, et al. Cyclosporine plasma levels in renal transplant patients. *Transplantation* 1985;39:132–137.

229. Veremis SA, Maddux MS, Pollak R, et al. Subtherapeutic cyclosporine concentrations during nafcillin therapy. *Transplantation* 1987;43:913–914.

230. Qureshi GD, Reinders TP, Somori GJ, et al. Warfarin resistance with nafcillin therapy. *Ann Intern Med* 1984;100:527–529.

231. Langhoff E, Madsen S. Rapid metabolism of cyclosporin and prednisone in kidney transplant patients on tuberculostatic treatment (Letter). *Lancet* 1983;2:1303.

232. McAllister WA, Thompson PJ, A-Habet SM, et al. Rifampicin reduces effectiveness and bioavailability of prednisolone. *Br J Med* 1983;286:923–925.

233. Daniels NJ, Dover JS, Schacter RK. Interaction between cyclosporin and rifampicin (Letter). *Lancet* 1984;2:639.

234. Van Buren D, Wideman CA, Ried M, et al. The antagonistic effect of rifampin upon cyclosporine bioavailability. *Transplant Proc* 1984;16:1642–1645.

235. Modry DL, Stinson EB, Oyer PE, et al. Acute rejection and massive cyclosporine requirements in heart transplant recipients treated with rifampin. *Transplantation* 1985;39:313–314.

236. Offermann G, Keller F, Molzahn M. Low cyclosporine A blood levels and acute graft rejection in a renal transplant recipient during rifampin treatment. *Am J Nephrol* 1985;5:385–387.

237. Howard P, Bixler TJ, Gill B. Cyclosporine-rifampicin drug interaction. *Drug Intell Clin Pharm* 1985;19:763–764.

238. Cassidy MJD, Van Zyl-Smit R, Pascoe MD, et al. Effects of rifampicin on cyclosporine A blood levels in a renal transplant recipient. *Nephron* 1985;41:207–208.

239. Allen RD, Hunnisett AG, Morris PJ. Cyclosporine and rifampicin in renal transplantation (Letter). *Lancet* 1985;1:980.

240. Wallwork J, McGregor CGA, Wells FC, et al. Cyclosporin and intravenous sulphadimidine and trimethoprim therapy (Letter). *Lancet* 1983;1:366–367.

241. Thompson JF, Chalmers DHK, Hinnisett AGW, et al. Nephrotoxicity of trimethoprim and cotrimoxazole in renal allograft recipients treated with cyclosporine. *Transplantation* 1983;36:204–206.

242. Jones KK, Hakim M, Wallwork J, et al. Serious interaction between cyclosporin A and sulphadimidine. *Br Med J* 1986;292:728–729.

243. Dossetor JB, Kovithavongs T, Salkie M, et al. Cyclosporine-associated lymphoproliferation, despite controlled cyclosporine blood concentrations, in a renal allograft recipient. *Proc Eur Dialysis Transplant Assoc* 1985;21:1021–1026.

244. Kreft-Jais C, Billaud EM, Gaudry C, et al. Effect of josamycin on plasma cyclosporine levels (Letter). *Eur J Clin Pharmacol* 1987;32:327–328.

245. Dieperink H, Moller J. Ketoconazole and cyclosporin (Letter). *Lancet* 1982;2:1217.

246. Ferguson RM, Sutherland DER, Simmons RL, et al. Ketoconazole, cyclosporin metabolism, and renal transplantation. *Lancet* 1982;2:882–883.

247. Smith J, Hows J, Donnelly P, et al. Interaction of cyclosporin A and ketoconazole. *Exp Hematol* 1983;11:176–178.

248. Shepard JH, Canafax DM, Simmons RL, et al. Cyclosporine-ketoconazole: a potentially dangerous drug-drug interaction (Letter). *Clin Pharmacy* 1986;5:468.

249. Girardet RE, Melo JC, Fox MS, et al. Concomitant administration of cyclosporine and ketoconazole for three and a half years in one heart transplant recipient. *Transplantation* 1989;48:887–890.

250. Charles BG, Ravenscroft PJ, Rigby RJ. The ketoconazole-cyclosporine interaction in an elderly renal transplant patient. *Aust N Z J Med* 1989;19:292–293.

251. Pochet JM, Pirson Y. Cyclosporine-diltiazem interaction (Letter). *Lancet* 1986;1:979.

252. Grino JM, Sebate I, Castelao AM, et al. Influence of diltiazem on cyclosporine clearance (Letter). *Lancet* 1986;1:1387.

253. Wagner K, Albrecht S, Newumayer H-H. Prevention of post-transplant acute tubular necrosis by the calcium antagonist diltiazem: a prospective randomized study. *Am J Nephrol* 1987;7:287–291.

254. Walz G, Kunzendorf U, Keller F, et al. Cyclosporine blood levels in diltiazem-treated kidney graft recipients. *Clin Tranplant* 1988;2:21–25.

255. Wagner K, Henkel M, Heinemeyer G, et al. Interaction of calcium channel blockers and cyclosporine. *Transplant Proc* 1988;20(suppl 2):561–568.

256. Wagner K, Heinemeyer G, Brockmuller F, et al. Interaction of cyclosporine and calcium antagonists. *Transplant Proc* 1989;21:1453–1456.

257. Bourbigot B, Guiserrix J, Airiau JM, et al. Nicardipine increases cyclosporin blood levels (Letter). *Lancet* 1986;1:1447.

258. Cantarovich M, Hiesse C, Lockiec F, et al. Confirmation of the interaction between cyclosporine and the calcium channel blocker nicardipine in renal transplant patients. *Clin Nephrol* 1987;28:190–193.

259. Kessler M, Netter P, Renoult E, et al. Influence of nicardipine on renal function and plasma cyclosporin in renal transplant patients. *Eur J Clin Pharmacol* 1989;36:637–638.

260. Lindholm AL, Henricsson S. Verapamil inhibits cyclosporin metabolism. *Lancet* 1987;1:1262-1263.

261. Angermann CE, Spes CH, Anthuber M, et al. Verapamil increases cyclosporine-A blood trough levels in cardiac transplant recipients [Abstract]. *J Am Coll Cardiol* 1988;11:206A.

262. Maggio TG, Bartels DW. Increased cyclosporine blood concentrations due to verapamil administration. *Drug Intell Clin Pharm* 1988;22:705–707.

263. Sabate I, Grino J, Castelao AM, et al. Evaluation of cyclosporine-verapamil interaction with observations on parent cyclosporine and metabolites. *Clin Chem* 1988;34:2151.

264. McNally P, Mistry N, Idle J, et al. Calcium channel blockers and cyclosporine metabolism. *Transplantation* 1989;48:1071.

265. Ptachcinski RJ, Carpenter BJ, Burchart GJ, et al. Effect of erythromycin on cyclosporine levels (Letter). *N Engl J Med* 1985;313:1416–1417.

266. Freeman DJ, Martell R, Carruthers SG, et al. Cyclosporin-erythromycin interaction in normal subjects. *Br J Clin Pharmacol* 1987;23:776–778.

267. Vereerstraeten P, Thiry P, Kinnaert P, et al. Influence of erythromycin on cyclosporine pharmacokinetics. *Transplantation* 1987;44:115–156.

268. Aoki FY, Yatscoff R, Jeffery J, et al. Effects of erythromycin on cyclosporine A kinetics in renal transplant patients [Abstract]. *Clin Pharmacol Ther* 1987;41:221.

269. Hourmant M, Lebigot JF, Vernillet L, et al. Coadministration of erythromycin results in an increase of blood cyclosporine to toxic levels. *Transplant Proc* 1985;17:2723–2727.

270. Murray BM, Edwards L, Morse GD, et al. Clinically important interaction of cyclosporine and erythromycin. *Transplantation* 1987;37:602–604.

271. Martell R, Heinrichs D, Stiller CR, et al. The effects of erythromycin in patients treated with cyclosporine. *Ann Intern Med* 1986;104:660–601.

272. Couet W, Istin B, Seniuta P, et al. Effect of ponsinomycin on cyclosporin pharmacokinetics. *Eur J Clin Pharmacol* 1990;39:165–167.

273. Ross WB, Roberts D, Griffin PJA, et al. Cyclosporine interaction with danazol and norethisterone (Letter). *Lancet* 1986;1:330.

274. Moller BB, Ekelund B. Toxicity of cyclosporine during treatment with androgens (Letter). *N Engl J Med* 1985;312:416.

275. Deray G, LeHoang P, Cacoub P, et al. Oral contraceptive interaction with cyclosporin. *Lancet* 1987;1:158–159.

276. Ged C, Rouillon JM, Pichard L, et al. The increase in urinary excretion of 6B-hydroxycortisol as a marker of human hepatic cytochrome P-450IIIA3 induction. *Br J Clin Pharmacol* 1989;28:373–387.

277. Pichard L, Gillet G, Fabre I, et al. Identification of the rabbit and human cytochromes P-450IIIA as the major enzymes involved in the N-demethylation of diltiazem. *Drug Metab Dispos* 1990;18:711–719.

278. Neumayer H-H, Wagner K. Diltiazem and economic use of cyclosporine (Letter). *Lancet* 1986;2:523.

279. Guengerich FP. Oxidation of 12a-ethynylestradiol by human liver cytochrome P-450. *Mol Pharmacol* 1988;33:500–508.

280. Wu YM, Venkataramanan R, Suzuki M, et al. Interaction between FK506 and cyclosporine in dogs. *Transplant Proc* 1991;23:2797–2799.

281. Bargetzi MJ, Aoyama T, Gonzalez FJ, et al. Lidocaine metabolism in human liver microsomes by cytochrome P450IIIA4. *Clin Pharmacol Ther* 1989;46:521–527.

282. Fabre G, Rahmani R, Placidi M, et al. Characterization of midazolam metabolism using human microsomal fractions and hepatocytes in suspension obtained by perfusing whole human livers. *Biochem Pharmacol* 1988;37:4389–4397.

283. Guengerich FP, Martin MV, Beaune PH, et al. Characterization of rat and human liver microsomal cytochrome P-450 forms involved in nifedipine oxidation, a prototype for genetic polymorphism in oxidative drug metabolism. *J Biol Chem* 1986;261:55051–55060.

284. Kiberd BA. Cyclosporine-induced renal dysfunction in human renal allograft recipients. *Transplantation* 1989;48:965–969.

285. Propper DJ, Whiting PH, Power DA, et al. The effect of nifedipine on graft function in renal allograft recipients treated with cyclosporine A. *Clin Nephrol* 1989;32:62–67.

286. Waxman DJ, Attisano C, Guengerich FP, et al. Human liver microsomal steroid metabolism: identification of the major microsomal steroid hormone 6B-hydroxylase cytochrome P-450 enzyme. *Arch Biochem Biophys* 1988;263:424–436.

287. Snyder DS. Interaction between cyclosporine and warfarin (Letter). *Ann Intern Med* 1988;108:311.

288. Watkins PB, Wrighton SA, Maurel P, et al. Identification of an inducible form of cytochrome P-450 in human liver. *Proc Natl Acad Sci U S A* 1985;82:6310–6314.

289. Nelson MV, Berchou RC, Kareti D, et al. Pharmacokinetic evaluation of erythromycin and caffeine administered with bromocriptine. *Clin Pharmacol Ther* 1990;47:694–697.

290. Couet W, Mathieu HP, Fourtillan JB. Effect of ponsinomycin on the pharmacokinetics of dihydroergotamine administered orally. *Fundam Clin Pharmacol* 1991;5:47–52.

291. Francis H, Tyndall A, Webb J. Severe vascular spasm due to erythromycin-ergotamine interaction. *Clin Rheumatol* 1984;3:243–246.

292. Kwan JTC, Foxall PJ, Davidson DGC, et al. Interaction of cyclosporin and itraconazole (Letter). *Lancet* 1987;2:282.

293. Trenk D, Brett W, Jahnchem E, et al. Time course of cyclosporin/itraconazole interaction. *Lancet* 1987;2:1335–1336.

294. Klintmalm G, Sawe J. High-dose methylprednisolone increases plasma cyclosporine levels in renal transplant patients (Letter). *Lancet* 1984; 1:731.

295. Ptachcinski RJ, Venkataramanan R, Burchart GJ, et al. Cyclosporine-high dose steroid interaction in renal transplant recipients: assessment by HPLC. *Transplant Proc* 1987;19:1728–1729.

296. Ost L. Impairment of prednisolone metabolism by cyclosporine treatment in renal graft recipients. *Transplantation* 1987;44:533–535.

297. Monahan BP, Ferguson CL, Killeavy ES, et al. Torsades de pointes occurring in association with terfenadine use. *JAMA* 1990;264:2788–2790.

298. Honig PK, Woosley RL, Zamani K, et al. Changes in the pharmacokinetics and electrocardiographic pharmacodynamics of terfenadine with concomitant administration of erythromycin. *Clin Pharmacol Ther* 1992;52:231–238.

Transplantation of the Liver, edited by Willis C. Maddrey, Eugene R. Schiff, and Michael F. Sorrell. Lippincott Williams & Wilkins, Philadelphia © 2001.

CHAPTER 13

Immunosuppressive Drugs

James Neuberger

In the early years of liver transplantation, immunosuppression was based on corticosteroids and azathioprine. The development and introduction into clinical practice of other classes of immunosuppressive agents has given the transplant clinician a powerful armamentarium of drugs for manipulating the immune system to control rejection and potentially to allow the development of tolerance. Inevitably, the increased availability of potent drugs with a wide spectrum of activity has brought challenges as well as benefits.

The aim of immunosuppression is to abrogate the host responses to the graft and permit graft acceptance with an absence of adverse effects. As our understanding of the processes of rejection become more clearly defined, it should become easier to develop strategies to achieve this aim. Nonetheless, there still remain significant problems to be overcome. Most centers currently adopt a combination of corticosteroids, azathioprine, and calcineurin inhibitors (either cyclosporine or tacrolimus). The introduction of newer agents, such as mycophenolate and sirolimus, has widened the choice of drugs available; however, it has proved difficult to develop a universally accepted baseline immunosuppressive regimen.

There are many problems with performing clinical studies comparing different immunosuppressive regimens. Most centers are currently achieving 5-year patient survival rates approaching or exceeding 80%; thus, the number of patients necessary to demonstrate a significant improvement in patient or graft survival is large, and funding for such trials may be difficult. Recruiting large numbers of patients requires multicenter studies, which bring additional methodologic and logistic difficulties. A second problem is selection of appropriate and clinically relevant end points. Most of the early studies used acute rejection as an end point. It is now clear that early acute rejection of the liver allograft has probably no long-term effects on graft survival or function.

More relevant end points are 5-year graft survival and the side effects of immunosuppression.

This need for long-term studies to assess immunosuppressive regimens brings a third problem: the introduction of new drugs and new formulations into clinical practice may mean that previous clinical trials are no longer clinically relevant. This is well illustrated by the clinical trials comparing cyclosporine-based and tacrolimus-based immunosuppression. Two large, well-conducted studies in Europe and North America compared tacrolimus with the galenic formulation of cyclosporine, Sandimmune. The introduction of the microemulsion preparation of cyclosporine, Neoral, which has a very different pharmacokinetic profile, means that the conclusions from these older trials may not be relevant to current practice. Because current trials are underway, the use of existing drugs may change; for example, it is now becoming common practice to reduce or withdraw corticosteroids in the first few months after transplantation. Where there is the potential for drug interaction, either pharmacologically or immunologically, extrapolation of clinical studies using older strategies may no longer be relevant.

The conclusion from these concerns is that it remains very difficult, if not impossible, to rely simply on an evidence-based approach to develop an immunosuppressive regimen.

DEVELOPING AN IMMUNOSUPPRESSIVE REGIMEN

Development of a logical immunosuppressive regimen is dependent on the understanding of the mechanism of rejection (discussed in Chapter 14); most currently used drugs have a relatively broad spectrum of action on the rejection response. Since rejection may be considered to be one aspect of inflammation, it is not surprising that these drugs will also predispose the patient to infection. If the processes of rejection can be disentangled from other aspects of inflammation, a more specific approach can be developed. As

J. Neuberger: Liver Unit, Queen Elizabeth Hospital, Birmingham B15 2TH, United Kingdom.

the processes of allograft rejection become clearer, it is evident that the development of acute rejection may not invariably be an adverse event and may actually promote tolerance. Thus there is a need to reevaluate the risks and benefits of powerful induction regimens.

Tailoring the Immunosuppressive Regimen

The immunosuppressive regimen needs to be modified according to various factors; for example, corticosteroids should be avoided in a patient with preexisting osteopenia. Some of the risk factors for acute and chronic allograft rejection are becoming identified; these include indication for transplantation, age of patient, renal function, and patient ethnicity. There are few data that show how immunosuppression should be tailored to these risk factors.

The indication for transplantation is an important consideration in selecting the immunosuppressant. For example, immunosuppression, especially with corticosteroids, is associated with increased hepatitis B viral replication; this may be because the hepatitis B virus genome has a glucocorticoid-responsive element. Thus, long-term use of prednisolone may be contraindicated in these patients. On the other hand, recurrence of autoimmune hepatitis may become apparent when corticosteroids are withdrawn. Other studies have suggested that in patients with primary biliary cirrhosis, recurrence of disease in the graft may occur earlier and more severely in those taking tacrolimus than in those taking cyclosporine.

Economic factors, too, will have an increasing influence in the choice of immunosuppressants. Balancing cost with efficacy is difficult, but such considerations are likely to play an increasing role in the next few years. During the next decade, it is possible that units will move away from a single approach to immunosuppression and adopt a variety of approaches tailored to the individual.

Tolerance

Tolerance remains the goal of the transplant clinician. There is evidence of tolerance from humans who have, for a variety of reasons, discontinued immunosuppression and have not developed graft damage. This observation has led some centers to withdraw immunosuppression from stable allograft recipients.[1] Freedom from immunosuppression can be achieved, but only in a small proportion of patients, and it is associated with risks of precipitating rejection and disease recurrence. Because late acute rejection is associated with an increased risk of chronic rejection and subsequent graft loss, this course of action is not without risk.

It is not yet possible to identify in advance those who will be tolerant of the graft. Strategies to develop tolerance in laboratory animals have been relatively successful, but extrapolation to humans has not yet been achieved. Strategies in animals include total body irradiation, costimulation blockade, development of chimerism, and lymphocyte depletion

using a variety of monoclonal and polyclonal antibodies, including Campath and diphtheria toxin–associated anti-CD3. Recently, Calne et al. have used Campath (a humanized antibody reacting with CD52) in renal allograft recipients and shown that the grafts can function well with minimal immunosuppression.[2] Whether this type of tolerance, termed *prope tolerance* (almost tolerance), is applicable to human liver allograft recipients is still to be determined.

General Complications of Immunosuppression

In addition to the side effects of the specific drugs used for immunosuppression, immunosuppression per se is associated with side effects and complications.

Malignancy

The association between immunosuppression and malignancy is well established. Penn[3] has established a registry of posttransplantation cancers. In a recent analysis comparing the reported incidence of cancers in liver and kidney allograft recipients, it was shown that whereas lymphomas account for over half the reported cases of *de novo* cancers in liver transplant recipients (57%), they accounted for only 12% of cancers in kidney recipients. Other cancers include cancers of the skin, uterus, cervix, and vulva. Most of the lymphomas occur within a mean of 14 months after transplantation, and other tumors occur at a mean of 27 months; these mean times are shorter than in renal allograft recipients but may reflect, in part, the longer period of follow-up for renal allograft recipients. Although some have suggested that, apart from skin cancers, liver allograft recipients are not at increased risk of nonlymphoid cancers compared with the general population,[4] this conclusion has not been confirmed by others.[5,6] The Pittsburgh group found significant increases in skin, oropharyngeal, and respiratory cancers but a lower incidence of breast and genitourinary malignancies in liver allograft recipients compared with an age- and sex-matched population.[5]

Infection

As indicated earlier, most immunosuppressive therapies are broad based and will therefore predispose the patient to an increased risk of infection—viral, bacterial, protozoal, and fungal. Maintaining a balance between the risks of underimmunosuppression (graft rejection) and overimmunosuppression (infection and malignancy) is difficult. It is usually safer to err on the side of underimmunosuppression because a rejected liver can be replaced whereas infection or malignancy may be fatal.

Neurologic Complications

In addition to the increased risk of infections affecting the central nervous system, immunosuppressed patients are at risk of leukoencephalopathy.[7] This form of multifocal necrotizing leukoencephalopathy is seen in patients with acquired immune deficiency syndrome (AIDS) and those who have received chemotherapy. There may be an infectious etiology, the condition is progressive. This type of neurologic complication must be distinguished from the complications caused by the calcineurin inhibitors.

Immunosuppression in Pregnancy and Breast Feeding

The management of women who wish to become pregnant following liver transplantation is difficult, and the potential for adverse effects of the immunosuppressive drugs on the fetus needs to be discussed with the mother. In general, experience is relatively limited. Our own practice is to avoid mycophenolate in women who wish to become pregnant, instead maintaining the woman on cyclosporine or tacrolimus, together with azathioprine or corticosteroids, or both, if indicated. There is little evidence to suggest that azathioprine is teratogenic. It should be noted that the manufacturers currently advise that tacrolimus is not indicated in women who wish to become pregnant.

Cyclosporine and tacrolimus are secreted into breast milk, so the mother should be advised to avoid breast feeding. At present there is little information about the use of mycophenolate, but the manufacturers advise against breast feeding. With respect to corticosteroids, if the mother is taking more than 10 mg per day of prednisolone (or equivalent), the possibility exists that the infant's adrenal function will be affected.

SPECIFIC DRUGS

Details of some of the drugs currently licensed for immunosuppression are provided in this section; please note that the list is not comprehensive and that not all drug interactions have been included. The recommended dose may vary. The product information leaflet should always be consulted.

Corticosteroids

Corticosteroids have been the mainstay of immunosuppression for many years both for the prevention of rejection and the treatment of acute rejection episodes. Recognition of the side effects of long-term therapy has led many centers to reevaluate their practices, and many centers are withdrawing corticosteroids during the first posttransplantation year.

Mode of Action

Corticosteroids act primarily on T-cell activation by inhibiting production of the T-cell cytokines that are required to augment the macrophage and lymphocyte response. Corticosteroids stimulate migration of circulating T cells from the intravascular compartment to lymphoid tissue.

Use in Liver Transplantation

Corticosteroids have, with azathioprine, long been the mainstay both of maintenance therapy and of treatment of acute rejection. Because of the long-term side effects of corticosteroids, many centers are starting to withdraw them during the first posttransplantation year, a process that can be done safely for the majority of patients. Some centers are evaluating immunosuppression without any use of corticosteroids; preliminary results are encouraging.

Dosage

Different corticosteroids have different activities; a comparison of doses is shown in Table 13.1. For treatment of acute rejection, the type, dose, and duration of corticosteroids used varies greatly between transplant units. There are no major studies evaluating the optimal treatment regimen. Our own unit uses 200 mg prednisolone daily for 3 days. The maintenance dose varies from 5 to 20 mg per day of prednisolone.

Side Effects

The many side effects associated with corticosteroids are listed in Table 13.2. Osteoporosis is a major potential problem; patients maintained on doses greater than 10 mg/kg per day (or equivalent) should be regularly screened for this complication and, where appropriate, offered treatment with either hormone replacement therapy or bisphosphonates such as etidronate or alendronate.

Drug Interactions

In general, drug interactions with corticosteroids are of limited clinical importance. Antacids will reduce the absorption of deflazacort. There is an interaction with cyclosporine: plasma concentrations of cyclosporine are increased by high-dose methylprednisolone, and cyclosporine increases the plasma concentration of prednisolone.

TABLE 13.1. *Equivalence of glucocorticoids*

Glucocorticoid	Dose (mg)
Cortisone acetate	25.0
Hydrocortisone	20.0
Deflazacort	6.0
Prednisolone	5.0
Prednisone	5.0
Methylprednisolone	4.0
Triamcinolone	4.0
Dexamethasone	0.75

TABLE 13.2. *Side effects of corticosteroids*

Cardiovascular	Sodium and fluid retention, hypertension
Endocrine	Carbohydrate intolerance, Cushingoid facies, growth retardation, secondary adrenocortical and pituitary hyporesponsiveness, menstrual irregularities
Ophthalmic	Posterior subcapsular cataracts, increased intraocular pressure, glaucoma, exophthalmos
Musculoskeletal	Osteoporosis, vertebral and femoral fractures, aseptic necrosis of femoral head, myopathy, muscle weakness
Neurologic	Altered mood, headaches, pseudotumor
Skin	Increased bruising, fragile skin, impaired wound healing
Gastrointestinal	Pancreatitis, peptic ulceration

Antimetabolites

Azathioprine

In humans, azathioprine is metabolized in the liver to 6-mercaptopurine (6-MP) and other metabolites. Intracellularly, 6-MP is converted into a variety of purine thioanalogues. 6-MP is eliminated primarily as the inactive, oxidized metabolite, thiouric acid. Oxidation of 6-MP is mediated by xanthine oxidase; variations in the phenotype of this enzyme explain, in part, the variability of side effects in patients. Those with the inherited deficiency of the enzyme thiopurine methyltransferase are particularly sensitive to the myelotoxic effects of azathioprine.

Mode of Action

Azathioprine acts by inhibition of DNA and RNA synthesis and thereby inhibits differentiation and proliferation of B and T lymphocytes. It also inhibits proliferation of promyelocytes, thus reducing the number of mononuclear cells in the peripheral blood.

Use in Liver Transplantation

Azathioprine has been used in liver transplantation for over three decades. Although there are no formal studies assessing its effects, two studies have shown that lack of azathioprine at 3 months is associated with a significant increase in chronic rejection.[8,9]

Dosage

The maintenance dose of azathioprine in liver allograft recipients lies between 1 and 2 mg/kg per day.

Side Effects

The most common side effect seen with azathioprine is bone marrow depression; patients should thus have their white cell count checked at least monthly after institution of azathioprine. The dose of azathioprine should be reduced when the total white cell count falls below 4×10^9/L and should be discontinued if the leukopenia persists. Nausea and vomiting may also be associated with azathioprine. Hepatotoxicity is seen in a small number of cases and is usually manifest by vascular disease (peliosis hepatis, regenerative nodular hyperplasia, venoocclusive disease, and hepatitis).[10] Other side effects are listed in Table 13.3.

Drug Interactions

Allopurinol should be avoided because of the increased risk of severe pancytopenia. Angiotensin-converting enzyme (ACE) inhibitors should be used with caution.

Mycophenolate Mofetil

Mycophenolate mofetil is a morpholinoethyl ester of mycophenolate developed by Allison and colleagues.[11] The ester is well absorbed and hydrolyzed to the active form, mycophenolic acid (MPA).

Mode of Action

The mode of action of MPA exploits the fact that both T and B lymphocytes require *de novo* synthesis of purines in order to proliferate, unlike other cell types, which have a salvage pathway. MPA is a potent, selective, reversible, and noncompetitive inhibitor of inosine monophosphate dehydrogenase. Inhibition of this enzyme blocks the *de novo* synthesis of guanosine nucleotide without incorporation of DNA. Thus, MPA has a powerful cytostatic effect on lymphocytes, inhibiting both mitogen- and alloantigen-induced stimulation. MPA inhibits antibody production by B cells and, by inhibiting glycosylation of monocyte and lymphocyte glycoproteins involved in adhesion to endothelial cells, may also inhibit mononuclear cell recruitment to the liver.

TABLE 13.3. *Side effects of azathioprine*

Bone marrow suppression
Megaloblastic changes
Acute pancreatitis
Alopecia
Liver damage
Peliosis hepatis
Nodular regenerative hyperplasia
Venoocclusive disease
Cholestatic hepatitis
Pneumonitis
Hypersensitivity reactions

The effects of MPA can be reversed by guanosine and deoxyguanosine.

Use in Liver Transplantation

Mycophenolate mofetil has been used in several studies for the treatment of acute rejection and for prevention of rejection.[12,13] Increasingly, centers are using mycophenolate in the routine immunosuppressive management of patients in place of azathioprine, with good effect.[14]

Dosage

The usual dosage is 2 to 3 g per day in two divided doses. The dosage should be reduced in cases of renal failure.

Side Effects

Neutropenia may affect up to 3% of patients receiving mycophenolate; if the white cell count does not rise on reducing the dosage, the drug should be discontinued. Gastrointestinal hemorrhage has been reported in up to 3% of patients. Diarrhea may affect up to 30% but usually responds to dose reduction. Other side effects attributed to mycophenolate include vomiting, tremor, renal damage, and hyperlipidemia. Because of the teratogenic potential, mycophenolate should be avoided in women who wish to or are likely to conceive. Use of the drug is not indicated in women who are breast feeding.

Drug Interactions

Concomitant use of acyclovir and of ganciclovir is associated with increased levels of both drugs. Absorption is decreased when mycophenolate is taken with antacids containing magnesium and aluminium hydroxide and with cholestyramine. Mycophenolate mofetil should not be given with other antimetabolites, such as azathioprine.

Calcineurin Inhibitors

The two calcineurin inhibitors currently in use in liver transplant recipients are cyclosporine and tacrolimus. The modes of action of the two agents are similar but not identical. Both drugs bind to intracellular proteins: cyclosporine binds to cyclophilin, and tacrolimus to the FK binding protein 12 (FKBP-12). It was initially believed that the mode of action of both cyclosporine and tacrolimus was a consequence of their interaction with these immunophilins, and that the immunosuppressive effects were mediated via the peptidyl prolyl cis-trans isomerase activity. It is now believed that the immunosuppressive effects are mediated by the complexing of the drug with immunophilin. The drug-protein complex binds to calcineurin with calmodulin and calcium, inhibiting the phosphatase activity of calcineurin. This results in inhibition of the dephosphorylation and translocation of the cytoplasmic unit of NF-AT (nuclear factor of activated T cells), which inhibits gene transcription for the formation of lymphokines such as interleukin 2 (IL-2).

Cyclosporine

Cyclosporine was introduced into clinical practice in the early 1980s and rapidly achieved widespread use. It is a neutral lipophilic cyclic endecapeptide extracted from the fungus *Tolypocladium inflatum Gams*.

Mode of Action

Cyclosporine acts by inhibiting T-cell activation. IL-2 synthesis and release is inhibited; this effect can be overcome by addition of external IL-2. Transcription of IL-2, IL-3, and interferon-γ is inhibited, the effect being greater on CD4+ cells than on CD8+ cells. Inhibition of IL-2 release results in inhibition of T-cell proliferation and lack of activation of macrophages and B cells.

Pharmacokinetics

Orally administered cyclosporine is incompletely absorbed; the extent of absorption is dependent on the formulation of cyclosporine and on the characteristics of individual patients. The metabolites have only limited immunologic activity. Most of the drug is excreted in bile, with about 5% being renally excreted. At present, three formulations of cyclosporine are available: a galenic preparation (Sandimmune), a microemulsion (Neoral), and a modified oral solution (SangCya). Rates of absorption vary between the three preparations, being greatest for the modified oral solution and lowest for the galenic preparation. Variations of absorption and the relationship between the area under the curve (AUC) and blood levels also differ between the three preparations. Thus, the preparations are not interchangeable without close monitoring of blood levels. High-fat meals will reduce absorption of cyclosporine.

Use in Liver Transplantation

Following initial positive results in studies with liver transplant recipients, cyclosporine became introduced into clinical practice and is now widely used. Because of the better absorption profile and reduced levels of rejection, Neoral has largely replaced Sandimmune.[15]

Dosage

Most centers will adjust the dosage of cyclosporine to achieve the target blood levels required. Immediately after transplantation, an average oral dose is between 8 to 10 mg/kg per day. There is no general agreement as to the optimum target range, and very little data on which to form a judgment.

Interpretation of blood levels of cyclosporine is dependent on the matrix used (blood, serum, or plasma) and the methods of assay used. Although measurement by high-performance liquid chromatography (HPLC) is the most reliable method, this is rarely practical for daily use. Other methods include monoclonal antibody radioimmunoassay (RIA), fluorescence polarization immunoassay (FPIA), and enzyme-multiplied immunoassay technique (EMIT). Most centers rely on the whole-blood trough levels measured by RIA; there is some indication that the 2-hour postdose level may correlate more closely with the AUC, but there are logistic difficulties in ensuring that blood is taken at the appropriate time after dosing.

Although it has been suggested that the target levels early after liver transplantation should be higher than when the patient is well, there is little evidence to support this approach. Target levels after 3 months will usually lie between 100 and 150 ng/mL. Levels must be interpreted in the light of graft function and evidence of side effects, especially renal function.

Side Effects

Cyclosporine is associated with many side effects (Table 13.4); of those that are specific to calcineurin inhibitors (rather than immunosuppressive drugs in general), renal failure has the greatest impact on a patient's quality of life. Other common side effects include hirsutism, gum hypertrophy, hypertension, and tremor. If the levels of cyclosporine are in the target therapeutic range and hypertension occurs, then either hypotensive therapy should be instituted (calcium channel antagonists such as nifedepine are the agents of choice) or cyclosporine discontinued. The calcium channel antagonists may affect the levels of cyclosporine and may increase the risk of developing gum hypertrophy. Gum hypertrophy may respond to increased dental hygiene; failing this, consideration should be given to dose reduction.

Renal failure is one of the greatest concerns in patients receiving long-term cyclosporine. McCauley found that only 23% of liver allograft recipients had normal renal function 39 months after liver transplantation.[16] Fisher, in a retrospective analysis, found that after 5 years posttransplantation, nearly 80% of patients had impaired renal function, as evidenced by a serum creatinine level greater than 125 μmol/L; of patients surviving at least 1 year, 4% had developed severe renal insufficiency (serum creatinine level greater than 250 μmol/L) and 2% had developed end-stage renal failure at a median of 5 years after transplantation.[17] The survival of patients with end-stage renal failure was reduced, with a median survival of 1.2 years. Dose reduction did little to improve poor renal function but may slow down rate progression of failure. The major factors identifying those at risk of developing renal failure include a high serum creatinine level at 3 months and a higher cumulative dose of cyclosporine. Brown, in a review of the NIDDK (National Institute of Diabetes and Digestive and Kidney Diseases) database, found that those with hepatorenal failure at the time of transplantation were more likely to require hemodialysis and develop severe renal insufficiency posttransplantation.[18]

It is probably not possible to define a regimen for cyclosporine administration that provides for adequate immunosuppression without the risk of nephrotoxicity.[19] General measures, such as aggressive treatment of hypertension, avoidance of those drugs that enhance the nephrotoxicity of cyclosporine, and maintenance of lowest effective doses of the drug, are the best option. Other strategies have been suggested:[20] Calcium channel antagonists may modify the metabolism of cyclosporine, allowing adequate immunosuppression but reducing the possibility of renal impairment by stimulating renal vasodilatation; dihydropyridine calcium channel blockers may slow the rate of interstitial fibrosis. Some centers are assessing the use of lower doses of cyclosporine in combination with other immunosuppressive agents.

Drug Interactions

Because cyclosporine is metabolized through the cytochrome P-450 system (cytochrome 3A4), drugs that affect the activity of this family of enzymes will affect drug levels (Table 13.5). Other drugs may enhance the nephrotoxic potential of cyclosporine. Although there is no need to avoid concomitant prescription of drugs that alter cyclosporine metabolism, levels must be closely monitored both when starting and discontinuing such medication. Cyclosporine will affect the metabolism of other drugs, notably digoxin, corticosteroids, lovastatin, and methotrexate. The combination of cyclosporine and statins may increase the risk of myopathy. Patients treated with ACE inhibitors must be monitored for hyerkalemia. Grapefruit juice increases the plasma concentration of cyclosporine.

Although there are no definitive studies in pregnancy, there are few reports of adverse effects in pregnancy. As with any prescription for a pregnant woman, the risks and benefits must be considered and discussed with the patient. Cyclosporine is secreted into breast milk.

TABLE 13.4. *Side effects of cyclosporine and tacrolimus*

Cardiovascular	Hypertension
Renal	Renal impairment and renal failure, hyperkalemia, hypomagnesemia
Nervous system	Headaches, cramps, tremor, paresthesia, confusion
Skin	Hirsutism, acne
Gastrointestinal	Gum hypertrophy, diarrhea, nausea and vomiting
Hepatic	Cholestasis
Hematologic	Hemolytic uremic syndrome
Breasts	Fibroadenosis
Metabolic	Diabetes mellitus, hyperlipidemia
Other	Bone pain

TABLE 13.5. *Drugs that interact with cyclosporine and tacrolimus*

Increase levels
Antifungals: fluconazole, ketoconazole, itraconazole
Antibiotics: erythromycin, clarithromycin
Glucocorticoids
Calcium channel blockers: diltiazem, nicardepine, verapamil
Others: danazol, metoclopramide, bromocriptine, cisapride, allopurinol, grapefruit juice
Decrease levels
Anticonvulsants: phenobarbitone, phenytoin, carbamazepine
Antibiotics: rifampin, nafcillin
Others: octreotide, ticlopidine, protease inhibitors
Increased nephrotoxicity
Antimicrobials: gentamicin, tobramycin, vancomycin, co-trimoxazole
Antifungals: ketoconazole, itraconazole, amphotericin B
Antiinflammatories: nonsteroidal antiinflammatory drugs

Cyclosporine and tacrolimus should not be taken together. This list is not exhaustive.

Tacrolimus

Tacrolimus (FK506) was introduced into clinical practice in the late 1980s and rapidly became, with cyclosporine, one of the mainstays of immunosuppressive regimens.

Mode of Action

The mode of action of tacrolimus is similar to that of cyclosporine (see previous discussion). The drug binds to FKBP and inhibits synthesis of IL-2.

Pharmacokinetics

Tacrolimus is absorbed from the gastrointestinal tract with a bioavailability of around 20%. There is variation between individuals. It is metabolized in the liver by the mixed function oxidase system, primarily cytochrome P-450 3A. Some of the metabolites do have immunologic activity. Clearance of tacrolimus is little affected by liver or renal insufficiency. Taking tacrolimus with food reduces absorption. Most drug is excreted in feces.

Use in Liver Transplantation

There have been many studies showing that tacrolimus is well tolerated in patients; it is now widely used in clinical practice.

Dosage

The recommended dosage of orally administered tacrolimus in patients undergoing liver transplantation is between 0.10 and 0.15 mg/kg per day given in two divided doses. The dosage needs to be adjusted in accordance with the blood levels, graft function, and evidence of side ef-

fects, such as renal impairment. The drug is measured using monoclonal antibodies either by enymze-linked immunosorbent assay (ELISA) or a microparticle enzyme immunoassay. The target trough whole-blood levels that should be achieved in liver allograft recipients have not been well defined, but most centers aim for levels between 10 and 15 ng/mL in the first few postoperative weeks and between 5 and 10 ng/mL when the patient is stable.

Side Effects

The side effects of tacrolimus are generally similar to those of cyclosporine, although hirsutism is not seen. There is no reason to believe that the nephrotoxicity of tacrolimus will be greatly different from that of cyclosporine.[19] There appears to be an increased risk of diabetes associated with the use of tacrolimus, but this may be transient. In liver allograft recipients, insulin-dependent diabetes mellitus occurs in 10% to 20% of patients receiving tacrolimus and is reversible in about half of these.

Myocardial hypertrophy has been reported in patients taking tacrolimus. This is detected by echocardiography showing concentric increases in the left ventricular posterior wall and the interventricular septum. The hypertrophy usually responds to dose reduction or treatment discontinuation.

Because of the teratogenic potential of tacrolimus, the drug is not indicated in women who are or may become pregnant, although there is little evidence that the adverse effects of tacrolimus are significantly different from those of cyclosporine.

Drug Interactions

The drug interactions with tacrolimus are similar to those noted with cyclosporine. There is a possible interaction with sex hormones, and the efficacy of oral contraceptives may be reduced (Table 13.5). The half-life of cyclosporine is prolonged by tacrolimus; in general, patients should not take the two drugs together.

Cyclosporine versus Tacrolimus

Several studies have compared cyclosporine-based immunosuppression with tacrolimus-based regimens.[21–23] Interpretation of these studies needs to be done with caution because some of these trials were initiated using a higher dose of tacrolimus than is currently used, thereby overestimating the side effects. Also, the preparation of cyclosporine tested was primarily the galenic form (Sandimmune), which has a less satisfactory efficacy than the microemulsion preparation (Neoral). In the multicenter studies, a fixed regimen of tacrolimus was compared with the current local practice, thereby adding another dimension of variability. Analysis by "intention to treat" may be misleading if a significant number of patients are switched from one therapy to the other. Finally, the choice of end points is problematic: Early acute rejection is not a good indicator of long-term graft or patient function and survival. Ductopenic rejection, which is associated with graft failure, is associated with many pretransplantation and posttransplantation variables (e.g., indication, donor and recipient cytomegalovirus serology matching); thus, randomization may not ensure that the two groups are similar.

Two major studies were done, in North America and in Europe. In the European study,[22,24] 545 patients were randomized in eight centers. Both the acute and chronic rejection rates were statistically significantly lower in those receiving tacrolimus: 40.5% and 1.5% for the tacrolimus group (acute and chronic rejection, respectively) compared with 49.8% and 5.3% for the cyclosporine group. Patient and graft survival were not significantly different in the two groups (82.9% and 77.5%, respectively, for tacrolimus, compared with 77.5% and 72.6% for cyclosporine). These findings were confirmed on long-term follow-up.[24] Similar findings were reported by the U.S. study, which involved 478 adults and 51 children.[25,26] However, this study found that there were more serious adverse events, requiring discontinuation of the drug, in those receiving tacrolimus than those taking cyclosporine. A longer-term comparison[26] showed a longer patient half-life for tacrolimus-treated patients (25 years) than for cyclosporine-treated patients (15 years). Similar findings were reported in comparative trials assessing the two regimens in children[23] and in patients with fulminant hepatic failure.[27]

Thus, although these findings suggest that tacrolimus may be more effective than Sandimmune, there are few data as yet to compare tacrolimus with Neoral, which is superior to Sandimmune.[15,28] Costs may be less with tacrolimus.[29] However, the availability of these two calcineurin inhibitors gives the clinician a wider choice of immunosuppressive agents; the decision which to use should not be viewed as based on competing alternatives but as allowing the clinician to tailor treatment to the individual.[30]

Sirolimus

Sirolimus (rapamycin) is a macrocyclic lactone isolated from *Streptomyces hygroscopicus*. Although sirolimus affects IL-2 production, there is no interaction with calcineurin.

Mode of Action

Sirolimus inhibits both B- and T-cell activity. Sirolimus reduces T-cell activation by inhibiting the IL-2–mediated signal transduction pathway. The progression to late G_1 phase is blocked, consistent with the finding that lymphocyte proliferation is blocked even when sirolimus is added 12 hours after initiation of stimulation. Rapamycin also inhibits B-cell stimulation, decreasing antibody production. Rapamycin interacts with FK-binding proteins but not cyclophilin.

Use in Liver Transplantation

There is only limited experience of the use of sirolimus with liver transplantation,[31] but, in combination with cyclosporine, there is powerful immunosuppression.

Dosage

In renal transplantation, the daily dose used in trials is between 2 and 5 mg per day. The target whole-blood trough levels in renal transplantation lie around 30 ng/mL in the early months after transplantation, falling to 15 ng/mL thereafter.

Side Effects

The most commonly observed side effects are hyperlipidemia (affecting both serum cholesterol and triglycerides), leukopenia, thrombocytopenia, apthous ulceration, and joint pains. Liver abnormalities are rarely seen.[32] No adverse renal side effects have been reported. The elevation in serum lipids may fall over time, and any long-term implications of elevated levels remain to be established.

Other Drugs

Several other agents that are effective in the prevention and treatment of human liver allograft rejection have not been extensively used or have not been widely licensed.

Deoxyspergualin

15-Deoxyspergualin (15-DSG) is a synthetic dehydroxylated form of spergualin, a product of *Bacillius lactosporos*. The intracellular binding protein is thought to be a member of the heat-shock protein family. In the cell nucleus, DSG may reduce the activity of DNA polymerase to inhibit DNA synthesis. Both *in vivo* and *in vitro* studies have shown that DSG and spergualin have similar efficacy but that the 15-deoxy form is more potent. DSG is effective *in vitro* in suppressing primary and secondary responses to thymus-dependent and thymus-independent antigens. The drug is also associated with suppression of IL-2 production and with interference with interferon stimulation of CD4 cells. DSG has an effect on B cells, inhibiting differentiation into plasma cells. In human liver allograft recipients, DSG appears to be effective in reversing established acute rejection and preventng acute rejection.[33,34] Toxicity is related to bone marrow suppression, paresthesia, hypotension, and anorexia.

Brequinar

Brequinar, a substituted four-quinoline carboxylic acid, is a potent anticancer drug with immunosuppressive activity. The drug inhibits the activity of dihydroorotate dehydrogenase and pyramidine synthesis. Animal studies suggest that brequinar may help in inducing tolerance and in preventing acute allograft rejection.

Leflunomide

Leflunomide, an isoxazol, inhibits dehydroorotate dehydrogenase and tyrosine kinase. This results in inhibition of *de novo* pyrimidine synthesis, thus blocking T- and B-cell proliferation and suppressing IgG and IgM synthesis. In animal studies, leflunomide is effective in prolonging graft survival and is synergistic with cyclosporine.[35] Leflunomide is metabolized to a number of derivatives, malononitrilamides (MNA), which also have immunosuppressive effects. The most assessed derivative is known as A771726, which, because of its very long half-life, may be of value in autoimmunity rather than transplantation. In animal models, MNAs are potent, dose-dependent immunosuppressives, well tolerated and possibly more effective than cyclosporine.[36,37] Use in humans is limited.

Ursodeoxycholic Acid

Ursodeoxycholic acid is a tertiary, naturally occurring bile acid that is used extensively in the treatment of patients with primary biliary cirrhosis and other cholestatic syndromes. Despite early reports of a beneficial effect in prevention of allograft rejection and a possible benefit in cardiac transplantation, its use in liver transplantation has not been shown.[38] Improvement may be associated with altered absorption of cyclosporine.

Enisoprost

Initial studies suggesting a beneficial effect of enisoprost have not been confirmed.

ANTIBODIES AND ANTILYMPHOCYTE PREPARATIONS

As the processes of the immune responses have become identified and understood, it has become possible to develop strategies to interfere with the immune response in a more specific way. Antilymphocyte preparations may be polyclonal or monoclonal.

Polyclonal Antilymphocyte Preparations

Polyclonal antilymphocyte preparations are obtained by immunizing animals with human lymphocytes and isolating and purifying the serum. These preparations may be antilymphocyte serum (ALS), antilymphocyte globulin (ALG), or antithymocyte globulin (ATG). There are concerns that standardization between batches may be poor. These polyclonal preparations contain antibodies with a much wider spectrum of activity than the monoclonal preparations. For example, ATG includes antibodies reacting not only with CD3 but also CD25, CD4, CD8, CD45, CD44, and HLA classes I and II.

These globulins are administered by intravenous injection. The dose will depend on the preparation and whether the treatment is being given for the prevention or treatment of acute rejection. Most manufacturers recommend prior testing for sensitization, often by intradermal injection. The white cell count falls rapidly, and full recovery may take weeks to months. There remains great variation in the use of these preparations. Although they are very effective, the risks of infections and, later, of malignancy are high.

Antibodies to the T-Cell Receptor

CD3, the T-cell receptor, plays a crucial role in T-cell interactions and antigen recognition. Blockade of this receptor prevents signal transduction. Administration of antibodies to CD3 is effective in the treatment of established rejection and is used in some centers in the induction process. Administration of these antibodies may be associated with a cytokine release syndrome (the "shake and bake syndrome") that may range from a mild, self-limiting illness to a severe shock-like syndrome. Other associated side effects include pyrexia, chest pain, diarrhea, wheezing, tachycardia, and hypertension. This syndrome can be prevented by prior administration of corticosteroids and indomethacin. Other side effects include neuropsychiatric syndromes, seizures, and headache. There is an increase in the risk of developing infections, especially cytomegalovirus and Epstein-Barr virus infections.

OKT3 is a monoclonal preparation containing antibodies directed against CD3. The agent is effective in lowering the total lymphocyte count and in the prevention and treatment of acute liver allograft rejection. In addition to the side effects listed above, aseptic meningitis may affect up to 3% of recipients. Fatal pulmonary edema is very rare.

Antibodies to the Interleukin-2 Receptor

The interleukin-2 receptor is implicated in clonal expansion and continued viability of activated T cells. The high-affinity IL-2 receptor is composed of three noncovalently bound chains, CD25 (a 55 kD α chain), a 75 kD β chain, and a 64 kD γ chain. While the β and γ chains are constitutively expressed on lymphocytes, CD25 is an activation complex present only on activated cells. Interaction with the IL-2 receptor is an attractive strategy for modulating the immune response for several reasons: Antigen stimulation in the absence of IL-2 may lead to anergy, and specific blockade of CD25 may lead to inhibition of those T cells responding to alloantigen. Because CD25 is not involved in transmembrane signaling, antibodies to the α chain will not result in agonist effects.[39] At present, two monoclonal antibodies to the α chain are licensed for clinical use. These antibodies are indicated for the prevention of rejection.

Basiliximab (Simulect) is a murine-human chimeric antibody that is specifically targeted to CD25. Binding to CD25 is maintained while serum levels exceed 25 µg/mL. The antibody can be given by central or peripheral administration, infused slowly in either 5% dextrose or 0.9% saline. The recommended administration for adults is 20 mg within 2 hours of surgery and 4 days after surgery.

Daclizumab (Zenapak) is a humanized monoclonal antibody that also reacts with CD25. The recommended dosage for renal allograft recipients is 1 mg/kg per dose for 5 doses; the initial dose is given within 24 hours of transplantation, the other four doses at 14-day intervals. The antibody is well tolerated; few patients develop human anti-mouse antibodies (HAMA). Several studies in renal allograft recipients show a reduction in the number of rejection episodes without significant adverse effects. At the time of writing, there are few published data concerning liver allograft recipients. The antibody may be more effective when administered with calcineurin inhibitors.

Other Antibodies

Several other antibodies have been used for the prevention and treatment of liver allograft rejection; these include anti-ICAM-1 and anti-LFA-1. Campath 1 (an antibody to CD52) has been used in allograft recipients. This antibody, which spares stem cells, has been implicated in the development of tolerance and may be of value in liver allograft recipients.[40] An alternative approach is to use CTLA4-Ig, a fusion protein that blocks CD28-mediated costimulatory responses and inhibits immune responses *in vivo* and *in vitro*.[41] Blocking costimulation in animals using monoclonal antibodies is an effective strategy yet to be demonstrated in man. Another approach has been to deliver cytotoxic therapy using monoclonal antibodies. Thus, a diphtheria toxin–related fusion protein in which the receptor-binding domain is replaced with a synthetic gene encoding human IL-2 has been used to target proliferating T cells. This has proved to be a very effective strategy in animals but has not yet been assessed in humans.[42]

In general, the efficacy of these techniques has been disappointing, but there seems little doubt that use of such approaches will prove to be a valuable addition to therapy in the future.[43]

REFERENCES

1. Mazariegos GV, Reyes J, Marino IR, et al. Weaning of immunosuppression in liver transplant recipients. *Transplantation* 1997;63:243–249.
2. Calne RY, Moffatt P, Friend P, et al. Prope (almost) tolerance using Campath 1H induction and low-dose cyclosporin monotherapy in 31 cadaveric renal allograft recipients, a follow-up of 7 to 21 months [Abstract]. *Transplantation* 1999;67:S560.
3. Penn I. Posttransplantation *de novo* tumors in liver allograft recipients. *Liver Transplant Surg* 1996;2:52–59.
4. Kelly DM, Emre S, Guy SR, et al. Liver transplant recipients are not at increased risk for nonlymphoid solid organ tumors. *Cancer* 1998;83:1237–1243.
5. Jain AB, Yee LD, Nalesnik MA, et al. Comparative incidence of *de novo* non-lymphoid malignancies after liver transplantation under tacrolimus using surveillance epidemiologic end result data. *Transplantation* 1998;66:1193–1200.
6. Jonas S, Rayes N, Neumann U, et al. *De novo* malignancies after liver transplantation using tacrolimus-based protocols or cyclosporine-based quadruple immunosuppression with an interleukin-3 receptor antibody or antithymocyte antibody. *Cancer* 1997;80:1141–1150.
7. Anders KH, Becker PS, Holden JK, et al. Multifocal necrotizing leukoencephalopathy with pontine predeliction in immunosuppressed patients. *Hum Pathol* 1993;24:897–904.
8. Van Hoek B, Wiesner RH, Krom RAF, et al. Severe ductopenic rejection following liver transplantation. *Semin Liver Dis* 1992;12:41–50.
9. Candinas D, Gunson BK, Nightingale P, et al. Sex mismatch as a risk factor for chronic rejection of liver allografts. *Lancet* 1995;34:1117–1121.
10. Slapak GI, Saxena R, Portmann B, et al. Graft and systemic disease in long-term survivors of liver transplantation. *Hepatology* 1997;25:195–202.
11. Platz KP, Sollinger HW, Hullet DA, et al. RS-61433—a new potent immunosuppressive agent. *Transplantation* 1991;51:27–31.
12. Hebert MF, Ascher NL, Lake JR, et al. Four-year follow-up of mycophenolate mofetil for graft rescue in liver allograft recipients. *Transplantation* 1999;67:707–712.
13. Klintmalm GB, Ascher NL, Busuttil RW. RS-61443 for treatment-resistant human liver rejection. *Transplant Proc* 1993;25:697–700.
14. Fisher RA, Ham JM, Marcos A, et al. A prospective randomized trial of mycophenolate mofetil with Neoral or tacrolimus after orthotopic liver transplantation. *Transplantation* 1998;66:1616–1621.
15. Mirza DF, Gunson BK, Soonawalla Z, et al. Reduced acute rejection after liver transplantation with Neoral-based triple immunosuppression. *Lancet* 1997;349:701–702.
16. McCauley J, Van Thiel DH, Starzl TE, et al. Acute and chronic renal failure in liver transplantation. *Nephron* 1990;55:121–128.
17. Fisher NC, Nightingale PG, Gunson BK, et al. Chronic renal failure following liver transplantation. *Transplantation* 1998;66:59–66.
18. Brown RS, Lombardero M, Lake JR. Outcome of patients with renal insufficiency undergoing liver or combined liver-kidney transplantation. *Transplantation* 1996;62:1788–1793.
19. Cohen DJ. Renal failure as a complication of non-renal transplantation. *Graft* 1999;2:S125–S132.
20. Bennett WM, DeMattos A, Mayer MM, et al. Chronic cyclosporin nephropathy: the Achilles' heel of immunosuppressive therapy. *Kidney Int* 1996;50:1089–1100.
21. Neuhaus P, Blumhardt G, Bechstein WO, et al. Comparison of FK506- and cyclosporine-based immunosuppression in primary orthotopic liver transplantation. A single center experience. *Transplantation* 1995;59:31–40.
22. European FK506 Multicentre Liver Study Group. Randomised trial comparing tacrolimus (FK506) and cyclosporin in prevention of liver allograft rejection. *Lancet* 1994;344:423–428.
23. McDiarmid SV, Busuttil RW, Ascher AL, et al. FK506 (tacrolimus) compared with cyclosporine for primary immunosuppression after pediatric liver transplantation. *Transplantation* 1995;59:530–536.
24. Williams R, Neuhaus P, Bismuth H, et al. Two-year data from the European multicentre tacrolimus (FK506) liver study. *Transplant Int* 1996;9(suppl 1):S144–S150.
25. The US Multicenter FK506 Study Group. A comparison of tacrolimus (FK506) and cyclosporine for immunosuppression in liver transplantation. *N Engl J Med* 1994;331:1110–1115.
26. Wiesner RH. A long-term comparison of tacrolimus (FK506) versus cyclosporine in liver transplantation: a report of the United States FK506 study group. *Transplantation* 1998;66:493–499.
27. Devlin J, Willimas R. Transplantation for fulminant hepatic failure: comparing tacrolimus versus cyclosporine for immunosuppression and the outcome in elective transplants. *Transplantation* 1996;62:1251–1255.
28. Van Buren D, Payne J, Geevarghese S, et al. Impact of Sandimmune, Neoral and Prograf on rejection incidence and renal function in primary liver transplant recipients. *Transplant Proc* 1998;30:1830–1832.

29. McKenna M, Alexander GJM, Jones M, et al. Economic analysis of tacrolimus (FK506) and cyclosporin in prevention of liver allograft rejection. *Eur Hosp Pharmacy* 1996;2.

30. Mueller AR, Klatz KP, Blumhardt G, et al. The optimal immunosuppression after liver transplantation according to diagnosis: cyclosporin A or FK506? *Clin Transpl* 1995;9:176–184.

31. Watson CJ, Friend PJ, Jamieson NV, et al. Sirolimus: a potent new immunosuppressant for liver transplantation. *Transplantation* 1999;67: 505–509.

32. Groth CG, Backman L, Morales J-M, et al. Sirolimus (rapamycin)-based therapy in human liver transplantation. *Transplantation* 1999; 67:1036–1042.

33. Groth CG, Ohlman S, Ericzon BH, et al. Deoxyspergualin for liver graft rejection. *Lancet* 1990;336:626.

34. Katoh H, Phkohchi N, Orii T, et al. Effectiveness of 15-deoxyspergualin on steroid-resistant acute rejection in living related liver transplantation *Transplant Proc* 1997;29:553–554.

35. Ostraat O, Qi ZQ, Tufveson G, et al. The effects of leflunomide and cyclosporin A on rejection of cardiac allografts in the rat. *Scand J Immunol* 1998;47:236–242.

36. Schorlemmer HU, Ruuth E, Kurrie R. Malononitrilamides synergistically prevent acute and treat ongoing skin allograft rejection with cyclosporin. *Transpl Int* 1998;11(suppl 1):S340–S344.

37. Lindner JK, Zantl N. Synergism of the malononitrilamides 279 and 715 with cyclosporin A in the induction of long-term cardiac allograft survival. *Transpl Int* 1998;11(suppl 1):S303–S309.

38. Pageaux GP, Blanc P, Perrigault P, et al. Failure of ursodeoxycholic acid to prevent acute cellular rejection after liver transplantation. *J Hepatol* 1995;23:119–122.

39. Vincenti F. Targetting the interleukin-2 receptor in clinical renal transplantation. *Graft* 1999;2:56–61.

40. Calne RY, Friend P, Moffatt S, et al. Prope tolerance, perioperative Campath 1H and low-dose cyclosporin monotherapy in renal allograft recipients. *Lancet* 1998;351:1701–1702.

41. Pearson TC, Alexander DZ, Winn KJ, et al. Transplantation tolerance induced by CTLA4-Ig. *Transplantation* 1994;57:1701–1706.

42. Parker KE, Giral M, Soulilou J-P. Fusion proteins in immunointervention. *Transplant Proc* 1992;24:2362–2365.

43. Adams DH. Adhesion molecules and liver transplantation: new strategies for therapeutic intervention. *J Hepatol* 1995;23:225–231.

Transplantation of the Liver, edited by Willis C. Maddrey, Eugene R. Schiff, and Michael F. Sorrell. Lippincott Williams & Wilkins, Philadelphia © 2001.

CHAPTER 14

The Immunology of Hepatic Allograft Rejection

Leslie B. Lilly, Jinwen Ding, and Gary A. Levy

Liver transplantation has become a recognized and effective form of therapy for patients with end-stage liver disease.[1,2] Today, over 5,000 liver transplants are performed annually in the United States, with 1-year and 5-year patient survival rates approaching 90% and 75%, respectively.[3] Although the incidence of acute cellular rejection remains at 40% to 50%, hepatic allograft loss directly related to chronic rejection has decreased to 3% to 5%.[3,4] Recent studies have suggested that a single episode of rejection may in fact be beneficial to long-term graft survival.[5]

The transplantation of an organ from a member of one species into a member of the same species (allotransplantation) elicits an allogeneic (nonself) immune response directed at the foreign antigens expressed on the donor organ tissues.[6,7] This immune response can be part of the innate immune system or the adaptive immune system.[8] The former system reflects the evolutionary experience of our species with the environment. It consists of antibodies, complement, natural killer (NK) cells, macrophages, and neutrophils.[9–11] The adaptive immune response reflects a finely tuned specific response orchestrated by macrophage T- and B-cell interactions.[12] The main targets of the adaptive response are the major histocompatibility complex (MHC) antigens designated as human leukocyte antigens (HLA) in man.[13,14] In addition, immune responses are directed toward minor histocompatibility antigens, which are derived from other polymorphic molecules that differ between donor and recipient.[15]

Rejection has been divided into hyperacute, acute, and chronic types (Table 14.1).[16] Hyperacute responses occur within minutes to hours, are antibody and complement mediated, and are generally irreversible.[17] Acute rejection is cell mediated, occurs over a period of days to months, and can be reversed using a variety of currently available drugs.[18] Chronic rejection generally occurs over a span of months, is unresponsive to current therapy, and continues to be a source of graft loss.[19]

The main focus of this chapter is a description of new insights into the mechanisms of cell-mediated liver transplant rejection and new avenues for therapy.

IMMUNE MECHANISMS

As part of the host's immune response, there are both innate and adaptive immune responses. Innate immunity has evolved over time to deal with noxious agents in a rapid manner. In general these responses consist of both humoral (antibody, complement, coagulation) and cellular elements (neutrophils and macrophages).[9–11] In contrast, a second learned, or adaptive, immune response has evolved that deals with the recognition of specific antigens via T- and B-cell receptors.[12] Both systems are involved in transplantation. With harvesting of an organ, leading to damage from ischemia and reperfusion, the innate immune system is evoked.[20] In classic transplantation rejection, the adaptive immune system is activated, which leads to cellular and humoral immunity (rejection) directed against transplantation antigens in a highly selective manner.[12]

Relationship of Injury and Rejection

During the process of organ harvesting, tissue injury occurs, which leads to the expression of molecules not normally expressed on the surface of tissues.[21–24] These "neo" antigens can elicit three types of immune responses. The first is the initiation of innate responses that consist of both cellular and humoral elements, including neutrophils, macrophages, cytokines, complement, and coagulation proteases. The second

L. B. Lilly, J. Ding, and G. A. Levy: Multi Organ Transplant Program, The Toronto General Hospital, University of Toronto, Toronto, Ontario, Canada.

TABLE 14.1. *Hepatic allograft rejection*

Type	Time of onset	Mechanism	Clinical outcome
Hyperacute	Minutes to hours	Anti-α-Gal, complement, platelets, thrombosis	Fatal
Acute	Days to weeks	T cells, macrophages, natural killer cells, B cells	Reversible
Chronic	Weeks to years	T cells, B cells, macrophages	Irreversible

and third responses constitute the adaptive immune response leading to production of specific T- and B-cell repertoires (Table 14.2).

Once an organ is damaged, endothelial cells become activated and increase expression of adhesion molecules, including P (platelet) and E (endothelial) selectins, vascular cell adhesion molecule 1 (VCAM-1), and hylauronate.[25,26] Leukocytes become activated by chemokines, including interleukin 8 (IL-8) and macrophage chemoattractant protein 1 (MCP-1). This leads to expression of the β_2 integrins, including lymphocyte function associated antigen 1 (LFA-1), Mac-1 (CD11bkD18), and very late antigen 4 (VLA-4), which bind to their counterligands on endothelial cells. This results in lymphocyte sticking and translocation of lymphoid cells from the blood into the interstitium. The differential expression of cytokines and adhesion molecules affects the nature and class of infiltrating lymphoid cells.[26] T helper 1 (T_H1) cells, in contrast to T helper 2 (T_H2) cells, bind to endothelium that expresses P- and E-selectins.[27] Furthermore, T_H1 cells respond to the chemokines macrophage inhibitory protein 1α (MIP1α), MIP1β, and RANTES, whereas T_H2 cells respond to eotaxin.[28,29]

Ischemic injury results in activation of the complement system, with production of C3a and C5a leading to further endothelial cell activation and recruitment of an intense inflammatory cell infiltrate. The C5b-9 membrane attack complex generated by alternative complement activation stimulates the production of IL-8 and platelet activating factor (PAF), which promote inflammation at the site of injury by activating platelets, neutrophils, and monocytes with release of PAF, chemokines, cytokines, and coagulation proteins.[8]

All of the above events, although nonspecific, constitute "nonmemory" aspects of the host's innate immune response; however, they can lead to more specific adaptive immune responses involving T cells, B cells, and macrophages. The importance of this innate response is exemplified by transplantation-induced ischemia, which is known to contribute to the rejection process. This is best demonstrated by the fact that living-related transplantations involving kidneys and livers have a markedly reduced incidence of ischemic injury, fewer occurrences of acute cellular rejection, and better graft outcomes, taking all other factors into consideration.[8]

The Cell-Mediated Immune Response to Organ Allografts

It is not possible to completely describe all of the immunology of transplantation in this chapter; however, prior to defining the role of the immune system specifically in liver transplantation, a brief presentation of the immune events involved will be undertaken.

In general, recipient donor T cells (CD4+) recognize donor HLA class II antigens in the transplanted organ and are subsequently activated to proliferate, differentiate, and secrete cytokines (Fig. 14.1).[30] These cytokines further increase the expression of HLA class II antigens on the vascular endothelium, stimulate B cells to produce high-titered and high-affinity antibodies against the allograft, and arm cytotoxic T cells, macrophages, and NK cells.

The Nature of the Alloantigen

The MHC locus on chromosome 12 encodes for molecules that are the primary target for the alloresponse.[31–33] The MHC encodes for two major classes of proteins: HLA class I and HLA class II. Class I molecules are expressed on the surface of all nucleated cells in the body, although at different densities, whereas class II molecules are exclusively expressed on B cells and cells of the macrophage lineage. Class II expression can be upregulated in a number of cell types, including the vascular endothelium, epithelium, and T lymphocytes.

MHC class II molecules present exogenous antigens to CD4+ T helper cells, leading to their activation as measured by cytokine production and by the production and secretion of antibodies by B cells. In contrast, endogenous antigens are presented in concert with MHC class I molecules to cytotoxic CD8+ T cells, resulting in elimination of viruses and tumor cells.[34] The MHC is highly polymorphic, allowing for increased collective immunity against pathogens. In 1974, Zinkernagel and Doherty demonstrated that CD8+ T cells are specific for both self and nonself (MHC restriction).[34]

TABLE 14.2. *Components of host immune response*

Type	Components	Target
Innate immunity	Macrophages, neutrophils, complement, coagulation cascade, NK cells, antibodies	Bacteria, xenoantigens
Adaptive immunity	T cells (T_H1, T_H2, CTL), B cells, macrophages, dendritic cells, chemokines, cytokines	Viruses, alloantigens

NK, natural killer; CTL, cytotoxic T lymphocytes.

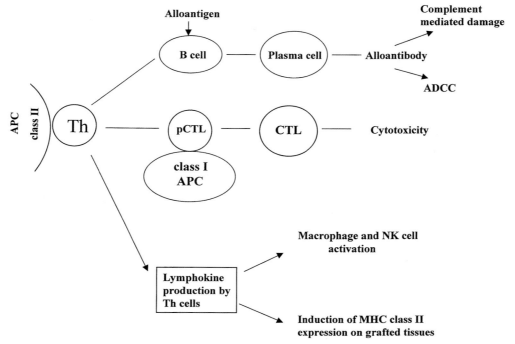

FIG. 14.1. Mechanism of activation of immune system in response to alloantigen. NK, natural killer; CTL, cytotoxic T lymphocyte; pCTL, precursor CTL; ADCC, antibody-dependent cell-mediated cytotoxicity; APC, antigen-presenting cell; Th, helper T cell.

More recently, it has been demonstrated that MHC class I molecules have peptide fragments of 8 to 10 amino acids within their peptide binding groove, whereas class II molecules have larger binding peptides (12 to 28 amino acids) resting on top of the groove in a more exposed manner.[35]

Class I and class II molecules have distinct pathways of antigen presentation. Class I molecules are transported to the surface of the cell with peptides produced by proteasomes on intracellular proteins. Peptide transporters move these peptides from the cytoplasm to the endoplasmic reticulum, where assembly of the class I peptide structure occurs. In contrast, class II molecules are exposed to peptides in acidic endosomal compartments. The MHC encoded heterodimer (HLA-DM) is found within this compartment and is essential for class II antigen presentation.[36]

In addition to major histocompatibility antigens, minor histocompatibility antigens are also important in allograft rejection. Multiple differences in the minor histocompatibility loci can be a strong immunogenic stimulus.[37]

Antigen-presenting Cells

Alloantigen presentation is accomplished by only a few specialized antigen-presenting cells (APCs). These APCs include dendritic cells, macrophages, B cells, and endothelial cells.[38] The most distinguishing feature of APCs is their unique display of costimulatory adhesion molecules. The adhesion molecules serve as ligands for counter-receptors

on T cells, as discussed previously. In addition to the expression of costimulatory molecules, other factors that influence APC function are the immune status of the responding T cell (naive versus memory) and proinflammatory mediators that may be present at the site of APC–T cell contact.[39,40]

When T cells encounter antigenic peptides displayed by competent APCs, they are activated to produce lymphokines, which allows them to acquire cytolytic activity and ultimately to proliferate. In general, CD4+ T cells survey peptides displayed by MHC class II molecules, whereas CD8+ T cells survey peptides displayed by MHC class I molecules. Proinflammatory cytokines such as IL-4 and interferon-γ influence the result of T-cell activation, including the pattern of cytokines secreted and the activity of cytolytic T cells.

Direct and Indirect Allorecognition

It has been proposed that two distinct routes of allorecognition exist.[38] In the first, the direct pathway, T cells recognize intact allo-MHC antigens on the surface of circulating donor cells. In the second, the indirect pathway, T cells recognize processed alloantigens in the context of self antigen-presenting cells.[41]

The T-cell response that results in early acute cellular rejection is caused mainly by the direct allorecognition pathway. T cells derived from the direct pathway constitute as many as 5% to 10% of the total T-cell peripheral pool. This strong response is due to the high density of MHC molecules on the donor graft and the large number of different peptides.

In the indirect pathway, donor alloantigens are shed from the graft, ingested by host antigen-presenting cells, and presented to CD4+ T cells. These activated T helper cells then secrete cytokines and provide the necessary signals for the growth and maturation of effector cytotoxic T cells and B cells. Indirect presentation is important in maintaining and amplifying the rejection response, especially in chronic rejection.[42]

Although dendritic cells, macrophages, and B cells are professional APCs, donor dendritic cells are probably the most potent stimulators of rejection. T-cell antigen recognition may occur peripherally or centrally. In rodents, depletion of dendritic cells from the donor allograft leads to prolonged graft survival; in humans, however, the dendritic cell may be less important where class II antigens are expressed on the endothelium.[43]

T-Cell Recognition

The T-Cell Receptor

Antigen specificity in allograft rejection is provided by clonally restricted T-cell receptors.[44] The T-cell receptor is composed of two chains, α and β, linked by disulfide bonds. The T-cell receptor (TCR) is associated with the CD3δ, C3Dε, and CD3γ chains and a τ-containing dimer.[44] The cytoplasmic domains of the invariant chains are much longer than those of the α and β chains and are responsible for coupling of the TCR to the intracellular signaling machinery. Within the cytoplasmic domain of the invariant chains exists a common domain that consists of a consensus sequence rich in paired leucines and tyrosines that interact with lck and fyn of the Src family of protein kinases, resulting in recruitment of ZAP-70 to the membrane receptor complex.

Coreceptors (CD4 and CD8)

CD4 binds to the β_2 segment of MHC class II molecules, whereas CD8 interacts with the α_3 segment of class I molecules. Both CD4 and CD8 bind to the cytoplasmic tyrosine kinase Lck, which brings Lck into close proximity with the TCR complex, where it acts early in the signal transduction pathway of activation of T cells. Later in the activation process, the CD4/Lck complex is anchored to the TCR complex. This process increases the avidity of the TCR-MHC interaction and increases the signaling process. CD45 is critical to T-cell receptor signaling, by dephosphorylating the negative regulatory site of Src family members.

T-Cell Activation

Following the engagement of the TCR, tyrosine phosphorylation of many proteins occurs (Fig. 14.2). Phos-

phorylation of phospholipase C-γ-1 increases its activity and induces cleavage of phosphatidylinositol bisphosphate, which leads to the production of the second messengers inositol 1,4,5-trisphosphate and diacylglycerol. Inositol 1,4,5-trisphosphate induces a sustained rise in intracellular calcium, whereas diacylglycerol activates protein kinase C. These two signals together induce and activate DNA binding factors needed for IL-2 gene transcription. The rise in intracellular calcium activates a calcium-dependent serine-threonine phosphatase, calcineurin, which modifies the constituitively expressed nuclear factor of activated T cells (NF-AT), dissociating its inhibitor (I-κB) and thus allowing it to translocate to the nucleus, where it induces transcription of IL-2. Cyclosporine and tacrolimus (FK506) bind to cytoplasmic proteins (immunophilins), which bind to calcineurin and inhibit its activation, thus preventing NF-AT cell function and IL-2 transcription.[45]

Tyrosine phosphorylation of Vav activates the *ras* signal transduction pathway. The oncogene *ras* interacts directly with the serine-threonine kinase Raf-1, which then regulates the activity of a kinase cascade that includes Mek and the mitogen-activated protein kinase (MAP kinase). This cascade leads to nuclear events involved in cell proliferation and differentiation by inducing c-*fos* and c-*jun* transcription factors. Expression of an activated form of *ras* potentiates IL-2 promoter activity. T-cell receptor stimulation in itself causes the nuclear factor of κB transcription factor to translocate to the nucleus and also regulates the mRNA stability of lymphokine mRNA by induction of RNA binding factors.

Costimulation

For maximal IL-2 production by T cells, antigen-presenting cells must also provide costimulatory signals (Fig. 14.3). There are a number of costimulatory molecules on APCs. The major costimulatory activity necessary for proliferation of T cells by IL-2 appears to be mediated by the interaction of the CD28 molecule on the T-cell surface with its ligands, members of the B7 family on APCs.[46] Engagement of the TCR in the absence of this costimulatory signal fails to induce an immune response, results in a state of anergy, and prevents transplant rejection.[47,48] Although the exact mechanism of costimulation is not known, it is postulated that CD28 engagement prevents lymphocyte death through enhanced expression of an intrinsic survival factor (Bcl-xl).[49]

In humans, more than 95% of resting CD4+ cells and 50% of resting CD8+ cells express CD28. Following activation, the expression of CD28 is markedly increased. Of interest, CD28 is structurally homologous to the cytolytic T-lymphocyte antigen 4 (CTLA-4). The expression of CTLA-4 is restricted to activated cytotoxic T lymphocytes and delivers a negative second signal modulating T-cell activation. Mice that lack this signal die from uncontrolled activation of T lymphocytes.[50] CD28 knockout mice lack a positive second signal, and T-cell responses

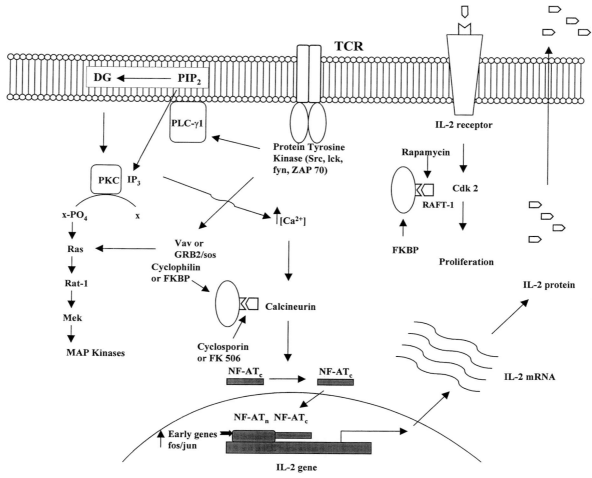

FIG. 14.2. Signal pathway for transcription of cytokine's genes and site of action of immunosuppressive drugs. TCR, T-cell receptor; PLC, phospholipase; PKC, protein kinase C; PIP2, phosphatidylinositol 4,5-bisphosphate; DG, diacylglycerol; IP3, inositol 1,4,5-triphosphate; FKBP, FK506 binding protein; NF-AT, nuclear factor of activated T cells.

are markedly diminished.[51] Blockade of this costimulatory pathway during engraftment may induce tolerance to the graft without the need for immunosuppressive drugs.

T-Cell Differentiation

Once an alloantigen interacts with a T-cell receptor as described previously, activation of genes leads to the development of differentiated effector T cells. The protooncogenes c-*myc* and c-*fos* are transcribed rapidly following T-cell activation. The products of these early-activation genes in concert with the effects of ongoing signal transduction initiate the next wave of gene activation, including the transcription of IL-2 and the IL-2 receptor. Subsequently, additional cytokines, including IL-3, IL-4, IL-5, IL-6, and interferon-γ, are produced. In response to these cytokines, and in particular IL-2 and IL-4, T cells take on differentiated functions that include immunoregulation and cy-

totoxicity. The genes coding for granzymes, perforins, and chemokines such as RANTES are then generated over the next 4 to 6 days. Within 7 to 14 days, late-activation molecules are produced, including the integrin supergene family.

CD4 T Cells and Cytokines

Activated CD4+ T cells secrete an array of cytokines that modulate and amplify the immune response. CD4+ T cells have been subdivided into T_H1 and T_H2 CD4+ T cells depending on the pattern of cytokine production. T_H1 cells predominately produce IL-2 and interferon-γ, whereas T_H2 cells produce IL-4, IL-5, IL-6, and IL-10.[52] T_H1 and T_H2 cells develop from a common precursor (T_H0) and can crossregulate each other. Interferon-γ inhibits the production of T_H2 cells, whereas IL-4 and IL-10 inhibit the production of T_H1 cells. Although human cells may not conform strictly to T_H1 and T_H2 cell phenotypes, rejecting

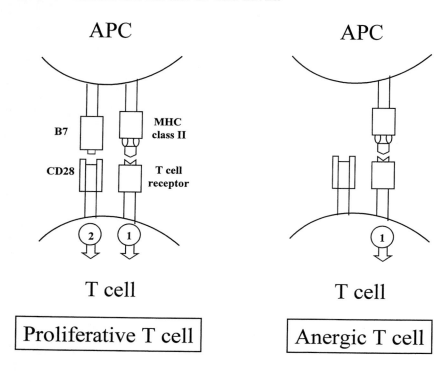

FIG. 14.3. Role of costimulatory molecules in lymphocyte activation. *1,* signal 1; *2,* signal 2. Both signal 1 and 2 are necessary for lymphocyte activation. APC, antigen-presenting cell; MHC, major histocompatibility complex.

allografts contain CD4+ cells that secrete predominately cytokines of the T_H1 phenotype.

The role of specific cytokines in rejection has been difficult to assess. For example, IL-2 knockout mice reject grafts. This may be because other T-cell growth factors, including IL-4, IL-10, IL-12, and IL-15, cause IL-2-independent cell proliferation.[52] Interferon-γ is an important cytokine in rejection because it recruits and activates macrophages, activates endothelial cells, and increases MHC antigen expression and transporter proteins associated with antigen presentation expression. In contrast, the role of IL-10 in rejection is controversial. It is a cytokine that is known to have both immunostimulatory and immunoregulatory activities. During the tolerance phase of allografts, IL-10 is present but may also contribute to acute and chronic allograft rejection.[53]

CD8 T Cells and Cytotoxicity

CD8+ T cells, also known as cytotoxic T lymphocytes (CTLs), are able to kill cells of an allograft either by the secretion of granzymes and perforins or by the induction of apoptosis through the Fas/Fas ligand pathway.[54,55]

Within activated CTLs are a number of cytolytic granules that contain a variety of cytolytic proteins, such as perforin, a complement-like protein, as well as a family of serine proteases called granzymes.[56] Perforins polymerize in the target cell membrane to produce large pores, leading to osmotic lysis of the cells. CD8+ T cells from perforin knockout mice are incapable of lysing virus-specific infected cells *in vitro* or clearing viral infections *in vivo.*

Granzymes are thought to induce apoptosis by deregulating normal control processes within the cell. Both granzyme

B and perforin transcripts are expressed in acute cellular rejection.[57] Binding of Fas ligand on activated CD8+ T cells to Fas antigen on target cells leads to apoptosis. Although Fas transcripts are expressed constitutively in syngeneic and allogeneic murine cardiac transplant recipients, Fas ligand is only detected in rejecting grafts.[58]

Leukocyte–Endothelial Cell Interactions

The migration of leukocytes across the endothelium into the allograft has been intensely studied, and their importance in a large number of liver diseases, including alcoholic hepatitis and cirrhosis, viral hepatitis, ischemic reperfusion injury, and acute and chronic rejection, has been well documented.[59] Migration of cells can be divided into four distinct phases: tethering, triggering, tight adhesion, and transendothelial cell migration. Cellular adhesion molecules are cell surface glycoproteins involved in cell-cell and cell-matrix interactions. These molecules are critical for leukocyte adhesion to the endothelium, transmigration, binding to target cells, and cytotoxicity. Three main family members of the cellular adhesion molecules participate in immune and inflammatory processes: the immunoglobulin gene superfamily, integrins, and selectins (Table 14.3).[59]

The initial tethering of leukocytes to endothelium is mediated by members of the selectin family.[60] The selectins are carbohydrate structures related to the sialyl Lewis antigen. L-selectin is expressed constitutively on most leukocytes, whereas E-selectin is expressed on endothelial cells in response to IL-1 and tumor necrosis factor α (TNF-α).

P-selectin is stored, preformed, in the Weibel-Palade bodies of endothelial cells and in the granules of platelets.[57]

TABLE 14.3. *Classification of adhesion molecules*

Molecule	Ligand	Tissue distribution
Integrins		
LFA-1 (CD11a/CD18)	ICAM-1, ICAM-2	KC, L, N, M, Mφ, DC
Mac-1 (CD11b/CD18)	ICAM-1, fibrinogen, iC3b	KC, N, M, Mφ
CR4 (CD11c/CD18)	iC3b	KC, N, M, Mφ
VLA-4 (CD49d/CD29)	VCAM-1, fibronectin	KC, α, N, M, Mφ
Immunoglobulin superfamily		
ICAM-1 (CD54)	LFA-1, Mac-1	L, KC, N, M, activated EC, DC
ICAM-2 (CD102)	LFA-1	L, KC, N, M, resting EC, DC
ICAM-3 (CD50)	LFA-1	L
VCAM-1 (CD106)	VLA-4	Resting and activated EC, KC
LFA-2 (CD2)	LFA-3	T cells
LFA-3 (CD58)	LFA-2	L, antigen-presenting cells
PECAM-1 (CD31)	PECAM-1	EC, L, N, P
Selectins		
L-selectin (CD62L)	Sulfated sialyl Lewis ^{x}, GlyCAM-1, CD34, MAdCAM-1	Naive and memory L, N, M, Mφ
P-selectin (CD62P)	Sialyl Lewis ^{x}, PSGL-1	Activated EC, P
E-selectin (CD62E)	Sialyl Lewis ^{x}	Activated EC

LFA, lymphocyte function associated antigen; ICAM, intercellular adhesion molecule; KC, Kupffer cells; L, lymphocytes; N, neutrophils; M, monocytes; Mφ, macrophages; DC, dendritic cells; VLA, very late antigen; VCAM, vascular cell adhesion molecule; EC, endothelial cells; P, platelets; PECAM, platelet endothelial cell adhesion molecule, PSGL; platelet slalylglyco lipid.

Once cells are activated, P-selectin is mobilized and is responsible for binding of neutrophils and monocytes. The rapid turnover of the selectins allows leukocyte–endothelial cell interaction to occur and can lead to further activation and tight cell adhesion. In the absence of further activation, however, cells disengage and move on.

Strong adhesion of leukocytes to the endothelium is mediated by the integrins.[61] Chemokines (chemoattractant cytokines) increase cell adhesion by activating the integrins on circulating leukocytes. Five integrins have been implicated as being important in lymphocyte–endothelial cell interactions: LFA-1, which binds intercellular adhesion molecule 1 (ICAM-1) and ICAM-2 on endothelium, and VLA-4, which binds VCAM-1.

After integrin-mediated attachment is established, leukocytes can then migrate through the endothelium and basement membrane to enter the tissue. This transmigration process is dependent on integrins and chemokines. At the same time, T cells secrete metalloproteases that digest the basement membrane, thus allowing cells to enter the tissue.

Release of inflammatory cytokines from macrophages, including IL-1, TNF-α and interferon-γ, induces changes in endothelium such as increased expression of MHC class II molecules and adhesion molecules, including E-selectin and ICAM-1.[62]

HEPATIC ALLOGRAFT REJECTION: IMMUNE TARGETS AND RESPONSES

Rejection of the transplanted liver is traditionally classified into three types: hyperacute, or antibody-mediated, rejection;

acute, or cellular, rejection; and chronic, or ductopenic, rejection. Each form reflects mobilization of a different pathway within the immune response and offers a distinct immunotherapeutic challenge. The hepatic allograft, however, is relatively resistant to progressive injury related to rejection, and organ loss attributable to drug-resistant rejection remains an uncommon occurrence following engraftment.

Hyperacute Rejection

Hyperacute rejection (HAR), a rare form of hepatic allograft rejection, is thought to be the result of the interaction of preformed recipient antibodies with the transplanted liver. Either preexisting antibodies exist in sufficient titers to produce massive necrosis, or a brief stimulus by donor antigen is sufficient to stimulate preprogrammed B cells to generate an immediate rise in titer.[63] When present, HAR becomes evident within hours to days of transplant surgery, resulting in hepatocyte necrosis that leads to rapid allograft failure. The only effective treatment is urgent retransplantation.[64–66]

The initial liver histopathology demonstrates sinusoidal congestion and hemorrhage;[67] subsequent examination reveals hepatocyte loss, largely mediated through ischemic injury.[68,69] Microvascular thrombosis is not generally recognized on routine histologic examination. The recipient antibodies produce damage through binding to endothelial cells, triggering activation and deposition of complement and activating the coagulation cascade. Massive fibrin deposition occurs, which, coupled with the production of vasospastic polypeptides, results in ischemia and further hepatocyte injury, ultimately resulting in organ failure with profound coagulopathy and hepatic encephalopathy.[63,67,70–72] Upregulation of endothelial cell adhesion molecule expression also occurs, promoting infiltration of leukocytes and increasing local cytokine release.

The identity of these preformed antibodies is controversial. HAR is recognized to occur during liver transplantation in humans in two situations: with ABO-incompatible grafts and in the presence of preformed, donor-specific, lymphocytotoxic antibodies.[73,74] These antibodies, which react against allogeneic HLA class I antigens, play an important pathogenetic role in renal allograft rejection; however, their role in liver transplantation is less certain. For this reason, and because of practical considerations, crossmatch results have largely been ignored in liver transplantation.[75,76] However, transplants done in the setting of a positive crossmatch have been associated with an increased blood transfusion requirement, an increase in the prothrombin time, and a fall in platelets, attributed to activation of the coagulation cascade and subsequent consumption of clotting factors. It is possible that even minor reperfusion injury to the liver results in an immediate increase in HLA class I antigen expression. It has been further suggested from animal studies that hepatic allografts are indeed inherently susceptible to such antibody-mediated injuries, but that recipient antibody titers may simply not be high enough to result in significant cellular injury.[77]

In ABO-incompatible liver transplants, the allograft may be lost in up to 50% of cases because of antibody-mediated mechanisms. In the ABO-nonidentical circumstance, however, a transient graft-versus-host-like disease has been described in which lymphocytes carried within the donor liver briefly produce antibodies directed against recipient erythrocytes, resulting in a hemolytic anemia that is typically observed 1 to 2 weeks following transplantation. This process is generally self-limited; when severe, the anemia can be treated with transfusion of donor, rather than recipient, blood.

Given how often preformed antibodies are present, it is remarkable that HAR is not more commonly seen.[78] The antibodies, directed toward HLA class I antigens on the endothelium of the donor liver, may be neutralized by high circulating amounts of soluble HLA class I antigens, which have been found in the serum of liver recipients immediately after reperfusion of the transplanted liver. Alternatively, the liver itself may act as a sponge, absorbing preformed antibodies or antigen-antibody complexes and thereby preventing endothelium-targeted injury from occurring. Resistance of the liver to antibody-mediated injury may also be related to its unique architecture. The liver has a dual blood supply, and the sinusoids are lined with discontinuous, or fenestrated, endothelium. Thus, any microthrombi formed by antibody binding and subsequent complement activation are less likely to result in occlusion and ischemia, such as one might see in a renal allograft. Indeed, immunohistochemical analysis of the endothelium in HAR has revealed deposition of immunoglobulin (Ig) G and IgM and complement components C1q and C3 in the sinusoids,

veins, and arteries of the allograft, similar to findings in renal allografts.[79]

HAR is occasionally recognized in the absence of either ABO incompatibility or a positive crossmatch, probably due to secondary immune mechanisms triggered by ischemia or a particularly severe reperfusion injury.[80]

Acute Rejection

Acute rejection (AcR), also known as cellular or reversible rejection, is typically first seen 5 to 7 days following transplantation; the majority of episodes occur within 90 days of transplant surgery.[64,74,81] Depending on whether protocol liver biopsies are carried out, AcR is seen in up to 75% of liver transplant recipients.[82,83] Although the clinical presentation is quite varied, it is typically characterized by a rise in the canalicular enzymes (alkaline phosphatase, γ-glutamyltransferase) and bilirubin, with a less substantial increase in the aminotransferases. It may, however, present as jaundice with significant transaminase elevations. Diagnosis is by liver biopsy, with three characteristic findings noted on histopathologic examination: (a) portal infiltration with expansion of the triads with a variety of cells, including predominantly lymphocytes; (b) bile duct invasion and injury; and (c) portal venous endophlebitis.[69] AcR is usually responsive to intravenous steroids alone or in conjunction with OKT3 and rarely results in graft loss. Steroid- and OKT3-unresponsive cases may benefit from switching cyclosporine to tacrolimus (or vice versa).

The targets of activated lymphocytes in AcR are the bile duct epithelial cells (BEC) and the endothelium of the veins and arteries within the liver. Direct hepatocyte involvement appears to be uncommon, particularly early. The portal infiltrate contains activated lymphoblastoid cells, both T cells and B cells, plasma cells, and, in lesser numbers, all other leukocyte populations. CD4+ cells are prominent and are thought to be the primary source of cytokines, which then act to upregulate HLA expression, increase cytotoxic T lymphocyte differentiation, and increase alloantibody production.[84] In the early phase of AcR, HLA class I–specific alloreactive T cells predominate; a mixture of class I–specific and class II–specific T cells is present in later phases.[84–86]

Normal hepatocytes constitutively express small amounts of HLA class I antigens, while exhibiting virtually no class II antigen expression.[87] This pattern is also seen in BEC and endothelial cells. Because the BEC are an important target in AcR, HLA class I and II expression has been extensively studied in these cells. During early episodes of AcR, class I and II expression are both enhanced.[88] Examination of liver biopsies in the clinically inapparent "prerejection" phase has shown augmentation in HLA-DR expression, with little or no increase in HLA-DP and HLA-DQ expression.

Upregulation of class II expression appears to occur for a number of reasons. First, allorecognition of HLA class I may result in the activation of recipient leukocytes (primarily CD8+ cells), with an increase in the secretion of proinflammatory cytokines (including IFN-γ), which then induce *de novo* expression of class II antigens on the surface of BEC. Class II expression is also increased by reperfusion injury to the bile ducts, since BEC appear to require higher oxygen tensions to maintain viability than do hepatocytes.[89] BEC infected by cytomegalovirus (CMV) have been shown to exhibit modified HLA expression as well as altered adhesion molecule expression. Finally, it has been suggested that BEC can act as "semiprofessional" antigen-presenting cells and essentially target themselves for allorecognition.

Enhanced HLA expression can also occur in the absence of rejection in the liver allograft. For example, increased class I and class II antigen expression has been noted in ischemia, cholestasis, bacterial cholangitis, and sepsis. Indeed, HLA overexpression is likely an important factor in the pathogenesis of a number of chronic liver diseases, including primary biliary cirrhosis.[89]

In an effort to determine whether AcR is most typical of a T_H1 or T_H2 response, bile collected during AcR has been analyzed for cytokine release.[90] This bile demonstrated significant increases in interleukins 4, 5, and 10 when compared with levels measured with no apparent ongoing rejection. This profile is typical of a T_H2 response (although both T_H1 and T_H2 cells may produce IL-10 in humans), complementing earlier data that had shown increased T_H2 cytokine gene expression at the site of liver allograft rejection.[91] However, the complex interactions between T_H1 and T_H2 responses make interpretation of this finding difficult. Higher absolute levels of T_H2 cytokines than T_H1 cytokines were noted, and it has been shown that T_H2 cytokines may augment, rather than inhibit, CTL differentiation. In addition, much lower absolute levels of T_H1 cytokines may be required to initiate CTL responses in rejection. IFN-χ, a T_H1 cytokine, can inhibit T_H2 cell development, thus favoring expansion of T_H1 cells, while IL-4 and IL-10 can, in turn, inhibit IFN-γ production. Thus, it has proved difficult to categorize AcR as either a pure T_H1 or T_H2 response. It has been further suggested that the infiltration of T_H2 cells may confer some benefit toward the achievement of long-term allograft survival.[92,93]

The mechanism of cell injury and death in AcR appears to be via accelerated apoptosis. The incidence of apoptotic hepatocytes roughly parallels the severity of acute rejection, although their injury probably occurs through indirect mechanisms. However, injured bile duct epithelial cells also display ultrastructural changes consistent with apoptosis, and it has been proposed that BEC apoptosis is the predominant mechanism of cell injury and death in AcR, whereas hepatocyte apoptosis assumes primary importance in chronic rejection.[94] It has already been demonstrated that apoptosis participates in tissue destruction during rejection in other solid organ transplants, including small intestinal, renal, and cardiac transplants.

Chronic Rejection

Chronic rejection (CR), often labeled with the more useful term ductopenic rejection, is first seen a few weeks follow-

ing transplantation, and may be diagnosed years later.[95] It is characterized by an ischemic injury to the bile ducts resulting in duct paucity, and is often considered one of the many "disappearing duct" syndromes.[96] Liver biochemistry is typically cholestatic, with little evidence of necroinflammatory activity. Response to therapy is variable and usually poor, and the disease progresses, often indolently, to allograft failure that necessitates retransplantation. Ductopenia has reverted spontaneously, and a recent multicenter trial confirmed that tacrolimus rescue therapy can reverse ductopenic CR in a significant number of patients. Fortunately, CR is uncommon, described in less than 5% of transplants in most large series.

An infiltrate is often noted early in CR, composed predominantly of activated CD8+ T lymphocytes. As duct necrosis evolves and duct paucity develops, the infiltrate resolves. A vasculopathy is also present, with intimal thickening and total or subtotal occlusion of hepatic arterial branches, resulting in ischemic loss of BEC. This may not be apparent on routine liver biopsy because it may involve larger ducts that are located somewhat remotely from the affected portal triads. Thus, duct loss results from a combination of duct-specific immune responses and arterial ischemic injury.[97] Hepatocytes may be specifically targeted, however. Studies looking at the incidence of apoptosis have demonstrated much higher parenchymal staining for apoptotic cells in CR than in AcR; it is difficult, however, to determine the role that ischemic injury might play in this observation.

A number of risk factors for CR have been proposed. The majority, but not the entire population, of patients who go on to develop CR have had an episode of AcR. Other studies, however, have shown that a single episode of AcR, if adequately treated, may actually have a protective effect and improve long-term graft survival.[98] It was suggested that patients who underwent transplantation for either primary biliary cirrhosis or primary sclerosing cholangitis were at increased risk of CR; however, larger longitudinal studies have cast some doubt on that observation. HLA mismatching may actually protect against, rather than promote, ductopenic rejection.[99] CMV infection does not appear to confer an increase in risk. Clearly, retransplantation for CR is a significant risk factor for the subsequent development of further CR, lending credence to the notion that it is recipient, rather than donor, factors that predominate.

PHARMACOLOGIC MANIPULATION OF THE IMMUNE SYSTEM

Greater understanding of the molecular mechanisms of activation of the immune system has led to the development of more selective immunosuppressive agents (Table 14.4).

Corticosteroids are powerful antiinflammatory agents that have been used to suppress the harmful effects of immune responses of autoimmune or allergic origin as well as those induced by graft rejection.[60] These agents are pharmacologic derivatives of members of the glucocorticoid family of steroid hormones that act through intracellular

TABLE 14.4. *Site of action of immunosuppressive drugs*

Drugs	Site of action
Corticosteroids	Cytotoxic to cells
Calcineurin inhibitors	
Tacrolimus	Inhibits NF-κB
Cyclosporin A	Inhibits transcription of IL-2
Rapamycin	Inhibits signal transduction through IL-2 receptor
Mycophenolate mofetil	Inhibits DNA synthesis
Azathioprine	Inhibits DNA synthesis
Antibodies to IL-2 receptor, CD40, and CTLA-4	Costimulation

NF-κB, nuclear factor of κB transcription factor; IL-2, interleukin 2; CTLA-4, cytolytic T-lymphocyte antigen 4.

receptors that are expressed in almost every cell of the body to regulate the transcription of specific genes (Table 14.5). Given the large number of genes regulated by corticosteroids, it is not surprising that the effects of these agents are very complex. The major beneficial effects are antiinflammatory. There are a number of adverse effects associated with their use, however, including fluid retention, weight gain, bone mineral loss, diabetes mellitus, and thinning of the skin. These agents continue to remain a mainstay in induction immunotherapy as well as in treatment of acute cellular rejection. They remain as one of the few agents that affect antigen presentation and macrophage activation.

Two cytotoxic agents commonly used as immunosuppressive agents are azathioprine (Imuran) and mycophenolate mofetil (CellCept). Both of these agents interfere with DNA synthesis and have their major pharmacologic effects on dividing cells. The use of azathioprine is limited by a range of toxic effects on tissues in the body, which have in common the property of continuous cell division. These effects include decreased immune function, leukopenia, anemia, thrombocytopenia, damage to intestinal epithelium, and hair loss. Mycophenolate mofetil is a more selective inhibitor of purine synthesis.[100] Its site of action is to inhibit inosine monophosphate dehydrogenase (IMPDH), an enzyme necessary for *de novo* purine synthesis in lymphocytes.[101] Its selectivity to lymphocytes results in fewer side effects than the use

of azathioprine, but gastrointestinal toxicity (diarrhea), leukopenia, and thrombocytopenia have limited its usefulness. In controlled clinical trials in renal allograft recipients, the use of mycophenolate mofetil has been associated with a marked reduction in the incidence of acute cellular rejection; controlled trials in liver transplant liver recipients are now being completed.[102,103] More recent studies have suggested that the use of this agent will allow for sparing of steroids.[104]

The systematic study of products from bacteria and fungi has led to the development of new immunosuppressive agents, including cyclosporin A, a cyclic decapeptide derived from the fungus *Tolypocladium inflatum Gams*,[105] tacrolimus (FK506),[106] a macrolide derived from the filamentous bacteria *Streptomyces tsukabaensis,* and rapamycin, a macrolide derived from *Streptomyces hygroscopicus*.[107] Cyclosporin A and tacrolimus block T-cell proliferation by reducing the expression (transcription) of several cytokine genes that are induced during T-cell activation.[108,109] These include IL-2, whose synthesis by T cells is an important growth signal for T lymphocytes. The mechanism of action of cyclosporin A and tacrolimus is now well understood.[110,111] Each binds to a different group of immunophilins: Cyclosporin A binds to the cyclophilins, and tacrolimus to the FK-binding proteins (FKBP). These immunophilins are peptidyl-prolyl cis-trans isomerases. The immunophilin-drug complexes inhibit the Ca^{2+}-activated serine-threonine phosphatase calcineurin, which, once activated following T-cell receptor binding, dephosphorylates the cytosolic component of the transcription factor NF-AT, allowing it to migrate to the nucleus, where it induces transcription of the IL-2 gene.[108-111]

Both Neoral (a microemulsion of cyclosporin A) and tacrolimus are effective immunosuppressive agents, but they have major toxicity profiles related to a narrow therapeutic window (efficacy dose versus toxicity dose). At present the most effective way of monitoring these agents is unclear.[112] Trough levels (C_{min}) have been used for both agents, but it is clear for both drugs that the relationship of C_{min} to exposure (area under the concentration/time curve, or AUC) and the relationship of dose to C_{min} are not sufficient to allow the use of trough levels as an effective and sensitive therapeutic monitoring tool. New strategies are now being studied, in-

TABLE 14.5. *Effects of corticosteroids*

Activity	Effect
Decreased IL-1, TNF-α, GM-CSF, IL-3, IL-4, IL-5, IL-8 activity	Decreased inflammation caused by cytokines
Decreased NOS activity	Decreased NO production
Decreased phospholipase A_2 activity, decreased cyclooxygenase type 2 activity	Decreased production of prostaglandins and leukotrienes
Increased lipocortin-1 activity	Decreased production of prostaglandins and leukotrienes
Decreased adhesion molecules	Reduced emigration of leukocytes from vessels
Induction of endonucleases	Induction of apoptosis in lymphocytes and eosinophils

IL, interleukin; TNF-α, tumor necrosis factor α; GM-CSF, granulocyte-monocyte colony-stimulating factor; NO, nitric acid, NOS; nitric oxide synthase.

cluding the use of AUC monitoring or surrogate markers for AUC such as C_2 (levels 2 hours postadministration).[113]

Rapamycin (sirolimus), like tacrolimus, binds to the FKBP family of immunophilins. However, the rapamycin-immunophilin complex has no effect on calcineurin activity but instead blocks the signal transduction pathway triggered by the ligation of IL-2 to the IL-2 receptor. It also inhibits lymphocyte proliferation driven by other growth factors, including IL-4 and IL-6. Recent evidence has suggested that rapamycin inhibits translation initiation by preventing formation of the cap structure present at the 5′ end of all cellular mRNAs.[114] The use of rapamycin has resulted in a dramatic reduction in the incidence of acute cellular rejection in renal transplant recipients and is now being studied in liver transplant recipients.

Antibodies to cell surface molecules have been used to remove specific lymphocyte subsets or to inhibit cell function. The potential of antibodies to remove unwanted lymphocytes is demonstrated by antilymphocyte globulins that have been employed to prevent or reverse acute cellular rejection. However, the first-generation antilymphocyte antibody preparations did not discriminate between useful lymphocytes and those lymphocytes responsible for rejection. More recently, monoclonal antibodies directed to specific molecular targets of lymphocyte activation have been designed and studied for their utility in transplantation.[115,116]

A potential target for more specific immunosuppressive therapy with monocolonal antibodies is the high-affinity interleukin 2 receptor (IL-2R) present on activated T cells but not resting T cells.[117] Two such anti–IL-2R monoclonal antibodies have now been approved for use in transplantation.[118,119] The first is daclizumab, a fully humanized antibody; the second is basiliximab, a chimeric anti–IL-2R monoclonal antibody. Both of these agents have been evaluated in renal transplant patients and have been shown to reduce the incidence of acute cellular rejection by 50%. Furthermore, their use allowed for the early sparing of calcineurin inhibitors at a time when renal function was most vulnerable to these agents. The toxicity profile of the IL-2R monoclonal antibodies was remarkably low, and no patients suffered major side effects. Preliminary studies in liver transplant patients have also shown these agents to be effective in reducing the incidence of acute cellular rejection and for sparing the need for calcineurin inhibitors early in the postoperative period.[120]

Additional monoclonal antibodies are now being examined that target the costimulatory molecules CD28-B7 and CD40-CD40L (signal 2 of T-cell activation).[121,122] These antibodies are being studied not only for their ability to reduce the incidence of acute cellular rejection but also for their ability to induce tolerance.[123] Preliminary studies in primates suggest that antibodies to CD40 have the potential to induce tolerance, and clinical trials are now being contemplated.[123]

An exciting new molecule that has been shown to prolong allograft survival of rodents is the novel immunosuppressant molecule FTY 720, whose action is to alter migration of antigen-specific lymphocytes between lymphoid tissues rather than to directly inhibit cellular function.[124] This agent does not synergize with cyclosporin A, tacrolimus, or rapamycin in vitro, but does synergize with cyclosporin A in vivo. FTY inhibits CD4 T-cell-dependent immune responses to a number of antigens, as well as T-cell-independent formation of antibody. It is now being examined in phase 1 trials in allotransplantation as well as for its potential use in xenotransplantation.

FUTURE DIRECTIONS

Tolerance Induction

The ability of the immune system to discriminate between self and nonself antigens through a variety of mechanisms is essential for preservation of host integrity. This nonreactivity of the immune system toward self or foreign antigens is called tolerance.[125] The intrathymic deletion of developing thymocytes that express potentially self-reactive T-cell receptors (central tolerance) is the major mechanism in the establishment of self-tolerance.[126] Thus, more than 95% of thymocytes do not enter the periphery but rather die within the thymus. This process can occur by apoptosis, in which the TCR displays an affinity extremely high for self antigens, or by neglect, in which the TCR displays little or no affinity.[127] Thus, only those cells carrying TCRs with moderate affinity for self MHC, which enables recognition of foreign peptide antigens in the context of self MHC class I or class II molecules, are positively selected during intrathymic development. These T cells leave the thymus and constitute the pool of mature CD4+ and CD8+ T cells in the periphery.

Several mechanisms have been proposed to explain how the immune system manages to mitigate potentially harmful mature peripheral T lymphocytes with reactivity against self antigens. The induction of peripheral tolerance has been hypothesized to occur by such mechanisms as clonal deletion, clonal ignorance, and clonal anergy as well as cytokine-mediated immune deviation or suppression.[128]

Prevention of immune responses against self antigens may be partially accounted for by a passive mechanism whereby self antigens are ignored by the immune system. Clonal ignorance may thus occur as a result of anatomical sequestration of self antigens away from immunocompetent lymphocytes. Alternatively, lymphocyte ignorance may result from inadequate T-cell triggering during antigen-lymphocyte interactions in the absence of a second signal.[129]

The maintenance of self-tolerance may also occur through the induction of clonal anergy. The two-signal hypothesis for T-cell activation was first proposed by Bretscher and Cohn to explain the paradox that lymphocyte antigen recognition can result in either clonal expansion or unresponsiveness.[130] The hypothesis predicted that antigen receptor occupancy alone would induce lymphocyte unresponsiveness, whereas antigen receptor occupancy plus a costimulatory signal would induce immunity.[131] Antigen recognition by T lymphocytes in the absence of a second-signal costimulation would then trigger cells to enter into a state of antigen-specific unresponsiveness, termed anergy. This phenomenon was first described by Schwartz using CD4+ T cell lines.[132] Engagement of antigen receptors without costimulation induced the cells to enter a state of functional unresponsiveness upon subsequent stimulation. An anergic T-cell state may also be induced under conditions that provide adequate costimulation but suboptimal antigen receptor signaling.[133] In an *in vivo* model of T-cell anergy, induction of an unresponsive state was thought to be mediated by interaction of CTLA-4 with B7. *In vivo* T-cell anergy may be induced not by the failure to provide costimulation but as a result of specific CTLA-4 signal transduction.[134] The regulatory function of CTLA-4 is most markedly illustrated by targeted disruption of the CTLA-4 gene in mice, which results in massive accumulation of activated lymphocytes in the spleen and lymph nodes, displaying manifestations of autoimmunity.[135]

An important mechanism of peripheral self-tolerance involves the elimination of mature self-reactive T cells by activation-induced cell death (apoptosis) due to coexpression of the Fas (CD95) death receptor and its ligand (FasL).[127] T cells become sensitive to apoptosis after activation by antigen and IL-2. Interleukin 2 potentiates the sensitization of cells to the Fas signal pathway by increasing transcription and cell surface expression of Fas ligand and suppressing transcription and expression of FLIP, the inhibitor of apoptosis.[136]

The stimulation of naive cells by antigen and second signals leads to their differentiation not only into effector cells, whose function is to eliminate the antigen, but also into regulatory cells.[137] CD4+ T helper lymphocytes can be divided into distinct subsets on the basis of their cytokine secretion pattern as defined earlier.[138] Regulatory T cells can be divided into T_H1 (IL-2 and interferon-γ), T_H2 (IL-10 and IL-44), and T_H3 (transforming growth factor β_1, or TGF-β_1) subsets; the cytokines produced by each of these T-cell subsets play a role in immune crossregulation. For example, TGF-β_1 plays a role in inhibiting T-cell proliferation,[139] and IL-10 inhibits T_H1 differentiation as well as macrophage activation and function.[140]

Tolerance Induction by the Liver

Immune privilege is a term applied to organs that have a unique relationship with the immune system. Specialized tissues or sites and the immune system cooperate in providing immune protection while preventing immunopathogenic tissue damage. The most prominent examples of these immune privileged sites are the eye, brain, and reproductive organs. The liver has long been known to display features of immune privilege. Spontaneous acceptance of a pig liver allograft in primates was first reported in 1969 by Calne et al.[141] In addition, it has been reported that some rat strains permanently accept allogeneic livers without the need for pharmacologic immunosuppressive agents, whereas these same animals reject other organs such as heart, kidney, or skin. The trans-

planted liver not only prevents its own rejection but can also induce donor-specific immune tolerance that provides immunoprotection against other subsequent transplanted organs or tissues in a donor-MHC-specific manner. As an example, orthotopic liver transplantation in mice abrogates the development of chronic rejection in subsequent aortic allotransplantation in a donor-specific manner.[142]

Clinical and experimental evidence from human organ transplantation also supports the notion that the liver is a specialized tissue that exhibits immunologic privilege. It has been recognized that patients receiving hearts or kidneys at the same time as a liver allograft have markedly less frequent and intense rejection episodes of the liver allografts.[142] Furthermore, successful withdrawal of immunosuppression has been accomplished in some liver transplant recipients.[143]

Although the mechanism for the immune privileged state of the liver has not been fully explained, a number of hypotheses have been put forward, including microchimerism caused by the existence of large numbers of dendritic cells within the donor liver that circulate and stably repopulate the recipient.[144] These cells then reprogram the host's immune system to accept donor antigens as self antigens (Table 14.6).[145]

An alternative explanation for this unique property of the liver is the existence of a unique T-cell population within the liver that expresses the NK1.1 marker. These cells are thought to deliver a death signal to circulating host T cells that migrate through the liver. Their existence may account for "oral tolerance"; it is known that performing a portocaval shunt results in loss of tolerance and development of T- and B-cell responses to food and bacterial antigens.[146] An additional explanation for the liver's resistance to rejection is that the large mass of the liver and donor antigen may lead to a state of immune tolerance caused by immune fatigue, as is reported when animals are injected with massive amounts of antigen.[147] Finally, the liver's regenerative capacity may mask an ongoing slow and mild rejection reaction.

Xenotransplantation

Xenotransplantation, the transplantation of cells, tissues, or organs between members of different species, has emerged as a potential solution to the shortage of human organs.[148] The concept of transplanting animal organs into humans is not new. The first attempt was by a Russian physician in 1682, who reportedly repaired the skull of a wounded nobleman by using a bone from the skull of a dog.[149] In 1964,

TABLE 14.6. *Possible mechanisms of tolerance induction by the liver*

Presence of tolerance-producing leukocytes and molecules
Anatomy of sinusoidal architecture
Decreased expression of MHC class I and class II molecules
Release of MHC class I molecules
Large mass and/or regeneration (masking rejection)

MHC, major histocompatibility complex.

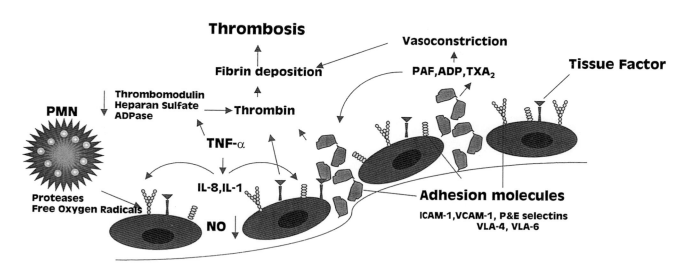

FIG. 14.4. Mechanism of hyperacute rejection in xenotransplantation. IgM, immunoglobulin M; TNF-α, tumor necrosis factor-α; IL, interleukin; NO, nitric oxide; PAF, platelet activating factor; PMN, polymorphonuclear cells; ADP, adenosine diphosphate, TXA$_2$, thromboxane A$_2$; ADPase, adenosine diphosphate degrading enzyme; ICAM-1, intercellular adhesion molecule 1; VCAM-1, vascular cellular adhesion molecule 1.

kidneys from nonhuman primates were transplanted into 13 patients.[150] Most died within days of the procedure, but one patient survived for 9 months on an immunosuppressive regimen of azathioprine, actinomycin C, and steroids. More recently, two patients received liver transplants using livers from baboons. One patient survived for more than 2 months, but ultimately both patients died of sepsis.[151]

The preferred source of the xenograft is a concordant species that is closely related to the recipient (e.g., a nonhuman primate). Discordant xenotransplantation (e.g., from pig to human) involves widely divergent species. Although it is immunologically much easier to achieve xenograft acceptance across concordant combinations, the widespread use of primates as donors poses a number of problems, including ethical issues, limited availability of the primate species, and the risk of infections (xenozoonosis).

The use of pigs as donors is attractive because of their similar size and physiology, their large litter size and short maturation period, and the fact that they are already used as a food source for humans. A disadvantage of performing pig-to-human discordant transplants is the occurrence

of hyperacute rejection due to the presence of preformed xenoreactive antibodies in humans, resulting in organ loss within minutes to hours of grafting.[152]

Hyperacute rejection is initiated by the binding of IgM and IgG antibodies present in humans to the carbohydrate epitope Gal-α-1,3-Gal, which is expressed as a terminal modification of glycoproteins on all cells of the pig (Fig. 14.4).[153] The binding of antibody results in activation of complement, which leads to platelet activation and massive thrombosis.[154] To overcome HAR, a number of approaches have been adopted, including the use of complement inhibitors such as cobra venom factor and the use of absorption columns to remove xenoreactive antibodies.[148] In general, these approaches have only modified HAR and not prevented it. The creation of pigs transgenic for human regulatory complement genes (decay accelerating factor, or DAF) has largely prevented HAR.[155] However, an additional hurdle that will need to be addressed will be strategies to prevent acute vascular rejection caused by antibody deposition and activation of macrophages, NK cells, and endothelial cells that results in loss of grafts at 14 to 30 days

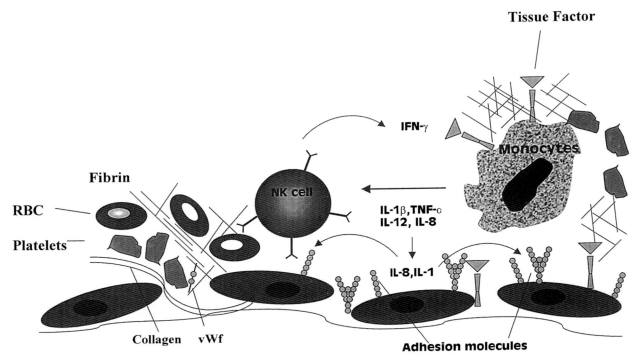

FIG. 14.5. Mechanism of delayed xenograft rejection. VWF, von Willebrand factor; IL, interleukin; TNF, tumor necrosis factor; IFN, interferon.

after transplantation due to thrombosis, a process termed delayed xenograft rejection (DXR) (Fig. 14.5).[156] To date, the use of organs from animals transgenic for DAF has demonstrated the ability to prevent HAR and modify DXR. Further preclinical work will be required prior to initiating clinical studies in humans.

Once these hurdles are overcome, the importance of acute cellular or humoral rejection will need to be evaluated, as well as the potential of present immunosuppressive regimens to prevent graft loss. An approach to reducing immunogenicity will be to induce tolerance by transfer of donor hematopoietic cells prior to or coincident with the transplant procedure to establish microchimerism as described previously.

As transplantation waiting lists continue to lengthen because of a shortage of donor organs, the death rates while on waiting lists continue to rise as well. Xenotransplantation offers the potential for an unlimited supply of healthy donor organs. The barriers to xenotransplantation, including HAR, DXR, cellular and humoral rejection, potential xenozoonosis, physiologic incompatibilies, and ethical concerns, will need to be addressed prior to successful implementation of this exciting new technology.

REFERENCES

1. Munoz SJ. Long-term management of the liver transplant recipient. *Med Clin North Am* 1996;90:1103–1120.
2. Maddrey WC, Van Thiel DH. Liver transplantation: an overview. *Hepatology* 1988;8:948–959.
3. Chung SW, Greig PD, Cattral M, et al. Evaluation of liver transplantation for high-risk indications. *Br J Surg* 1997;84:189–195.
4. Wiesner RH for the U.S. FK506 Study Group. A long-term comparison of tacrolimus (FK506) versus cyclosporine in liver transplantation. *Transplantation* 1998;66:493–499.
5. Wiesner RH, Demetris AJ, Belle SH, et al. Acute hepatic allograft rejection: incidence, risk factors, and impact on outcome. *Hepatology* 1998;28:638–645.
6. Wiesner RH, Ludwig J, van Hoek B, et al. Current concepts in cell-mediated hepatic allograft rejection leading to ductopenia and liver failure. *Hepatology* 1991;14:721–729.
7. Krams SM, Ascher NL, Martinez OM. New immunologic insights into mechanisms of allograft rejection. *Gastroenterol Clin North Am* 1993;22:381–400.
8. Lu CY, Penfield JG, Kielar M, et al. Does the injury of transplantation initiate acute rejection? *Graft* 1999;2(2):S36–S41.
9. Bendelac A, Fearon DT. Innate pathways that control acquired immunity. *Curr Opin Immunol* 1997;9:1–3.
10. Medzhitov R, Janeway CA Jr. Innate immunity: impact on the adaptive immune response. *Curr Opin Immunol* 1997;9:4–9.
11. Ibrahim MAA, Chain BM, Katz DR. The injured cell: the role of the dendritic cell system as a sentinel receptor pathway. *Immunol Today* 1995;16:181–186.
12. Pattison JM, Krensky AM. New insights into mechanisms of allograft rejection. *Am J Med Sci* 1997;313:257–263.
13. Hansen TH, Carreno BM, Sachs DH. *The major histocompatibility complex*. New York: Raven Press, 1993:577–628.
14. Germain RN. MHC-dependent antigen processing and peptide presentation. Providing ligands for T cell activation. *Cell* 1994;76:288–299.
15. Scott DM, Ehrmann IE, Ellis PS, et al. Identification of a mouse male-specific transplantation antigen H-Y. *Nature* 1995;376:695–698.
16. Ludwig J. Terminology of hepatic allograft rejection. *Semin Liver Dis* 1992;12:89–92.
17. Platt JL, Fischel RJ, Matas AJ, et al. Immunopathology of hyperacute xenograft rejection in a swine-to-primate model. *Transplantation* 1991;52:214–220.
18. Suthanthiran M, Strom TB. Renal transplantation. *N Engl J Med* 1994;331:365–376.

19. Halloran PF, Melk A, Barth C. Rethinking chronic allograft nephropathy: the concept of accelerated senescence. *J Am Soc Nephrol* 1999; 10:167–181.
20. Paller MS. The cell biology of reperfusion injury in the kidney. *J Invest Med* 1994;42:632–639.
21. Lefer AM. Role of selectins in myocardial ischemia-reperfusion injury. *Ann Thorac Surg* 1995;60:773–777.
22. Entman ML, Smith CW. Post-reperfusion inflammation: a model for reaction to injury in cardiovascular disease. *Cardiovasc Res* 1994;28: 1301–1311.
23. Ibrahim S, Jacobs F, Zukin Y, et al. Immunohistochemical manifestations of unilateral kidney ischemia. *Clin Transplant* 1996;10:646–652.
24. Goes N, Hobart M, Ramassar V, et al. Many forms of renal injury induce a stereotyped response with increased expression of MHC, IFN-gamma, and adhesion molecules. *Transplant Proc* 1997;29:1085.
25. Pober JS, Cotran RS. The role of endothelial cells in inflammation. *Transplantation* 1990;50:537–544.
26. Springer TA. Traffic signals for lymphocyte recirculation and leukocyte emigration. *Cell* 1994;76:301.
27. Austrup F, Vestweber D, Borges E, et al. P- and E-selectin mediate recruitment of T-helper-1, but not T-helper-2 cells into inflamed tissues. *Nature* 1997;385:81–86.
28. Simon DI, Mullins ME, Jia L, et al. Polynitrosylated proteins: characterization, bioactivity and functional consequences. *Proc Natl Acad Sci U S A* 1996;93:4736–4741.
29. Siveke JT, Hamann A. T helper 1 and T helper 2 cells respond differentially to chemokines. *J Immunol* 1998;160:550–554.
30. Krensky AM, Weiss A, Crabtree G, et al. T-lymphocyte-antigen interactions in transplant rejection. *N Engl J Med* 1990;322:510–517.
31. Hansen TH, Carreno BM, Sachs DH. The major histocompatibility complex. In: Paul WE, ed. *Fundamental immunology.* New York: Raven Press, 1993:577–628.
32. Markus BH, Duquesnoy RJ, Blaheta RA, et al. Role of HLA antigens in liver transplantation with special reference to cellular immune reactions. *Langenbecks Arch Surg* 1998;383:87–94.
33. Chitilian HV, Auchincloss H Jr. Studies of transplantation immunology with major histocompatibility complex knockout mice. *J Heart Lung Transplant* 1997;16:153–159.
34. Zinkernagel RM, Doherty PC. Restriction of *in vitro* T cell-mediated cytotoxicity in lymphocytic choriomeningitis within a syngeneic or semiallogeneic system. *Nature* 1974;248:701–702.
35. Bjorkman PJ, Saper MA, Samraoul B, et al. Structure of the human class I histocompatibility antigen, HLA-A2. *Nature* 1987;329:506–512.
36. Sanderson F, Kleijmeer N, Kelly A, et al. Accumulation of HLA-DM, a regulator of antigen presentation, in MHC class II compartments. *Science* 1994;266:1566–1569.
37. Scott DM, Ehrmann IE, Ellis PS, et al. Identification of a mouse male-specific transplantation antigen, H-Y. *Nature* 1995;376:695–698.
38. Germain RN. Antigen processing and presentation. In: Paul WE, ed. *Fundamental immunology.* New York: Raven Press, 1993:629–670.
39. Dubey C, Croft M, Swain SL. Naive and effector CD4 T cells differ in their requirements for T cell receptor versus costimulatory signals. *J Immunol* 1996;157:3280–3289.
40. Hintzen RQ, Lens SMA, Lammers K, et al. Engagement of CD27 with its ligand CD70 provides a second signal for T cell activation. *J Immunol* 1995;154:2612–2623.
41. Lechler R, Batchelor J. Restoration of immunogenicity to passenger cell depleted kidney allografts by the addition of donor strain dendritic cells. *J Exp Med* 1982;155:31–41.
42. Fangmann J, Dalchau R, Fabre JW. Rejection of skin allografts by indirect allorecognition of donor Class I major histocompatibility complex peptides. *J Exp Med* 1992;175:1521–1529.
43. Pober JS, Orosz G, Rose ML, et al. Can graft endothelial cells initiate a host anti-graft immune response? *J Exp Med* 1996;61:343–349.
44. Weiss A, Littman DR. Signal transduction by lymphocyte antigen receptors. *Cell* 1994;76:263–274.
45. Clysstene NA, Crabtree GR. Calcineurin is a key signaling enzyme in T lymphocyte activation and the target of the immunosuppressive drugs cyclosporin A and FK506. *Ann N Y Acad Sci* 1993;696:200–230.
46. Linsley PS, Ledbetter JA. The role of CD28 receptor during T cell responses to antigen. *Ann Rev Immunol* 1993;11:191–212.
47. Boussiotis VA, Gribben JG, Freeman GJ, et al. Blockade of the CD28 co-stimulatory pathway: a means to induce tolerance. *Curr Opin Immunol* 1994;6:797–807.
48. Lenschow DJ, Zeng Y, Thistlewaite JR, et al. Long term survival of xenogeneic pancreatic islet grafts induced by CTLA4Ig. *Science* 1992;257:789–792.
49. Boise LH, Noel PJ, Thompson CB. CD28 and apoptosis. *Curr Opin Immunol* 1995;7:620–625.
50. Waterhouse P, Penninger JM, Timmins E, et al. Lymphoproliferative disorders with early lethality in mice deficient in CTLA-4. *Science* 1995;270:985–988.
51. Shahinian A, Pfeffer K, Lee KP, et al. Differential T-cell costimulatory requirements in CD28-deficient mice. *Science* 1993;261:609–612.
52. Mosmann TR, Coffman RL. Th1 and Th2 cells: different patterns of lymphokine secretion lead to different functional properties. *Ann Rev Immunol* 1989;7:145–173.
53. Zheng XX, Steele AW, Nickerson PW, et al. Administration of noncytolytic IL-10/Fc in murine models of lipopolysaccharide-induced septic shock and allogeneic islet transplantation. *J Immunol* 1995;154: 5590–5600.
54. Cohen JJ, Duke RC, Fadok VA, et al. Apoptosis and programmed cell death in immunity. *Ann Rev Immunol* 1992;10:267–293.
55. Kabelitz D, Pohl T, Pechold K. Activation-induced cell death (apoptosis) of mature peripheral T lymphocytes. *Immunol Today* 1993;14: 338.
56. Solary E, Eymin B, Droin N, et al. Proteases, proteolysis and apoptosis. *Cell Biol Toxicol* 1998;14:121–132.
57. Lipman ML, Stevens AC, Strom TB. Heightened intragraft CTL gene expression in acutely rejecting renal allografts. *J Immunol* 1994;152: 5120–5127.
58. Larsen CF, Alexander DZ, Hendrix R, et al. Fas-mediated cytotoxicity. *Transplantation* 1996;60:221–224.
59. Jaeschke H. Cellular adhesion molecules: regulation and functional significance in the pathogenesis of liver diseases. *Am J Physiol* 1997; 273:G602-G611.
60. McEver RP, Moore KL, Cummings RD. Leukocyte trafficking mediated by selectin-carbohydrate interactions. *J Biol Chem* 1995;270: 11025–11028.
61. Ruoslahti E. Integrins. *J Clin Invest* 1991;87:1–5.
62. Briscoe DM, Yeung A, Schoen EL, et al. Predictive value of inducible endothelial cell adhesion molecule expression for acute rejection of human cardiac allografts. *Transplantation* 1995;59:204–211.
63. Bird G, Friend P, Donaldson P, et al. Hyperacute rejection in liver transplantation: a case report. *Transplant Proc* 1989;21:3742–3744.
64. Mor E, Solomon H, Gibbs JF, et al. Acute cellular rejection following liver transplantation: clinical pathologic features and effect on outcome. *Semin Liver Dis* 1992;12:28–40.
65. Ratner LE, Phelan D, Brunt EM, et al. Probable antibody-mediated failure of two sequential ABO-incompatible hepatic allografts in a single recipient. *Transplantation* 1993;55:814–819.
66. Imagawa DK, Noguchi K, Iwaki Y, et al. Hyperacute rejection following ABO-compatible orthotopic liver transplantation—a case report. *Transplantation* 1992;54:1114–1117.
67. Hubscher SG, Adams DH, Neuberger IM, et al. Massive hemorrhagic necrosis of the liver after transplantation. *J Clin Pathol* 1989;42: 360–370.
68. International panel comprised of Demetris AJ, Batts KP, Dhillon AP, et al. Banff schema for grading liver allograft rejection: an international consensus document. *Hepatology* 1997;25:658–663.
69. Ayres R, Adams D. Acute rejection of human liver allografts. In: Neuberger J, Adams D, eds. *Immunology of liver transplantation.* London: Edward Arnold, 1993:197–215.
70. Guggenheim J, Samuel D, Reynes M, et al. Liver transplantation across ABO blood group barriers. *Lancet* 1990;336:519–523.
71. Demetris AJ, Jaffe R, Tzakis A, et al. Antibody mediated rejection of human orthotopic liver allografts: a study of liver transplantation across ABO blood barriers. *Am J Pathol* 1988;132:489–502.
72. Starzl TE, Demetris AJ, Todo S, et al. Evidence for hyperacute rejection of human liver grafts: the case of the canary kidney. *Clin Transplant* 1989;3:37–45.
73. Gubernatis G, Lauchart W, Jonker M, et al. Signs of hyperacute rejection of liver grafts in rhesus monkeys after donor-specific presensitization. *Transplant Proc* 1987;19:1082–1083.
74. Demetris AJ, Qians S, Hong S, et al. Liver allograft rejection: an overview of morphologic findings. *Am J Surg Pathol* 1990;14:49–63.
75. Gordon RD, Fung JJ, Markus B, et al. The antibody crossmatch in liver transplantation. *Surgery* 1986;100:705–715.

76. Moore SB, Wiesner RH, Perkins JD, et al. A positive lymphocyte crossmatch and major histocompatibility complex mismatching do not predict early rejection of liver transplants in patients treated with cyclosporine. *Transplant Proc* 1987;19:2390–2391.

77. Donaldson PT, Underhill JA, O'Grady JA, et al. Influence of tissue typing on rejection and outcome. In: Rodes J, Arroyo V, eds. *Therapy in liver diseases.* Barcelona: Ediciones Doyma, 1991:189–196.

78. Demetris AJ, Markus BH. Immunopathology of liver transplantation. *CRC Crit Rev Immunol* 1989;2:67–92.

79. Demetris AJ, Murase N, Nakamura K, et al. Immunopathology of antibodies as effectors of orthotopic liver allograft rejection. *Semin Liver Dis* 1992;12:51–59.

80. Ludwig J. Terminology of hepatic allograft rejection [Glossary]. *Semin Liver Dis* 1992;12:89–92.

81. Wiesner RH, Ludwig J, van Hoek B, et al. Current concepts in cell-mediated hepatic allograft rejection leading to ductopenia and liver failure. *Hepatology* 1991;14:721–729.

82. Ludwig J, Batts KP, Ploch M, et al. Endothelitis in hepatic allografts. *Mayo Clin Proc* 1989;64:545–554.

83. Snover DC, Freese DK, Sharp HL, et al. Liver allograft rejection. Analysis of the use of biopsy in determining outcome of rejection. *Am J Surg Pathol* 1987;11:1–10.

84. Krams SM, Martinez OM. Apoptosis as a mechanism of tissue injury in liver allograft rejection. *Semin Liver Dis* 1998;18:153–167.

85. Molajoni ER, Cinti P, Orlandini A, et al. Mechanisms of liver allograft rejection: the indirect recognition pathway. *Hum Immunol* 1997;53: 57–63.

86. Fleming KA, McMichael A, Morton JA, et al. Distribution of HLA class I antigens in normal human tissue and in mammary cancer. *J Clin Pathol* 1981;34:779–784.

87. Steinhoff G, Wonigeit K, Pichlmayr R. Analysis of sequential changes in major histocompatibility complex expression in human liver grafts after transplantation. *Transplantation* 1988;45:394–401.

88. Hubscher SG, Adams DH, Elias E. Changes in expression of major histocompatibility class II antigens in liver allograft rejection. *Transplant Proc* 1990;22:1828–1829.

89. Scholz M, Auth MKH, Markus BH. The immunological role of biliary epithelial cells in human liver transplant rejection. *Transplant Immunol* 1997;5:142–151.

90. Lang T, Krams SM, Berquist W, et al. Elevated biliary interleukin 5 as an indicator of liver allograft rejection. *Transplant Immunol* 1995; 3:291–298.

91. Martinez OM, Krams SM, Sterneck M, et al. Intragraft cytokine profile during human liver allograft rejection. *Transplantation* 1992;53: 449–456.

92. Takeuchi T, Lowry RP, Konieczny B. Heart allografts in murine systems. The differential activation of Th2-like effector cells in peripheral tolerance. *Transplantation* 1992;53:1281–1294.

93. Ferraresso M, Tian L, Ghobrial R, et al. Rapamycin inhibits production of cytotoxic but not noncytotoxic antibodies and preferentially activated T helper 2 cells that mediate long-term survival of heart allografts in rats. *J Immunol* 1994;153:3307–3318.

94. Afford SC, Hubscher S, Strain AJ, et al. Apoptosis in the human liver during allograft rejection and end-stage liver disease. *J Pathol* 1995; 176:373–380.

95. Ludwig J, Wiesner RH, Batts KP, et al. The acute vanishing bile duct syndrome (acute irreversible rejection) after orthotopic liver transplantation. *Hepatology* 1987;7:476–483.

96. Woolf GM, Vierling JM. Disappearing intrahepatic bile ducts: the syndromes and their mechanisms. *Semin Liver Dis* 1993;13:261–275.

97. Lowes JR, Hubscher SG, Neuberger JM. Chronic rejection of the liver allograft. *Gastroenterol Clin North Am* 1993;22:401–420.

98. Demetris AJ, Murase N, Delancy CP, et al. The liver allograft, chronic (ductopenic) rejection, and microchimerism: what can they teach us? *Transplant Proc* 1995;27:67–70.

99. Donaldson P, Underhill J, Doherty D, et al. Influence of human leukocyte antigen matching on liver allograft survival and rejection: "the dualistic effect." *Hepatology* 1993;17:1008–1015.

100. Engui EM, Allison AC. Immunosuppressive activity of mycophenolate mofetil. *Ann N Y Acad Sci* 1993;685:308–329.

101. Allison AC, Engui EM. Purine metabolism and immunosuppressive effects of mycophenolate mofetil (MMF). *Clin Transplant* 1996; 10:77–84.

102. Sollinger HW for the US Renal Transplant Mycophenolate Mofetil Study Group. Mycophenolate mofetil for the prevention of acute rejection in primary cadaveric renal allograft recipients. *Transplantation* 1995;60:225–232.

103. Tricontinental Mycophenolate Mofetil Study Group. A blinded randomized clinical trial of mycophenolate mofetil for the prevention of acute rejection in cadaveric renal transplantation. *Transplantation* 1996;61:1029–1037.

104. Cole E, Landsberg D, Russell D, et al. for the Canadian Zenapax/MMF Renal Study Group. Renal transplantation without steroids—a multicentre Canadian pilot study [Abstract]. *Transplantation* 1999; 67(7):S239.

105. Borel JF, Baumann G, Chapman I, et al. *In vivo* pharmacological effects of ciclosporin and some analogues. *Adv Pharmacol* 1996; 35:115–246.

106. The U.S. Multicenter FK506 Liver Study Group. A comparison of tacrolimus (FK506) and cyclosporine for immunosuppression in liver transplantation. *N Engl J Med* 1994;331:1110–1115.

107. Strepkowski SM. Sirolimus, a potent new immunosuppressive drug for organ transplantation. *Ann Transplant* 1996;1(3):19–25.

108. Kronke M, Leonard WJ, Depper JM, et al. Cyclosporin A inhibits T-cell growth factor gene expression at the level of mRNA transcription. *Proc Natl Acad Sci U S A* 1984;81:5214–5218.

109. Bierer BE. Biology of cyclosporin A and FK506. *Prog Clin Biol Res* 1994;390:203–223.

110. O'Keefe SJ, Tamura J, Kincaid RL, et al. FK-506- and CsA-sensitive activation of the interleukin-2 promoter by calcineurin. *Nature* 1992; 357:692–694.

111. Baumann G, Geisse S, Sullivan M. Cyclosporin A and FK-506 both affect DNA binding of regulatory nuclear proteins to the human interleukin-2 promoter. *New Biol* 1991;3:270–278.

112. Keown P, Kahan BD, Johnston A, et al. Optimization of cyclosporine therapy with new therapeutic drug monitoring strategies. Report from the International Neoral TDM Advisory Consensus Meeting. *Transplant Proc* 1998;30(5):1645–1649.

113. Grant D, Kneteman N, Tchervenkov J, et al. Peak cyclosporine levels (C$_{max}$) correlate with freedom from liver graft rejection. *Transplantation* 1999;67:1133–1177.

114. Klagehpour K, Pyronnet S, Gingras AC, et al. Translational homeostasis: eukaryotic translation initiation factor 4E control of 4E-binding protein 1 and p70 s6 kinase activities. *Mol Cell Biol* 1999;19:4302–4310.

115. Vincenti F. Targeting the interleukin-2 receptor in clinical renal transplantation. *Graft* 1999;2(2):56–61.

116. Waldman TA, Goldman CK. The multichain interleukin-2 receptor: a target for immunotherapy of patients receiving allografts. *Am J Kidney Dis* 1989;14:45–53.

117. Taniguchi T, Minami Y. The IL-2 receptor system: a current overview. *Cell* 1993;75:5–8.

118. Vincenti F, Kirman R, Light S, et al. Interleukin-2-receptor blockade with daclizumab to prevent acute rejection in renal transplantation. *N Engl J Med* 1998;338:161–165.

119. Nashan B, Moor R, Amlot P, et al. Randomised trial of basiliximab versus placebo for control of acute cellular rejection in renal allograft recipients. *Lancet* 1997;350:1193–1198.

120. Koch M, Niemeyer G, Nashan B. Pharmacokinetic and pharmacodynamic evaluation of a two dose daclizumab regimen in liver transplantatation [Abstract]. *Transplantation* 1999;57(7):S31.

121. Lenschow DJ, Zeng Y, Hathcock KS, et al. Inhibition of transplant rejection following treatment with anti-B7–2 and anti-B7–1 antibodies. *Transplantation* 1995;60:1171–1178.

122. Guerette B, Gingras M, Wood K, et al. Immunosuppression with monoclonal antibodies and CTLA4-Ig after myoblast transplantation in mice. *Transplantation* 1996;62:962–967.

123. Kirk AD, Harlan DM, Armstrong NN, et al. CTLA4-Ig and anti-CD40 ligand prevent renal allograft rejection in primates. *Proc Natl Acad Sci U S A* 1997;94:8789–8794.

124. Chiba K, Yanagawa Y, Kataoka H, et al. FTY 720 a novel immunosuppressant induces sequestration of circulating lymphocytes by acceleration of lymphocyte homing. *Transplant Proc* 1999;31: 1230–1233.

125. Kabelitz D. Apoptosis, graft rejection and transplantation tolerance. *Transplantation* 1998;65:869–875.

126. Kisielow P, von Boehmer H. Development and selection of T cells: facts and puzzles. *Adv Immunol* 1995;58:87–209.

127. Dhein J, Walczak H, Baumler C, et al. Autocrine T cell suicide mediated by Apol/(Fas/CD95). *Nature* 1995;373:438–441.

128. Van Parijs, Abbas AK. Homeostasis and self-tolerance in the immune system: turning lymphocytes off. *Science* 1998;280:243–248.
129. Ohashi PS, Oehen S, Buerki K, et al. Ablation of "tolerance" and induction of diabetes by virus infection in viral antigen transgenic mice. *Cell* 1991;65:305–317.
130. Bretscher P, Cohn M. A theory of self-non-self discrimination. *Science* 1970;169:1042–1049.
131. Linsley PS, Ledbetter JA. The role of the CD28 receptor during T cell responses to antigen. *Annu Rev Immunol* 1993;11:191–212.
132. Schwartz RH. A cell culture model for T lymphocyte clonal anergy. *Science* 1990;248:1349–1356.
133. Sloan-Lancaster J, Evavold BD, Allen PM. Induction of T-cell anergy by altered T-cell-receptor ligand on live antigen-presenting cells. *Nature* 1993;363:156–159.
134. Perez VL, Van Parijs L, Biuckians A, et al. Induction of peripheral T cell tolerance *in vivo* requires CTLA-4 engagement. *Immunity* 1997;6(4):411–417.
135. Tivol EA, Borriello F, Schweitzer AN, et al. Loss of CTLA-4 leads to massive lymphoproliferation and fatal multiorgan tissue destruction, revealing a critical negative regulatory role of CTLA-4. *Immunity* 1995;3(5):541–547.
136. Van Parijs L, Biuckians A, Ibragimov A, et al. Functional responses and apoptosis of CD25 (IL-2R alpha)-deficient T cells expressing a transgenic antigen receptor. *J Immunol* 1997;158:3738–3745.
137. Mosmann TR, Sad S. The expanding universe of T-cell subsets: Th1, Th2 and more. *Immunol Today* 1996;17:138–146.
138. Seder RA, Paul WE. Acquisition of lymphokine-producing phenotype by CD4+ T cells. *Annu Rev Immunol* 1994;12:635–673.
139. Wahl SM. Transforming growth factor beta: the good, the bad and the ugly. *J Exp Med* 1994;180:1587–1590.
140. Groux H, O'Garra A, Bigler M, et al. A CD4+ T-cell subset inhibits antigen-specific T-cell responses and prevents colitis. *Nature* 1997;389:737–742.
141. Calne RY, Sells RA, Pena JR, et al. Induction of immunological tolerance by porcine liver allografts. *Nature* 1969;223:472–476.
142. Kamada N. The immunology of experimental liver transplantation in the rat. *Immunology* 1985;55(3):369–389.
143. Kamei T, Callery MP, Flye MW. Pretransplant portal venous administration of donor antigen and portal venous allograft drainage synergistically prolong rat cardiac allograft survival. *Surgery* 1990;108:415–421.
144. Starzl TE, Demetris AJ, Murase N, et al. Cell migration, chimerism and graft acceptance. *Lancet* 1992;339:1579–1582.
145. Buckingham WJ, Grailer AP, Fechner JH Jr, et al. Microchimerism linked to cytotoxic T lymphocyte functional unresponsiveness (clonal anergy) in a tolerant renal transplant recipient. *Transplantation* 1995;59:1147–1155.
146. Crispe IN, Mehal WZ. Strange brew: T cells in the liver. *Immunol Today* 1996;17:522–525.
147. Bishop GA, Sun J, Sheil AG, et al. High-dose/activation-associated tolerance: a mechanism for allograft tolerance. *Transplantation* 1997;64:1377–1382.
148. Sim KH, Marinov A, Levy GA. Xenotransplantation: a potential solution to the critical organ donor shortage. *Can J Gastroenterol* 1999;13:311–318.
149. Lanza RP, Cooper DKC, Chick WL. Xenotransplantation. *Sci Am* 1997;8:54–59.
150. Reemstra K, McCracken BH, Schlegel JU. Renal heterotransplantation in man. *Ann Surg* 1964;160:384–410.
151. Starzl T, Demetris A, Murase N, et al. Cell migration, chimerism and graft acceptance. *Lancet* 1992;339:1579–1582.
152. Nagayasu T, Platt JL. A perspective on xenotransplantation. *Graft* 1999;2(2):S152–S158.
153. Galili U, Clark MR, Shohet SB, et al. Evolutionary relationship between the natural anti-Gal antibody and the Gal α-1–3Gal epitope in primates. *Proc Natl Acad Sci U S A* 1987;84:1369–1373.
154. Platt JL, Fischel RJ, Matas AJ, et al. Immunopathology of hyperacute xenograft rejection in a swine-to-primate model. *Transplantation* 1991;52:214–220.
155. McCurry KR, Kooyman DL, Alvarado CG, et al. Human complement regulatory proteins protect swine-to-primate cardiac xenografts from humoral injury. *Nat Med* 1995;1:423–427.
156. Leventhal JR, Matas AJ, Sun LH, et al. The immunopathology of cardiac xenograft rejection in the guinea pig to rat model. *Transplantation* 1993;56:1–8.

Transplantation of the Liver, edited by Willis C. Maddrey, Eugene R. Schiff, and Michael F. Sorrell. Lippincott Williams & Wilkins, Philadelphia © 2001.

CHAPTER 15

Histopathology of the Liver following Transplantation

Jurgen Ludwig and Jay H. Lefkowitch

As the number of centers offering orthotopic liver transplantation (OLT) has grown, so has our understanding of the spectrum of liver transplant histopathology. Acute rejection continues to be the most common postoperative complication, with 65% of a large cohort of recipients in a recent study developing a first episode within a year of transplantation, usually during the first 6 weeks after surgery.[1] However, other disease processes, including recurrence of the original disease, intercurrent infections, biliary anastomotic problems, and hepatic artery thrombosis, may be present or superimposed on acute rejection, providing the pathologist with significant interpretive challenges (Fig. 15.1).

This chapter reviews the salient liver pathology with which pathologists and clinicians involved in liver transplantation need to be familiar. It incorporates the observations of the senior author (J. L.) based on biopsy findings in 349 patients who underwent 400 liver transplant procedures from 1985 to 1992 at the Mayo Clinic (Rochester, Minnesota).

BIOPSY SCHEDULES

After OLT, liver biopsies are done in all centers whenever needed for the diagnosis of complications or the evaluation of treatment results. In addition, most groups also adhere to a schedule of protocol biopsies to (a) identify conditions that may not have produced clinical symptoms, (b) obtain baseline material for comparison with subsequent evaluations, and (c) study posttransplantation tissue pathology as part of ongoing research projects. In most instances both protocol and nonprotocol specimens are obtained percuta-

neously, but occasionally material is obtained during laparotomies or even through a midline skin window.[2]

At the Mayo Clinic, protocol biopsies are done before removal of the donor liver, at the end of the transplant procedure (day 0), 1 week, 3 weeks, 4 months, and 12 months after transplantation, and then on a yearly basis. The biopsy of the donor liver and the day 0 biopsy are done to record the microscopic appearance of the graft before and after the ischemic phase. Obtaining a biopsy after revascularization can be helpful in assessing possible preservation injury.[3]

METHODS OF SPECIMEN PREPARATION

Biopsy Specimens

All specimens are used for routine light microscopy, but many samples are also submitted for virologic and other microbiological studies. In addition, specimens can be studied immunohistologically, histochemically, and electron microscopically. If only a small specimen has been obtained, routine light microscopy is generally the only examination that should be done; microbiological study is usually the second most important diagnostic method. If sufficient tissue is available, snap-frozen material should be saved in liquid nitrogen for immunochemical or other special studies.

Tissue samples should be subdivided for the described purposes immediately after they have been obtained. As a rule, one sterile portion should be submitted for microbiological study—most commonly for viral cultures. The main portion of the remaining specimen is used for light microscopic study and thus is placed in an all-purpose fixative such as neutral-buffered formalin; another piece can be placed in Zeus' solution (Zeus Scientific, Inc., Raritan, NJ) if preparation of frozen sections for immunostaining is desired. A few additional small samples can be submerged in

J. Ludwig: 25007 Pinewater Cove Lane, Bonita Springs, Florida 34134.

J. H. Lefkowitch: Department of Pathology, College of Physicians and Surgeons of Columbia University, New York, New York 10032.

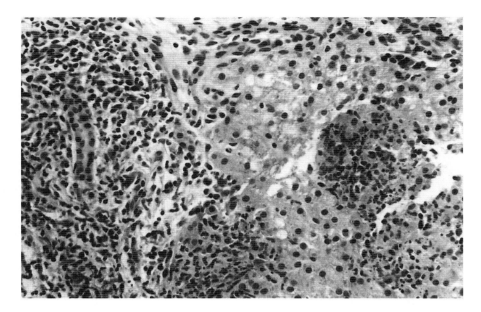

FIG. 15.1. Several pathologic processes are present in this liver biopsy taken from a child several weeks after receiving a pediatric cadaveric liver transplant. The portal tract at left shows acute rejection, with a mononuclear cell infiltrate surrounding and infiltrating the bile duct. At right, a focus of parenchymal necrosis with cellular debris and neutrophils was attributed to adenovirus infection.

refrigerated Trumps' formaldehyde-glutaraldehyde solution or some other fixative suitable for electron microscopic study. Once these samples are embedded for electron microscopy, the actual examination of grids can be deferred to a later time. For the management of transplant patients, routine light microscopy of paraffin-embedded sections will suffice in most instances. Special stains and immunohistochemical stains also have specific indications (Table 15.1).

At the Mayo Clinic and elsewhere, clinicians review all transplant biopsy specimens with their pathologist. In urgent cases, this is done as soon as the specimens are available, before treatment decisions are made. If biopsy diagnoses are needed with special urgency, specimens are prepared with a 2-hour cycle in the Autotechnicon Ultra machine (Technicon Instruments, Tarrytown, NY), resulting in an overall turnaround time of approximately 5 hours. The quality of the preparations is sufficient, but this service is work-intensive

and thus costly. Normally, reports are generated the day after the biopsy procedure.

Frozen sections may be requested for evaluating the suitability of donor livers for transplantation. If large droplet (macrovesicular) fat is present, the pathologist should indicate the degree: mild (30% or less), moderate (30% to 60%) or marked (more than 60%). Livers with marked macrovesicular fat are usually not used because of the high risk of primary graft dysfunction.[4-6] In contrast, small droplet (microvesicular) fatty liver can be used for transplantation.[7] Frozen-section techniques cannot be recommended for other purposes; the slides often do not yield sufficient detail.

Excised Recipient Livers (Native or Explant Livers)

Material for microbiological study should be obtained in the operating room. If preparation of specimen cholangiog-

TABLE 15.1. *Role of special stains in transplant pathology*

Staining method	Posttransplantation lesion sought
Trichrome	Perivenular fibrosis (rejection arteriopathy effect)
	Fibrosing cholestatic hepatitis (portal and periportal fibrosis)
	Portal or periportal fibrosis in recurrent chronic viral hepatitis B or C
Reticulin	Perivenular necrosis (severe rejection or rejection arteriopathy effect)
Iron	Transfusional or hemolytic iron in Kupffer cells; highlights minimal cholestasis that may not be well seen on H&E stain
Victoria blue (or orcein)	Hepatitis B surface antigen
Gomori's methenamine silver	Fungal infections
Immunoperoxidase	
Anti-HBs	Hepatitis B surface antigen
Anti-HBc	Hepatitis B core antigen
Anti-CMV	Cytomegalovirus hepatitis
Anti-HSV	Herpesvirus hepatitis
Antiadenovirus	Adenovirus hepatitis
Anticytokeratin	Bile duct epithelium in possible chronic (ductopenic) rejection

H&E, hemotoxylin and eosin; CMV, cytomegalovirus; HSV, herpes simplex virus.

raphy or angiography is intended, microbiological material should not be excised but should be removed with a biopsy needle because artifactual shunts can easily be created. The specimen is then photographed, weighed, measured, and sliced by the pathologist at intervals of 0.5 to 1.0 cm to optimize identification of unusually large (0.8 cm or greater diameter) nodular lesions that may prove to be macroregenerative nodules (large regenerative nodules), dysplastic nodules, or hepatocellular carcinoma. Tissue from the explant liver or focal lesions may be snap frozen, submitted to institutional tissue banks, and processed for routine histopathologic evaluation.

To prepare formalin-fixed surgical specimens for permanent storage, at the Mayo Clinic a perfusion method for entire livers has been developed.[8] For this procedure, the portal vein, hepatic artery, and hepatic duct are cannulated at the hilum and perfused for 3 days with neutral-buffered formalin solution. It is very helpful if the artery and duct cannulation is done by the surgeon just before the recipient livers are removed; these structures often are transected deep in the hilum and may be difficult to identify in the laboratory. The perfusion should be begun as soon as possible after the specimen has been obtained from the operating room. Good success has been achieved with an apparatus that had been used at the Mayo Clinic for years to perfuse lungs;[9] a pump provides a constant perfusion pressure of 25 to 30 cm of water via a set of stacked plastic formalin containers. The specimen shown in Fig. 15.9B illustrates the results of this method.

Before or after the perfusion procedure, cholangiography or angiography can be done with contrast media such as diatrizoate meglumine and diatrizoate sodium (Renovist II, Squibb & Sons, Princeton, NJ). As mentioned, cross-filling of other systems can occur if artifactual shunts were created during surgery or biopsy.

After fixation the livers are sliced. To obtain smooth and even cut surfaces, a knife with an extra-long blade (e.g., 78 cm) permits most livers to be cut with an uninterrupted pulling motion. The quality of the fixed specimens is excellent and is suitable even for techniques such as scanning electron microscopy.[8]

HISTOLOGIC FINDINGS

Normal Specimens and Minimal Changes

Biopsy specimens from donor livers prior to removal of the graft are normal in most instances. At the end of the transplant procedure (day 0 biopsy), focal liver cell necroses with accumulation of neutrophils ("surgical hepatitis" or "surgical neutrophils"[10]) are often present (see the section entitled "Differential Diagnosis of Histologic Findings after Orthotopic Liver Transplantation"). In a few patients nearly normal specimens are obtained postoperatively and during the following months and years, with only minimal changes found, such as mild ductular proliferation, a

slightly increased number of T cells in the sinusoids and the portal tracts, or an occasional apoptotic (acidophilic or Councilman) body.

The state of tolerance to the engrafted liver in some of these patients can be predicted if there is a low incidence of early rejection and if transplantation has been performed for a nonimmunologic disease.[11] Tolerance is also associated with fewer CD8 and CD3 lymphocytes within the lobules in posttransplantation biopsies.[12] Unfortunately, prolonged absence of important pathologic abnormalities is the exception, found in only 10% to 20% of Mayo Clinic cases.

Bile Flow Impairment

In nonallograft livers, bile flow impairment is nearly always the result of large-duct biliary obstruction. Conditions of this type certainly also occur in allografts, for example, after biliary strictures have developed. However, cholangiographically normal allografts also may show histologic evidence of bile flow impairment, most commonly in the presence of bile leaks or in ischemic cholangitis,[13] preservation injury,[14] and ABO incompatibility.[15,16] Thus, *bile flow impairment* serves as a collective term for both mechanical biliary obstruction and the aforementioned cholangiographically nondiagnostic conditions. They all share the same biopsy manifestations, namely, portal edema, ductular proliferation, and often hepatocanalicular cholestasis, primarily in zone 3.

The histologic diagnosis of bile flow impairment may be complicated by the presence of cellular rejection (see the section "Rejection"). This association was a rather common observation in Mayo Clinic material;[13] it appears that biliary obstruction and possibly other conditions may initiate the immunologic events that lead to rejection (better described as secondary rejection). The diagnosis of bile flow impairment may be complicated further by the presence of functional cholestasis (see the next section). Thus, the bile flow problem may be much less severe than it appears on biopsy. Finally, bile flow impairment may coexist with cholestatic hepatitis of unknown cause; the affected patients often have septicemia and are on multiple drugs. It is often impossible to pinpoint the pathogenetic mechanisms in cases of this type. The presence of bile plugs in the ductules (cholangioles) is rarely a feature of obstruction or rejection but may suggest systemic infection[17,18] or another extrahepatic abnormality.

Functional Cholestasis

Definition

Functional cholestasis is the presence of bile in lobules, with or without feathery degeneration of hepatocytes, occurring in the early posttransplantation period and in the absence of a documented cause such as biliary obstruction or viral infection.

Histologic Findings

Typically, the cholestasis is canalicular and hepatocellular, often with prominent feathery degeneration of the hepatocytes, which may also contain a few Mallory bodies. The cholestasis involves primarily zones 2 and 3 (Fig. 15.2). Because of the associated feathery degeneration, these zones may appear sharply delineated from the uninvolved zone 1 parenchyma. Portal tracts are normal or show mild abnormalities. Rejection changes, if present, do not appear to be related to the cholestasis.

Incidence and Pathogenesis

Cholestasis of this type is common in the first 2 or 3 weeks after OLT. At the Mayo Clinic it was found in 25% of cases. The term *functional cholestasis*[18] has been coined for this condition to connote the transient nature of the findings. The change may reflect a functional adaptation after the graft was damaged by ischemia.[19,20] This condition must not be confused with obstructive cholestasis, a misdiagnosis that might lead to unnecessary invasive procedures.

Unexplained centrilobular cholestasis may also occur months after OLT. Whether the origin of this condition has anything in common with the cause of the early functional cholestasis is not clear.

Ischemic Lesions

Definition

Ischemic lesions consist of bile duct necrosis, nonzonal coagulation necrosis of hepatic tissue, or zonal necrosis, generally involving zone 3 of the lobules. These lesions are caused by impaired blood circulation or unknown mechanisms resulting in or simulating hypoperfusion.

Manifestations of Hepatic Artery Thrombosis and Other Conditions Causing Low Perfusion

Hepatic artery thrombosis occurs in approximately 25% of patients who undergo liver transplantation. Causes include surgical technical problems, preservation-related damage, and vascular rejection. Other livers appear to compensate for the perfusion impairment of the parenchyma but later develop ischemic cholangitis with duct wall necrosis, strictures, or cholangiectases.[13] These lesions may occur alone or in any combination; biopsy specimens from affected patients often show features of bile flow impairment (see previous discussion).

Bile duct necrosis and strictures also may develop after vasoconstriction, arteritis, or arterial thrombosis in humoral (antibody-mediated) rejection (see "Rejection"). The speed with which ischemia develops may affect the types of injury observed. Indeed, in a few patients with hepatic artery thrombosis or stenosis, no evidence of graft damage can be found.

Small subcapsular anemic infarctions are a common finding[21] (Fig. 15.3) and in most instances are inconsequential. Thus, biopsy evidence of infarcted hepatic tissue does not necessarily imply that the graft is doomed. Nevertheless, multilobular anemic or hemorrhagic infarctions are always alarming findings, and their presence is an indication for further clinical studies.

Primary Graft Dysfunction

Primary graft dysfunction (PGD) usually occurs in the first week after OLT, generally in the absence of demonstrable vascular occlusions or other obvious causes. The presence of hypertensive arteriopathy in the donor liver may be an exception in this regard.[22] The degree of graft dysfunction varies from minor abnormalities to primary nonfunction.[5]

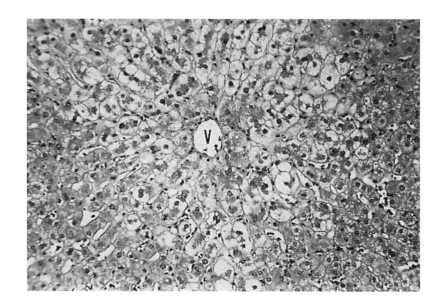

FIG. 15.2. Functional cholestasis with prominent feathery degeneration of hepatocytes in zones 2 and 3 of the acinus, 7 days after orthotopic liver transplantation. Zone 1, at the sides of the figure, appears normal. This lesion is usually transient. *V* indicates the terminal hepatic vein (central vein).

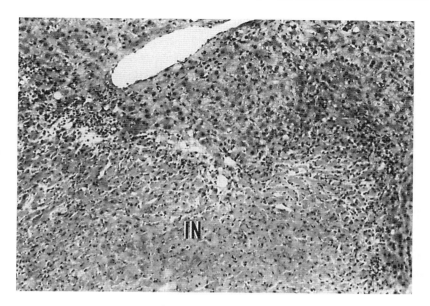

FIG. 15.3. Ischemic infarction (*IN*) with loss of nuclear staining of hepatocytes, 1 month after orthotopic liver transplantation. Note inflammatory cells at the edge of the lesion. Such infarctions may be an incidental finding.

In the most severe cases, the mortality rate without retransplantation is in the neighborhood of 80%. PGD is reported to occur in up to 7% of transplants.[5]

Biopsy specimens are reminiscent of diffuse ischemic coagulation necrosis, but the degree of necrosis tends to be lower than in anemic infarctions (Fig. 15.4), and the portal tracts remain intact. Again, imaging procedures are required to reliably distinguish localized infarctions from subtotal infarctions or massive necrosis of unknown cause.

The pathogenesis of PGD is related to a number of factors, including, prominently, ischemia-reperfusion injury with resulting production of reactive oxygen species; cytokine release through neutrophil, Kupffer cell, and endothelial interactions; and the type of graft perfusate solution used.[5] A significant correlation appears to exist between increasing donor age and increasing incidence of primary graft dysfunction. Intraoperative coagulopathy, metabolic acidosis, and bicarbonate administration also appear to increase the likelihood of early graft failure.[23]

Rejection

Allograft rejection is the most common indication for liver biopsy after OLT. The histopathologic features of the condition are well recognized.[24–38] An international working party that met at the World Congress of Gastroenterology in 1994 published a summary document describing the terminology, histopathologic lesions, and clinical and laboratory findings

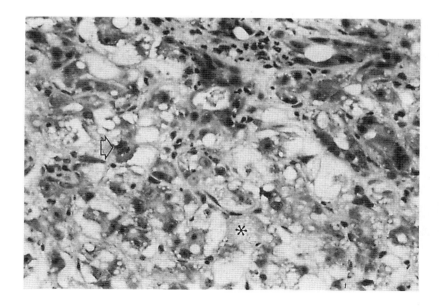

FIG. 15.4. Massive hepatic necrosis (primary nonfunction of the graft) with early regenerative changes, including formation of neocholangioles and the presence of hepatocellular mitoses (*arrow*). Necrotic hepatocytes with vacuolated cytoplasm and lysed nuclei are still present (*asterisk*). The cause of the necrosis is not clear. Postmortem liver biopsy specimen, 6 days after orthotopic liver transplantation.

seen in the three major forms of rejection: humoral (antibody-mediated), acute (cellular), and chronic (ductopenic) rejection.[39] All types of allograft rejection are clinical and pathologic conditions that result from immune responses of the host against the graft. Bile duct epithelial cells and endothelium are the main targets of the immune response. The process of rejection leads to graft dysfunction or failure by complex mechanisms.[29]

Humoral (Antibody-Mediated) Rejection

Humoral rejection occurs either immediately (hyperacute rejection) or within the first week after transplantation. Specimens typically show coagulative and hemorrhagic necrosis. Fibrin thrombi are found in arteries and veins in some instances, but neutrophilic or necrotizing arteritis may also be present. Immunofluorescence and immunoperoxidase studies show linear deposits of immunoglobulin (Ig) G or IgM in arteries, veins, and portal endothelium (although only IgG deposits appear to be of importance[31]). C3, C4, and C1q may be demonstrable by the same methods.

The diagnosis can be confirmed by demonstrating donor-specific antibodies in the grafts; in rejection-unrelated primary graft dysfunction, these antibodies are not demonstrable. The antibodies are either preformed or develop after transplantation and may be directed against HLA antigens, ABO antigens, or endothelium.[39] It should be noted that some presensitized (crossmatch-positive) patients respond only mildly, despite the presence of the preformed IgG donor lymphocytotoxic antibodies. In these cases, specimens show mixed inflammatory infiltrates in portal tracts with venulitis and cholangiolitis; platelet margination

is found in terminal hepatic veins and sinusoids. Swelling of centrilobular hepatocytes, as in functional cholestasis (see previous discussion) may develop, and cellular rejection may also ensue.[31]

Acute (Cellular) Rejection

Acute rejection is an immune cell-mediated injury characterized by the triad of (a) portal inflammatory infiltrates, (b) nonsuppurative cholangitis, and (c) endotheliitis or phlebitis of the portal or hepatic vein branches (Figs. 15.5 through 15.7). Endotheliitis is not present in all cases. The inflammatory infiltrates typically consist of CD4 and CD8 lymphocytes, a few B lymphocytes, plasma cells, and large granular lymphocytes; neutrophils may abound (Fig. 15.6B). In many instances eosinophils are a conspicuous component and are helpful diagnostic evidence that an acute rejection infiltrate is present.[32,40,41] Inflammatory cells in mitosis may also be found. If inflammatory cells accumulate in the sinusoids, they are usually CD8 cells.

In most instances of acute rejection, interlobular bile ducts display features of nonsuppurative cholangitis (Fig. 15.5). The bile duct epithelial changes range from mild reactive nuclear pleomorphism to altered cell polarity, pyknosis and cytoplasmic vacuolization, increased mitotic activity, and, in the most severe cases, bile duct destruction. Inflammatory cells are present in close proximity to bile duct epithelium or invade the epithelium through the basement membrane.

Portal veins as well as terminal hepatic veins (central veins), intercalated veins, and interlobular veins may show adherence of lymphocytes and sometimes of other

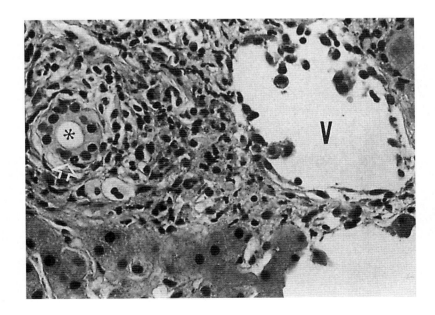

FIG. 15.5. Portal tract with characteristic features of acute rejection, 13 days after orthotopic liver transplantation. Note the mixed inflammatory infiltrates, the nonsuppurative cholangitis, and the endotheliitis. The interlobular bile duct (*asterisk*) shows pyknosis and cytoplasmic vacuolation of epithelial cells. The wall has been invaded by a neutrophil and a lymphocyte (*arrow*). The portal vein (*V*) shows typical endotheliitis (compare with Fig. 15.7).

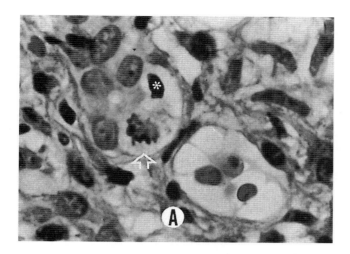

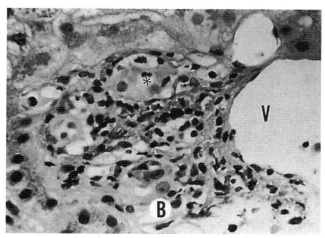

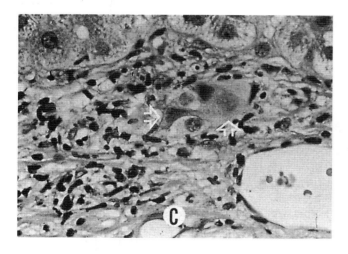

FIG. 15.6. Interlobular bile ducts with features of rejection cholangitis. **A:** Note mitosis of one epithelial cell (*arrow*), and cytoplasmic vacuolation with pyknosis (*asterisk*) of the adjacent cell. Four and a half months after orthotopic liver transplantation (OLT). **B:** Vacuolation and pyknosis of ductal epithelial cells and invasion of the duct wall by inflammatory cells (*asterisk*). Note the neutrophils in and around the duct; this feature may make it difficult to distinguish rejection from biliary obstruction (see Fig. 15.12) or infection. *V* indicates the portal vein. Two months after OLT. **C:** Duct destruction with pyknosis and lytic necrosis of epithelial cells (*arrows*). The lesions are from the same specimen as **(B),** but obtained 1 week after OLT.

inflammatory cells to the endothelial surfaces (Figs. 15.5 and 15.7A, C, and D). This condition has been named *endotheliitis*. If inflammatory cells have invaded the wall of the vein, phlebitis is present (Fig. 15.7B). Each condition may occur with or without the other. Immunocytes attach themselves to the endothelium with a single stalk

(Fig. 15.7A and C) or with pseudopods (Fig. 15.7D), or they accumulate just under the endothelial cells; even eosinophils can be found at this site. Endotheliitis is not diagnostic of only rejection, but can be seen in acute and chronic viral hepatitis and other conditions as well[33] (Fig. 15.7E). Arteritis at the level of the interlobular bile ducts

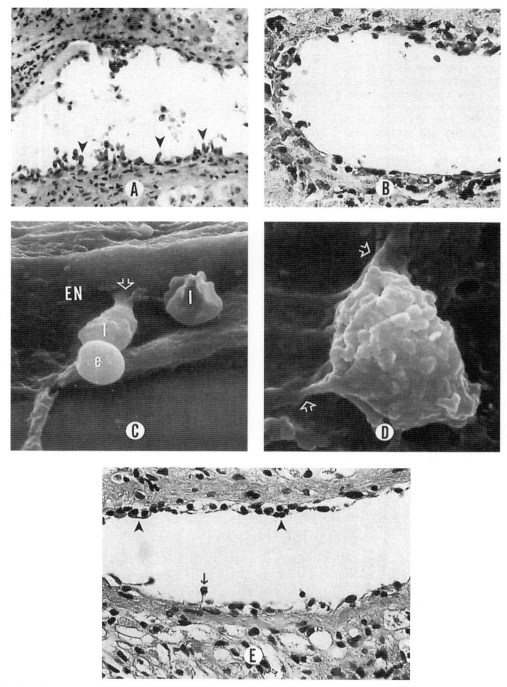

FIG. 15.7. Rejection **(A–D)** and nonrejection **(E)** endotheliitis and phlebitis. **A:** Interlobular vein with characteristic features of rejection endotheliitis. Note immunocytes (*arrowheads*) that have attached themselves to the endothelial lining of the vein. Many immunocytes appear elongated, with their longest axis perpendicular to the wall of the vein. Two weeks after orthotopic liver transplantation (OLT). **B:** Interlobular vein with endotheliitis/phlebitis. Note that most immunocytes have invaded the subendothelial layer of the wall (phlebitis). Only a few cells have remained attached to the luminal side of the endothelium (endotheliitis). This process is probably more advanced than the condition shown in **(A)**. Three months after OLT. **C:** Scanning electron micrograph of immunocytes (*I*) in endotheliitis, 2 months after OLT. Note the polypoid shape of the elongated immunocyte attached to the endothelium (*EN*) by a narrow stalk (*arrow*); these cells closely resemble those shown in **(A)**. One immunocyte is partially obscured by an erythrocyte (*e*). Original magnification, ×3000. **D:** Scanning electron micrograph of immunocyte with pseudopodia (*arrows*) that are anchored to the endothelium. Breakage lines in pseudopodia (top and bottom) are artifacts. Original magnification, ×10,000. **E:** Nonrejection endotheliitis/phlebitis in the native liver at the time of transplantation for subfulminant viral hepatitis. Note the presence of lymphocytes and possibly other mononuclear cells attached to (*arrow*) and under (*arrowheads*) the endothelial lining.

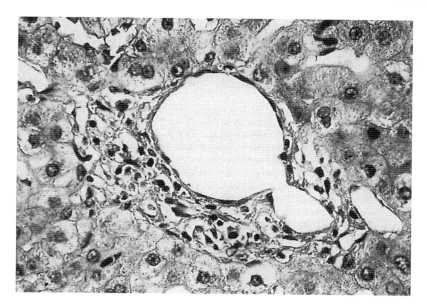

FIG. 15.8. Chronic (ductopenic) rejection, 6 weeks after orthotopic liver transplantation. This portal tract shows only very mild inflammation, but neither a bile duct nor an artery branch can be identified (ductopenia and arteriopenia, respectively). The portal vein appears distended. Note the absence of endotheliitis. Retransplantation was required shortly thereafter.

may rarely be found and may be associated with a poor prognosis.[24]

Chronic (Ductopenic) Rejection

Chronic rejection is characterized in the majority of cases by loss of interlobular bile ducts in 50% or more of portal tracts (Fig. 15.8) accompanied by arteriopathy affecting hepatic artery branches at the hilum (Fig. 15.9). In less than 15% of cases of chronic rejection, either ductopenia or arteriopathy is present independently.[42] Rare cases of recovery from chronic rejection may occur.[43] Cytokeratin immunostaining may be necessary in attempting to identify bile duct epithelium amidst portal tract inflammatory infiltrates.[27] Atrophy and pyknosis of bile duct epithelium are also features of chronic rejection.[44] In advanced chronic rejection, inflammatory infiltrates tend to fade, and absence of bile duct epithelium in proximity to hepatic artery branches is conspicuous. The term *vanishing bile duct syndrome* has been used as a synonym in this context. The parenchyma usually shows severe cholestasis. Chronic rejection usually develops 60 days or later following transplantation, but may rarely occur after only a few weeks. Ductopenia and vascular rejection have also been reported in association with venoocclusive lesions and massive hemorrhagic necrosis of the allograft.[37]

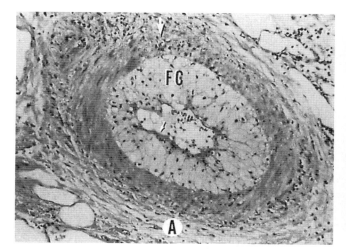
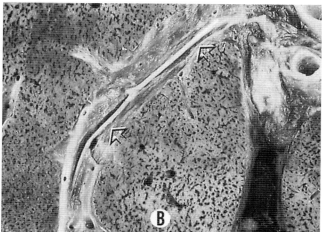

FIG. 15.9. Rejection arteriopathy. **A:** Septal artery, 3 months after orthotopic liver transplantation. Note the accumulation of foam cells (*FC*) in the intima. Mild arteritis with a few inflammatory cells can be identified near the endothelium and in the media (*arrows*). **B:** Segmental hepatic artery in a formalin-perfused recipient liver after retransplantation for chronic rejection. The vessel measured approximately 1.5 mm in diameter and is bright yellow (*arrows*) because of the accumulation of foam cells. This graft had been implanted only 2 months earlier.

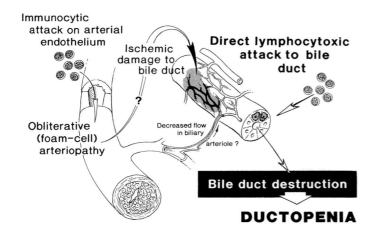

FIG. 15.10. Mechanisms of bile duct destruction leading to chronic rejection. The immunologic attack on the right is a proven feature, whereas the role of ischemia is still controversial; it may be an important factor in some instances. (From Wiesner RH, Ludwig J, Van Hoei B, et al. Current concepts in cell-mediated hepatic allograft rejection leading to ductopenia and liver failure. *Hepatology* 1991;14:725, with permission.)

Rejection arteriopathy is characterized by the accumulation of foam cells (lipid-laden macrophages) in the intima of the affected vessels. The process often leads to extreme narrowing of the vascular lumina. Inflammatory cells may be found in the wall and near the endothelial surface (Fig. 15.9A), but in other instances no arteritic changes can be identified. Because of the lipid, the affected arteries appear bright yellow (Fig. 15.9B). Rejection arteriopathy is rarely recognized clinically because the affected arteries are generally too large to be seen in biopsy specimens and too small to be identified in arteriograms. Its presence may be inferred when zone 3 necrosis or fibrosis, or both, is present on biopsy in the appropriate time frame for chronic rejection. Apart from its prognostic significance, vascular rejection might be important because of its possible role in the development of bile duct ischemia and necrosis.[13,25] Also, vascular rejection might be responsible for the arteriopenia found in small portal tracts of some allografts with the features of vanishing bile duct syndrome.[30,38] The possible effect of rejection arteriopathy on a bile duct is shown in Fig. 15.10. Figure 15.11 summarizes the possible outcomes of rejection cholangitis.

Grading of Acute Rejection

A meeting of an international panel of hepatologists and pathologists in Banff, Canada, in 1995 resulted in the 1997 publication of a schema for grading acute rejection[45] that has been widely adopted for use. By assigning scores of 1, 2, or 3, in order of increasing severity, for each of the components of the rejection triad, a total Rejection Activity Index (RAI) can be reported for a given biopsy specimen showing acute rejection (Table 15.2). The descriptive terms of mild, moderate, or severe rejection can be combined with the semiquantitative score and its subcomponents in the diagnostic formulation (e.g., "Mild acute rejection, Banff RAI = 4 [2 + 1 + 1]").

Bile Duct Obstruction

Postoperative obstruction of the bile duct anastomosis may result in fever and rising serum bilirubin and alkaline phosphatase levels. Liver biopsy in such cases shows portal edema, proliferating bile ductules, and neutrophil infiltrates (Fig. 15.12). Superimposed infiltrates of acute rejection may also be present, but the proliferating bile duct structures should alert the pathologist that the status of the bile duct anastomosis needs to be evaluated cholangiographically.

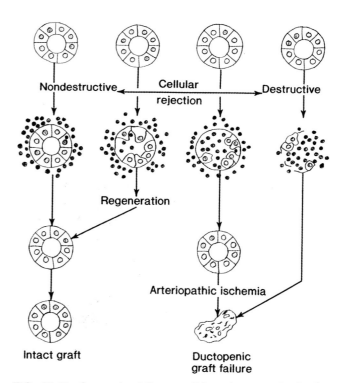

FIG. 15.11. Synopsis of the possible outcomes of rejection cholangitis. The two sequences on the left illustrate mild and moderately severe rejection cholangitis with recovery. The third sequence shows temporary recovery of the duct with subsequent ischemic necrosis, as illustrated in Fig. 15.10. As indicated in the text, this sequence is hypothetical. The sequence on the right shows irreversible immunocytic destruction of the bile duct, without an ischemic component.

TABLE 15.2. *Banff scoring system for acute rejection*

Category	Criteria	Score
Portal inflammation	Mostly lymphocytic inflammation involving, but not noticeably expanding, a minority of the triads.	1
	Expansion of all or most of the triads by a mixed infiltrate containing lymphocytes with occasional blasts, neutrophils, and eosinophils.	2
	Marked expansion of most or all of the triads by a mixed infiltrate containing numerous blasts and eosinophils with inflammatory spillover into the periportal parenchyma.	3
Bile duct inflammation damage	A minority of the ducts are cuffed and infiltrated by inflammatory cells and show only mild reactive changes such as increased nuclear-to-cytoplasmic ratio of the epithelial cells.	1
	Most or all of the ducts are infiltrated by inflammatory cells. More than an occasional duct shows degenerative changes such as nuclear pleomorphism, disordered polarity, and cytoplasmic vacuolization of the epithelium.	2
	Same as for a score of 2, with most or all of the ducts showing degenerative changes or focal luminal disruption.	3
Venous endothelial inflammation	Subendothelial lymphocytic infiltration involving some, but not a majority, of the portal and/or hepatic venules.	1
	Subendothelial infiltration involving most or all of the portal and/or hepatic venules.	2
	Same as for a score of 2, with moderate or severe perivenular inflammation that extends into the perivenular parenchyma and is associated with perivenular hepatocyte necrosis.	3

Total score equals the sum of the components.

From Demetris AJ, Batts KP, Dhillon AP, et al. Banff schema for grading liver allograft rejection: an international consensus document. *Hepatology* 1997;25:658–663, with permission.

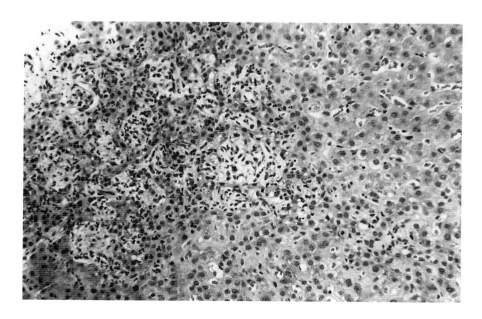

FIG. 15.12. Large bile duct obstruction after liver transplantation. The portal tract at left is expanded by edema and inflammatory cells, predominantly neutrophils. Note the many proliferating bile ductular structures. The integrity of the surgical biliary anastomosis in this case had been of clinical concern prior to this biopsy.

Infection

Infection is the most common fatal complication of liver transplantation, particularly in the first 3 months postoperatively. However, in most instances the infections affect extrahepatic sites,[46] not the allograft.

Viral Infections

By far the most common biopsy finding in this category is cytomegalovirus (CMV) hepatitis, typically characterized by the presence of inclusion bodies in epithelial (Fig. 15.13) or mesenchymal cells. If inclusions cannot be identified, the next best diagnostic method for the detection of CMV antigen is probably immunohistochemistry; a third choice is *in situ* DNA hybridization.[47]

The greatest risk for developing CMV hepatitis exists for recipients who are CMV negative and who receive CMV-infected allografts. Treatment with antilymphocytic sera is another risk factor.[48] Although the role of CMV infection in chronic rejection has been debated,[49,50] *in situ* DNA hy-

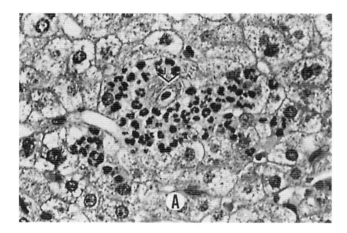

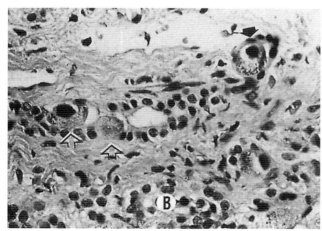

FIG. 15.13. Cytomegalovirus hepatitis. **A:** Swollen hepatocyte with nuclear inclusion body (*arrow*) surrounded by a cluster of neutrophils, 3 weeks after orthotopic liver transplantation (OLT). **B:** Interlobular bile duct with nuclear inclusion bodies (*arrows*), 2 months after OLT.

bridization studies for the CMV genome in allografts removed for chronic rejection have shown persistent CMV infection in bile duct epithelium and in endothelium.[51]

Adenoviral infections must also be considered, but only in pediatric liver transplant patients.[52] Nonzonal necroses (Fig. 15.1), mixed inflammatory infiltrates, and intranuclear viral inclusion bodies are found. Immunostains may be helpful.

Epstein-Barr virus (EBV) infection of the allograft may also cause hepatitis with persistent graft dysfunction.[53–56] Typically, portal tracts and random areas within the acini are infiltrated by rather monotonous-appearing immunoblasts, with or without intermixed plasma cells and macrophages (Fig. 15.14). Cholangitis may be present but tends to be mild,[53,54] which helps distinguish this condition from cellular rejection. This is particularly important because endotheliitis may also be a feature of EBV hepatitis. If immunosuppressive treatment is not reduced in a patient with EBV hepatitis, a lymphoproliferative disorder with features of non-Hodgkin's lymphoma may develop; the tumor cells generally have B-cell markers. All transitions within the spectrum of EBV hepatitis and frank lymphoma can be observed.[57] Semiquantitative polymerase chain reaction for EBV DNA, *in situ* hybridization for EBV RNA, and immunoperoxidase for EBV latent membrane protein are available for excluding EBV infection; the first two tests are the most sensitive.[58]

Finally, hepatitis B and C may affect allografts, either as *de novo* infections or, more often, as recurrent disease. As with CMV, the transplanted graft can transmit hepatitis B or C.[59] These conditions are discussed later, in the section "Recurrence of Pretransplantation Liver Disease."

Bacterial Infections

Most bacterial infections are extrahepatic and caused by Enterobacteriaceae.[46] In the liver, bile ducts are the most likely site of infection. However, bacterial cholangitis, with or without cholangitic abscesses, is no longer a common finding, except in patients who developed ischemic cholangitis.[13] Thus, evidence of bacterial cholangitis may be a manifestation of hepatic artery thrombosis or other vascular abnormalities. Neutrophilic cholangitis and portal edema are characteristic biopsy findings. Hepatic infarcts, in the same setting, may also become the site of bacterial superinfection. Metastatic abscesses in septicemia are generally autopsy findings, not biopsy features.

Fungal Infections

Fungal infections are common in immunosuppressed patients but quite rare in biopsy specimens from allografts. However, systemic fungal infections have been described in many patients who died, particularly in the first months after OLT. The most common organisms in this setting were *Aspergillus fumigatus* and *Candida* species, in that order.[46,60]

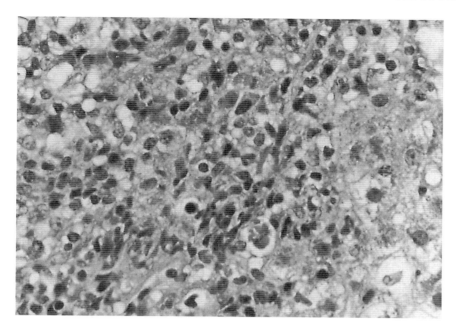

FIG. 15.14. Epstein-Barr virus hepatitis, 1 year 4 months after orthotopic liver transplantation. An immunoblastic intralobular infiltrate is intermixed with plasma cells and macrophages. The vacuolation in the background was caused by (unrelated) focal fatty change of the hepatocytes.

Recurrence of Pretransplantation Liver Disease

Hepatic allografts are subject to recurrence of many of the liver diseases for which transplantation was undertaken.[61] In some of these conditions, such as primary biliary cirrhosis and chronic hepatitis C, the histopathologic features overlap with lesions seen in acute rejection. This poses diagnostic challenges for the pathologist.

Viral Hepatitis

Hepatitis B

Hepatitis B recurs in the majority of patients who have had OLT because of chronic hepatitis B, although immunopro-

phylaxis has improved the rate and severity of recurrence.[62] The most severe forms of recurrent hepatitis B are observed in the first year after OLT and sometimes as early as the second month after transplantation. In fibrosing cholestatic hepatitis, biopsy specimens show abundant hepatitis B surface antigen and hepatitis B core antigen, together with lobular inflammation, cholestasis, bridging necrosis, and fibrosis.[63–68] In most instances, this leads to graft loss. After retransplantation the process may repeat itself at an accelerated pace (subfulminant recurrent hepatitis B[62]). The cases of recurrent hepatitis B that usually occur in the second year after OLT generally do not differ from those in nontransplantation patients. The recurrent hepatitis may be mild or severe, with or without cirrhosis. Carrier states (Fig. 15.15)

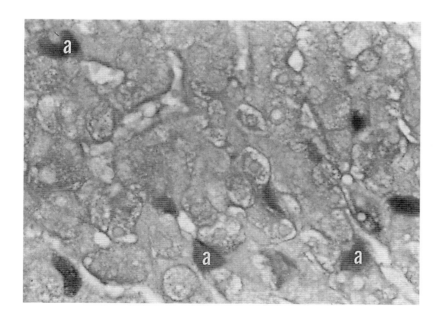

FIG. 15.15. Carrier state for hepatitis B virus. Note the hepatitis B surface antigen (*a*) in the cytoplasm of hepatocytes, in the absence of any inflammatory changes. This infection was acquired after orthotopic liver transplantation for primary sclerosing cholangitis 1 year earlier. Shikata's orcein stain.

with stainable antigen but without hepatitis may occur.[69] At the Mayo Clinic, carrier states have been observed mostly in patients who became infected in the posttransplantation period.

Hepatitis B and D

The hepatitis D virus (HDV) tends to reinfect the graft within weeks or a few months after OLT, but appreciable hepatitis with abundant immunostainable HDV antigen develops only after hepatitis B virus has become detectable. The coinfection with HDV often seems to improve the prognosis of recurrent hepatitis B.[70]

Hepatitis C

Most allografts of patients transplanted for end-stage liver disease due to hepatitis C virus (HCV) become reinfected with the virus, but in comparison with hepatitis B, recurrent hepatitis C is a much milder disease.[71–73] It often appears only toward the end of the first year or in the second year after OLT. Mild periportal hepatitis with lymphoid aggregates, with or without fatty change, is the most common biopsy presentation (Fig. 15.16). Fatty change alone may be an early marker of recurrence.[74] Lymphoid cholangitis and endotheliitis may also be found, and in these instances recurrent hepatitis C may be difficult to distinguish from acute rejection. In difficult cases, polymerase chain reaction allows identification of HCV RNA in biopsy tissue. This test is particularly important in cases without hepatitis C antibodies.[75] A small subgroup of patients with recurrent hepatitis C with unusually severe cholestatic disease has been reported.[76,77] The hepatic lesions in such cases include confluent necrosis, hepatocellular ballooning, bridging fibrosis, bile ductular proliferation, and cirrhosis. If HCV infection is acquired with the transplant,[59] the biopsy changes also tend to be mild.[78,79]

Primary Biliary Cirrhosis

Primary biliary cirrhosis (PBC) probably recurs in 10% to 20% of patients who undergo transplantation, but the course of the disease is quite mild. A few instances of recurrent cirrhosis have been reported,[80] but in the Mayo Clinic experience actual cirrhosis has not yet been encountered in any of these patients. Because chronic nonsuppurative destructive cholangitis of PBC shares many features with rejection, the presence of granulomatous cholangitis (florid duct lesion) is the only morphologically confirmatory finding (Fig. 15.17). It should be noted that mitochondrial antibodies may persist after transplantation for PBC, without evidence of recurrent disease. Several patients who underwent transplantation for PBC have later developed autoimmune hepatitis, with positive serum autoantibodies and lymphoplasmacytic periportal hepatitis on biopsy.[81]

Primary Sclerosing Cholangitis

Following transplantation, cholangiograms may suggest recurrence of primary sclerosing cholangitis (PSC), but other conditions, such as anastomotic obstruction or ischemia, may produce similar changes. However, using strict inclusion and exclusion criteria, a recent Mayo Clinic series found a PSC recurrence rate of 20%.[82] The most reliable

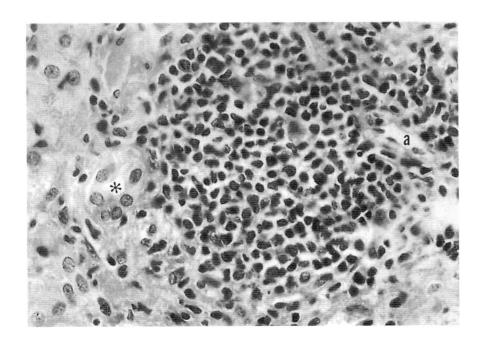

FIG. 15.16. Recurrent hepatitis C, 4 years 9 months after orthotopic liver transplantation. Note the typical lymphoid aggregate in the portal tract. The hepatic artery branch (*a*) is partially obscured by the infiltrate, but the interlobular bile duct (*asterisk*) appears to be intact. The intralobular fatty change cannot be appreciated in this field.

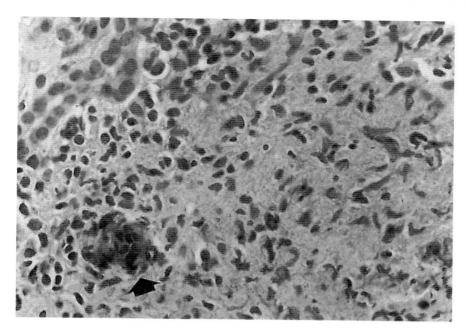

FIG. 15.17. Recurrent primary biliary cirrhosis, 3 years 2 months after orthotopic liver transplantation. Portal tract with noncaseating epithelioid cell granuloma is seen adjacent to an inflamed interlobular bile duct (*arrow*) with severely damaged epithelium. An intact ductule (cholangiole) is visible to the left of the granulomatous cholangitis (florid duct lesion).

histopathologic evidence of recurrent PSC is fibroobliterative cholangitis.

Autoimmune Hepatitis

Although uncommon, autoimmune hepatitis may recur after OLT.[61] Elevated serum globulins, serum autoantibodies, and aminotransferase levels are important in establishing the diagnosis. In children, recurrent autoimmune hepatitis can be especially aggressive, leading to cirrhosis within a year of transplantation.[83] The presence of periportal lymphoplasmacytic hepatitis on liver biopsy is consistent with recurrent disease, particularly if serologic markers of hepatitis virus infection are negative. In some cases, lobular hepatitis may be the first sign of recurrent autoimmune hepatitis.[84]

Metabolic Diseases

If the enzyme defect is situated in the liver, OLT will cure the disease without recurrence. Examples are α_1-antitrypsin deficiency, Wilson's disease, type 1 hyperoxaluria, hemophilias A and B, and tyrosinemia.[31] In contrast, OLT does not effect a complete cure in type IV glycogen storage disease, familial hypercholesterolemia, and erythropoietic protoporphyria. Indeed, in erythropoietic protoporphyria, protoporphyrin should be expected to reaccumulate in the graft.[85,86] The data are not entirely clear for hereditary hemochromatosis,[87] but because the protein product of the mutated gene for the disease (HFE gene) is expressed on intestinal epithelium,[88] abnormalities in iron absorption could be anticipated to persist following liver transplantation. Moreover, iron reaccumulation on liver biopsy was noted in

a study of patients with hemochromatosis who underwent liver transplantation.[89]

Tumor Recurrence

Hepatocellular carcinoma recurs in 60% to 80% of cases if the tumor was large or otherwise symptomatic.[90] If the tumor was an incidental finding, the prognosis is quite good. The liver and the lungs are the most common sites of recurrent hepatocellular carcinoma. Cholangiocarcinomas recur so commonly that the diagnosis is generally considered a contraindication to transplantation. OLT occasionally is also done for uncommon malignancies, including metastatic carcinoid tumors. In the latter instance recurrence is inevitable, but patients may still have a good quality of life for some time.[91] The histologic findings in all these cases do not differ from those in nonallografts.

Hepatic Vein Thrombosis (Budd-Chiari Syndrome)

OLT is an important therapeutic option in Budd-Chiari syndrome, although recurrence and death have occurred in a few instances.[92] The histologic findings in the allograft generally show more acute disease than is found in the native liver.

DIFFERENTIAL DIAGNOSIS OF HISTOLOGIC FINDINGS AFTER ORTHOTOPIC LIVER TRANSPLANTATION

The pathologist is faced with distinguishing the histologic changes of acute or chronic rejection from other lesions seen after liver transplantation. These distinctions are discussed in this section and provided in synopsis in Table 15.3.

TABLE 15.3. *Synopsis of common biopsy findings after orthotopic liver transplantation*

Histologic findings	Suspected etiologic mechanisms			
	Rejection	Biliary obstruction	Ischemia	Other causes and remarks
Portal changes				
Inflammation	Mononuclear cells, eosinophils, and neutrophils	Neutrophils with edema	May resemble obstruction	Hepatitis B or C; many other causes
Cholangitis	Mononuclear more than neutrophilic; may be destructive	Neutrophilic more than mononuclear; not destructive	May resemble obstruction; may be destructive	Cholangitis in CMV infection (inclusions!) or hepatitis C; neutrophilic cholangitis in systemic infections
Endotheliitis/phlebitis	Near-diagnostic if present	No	No	Nonspecific endotheliitis is rare in allografts
Arteritis or arteriopathy	Near-diagnostic if present	No	No	Lesions are rarely identified in biopsy specimens
Lobular changes				
Lobular hepatitis	Sinusoidal endotheliitis	Not prominent	Not prominent	Hepatitis B or C; systemic viral infection (EBV); possibly drug-induced hepatitis
Cholestasis	Common in severe cases	Yes	Common	Functional cholestasis in the early posttransplantation period; cholestasis in sepsis (all zones or ductal)
Necrosis (centrilobular)	Common in severe cases	No	Common	Adverse drug effects (?)
Endotheliitis/phlebitis (hepatic vein branches)	Near-diagnostic if present	No	No	Nonspecific endotheliitis/phlebitis rare but may be associated with severe lobular hepatitis

CMV, cytomegalovirus; EBV, Epstein-Barr virus.

Portal Changes

Abnormalities of portal tracts in allografts often reveal diagnostic features, whereas the lobular changes are less specific. In this respect allografts do not differ from nonallografts. Diagnostic changes may affect all structures within the portal tract.

Portal and Periportal Hepatitis

If the inflammation is not associated with other diagnostic features, such as cholangitis or endotheliitis, portal hepatitis may represent nonspecific inflammation, rejection, recurrent hepatitis C, and other conditions that cannot be diagnosed without additional studies. Periportal hepatitis is an uncommon finding. Most affected patients have either severe acute rejection or chronic, usually recurrent, viral or autoimmune hepatitis. Bridging necrosis may be present in these instances.

Cholangitis

In most instances the cholangitis is nonsuppurative and is caused by acute rejection. Typically, the ducts are surrounded and often also infiltrated by mixed inflammatory cells, as discussed earlier. T lymphocytes predominate, but neutrophils, plasma cells, and eosinophils may be plentiful. The predominance of neutrophils in this type of pleomorphic cholangitis[93] may give rise to the erroneous diagnosis of biliary obstruction. This situation is complicated by the fact that rejection cholangitis and cholangitis associated with biliary obstruction or ischemia occur together in many instances, probably more often than one would expect by chance. In these instances the rejection may be secondary.[13]

In rejection cholangitis, immunocytes can be seen inside the basement membrane, between ductal epithelial cells, and sometimes within the lumen. The ductal epithelial cells may show pyknosis, cytoplasmic vacuolation, ballooning, and other degenerative changes. In severe cases duct destruction occurs (Fig. 15.8). If ductopenia involves the majority of portal tracts, the process is probably irreversible and the graft should be expected to fail.[30] Rejection-related duct loss affects only interlobular and adjacent septal bile ducts, whereas the inflammation also appears to involve larger ducts.

Obstructive or infective cholangitis is usually associated with portal edema, ductular proliferation, and predominance of neutrophils (Fig. 15.12), particularly with neutrophils in the lumina of the ducts. Unless suppuration occurs, the cholangitis is nondestructive. Ischemic cholangitis should also be considered in this context.[13] Although this condition tends to affect large bile ducts, it often manifests itself in biopsy specimens by showing features of biliary obstruction or infection (Table 15.4). Neutrophilic or mixed-cell cholangitis may also occur in systemic infections, without evidence of primary liver disease.[94]

Other types of cholangitis include CMV cholangitis (Fig. 15.13B) and cholangitis associated with hepatitis C.[95,96] As indicated previously, granulomatous cholangitis (florid duct lesion) is near-diagnostic for recurrent PBC.

Arteritis, Arteriopathy, and Loss of Arteries

Rejection arteritis and arteriopathy are important diagnostic and prognostic features.[34] The diagnosis of rejection arteritis is often difficult because it is frequently associated with dense portal inflammation, which tends to obscure the arterial changes. Rejection arteriopathy, which is characterized by the presence of lipid-laden macrophages in the intima, is readily diagnosable (Fig. 15.9A) whether or not it is associated with arteritis. The term *vascular rejection* is a synonym for rejection arteriopathy. The diagnostic usefulness of arteriopathy is limited, because the condition involves primarily large septal hepatic artery branches (Fig. 15.9B)

or branches near the hilum and thus cannot be identified in most needle-biopsy specimens. Occasionally, portal arteriosclerosis and arteriolosclerosis may be difficult to distinguish from rejection arteriopathy. Finally, as mentioned earlier, loss of hepatic artery branches may occur in the setting of chronic irreversible rejection with duct loss.[30,38] The cause of this "arteriopenia" is not clear, but it might be due to arteriopathic occlusion upstream.

Portal Endotheliitis, Phlebitis, and Phlebothrombosis

Attachment of lymphocytes, primarily CD4 and CD8 cells, to the endothelium is an important sign of rejection. This putative immune attachment of immunocytes cannot be clearly distinguished from presumably nonspecific attachment in other inflammatory disorders of the liver (Fig. 15.7E).[33] However, in hepatic allografts, prominent accumulations of lymphocytes and other mononuclear cells on the endothelium (Fig. 15.7A–D) may be considered rejection endotheliitis. A cytoplasmic stalk sometimes gives the attached immunocytes a polypoid shape; this probably results from the pull exerted by the bloodstream and would suggest that the attachment is rather firm. In rejection endotheliitis, inflammatory cells often penetrate the endothelial layer and then accumulate in the immediate subendothelial space, or infiltrate the wall of the vein. This feature of rejection is best described as portal endotheliitis/phlebitis. The same condition also occurs in the terminal hepatic (central) veins. Portal and central endotheliitis/phlebitis often coexist; in the presence of prominent portal inflammation, central endotheliitis is easier to identify. Sinusoidal endotheliitis also may be seen (see the following section).

Portal thrombosis and thrombophlebitis in allografts may develop as surgical or nonsurgical complications. However, these conditions are quite uncommon in biopsy material.

Lobular Changes

Any insult to the hepatic allograft may lead to lobular abnormalities. Increased mononuclear cells in sinusoids often represent a nonspecific response—primarily Kupffer cell proliferation. However, immune adherence also seems to occur at these sites. This sinusoidal endotheliitis (Fig. 15.18) appears to have the same diagnostic and prognostic significance that can be ascribed to portal and central endotheliitis/phlebitis. The presence of sinusoidal endotheliitis should be suspected if portal or central endotheliitis is present and if hepatocellular changes are minimal, so that a nonspecific inflammatory response to lobular hepatitis with hepatocellular injury appears unlikely. Nevertheless, this distinction is not always possible. A response to antirejection treatment is probably the most reliable proof that sinusoidal endotheliitis indeed has been present. Immunostaining in these instances reveals a predominance of CD4 cells.

Rejection-related centrilobular hepatitis with HLA-DR expression is much more prominent in patients who have

TABLE 15.4. *Possible consequences of hepatic artery thrombosis and associated liver biopsy findings*

Pathogenic events		Possible liver biopsy findings
Hepatic artery thrombosis	→	Normal liver or infarcts or centrilobular necrosis
↓		
Ischemic cholangitis	→	As above and/or features of bile flow impairment or cellular rejection or both
↓		
Infective cholangitis	→	As above and/or cholangitis abscesses

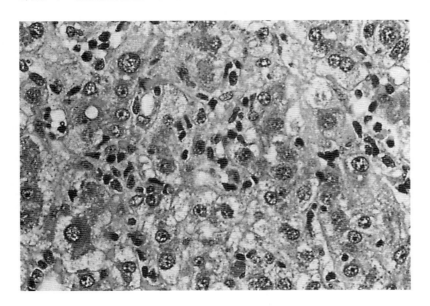

FIG. 15.18. Sinusoidal endotheliitis in advanced rejection with duct loss (vanishing bile duct syndrome), 5 weeks after orthotopic liver transplantation. Most of the lymphocytes in the sinusoids were CD4 positive. (From Ludwig J, Wiesner RH, Batts KP, et al. The acute vanishing bile duct syndrome (acute irreversible rejection) after orthotopic liver transplantation. *Hepatology* 1987;7: 481, with permission.)

been immunosuppressed with FK506 than in controls treated with cyclosporin A.[97] For other rejection-related centrilobular changes, see the next section.

Endotheliitis and Phlebitis of Terminal Hepatic Veins; Centrilobular Necroses

Rejection-related centrilobular endotheliitis and phlebitis often coexist with the same process in the portal veins, as discussed earlier. Intercalated and interlobular veins may also be affected in these instances. The relationship between centrilobular endotheliitis/phlebitis and the pathogenesis of centrilobular necroses is not clear, but the presence of these necroses (Fig. 15.19) is a feature of more severe acute rejection and for some patients may be an ominous prognostic sign.[34] In these instances terminal hepatic veins may appear sclerotic or even obliterated, and small peliosis-type lesions may develop. In these lesions, as in dilated sinusoids in the vicinity of centrilobular necroses, clusters of hematopoietic cells may be found (Fig. 15.20). Such clusters can also be found in a random distribution in otherwise normal allografts. More commonly, only a few isolated megakaryocytes are found in such specimens. It is still not known whether these hematopoietic cells are donor cells or host cells.

Sinusoidal infiltrates resembling sinusoidal endotheliitis may be found in EBV hepatitis and posttransplantation lymphoproliferative disease, as mentioned earlier. Irregular clusters of immunoblasts in the sinusoids should bring EBV hepatitis into consideration. *In situ* hybridization, polymerase chain reaction, and serologic testing generally establish the

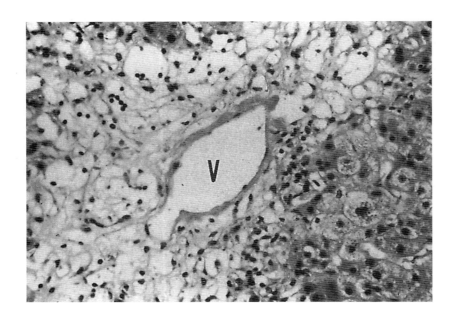

FIG. 15.19. Centrilobular necrosis in rejection with duct loss (chronic rejection), 2 months after orthotopic liver transplantation. Note the dropout of hepatocytes from the mesenchymal framework surrounding the terminal hepatic vein (*V*). Most of the inflammatory cells at the edge of the necrosis (*arrow*) were CD4 and CD8 positive.

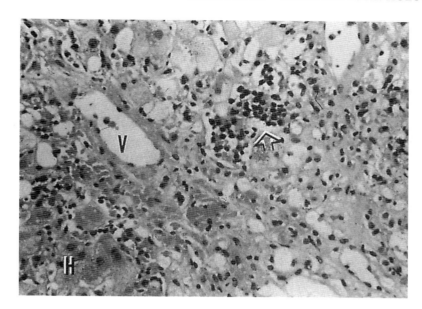

FIG. 15.20. Extramedullary hematopoiesis in a hepatic allograft with zone 3 necrosis, 2 months after orthotopic liver transplantation. Note the cluster of hematopoietic cells (*arrow*) in the dilated sinusoid near the terminal hepatic vein (*V*). Most parenchymal cells have disappeared from this area, but a few hepatocytes (*H*) are still identifiable.

diagnosis. In advanced posttransplantation lymphoproliferative diseases, monomorphic and monoclonal cells with the features of a B-cell non-Hodgkin's lymphoma may be found. In other instances, both polyclonal and monoclonal populations are present.[57]

Multiple apoptotic (acidophilic or Councilman) bodies may appear in both rejection and recurrent viral hepatitis, such as hepatitis C. In the latter instance polymerase chain reaction may detect the presence of HCV,[75] and immunohistochemical methods[98,99] may even locate the antigen. The immunohistochemical detection of hepatitis B antigens is now routinely available.

Clusters of neutrophils in the sinusoids or associated with minute necroses are common findings in biopsy specimens obtained at the end of the transplantation procedure or shortly thereafter (Fig. 15.21). This is a familiar feature of many surgical specimens, not just allografts; the changes are a result of mechanical trauma,[10] hypoxia,[100] or both. These infiltrates have little, if any, prognostic significance and must not be mistaken for a sign of infection. If focal necroses and clusters of neutrophils are found in follow-up specimens, a careful search for CMV viral inclusion bodies should be made and immunohistochemical staining for CMV should be ordered. Smaller collections of neutrophils unrelated to CMV infection are occasionally seen several months after transplantation in "mini-microabscesses" that do not appear to adversely affect the graft.[101]

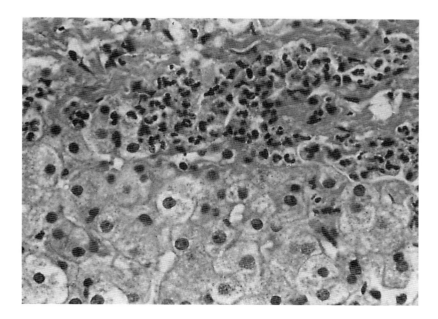

FIG. 15.21. Subcapsular cluster of neutrophils with focal necrosis in a day 0 biopsy specimen, obtained at the end of the transplant procedure. This is a reversible nonspecific feature ("surgical neutrophils" or "surgical hepatitis"), not a sign of infection.

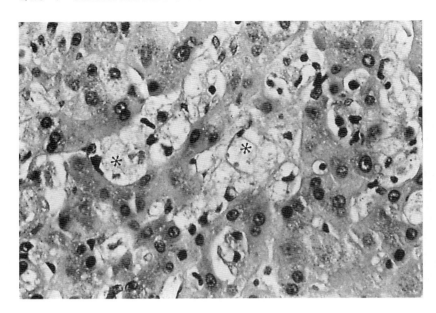

FIG. 15.22. Perisinusoidal lipid-laden macrophages (*asterisks*) in chronic rejection with ductopenia and vascular arteriopathy. This change is usually accompanied by cholestasis.

Cholestasis is the most common important lobular change. Particularly in the first 1 to 3 weeks, centrilobular and midzonal cholestasis with much feathery degeneration, but without other changes, may be present. This functional cholestasis was discussed earlier in this chapter. In specimens with features of rejection, the presence of cholestasis generally reflects more severe disease than rejection with absence of this feature. In irreversible ductopenic rejection, cholestasis is often quite severe. Perisinusoidal lipid-laden macrophages often accompany prominent hepatocanalicular cholestasis (Fig. 15.22). Other causes of lobular hepatocanalicular cholestasis include large-duct biliary obstruction or viral hepatitis (e.g., subfulminant recurrent hepatitis B; see "Recurrence of Pretransplantation Liver Disease") and drug-induced hepatitis. The last condition may be common, but specific examples are exceedingly difficult to prove in the posttransplantation setting. In any event, many cases of unexplained lobular cholestasis in allografts do not appear to be drug induced. Ductular cholestasis (cholestasis in cholangioles) is occasionally found near the limiting plates of portal tracts. This feature is rather nonspecific and occurs with sepsis or other systemic conditions, but in some instances biliary obstruction or rejection is also complicated by this finding.

Nonzonal ischemic necrosis and infarctions (Fig. 15.3) are rather common biopsy findings in allografts.[21] As indicated earlier, such lesions in biopsy specimens do not necessarily represent catastrophic graft damage.

In the rare condition termed lipopeliosis,[102] sinusoids engorged with lipid vacuoles are found. This has been described in cases where a steatotic donor liver suffered preservation injury with subsequent rupture of damaged fatty hepatocytes.

Time Relationships of Histologic Findings

The length of the posttransplantation interval is often the most important information needed for correct biopsy interpretation. For instance, widespread necrosis in the first 2 weeks after OLT might suggest primary graft dysfunction or antibody-mediated rejection. Functional cholestasis, bile flow impairment, and acute rejection are most commonly found in the first month after OLT. CMV hepatitis usually appears in the second and third months. Hepatic artery thrombosis and ischemic cholangitis may cause biopsy changes during this same interval but also at any time thereafter, well into the second year. Subfulminant recurrent hepatitis B often appears in or after the third month. The first cases of chronic rejection and vanishing bile duct syndrome tend to appear in the third week after OLT, but many cases require several months to develop.

Late-onset chronic rejection (i.e., in the second year) is rare in the Mayo Clinic experience.[25] Hepatocellular carcinomas often recur late in the first year after OLT or in the second year. Other conditions commonly encountered in the second year include recurrent hepatitis B and C and acquired hepatitis C. Rare cases of recurrent PBC or posttransplantation lymphoproliferative disease may be encountered in the third or subsequent years. In rare instances, posttransplantation lymphoma can develop as early as 2 months after OLT.[103] Carcinoid tumors tend to recur in the second and third years.

REFERENCES

1. Wiesner RH, Demetris AJ, Belle SH, et al. Acute hepatic allograft rejection: incidence, risk factors and impact on outcome. *Hepatology* 1998;28:638–645.

2. Williams JW, Vera SR, Peters TG. A technique for safe, frequent biopsy of the liver after hepatic transplantation. *Surg Gynecol Obstet* 1986;162:592–594.

3. Gaffey MJ, Boyd JC, Traweek ST, et al. Predictive value of intraoperative biopsies and liver function tests for preservation injury in orthotopic liver transplantation. *Hepatology* 1997;25:184–189.

4. Ploeg RJ, D'Allessandro AM, Knechtle SJ, et al. Risk factors for primary dysfunction after liver transplantation—a multivariate analysis. *Transplantation* 1993;55:807–813.

5. Bzeizi KI, Jalan R, Plevris JN, et al. Primary graft dysfunction after liver transplantation: from pathogenesis to prevention. *Liver Transplant Surg* 1997;3:137–148.

6. Trevisani F, Colantoni A, Caraceni P, et al. The use of donor fatty liver for liver transplantation: a challenge or a quagmire? *J Hepatol* 1996; 24:114–121.

7. Fishbein TM, Fiel MI, Emre S, et al. Use of livers with microvesicular fat safely expands the donor pool. *Transplantation* 1997;64:248–251.

8. Ludwig J, MacCarty RL, LaRusso NF, et al. Intrahepatic cholangiectases and large-duct obliteration in primary sclerosing cholangitis. *Hepatology* 1986;6:560–568.

9. Ludwig J, Ottman DM, Eichmann TJ. Methods in pathology: the preparation of native livers for morphologic studies. *Mod Pathol* 1994;7.

10. Christoffersen P, Poulsen H, Skeie E. Focal liver cell necroses accompanied by infiltration of granulocytes arising during operation. *Acta Hepato–Splenol* 1970;17:240-245.

11. Devlin J, Doherty D, Thomson L, et al. Defining the outcome of immunosuppression withdrawal after liver transplantation. *Hepatology* 1998;27:926–933.

12. Wong T, Nouri-Aria T, Devlin J, et al. Tolerance and latent cellular rejection in long-term liver transplant recipients. *Hepatology* 1998;28: 443–449.

13. Ludwig J, Batts KP, MacCarty RL. Ischemic cholangitis in hepatic allografts. *Mayo Clin Proc* 1992;67:519–526.

14. Li S, Stratta RJ, Langnas AN, et al. Diffuse biliary tract injury after orthotopic liver transplantation. *Am J Surg* 1992;164:536–540.

15. Sanchez-Urdazpal L, Sterioff S, Janes C, et al. Increased bile duct complications in ABO incompatible liver transplant recipients. *Transplant Proc* 1991;23:1440.

16. Woster A, Ghent C. Cholangiographic appearances of ductular rejection of ABO-incompatible liver transplants. *J Clin Gastroenterol* 1992;15:222–224.

17. Lefkowitch JH. Bile ductular cholestasis: an ominous histopathologic sign related to sepsis and "cholangitis lenta." *Hum Pathol* 1982;13: 19–24.

18. Wight DGD. Differential diagnosis of cholestasis in liver allografts. *Transplant Proc* 1986;18:152–156.

19. Ng IOL, Burroughs AK, Rolles K, et al. Hepatocellular ballooning after liver transplantation: a light and electronmicroscopic study with clinicopathological correlation. *Histopathology* 1991;18:323–330.

20. Goldstein NS, Hart J, Lewin KJ. Diffuse hepatocyte ballooning in liver biopsies from orthotopic liver transplant patients. *Histopathology* 1991;18:331–338.

21. Russo PA, Yunis EJ. Subcapsular hepatic necrosis in orthotopic liver allografts. *Hepatology* 1986;6:708–713.

22. Wisecarver J, Radio S, Shaw B Jr, et al. Intrahepatic arteriopathy associated with primary non-function of liver allografts. *Mod Pathol* 1993;6:115A.

23. Shayeb J, Plevak D, Rettke S, et al. Predictors of primary nonfunction (PNF)—is donor liver fat content (DLFC) important? *Transplant Proc* 1993;25:1974.

24. Demetris AJ, Qian S, Sun H, et al. Liver allograft rejection: an overview of morphologic findings. *Am J Surg Pathol* 1990;14:49–63.

25. Wiesner RH, Ludwig J, van Hoek B, et al. Current concepts in cell-mediated hepatic allograft rejection leading to ductopenia and liver failure. *Hepatology* 1991;14:721–729.

26. Demetris A, Belle S, Hart J, et al. Intraobserver and interobserver variation in the histopathological assessment of liver allograft rejection. *Hepatology* 1991;14:751–755.

27. Freese DK, Snover DC, Sharp HL, et al. Chronic rejection after liver transplantation: a study of clinical, histopathological and immunological features. *Hepatology* 1991;13:882–891.

28. Ludwig J. Terminology of hepatic allograft rejection. *Semin Liver Dis* 1992;12:89–92.

29. Demetris AJ, Markus B. Immunopathology of liver transplantation. *Crit Rev Immunol* 1991;9:67–92.

30. Ludwig J, Wiesner RH, Batts KP, et al. The acute vanishing bile duct syndrome (acute irreversible rejection) after orthotopic liver transplantation. *Hepatology* 1987;7:476–483.

31. Demetris AJ, Nakamura K, Yagihashi A, et al. A clinicopathological study of human liver allograft recipients harboring preformed IgG lymphocytotoxic antibodies. *Hepatology* 1992;16:671–681.

32. Foster PF, Bhattacharyya A, Sankary HN, et al. Eosinophil cationic protein's role in human hepatic allograft rejection. *Hepatology* 1991; 13:1117–1125.

33. Nonomura A, Mizukami Y, Matsubara F, et al. Clinicopathological study of lymphocyte attachment to endothelial cells (endothelialitis) in various liver diseases. *Liver* 1991;11:78–88.

34. Ludwig J, Gross JB, Perkins JD, et al. Persistent centrilobular necroses in hepatic allografts. *Hum Pathol* 1990;21:656–661.

35. Itoh S, Ishida Y, Matsuo S. Mallory bodies in a patient with type Ia glycogen storage disease. *Gastroenterology* 1987;92:520–523.

36. Seki K, Minami Y, Nishikawa M, et al. "Nonalcoholic steatohepatitis" induced by massive doses of synthetic estrogen. *Gastroenterol Japon* 1983;18:197–203.

37. Hubscher SG, Adams DH, Buckels JAC, et al. Massive hemorrhagic necrosis of the liver after transplantation. *J Clin Pathol* 1989;42:360–370.

38. Oguma S, Belle S, Starzl TE, et al. A histometric analysis of chronically rejected human liver allografts: insights into the mechanisms of bile duct loss: direct immunologic and ischemic factors. *Hepatology* 1989;9:204–209.

39. International Working Party. Terminology for hepatic allograft rejection. *Hepatology* 1995;22:648–654.

40. DeGroen PC, Kephart GM, Gleich GJ, et al. The eosinophil as an effector cell of the immune response during hepatic allograft rejection. *Hepatology* 1994;20:654–662.

41. Nagral A, Ben-Ari Z, Dhillon AP, et al. Eosinophils in acute cellular rejection in liver allografts. *Liver Transplant Surg* 1998;4:355–362.

42. McCaughan GW, Bishop GA. Atherosclerosis of the liver allograft. *J Hepatol* 1997;27:592–598.

43. Noack KB, Wiesner RH, Batts K, et al. Severe ductopenic rejection with features of vanishing bile duct syndrome: clinical, biochemical, and histologic evidence for spontaneous resolution. *Transplant Proc* 1991;23:1448–1451.

44. Demetris AJ, Seaberg EC, Batts KP, et al. Chronic liver allograft rejection. A National Institute of Diabetes and Digestive and Kidney Diseases interinstitutional study analyzing the reliability of current criteria and proposal of an expanded definition. *Am J Surg Pathol* 1998;22:28–39.

45. Demetris AJ, Batts KP, Dhillon AP, et al. Banff schema for grading liver allograft rejection: an international consensus document. *Hepatology* 1997;25:658–663.

46. Markin RS, Stratta RJ, Woods GL. Infection after liver transplantation. *Am J Surg Pathol* 1990;14:64–78.

47. Theise N, Birks E, Grundy J, et al. Detection of cytomegalovirus in liver allografts in the early posttransplant period: a study and review of the literature. *Eur J Gastroenterol Hepatol* 1992;4:727–732.

48. Stratta RJ, Shaeffer M, Markin R, et al. Cytomegalovirus infection and disease after liver transplantation: an overview. *Dig Dis Sci* 1992; 37:673–688.

49. Arnold J, Portmann B, O'Grady J, et al. Cytomegalovirus infection persists in the liver graft in the vanishing bile duct syndrome. *Hepatology* 1992;16:285–292.

50. Paya C, Wiesner R, Hermans P, et al. Lack of association between cytomegalovirus infection, HLA matching and the vanishing bile duct syndrome after liver transplantation. *Hepatology* 1992;16:66–70.

51. Lautenschlager I, Höckerstedt K, Jalanko H, et al. Persistent cytomegalovirus in liver allografts with chronic rejection. *Hepatology* 1997;25:190–194.

52. Koneru B, Jaffe R, Esquivel CO, et al. Adenoviral infections in pediatric liver transplant recipients. *JAMA* 1987;258:489–492.

53. Markin RS. Manifestations of Epstein-Barr virus-associated disorders in liver. *Liver* 1994;14:1–13.

54. Hubscher SG, Williams A, Davison SM, et al. Epstein-Barr virus in inflammatory diseases of the liver and liver allografts: an *in situ* hybridization study. *Hepatology* 1994;20:899–907.

55. Langnas AN, Markin RS, Inagaki M, et al. Epstein-Barr virus hepatitis after liver transplantation. *Am J Gastroenterol* 1994;89:1066–1070.

56. Alshak NS, Jiminez AM, Gedebou M, et al. Epstein-Barr virus infection in liver transplantation patients: correlation of histopathology and semiquantitative Epstein-Barr virus DNA recovery using polymerase chain reaction. *Hum Pathol* 1993;24:1306–1312.
57. Craig FE, Gulley ML, Banks PM. Posttransplant lymphoproliferative disorders. *Am J Clin Pathol* 1993;99:265–276.
58. Lones MA, Shintaku IP, Weiss LM, et al. Posttransplant lymphoproliferative disorder in liver allograft biopsies: a comparison of three methods for the demonstration of Epstein-Barr virus. *Hum Pathol* 1997;28: 533–539.
59. Pereira P, Milford E, Kirkman R, et al. Transmission of hepatitis C virus by organ transplantation. *N Engl J Med* 1991;325:454–460.
60. Cuervas-Mons V, Martinez AJ, Dekker A, et al. Adult liver transplantation: an analysis of the early causes of death in 40 consecutive cases. *Hepatology* 1986;6:495–501.
61. Davern TJ, Lake JR. Recurrent disease after liver transplantation. *Semin Gastrointest Dis* 1998;9:86–109.
62. Todo S, Demetris AJ, Van Thiel D, et al. Orthotopic liver transplantation for patients with hepatitis B virus-related liver disease. *Hepatology* 1991;13:619–626.
63. Davies SE, Portmann BC, O'Grady JG, et al. Hepatic histological findings after transplantation for chronic hepatitis B virus infection, including a unique pattern of fibrosing cholestatic hepatitis. *Hepatology* 1991;13:150–157.
64. O'Grady JG, Smith HM, Davies SE, et al. Hepatitis B virus reinfection after orthotopic liver transplantation. Serological and clinical implications. *J Hepatol* 1992;14:104–111.
65. Benner KG, Lee RG, Keeffe EB, et al. Fibrosing cytolytic liver failure secondary to recurrent hepatitis B after liver transplantation. *Gastroenterology* 1992;103:1307–1312.
66. Lau JYN, Bain VG, Davies SE, et al. High-level expression of hepatitis B viral antigens in fibrosing cholestatic hepatitis. *Gastroenterology* 1992;102:956–962.
67. Phillips MJ, Cameron R, Flowers MA, et al. Post-transplant recurrent hepatitis B viral liver disease. Viral burden, steatoviral, and fibroviral hepatitis B. *Am J Pathol* 1992;140:1295–1308.
68. Lucey MR, Graham DM, Martin P, et al. Recurrence of hepatitis B and delta hepatitis after orthotopic liver transplantation. *Gut* 1992;33: 1390–1396.
69. Hart J, Remotti H, Lewin KJ. Histologic spectrum of recurrent chronic hepatitis B (CHB) following liver transplantation. *Mod Pathol* 1992; 5:97A.
70. O'Grady J, Smith H, Davies S, et al. Hepatitis B virus reinfection after orthotopic liver transplantation. *J Hepatol* 1992;14:104–111.
71. König V, Bauditz J, Lobeck H, et al. Hepatitis C virus reinfection in allografts after orthotopic liver transplantation. *Hepatology* 1992;16: 1137–1143.
72. Ferrell LD, Wright TL, Roberts J, et al. Hepatitis C viral infection in liver transplant recipients. *Hepatology* 1992;16:865–876.
73. Böker KHW, Dalley G, Bahr MJ, et al. Long-term outcome of hepatitis C virus infection after liver transplantation. *Hepatology* 1997;25: 203–210.
74. Baiocchi L, Tisone G, Palmieri G, et al. Hepatic steatosis: a specific sign of hepatitis C reinfection after liver transplantation. *Liver Transplant Surg* 1998;4:441–447.
75. Poterucha JJ, Rakela J, Lumeng L, et al. Diagnosis of chronic hepatitis C after liver transplantation by the detection of viral sequences with polymerase chain reaction. *Hepatology* 1992;15:42–45.
76. Taga SA, Washington MK, Terrault N, et al. Cholestatic hepatitis C in liver allografts. *Liver Transplant Surg* 1998;4:304–310.
77. Schluger LK, Sheiner PA, Thung SN, et al. Severe recurrent cholestatic hepatitis C following orthotopic liver transplantation. *Hepatology* 1996;23:971–976.
78. Wright T, Donegan E, Hsu H, et al. Recurrent and acquired hepatitis C viral infection in liver transplant recipients. *Gastroenterology* 1992; 103:317–322.
79. Shah G, Demetris A, Gavaler J, et al. Incidence, prevalence, and clinical course of hepatitis C following liver transplantation. *Gastroenterology* 1992;103:323–329.
80. Hubscher SG, Buckels JAC, Elias E, et al. Does primary biliary cirrhosis recur after transplantation? *Hepatology* 1992;16:545A.
81. Jones DEJ, James OFW, Portmann B, et al. Development of autoimmune hepatitis following liver transplantation for primary biliary cirrhosis. *Hepatology* 1999;30:53–57.
82. Graziadei IW, Wiesner RH, Batts KP, et al. Recurrence of primary sclerosing cholangitis following liver transplantation. *Hepatology* 1999;29:1050–1056.
83. Birnbaum AH, Benkov KJ, Pittman NS, et al. Recurrence of autoimmune hepatitis in children after liver transplantation. *J Pediatr Gastroenterol Nutr* 1997;25:20–25.
84. Pessoa MG, Terrault NA, Ferrell LD, et al. Hepatitis after liver transplantation: the role of the known and unknown viruses. *Liver Transplant Surg* 1998;4:461–468.
85. Mion F, Faure J, Berger F, et al. Liver transplantation for erythropoietic protoporphyria. Report of a new case with subsequent medium-term follow-up. *J Hepatol* 1992;16:203–207.
86. Nordmann Y. Erythropoietic protoporphyria and hepatic complications. *J Hepatol* 1992;16:4–6.
87. Powell LW. Does transplantation of the liver cure genetic hemochromatosis? *J Hepatol* 1992;16:259–261.
88. Bacon BR. Diagnosis and management of hemochromatosis. *Gastroenterology* 1997;113:995–999.
89. Farrell FJ, Nguyen M, Woodley S, et al. Outcome of liver transplantation in patients with hemochromatosis. *Hepatology* 1994;20:404–410.
90. Iwatsuki S, Gordon RD, Shaw BW Jr, et al. Role of liver transplantation in cancer therapy. *Ann Surg* 1985;202:401–407.
91. Arnold JC, O'Grady JG, Bird GL, et al. Liver transplantation for primary and secondary apudomas. *Br J Surg* 1989;76:248–249.
92. Halff G, Todo S, Tzakis AG, et al. Liver transplantation for the Budd-Chiari syndrome. *Ann Surg* 1990;21:43–49.
93. Ludwig J, Czaja AJ, Dickson ER, et al. Manifestations of nonsuppurative cholangitis in chronic hepatobiliary diseases: morphologic spectrum, clinical correlations and terminology. *Liver* 1984;4:105–116.
94. Vyberg M, Poulsen H. Abnormal bile duct epithelium accompanying septicemia. *Virchows Archiv A Pathol Anat Histopathol* 1984;402: 451–458.
95. Bach N, Thung SN, Schaffner F. The histological features of chronic hepatitis C and autoimmune chronic hepatitis: a comparative analysis. *Hepatology* 1992;15:572–577.
96. Lefkowitch JH, Schiff ER, Davis GL, et al. Pathological diagnosis of chronic hepatitis C: a multicenter comparative study with chronic hepatitis B. *Gastroenterology* 1993;104:595–603.
97. Hytiroglou P, Lee R, Sharma K, et al. Histologic differences of acute cellular rejection in liver transplant recipients on FK 506 and cyclosporin A. *Mod Pathol* 1992;5:97A.
98. Nuovo GJ, Lidonnici K, Lane B. Histological correlation of hepatitis cDNA in liver biopsies as detected by RT *in situ* PCR hybridization. *Mod Pathol* 1993;6:51A.
99. Cartun RW, Siles FJ, Pedersen CA, et al. Immunocytochemical detection of a hepatitis C virus-related antigen in formalin-fixed liver tissue. *Mod Pathol* 1993;6:108A.
100. McDonald GSA, Courtney MG. Operation-associated neutrophils in a percutaneous liver biopsy: effect of prior transjugular procedure. *Histopathology* 1986;10:217–222.
101. MacDonald GA, Greenson JK, DelBuono EA, et al. Mini-microabscess syndrome in liver transplant patients. *Hepatology* 1997;26:192–197.
102. Cha I, Bass N, Ferrell LD. Lipopeliosis. An immunohistochemical and clinicopathologic study of five cases. *Am J Surg Pathol* 1994;18: 789–795.
103. Palazzo J, Lundquist K, Mitchell D, et al. Rapid development of lymphoma following liver transplantation in a recipient with hepatitis B and primary hemochromatosis. *Am J Gastroenterol* 1993;88:102–104.

Transplantation of the Liver, edited by Willis C. Maddrey, Eugene R. Schiff, and Michael F. Sorrell. Lippincott Williams & Wilkins, Philadelphia © 2001.

CHAPTER 16

Preservation of the Liver

John J. Lemasters, Hartwig Bunzendahl, and Ronald G. Thurman

CLINICAL ISSUES IN LIVER PRESERVATION FOR TRANSPLANTATION SURGERY

Transplantation of the liver is an accepted therapy for children and adults with end-stage liver disease; it provides good long-term survival and resumption of a nearly normal life style. With the advent of University of Wisconsin (UW) cold storage solution,[1] livers can now be preserved clinically for up to 24 hours by simple cold ischemic storage.[2,3] Use of UW solution during storage also improves postoperative liver function and decreases graft-threatening surgical complications such as hepatic artery thrombosis.[3,4] Animal studies and clinical trials suggest that preservation can also be improved by flushing livers at the end of storage with a rinse solution that is distinct from the storage solution.[5–8] The efficacy of rinse solutions underscores the importance of reperfusion injury in limiting liver preservation for transplantation. This reperfusion injury specifically involves sinusoidal endothelial and Kupffer cells (see "Structural and Functional Changes during Cold Storage and after Reperfusion," later in this chapter).

Increased time of storage has several important benefits. Longer preservation time improves donor liver procurement and utilization, increases time for the preoperative preparation of recipients, and generally expands the availability of transplantation therapy. In 1988, 58 centers performed liver transplantations in the United States. By 2000, this number had increased to 125. Clearly, improvements in surgical techniques and immunosuppression contributed to this expansion, but perhaps the most important factor favoring this expansion was the improved donor liver preservation afforded by UW solution. With UW solution, liver transplantation surgery no longer has to be performed on an emergency basis, often in the middle of the night. For the first time, liver transplantations can be scheduled a day in advance, and 24-hour stand-by availability is no longer required of surgeons, support staffs, and operating facilities. In addition, the longer preservation times provided by UW solution permit lengthy back-table procedures to reduce liver size in pediatric cases, where size-matched organs are particularly difficult to find, and to split livers, allowing one donor liver to rescue two patients from terminal liver disease.[9–11]

Method of Preservation of Human Livers

Details of the donor operation in clinical liver transplantation are provided in Chapter 4. Briefly, in brain-dead human donors, preservation is initiated by aortic infusion of cold UW solution. Some centers also infuse storage solution directly into the liver by a cannula in the portal vein. The liver is then removed, often flushed again with cold storage medium, placed in a sterile plastic bag surrounded by storage medium, and stored in ice slush. Storage temperature in the ice-water bath is very close to 0°C, although a temperature of 4°C is often incorrectly stated in the literature. The liver should be fully immersed in the ice-water bath to remain equilibrated at this storage temperature. As a practical matter, some livers warm during transport to 10° or 12°C by the time they arrive at a transplantation center. The deleterious clinical effects of such fluctuations of temperature, if any, are not known, although studies in rats indicate that storage temperature should be maintained at 4°C or below.[12,13]

At the time of implantation, attempts are made to keep the liver cold with surface cooling. Before recirculation, storage solution in the stored liver is flushed out with 300 to 500 mL of blood or Ringer's solution. Effluent from this flush is discarded to avoid sudden systemic hyperkalemia. Prompt resumption of bile flow is an early indication of a successful graft. Inadequately preserved livers usually fail 1 to 2 days after transplantation, whereas immunologic rejection does not begin for about a week or more. Biopsies taken shortly

J. J. Lemasters, H. Bunzendahl, and R. G. Thurman: Departments of Cell Biology & Anatomy, Surgery and Pharmacology, School of Medicine, University of North Carolina, Chapel Hill, North Carolina 27599–7090.

after transplantation show hepatocellular ballooning with a slight centrilobular predominance.[14] This contrasts with acute immunologic rejection, in which portal inflammation, endothelialiitis, and bile duct damage predominate.[15,16] Although experiments utilizing continuous perfusion for liver preservation are promising,[17] practical reservations remain concerning sterility, oxygenation, transportation, the expense of the perfusion equipment, and the need for specially trained technicians to run the equipment. For these reasons, cold ischemic storage of livers predominates for human transplantation.

Primary Graft Nonfunction and Dysfunction

A major problem in liver preservation is primary graft nonfunction, which still occurs in 5% to 10% of patients.[18,19] Primary nonfunction is characterized by metabolic failure of the newly implanted graft, rapidly rising levels of serum transaminases, lack of bile formation, and severe coagulopathy. The clinical course progresses quickly to hypoglycemia, hepatic encephalopathy, acute renal failure, disseminated intravascular coagulation, and death unless retransplantation is performed within 3 to 4 days. The failing graft may actually accelerate clinical deterioration, and removal of the failing graft or diversion of its blood flow stabilizes cardiovascular and pulmonary function until retransplantation takes place.[20] Because every retransplantation means that another patient on the waiting list may die, innovative approaches are urgently needed to salvage nonfunctioning grafts as well as to expand the donor pool to include donor organs that are not presently being used.

Alterations of liver function and histology attributed to storage/reperfusion injury occur even to grafts that survive and eventually perform well. Sharp elevations of serum transaminases typically occur 1 to 3 days postoperatively, sometimes followed by a syndrome of functional cholestasis with sustained high bilirubin level, diminished bile flow, and centrilobular hepatocellular ballooning and feathery degeneration.[14] If severe, this phenomenon is called primary graft dysfunction or initial poor function, as distinguished from primary nonfunction.[21] In various series, moderate to severe primary graft dysfunction occurred in 7% to 31% of liver transplant recipients.[18,19,21–23] The reversible disturbances of primary graft dysfunction usually resolve within 3 weeks, but are associated with 2- to 4-fold greater graft loss, longer stays in the intensive care unit (ICU) and hospital, and increased overall mortality. Nonanastomotic biliary strictures may also develop in some transplant patients after several weeks.[24,25] The incidence of such strictures rises with increasing storage time, suggesting a role of cold ischemia in their etiology.

Variables Influencing the Development of Primary Nonfunction

Several observations suggest that the etiology of primary nonfunction is, at least in part, related to storage/reperfusion injury. In animal models, liver graft failure from storage/reperfusion injury is essentially identical to graft failure in clinical primary nonfunction. Further, the clinical incidence of primary nonfunction is strongly dependent on the storage time, with primary nonfunction and early retransplantation occurring nearly 4 times more often after 20 hours or more of storage than after less than 10 hours.[26] Similarly, primary graft dysfunction and ischemic biliary strictures occur more frequently after prolonged cold ischemic storage.[18,19,21–25] In the absence of steatosis, the histology of biopsies taken just prior to reperfusion does not discriminate viable grafts from nonviable grafts, consistent with the idea that a critical injury leading to primary nonfunction occurs during or after reperfusion.[26,27]

Although many aspects of primary nonfunction appear related to liver preservation, others are not. Fatty livers from alcoholic and obese donors tend to do poorly after transplantation.[28,29] Graft survival of livers from female donors transplanted into male recipients is decreased in comparison with grafts from male donors,[30–32] and grafts from older donors tend to perform more poorly.[30,32,33] Nutrition of the donor is also important. Glycogen superloading of livers by carbohydrate infusion into donors reduces injury to stored rat livers.[34] High donor liver glycogen content also seems to correlate with good graft function after human transplantation.[35] In rats, liver storage and transplantation severely deplete glycogen stores, which makes grafts more vulnerable to hypoxic hepatocellular injury.[36] By contrast, prolonged donor fasting (4 days) improves survival after orthotopic rat liver transplantation.[37,38] However, a 4-day fast is a very severe stress to rats, and many rats do not survive a 5-day fast.

Marginal Livers

Livers stressed *in vivo* prior to storage by hypoxia, ischemia, or other metabolic perturbations are called marginal livers because of doubts concerning their suitability as donor organs. Suspicion is raised if heart-beating cadaveric donors experience prolonged episodes of hypotension or require pressor agents to maintain blood pressure, or if the donor liver simply "looks bad" at the time of harvest. Excessive use of vasopressors has been shown to decrease the energy charge of transplanted livers.[39,40] Other factors, such as donor age over 60, are also used to exclude potential donor livers, but because of the continuing organ shortage, livers from older donors are increasingly being utilized with apparent success.[41–43] However, livers from older donors are at greater risk for storage/reperfusion injury.[44] Therefore, only livers in good condition should be utilized from older donors, as assessed at harvest from donor hemodynamic stability, good donor liver function, low liver fat content, short cold ischemia time, and soft consistency of the donor liver.

The criteria for accepting or rejecting marginal livers remain largely based on the clinical experience of the individual surgeon. Livers are recovered from about 80% of all organ donors (about 4,800 livers from 5,800 donors yearly in the United States). Thus, the decision is made to not use 1,000 livers by one exclusion criterion or another. Given the imprecision of the exclusion criteria, many rejected livers might, in fact, be suitable for transplantation.

Tests to Predict Posttransplantation Graft Performance

A reliable test to predict whether a given stored liver will be viable as a graft would permit surgeons to avoid using livers that will fail immediately after transplantation and to use marginal livers that otherwise would be discarded. Unfortunately, histology prior to implantation does not discriminate viable from nonviable livers.[26,27] Another approach is to assess donor liver function *in vivo* prior to storage. The MEGX test assesses the hepatic metabolism of lidocaine to monoethylglycinexylidide (MEGX) in a cytochrome P-450–dependent reaction.[45] Several studies have indicated that low donor MEGX scores predict poor graft function postoperatively.[45,46] Unfortunately, other studies report that MEGX scores do not accurately predict graft outcome.[47–50] Similarly, donor measurements of the ratio of serum acetoacetate to β-hydroxybutyrate as a measure of hepatic function do not consistently predict graft success or failure.[51] The inability of such tests to predict graft performance is probably because one major form of injury leading to primary nonfunction and failure of liver grafts is reperfusion injury after storage.

Surgical Variables Influencing Storage/Reperfusion Injury

During bench procedures to prepare transplants for implantation, warming of preserved livers is virtually unavoidable. In addition, during the actual implantation procedure, the donor organ warms as it sits in the abdominal cavity, despite efforts to provide external cooling. Dilution of UW cold storage solution with chilled saline or Ringer's solution may also be a neglected source of graft damage.[52] Even after circulation is restored, reflow of blood may be inhomogeneous and slow in areas of the liver, allowing warm ischemic/hypoxic injury to continue.

Human and Economic Impact of Primary Nonfunction and Early Retransplantation

Lack of donor organs and primary graft nonfunction are major obstacles to the more widespread application of liver transplantation surgery. It is estimated that nearly 5,000 human liver transplantations will be performed in the United States in 2000 at a total cost of more than $1 billion.[53] In 1997, the most recent year for which complete data are available, 9,647 patients were listed for liver transplantation surgery, and the average waiting period was about 16 months.[54] Each year, hundreds of these patients tragically die before a suitable donor liver can be found. If rates of primary nonfunction and early retransplantation could be reduced by half, an annual savings of more than $50 million would be achieved, and another 250 patients would receive livers.

In addition, if marginal donor livers now rejected as unsuitable could be used, the donor liver pool would be increased, and both waiting lists and waiting periods would be shortened. The unfortunate fact for most transplant candidates is that their underlying disease worsens while they await a donor liver. Progression of disease can increase the risk of surgery or even contraindicate it. Thus, any measure decreasing waiting times benefits the transplant candidate. These several humanitarian concerns and economic reasons continue to motivate research efforts to better understand the mechanisms underlying injury to livers stored for transplantation surgery.

PRESERVATION SOLUTIONS

Euro-Collins Solution

In early studies, livers were stored in blood plasma or a physiologic saline, such as Ringer's solution, prior to transplantation surgery. Subsequently, Euro-Collins solution (Table 16.1) was shown to provide superior preservation of livers for transplantation surgery, permitting up to 8 hours of preservation.[55] Euro-Collins solution, a derivative of storage solutions originally developed by Geoffrey Collins for kidney preservation,[56,57] was designed to match the ionic composition of cytosol. During cold ischemic storage, energy-dependent gradients of Na^+, K^+, and other ions develop across the plasma membrane collapse, causing cellular K^+ depletion and Na^+ and Ca^{2+} loading. Euro-Collins solution is high in K^+ and low in Na^+ and Ca^{2+} in order to prevent disruption of intracellular ions. Euro-Collins solution is also high in glucose to support anaerobic glycolysis.

University of Wisconsin Cold Storage Solution

The next advance in liver preservation came with the development of University of Wisconsin cold storage solution (Table 16.2) by Folkert Belzer, James Southard, and their

TABLE 16.1. *Composition of Euro-Collins solution*

Ingredient	Concentration (mM)
KH_2PO_4	15
K_2HPO_4	43
KCl	15
$NaHCO_3$	10
Glucose	200
Total Na^+	10
Total K^+	116
Total Cl^-	15
pH	7.2
Osmolarity (mOs)	355

Data are from Dreikron K, Horsch R, Rohl L. 48 to 96 hour preservation of canine kidneys by initial perfusion and hypothermic storage using the Euro-Collins solution. *Eur Urol* 1980;6:221–224.

TABLE 16.2. *Composition of University of Wisconsin solution*

Ingredient	Concentration
K-lactobionate	100 mM
Na KH$_2$PO$_4$	25 mM
Adenosine	5 mM
MgSO$_4$	5 mM
Glutathione	3 mM
Raffinose	30 mM
Allopurinol	1 mM
Hydroxyethyl starch	50 g/L
Dexamethasone	8 mg/L
Insulin	100 U/L
Bactrim	0.5 mL/L
Total Na$^+$	30 mM
Total K$^+$	120 mM
pH	7.4
Osmolarity (mOs)	310–330

Data are from Belzer FO, Southard JH. Principles of solid-organ preservation by cold storage. *Transplantation* 1988; 45:673–676; and Jamieson NV, Sundberg R, Lindell S, et al. Preservation of the canine liver for 24–48 hours using simple cold storage with UW solution. *Transplantation* 1988;46:517–522.

colleagues.[1,58] With UW solution, clinical preservation of livers by cold ischemic storage was extended to 24 hours, a tripling of preservation time.[1–3] UW solution, or a similar variant, is now used throughout the world as the preferred storage solution in clinical liver transplantation.

UW solution was designed to counter several potential mechanisms contributing to storage injury to the liver.[1] As in Euro-Collins solution, K$^+$ is high and Na$^+$ and Ca^{2+} are low to maintain intracellular ions. Mg^{2+} is also high. Similarly, phosphate is the principal buffer. Raffinose and lactobionate replace the more permeant glucose and Cl$^-$ to prevent cell swelling during storage. Hydroxyethyl starch, a high molecular weight solute, is included to reduce interstitial edema. Allopurinol, an inhibitor of superoxide-generating xanthine oxidase, and glutathione provide antioxidant protection.

Adenosine triphosphate (ATP) hydrolysis during ischemia generates adenosine, which is then degraded to inosine and hypoxanthine, neither of which can be directly phosphorylated to reform ATP after reperfusion. Accordingly, adenosine is included in UW solution to facilitate regeneration of ATP, and insulin is added to stimulate glycolysis. Finally, dexamethasone is used to stabilize lysosomal membranes, and penicillin combats microbial growth.

Components Required for Efficacy in Liver Preservation

One of the most important components of UW solution is lactobionate, which has the effect of reducing cell swelling during storage.[59–61] Lactobionate also chelates Ca^{2+} and possibly free Fe^{3+}, a property that may also contribute to its beneficial effect. By contrast, raffinose seems unnecessary.[59,61,62]

Glutathione is important in UW solution, and its removal decreases survival of liver grafts after transplantation.[59,63] Reduced glutathione (GSH) is more effective than oxidized glutathione (GSSH).[64] The glutathione used in commercial UW solution is GSH, but GSH rapidly oxidizes to GSSH after manufacture.[65] For this reason, many surgeons will supplement commercial UW solution with fresh GSH from powder just prior to organ storage.

Adenosine also contributes to the efficacy of UW solution, although not to the same extent as lactobionate.[59,60] Adenosine also contributes to kidney preservation.[66] Adenosine is a cardioactive compound; when washed out of a stored organ into the circulation, it can cause transient bradyarrhythmias.[67] Because of the high adenosine and K$^+$ content of UW solution, surgeons flush liver implants with saline or blood to remove UW solution remaining inside the graft vasculature prior to reestablishing connection to the patient's circulation.

Because of patent and manufacturing considerations, hydroxyethyl starch is the ingredient adding most to the cost of commercial UW solution, which is about $300 per liter. Efforts to simplify UW solution, and thereby reduce its cost, generally begin with the elimination of hydroxyethyl starch. Some studies in liver indicate that hydroxyethyl starch does not add to the overall utility of UW solution,[58,59,68] whereas other studies suggest that hydroxyethyl starch is beneficial.[69–71] In stored pancreas and heart, hydroxyethyl starch is very important for success.[72,73] Overall, some benefit of hydroxyethyl starch to the liver seems likely. Nonetheless, hydroxyethyl starch may be the source of undesirable particulates in some manufactured lots of UW solution, necessitating filtration before use.[74]

Other components are less critical to the success of UW solution. Na$^+$/K$^+$ ratios can be reversed without ill effect or even with some improvement.[75–77] Similarly, allopurinol, Mg^{2+}, and insulin are not necessary ingredients.[60]

Other Storage Solutions

In some centers internationally, simplified UW solutions lacking hydroxyethyl starch and some other components have been placed in clinical use.[78–80] The motivation for using a simplified solution is cost savings, rather than improvement of performance. This may be a false economy, since an increase in the rate of primary nonfunction of even a fraction of a percent would wipe out any savings from use of a less expensive but less effective preservation solution. Because no solution has consistently demonstrated superior performance, the original UW solution remains preferred for liver storage in most of the world.

Nonetheless, other storage solutions show promise in experimental studies. These include HTK solution,[81] SLS solution,[82] and Celsior.[83] HTK solution contains histidine, tryptophan, and α-ketoglutarate and is designed to provide higher buffering capacity than other storage solu-

TABLE 16.3. *Composition of HTK solution*

Ingredient	Concentration (mM)
Histidine	180
Histidine HCl	18
Mannitol	30
NaCl	15
KCl	8
MgCl$_2$	4
Tryptophan	2
K-α-ketoglutarate	1
Total Na$^+$	15
Total K$^+$	9
Total Cl$^-$	49
pH	7.3
Osmolarity (mOs)	310

Data are from Bretschneider HJ, Helmchen U, Kehrer G. Nierenprotektion [in German]. *Klin Wochenschr* 1988;66:817–827.

TABLE 16.5. *Composition of Celsior solution*

Ingredient	Concentration (mM)
Mannitol	60
Na-lactobionate	80
Na-glutamate	20
CaCl$_2$	0.25
KCl	15
MgCl$_2$	13
Histidine	30
Glutathione	3
Total Na$^+$	100
Total K$^+$	15
Total Cl$^-$	26.5
pH	7.3
Osmolarity (mOs)	320

Data are from Menasche P, Termignon JL, Pradier F, et al. Experimental evaluation of Celsior, a new heart preservation solution. *Eur J Cardiothorac Surg* 1994;8: 207–213.

tions (Table 16.3). Several experimental and clinical studies show that HTK solution is about as effective as UW solution for shorter periods of cold ischemic liver storage.[84–86] After longer storage, HTK solution appears to be less effective than UW solution.[70,87] The efficacy of HTK may be due less to its buffering capacity than to the fact that histidine is an impermeant solute like lactobionate.

SLS solution contains lactobionate, sucrose, chlorpromazine, and high Na$^+$ (Table 16.4). In rat liver transplantation, including the harvest of livers from non–heart-beating rat donors, SLS was superior to UW solution, an effect attributed in part to the deletion of the highly viscous hydroxyethyl starch.[82,88,89] In canine liver transplantation, in contrast, UW solution was superior.[90] A nonprospective, nonrandomized human clinical study showed slightly better graft survival with SLS solution.[91] Overall, no clear advantage of HTK or SLS solutions over UW solution has yet been established.

TABLE 16.4. *Composition of SLS solution*

Ingredient	Concentration
Na$^+$	155 mM
K$^+$	5 mM
Mg^{2+}	5 mM
Phosphate	25 mM
Sucrose	75 mM
Lactobionate	100 mM
Glutathione	3 mM
Chlorpromazine	1–10 mg/L
pH	7.4
Osmolarity (mOs)	370

Data are from Tokunaga Y, Wicomb WN, Concepcion W, et al. Successful 20-hour rat liver preservation with chlorpromazine in sodium lactobionate sucrose solution. *Surgery* 1991;110:80–86.

Celsior is a new solution developed as a cardioplegic solution for cardiac ischemic arrest and as a preservation solution for heart transplantation.[83] Marketed in Europe, Celsior also shows good results in lung transplantation.[92] Celsior combines nonpermeant solutes (mannitol, lactobionate), extracellular cations (Mg^{2+}, Ca^{2+}, high Na$^+$/K$^+$ ratio), pH buffering (histidine), and antioxidant protection (glutathione) (Table 16.5). Lacking hydroxyethyl starch, Celsior has a low viscosity, which decreases intravascular pressure at high flow rates and reduces damage to the microvasculature. In preliminary studies, Celsior is as effective as UW solution in liver storage.[93,94] Because Celsior is superior to UW solution for combined heart and lung transplantation, increased use of Celsior for multiorgan harvesting will likely result in the greater use of Celsior for human liver preservation.

STRUCTURAL AND FUNCTIONAL CHANGES DURING COLD STORAGE AND AFTER REPERFUSION

The understanding of cellular mechanisms of storage/reperfusion injury in liver has advanced considerably in the past several years and now guides the development of new strategies to improve liver preservation for transplantation. Most of our detailed knowledge comes from studies of animal livers, especially in the rat, but major findings from animal models have since been confirmed in human livers. What has emerged is that reperfusion injury is the key event leading to graft failure after prolonged cold ischemic storage. Although changes do occur during storage, such as hepatocellular swelling and blebbing, reperfusion-induced loss of viability of endothelial cells and activation of Kupffer cells is the probable basis for graft failure after transplantation (summarized in Fig.

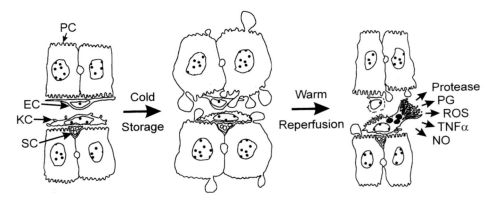

FIG. 16.1. Scheme of storage/reperfusion injury to liver. During cold ischemic storage, parenchymal cells (PC) swell and bleb. Endothelial cells (EC) and Kupffer cells (KC) show some rounding and retraction of cytoplasmic processes. After warm reperfusion, hepatocytes resorb or shed their blebs, and endothelial cells lose viability. Additionally, Kupffer cells ruffle and release inflammatory mediators, including prostaglandins (PG), proteases, reactive oxygen species (ROS), nitric oxide (NO), tumor necrosis factor α (TNFα), and other cytokines. Stellate cells (fat-storing or Ito cells, SC) show little change during storage and reperfusion.

16.1). Because liver injury during storage and reperfusion is quite cell specific, each hepatic cell type is discussed separately here.

Hepatocytes

Hepatocytes of normal liver display three distinct surfaces as viewed by scanning electron microscopy: the subsinusoidal, intercellular, and canalicular domains (Fig. 16.2).[95]

Subsinusoidal surfaces have extensive microvilli that fill the space of Disse. Microvilli also extend into recesses between adjacent hepatocytes. Smooth intercellular domains form where hepatocytes abut one another. They are featureless except for occasional peglike interdigitations and plaques of torn membrane corresponding to gap junctions. Bile canaliculi form in the middle of the intercellular domains between adjacent hepatocytes. The canalicular domains are covered with numerous microvilli.

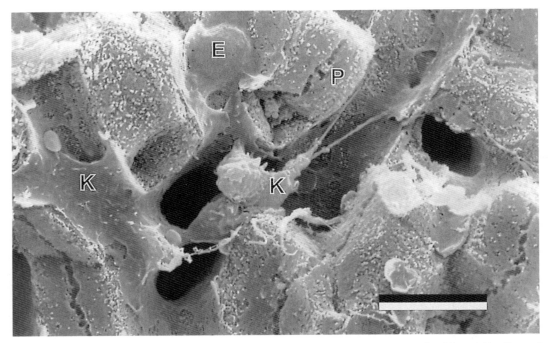

FIG. 16.2. Scanning electron micrograph of normal rat liver. Note endothelial cells *(E)* and Kupffer cells *(K)* in the wall of the sinusoids, and parenchymal cells *(P)* with canaliculi. Bar is 10 μm.

OF

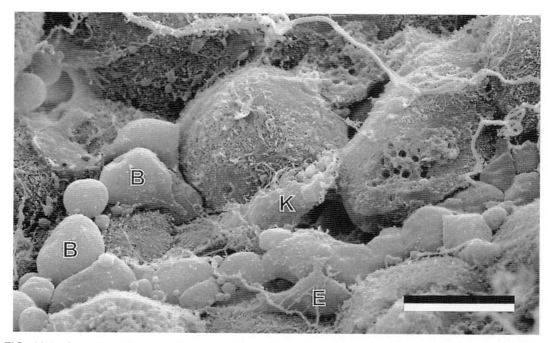

FIG. 16.3. Scanning electron micrograph of a rat liver stored for 16 hours in Euro-Collins solution. Large blebs *(B)* fill the sinusoids, obscuring observation of nonparenchymal cells lining the sinusoids. Where they can be seen, endothelial cells *(E)* are retracted but still generally flattened and adherent to underlying hepatocytes. Kupffer cells *(K)* are also retracted and show blunted ruffling. Bar is 10 μm.

During cold ischemic storage, hepatocytes swell and form surface protrusions called blebs (Fig. 16.3).[96–99] These blebs form on the subsinusoidal surfaces of hepatocytes and protrude into sinusoids through fenestrations in the sinusoidal endothelium. The plasma membrane covering the blebs seems to originate from microvilli, which disappear. A similar pattern of blebbing develops during warm hypoxia/ischemia but progresses much more rapidly.[95] After 16 hours of cold ischemic storage in Euro-Collins solution, hepatocellular blebs literally fill the sinusoids. The combined effect of bleb formation and hepatocellular swelling is to occlude the sinusoidal lumina. Swelling and bleb formation are less severe after shorter periods of storage, and both occur more slowly in UW cold storage solution. Even macroscopically, the reduction of tissue swelling with UW solution compared with Euro-Collins solution is quite dramatic.

Upon reperfusion with warm buffer or blood, bleb formation and swelling reverse (Fig. 16.4). Initially, the volume correction overshoots, and hepatocellular volume becomes less than before storage. These observations indicate that storage-induced changes to hepatocytes are reversible. Even after 96 hours of storage in Euro-Collins solution, long past the point when liver grafts will fail from storage injury, little hepatocellular death and lactate dehydrogenase release occur after reperfusion (Fig. 16.5).[100] Similarly, rates of oxygen consumption and carbohydrate metabolism remain within normal limits.[96,100,101] These findings strongly suggest that primary nonfunction and graft failure from cold storage injury are not caused by damage to hepatocytes.

Storage/Reperfusion Injury to Endothelial Cells

Hepatic sinusoids are lined by endothelial cells forming a fenestrated sieve plate separating the vascular space from the subsinusoidal surface of the hepatocytes (Fig. 16.2). During storage, endothelial cells show rounding and retraction of their extended sheetlike cytoplasm (Fig. 16.3). After shorter periods of storage, these changes to endothelial cells are reversed after reperfusion, at least in part, and the rounded endothelial cells spread out. *In vivo,* the sinusoidal lining is fully recovered within 24 hours. However, after times of storage associated with graft failure, reperfusion leads to destruction of the sinusoidal lining (Fig. 16.4).[96–100,102–104] In rats, after more than 8 hours in Euro-Collins solution or 16 hours in UW solution, reperfusion initiates a sequence of nuclear membrane vacuolization, mitochondrial swelling and lysis, plasma membrane breaks, cytoplasmic rarefaction, ball-like rounding, and nuclear condensation, culminating in trypan blue uptake and cell death (Figs. 16.6 and 16.7).[96,99,100] Shredded, stringlike fragments are all that remain of the sieve plates, and remnants of nuclear regions of the endothelial cells are covered by a perforated plasma membrane (Fig. 16.4).

After 24 hours in Euro-Collins solution and brief reperfusion, 35% to 40% of nonparenchymal cells lose viability, as

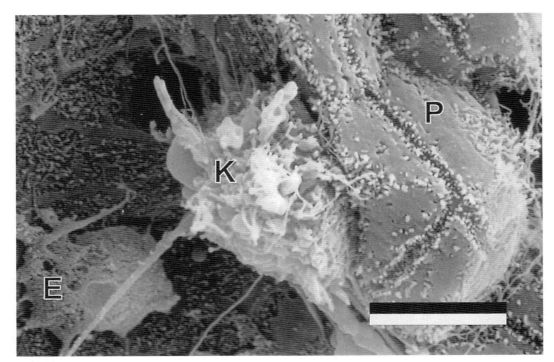

FIG. 16.4. Scanning electron micrograph showing Kupffer cell activation and endothelial cell killing after 24 hours of cold storage in Euro-Collins solution and brief reperfusion. Note rounding and ruffling of the Kupffer cell *(K)* and the rough irregular surface of the remnant of an endothelial cell *(E)*, indicative of loss of cell viability. Hepatic parenchymal cells *(P)* show normal features. Bar is 5 μm.

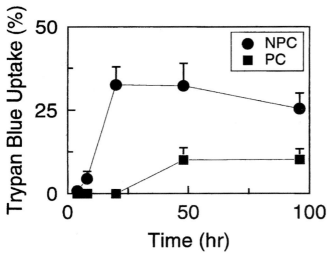

FIG. 16.5. Trypan blue uptake in hepatic nonparenchymal cells (NPC) and parenchymal cells (PC) after cold ischemic storage and reperfusion. Rat livers were stored 4 to 96 hours in cold Euro-Collins solution and reperfused for 15 minutes with warm Krebs-Henseleit bicarbonate buffer. Viability of parenchymal and nonparenchymal cells was determined by trypan blue exclusion. (From Caldwell-Kenkel JC, Thurman RG, Lemasters JJ. Selective loss of nonparenchymal cell viability after cold, ischemic storage of rat livers. *Transplantation* 1988;45:834–837, with permission.)

assessed by nuclear staining with trypan blue (Figs. 16.5 and 16.7). This corresponds to virtually 100% of endothelial cells. Trypan blue is a DNA-intercalating dye that gains entrance to cells only after viability has been lost, and its staining provides a specific indicator of cell death in tissue sections of livers briefly perfused with the dye. Cell killing is also indicated by release of the BB isozyme of creatine kinase, an enzyme localized to hepatic nonparenchymal cells.[105] Purine nucleoside phosphorylase release has also been proposed as an indicator of endothelial cell killing,[106,107] but this enzyme is also found in hepatocytes and is not exclusively localized to nonparenchymal cells as originally thought.[108]

Plasma hyaluronic acid is cleared solely by hepatic sinusoidal endothelial cells.[109] Accordingly, serum hyaluronic acid levels and hepatic hyaluronic acid clearance are indices of sinusoidal endothelial cell function and viability.[110] After various times of cold storage of rat livers, hyaluronic acid clearance decreases and serum hyaluronic acid levels increase after reperfusion and transplantation.[111–113] These changes parallel loss of endothelial cell viability. In clinical liver transplantation, measures of serum hyaluronic acid levels, hepatic hyaluronic acid clearance, and hyaluronic acid content in the initial effluent after reperfusion of stored livers show promise as early predictors of liver graft function.[110,114,115]

Loss of endothelial cell viability first occurs after about 8 hours of storage in Euro-Collins solution and reaches a maximum after 24 hours (Fig. 16.5). If stored livers are reperfused with cold storage solution containing trypan

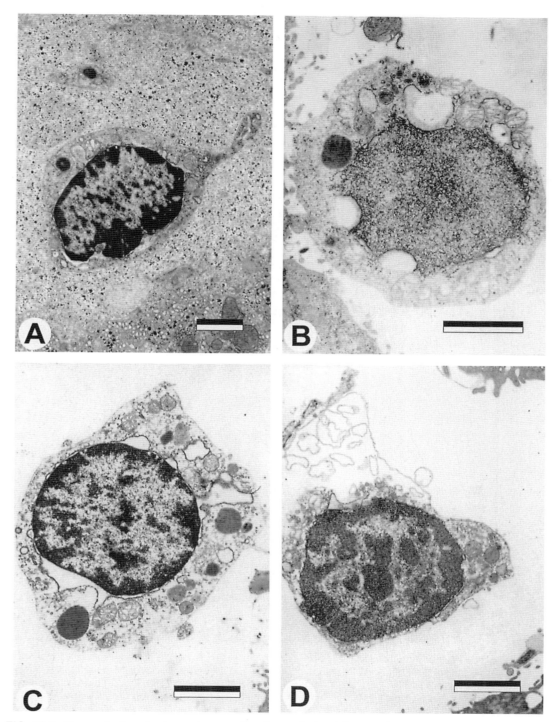

FIG. 16.6. Transmission electron micrographs of reperfusion injury to sinusoidal endothelial cells. Rat livers were stored for 24 hours in Euro-Collins solution and reperfused for 0 **(A)**, 2 **(B)**, 6 **(C)**, and 30 minutes **(D)**. Each panel depicts a representative endothelial cell. Note progressive swelling and disintegration of the endothelial cells. Bars are 2 μm.

blue, rather than with warm physiologic buffer, labeling of endothelial nuclei is greatly reduced. Since trypan blue labels nonviable cells in a temperature-independent fashion, this finding indicates that lethal endothelial cell injury does not occur until after reperfusion; that is, endothelial cell

killing is a reperfusion injury. Previously, some question existed as to whether lethal injury to sinusoidal endothelial cells after liver storage was truly a reperfusion injury. Most findings now support the idea of reperfusion injury, as originally proposed.[100,104] However, it is important to emphasize

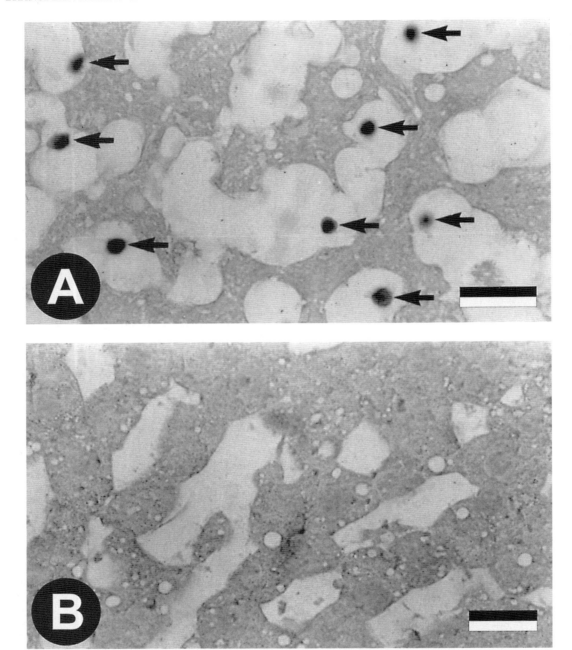

FIG. 16.7. Loss of endothelial cell viability after reperfusion and protection by reperfusion with Carolina rinse solution. Rat livers were stored 24 hours in UW solution and reperfused for 15 minutes with Krebs-Henseleit bicarbonate buffer **(A)** or Carolina rinse solution without glycine **(B)**. Trypan blue was added to the reperfusion solutions to identify nuclei of nonviable cells (*arrows* in **A**). Bars are 20 μm.

that changes during cold ischemia make the tissue vulnerable to the reperfusion injury.

Liver preservation in UW cold storage solution delays the onset of lethal reperfusion injury to endothelial cells. The delay of endothelial cell killing parallels the improvement of graft survival after transplantation. During warm anoxic injury to livers, nutritional state (fed versus fasted) strongly influences the extent of hepatocellular damage:

livers from fasted animals are much more vulnerable to lethal cell injury than livers from fed animals.[116,117] By contrast, storage/reperfusion injury to endothelial cells is not different in fed and fasted livers,[96] although another study reports that glycogen superloading of livers reduces endothelial cell injury.[118]

Cytochemistry and electron microscopy confirm the original light microscopic findings that nonparenchymal cells losing viability after liver storage and reperfusion are sinusoidal endothelial cells.[96,97,99] Similar changes to endothelial cells also occur in human livers after storage and reperfusion.[119,120] Kupffer cells, stellate (fat-storing or Ito) cells, and bile duct epithelial cells escape lethal storage/reperfusion injury.

Storage/Reperfusion Activation of Kupffer Cells

In normal livers, Kupffer cells rest on the luminal side of the sinusoidal endothelial lining (Fig. 16.2). Most are flattened, with sparse microvilli on an otherwise smooth cellular surface. Other Kupffer cells may be more rounded and irregular in shape. During cold storage, relatively minor structural changes occur to Kupffer cells, notably some rounding and blunted ruffling.[99]

In contrast to the minor changes to Kupffer cells during storage, reperfusion with warm oxygenated buffer or blood initiates a rapid and marked activation of these macrophages, as first suggested by light microscopy and subsequently corroborated by electron microscopy (Figs. 16.4 and 16.8).[96,97,99] Vacuolization, cell surface ruffling, formation of wormlike densities, and degranulation all occur within minutes after reperfusion. Particle phagocytosis, superoxide production, and release of hydrolytic enzymes by

Kupffer cells are also all increased by storage and reperfusion.[99,121,122] After 24 hours in Euro-Collins solution, virtually every Kupffer cell becomes activated after reperfusion.

Reperfusion-induced activation of Kupffer cells and endothelial cell killing occur in parallel, and both are diminished by storage in UW solution.[96,99] In general, graft failure after transplantation correlates well with the severity of reperfusion injury to Kupffer and endothelial cells after various periods of storage. Kupffer cell activation and endothelial cell killing can be documented *in vivo* in rat liver grafts that are failing from storage/reperfusion injury,[123,124] as well as in human clinical specimens.[119,120] In grafts stored under survival conditions, nonparenchymal injury *in vivo* is greatly reduced.

Kupffer cell activation also occurs in reperfusion injury after warm ischemic/hypoxic injury to liver.[125,126] In isolated perfused rat livers, reoxygenation after low-flow hypoxia produces a 3-fold increase in particle phagocytosis and structural alterations to Kupffer cells characteristic of activation.[125] Oxygen free radical formation is also increased in Kupffer cells isolated from ischemic livers and in cultured Kupffer cells after anoxia followed by reoxygenation *in vitro*.[127,128] Levels of tumor necrosis factor α (TNF-α) in the serum increase after warm hepatic ischemia/reperfusion *in vivo*. Increased TNF-α is also released after cold ischemic

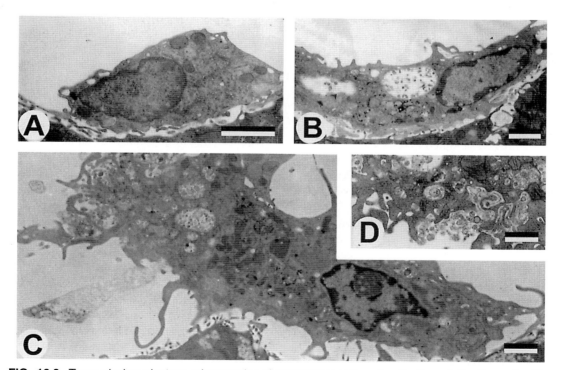

FIG. 16.8. Transmission electron micrographs of reperfusion-induced activation of Kupffer cells. The panels depict representative Kupffer cells from a normal rat liver **(A)** and from rat livers stored for 8 hours **(B)** or 24 hours **(C, D)** in Euro-Collins solution and reperfused briefly. Note the multiple invaginations, vacuolization, surface ruffling, and degranulation after 24 hours of storage. In **(D),** note the presence of free granules in the extracellular space and wormlike densities within the plasma membrane invaginations. Bars are 2 μm in **(A), (B),** and **(C)** and 1 μm in **(D).**

liver storage.[129] This cytokine likely originates from Kupffer cells and contributes to pulmonary interstitial edema and infiltration.[130] Similar pulmonary changes occur after orthotopic rat liver transplantation and are reduced by anti–TNF-α antibodies,[131–133] although graft survival may not be improved.[134]

Late Reperfusion Injury to Hepatocytes

After orthotopic rat liver transplantation, 10% to 15% of hepatocytes in the transplanted graft are nonviable 24 hours postoperatively.[135] Lethal hepatocellular injury is not observed early postoperatively (0 to 2 hours). In liver explants reperfused with anoxic rather than oxygenated buffer just prior to implantation, hepatocellular injury is diminished. Increased cell viability is associated with better microcirculation when blood flow is initially reestablished. These findings demonstrate that an oxygen-dependent reperfusion injury to liver grafts occurs even when the ultimate outcome of transplantation is not primary nonfunction and graft failure.

Mechanisms of Graft Failure from Storage/Reperfusion Injury

Reperfusion-induced activation of Kupffer cells and killing of sinusoidal endothelial cells occurs after storage of livers for times associated with graft failure after transplantation. In such livers, the interaction of damaged sinusoids with blood leads to microcirculatory disturbances characterized by leukocyte margination, platelet adhesion, hemostasis, inflammation, and ischemia.[124] Even in successful liver grafts that survive, microcirculatory disturbances occur early after reperfusion and appear to lead to foci of necrosis 24 hours later.[135]

Platelet trapping, fibrin deposition, and leukocyte margination after reperfusion of stored livers increase with increasing time of storage.[124,136–138] Clinically, platelet trapping seems to predict poorer outcomes after liver transplantation.[119,139] Sinusoidal blood flow decreases and leukocyte sticking increases in vivo after orthotopic rat liver transplantation.[124] In normal livers, leukocyte movement in hepatic sinusoids is smooth and rapid with negligible margination.[124,140] In livers transplanted under survival conditions, leukocyte velocity decreases 2-fold to 3-fold, and margination increases to 10% of cells. In liver grafts failing from storage/reperfusion injury, leukocyte margination rises to 40% and flow decreases more. In addition, phagocytosis of latex beads by Kupffer cells is enhanced. After about 4 hours, hepatocytes begin to lose viability. These events likely underlie the progression to primary graft nonfunction and failure from storage/reperfusion injury.

Activated Kupffer cells can release superoxide radicals, nitric oxide, proteases, eicosinoids, TNF-α, and other cytokines directly into the blood.[141] Because Kupffer cells constitute 80% to 90% of all tissue macrophages,[142] the relative magnitude of these secretions can be very large and produce profound physiologic alterations both locally in the liver itself and distally in other organs. Products released by Kupffer cells likely intensify inflammatory responses and microcirculatory disturbances already created by damage to the sinusoidal endothelium. Free radical formation in vivo and in situ is revealed with spin trapping techniques and nitroblue tetrazolium cytochemistry after storage and reperfusion.[122,143] Free radicals may stimulate neutrophil margination and increase inflammation, since superoxide dismutase decreases neutrophil infiltration into reperfused liver after both warm and cold ischemia.[144,145] In addition to these local effects, systemic release of inflammatory mediators by activated Kupffer cells may be the cause of adult respiratory distress syndrome and multiple organ failure associated with liver failure.[146]

The improved survival of livers from fasted donors appears linked to effects on Kupffer cells. Prolonged fasting decreases Kupffer cell particle phagocytosis, TNF-α formation, and the Kupffer cell–dependent increase of hepatic oxygen uptake after liver storage.[147–149] By contrast, treatments that activate Kupffer cells, such as donor treatment with lipopolysaccharide (LPS) or physical manipulation of the explanted liver, dramatically decrease graft survival after orthotopic rat liver transplantation.[150–152]

Increased intracellular calcium activates Kupffer cells and other macrophages.[153] Nisoldipine and other calcium channel blockers decrease particle phagocytosis by stored rat livers and improve long-term graft survival when included in the storage solution.[121] Other calcium antagonists, including nifedipine, verapamil, lidoflazine, and chlorpromazine, also improve liver preservation,[82,154–157] in confirmation of earlier studies of warm hypoxic/ischemic injury to liver.[158] The site of action of nisoldipine is an L-type voltage-sensitive calcium channel in the plasma membranes of Kupffer cells,[159] although Ito cells and possibly endothelial cells also possess voltage-gated calcium channels.[160–162] Methylpalmitate, an inhibitor of phagocytosis by Kupffer cells, also improves graft survival, but to a lesser extent than nisoldipine.[163]

Nisoldipine inhibits TNF-α release by LPS-stimulated cultured Kupffer cells.[164] Other compounds that improve graft survival, including pentoxifylline, adenosine, and prostaglandin E₁, also suppress LPS-stimulated TNF-α formation by cultured Kupffer cells.[164] Suppression by adenosine is by a cAMP-dependent adenosine A₂ receptor mechanism.[165] Pentoxifylline treatment of recipients or donors, or both, improves survival after rat liver transplantation after prolonged cold ischemic storage and decreases Kupffer cell TNF-α and superoxide formation.[134,166,167] Pentoxifylline also decreases liver damage, diminishes leukocyte margination, and improves survival after warm hepatic ischemia/reperfusion in vivo.[168–170] Improvement of graft survival by recipient treatment with pentoxifylline occurs without reduction of reperfusion-induced injury to the sinusoidal endothelium.[166] Thus, pentoxifylline is therapeutically effective after storage/reperfusion injury has already occurred. Poor early graft function in clinical transplantation is associated with prolonged release of proinflammatory cytokines.[171] Continuing release of cytokines from transplanted liver grafts may exacerbate and extend tissue damage from storage/reperfusion injury.

Kupffer cells degranulate and release hydrolytic enzymes after cold storage and reperfusion.[99] Proteases are among these hydrolytic enzymes, and protease inhibitors show some efficacy in decreasing storage/reperfusion injury.[121,172] Protease, and specifically calpain, activity increases in liver tissue during cold ischemia and after warm reperfusion.[172–174] As a consequence of protease activity, amino acids in the initial reperfusion effluents of stored livers increase with increasing times of storage.[175] However, protease inhibition at best provides a temporary benefit against graft failure and fails to improve long-term graft survival.[121,176] Thus, protease activation alone cannot account for the loss of graft viability from storage/reperfusion injury. A combination of factors from Kupffer cells, including release of reactive oxygen species, proinflammatory cytokines, and hydrolytic enzymes such as proteases and possibly other toxic mediators, probably contributes to loss of graft viability.

pH Paradox in Reperfusion Injury to Endothelial Cells

Lethal endothelial cell injury after reperfusion of stored livers occurs in parallel with activation of Kupffer cells, but is not reduced by the antioxidants allopurinol, desferrioxamine, superoxide dismutase, and catalase, or by washout with anoxic buffer.[122] Thus, lethal reperfusion injury to sinusoidal endothelial cells is not mediated by oxygen free radicals. These findings indicate, therefore, that oxygen-independent mechanisms contribute to the primary injury to endothelial cells. However, subsequent alterations after transplantation, probably involving Kupffer cells, are oxygen dependent and likely involve free radical formation.

Ischemic tissues become anoxic and acidotic. After reperfusion, reoxygenation and a return to physiologic pH occur simultaneously. Although much interest has focused on the possible role of oxygen free radicals in reperfusion injury, evidence in several cell types indicates that changes of pH play an important role in ischemia/reperfusion injury. First, the acidosis that occurs naturally during ischemia is quite protective against the onset of necrotic cell death in both hepatocytes and sinusoidal endothelial cells.[177–179] Hypoxic ATP-depleted cells survive much longer at an acidotic pH (pH < 7.0) than at a normal pH of 7.4. Second, the return from acidotic pH to normal pH during reperfusion is a stress that actually precipitates lethal cell injury and accounts for a large part of reperfusion-induced cell killing.[177,178,180] This phenomenon is called a pH paradox. A pH paradox contributes to lethal storage/reperfusion injury to sinusoidal endothelial cells, since reperfusion with acidotic buffer (pH 6.5–6.8) greatly reduces endothelial cell killing after cold ischemic storage.[122] pH-dependent loss of cell viability is linked to the recovery of intracellular pH after reperfusion.[180–182]

A phenomenon known as the mitochondrial permeability transition (MPT) underlies the pH paradox. The MPT occurs when a permeability transition (PT) pore conducting solutes of molecular mass up to 1,500 Da opens in the mitochondrial inner membrane.[183] Increased Ca^{2+} and generation of reactive oxygen species promote PT pore opening, which in turn causes mitochondrial depolarization, large-amplitude mitochondrial swelling, and uncoupling of oxidative phosphorylation. Necrotic cell death then follows as a consequence of ATP depletion. Cyclosporin A at nanomolar concentrations inhibits the MPT, but this effect is unrelated to the immunosuppressive action of cyclosporin A. Acidic pH also blocks PT pore conductance. In cultured hepatocytes, nonspecific mitochondrial membrane permeability abruptly increases as acidotic intracellular pH recovers toward normal during reperfusion.[182] Reperfusion at acidotic pH or with cyclosporin A prevents this increase of mitochondrial membrane permeability, which allows mitochondrial repolarization to occur and prevents cell death.[182] Cyclosporin A also decreases sinusoidal endothelial cell killing after warm anoxia and reoxygenation,[184] and pH-dependent killing of sinusoidal endothelial cells is associated with mitochondrial depolarization.[179] Cyclosporin A also seems to minimize reperfusion injury to livers after warm and cold ischemia[185–187] and specifically to decrease damage to sinusoidal endothelial cells,[188] but involvement of the MPT in cold ischemic injury has not yet been directly demonstrated.

Changes Leading to Necrotic Death of Sinusoidal Endothelial Cells

Onset of the MPT causes uncoupling of oxidative phosphorylation. Uncoupling is a more severe derangement than the simple respiratory inhibition that occurs during ischemia. Uncoupled mitochondria actively hydrolyze ATP, including ATP generated by other metabolic pathways such as glycolysis.[189] The consequence is profound ATP depletion. After ATP depletion, changes in cellular structure and membrane function begin to occur that culminate in cellular lysis, the hallmark of necrotic cell death. In hepatocytes, one of the earliest changes after both normothermic and hypothermic ATP depletion is plasma membrane bleb formation.[95,99,190] Additionally, cells increase in volume by 30% to 50%, the cisternae of endoplasmic reticulum dilate, and moderate mitochondrial swelling occurs.

To this point, cell injury can be reversed. Irreversible injury develops when a plasma membrane bleb physically ruptures, an event that leads to failure of the plasma membrane permeability barrier, release of intracellular enzymes and metabolites, and collapse of all electrical and ionic gradients across the plasma membrane.[190,191] In hepatocytes, myocytes, and sinusoidal endothelial cells during normothermic hypoxic stress, a metastable state precedes this abrupt failure of the plasma membrane.[191–194] The metastable state begins with mitochondrial depolarization and onset of the MPT. Subsequently, lysosomes disintegrate, blebs coalesce, and cell swelling accelerates. As this occurs, the plasma membrane becomes permeable to low molecular weight organic anions. Continued cellular swelling culminates with rupture of a plasma membrane bleb and consequent equilibration of intracellular and extracellular solutes.

In cultured rat sinusoidal endothelial cells, accelerated swelling in the metastable state seems initiated by opening of channels in the plasma membrane that are selectively permeable to anions, including organic anions up to a molecular weight of at least 600 Da.[195] The cytoprotective amino acid glycine inhibits these so-called death channels. After death channels open, colloid osmotic forces and the entry of cations (K^+ and Na^+) through open cation channels[196-198] drive the rapid swelling associated with the metastable state. Swelling continues until a plasma membrane bleb ruptures. After rupture, the driving force for swelling is lost and further volume growth ceases abruptly. Since mitochondrial membrane permeabilization and lysosomal disintegration precede onset of the metastable state, a hydrolytic enzyme or factor released or activated by these organelles may be important for death-channel opening. Opening of a glycine-sensitive plasma membrane channel of somewhat different properties is also described in renal cells preceding necrotic cell death.[199]

Apoptosis in Storage/Reperfusion Injury

Classically, ischemia/reperfusion injury is associated with necrotic cell death in which cell lysis occurs after breakdown of the plasma membrane. Apoptosis, or programmed cell death, by contrast, is a morphologically and biochemically distinct form of cell death characterized by cell shrinkage, nuclear fragmentation, DNA degradation, and the activation of cysteine-aspartate proteases (caspases) and other degradative enzymes.[200] In transplantation biology, cell death during immunologic graft rejection occurs principally by apoptosis,[201,202] and early allograft dysfunction and failure are linked to accelerated apoptosis in human clinical liver transplantation.[203,204] Apoptosis is also a feature of warm ischemia/reperfusion injury in many tissues.[202,205,206] Apoptosis also occurs in parenchymal and nonparenchymal cells after rat liver transplantation and increases with increasing times of cold ischemic storage.[207,208] Apoptosis detected by the terminal deoxynucleotide transferase-mediated UTP nick end labeling (TUNEL) technique peaks within 12 hours after transplantation in nonparenchymal cells and within 48 hours for parenchymal cells. Substantial increases (greater than 10-fold) in apoptosis occur in the absence of primary graft failure and may underlie the delayed oxygen-dependent parenchymal cell killing reported previously.[135]

Apoptosis after storage/reperfusion is associated with activation of caspase 3 and other proteases.[209,210] The caspase inhibitor IDN-1965 decreases apoptosis by nearly two-thirds when given to donor animals and added to the storage and reperfusion solutions. Treatment with this protease inhibitor delays graft failure from storage/reperfusion injury by several hours but does not improve long-term graft survival, as observed for other protease inhibitors.[121,210] Thus, apoptosis should be considered as one of many factors leading to liver graft failure from storage/reperfusion injury.

A powerful event initiating apoptosis is the MPT.[211,212] Large-amplitude mitochondrial swelling after onset of the MPT breaks the mitochondrial outer membrane and releases cytochrome c and other proapoptotic factors into the cytosol. The interaction of cytochrome c with apoptosis-activating factor 1 (APAF-1) and ATP (or dATP) then activates caspase 9, which in turn activates caspase 3, the principal "executioner" caspase whose activity leads directly to the outward manifestations of apoptosis, such as internucleosomal DNA fragmentation.[213,214] Thus, the MPT is in the peculiar position of initiating both apoptosis and necrosis.

What determines which form of cell death occurs after the MPT? A deciding factor may be levels of cellular ATP. If ATP is profoundly depleted, then cytochrome c cannot activate caspase 3 through the APAF-1/caspase 9 pathway.[213] Instead, cells must die a necrotic death, which occurs rapidly in aerobic cells. However, if glycolysis or a subpopulation of functional mitochondria maintains ATP levels above 10% to 20% of normal, then necrotic cell death is averted and apoptosis progresses instead.[215] Thus, ATP acts a switch between apoptosis and necrosis.[216-218] As long as ATP is maintained, the apoptotic pathway progresses, but when ATP becomes profoundly depleted, necrosis develops instead. In this way, the MPT represents a shared pathway leading to both apoptotic and necrotic cell death. In ischemia/reperfusion injury, the features of apoptosis and necrosis coexist. Rather than being totally distinct phenomena, pure apoptosis and pure necrotic cell death may in fact represent extremes in a continuous spectrum of cellular changes in dying cells. Recently, the term *necrapoptosis* was introduced to emphasize that apoptosis and necrosis share common pathways and may not be the distinct entities first proposed.[219]

CAROLINA RINSE SOLUTION

Reperfusion after restoration of circulation to liver grafts causes endothelial cell killing and Kupffer cell activation. In an attempt to reduce this reperfusion injury, a new solution, called Carolina rinse solution, was devised at the University of North Carolina to counter potential mechanisms contributing to reperfusion injury (Table 16.6).[5] Carolina rinse solution contains electrolytes similar to Ringer's solution, antioxidants (glutathione, desferrioxamine, allopurinol), substrates to regenerate ATP (fructose, glucose, insulin, and adenosine), a calcium channel blocker (nicardipine), colloid osmotic support against interstitial edema (hydroxyethyl starch), and mildly acidic pH (MOPS buffer, pH 6.5). Adenosine and nicardipine are also vasodilators and may improve microcirculation. Reperfusion of rat livers with Carolina rinse solution almost completely prevents endothelial cell killing after

TABLE 16.6. *Composition of Carolina rinse solution-glycine*

Ingredient	Concentration
NaCl	115 mM
KCl	5 mM
$CaCl_2$	1.3 mM
KH_2PO_4	1 mM
$MgSO_4$	1.2 mM
Hydroxyethyl starch	50 g/L
Allopurinol	1 mM
Desferrioxamine	1 mM
Glutathione	3 mM
Fructose	10 mM
Glucose	10 mM
Glycine[a]	5 mM
Adenosine	200 μM
Nicardipine	2 μM
Insulin	100 U/L
3-[N-morpholino]propanesulfonic acid (MOPS)	20 mM
Total Na+	115 mM
Total K+	6 mM
Total Cl−	122 mM
pH	6.5
Osmolarity (mOs)	290–305

[a]Earlier versions of Carolina rinse solution did not contain glycine.

Data are from Bachmann S, Peng X-X, Currin RT, et al. Glycine in Carolina rinse solution reduces reperfusion injury, improves graft function and increases graft survival after rat liver transplantation. *Transplant Proc* 1995;27:741–742; and Currin RT, Caldwell-Kenkel JC, Lichtman SN, et al. Protection by Carolina rinse solution, acidotic pH and glycine against lethal reperfusion injury to sinusoidal endothelial cells of rat livers stored for transplantation. *Transplantation* 1996;62: 1549–1558.

24 hours of storage in UW solution (Fig. 16.7).[5] Carolina rinse solution also reduces activation of Kupffer cells, as measured by particle phagocytosis, electron microscopy, and free radical formation.[220] It improves early excretory hepatocellular function and microvascular perfusion and reduces leukocyte accumulation.[220,221]

When stored rat livers are flushed with Carolina rinse solution just prior to implantation, graft failure from storage/reperfusion injury is markedly reduced. After orthotopic rat liver transplantation without arterialization, Carolina rinse solution increases long-term graft survival from 4% to 56% after 12 hours of cold storage in UW solution.[6] With arterialization after 15 hours of storage, survival increases from 8% to 40%.[222] Carolina rinse solution has also been reported to improve the survival of canine kidney grafts after prolonged storage.[223] Controversy has existed over whether endothelial cell killing in stored livers is a reperfusion injury, as described here, or whether irreversible damage occurs during storage prior to reperfusion. Protection by Carolina rinse solution *in vitro* and *in vivo* is compelling evidence that the irreversible event leading to endothelial cell killing and graft failure is the consequence of reperfusion. Two small clinical trials confirm the efficacy of flushing with Carolina rinse solution at the end of storage to decrease graft injury after implantation.[224,225] Acceptance of Carolina rinse solution for general use, however, awaits confirmation of these results in a large multicenter trial.

Components Required for Efficacy

Carolina rinse solution and UW solution both contain adenosine. In rats, reduction of adenosine in Carolina rinse solution from 1 mM to 100 to 200 μM increases graft survival, but if adenosine is removed entirely, the benefit is lost.[6,220,222] Carolina rinse solution also loses efficacy when the antioxidants (glutathione, allopurinol, desferrioxamine) are removed or if pH is raised to pH 7.4.[134] A simplified Carolina rinse solution containing adenosine and antioxidants in Ringer's solution at low pH also has efficacy.[220]

Carolina rinse solution and adenosine suppress LPS-stimulated TNF release by cultured Kupffer cells, an effect mediated by adenosine A_2 receptors.[164,165] Thus, suppression of Kupffer cell cytokine release may be one of the mechanisms by which Carolina rinse solution improves graft survival after storage/reperfusion injury. Adenine and ribose, metabolic precursors of adenosine, do not improve survival.[220] This finding also supports the concept that adenosine acts via a receptor, rather than by promoting resynthesis of ATP.

Temperature Dependence

Higher temperature decreases vascular resistance in isolated perfused organs.[226] After orthotopic rat liver transplantation, liver grafts stored for 8 hours in Euro-Collins solution and rinsed with cold Ringer's solution just prior to implantation fail in 3 days. In contrast, the same grafts survive after rinsing with warm (37°C) Ringer's solution.[131] Warm rinsing reduces vascular resistance, improves blood flow, and decreases Kupffer cell activation after graft revascularization.[131,227] Warm treatment also decreases subsequent lung injury. The benefit of Carolina rinse solution is increased by using it warm (30°C) rather than cold (1° to 4°C).[222] After 18 hours of cold storage in UW solution, long-term survival increases from 0% to 80% when grafts are rinsed with warm rather than cold Carolina rinse solution. The principal benefit of warm temperature seems to be improvement of the microcirculation, allowing more rapid and more homogenous perfusion.

The viability of hepatocytes stored in UW solution, Ringer's solution, and Carolina rinse solution is also temperature dependent. During treatment with cyanide to mimic anoxia-induced ATP depletion during organ storage, relative cell survival in various solutions at 0°C to 1°C is greatest in UW solution, followed by Carolina rinse solution and then Ringer's solution.[228] As temperature increases above 12°C, the rank order of cell survival in different solutions changes, with Carolina rinse solution demonstrating much higher survival than Ringer's solution, which shows higher cell survival than UW solution. At 37°C, almost no cell killing occurs in Carolina rinse solution at times when cell killing is virtually 100% in UW and Ringer's solution. Notably, at room temperature and above, cell killing in UW solution is greater than in ordinary Ringer's solution. This acceleration of lethal hypoxic injury in UW solution at warm temperatures implies that UW solution should be avoided when rewarming liver explants.

Carolina Rinse Solution and Glycine

Glycine is a cytoprotective amino acid that protects kidney cells, hepatocytes, and sinusoidal endothelial cells against hypoxic injury.[179,182,229–232] In a normothermic low-flow, reflow model of liver injury, glycine prevents enzyme release, peroxidation, and loss of hepatocellular viability after reoxygentation.[232] Glycine also prevents reperfusion-induced endothelial cell killing after liver storage.[233,234] Protection by Carolina rinse solution and glycine are synergistic. Thus, after 48 hours of storage in UW solution when neither Carolina rinse solution nor glycine fully protects against reperfusion-induced endothelial cell killing, the combination of 5 mM glycine in Carolina rinse solution virtually eliminates all lethal cell injury. *In vivo* after orthotopic rat liver transplantation, glycine also adds to the efficacy of Carolina rinse solution. After longer periods of storage (e.g., 24 hours), Carolina rinse–glycine improves graft survival from 0% to 50% compared with Carolina rinse solution alone. After shorter periods of storage when all grafts survive regardless of the rinse solution, Carolina rinse–glycine nonetheless decreases reperfusion injury as assessed by postoperative elevations of hepatic enzymes in the serum.

One important effect of glycine is to block a chloride channel in Kupffer cells.[235] Chloride channel blockade produces resistance to plasma membrane depolarization, which inhibits opening of the voltage-dependent calcium channel and Kupffer cell activation. During the donor operation of orthotopic rat liver transplantation, physical manipulation of the donor organ causes Kupffer cell activation, which leads to decreased graft survival. Inactivation of Kupffer cells by treatment of donor rats with dietary glycine restores survival from 30% to 100% after transplantation and decreases postoperative transaminases.[152] Intravenous glycine given to donors, and possibly recipients, is also beneficial.[236–238]

NEW DIRECTIONS FOR IMPROVING GRAFT QUALITY AND EXPANDING THE DONOR POOL

Fatty Livers

Brain-dead accident and suicide victims constitute a large proportion of the human organ donor pool. Suicides and vehicular accidents are overwhelmingly associated with alcohol consumption. Thus, a high percentage of organ donors are alcohol consumers who are at high risk for fatty liver.

Hepatic steatosis in livers from obese and alcoholic donors is strongly associated with primary graft nonfunction.[239] In experimental transplantation of fatty livers, graft failure is accompanied by disturbed microcirculation and increased leukocyte and platelet margination.[240–242] Additionally, a carbon-centered free radical is formed after transplantation of fatty livers from ethanol-treated donor rats.[243]

Gadolinium chloride pretreatment, which selectively ablates Kupffer cells, blocks radical formation and improves graft survival to nearly control levels.[244] Other antioxidants, including allopurinol (a xanthine oxidase inhibitor), catechin (a free radical scavenger), and Carolina rinse solution, also suppress free radical generation.[245] Similarly, organic radicals form during normothermic low-flow, reflow injury to perfused rat livers.[246] Ethanol contributes independently of fat to radical formation and enzyme release in a fashion blocked by gadolinium chloride.[247] These results indicate that ethanol increases free radical formation in fatty grafts after transplantation by activation of Kupffer cells, although adherent leukocytes also contribute to free radical generation.[248] Thus, measures preventing Kupffer cell activation after transplantation might allow the use of moderately steatotic livers for clinical transplantation.

Non–heart-beating Donors

Organs for human liver transplantation are made available by living-related liver donation and cadaver donation. Living-related donation by partial hepatectomy is increasingly used for pediatric liver transplantation, which has eased the very short supply of donor livers for pediatric cases considerably.[11] For adults, the number of heart-beating cadavers suitable for liver donation remains the key limiting factor for liver transplantation therapy. In human kidney transplantation, organ donation from non–heart-beating cadavers is now employed successfully at many centers.[249] Organ donors are terminally ill patients who do not meet the criteria of brain death and whose life support is withdrawn at the request of the family. After cardiac arrest occurs and death is pronounced several minutes later, the organs are harvested. Thus, organs from non–heart-beating cadaveric donors experience at least 10 minutes of warm ischemia prior to cold preservation. However, clinical results with livers from non–heart-beating donors remain poor, and 2-month graft survival was only 50% even for donors who were extubated in an operating room setting.[250]

In animal models, livers can be stored and transplanted after short periods of warm ischemia, but graft viability decreases rapidly as the time of warm ischemia increases (Fig. 16.9).[251,252] In rats, 50% graft failure occurs after about 60 minutes of warm *in situ* ischemia. The nature of the injury is also different. Unlike cold ischemia/reperfusion injury, liver damage after warm ischemia occurs primarily to parenchymal rather than nonparenchymal cells (Fig. 16.9). Moreover, tissue damage is not a reperfusion injury. Instead, hepatocytes lose viability during warm ischemia

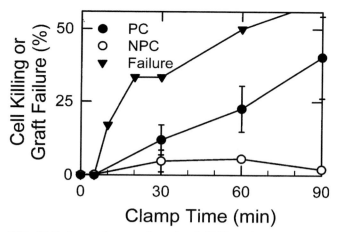

FIG. 16.9. Loss of parenchymal cell (PC) and nonparenchymal cell (NPC) viability in relation to graft survival after *in situ* warm ischemia. Rat aortas were clamped for 0 to 90 minutes. After clamping, livers were immediately infused with cold UW solution containing trypan blue and fixed for assessment of cell killing by nuclear trypan blue staining. In parallel experiments, aortas were clamped, and livers were harvested and transplanted after 2 hours of storage in cold UW solution. Warm ischemia caused predominantly parenchymal cell killing that increased with increasing clamp times. Nonparenchymal cell killing was modest. Graft viability decreased as parenchymal cell killing increased. No graft survived after 120 minutes of aortic clamping. (From Currin RT, Peng X-X, Thurman RG, et al. Loss of hepatocyte viability during warm ischemia causes graft failure of livers from non-heart beating donors. *Hepatology* 1999;30:275a, with permission.)

prior to reperfusion. Consequently, new and different strategies will be needed to block warm ischemic injury in this context and to improve the outcome of non–heart-beating cadaveric donation in liver transplantation. Moreover, harvesting of organs from non–heart-beating cadavers may require machine perfusion preservation in order to monitor functional parameters prior to implantation.[249]

Preconditioning of Donor Livers

One strategy to improve the quality of organ donation is to pretreat donors in a fashion that produces resistance to harvest, storage, and reperfusion injury. In heart and other organs, including liver, brief periods of ischemia followed by reperfusion confer protection against subsequent prolonged ischemia, a phenomenon called ischemic preconditioning.[253–255] Ischemic preconditioning of donor rat livers also decreases endothelial cell killing, Kupffer cell activation, and liver graft failure from prolonged cold storage.[256–258] Adenosine release during ischemic preconditioning mediates cytoprotection by an adenosine A_2 receptor mechanism.[259] Both Kupffer cells and sinusoidal endothelial cells contain cAMP-coupled adenosine A_2 receptors,[165,260] and treatment of donor livers with a membrane-permeant cAMP

analogue prior to storage provides the same protection as ischemic preconditioning.[260]

Similarly, donor pretreatment with prostaglandin analogues such as dimethylprostaglandin E_2 decreases endothelial cell killing after cold storage and reperfusion and improves graft success after transplantation.[261] Kupffer cells and sinusoidal endothelial cells also contain cAMP-linked prostaglandin receptors, which presumably account for prostaglandin-mediated protection. Ischemic preconditioning against warm ischemia/reperfusion injury may also involve increased formation of nitric oxide, a vasodilator that likely improves microcirculation after ischemia/reperfusion and prevents the no-reflow phenomenon.[255] Overall, these new developments indicate that pretreatment of donors prior to organ harvest can substantially improve graft function and viability after transplantation.

Gene Therapy

Another strategy to make donor livers resistant to storage/reperfusion injury is genetic modification. Recent work indicates that adenovirus-mediated transfer of genes for bcl_2, an antiapoptotic protooncogene, and superoxide dismutase, an antioxidant enzyme, into donor livers prior to storage decreases graft injury and improves graft survival after transplantation.[262,263] By contrast, suppression of activation of nuclear factor-κB (NF-κB) with an adenovirus carrying a modified gene for IκB, the natural inhibitor of NF-κB, increases graft injury after storage/reperfusion.[264]

CONCLUSION

Advances made in research on liver preservation for transplantation illustrate how the understanding of basic mechanisms yields practical new strategies to extend the time and quality of liver storage. The mechanisms underlying storage/reperfusion injury are multifactorial, and we are no longer so naive as to think that some single mechanism will account for loss of graft viability. Indeed, the consequences of reperfusion-induced endothelial injury and Kupffer cell activation are not only hemostasis and inflammation within the liver itself but also systemic reactions resulting in adult respiratory distress, clotting disorders, and multiple organ failure.

As we come to better understand the mechanisms of storage/reperfusion injury, we should be able to develop additional strategies, like UW solution and Carolina rinse solution, to further minimize injury after liver storage, reperfusion, and implantation. Such advances are needed to reduce the still-high incidence of primary nonfunction and dysfunction in transplanted livers and to allow increased use of livers from marginal donors now considered too risky for human use. Liver transplantation is very severely limited by the number of suitable organ donors. Advances in our understanding of storage/reperfusion injury may also one day allow us to use previously untapped organ donor pools, such as non–heart-beating cadavers.

ACKNOWLEDGMENTS

This work was supported in part by NIH grants DK37034 and AA09156 and NIH grant P30 DK34987 to the Center for Gastrointestinal Biology and Disease at the University of North Carolina.

REFERENCES

1. Belzer FO, Southard JH. Principles of solid-organ preservation by cold storage. *Transplantation* 1988;45:673–676.
2. Kalayoglu M, Hoffman RM, D'Alessandro AM, et al. Clinical results in liver transplantation using UW solution for extended preservation. *Transplant Proc* 1989;21:3487–3488.
3. Todo S, Nery J, Yanaga K, et al. Extended preservation of human liver grafts with UW solution. *JAMA* 1989;261:711–714.
4. Howard TK, Klintmalm GB, Cofer JB, et al. The influence of preservation injury on rejection in the hepatic transplant recipient. *Transplantation* 1990;49:103–107.
5. Currin RT, Thurman RG, Toole JG, et al. Evidence that Carolina rinse solution protects sinusoidal endothelial cells against reperfusion injury after cold ischemic storage of rat liver. *Transplantation* 1990;50:1076–1078.
6. Gao W, Takei Y, Marzi I, et al. Carolina rinse solution—a new strategy to increase survival time after orthotopic liver transplantation in the rat. *Transplantation* 1991;52:417–424.
7. Sanchez-Urdazpal L, Gores GJ, Lemasters JJ, et al. Carolina rinse solution decreases liver injury during clinical liver transplantation. *Transplant Proc* 1993;25:1574–1575.
8. Bachmann S, Bechstein WO, Keck H, et al. Pilot study: Carolina rinse solution improves graft function after orthotopic liver transplantation in humans. *Transplant Proc* 1996;29:390–392.
9. Broelsch CE, Emond JC, Thistlethwaite JR, et al. Liver transplantation with reduced-size donor organs. *Transplantation* 1988;45:519–524.
10. Malago M, Rogiers X, Broelsch CE. Liver splitting and living donor techniques. *Br Med Bull* 1997;53:860–867.
11. Reyes J, Mazariegos GV. Pediatric transplantation. *Surg Clin North Am* 1999;79:163–189.
12. Okouchi Y, Tamaki T, Kozaki M. The optimal temperature for hypothermic liver preservation in the rat. *Transplantation* 1992;54:1129–1130.
13. Hertl M, Chartrand PB, West DD, et al. The effects of hepatic preservation at 0°C compared to 5°C: influence of antiproteases and periodic flushing. *Cryobiology* 1994;31:434–440.
14. Williams JW, Vera S, Peters PG, et al. Cholestatic jaundice after hepatic transplantation. A nonimmunologically mediated event. *Am J Surg* 1986;151:65–70.
15. Snover DC, Sibley RK, Freese DK, et al. Orthotopic liver transplantation: a pathological study of 63 serial liver biopsies from 17 patients with special reference to the diagnostic features and natural history of rejection. *Hepatology* 1984;4:1212–1222.
16. Demetris AJ, Batts KP, Dhillon AP, et al. Banff schema for grading liver allograft rejection: an international consensus document. *Hepatology* 1997;25:658–663.
17. Pienaar BH, Lindell SL, van Gulik TM, et al. Seventy-two-hour preservation of canine liver by machine perfusion. *Transplantation* 1990;49:258–260.
18. Porte RJ, Ploeg RJ, Hansen B, et al. Long-term graft survival after liver transplantation in the UW era: late effects of cold ischemia and primary dysfunction. European Multicentre Study Group. *Transpl Int* 1998;11(suppl 1):S164-S167.
19. Rosen HR, Martin P, Goss J, et al. Significance of early aminotransferase elevation after liver transplantation. *Transplantation* 1998;65:68–72.
20. Oldhafer KJ, Bornscheuer A, Fruhauf NR, et al. Rescue hepatectomy for initial graft non-function after liver transplantation. *Transplantation* 1999;67:1024–1028.
21. Ploeg RJ, D'Alessandro AM, Knechtle SJ, et al. Risk factors for primary dysfunction after liver transplantation—a multivariate analysis. *Transplantation* 1993;55:807–813.
22. Katz E, Mor E, Patel T, et al. Association between preservation injury and early rejection in clinical liver transplantation: fact or myth? *Transplant Proc* 1993;25:1907–1908.
23. Deschenes M, Belle SH, Krom RA, et al. Early allograft dysfunction after liver transplantation: a definition and predictors of outcome. National Institute of Diabetes and Digestive and Kidney Diseases Liver Transplantation Database. *Transplantation* 1998;66:302–310.
24. Sanchez-Urdazpal L, Gores GJ, Ward EM, et al. Ischemic-type biliary complications after orthotopic liver transplantation. *Hepatology* 1992;16:49–53.
25. Porayko MK, Kondo M, Steers JL. Liver transplantation: late complications of the biliary tract and their management. *Semin Liver Dis* 1995;15:139–155.
26. Furukawa H, Todo S, Imventarza O, et al. Effect of cold ischemia time on the early outcome of human hepatic allografts preserved with UW solution. *Transplantation* 1991;51:1000–1004.
27. Gaffey MJ, Boyd JC, Traweek ST, et al. Predictive value of intraoperative biopsies and liver function tests for preservation injury in orthotopic liver transplantation. *Hepatology* 1997;25:184–189.
28. D'Alessandro AM, Kalayoglu M, Sollinger HW, et al. The predictive value of donor liver biopsies for the development of primary nonfunction after orthotopic liver transplantation. *Transplantation* 1991;51:157–163.
29. Marsman WA, Wiesner RH, Rodriguez L, et al. Use of fatty donor liver is associated with diminished early patient and graft survival. *Transplantation* 1996;62:1246–1251.
30. Marino IR, Doyle HR, Aldrighetti L, et al. Effect of donor age and sex on the outcome of liver transplantation. *Hepatology* 1995;22:1754–1762.
31. Brooks BK, Levy MF, Jennings LW, et al. Influence of donor and recipient gender on the outcome of liver transplantation. *Transplantation* 1996;62:1784–1787.
32. Marino IR, Doria C, Doyle HR, et al. Matching donors and recipients. *Liver Transplant Surg* 1998;4(suppl 1):S115–S119.
33. Deschenes M, Forbes C, Tchervenkov J, et al. Use of older donor livers is associated with more extensive ischemic damage on intraoperative biopsies during liver transplantation. *Liver Transplant Surg* 1999;5:357–361.
34. Morgan GR, Sanabria JR, Clavien PA, et al. Correlation of donor nutritional status with sinusoidal lining cell viability and liver function in the rat. *Transplantation* 1991;51:1176–1183.
35. Cywes R, Greig PD, Sanabria JR, et al. Effect of intraportal glucose infusion on hepatic glycogen content and degradation, and outcome of liver transplantation. *Ann Surg* 1992;216:235–246.
36. Savier E, Lindert K, Lemasters JJ, et al. Liver transplantation depletes hepatic carbohydrate reserves and increases sensitivity to hypoxia [Abstract]. *Hepatology* 1990;12:864.
37. Sumimoto R, Southard JH, Belzer FO. Livers from fasted rats acquire resistance to warm and cold ischemia injury. *Transplantation* 1993;55:728–732.
38. Lindell SL, Hansen T, Rankin M, et al. Donor nutritional status—a determinant of liver preservation injury. *Transplantation* 1996;61:239–247.
39. Okamoto R, Yamamoto Y, Lin H, et al. Influence of dopamine on the liver assessed by changes in arterial ketone body ratio in brain-dead dogs. *Surgery* 1990;107:36–42.
40. Osaki N, Ringe B, Bunzendahl H, et al. Postoperative recovery of mitochondrial function of the human liver graft procured and preserved with University of Wisconsin (UW) solution. *Transpl Int* 1990;3:128–132.
41. Emre S, Schwartz ME, Altaca G, et al. Safe use of hepatic allografts from donors older than 70 years. *Transplantation* 1996;62:62–65.
42. Hoofnagle JH, Lombardero M, Zetterman RK, et al. Donor age and outcome of liver transplantation. *Hepatology* 1996;24:89–96.
43. Jimenez-Romero C, Moreno-Gonzalez E, Colina-Ruiz F, et al. Use of octogenarian livers safely expands the donor pool. *Transplantation* 1999;68:572–575.
44. Deschenes M, Forbes C, Tchervenkov J, et al. Use of older donor livers is associated with more extensive ischemic damage on intraoperative biopsies during liver transplantation. *Liver Transplant Surg* 1999;5:357–361.
45. Oellerich M, Raude E, Burdelski M, et al. Monoethylglycinexylidide formation kinetics: a novel approach to assessment of liver function. *J Clin Chem Clin Biochem* 1987;25:845–853.
46. Oellerich MM, Burdelski B. Ringe P, et al. Lignocaine metabolite formation as a measure of pre-transplant liver function. *Lancet* 1989;25:640–642.
47. Adam R, Azoulay D, Astarcioglu I, et al. Limits of the MEGX test in the selection of liver grafts for transplantation. *Transplant Proc* 1993;25:1653–1654.

48. Reding R, Wallemacq P, de Ville de Goyet J, et al. The unreliability of the lidocaine/monoethylglycinexylidide test for assessment of liver donors. *Transplantation* 1993;56:323–326.

49. Zotz RB, von Schonfeld J, Erhard J, et al. Value of an extended monoethylglycinexylidide formation test and other dynamic liver function tests in liver transplant donors. *Transplantation* 1997;63:538–541.

50. Woodside KJ, Merion RM, Williams TC. Prospective multivariate analysis of donor monoethylglycine xylidide (MEGX) testing in liver transplantation. Transplantation Society of Michigan Scientific Studies Committee. *Clin Transplant* 1998;12:43–48.

51. Yamaoka Y, Taki Y, Gubernatis G, et al. Evaluation of the liver graft before procurement. Significance of arterial ketone body ratio in brain-dead patients. *Transpl Int* 1990;3:78–81.

52. Shaw BW. Starting a liver transplant program. *Semin Liver Dis* 1989;9:159–167.

53. Showstack J, Katz PP, Lake JR, et al. Resource utilization in liver transplantation: effects of patient characteristics and clinical practice. NIDDK Liver Transplantation Database Group. *JAMA* 1999;281:1381–1386.

54. Annual report of the U.S. Scientific Registry for Organ Transplantation and the Organ Procurement and Transplantation Network. Richmond, VA: United Network for Organ Sharing, 1998.

55. Benichou J, Halgrimson CG, Weil R, et al. Canine and human liver preservation for 6–18 hours by cold infusion. *Transplantation* 1977;24:407–411.

56. Collins GM, Bravo-Sugarman M, Terasaki PI. Kidney preservation for transportation. *Lancet* 1969;1:1219–1222.

57. Dreikron K, Horsch R, Rohl L. 48 to 96 hour preservation of canine kidneys by initial perfusion and hypothermic storage using the Euro-Collins solution. *Eur Urol* 1980;6:221–224.

58. Jamieson NV, Sundberg R, Lindell S, et al. Preservation of the canine liver for 24–48 hours using simple cold storage with UW solution. *Transplantation* 1988;46:517–522.

59. Yu W, Coddington D, Bitter-Suermann H. Rat liver preservation I. The components of UW solution that are essential to its success. *Transplantation* 1990;49:1060–1066.

60. Marshall VC, Howden BO, Jablonski P, et al. Analysis of UW solution in a rat liver transplant model. *Transplant Proc* 1990;22:503–505.

61. Sumimoto R, Kamada N. Lactobionate as the most important component in UW solution for liver preservation. *Transplant Proc* 1990;22:2198–2199.

62. Kobayashi T, Sumimoto R, Shimada H, et al. Effect of sugars in the preservation solution on liver storage in rats. *Cryobiology* 1991;28:428–435.

63. Sumimoto R, Jamieson NV, Kobayashi T, et al. The need for glutathione and allopurinol in HL solution for rat liver preservation. *Transplantation* 1991;52:565–567.

64. Boudjema K, van Gulik TM, Lindell SL, et al. Effect of oxidized and reduced glutathione in liver preservation. *Transplantation* 1990;50:948–951.

65. Evans PJ, Tredger JM, Dunne JB, et al. Catalytic metal ions and the loss of reduced glutathione from University of Wisconsin preservation solution. *Transplantation* 1996;62:1046–1049.

66. Biguzas M, Jablonski P, Howden BO, et al. Evaluation of UW solution in rat kidney preservation. *Transplantation* 1990;49:1051–1055.

67. Prien T, Dietl KH, Zander J, et al. Bradyarrhythmia with University of Wisconsin preservation solution. *Lancet* 1989;1:1319–1320.

68. Howden BO, Jablonski P, Thomas AC, et al. Liver preservation with UW solution I. Evidence that hydroxyethyl starch is not essential. *Transplantation* 1990;49:869–872.

69. Adam R, Settaf A, Fabiani B, et al. Comparative evaluation of Euro-Collins, UW solution, and UW solution without hydroxyethyl starch in orthotopic liver transplantation in the rat. *Transplant Proc* 1990;22:499–502.

70. den Butter G, Saunder A, Marsh DC, et al. Comparison of solutions for preservation of the rabbit liver as tested by isolated perfusion. *Transpl Int* 1995;8:466–471.

71. Neveux N, De Bandt JP, Charrueau C, et al. Deletion of hydroxyethyl-starch from University of Wisconsin solution induces cell shrinkage and proteolysis during and after cold storage of rat liver. *Hepatology* 1997;25:678–682.

72. Ploeg RJ, Boudjema K, Marsh D, et al. The importance of a colloid in canine pancreas preservation. *Transplantation* 1992;53:735–741.

73. Wicomb WN, Collins GM. 24-hour rabbit heart storage with UW solution. *Transplantation* 1989;48:6–9.

74. Walcher F, Marzi I, Schafer W, et al. Undissolved particles in UW solution cause microcirculatory disturbances after liver transplantation in the rat. *Transpl Int* 1995;8:161–162.

75. Moen J, Claesson K, Pienaar H, et al. Preservation of dog liver, kidney, and pancreas using the Belzer-UW solution with high-sodium and low-potassium content. *Transplantation* 1989;47:940–945.

76. Sumimoto R, Jamieson NV, Wake K, et al. 24-hour rat liver preservation using UW solution and some simplified variants. *Transplantation* 1989;48:1–5.

77. Ben Abdennebi H, Steghens JP, Margonari J, et al. High-Na+ low-K+ UW cold storage solution reduces reperfusion injuries of the rat liver graft. *Transpl Int* 1998;11:223–230.

78. Jamieson NV. A new solution for liver preservation. *Br J Surg* 1989;76:107–108.

79. Muhlbacher F, Langer F, Mittermayer C. Preservation solutions for transplantation. *Transplant Proc* 1999;31:2069–2070.

80. Krishnan H, Hannon MF, Bawa SM, et al. Comparison of the efficacy of University of Wisconsin solution and Newcastle organ perfusion fluid in the preservation of livers for transplantation. *Transpl Int* 1998;11(suppl 1):S387-S389.

81. Bretschneider HJ, Helmchen U, Kehrer G. Nierenprotektion [in German]. *Klin Wochenschr* 1988;66:817–827.

82. Tokunaga Y, Wicomb WN, Concepcion W, et al. Successful 20-hour rat liver preservation with chlorpromazine in sodium lactobionate sucrose solution. *Surgery* 1991;110:80–86.

83. Menasche P, Termignon JL, Pradier F, et al. Experimental evaluation of Celsior, a new heart preservation solution. *Eur J Cardiothorac Surg* 1994;8:207–213.

84. Erhard J, Lange R, Scherer R, et al. Comparison of histidine-tryptophan-ketoglutarate (HTK) solution versus University of Wisconsin (UW) solution for organ preservation in human liver transplantation. A prospective, randomized study. *Transpl Int* 1994;7:177–181.

85. Hatano E, Kiuchi T, Tanaka A, et al. Hepatic preservation with histidine-tryptophan-ketoglutarate solution in living-related and cadaveric liver transplantation. *Clin Sci* 1997;93:81–88.

86. Spiegel HU, Schleimer K, Kranz D, et al. Organ preservation with EC, HTK, and UW solutions in orthotopic liver transplantation in syngeneic rats. Part I: Functional parameters. *J Invest Surg* 1998;11:49–56.

87. Peng X-X, Currin RT, Bachmann S, et al. Superiority of UW solution over HTK solution for graft survival and nonparenchymal cell viability after liver preservation for transplantation. In: Wisse E, Knook DL, Balabaud C, eds. *Cells of the hepatic sinusoid*, vol. 6. Leiden, The Netherlands: The Kupffer Cell Foundation, 1997:210–212.

88. Egawa H, Esquivel CO, Wicomb WN, et al. Significance of terminal rinse for rat liver preservation. *Transplantation* 1993;56:1344–1347.

89. Tojimbara T, Wicomb WN, Garcia-Kennedy R, et al. Liver transplantation from non-heart beating donors in rats: influence of viscosity and temperature of initial flushing solutions on graft function. *Liver Transpl Surg* 1997;3:39–45.

90. Zhu Y, Furukawa H, Nakamura K, et al. Sodium lactobionate sucrose solution for canine liver and kidney preservation. *Transplant Proc* 1993;25:1618–1619.

91. Nakazato PZ, Itasaka H, Concepcion W, et al. Effects of abdominal en bloc procurement and of a high sodium preservation solution in liver transplantation. *Transplant Proc* 1993;25:1604–1606.

92. Roberts RF, Nishanian GP, Carey JN, et al. A comparison of the new preservation solution Celsior to Euro-Collins and University of Wisconsin solutions in lung reperfusion injury. *Transplantation* 1999;67:152–155.

93. Cascales P, Fernandez-Cornejo V, Sanchez-Del Campo F, et al. Evaluation of Celsior solution in experimental liver preservation using *ex situ* isolated rat liver perfusion. *Transplant Proc* 1999;31:2437–2438.

94. Valero R, Almenara R, Garcia-Valdecasas JC, et al. Usefulness of Celsior in graft preservation of livers obtained from non heart beating donors in experimental (pigs) liver transplantation: comparative study with University of Wisconsin solution. *Transplant Proc* 1999;31:2433–2434.

95. Lemasters JJ, Stemkowski CJ, Ji S, et al. Cell surface changes and enzyme release during hypoxia and reoxygenation in the isolated, perfused rat liver. *J Cell Biol* 1983;97:778–786.

96. Caldwell-Kenkel JC, Currin RT, Tanaka Y, et al. Reperfusion injury to endothelial cells following cold ischemic storage of rat livers. *Hepatology* 1989;10:292–299.

97. Lemasters JJ, Caldwell-Kenkel JC, Currin RT, et al. Endothelial cell killing and activation of Kupffer cells following reperfusion of rat livers stored in Euro-Collins solution. In: Wisse E, Knook DL, Decker K, eds. *Cells of the hepatic sinusoid,* vol. 2. Rijswijk, The Netherlands: Kupffer Cell Foundation, 1989:277–280.

98. Momii S, Koga A, Eguchi M, et al. Ultrastructural changes in rat liver sinusoids during storage in cold Euro-Collins solution. *Virchows Arch B* 1989;57:393–398.

99. Caldwell-Kenkel JC, Currin RT, Tanaka Y, et al. Kupffer cell activation and endothelial cell damage after storage of rat livers: effects of reperfusion. *Hepatology* 1991;13:83–95.

100. Caldwell-Kenkel JC, Thurman RG, Lemasters JJ. Selective loss of nonparenchymal cell viability after cold, ischemic storage of rat livers. *Transplantation* 1988;45:834–837.

101. Marzi I, Zhong Z, Lemasters JJ, et al. Evidence that graft survival is not related to parenchymal cell viability in rat liver transplantation: the importance of nonparenchymal cells. *Transplantation* 1989;48:463–468.

102. Myagkaya GL, van Veen HA, James J. Ultrastructural changes in the rat liver during Euro-Collins storage, compared with hypothermic *in vitro* ischemia. *Virchows Arch B* 1987;53:176–182.

103. McKeown, CMB, Edwards V, Phillips MJ, et al. Sinusoidal lining cell damage: the critical injury in cold preservation of liver allografts in the rat. *Transplantation* 1988;46:178–191.

104. Lemasters JJ, Thurman RG. Reperfusion injury after liver preservation for transplantation. *Ann Rev Pharmacol Toxicol* 1997;37:327–338.

105. Vaubourdolle M, Chazouilleres O, Poupon R, et al. Creatine kinase-BB: a marker of liver sinusoidal damage in ischemia-reperfusion. *Hepatology* 1993;17:423–428.

106. Rao PN, Walsh TR, Makowka L, et al. Purine nucleoside phosphorylase: a new marker for free oxygen radical injury to the endothelial cell. *Hepatology* 1990;11:193–198.

107. Brass CA, Mody MG. Evaluation of purine nucleoside phosphorylase release as a measure of hepatic endothelial cell injury. *Hepatology* 1995;21:174–179.

108. Leser H, Holstege A, Gerok W. The role of nonparenchymal and parenchymal liver cells in the catabolism of extracellular purines. *Hepatology* 1989;10:66–71.

109. Eriksson S, Fraser JR, Laurent TC, et al. Endothelial cells are a site of uptake and degradation of hyaluronic acid in the liver. *Exp Cell Res* 1983;144:223–228.

110. Smedsrod B. Non-invasive means to study the functional status of sinusoidal liver endothelial cells. *J Gastroenterol Hepatol* 1995;10(suppl 1):S81-S83.

111. Shimizu H, He W, Guo P, et al. Serum hyaluronate in the assessment of liver endothelial cell function after orthotopic liver transplantation in the rat. *Hepatology* 1994;20:1323–1329.

112. Reinders ME, van Wagensveld BA, van Gulik TM, et al. Hyaluronic acid uptake in the assessment of sinusoidal endothelial cell damage after cold storage and normothermic reperfusion of rat livers. *Transpl Int* 1996;9:446–453.

113. Wang L, Zhao D, Suehiro T, et al. Assessment of damage and recovery of sinusoidal endothelial cell function by *in vivo* hyaluronic acid uptake in cold-preserved and transplanted rat livers. *Transplantation* 1996;62:1217–1221.

114. Rao PN, Bronsther OL, Pinna AD, et al. Hyaluronate levels in donor organ washout effluents: a simple and predictive parameter of graft viability. *Liver* 1996;16:48–54.

115. Suehiro T, Boros P, Emre S, et al. Assessment of liver allograft function by hyaluronic acid and endothelin levels. *J Surg Res* 1997;73:123–128.

116. Bradford BU, Marotto M, Lemasters JJ, et al. New simple models to evaluate zone-specific damage to hypoxia in the perfused rat liver: time course and effect of nutritional state. *J Pharmacol Exp Ther* 1986;236:263–268.

117. Marotto ME, Thurman RG, Lemasters JJ. Early midzonal cell death during low-flow hypoxia in the isolated, perfused rat liver: protection by allopurinol. *Hepatology* 1988;8:585–590.

118. Morgan GR, Sanabria JR, Clavien PA, et al. Correlation of donor nutritional status with sinusoidal lining cell viability and liver function in the rat. *Transplantation* 1991;51:1176–1183.

119. Carles J, Fawaz R, Neaud V, et al. Ultrastructure of human liver grafts preserved with UW solution. Comparison between patients with low and high postoperative transaminases levels. *J Submicrosc Cytol Pathol* 1994;26:67–73.

120. Carles J, Fawaz R, Hamoudi NE, et al. Preservation of human liver grafts in UW solution. Ultrastructural evidence for endothelial and Kupffer cell activation during cold ischemia and after ischemia-reperfusion. *Liver* 1994;124:50–56.

121. Takei Y, Marzi I, Kauffman FC, et al. Increase in survival time of liver transplants by protease inhibitors and a calcium channel blocker, nisoldipine. *Transplantation* 1990;50:14–20.

122. Caldwell-Kenkel JC, Currin RT, Coote A, et al. Reperfusion injury to endothelial cells after cold storage of rat livers: protection by mildly acidic pH and lack of protection by antioxidants. *Transpl Int* 1995;8:77–85.

123. Caldwell-Kenkel JC, Currin RT, Gao W, et al. Reperfusion injury to livers stored for transplantation: endothelial cell killing and Kupffer cell activation. In: Wisse E, Knook DL, Decker K, eds. *Cells of the hepatic sinusoid,* vol. 3. Rijswijk, The Netherlands: Kupffer Cell Foundation, 1989:376–380.

124. Takei Y, Marzi I, Gao W, et al. Leukocyte adhesion and cell death following orthotopic liver transplantation in the rat. *Transplantation* 1991;51:959–965.

125. Jaeschke H, Farhood A. Neutrophil and Kupffer cell-induced oxidant stress and ischemia-reperfusion injury in rat liver. *Am J Physiol* 1991;260:G355-G362.

126. Lindert KA, Caldwell-Kenkel JC, Nukina S, et al. Activation of Kupffer cells on reperfusion following hypoxia: particle phagocytosis in a low-flow, reflow model. *Am J Physiol* 1992;262:G345–G350.

127. Jaeschke H, Bautista AP, Spolarics Z, et al. Superoxide generation by Kupffer cells and priming of neutrophils during reperfusion after hepatic ischemia. *Free Radical Res Commun* 1991;15:277–284.

128. Rymsa B, Wang JF, de Groot H. O_2-release by activated Kupffer cells upon reoxygenation. *Am J Physiol* 1991;261:G602–G607.

129. Arii S, Monden K, Adachi Y, et al. Pathogenic role of Kupffer cell activation in the reperfusion injury of cold-preserved liver. *Transplantation* 1994;58:1072–1077.

130. Colletti LM, Remick DG, Burtch GD, et al. The role of tumor necrosis factor alpha in the pathophysiologic alterations following hepatic ischemia/reperfusion injury. *J Clin Invest* 1990;85:1936–1943.

131. Takei Y, Gao W, Hijioka T, et al. Increase in survival of liver grafts after rinsing with warm Ringer's solution due to improvement of hepatic microcirculation. *Transplantation* 1991;52:225–230.

132. Goto M, Takei Y, Kawano S, et al. Tumor necrosis factor and endotoxin in the pathogenesis of liver and pulmonary injuries after orthotopic liver transplantation in the rat. *Hepatology* 1992;16:487–493.

133. Savier E, Shedlofsky SI, Swim AT, et al. The calcium channel blocker nisoldipine minimizes the release of tumor necrosis factor and interleukin-6 following rat liver transplantation. *Transpl Int* 1992;5:S398–S402.

134. Bachmann S, Caldwell-Kenkel JC, Currin RT, et al. Protection by pentoxifylline against graft failure from storage injury after orthotopic rat liver transplantation with arterialization. *Transpl Int* 1992;5(suppl 1):S345–S350.

135. Thurman RG, Marzi I, Seitz G, et al. Hepatic reperfusion injury following orthotopic liver transplantation in the rat. *Transplantation* 1988;46:502–506.

136. Clavien PA, Harvey PR, Sanabria JR, et al. Lymphocyte adherence in the reperfused rat liver: mechanisms and effect. *Hepatology* 1993;17:131–142.

137. Arai M, Mochida S, Ohno A, et al. Blood coagulation in the hepatic sinusoids as a contributing factor for liver injury following orthotopic liver transplantation in the rat. *Transplantation* 1996;62:1398–1401.

138. Cywes R, Packham MA, Tietze L, et al. Role of platelets in hepatic allograft preservation injury in the rat. *Hepatology* 1993;18:635–647.

139. Cywes R, Brendan J, Mullen M, et al. Prediction of the outcome of transplantation in man by platelet adherence in donor liver allografts. *Transplantation* 1993;56:316–323.

140. Post S, Gonzalez AP, Palma P, et al. Assessment of hepatic phagocytic activity by *in vivo* microscopy after liver transplantation in the rat. *Hepatology* 1992;16:803–809.

141. Smedsrod B, De Bleser PJ, Braet F, et al. Cell biology of liver endothelial and Kupffer cells. *Gut* 1994;35:1509–1516.

142. Biozzi G, Stiffel C. The physiopathology of the reticuloendothelial cells of liver and spleen. *Progr Liver Dis* 1965;2:166–191.

143. Connor HD, Gao W, Nukina S, et al. Evidence that free radicals are involved in graft failure following orthotopic liver transplantation in the rat—an electron paramagnetic resonance spin trapping study. *Transplantation* 1992;54:199–204.

144. Koo A, Komatsu H, Tao G, et al. Contribution of no-reflow phenomenon to hepatic injury after ischemia-reperfusion: evidence for a role for superoxide anion. *Hepatology* 1992;15:507–514.

145. Marzi I, Knee J, Buhren V, et al. Reduction by superoxide dismutase of leukocyte-endothelial adherence after liver transplantation. *Surgery* 1992;111:90–97.

146. Matuschak GM, Rinaldo JE, Pinsky MR, et al. Effect of end stage liver failure on the incidence and resolution of adult respiratory distress syndrome. *J Crit Care* 1987;2:162–173.

147. Fusaoka T, Hunt KJ, Lemasters JJ, et al. Evidence that activation of Kupffer cells increases oxygen uptake after cold storage. *Transplantation* 1994;58:1067–1071.

148. Sankary HN, Chong A, Foster P, et al. Inactivation of Kupffer cells after prolonged donor fasting improves viability of transplanted hepatic allografts. *Hepatology* 1995;22:1236–1242.

149. Lindell SL, Hansen T, Rankin M, et al. Donor nutritional status—a determinant of liver preservation injury. *Transplantation* 1996;61: 239–247.

150. Peng X-X, Currin RT, Musshafen TL, et al. Lipopolysaccharide treatment of donor rats causes graft failure after orthotopic liver transplantation. In: Wisse E, Knook DL, Decker K, eds. *Cells of the hepatic sinusoid,* vol. 5. Leiden, The Netherlands: Kupffer Cell Foundation, 1995:234–235.

151. Azoulay D, Astarcioglu I, Lemoine A, et al. The effects of donor and recipient endotoxemia on TNF alpha production and mortality in the rat model of syngenic orthotopic liver transplantation. *Transplantation* 1995;59:825–829.

152. Schemmer P, Schoonhoven R, Swenberg JA, et al. Gentle *in situ* liver manipulation during organ harvest decreases survival after rat liver transplantation: role of Kupffer cells. *Transplantation* 1998;65: 1015–1020.

153. Wake K, Decker K, Kirn A, et al. Cell biology and the kinetics of Kupffer cells in the liver. *Int Rev Cytol* 1989;118:173–229.

154. ArRajab A, Ahren B, Bengmark S. Improved liver preservation for transplantation due to calcium channel blockade. *Transplantation* 1991;51:965–967.

155. Cheng S, Ragsdale JR, Sasaki AW, et al. Verapamil improves hepatic preservation with UW solution. *J Surg Res* 1991;50:560–564.

156. Jacobsson J, Sundberg R, Valdivia LA, et al. Liver preservation with lidoflazine and the University of Wisconsin solution: a dose-finding study. *Transplantation* 1993;56:472–475.

157. Huntress JD, Papadakos PJ. The role of calcium-channel antagonists in solid organ transplantation. *New Horizons* 1996;4:129–133.

158. Thurman RG, Apel E, Badr M, et al. Protection of liver by calcium entry blockers. *Ann N Y Acad Sci* 1988;522:757–770.

159. Hijioka T, Rosenberg RL, Lemasters JJ, et al. Kupffer cells contain voltage-dependent calcium channels. *Molec Pharmacol* 1992;41: 434–440.

160. Oide H, Thurman RG. Hepatic Ito cells contain calcium channels: increases with transforming growth factor-beta 1. *Hepatology* 1994;20: 1009–1014.

161. Gatmaitan Z, Varticovski L, Ling L, et al. Studies on fenestral contraction in rat liver endothelial cells in culture. *Am J Pathol* 1996; 148:2027–2041.

162. Bataller R, Nicolas JM, Gines P, et al. Contraction of human hepatic stellate cells activated in culture: a role for voltage-operated calcium channels. *J Hepatol* 1998;29:398–408.

163. Marzi I, Cowper KB, Takei Y, et al. Methyl palmitate prevents Kupffer cell activation and improves survival after orthotopic liver transplantation in the rat. *Transpl Int* 1991;4:215–220.

164. Currin RT, Reinstein LJ, Lichtman SN, et al. Inhibition of tumor necrosis factor release from cultured rat Kupffer cells by agents that reduce graft failure from storage injury. *Transplant Proc* 1993;25: 1631–1632.

165. Reinstein LJ, Lichtman SN, Currin RT, et al. Suppression of lipopolysaccharide-stimulated release of tumor necrosis factor by adenosine: evidence for A₂ receptors on rat Kupffer cells. *Hepatology* 1994;19:1445–1452.

166. Bachmann S, Caldwell-Kenkel JC, Currin RT, et al. Ultrastructural correlates of liver graft failure from storage injury: studies of graft protection by Carolina rinse solution and pentoxifylline. *Transplant Proc* 1993;25:1620–1624.

167. Kozaki K, Egawa H, Bermudez L, et al. Effects of pentoxifylline pretreatment on Kupffer cells in rat liver transplantation. *Hepatology* 1995;21:1079–1082.

168. Peng X-X, Currin RT, Thurman RG, et al. Protection by pentoxifylline against normothermic liver ischemia/reperfusion in rats. *Transplantation* 1995;59:1537–1541.

169. Fabia R, Travis DL, Levy MF, et al. Effect of pentoxifylline on hepatic ischemia and reperfusion injury. *Surgery* 1997;121:520–525.

170. Muller JM, Vollmar B, Menger MD. Pentoxifylline reduces venular leukocyte adherence ("reflow paradox") but not microvascular "no reflow" in hepatic ischemia/reperfusion. *J Surg Res* 1997;71:1–6.

171. Boros P, Suehiro T, Curtiss S, et al. Differential contribution of graft and recipient to perioperative TNF-alpha, IL-1 beta, IL-6 and IL-8 levels and correlation with early graft function in clinical liver transplantation. *Clin Transplant* 1997;11:588–592.

172. Clavien PA, Sanabria JR, Upadhaya A, et al. Evidence of the existence of a soluble mediator of cold preservation injury. *Transplantation* 1993;56:44–53.

173. Ferguson DM, Gores GJ, Bronk SF, et al. An increase in cytosolic protease activity during liver preservation. Inhibition by glutathione and glycine. *Transplantation* 1993;55:627–633.

174. Aguilar HI, Steers JL, Wiesner RH, et al. Enhanced liver calpain protease activity is a risk factor for dysfunction of human liver allografts. *Transplantation* 1997;63:612–614.

175. von Frankenberg M, Stachlewitz RF, Forman DT, et al. Amino acids in rinse effluents as a predictor of graft function after transplantation of fatty livers in rats. *Transpl Int* 1999;12:168–175.

176. Kohli V, Gao W, Camargo CA Jr, et al. Calpain is a mediator of preservation-reperfusion injury in rat liver transplantation. *Proc Natl Acad Sci U S A* 1997;94:9354–9359.

177. Gores GJ, Nieminen A-L, Fleishman KE, et al. Extracellular acidosis delays onset of cell death in ATP-depleted hepatocytes. *Am J Physiol* 1988;255:C315-C322.

178. Currin RT, Gores GJ, Thurman RG, et al. Protection by acidotic pH against anoxic cell killing in perfused rat liver: evidence for a "pH paradox." *FASEB J* 1991;5:207–210.

179. Nishimura Y, Romer LH, Lemasters JJ. Mitochondrial dysfunction and cytoskeletal disruption during chemical hypoxia to cultured rat hepatic sinusoidal endothelial cells: the pH paradox and cytoprotection by glucose, acidotic pH and glycine. *Hepatology* 1998; 27:1039–1049.

180. Bond JM, Herman B, Lemasters JJ. Protection by acidic pH against anoxia/reoxygenation injury to rat neonatal cardiac myocytes. *Biochem Biophys Res Commun* 1991;179:798–803.

181. Harper IS, Bond JM, Chacon E, et al. Inhibition of Na⁺/H⁺ exchange preserves viability, restores mechanical function, and prevents the pH paradox in reperfusion injury to rat neonatal myocytes. *Basic Res Cardiol* 1993;88:430–442.

182. Qian T, Nieminen A-L, Herman B, et al. Mitochondrial permeability transition in pH-dependent reperfusion injury to rat hepatocytes. *Am J Physiol* 1997;273:C1783–C1792.

183. Bernardi P. Mitochondrial transport of cations: channels, exchangers, and permeability transition. *Physiol Rev* 1999;79:1127–1155.

184. Fujii Y, Johnson ME, Gores GJ. Mitochondrial dysfunction during anoxia/reoxygenation injury of liver sinusoidal endothelial cells. *Hepatology* 1994;20:177–185.

185. Goto S, Kim YI, Shimada T, et al. The effects of pretransplant cyclosporine therapy on rats grafted with twelve-hour cold-stored livers with special reference to reperfusion injury. *Transplantation* 1991;52: 615–621.

186. Kawano K, Kim YI, Ono M, et al. Evidence that both cyclosporin and azathioprine prevent warm ischemia reperfusion injury to the rat liver. *Transpl Int* 1993;6:330–336.

187. Shimizu S, Kamiike W, Hatanaka N, et al. Beneficial effects of cyclosporine on reoxygenation injury in hypoxic rat liver. *Transplantation* 1994;57:1562–1566.

188. Kai T, Kim YI, Kitamura H, et al. Attenuation of cold ischemic liver injury by cyclosporine in association with endotoxemia and chemokine release. *Transplant Proc* 1994;26:2370–2374.

189. Nieminen A-L, Saylor AK, Herman B, et al. ATP depletion rather than mitochondrial depolarization mediates hepatocyte killing after metabolic inhibition. *Am J Physiol* 1994;267:C67–C74.

190. Lemasters JJ, DiGuiseppi J, Nieminen A-L, et al. Blebbing, free Ca⁺⁺ and mitochondrial membrane potential preceding cell death in hepatocytes. *Nature* 1987;325:78–81.

191. Nieminen A-L, Gores GJ, Wray BE, et al. Calcium dependence of bleb formation and cell death in hepatocytes. *Cell Calcium* 1988; 9:237–246.

192. Gores GJ, Nieminen A-L, Wray BE, et al. Intracellular pH during 'chemical hypoxia' in cultured rat hepatocytes: protection by intracellular acidosis against the onset of cell death. *J Clin Invest* 1989; 83:386–396.

193. Herman B, Nieminen A-L, Gores GJ, et al. Irreversible injury in anoxic hepatocytes precipitated by an abrupt increase in plasma membrane permeability. *FASEB J* 1988;2:146–151.

194. Zahrebelski G, Nieminen A-L, Al-Ghoul K, et al. Progression of subcellular changes during chemical hypoxia to cultured rat hepatocytes: a laser scanning confocal microscopic study. *Hepatology* 1995;21: 1361–1372.

195. Nishimura Y, Lemasters JJ. Plasma membrane permeability changes in cultured sinusoidal endothelial cells exposed to cyanide monitored by negative contrast confocal microscopy. *Cell Vision – J Anal Morphol* 1997;4:174–175.

196. Carini R, Bellomo G, Grazia De Cesaris M, et al. Glycine protects against hepatocyte killing by KCN or hypoxia by preventing intracellular Na+ overload in the rat. *Hepatology* 1997;26:107–112.

197. Ju Y-K, Saint DA, Gage PW. Inactivation-resistant channels underlying the persistent sodium current in rat ventricular myocytes. *Proc R Soc Lond B* 1994;456:2–8.

198. Haddad GG, Jiang C. Mechanisms of neuronal survival during hypoxia: ATP-sensitive K+ channel. *Biol Neonate* 1994;65:160–165.

199. Dong Z, Patel Y, Saikumar P, et al. Development of porous defects in plasma membranes of adenosine triphosphate-depleted Madin-Darby canine kidney cells and its inhibition by glycine. *Lab Invest* 1998;78:657–668.

200. Nunez G, Benedict MA, Hu Y, et al. Caspases: the proteases of the apoptotic pathway. *Oncogene* 1998;17:3237–3245.

201. Afford SC, Hubscher S, Strain AJ, et al. Apoptosis in the human liver during allograft rejection and end-stage liver disease. *J Pathol* 1995; 176:373–380.

202. Patel T, Gores GJ. Apoptosis in liver transplantation: a mechanism contributing to immune modulation, preservation injury, neoplasia, and viral disease. *Liver Transplant Surg* 1998;4:42–50.

203. Borghi-Scoazec G, Scoazec JY, Durand F, et al. Apoptosis after ischemia-reperfusion in human liver allografts. *Liver Transplant Surg* 1997;3:407–415.

204. Kuo PC, Drachenberg CI, de la Torre A, et al. Apoptosis and hepatic allograft reperfusion injury. *Clin Transplant* 1998;12:219–223.

205. Schumer M, Colombel MC, Sawczuk IS, et al. Morphologic, biochemical, and molecular evidence of apoptosis during the reperfusion phase after brief periods of renal ischemia. *Am J Pathol* 1992;140:831–838.

206. Gottlieb RA, Burleson KO, Kloner RA, et al. Reperfusion injury induces apoptosis in rabbit cardiomyocytes. *J Clin Invest* 1994;94: 1621–1628.

207. Gao W, Bentley RC, Madden JF, et al. Apoptosis of sinusoidal endothelial cells is a critical mechanism of preservation injury in rat liver transplantation. *Hepatology* 1998;27:1652–1660.

208. Currin RT, Peng X-X, Arai M, et al. Progression of apoptosis after liver preservation and transplantation [Abstract]. *Hepatology* 1997;26:496A.

209. Natori S, Selzner M, Valentino KL, et al. Apoptosis of sinusoidal endothelial cells occurs during liver preservation injury by a caspase-dependent mechanism. *Transplantation* 1999;68:89–96.

210. Sindram D, Kohli V, Madden JF, et al. Calpain inhibition prevents sinusoidal endothelial cell apoptosis in the cold ischemic rat liver. *Transplantation* 1999;68:136–140.

211. Kroemer G, Petit P, Zamzami N, et al. The biochemistry of programmed cell death. *FASEB J* 1995;9:1277–1287.

212. Bradham CA, Qian T, Streetz K, et al. The mitochondrial permeability transition is required for TNFα-mediated apoptosis and cytochrome *c* release. *Molec Cell Biol* 1998;18:6353–6364.

213. Liu X, Kim CN, Yang J, et al. Induction of apoptotic program in cell-free extracts: requirement for dATP and cytochrome *c*. *Cell* 1996;86: 147–157.

214. Li P, Budihardjo NDI, Srinivasula SM, et al. Cytochrome *c* and dATP-dependent formation of Apaf-1/caspase 9 complex initiates an apoptotic protease cascade. *Cell* 1997;91:479–489.

215. Qian T, Herman B, Lemasters JJ. The mitochondrial permeability transition mediates both necrotic and apoptotic death of hepatocytes exposed to Br-A23187. *Toxicol Appl Pharmacol* 1999;154:117–125.

216. Richter C, Schweizer M, Cossarizza A, et al. Control of apoptosis by the cellular ATP level. *FEBS Lett* 1996;378:107–110.

217. Leist M, Single B, Castoldi AF, et al. Intracellular adenosine triphosphate (ATP) concentration: a switch in the decision between apoptosis and necrosis. *J Exp Med* 1997;185:1481–1486.

218. Eguchi Y, Shimizu S, Tsujimoto Y. Intracellular ATP levels determine cell death fate by apoptosis or necrosis. *Cancer Res* 1997;57: 1835–1840.

219. Lemasters JJ. Mechanisms of hepatic toxicity. V. Necrapoptosis and the mitochondrial permeability transition: shared pathways to necrosis and apoptosis. *Am J Physiol* 1999;276:G1–G6.

220. Gao W, Hijioka T, Lindert KA, et al. Evidence that adenosine is a key component in Carolina rinse responsible for reducing graft failure after orthotopic liver transplantation in the rat. *Transplantation* 1991;52:992–998.

221. Post S, Rentsch M, Gonzalez AP, et al. Effects of Carolina rinse and adenosine rinse on microvascular perfusion and intrahepatic leukocyte-endothelium interaction after liver transplantation in the rat. *Transplantation* 1993;55:972–977.

222. Bachmann S, Caldwell-Kenkel JC, Oleksi I, et al. Warm Carolina rinse solution prevents graft failure from storage injury after orthotopic rat liver transplantation with arterialization. *Transpl Int* 1992;5:108–114.

223. Sato E, Hachisuka T, Yokoyama I, et al. Protective effects of Carolina rinse solution against reperfusion injury in canine auto-transplantation. *Eur Surg Res* 1993;25:254–260.

224. Sanchez-Urdazpal L, Gores GJ, Lemasters JJ, et al. Carolina rinse solution decreases liver injury during clinical liver transplantation. *Transplant Proc* 1993;25:1574–1575.

225. Bachmann S, Bechstein WO, Keck H, et al. Pilot study: Carolina rinse solution improves graft function after orthotopic liver transplantation in humans. *Transplant Proc* 1997;29:390–392.

226. Blide T. Vascular resistance in hypothermically perfused kidneys damaged by warm ischemia. *Scand J Urol Nephrol* 1976;10:43–48.

227. Rentsch M, Post S, Palma P, et al. Intravital studies on beneficial effects of warm Ringer's lactate rinse in liver transplantation. *Transpl Int* 1996;9:461–467.

228. Currin RT, Thurman RG, Lemasters JJ. Carolina rinse solution protects ATP-depleted hepatocytes against lethal cell injury. *Transplant Proc* 1991;23:645–647.

229. Weinberg JM, Davis JA, Abarzua M, et al. Cytoprotective effects of glycine and glutathione against hypoxic injury to renal tubules. *J Clin Invest* 1987;80:1446–1454.

230. Dickson RC, Bronk SF, Gores GJ. Glycine cytoprotection during lethal hepatocellular injury from adenosine triphosphate depletion. *Gastroenterology* 1992;102:2098–2107.

231. Marsh DC, Vreugdenhil PK, Mack VE, et al. Glycine protects hepatocytes from injury caused by anoxia, cold ischemia and mitochondrial inhibitors, but not injury caused by calcium ionophores or oxidative stress. *Hepatology* 1993;17:91–98.

232. Zhong Z, Jones S, Thurman RG. Glycine minimizes reperfusion injury in a low-flow, reflow liver perfusion model in the rat. *Am J Physiol* 1996;270:G332–G338.

233. Bachmann S, Peng X-X, Currin RT, et al. Glycine in Carolina rinse solution reduces reperfusion injury, improves graft function and increases graft survival after rat liver transplantation. *Transplant Proc* 1995;27:741–742.

234. Currin RT, Caldwell-Kenkel JC, Lichtman SN, et al. Protection by Carolina rinse solution, acidotic pH and glycine against lethal reperfusion injury to sinusoidal endothelial cells of rat livers stored for transplantation. *Transplantation* 1996;62:1549–1558.

235. Ikejima K, Qu W, Stachlewitz RF, et al. Kupffer cells contain a glycine-gated chloride channel. *Am J Physiol* 1997;272:G1581–G1586.

236. den Butter G, Lindell SL, Sumimoto R, et al. Effect of glycine in dog and rat liver transplantation. *Transplantation* 1993;56:817–822.

237. Schemmer P, Bradford BU, Rose ML, et al. Intravenous glycine improves survival in rat liver transplantation. *Am J Physiol* 1999;276: G924–G932.

238. Thurman RG, Schemmer P, Zhong Z, et al. Kupffer cell-dependent reperfusion injury in liver transplantation: new clinically relevant use of glycine. *Langenbecks Archiv Chir* 1998;115:185–190.

239. Todo S, Demetris AJ, Makowa L, et al. Primary nonfunction of hepatic allografts with preexisting fatty infiltration. *Transplantation* 1989;47:903–905.

240. Teramoto K, Bowers JL, Kruskal JB, et al. Hepatic microcirculatory changes after reperfusion in fatty and normal liver transplantation in the rat. *Transplantation* 1993;56:1076–1082.

241. Hayashi M, Tokunaga Y, Fujita T, et al. The effects of cold preservation on steatotic graft viability in rat liver transplantation. *Transplantation* 1993;56:282–287.
242. Lemasters JJ, Gao W, Currin RT, et al. Ultrastructure of livers from alcohol-treated rats following orthotopic liver transplantation [Abstract]. *Toxicologist* 1994;14:284.
243. Gao W, Connor HD, Lemasters JJ, et al. Primary nonfunction of fatty livers produced by alcohol is associated with a new, antioxidant-insensitive free radical species. *Transplantation* 1995;59:674–679.
244. Zhong Z, Connor H, Mason RP, et al. Destruction of Kupffer cells increases survival and reduces graft injury after transplantation of fatty livers from ethanol-treated rats. *Liver Transplant Surg* 1996;2:383–387.
245. Zhong Z, Connor H, Stachlewitz RF, et al. Role of free radicals in primary non-function of marginal fatty grafts from rats treated acutely with ethanol. *Mol Pharmacol* 1997;52:912–919.
246. Zhong A, Connor HD, Mason RP, et al. Role of Kupffer cells in reperfusion injury in fat-loaded livers from ethanol-treated rats. *J Pharmacol Exp Ther* 1995;275:1512–1517.
247. Zhong Z, Arteel GE, Connor HD, et al. Binge drinking disturbs hepatic microcirculation after transplantation: prevention with free radical scavengers. *J Pharmacol Exp Ther* 1999;290:611–620.
248. Stachlewitz RF, Gao W, Zhong Z, et al. Generation of lipid free radicals by adherent leukocytes from transplanted rat liver. *Transpl Int* 1998;11:353–360.
249. Stubenitsky BM, Booster MH, Nederstigt AP, et al. Kidney preservation in the next millenium. *Transpl Int* 1999;12:83–91.
250. Casavilla A, Ramirez C, Shapiro R, et al. Experience with liver and kidney allografts from non-heart-beating donors. *Transplantation* 1995;59:197–203.
251. Harvey PR, Iu S, McKeown CM, et al. Adenine nucleotide tissue concentrations and liver allograft viability after cold preservation and warm ischemia. *Transplantation* 1988;45:1016–1020.
252. Currin RT, Peng X-X, Thurman RG, et al. Loss of hepatocyte viability during warm ischemia causes graft failure of livers from non-heart beating donors [Abstract]. *Hepatology* 1999;30:275A.
253. Carroll R, Yellon DM. Myocardial adaptation to ischaemia—the preconditioning phenomenon. *Int J Cardiol* 1999;68(suppl 1):S93–S101.
254. Kume M, Yamamoto Y, Saad S, et al. Ischemic preconditioning of the liver in rats: implications of heat shock protein induction to increase tolerance of ischemia-reperfusion injury. *J Lab Clin Med* 1996;128:251–258.
255. Peralta C, Hotter G, Closa D, et al. Protective effect of preconditioning on the injury associated to hepatic ischemia-reperfusion in the rat: role of nitric oxide and adenosine. *Hepatology* 1997;25:934–937.
256. Yin DP, Sankary HN, Chong ASF, et al. Protective effect of ischemic preconditioning on liver preservation-reperfusion injury in rats. *Transplantation* 1998;66:152–157.
257. Arai M, Lemasters JJ. Improvement of recipient survival and suppression of Kupffer cell activation by ischemic preconditioning after rat liver transplantation [Abstract]. *Gastroenterology* 1998;114:A1205.
258. Arai M, Thurman RG, Lemasters JJ. Involvement of Kupffer cells and sinusoidal endothelial cells in ischemic preconditioning to rat livers stored for transplantation. *Transplant Proc* 1999;31:425–427.
259. Arai M, Lemasters JJ. Contribution of adenosine receptors to sinusoidal endothelial cell protection by ischemic preconditioning. In: Wisse E, Knook DL, *Cells of the hepatic sinusoid,* vol. 7. Leiden, The Netherlands: The Kupffer Cell Foundation, 1999:121–122.
260. Arai M, Thurman RG, Lemasters JJ. cAMP mediates protective preconditioning of sinusoidal endothelial cells against storage/reperfusion injury [Abstract]. *Hepatology* 1999;30:312A.
261. Arai M, Peng X-X, Currin RT, et al. Protection of sinusoidal endothelial cells against storage/reperfusion injury by prostaglandin E2 derived from Kupffer cells. *Transplantation* 1999;68:440–445.
262. Bilbao G, Contreras JL, Gomez-Navarro J, et al. Genetic modification of liver grafts with an adenoviral vector encoding the Bcl-2 gene improves organ preservation. *Transplantation* 1999;67:775–783.
263. Lehmann TG, Wheeler MD, Schoonhoven R, et al. Adenoviral gene delivery of Cu/Zn-superoxide dismutase minimizes liver injury and improves survival after liver transplantation in the rat [Abstract]. *Hepatology* 1999;30:298A.
264. Bradham CA, Schemmer P, Stachlewitz RF, et al. Activation of nuclear factor-kappa B during orthotopic liver transplantation in rats is protective and does not require Kupffer cells. *Liver Transplant Surg* 1999;5:282–293.

Transplantation of the Liver, edited by Willis C. Maddrey, Eugene R. Schiff, and Michael F. Sorrell. Lippincott Williams & Wilkins, Philadelphia © 2001.

CHAPTER 17

Infectious Disease Problems

Robert H. Rubin

Over the past two decades, liver transplantation has evolved from a desperate experimental approach for treating end-stage liver disease to a practical, accepted therapy that is carried out on a daily basis at transplant centers throughout the world. At the present time, because of improvements in surgical techniques, medical management, and immunosuppressive therapy, 1-year allograft and patient survival rates of more than 85% are being achieved at the leading transplant centers.[1]

Despite these advances, infection continues to be a major problem; invasive infection remains the major cause of death following liver transplantation, with an incidence far greater than that observed in either or both kidney and heart transplantation. Because the donors of these organs tend to be the same, and because the immunosuppressive regimens used in these three forms of organ transplantation are quite similar, the higher rate of infection in liver transplantation must be due to other factors. The two most likely explanations for this difference are the advanced state of debility of many patients with end-stage liver disease prior to transplantation (a problem exacerbated by the continuing shortage of organs, which often delays the time of transplantation for many individuals beyond the point of optimal health for withstanding the operation) and the technical complexity of the surgery. Since the first experimental studies of liver transplantation, it has been clear that liver injury secondary to the technical aspects of organ procurement and transplantation is a major factor in the pathogenesis of approximately 75% of the cases of lethal infection.[1–8]

Thus, it may be said that the liver transplant patient is at risk for the same infectious disease complications resulting from environmental exposures and immunosuppression as

R. H. Rubin: Surgical and Transplant Infectious Disease Department, Massachusetts General Hospital; Center for Experimental Pharmacology and Therapeutics, Harvard-Massachusetts Institute of Technology Division of Health Sciences and Technology; Department of Medicine, Harvard Medical School, Boston, Massachusetts 02114.

renal and heart transplant patients are. In addition, however, the liver transplant recipient has the burden of several technical complications unique to liver transplantation: the surgical demands of the native hepatectomy and the biliary and vascular anastomoses required for the new liver, the propensity for intraabdominal bleeding due to a profound coagulopathy and the need to operate in the face of portal hypertension, and the frequent need for prolonged ventilatory support because of postoperative encephalopathy.[1–8]

In addition to the technical challenges involved with liver transplantation, a number of special hurdles face the clinician when dealing with the infectious disease problems of the transplant recipient. For instance, the combination of a vascularized organ that differs from the recipient at both major and minor histocompatibility loci, the lifetime requirement for immunosuppression, and the presence of chronic infection with a group of viruses that are both modulated by and themselves contribute to the net state of immunosuppression has created a series of clinical syndromes hitherto unknown in human medicine and biology.[1,2]

The key factor in successfully treating most infections in the transplant patient is early recognition and initiation of effective therapy. This task is frequently rendered difficult because of the impaired inflammatory response that is typical of the transplant recipient who is in an immunosuppressed state. Immunosuppression can result in a blunting of many of the symptoms and physical findings of infection until very late in the patient's course, thus rendering early diagnosis quite challenging. For this reason, the approach of the clinician must be quite aggressive: biopsying unexplained skin lesions, even if innocuous in appearance; performing computed tomographic (CT) scans or magnetic resonance imaging (MRI) of the brain as well as a lumbar puncture in a patient with an unexplained headache; or performing chest CT scans in patients with unexplained cough, even in the presence of a normal chest x-ray.[1,2]

Because of the potential impact of infection on these patients, the emphasis must be placed on prevention. Thus, an important principle that warrants particular emphasis is that the therapeutic prescription for the organ transplant patient has two components: an immunosuppressive program to prevent and treat rejection, and an antimicrobial strategy to make this regimen safe.[1,2,9]

RISK OF INFECTION

The risk of infection in the liver transplant recipient is largely determined by the interaction among factors in three categories: technical and anatomic factors related to the transplant operation and the postoperative care; the epidemiologic exposures the patient encounters; and the net state of immunosuppression. Technical and anatomic factors are the primary driving force in the pathogenesis of infections that occur in the first month posttransplantation; after that, it is the semiquantitative interaction between epidemiologic exposure and the net state of immunosuppression that is the primary determinant of infection. This interaction is a useful concept for the clinician in the assessment of the individual patient. Thus, if the patient's net state of immunosuppression is deemed to be relatively low and opportunistic infection occurs, this is prima facie evidence of an excessive epidemiologic exposure (with possible epidemic potential). Conversely, if the patient's net state of immunosuppression is high, then he or she needs to be protected from even trivial exposure to potential pathogens.[1,2]

The technical and anatomic factors of importance in the pathogenesis of infection in the liver transplant patient can be divided into two categories: (a) those related to technical mishaps during the operation that result in devitalized tissue, fluid collections or hematomas that require indwelling drains and catheters, bacterial contamination of the operative field from endogenous sources (e.g., the bowel in the case of a choledochojejunostomy or a previously colonized biliary tract) or a biliary leak; and (b) those related to postoperative care that lead to infection by damaging the primary mucocutaneous barriers to infection. The prime examples of this latter category are vascular access catheters, drainage catheters, and prolonged endotracheal intubation.[1–8]

The epidemiologic exposures of importance for the transplant patient can be divided into two general categories: those occurring within the community and those occurring within the hospital. In the community the major concerns are *Mycobacterium tuberculosis,* the geographically restricted systemic mycoses (especially *Coccidioides immitis* and *Histoplasma capsulatum*), *Strongyloides stercoralis,* and such common community-acquired infections as those caused by influenza, respiratory syncytial virus and other common respiratory viruses, and such food-borne pathogens as *Listeria monocytogenes, Salmonella* species, and *Campylobacter jejuni.*[1,2,9]

Mycobacterium tuberculosis infection and the systemic mycoses share several characteristics in common, with three patterns of disease being observed in all of these: *progressive primary infection* following inhalation exposure, with progressive pulmonary infection or systemic dissemination, or both, because of the patient's immunosuppressed state; *reactivation* of a dormant site of old infection, again with systemic dissemination because of the immunosuppressive therapy; and, finally, attenuation of established immunity because of immunosuppression, followed by *reinfection* and dissemination on repeat exposure. The emphasis is on progressive infection and disseminated disease, with the following clinical syndromes being suggestive of one of these infections: fever of unknown origin, progressive or miliary pulmonary infection, or clinically evident infection at sites of metastatic disease [e.g., skin for blastomycosis; central nervous system (CNS) for coccidioidomycosis; mucocutaneous sites or CNS for histoplasmosis; and miliary, skeletal, renal, or CNS sites for tuberculosis].[1,2,9]

Strongyloides stercoralis is an intestinal nematode that is endemic in many areas of the world, including the southern regions of the United States. The organism's complex life cycle includes an autoinfection aspect that allows the organism to be maintained in the gastrointestinal tract of a human host for decades—long after the host may have left the endemic area. In such individuals the organism is kept in check by an intact cell-mediated immune system, so that nonimmunosuppressed patients may be infested with *S. stercoralis* but be asymptomatic. After the initiation of immunosuppressive therapy, a life-threatening hyperinfection syndrome or disseminated strongyloidiasis can develop. The hyperinfection syndrome represents an exaggeration of the normal life cycle of the parasite, including a severe ulcerating, hemorrhagic enterocolitis and pneumonia. Disseminated strongyloidiasis is characterized by extension of the process outside its normal domain, with the filariform larvae invading all portions of the body. These larvae may have adherent gut bacteria. Thus, the clinical presentation can be gram-negative sepsis or meningitis that is unresponsive to therapy unless the *Strongyloides* component is also treated.[10–17]

Although therapy of an established *S. stercoralis* infection in transplant patients is possible with thiabendazole or ivermectin plus systemic antibacterial drugs aimed at the complicating bacterial infection, the mortality rate is greater than 50%. Thus, it is far better to eradicate asymptomatic infection prior to the transplant procedure. Any patient with a history of residence in an area of the world with endemic *Strongyloides* infection should undergo serologic testing for this organism, with all persons found to be positive then undergoing preemptive therapy with ivermectin or thiabendazole. Alternatively, duodenal intubation can be carried out to obtain specimens for parasite identification. It is important to recognize that a routine stool ova and parasite examination in asymptomatic carriers has a sensitivity of less than 30%.[1,2,10–17]

Because transplant patients are being rehabilitated and returned to normal life in larger numbers than in the past, such common infections as those due to influenza, parainfluenza, respiratory syncytial virus, and adenoviruses have a particularly striking impact whenever there is significant circulation of these viruses in the community. These respiratory viruses have a more prolonged course, a higher rate of pneumonia, and an increased rate of bacterial and fungal superinfection in the transplant recipient than in the nontransplant community.[1,2,18–20]

In sum, the clinician must be concerned about both recent and remote epidemiologic exposures. The transplant patient can be compared to a "sentinel chicken" who will reflect any excess traffic in microorganisms that is present in the environment with clinically important infection.[21]

Exposure to excessive numbers of microorganisms within the hospital environment is even more common than community exposure. Person-to-person spread, often on the hands of medical personnel, of such antimicrobial-resistant infections as those caused by vancomycin-resistant *Enterococcus faecium,* methicillin-resistant *Staphylococcus aureus, Clostridium difficile,* antibiotic-resistant gram-negative bacilli, and azole-resistant *Candida* species is a growing problem among transplant recipients. Inhalation of air contaminated with *Aspergillus* species, *Pseudomonas aeruginosa,* and other organisms can lead to life-threatening pulmonary infection or to wound contamination and invasive infection. Exposure to potable water colonized with *Legionella* species can also lead to devastating pulmonary infection. Although all these infections can occur in other hospitalized patient populations, transplant patients have been particularly affected by these environmental hazards over the years—the sentinel chicken analogy applies even more to the hospital environment than the community environment.[1,2,21–27]

Two patterns of nosocomial exposure have been identified:

1. Domiciliary, in which the exposure occurs on the ward or within the room where the patient is housed
2. Nondomiciliary, in which the exposure occurs when the patient is taken from his or her room through the hospital to the operating room endoscopy facility, or the radiology suite for an essential procedure

Outbreaks caused by domiciliary exposure are usually identifiable by the clustering of cases in time and space, and can be effectively prevented by the provision of a high-efficiency particulate-arresting filtered air supply. Nondomiciliary outbreaks are both more common and more difficult to identify than domiciliary outbreaks because of the lack of clustering of cases on a particular ward. The clue to a nondomiciliary problem is the occurrence of opportunistic infection when the net state of immunosuppression is not at a level that such infection should appear unless an intensive microbial challenge has occurred.[1,2,21,25–27]

The net state of immunosuppression is a complex function determined by the interaction of a number of factors. The most important of these is the immunosuppressive program that is in place; that is, the dose, duration, and temporal sequence in which these drugs are administered. The presence of acquired abnormalities adds significantly to the net state of immunosuppression. These abnormalities include damage to the mucocutaneous surfaces of the body; devitalized tissue; undrained collections of blood, lymph, ascites, bile, or urine; indwelling foreign bodies such as bladder, biliary, and drainage catheters, endotracheal tubes, and vascular access devices; and neutropenia, particularly that associated with cytomegalovirus (CMV) infection. A third group of factors that help determine the risk of infection are such metabolic ones as protein malnutrition, uremia, and, perhaps, hyperglycemia. Although these are not themselves sufficiently potent to measurably increase the rate of infection in most individuals, in the liver transplant patient they do intensify the risk significantly.

The final factor in determining the net state of immunosuppression is the presence of infection with one of the immunomodulating viruses: CMV, Epstein-Barr virus (EBV), human herpesvirus 6 (HHV-6), hepatitis B (HBV) and C (HCV) viruses, and human immunodeficiency virus (HIV). The importance of these viruses in determining the net state of immunosuppression is illustrated by the following statistic: over the past two decades, more than 90% of the transplant patients at our institution who developed opportunistic infection with such organisms as *Aspergillus* species, *Pneumocystis carinii, Nocardia asteroides,* and *Cryptococcus neoformans* did so in the setting of immunomodulating viral infection. In fact, the patients who were exceptions all acquired their infections because of exposure to a previously unrecognized environmental hazard.[1,2]

TIMETABLE OF INFECTION

A standard pattern or timetable delineates when different infections occur in the posttransplantation period (Fig. 17.1, Table 17.1). Although such clinical syndromes as fever of obscure origin, pneumonia, or CNS infection can occur at any point in the posttransplantation course, the microbial causes of these clinical conditions are very different at different time points. We find this timetable to be useful in three ways in the management of transplant recipients: (a) in the differential diagnosis of the individual patient with a clinical infectious disease syndrome; (b) as an epidemiologic tool, because exceptions to the timetable are usually due to excessive environmental exposures; and (c) as the basis for designing focused, cost-effective preventive strategies. The posttransplantation course can be divided into three different time periods for the purposes of this timetable: the first month, the period 1 to 6 months posttransplantation, and the late period (more than 6 months posttransplantation).[1,2,28]

Infection in the First Month Posttransplantation

In the first month posttransplantation, the infectious disease problems of the liver transplant recipient are of three types: (a) infection that was present in the allograft recipient prior to transplantation and that continues posttransplantation, perhaps exacerbated by the surgical procedure or the posttransplantation immunosuppression; (b)

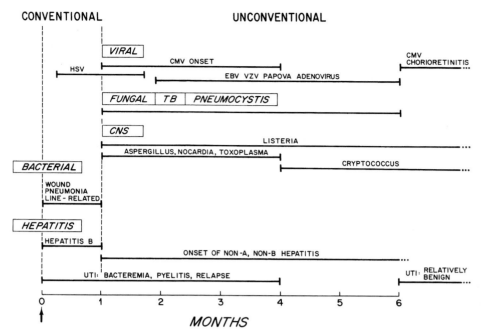

FIG. 17.1. Timetable for the occurrence of infection in the liver transplant patient. Any exception to this timetable should initiate a search for an unusual epidemiologic hazard. CMV, cytomegalovirus; HSV, herpes simplex virus; EBV, Epstein-Barr virus; VZV, varicella-zoster virus; PAPOVA, papovavirus; TB, tuberculosis; CNS, central nervous system; UTI, urinary tract infection. (Modified from Rubin RH, Wolfson JS, Cosimi AB, et al. Infection in the renal transplant recipient. *Am J Med* 1981;70:405–411, with permission of the *American Journal of Medicine*.)

TABLE 17.1. *Infection in the liver transplant recipient at different times in the posttransplantation course*

First month posttransplantation
Infection present in recipient prior to transplantation (e.g., hepatitis, strongyloidiasis, tuberculosis, smoldering bacterial infection)
Infection transmitted with the allograft (e.g., hepatitis, human immunodeficiency virus, acute bacterial and candidal infections)
Infection related to technical complications of the transplant procedure (e.g., pneumonia, wound infection, liver abscess, biliary sepsis)
1–6 months posttransplantation
Lingering effects of infection acquired earlier
Viral infection (e.g., from cytomegalovirus, Epstein-Barr virus, hepatitis)
Opportunistic infection (e.g., from *Pneumocystis, Listeria, Nocardia*)
More than 6 months posttransplantation
Patients with chronic cytomegalovirus, Epstein-Barr virus, or hepatitis virus infection are at risk for progressive chorioretinitis, B-cell lymphoproliferative disease, hepatocellular carcinoma, or cirrhosis
Patients with good graft function and minimal immunosuppression have a minimal risk of opportunistic infections but remain at risk for community-acquired infections (e.g., influenza, pneumococcal pneumonia)
Patients with chronic rejection and a history of excessive acute and chronic immunosuppression are at high risk for opportunistic infections (e.g., from *Cryptococcus, Listeria, Pneumocystis*)

infection conveyed with the allograft; and (c) the same bacterial and candidal infections that occur in nonimmunosuppressed patients undergoing comparable surgery and which are related to surgical wounds and pulmonary, biliary, urinary tract, and intravenous access. This last group accounts for more than 95% of the infections that arise in the first month posttransplantation. The incidence of such infections is largely determined by the technical skill with which the surgery is accomplished, the endotracheal tube managed, and the drainage catheters and vascular access devices utilized.[1,2,28]

Notable by their absence in this period are opportunistic infections caused by such pathogens as *Aspergillus* species, *Legionella* species, *Nocardia asteroides,* and others, which are rarely seen during this first-month "golden period." Indeed, a single case of opportunistic infection in this period is usually a tip-off to an excessive nosocomial hazard that has the potential for causing a generalized epidemic, and should trigger an intensive epidemiologic investigation. This observation is particularly striking considering that the actual daily doses of immunosuppressive drugs administered are at their highest level during this period. This fact emphasizes that, in the absence of a particular epidemiologic hazard, the *duration* of immunosuppression (i.e., the area under the curve) is a more important determinant of infection risk than the individual daily doses of drugs.

Infection 1 to 6 Months Posttransplantation

The infections occurring in the liver transplant patient during this time period can be divided into three general categories: (a) the residual effects of technical problems and ensuing infection that occurred earlier (e.g., liver abscess secondary to problems with the vascular anastomosis, intraperitoneal infection due to infected fluid collections, or cholangitis secondary to biliary complications), (b) infection with the immunomodulating viruses (particularly CMV, the most important cause of infection in this time period, but also EBV, HHV-6, HBV, HCV, and HIV), and (c) opportunistic infection (with such organisms as *Pneumocystis carinii, Listeria monocytogenes,* and *Aspergillus* species) made possible by the combined contributions of immunomodulating viral infection and sustained immunosuppressive therapy. The net state of immunosuppression is now at a level to permit such opportunistic infection to occur without a particularly intense epidemiologic exposure.[1,2,28]

Infection More Than 6 Months Posttransplantation

In this late period, transplant patients can be divided into three different categories in terms of infectious disease risks and consequences. The 80% of patients who have had a good outcome from their transplant, who are free of chronic viral infection, and who are on baseline immunosuppression are primarily at risk for community-acquired respiratory viral infection (e.g., influenza, respiratory syncytial virus, and adenovirus infection) and its consequences. The 10% of patients with chronic viral infection, particularly with the hepatitis viruses, will have progressive organ dysfunction unless antiviral therapy can be made to work for the individual. (In the case of HBV and HCV infection, there can be the inexorable progression to end-stage liver disease or carcinoma.) Finally, the 10% of patients who have poor allograft function, excessive immunosuppression, and often chronic viral infection (the "chronic ne'er-do-wells") are the transplant patients at highest risk of opportunistic infection with such organisms as *Cryptococcus neoformans, Pneumocystis carinii, Listeria monocytogenes,* and *Nocardia asteroides.*[1,2,28]

INFECTION IN THE FIRST MONTH POSTTRANSPLANTATION

Preexisting Infection in the Allograft Recipient

As in all forms of transplantation, it is essential that the liver transplant recipient be free of active infection prior to the time of transplantation and the initiation of immunosuppression. This is particularly important in liver transplantation for several reasons. First, the extensive upper abdominal surgery, prolonged anesthesia, and underlying encephalopathy mandate extended endotracheal intubation and ventilatory support, which will impede the ability to treat pneumonia (indeed, preexisting lung injury is prone to sequential posttransplantation superinfection with antibiotic-resistant

gram-negative bacilli and a variety of fungal species). Second, the multiple vascular and biliary anastomoses require the patient to be free of both intravascular and intraperitoneal infections at the time of surgery. Finally, any undetected site of infection will be further obscured by the major metabolic, hemodynamic, and immunologic changes present in the peritransplantation period. An axiom of liver transplantation is that if significant infection, particularly in the lungs, is present at the time of surgery, it is nearly impossible to "catch up" posttransplantation, and the patient will usually succumb to progressive infection.[1,2]

The need for the allograft recipient to be free of infection places a special emphasis on choosing the appropriate time for transplantation. Whereas with kidney transplantation, peritoneal dialysis and hemodialysis may be used to support and improve the condition of a patient with end-stage renal disease awaiting surgery, no such life support system is available for end-stage liver disease patients. Thus, the clinician caring for the patient with liver disease is caught between the concerns of too early transplantation, particularly in someone whose native liver might regenerate (as in certain cases of acute liver failure), and too late transplantation, when complications have occurred that are irreversible.

As far as infection is concerned, we have seen three types of complications develop from delaying the performance of liver transplantation too long.[1,2] First, because of increasing hepatic encephalopathy, the patient is unable to protect the airway and develops aspiration pneumonia, often with antibiotic-resistant intensive care unit flora. Such lung injury and infection carries an extra risk during the peritransplantation period because progressive superinfection is frequent, with death resulting from pulmonary sepsis and progressive respiratory insufficiency. Such pneumonias are best prevented. Ideally, transplantation should be carried out before encephalopathy becomes so deep or constant that airway protection cannot be maintained. In patients in whom this is not possible, early intubation to protect the lungs is indicated. Once such intubation is performed, transplantation should be carried out as soon as possible. After 72 hours of intubation, the risk of pneumonia in these patients begins to increase precipitously.

Second, spontaneous bacterial peritonitis is a constant risk in patients with ascites due to end-stage liver disease. Such infections must be completely eradicated before transplantation. Oral prophylaxis with fluoroquinolones in patients with ascites due to end-stage liver disease offers significant protection (particularly as "secondary" prophylaxis, after a first bout of spontaneous bacterial peritonitis).

Third, intravenous or intraarterial line–related sepsis becomes an increasing problem as the degree of illness increases and the patient requires intensive care prior to transplantation.

Because of these concerns and the increasing success of liver transplantation, we favor relatively early transplantation for patients with irreversible liver disease—preferably weeks to months before the final downhill spiral requiring intensive care occurs and the risk of pretransplantation infection begins to escalate. Unfortunately, the continuing shortage in donor organs renders this strategy difficult to carry out.

Posttransplantation Infection of Donor Origin

Although it has been less well documented in liver transplant recipients, the experience with renal and cardiac transplantation has led to the recognition that the allograft may carry infection to the recipient. Such infections can be divided into two general categories: chronic infection, such as HBV, HCV, and HIV, which can be transmitted by an allograft from an infected donor; and acute infection associated with the terminal illness. Bloodstream infection with bacteria or *Candida* species can affect the allograft, threatening vascular suture lines in the transplant recipient. The end result of vascular suture line infection is a mycotic aneurysm, with a high risk of rupture, as well as systemic sepsis.

To guard against these possibilities, the following guidelines for evaluating a prospective cadaveric donor have been suggested.[1,2,29]

Careful assessment of the potential donor for possible sepsis should be carried out. Donors with diagnosed infection due to easily treatable organisms with little potential for vascular infection (e.g., pneumococcal or meningococcal meningitis) who have received 72 hours or more of effective antibiotics may still be acceptable. In contrast, certain donors should be regarded as suspect: those with possible systemic infection with such organisms as *Staphylococcus aureus, Salmonella* species, *Pseudomonas aeruginosa,* or other bacteria with a high potential for metastasizing or for which antimicrobial therapy is less than optimal (e.g., vancomycin-resistant enterococci, methicillin-resistant *Staphylococcus aureus,* highly resistant gram-negative bacilli, and fungi); victims of drowning; burn victims; and patients who have been maintained on a respirator with indwelling lines and catheters for a period of more than 7 days.[30]

Careful culturing of the donor (including preterminal blood cultures) should be carried out, with intensive bactericidal antimicrobial therapy administered to the recipient if positive cultures for potential pathogens are noted.

Rarely, dormant fungal or mycobacterial infection that has asymptomatically metastasized to the liver of the donor during a recognized or unrecognized primary infection may be reactivated following the institution of posttransplantation immunosuppression. Therefore, a complete history of the prospective donor's exposures and illnesses should be obtained.

An important technical issue in liver transplantation that will have profound effects not only on the outcome of a particular transplantation but also on the incidence of infection in the first month posttransplantation is the condition of the allograft at the completion of the operation. Prolonged allograft nonfunction, usually due to prolonged ischemia in association with transplantation, has systemic consequences that lead to coagulopathy, bleeding, metabolic derangement, and encephalopathy. As a result, intraabdominal bleeding and a prolonged need for ventilatory support will greatly increase the risk of infection, both intraabdominally and in the lungs.[1]

New Infections Arising in the First Month Posttransplantation

As previously mentioned, the major infectious disease problems in the first month following liver transplantation are those related to the technical aspects of the transplant procedure and perioperative care.

Infections Related to Vascular Anastomotic Problems

Four vascular anastomoses must be successfully accomplished during the liver transplant operation: the suprahepatic vena caval anastomosis, the infrahepatic vena caval anastomosis, the portal vein anastomosis, and, finally, reconstruction of the hepatic artery. Vascular patency is of critical importance to both graft and patient survival, with portal vein thrombosis, hepatic artery thrombosis, and hepatic vein occlusion developing in the first few days posttransplantation being well-recognized complications. Rarely, late thromboses have also been documented, often after cessation of anticoagulant therapy in individuals at increased risk for clotting or after severe hypotension from another cause. Because of the size of the vessels involved, vascular occlusion, especially of the hepatic artery, is a particular problem in pediatric liver transplantation. Manifestations of these vascular catastrophes include ascites, variceal bleeding, and significant deterioration in liver function. Not uncommonly, however, fever and bacteremia may be the major clues.

Sepsis is particularly common following interruption in the hepatic arterial circulation, the most common vascular complication, with secondary infection of the hepatic infarct leading to areas of hepatic gangrene, abscess formation, and fulminant sepsis due to bowel bacterial flora or candidal species. Indeed, unexplained sepsis may be the first clue to a problem with the hepatic circulation. Although angiography remains the gold standard for diagnosing vascular difficulties, with early diagnosis before the onset of secondary sepsis offering the possibility of operative salvage or retransplantation, duplex (combined real-time and pulsed Doppler) sonography, spiral CT and magnetic resonance angiography are increasingly playing a role in the assessment of the allograft's vasculature.[1,3–8,31–37]

A more insidious consequence of vascular insufficiency can result when the vascular supply to the liver parenchyma remains intact but the biliary anastomosis is rendered ischemic. This results in a breakdown of the biliary anastomosis, a bile leak, and secondary infection. Alternatively, postischemic scarring can result in stricture formation (usually later in the posttransplantation course), again with a high incidence of secondary infection. Such secondary infection may take the form of deep wound infection, cholangitis, liver abscess, or bacteremia, with the microorganisms causing this again derived from the normal flora of the small bowel—

streptococci, Enterobacteriaceae, bowel anaerobes, and *Candida* species. Polymicrobial infection is common in these circumstances. This form of vascular insufficiency affecting the biliary anastomosis is analogous to the urine leaks and ureteral strictures developing after renal transplantation as a result of vascular insufficiency of the ureter.[1–8,31–37]

Infections Related to Biliary Anastomotic Problems

With increasing surgical experience, vascular problems have become less prevalent in liver transplant patients; the major technical barrier to successful liver transplantation is now the biliary anastomosis. Whenever possible, the anastomosis of choice is a choledochocholedochostomy, which maintains the native sphincter of Oddi intact. When this is not possible, a choledochojejunostomy constructed with a Roux-en-Y technique that offers protection against microbial contamination from the gastrointestinal tract can be utilized. Although a biliary leak can develop with either anastomosis, obstruction is the major concern with the choledochocholedochostomy procedure, whereas reflux of organisms is the weakness of the choledochojejunostomy procedure.[1,32–36,38]

The cardinal rule in the first few weeks following liver transplantation is that any episode of unexplained fever or bacteremia should be regarded as a manifestation of a technical problem involving the vascular tree, the biliary anastomosis, or deep wound infection until proven otherwise.

Accordingly, in addition to instituting broad-spectrum antimicrobial therapy aimed at upper small bowel flora (e.g., an advanced spectrum β-lactam, imipenem, or β-lactam–β-lactamase inhibitor with or without an aminoglycoside), an extensive radiological evaluation is indicated. This evaluation should include sonographic studies, CT scanning, cholangiography, and some assessment of the patency of the hepatic vessels. Prompt surgery or endoscopic placement of a biliary stent, under antimicrobial coverage, in patients with biliary anastomotic problems can often salvage the situation.[1]

Bacterial colonization of the bile of liver transplant patients is common, caused in large part by the presence of a T tube in the biliary tree for many weeks posttransplantation. In our transplant program, in which long-term trimethoprim-sulfamethoxazole prophylaxis is maintained indefinitely, innocuous colonization of the biliary tree with enterococci or *Staphylococcus epidermidis* is the rule. Such colonization itself requires no therapy, although colonization plus obstruction, tissue injury, or necrosis can lead to serious clinical infection (Fig. 17.2).[1]

Wound Infections Posttransplantation

Extensive experience with renal, cardiac, and hepatic transplantation has demonstrated that the incidence of wound infections following surgery in these patients is directly related to the occurrence of such technical complications as

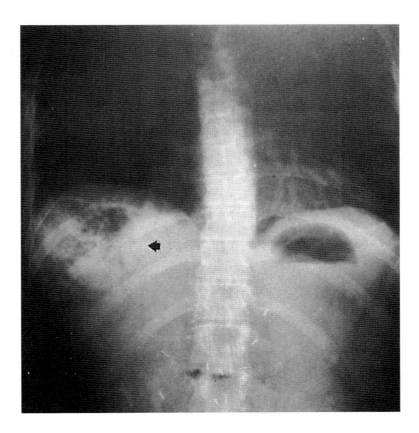

FIG. 17.2. An abdominal x-ray demonstrating a large liver abscess developing in the right lobe of the hepatic allograft following liver biopsy. (The *arrow* indicates the abscess cavity.)

leaks or hematoma formation. The signs of such infections are frequently obscured by the antiinflammatory effects of the immunosuppressive therapy being administered. Therefore, prompt use of CT and ultrasonic scans and blind needle aspirations of a suspicious wound in any patient with a fever in the first month posttransplantation is indicated.

By its nature, liver transplantation is particularly likely to be associated with such problems—first, because of the occurrence of bile leaks, and second, because of bleeding problems at the time of surgery. Whenever large volumes of blood are required intraoperatively and perioperatively, intraabdominal hematomas with a risk of secondary infection are important considerations. Thus, it is not surprising that the rate of deep wound infection is probably on the order of 5% to 15%, which is increased further if reexploration for bleeding or retransplantation is required or a biliary leak develops. Of particular concern have been the reports of a relatively high incidence of fungal infection in these patients, including a 16% incidence of candidemia in one of these studies.[1–8,31,36,39–43]

There is both intense interest and intense controversy regarding antimicrobial strategies to prevent infection, particularly deep wound or intraabdominal infection in the first month following liver transplantation. Most groups prescribe a cephalosporin (cefazolin or cefotaxime), with or without broader gram-negative coverage, as perioperative systemic prophylaxis, beginning on call to the operating room and continuing for 3 to 5 days posttransplantation. Other groups have utilized the concept of selective bowel decontamination, using a regimen of oral gentamicin, polymyxin, and nystatin begun at least 1 week before likely transplantation and continued for the first 21 days posttransplantation. This regimen has been associated with a low incidence of infection, particularly fungal infection. Initiating the regimen at the time of transplantation appears to offer little protection.[1,2,9,44–51]

At the Massachusetts General Hospital, we use elements of both approaches and have a low rate of wound infection and postoperative candidal infection (3% and 1%, respectively). Antibacterial prophylaxis is accomplished with 3 days of peritransplantation cefazolin, followed by 6 months (or longer) of trimethoprim-sulfamethoxazole therapy. Antifungal prophylaxis is begun approximately 3 weeks prior to expected transplantation, with the administration of oral clotrimazole 10 mg twice daily. This is continued for the first 10 days posttransplantation unless one of the following circumstances is present: a choledochojejunostomy biliary anastomosis, the presence of diabetes in the recipient, a history of broad-spectrum antibacterial therapy immediately prior to transplantation, or the need for reexploration. In all of these circumstances, the risk of deep wound or intraabdominal infection with *Candida* is increased, and systemic fluconazole (200 mg per day) is substituted for the clotrimazole.[1]

Pneumonia and Intravascular Line–Related Sepsis

Pulmonary difficulties following liver transplantation are common because of the interplay of a number of factors, such as the chronic pulmonary difficulties associated with long-standing cirrhosis, fluid overload, a distended abdomen causing poor respiratory mechanics, and obtundation. When these are coupled with aspiration of pharyngeal flora, postoperative atelectasis, and a need for prolonged intubation, the risk of pneumonia is great. The incidence of pneumonia is further increased if significant lung injury due to aspiration occurred within 2 weeks preoperatively or if attempted extubation failed and the patient had to be reintubated because of respiratory failure. The occurrence of pneumonia posttransplantation can be decreased by aggressive chest physiotherapy to prevent atelectasis and to mobilize secretions, by assuring the quality of the air to which the patient is exposed (especially while intubated), and by early extubation.[1,52–54]

Any immunocompromised patient is at high risk for systemic sepsis caused by contaminated vascular access devices. In the liver transplant patient, fluid management is sufficiently complicated that such invasive monitoring tools as central lines or Swan-Ganz lines are required both intraoperatively and in the immediate postoperative period. However, every effort must be made to discontinue their use as quickly as possible or if any unexplained fever occurs.[1]

INFECTION 1 TO 6 MONTHS POSTTRANSPLANTATION

Other than the lingering effects of infection related to technical problems that have occurred earlier, the dominant causes of infectious disease problems in this period are the immunomodulating viruses. The potential clinical effects of these infections are very broad and should be considered in four different categories:[1,2]

1. The production of clinical infectious disease syndromes (e.g., fever, pneumonia, hepatitis, mononucleosis, gastroenteritis, etc.) by the virus itself
2. The production of an immunosuppressed state by the virus that contributes significantly to the net state of immunosuppression and thus predisposes the patient to potentially lethal opportunistic superinfection
3. The participation of the virus in the production of allograft injury through mechanisms different from those involved in classic rejection
4. The participation of the virus in the processes of oncogenesis

The last three of these consequences of viral replication are thought to be "indirect" effects, that is, effects caused by cytokines, chemokines, and growth factors elaborated by the host in response to the viral replication.[1,2,55]

Herpesviruses

The single most important group of infections that affect the transplant patient are the herpesviruses: CMV, EBV, herpes simplex viruses 1 and 2 (HSV-1 and HSV-2), varicella-zoster virus (VZV), and human herpesviruses 6, 7, and 8 (HHV-6,

HHV-7, and HHV-8). These viruses cause both direct and indirect effects, appear to modulate each other's activity, and exert their greatest impact during the time period 1 to 6 months posttransplantation. These viruses share a number of characteristics that help explain their great impact on transplant patients.[1,2,56,57]

Latency

All herpesviruses exhibit the property of latency; that is, once infected with the virus, latent infection, capable of being reactivated, remains after all evidence of replicating virus has disappeared. The laboratory marker for the presence of latent infection is circulating antibody to the virus (seropositivity). The herpesviruses differ in terms of the stability of their latency. CMV and VZV latencies are quite stable, whereas EBV and HSV latencies are not (HHV-6, -7, and -8 are less clearly understood). In the case of CMV, the major signaling pathway for viral reactivation is through tumor necrosis factor (TNF), thus explaining the role of other infections, antilymphocyte antibodies, and allogeneic reactions in viral reactivation: These are all situations in which TNF is elaborated both locally and systemically. Other pathways can also result in viral reactivation. The stress mediators epinephrine and norepinephrine, as well as certain prostaglandins through cAMP-dependent signaling pathways, can reactive CMV.[58–61]

Cell Association

All the herpesviruses are highly cell associated, meaning that transmission requires intimate mucosal-to-mucosal contact or the transfer of infected (either latently or productively) cells from one individual to another—as with a transfusion or a transplant from a seropositive donor. Once replicating virus is present, systemic dissemination and amplification of the extent of the infection also occur on a cell-to-cell basis. This renders humoral immunity inefficient and cell-mediated immunity critical in terms of host defense against these viruses. In particular, virus-specific major histocompatibility complex (MHC)-restricted cytotoxic T cells are the critical host defense against these viruses. This is precisely the aspect of host defense most inhibited by modern immunosuppressive programs.[1,2,56,57]

Oncogenesis

All the herpesviruses should be considered potentially oncogenic. Clear-cut relationships have been demonstrated between EBV and posttransplantation lymphoproliferative disease (PTLD)[1,2,62] and between HHV-8 and Kaposi's sarcoma.[63–66] However, it is also clear that the relationship between these viruses and certain malignancies is more complex than a one-to-one relationship. Thus, patients with symptomatic CMV disease have a 7-fold to 10-fold increased risk for EBV-associated PTLD. It is believed that cytokines, growth factors, and chemokines elaborated by the transplant recipient

in response to the replication of one virus can modulate the biologic effects of other viruses—in this case, the pathogenesis of EBV-associated PTLD.[2,67,68]

Influence of Immunosuppression

All the herpesviruses appear to be similarly affected by different components of the immunosuppressive regimen. Whereas antilymphocyte antibodies that induce a cytokine response (manifested as fever and chills) are extremely potent in reactivating these viruses (presumably due to the TNF release engendered by such agents as antithymocyte globulin and OKT3), other potent immunosuppressive agents such as cyclosporine, tacrolimus, rapamycin, and corticosteroids have no ability to reactivate latent virus. Cytotoxic agents such as azathioprine, mycophenolate, and cyclophosphamide have moderate virus-reactivating effects. Once replicating virus is present, however, drugs such as cyclosporine and tacrolimus are extremely potent in blocking the host's response to the replicating virus, thus amplifying the extent and the clinical effects of these viruses on the host. Indeed, we refer to cyclosporine and tacrolimus as having "an *in vivo* polymerase chain reaction (PCR) effect" on these viruses.[1,2]

Cytomegalovirus Infection

Of all infections that can occur in the liver transplant recipient, CMV is both the most common and has the most diverse effects. An estimated 50% to 75% of liver transplant patients will have some evidence of CMV replication posttransplantation, with less than half of these having clinically overt disease (the exact percentages will depend on the variety of factors outlined in Table 17.2). Unless antiviral prophylaxis is employed, the great majority of CMV infections have their origins in the time period 3 weeks to 4 months posttransplantation. Three major epidemiologic patterns of infection are observed: primary infection, reactivation infection, and superinfection.[1,2]

Primary Infection

Primary CMV infection occurs when the transplant patient has had no pretransplantation experience with CMV (and is CMV seronegative) and is infected with virus carried latently in cells from a seropositive latently infected donor. In liver transplantation there are two major sources of these cells: the liver allograft itself and viable leukocyte-containing blood products. The importance of transfusion-related CMV disease is underlined by the observation that 16% of seronegative individuals receiving liver allografts from seronegative donors developed symptomatic CMV from blood products, although transfusion-related primary disease tends to be milder than that acquired from the allograft.[69] This source of CMV can be eliminated either by the use of blood products from seronegative donors or by the use of leukocyte filters when red cell or platelet transfusions are administered. Approximately 10% to 15% of transplant patients are at risk for primary infection

TABLE 17.2. *Incidence of clinical disease due to cytomegalovirus in transplant patients with differing exposure to latent virus and immunosuppression*

Donor serologic status[a]	Recipient serologic status[a]	Immunosuppression[b]	Incidence of clinical CMV disease (%)
Positive	Negative	CyA, MMF, Pred	50–60
Negative	Positive	CyA, MMF, Pred	10–15
Positive	Positive	CyA, MMF, Pred	20–25
Either	Positive	ATG or OKT3 induction	25–30
Either	Positive	ATG or OKT3 antirejection therapy	50–75
Negative	Negative	CyA, MMF, Pred, OKT3 or ATG	0

[a]Only cytomegalovirus-negative blood products are assumed as being administered.

[b]Standard immunosuppression is with cyclosporine (CyA), mycophenolate mofetil (MMF), and prednisone (Pred). Available evidence suggests similar results if tacrolimus is substituted for cyclosporine or if azathioprine is substituted for mycophenolate.

CMV, cytomegalovirus; ATG, antithymocyte globulin; OKT3, anti–T-cell monoclonal antibody.

(donor seropositive and recipient seronegative, D+R−), with 50% to 60% of these developing clinical infectious disease syndromes as a consequence of CMV replication.[1,2]

Reactivation Infection

Reactivation CMV infection occurs when a transplant patient who has been infected with CMV previously (and who is seropositive for CMV pretransplantation) reactivates endogenous latent virus. Approximately 75% of transplant patients are seropositive prior to transplantation. The incidence of symptomatic CMV disease in these patients is dependent on the nature of the immunosuppressive therapy administered: 10% to 15% if a regimen of cyclosporine (or tacrolimus), azathioprine, and prednisone is utilized; 25% to 30% if induction antilymphocyte antibody therapy is employed; and 50% to 60% if antirejection antilymphocyte antibody therapy is required.[1,2,70,71]

Superinfection

CMV superinfection occurs when an individual who is seropositive for CMV prior to transplantation develops active infection due to a virus of donor rather than endogenous origin. Studies in renal transplant patients have suggested that superinfection occurs in as many as 50% of renal transplants in which both the donor and the recipient are seropositive pretransplantation. Currently available evidence suggests that patients with superinfection are probably at higher risk for clinical disease than those with reactivation infection, although the exact extent of this effect in liver transplant patients needs further study.[1,2]

Clinical Impact of Cytomegalovirus Infection

The major clinical effects of CMV infection in liver transplant patients are outlined in Table 17.3. By far the most common effect is the development of fever, usually associated with constitutional symptoms of anorexia, malaise, myalgias, arthralgias, and a low-grade (5%–10%) atypical lymphocytosis and moderate leukopenia (2000–4000/mm^3) and thrombocytopenia (50,000–100,000/mm^3). Indeed, CMV is the most important cause of fever in the time period 1 to 4 months posttransplantation. CMV hepatitis is an important manifestation of CMV disease in liver transplant recipients, clinically mimicking allograft rejection. Figure 17.3 shows the liver biopsy of a patient with CMV hepatitis, with the typical CMV-induced inclusions on histologic examination. Clinically significant CMV hepatitis can be present in the absence of these inclusions, however, and immunoperoxidase staining of the biopsy specimen can add considerably to the diagnostic yield of the biopsy procedure.[1,2,72–76]

Infection of the gastrointestinal tract with CMV can take on a variety of forms, ranging from frank ulcerations and hemorrhage to nonspecific findings of altered gastric motility (as manifested by nausea, vomiting, and anorexia). Gastrointestinal effects of CMV can occur in the absence of fever, leukopenia, or other manifestations of CMV disease. The other life-threatening effects of

TABLE 17.3. *Major clinical effects of cytomegalovirus infection in liver transplant recipients*

Direct effects
Fever, mononucleosis-like syndrome
Hepatitis
Neutropenia and/or thrombocytopenia
Pneumonia
Inflammation and necrosis of gastrointestinal mucosa
Chorioretinitis
Indirect effects
Global depression in host defenses
Contributing role in pathogenesis of allograft injury
Increased risk of EBV-associated PTLD

EBV, Epstein-Barr virus; PTLD, posttransplantation lymphoproliferative disease.

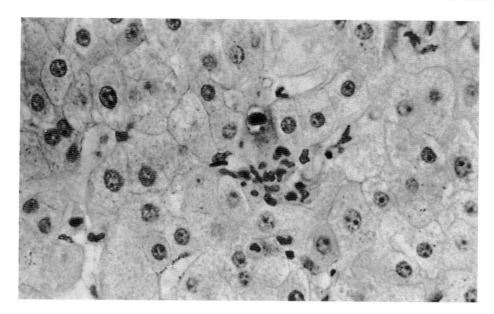

FIG 17.3. A liver biopsy of a patient with low-grade fever and deteriorating findings on liver function tests 4 weeks after orthotopic liver transplantation. The biopsy revealed evidence of cytomegalovirus infection (typical inclusion bodies). The patient was treated with a decrease in immunosuppresive therapy, and the fever and liver function abnormalities resolved.

CMV are far less common and include pneumonia and severe leukopenia and thrombocytopenia (Fig. 17.4). Chorioretinitis, beginning more than 4 months posttransplantation, is the major late effect of CMV and can either follow more typical early disease or be the first clinical manifestation of CMV replication.[1,2,72–84]

Of major importance is the broad-based depressant effect that CMV has on host defenses, thus facilitating superinfection with opportunistic pathogens such as *Pneumocystis carinii, Listeria monocytogenes,* and *Aspergillus fumigatus.* In addition, there is increasing evidence that CMV plays an important role in the pathogenesis of acute and chronic allograft injury; that is, injury that is caused not by the lytic viral infection but rather by the cytokines, chemokines, and growth factors elaborated by the donor in response to CMV infection. These, in turn, cause activation of leukocytes, endothelial cells, and an increase in display of MHC and other antigens on the allograft, thus facilitating the processes of allograft injury. An important unanswered question is whether all CMV replication is detrimental to the outcome of transplantation or only that which results in clinical infectious disease syndromes.[1,2,55]

Diagnosis

Major changes have occurred in the diagnostic approach to CMV disease, in large part because of the availability of useful antiviral strategies. The following principles underline the strategy employed by the leading centers today.[85,86]

Serologic tests are useful prior to transplantation in assessing the donor and recipient for the presence of latent virus. Posttransplantation serologic testing, including measurements of anti-CMV IgM titers, has no significant role in the management of patients because it is too insensitive for making timely decisions regarding antiviral therapy.

The demonstration of viremia, as opposed to peripheral excretion of virus in urine or respiratory secretions, is the single most useful laboratory test available for assessing CMV infection. The question is the best way to accomplish this demonstration. Classic tissue culture with the end point being a cytopathic effect has long been the gold standard, but because it can require 4 to 6 weeks for definitive results, it does not give the timely information needed to guide therapy. The shell vial technique, which relies on an immunofluorescent end point, can yield answers in 24 to 48 hours, is timely and specific, but can have a sensitivity of only 50%. Antigenemia assay, although labor intensive, can yield a semiquantitative assessment of viral load in 24 hours and has become the most commonly used assay (it should be noted, however, that significant gastrointestinal CMV disease can be present despite a negative antigenemia assay). Polymerase chain reaction (PCR), usually qualitative as a screening test and then quantitative to assess viral load, is clearly the test of the future.

Demonstration of virus in tissue biopsies by immunofluorescence, as well as routine histology, remains the standard for diagnosing tissue-invasive disease.

Management

Intravenous ganciclovir, at a dose of 5 mg/kg twice daily (with dosage adjustment for renal dysfunction) for a minimum period of 2 to 3 weeks is the standard of care for the treatment of symptomatic CMV disease. Our preference is to treat with intravenous ganciclovir until the antigenemia assay or the PCR assay shows total clearance from the blood. Patients with primary disease, those in whom a six-antigen MHC mismatch between donor and recipient is present, and those in whom high-dose immunosuppression continues to be required are at high risk for relapse. Patients

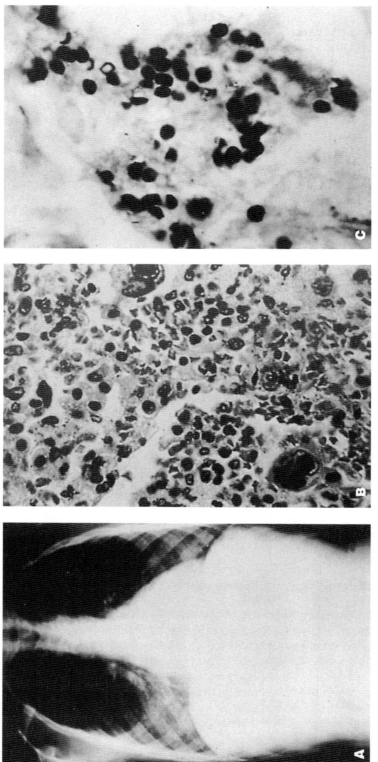

FIG 17.4. A: A chest x-ray taken 5 weeks posttransplantation because of fever and increasing dyspnea revealed bilateral interstitial pneumonia. A lung biopsy of this patient revealed evidence of both **B:** cytomegalovirus and **C:** *Pneumocystis* infection.

with relapsing infection in these circumstances not infrequently develop ganciclovir-resistant infection, necessitating the use of foscarnet, an extremely nephrotoxic drug in this circumstance. Although there are no controlled studies establishing the merits of the approach, many authorities advocate the use of anti-CMV hyperimmune globulin in addition to the intravenous ganciclovir for patients with relapsing or tissue-invasive infection, or both. Oral ganciclovir has no role in the treatment of symptomatic disease or in patients with persistent viremia; because of its relatively poor bioavailability, oral ganciclovir increases the risk of resistant infection in these patients whose viral load is high. Oral ganciclovir can be useful, however, as an adjunctive therapy once viremia has been cleared. It is our policy to administer oral ganciclovir (1 g three times daily) for 3 months after intravenous therapy in the patient groups at high risk for relapse.[1,9,86]

A variety of preventive strategies, using a variety of drugs, have been used against CMV. Virtually all of the published reports have focused on the prevention of the direct infectious disease effects of CMV rather than the indirect effects; the best way to prevent the latter remains to be determined. Because the risk of CMV disease is different in different patient populations, we advocate a stratified approach:[1,9,86]

1. For patients at risk for primary disease (D+R−), the incidence of CMV disease is high enough (more than 50%) to justify prophylaxis. The most cost-effective prophylaxis program currently available is 7 days of intravenous ganciclovir followed by oral ganciclovir for 3 months. Alternatively, intravenous ganciclovir can be continued for 6 months through an indwelling vascular access device. Oral valacyclovir has been shown to be promising for D+R− renal transplant patients, but there is as yet no information in liver transplant recipients.[87]
2. For seropositive patients requiring antilymphocyte antibody therapy, intravenous ganciclovir for the duration of the antibody therapy, followed by oral ganciclovir for 3 months, will essentially eliminate the risk of symptomatic CMV disease.[88]
3. For seropositive patients not receiving antilymphocyte antibody therapy, three choices are available: prophylaxis with oral ganciclovir; prophylaxis with valacyclovir; or no prophylaxis, but weekly viremia monitoring by antigenemia or quantitative PCR, with preemptive intravenous ganciclovir initiated once these assays become positive.

Epstein-Barr Virus Infection

The full range of effects of EBV in the liver transplant patient has been difficult to delineate because of the ubiquity of CMV and HHV-6 infection and the likelihood that similar clinical infectious disease syndromes can be caused by these related herpesviruses. It is now apparent, however, that a mononucleosis-like syndrome clearly can be caused by EBV in these patients. This syndrome differs from what is observed in the normal host by the absence of a heterophil antibody response and the infrequency of either pharyngitis or splenomegaly in the transplant patient. Liver transplant patients with chronic hepatic allograft dysfunction due to primary EBV infection possibly acquired from the allograft have also been described.[1,2,62,67]

The most important effects of EBV in the transplant patient have to do with its role in the pathogenesis of EBV-associated PTLD. The epithelial cells of the upper respiratory tract, where lytic infection occurs, are the natural reservoir for EBV infection, resulting in the pharyngitis that is common in infectious mononucleosis and the presence of virus-laden saliva, which is the natural transmitter of EBV in the community. Secondary infection of B lymphocytes traversing the lymphoid tissue of the oral cavity then occurs, resulting in latent infection but also in transformation and immortalization of these cells. EBV-seropositive individuals (more than 90% of adults are seropositive) harbor B lymphocytes latently infected with EBV that have the potential for unlimited growth. Lymphoproliferation does not occur in the immunologically normal individual because of an active surveillance mechanism based primarily on MHC-restricted, EBV-specific, cytotoxic T cells. Cyclosporine and tacrolimus inhibit this surveillance mechanism in a dose-related fashion, thus encouraging the outgrowth of the transformed lymphocytes. Antilymphocyte antibody therapy adds to the problem by inducing viral reactivation and a high level of replication, thus increasing the opportunity for B cells to be infected and transformed. Primary EBV infection, which is relatively frequent in pediatric liver allograft recipients, is another significant risk factor for PTLD.[1,2,62,67,89–95]

The incidence of PTLD has been reported to be 2% to 5% among liver transplant recipients. The clinical presentation can be quite variable, and includes one or more of the following: unexplained fever; a mononucleosis-type syndrome with fever, malaise, lymphadenopathy, and tonsillitis; a gastrointestinal presentation that can include bleeding, abdominal pain, gut perforation, or obstruction; hepatocellular dysfunction; and CNS dysfunction. Not uncommonly, the allograft itself is particularly involved in the process. Pathologically, PTLD encompasses a range of histology (nonspecific reactive hyperplasia, polymorphic B-cell hyperplasia, polymorphic B-cell lymphoma, immunoblastic sarcoma) and clonality, from the reactive to the frankly malignant, with a frequent lack of uniformity from site to site within the individual patient. Diagnosis is made by histology, although there is increasing evidence that high EBV loads by PCR assay can be informative. Unlike the typical B-cell lymphoma in a nonimmunosuppressed patient, PTLD can be totally extranodal, with florid disease in the face of negative CT scans from head to toe.[1,2,62,67,89–95]

At present, optimal management of PTLD remains to be defined. It is hoped that preventive antiviral strategies aimed at both CMV and EBV, particularly at times of intensive immunosuppression, will decrease the incidence of PTLD. Once PTLD is present, approximately 25% of patients will improve with the cessation of immunosuppression (with or without antiviral therapy). However, for the majority of patients in whom PTLD is discovered, further therapy is needed. Possibilities include surgery or radiation therapy for localized disease, antilymphoma chemotherapy, an anti–B-cell monoclonal antibody, and the combination of interferon and intravenous immunoglobulin G. Clearly, prevention is preferred.[1,2,62,67,89–95]

Human Herpesvirus 6 Infection

HHV-6 infection is prevalent in humans, with childhood infections resulting in a near 100% seropositivity rate by age 3. The primary target of this virus is CD4+ lymphocytes, although the virus can replicate in CD8+ cells, natural killer cells, and macrophages. Infection of these cells results in the elaboration of large amounts of cytokines; it is currently believed that this accounts for the modulating effects HHV-6 has on host defenses, allograft rejection, and the course of infection with such other viruses as CMV and EBV. In normal children HHV-6 is the cause of exanthem subitum and of febrile convulsions.[96–99] Approximately 30% of liver transplant patients have evidence of replicating HHV-6 infection posttransplantation, virtually all due to reactivation infection (although the possibility of transmission via the allograft has been reported).

The clinical significance of HHV-6 is still being deciphered, but it is likely that the following effects are important: HHV-6 and CMV replication often occur together, and it appears that dual infection may be clinically more severe than infection with either virus alone; HHV-6 may be a cause of encephalitis, interstitial pneumonia, and bone marrow dysfunction; and HHV-6 has been associated with increased length of hospital stay due to rejection or opportunistic infection, or both. In sum, the effects of HHV-6 appear to be similar to those of CMV.[100–102]

Diagnosis of HHV-6 infection is by culture (preferably by a rapid shell vial assay) or PCR; the latter method is most often used. An issue arises similar to that seen with other herpesviruses, namely, how one distinguishes between clinically important viral infection and trivial, subclinical viral shedding. This question is likely to become even more important because both ganciclovir and foscarnet are quite active against this virus, although acyclovir is not. It is likely that future studies of antiviral strategies for CMV and EBV will also, by necessity, monitor the effects on HHV-6.

Varicella-Zoster Virus Infection

Unless sustained antiviral therapy is being administered, approximately 10% of liver transplant patients develop clinical zoster, which represents reactivation infection and rarely disseminates. This form of VZV infection does not necessarily require changes in the immunosuppressive regimen, and, although extradermatomal cutaneous dissemination can occur in 20% to 30% of individuals, rarely causes visceral disease.

Treatment with oral fanciclovir or valacyclovir hastens lesion healing and may shorten the duration and decrease the intensity of neuralgic pain.[1]

Far more important is primary VZV infection, which produces a disseminated infection characterized by hemorrhagic pneumonia and skin lesions, encephalitis, disseminated intravascular coagulation, pancreatitis, gastrointestinal disease, and hepatitis. Because of the prohibitive mortality associated with primary VZV infection in transplant patients, we advocate the following steps. All transplant candidates should be screened for antibody to VZV prior to transplantation. Seronegative individuals, predominantly children, should receive the VZV vaccine, and seroconversion should be documented. Those who are seronegative posttransplantation should likewise receive the vaccine, although the rate of seroconversion is less than 50% in these individuals; we advocate the use of zoster immune globulin following exposures for these individuals if seroconversion has not occurred. The occurence of primary VZV should be deemed a medical emergency in a transplant patient, requiring high-dose intravenous acyclovir therapy immediately (10 mg/kg every 8 hours, with dosage adjustments for renal dysfunction).[1]

Human Immunodeficiency Virus Infection

Liver transplantation is an extremely efficient means of transmitting HIV infection, with an approximately 100% rate of transmission when an allograft from an HIV-infected donor is placed into an uninfected individual. The first step in protecting transplant patients from HIV infection is the appropriate testing of all organ and blood donors. Care must be taken not only in the actual testing, but also in ensuring that an appropriate blood sample is tested. HIV testing can be falsely negative if the donor has received multiple units of blood in a futile attempt to correct a bleeding diathesis, in which case the specimen drawn represents blood bank blood rather than the donor's. When this has occurred, all recipients of organs were infected with HIV.[1,103–107]

Although appropriate testing is extremely effective in protecting the recipient, it is important to note that HIV has been transmitted by an allograft from a donor who was seronegative for HIV by conventional testing for antibody to HIV.[108] Presumably, this donor was in the window period when replicating virus is present but an antibody response has not yet appeared. Although these events are rare, we still advocate the rejection of a potential donor with significant risk factors for HIV (e.g., history of homosexual activity in a male with multiple partners, history of intravenous drug abuse with shared needles, hemophilia, or incarceration in a prison with a high incidence of HIV).[1]

When primary HIV infection is acquired posttransplantation, it often produces a mononucleosis-like syndrome, akin to that produced by CMV or EBV, approximately 6 weeks posttransplantation, with seroconversion occurring in association with this event. However, we have reported a liver transplant patient who died of acquired immunodeficiency syndrome (AIDS) but who did not seroconvert for 3 years after acquiring the infection at the time of transplantation. The mean time to the development of overt AIDS in patients who acquire primary HIV infection at the time of transplantation has been approximately 3 years.[1,103–108]

For the last 15 years, with the recognition that posttransplantation immunosuppression amplified the HIV viral load and accelerated the course of HIV infection, there has been a virtual moratorium on performing transplant procedures in patients with end-stage liver disease who are infected with this virus. In recent years, with the advent of highly active antiretroviral therapy (HAART), there is once again interest, appropriately, in addressing this problem. If transplantation were to be undertaken, the following guidelines would appear to be a reasonable place to start:

1. The patient should, other than the HIV infection, be an ideal candidate for liver transplantation.
2. The patient should be on a stable HAART regimen that has reduced the viral load in the blood to a level undetectable by sensitive PCR assay.
3. The CD4 lymphocyte count should be greater than 300/mm³.
4. The patient should have been free of any opportunistic infection for at least 18 months, and should be tolerating an effective anti-*Pneumocystis* prophylactic regimen.

Hepatitis

Since the earliest days of clinical liver transplantation, it has been recognized that hepatitis viruses have a significant impact on liver transplant patients, both as a major cause of end-stage liver disease necessitating transplantation and as a cause of significant recurrent disease posttransplantation. Although hepatitis A can be an uncommon cause of fulminant hepatic failure, it does not recur posttransplantation. In contrast, hepatitis B and C have been and continue to be significant problems both pre- and posttransplantation. There is nearly 100% transmission of both HBV and HCV with allografts from donors who have active replicating infection with both these viruses. The replication of both viruses is upregulated by immunosuppression, particularly prednisone.[1,109]

Hepatitis B

HBV is a frequent cause of all three forms of liver disease that commonly bring patients to liver transplantation: fulminant hepatic failure, progressive hepatic failure with cirrhosis, and hepatocellular carcinoma. Until the development of treatment strategies, the outcome of liver transplantation for hepatitis B was significantly worse than for other forms of liver disease caused by recurrent disease. Patients with active viral replication [detectable HBV DNA or hepatitis B core antigen (HBcAg), or both, in the serum] had a distinctly worse outcome from transplantation, whereas those with

fulminant disease or coinfection with hepatitis D virus had a distinctly better prognosis.[110,111]

The management of HBV-infected individuals as they approach transplantation is receiving increasing attention. On the one hand, it is believed that if antiviral therapy could change the HBV infection to a nonreplicative state (e.g., serology becoming negative for HBV DNA and HBcAg), the risk of posttransplantation infection would be significantly decreased. Unfortunately, currently available therapy with interferon or lamivudine has its drawbacks. Interferon therapy can precipitate life-threatening decompensation, whereas lamivudine presents the possibility of the emergence of premature resistance. Thus, at present, pretransplantation therapy is offered to the minority of patients.[112–116]

The first major advance in the management of HBV-infected patients with end-stage liver disease was the development of immunoprophylaxis with hepatitis B immune globulin (HBIG). Regimens in which 10,000 U of HBIG are given during the anhepatic phase of the transplant operation, daily for 1 week, and then monthly—with monitoring to ensure that the antibody to hepatitis B surface antigen (anti-HBs) titer remains more than 500 IU/mL—have greatly improved the outcome for HBV-infected individuals posttransplantation. Indeed, survival rates in these patients are now comparable with those achieved for other forms of liver disease. However, breakthrough recurrences occur in 20% to 50% of individuals over time.[109,117–119]

For patients with clinical disease posttransplantation, lamivudine offers significant clinical and laboratory benefit. Unfortunately, over time, resistance develops because of mutations at the YMDD locus of the viral polymerase (e.g., 14 of 67 patients after 8 months in one series developed resistance). Other anti-HBV drugs are currently in development, and it is likely that multidrug therapy akin to that employed for tuberculosis will be the treatment of the future.[109,120]

For those patients free of HBV infection, it is important to avoid the transmission of HBV at the time of transplantation. It is now apparent that livers from donors who are hepatitis B surface antigen (HBsAg) negative but HBcAg positive have a 20% or more risk of harboring clinically important levels of virus that will emerge, causing clinical disease, posttransplantation. Our approach is to restrict the use of livers from donors positive for antibody to HBcAg to recipients who are positive for HBsAg as well as to critically ill patients requiring immediate transplantation. In the latter group, HBIG and lamivudine therapy is employed peri- and posttransplantation.[109,121,122]

Hepatitis C

Hepatitis C is a growing problem in liver transplantation. Some 30% to 40% of patients coming to liver transplantation are infected with this virus (often in the presence of such other forms of liver disease as alcoholic liver disease). The rate of recurrence posttransplantation approaches 100%. However, the course of HCV posttransplantation is usually relatively slow, with only moderate cirrhosis being observed 3 to 5 years posttransplantation in approximately 30% of individuals. United Network for Organ Sharing (UNOS) data in the United States suggest that 5-year graft survival, but not patient survival, was significantly lower for HCV patients than for those with alcoholic liver disease.[109,123–126]

Treatment of HCV posttransplantation is in its infancy. Interferon alone has a low rate of success. The combination of ribavirin and interferon, although complicated by side effects (hemolytic anemia with the ribavirin, and leukopenia, fever, and malaise with or without allograft rejection with the interferon), appears to offer measurable benefit in as many as 50% of patients.[109,127–130]

Because of the limitations of therapy, prevention remains the best strategy. In particular, an area of continuing concern is the evaluation of a donor for HCV infection. Approximately 4% to 5% of donors are anti-HCV positive; half of these have replicating virus. Livers from this half are highly efficient in transmitting the virus. Because of the shortage of donors, there has been considerable controversy about the appropriate approach to anti-HCV–positive donors, particularly since for the first 5 years posttransplantation, HCV acquisition does not have a significant effect on morbidity or mortality.[109,131–134] Because of concerns about longer-term outcomes, our policy has been to restrict the use of livers from anti-HCV–positive donors to patients in extremis, those with cancer, and the elderly. In particular we have avoided the use of these organs for children and younger adults.

INFECTIOUS DISEASE PROBLEMS OF PARTICULAR IMPORTANCE

Central Nervous System Infection

Infection of the central nervous system is a major cause of morbidity and mortality in chronically immunosuppressed patients, such as liver transplant recipients. Four distinct patterns of CNS infection are noted:[1,135]

1. Acute meningitis, usually caused by *Listeria monocytogenes,* is the most common cause of bacterial CNS infection in transplant patients.
2. Subacute to chronic meningitis is usually caused by *Cryptococcus neoformans.*
3. Focal brain infection with focal neurologic abnormalities is most commonly caused by *Aspergillus* infection metastatic from a site of active pulmonary infection, but on occasion can be caused by *Listeria, Toxoplasma gondii, Nocardia asteroides,* and PTLD.
4. Progressive dementia is due to progressive multifocal leukoencephalopathy caused by the papovavirus JC virus.

Together, *L. monocytogenes, C. neoformans,* and *Aspergillus* species account for more than three-quarters of the CNS infections occurring in transplant patients. Like the other forms of infection previously discussed, each of these infections tends to occur at a particular time posttransplan-

tation. The first month is essentially free of CNS infection. *Listeria* infection occurs especially frequently in the middle and late periods. Toxoplasmosis, aspergillosis, and nocardial infections occur almost exclusively in association with viral infection, or in the "chronic ne'er do wells" in the late period. Cryptococcal infection appears almost exclusively in the late period, again in "ne'er do wells."[1,135]

The final point concerning CNS infection in the transplant patient that bears emphasis is that such classic signs of CNS infection as meningismus and altered consciousness may be absent in these chronically immunosuppressed patients. Indeed, the most frequent clinical presentation is an unexplained headache, the presence of which should trigger a neurologic evaluation (including CT scan and lumbar puncture, with an MRI scan being performed in patients with a high suspicion of disease).[1,135]

Dermatologic Manifestations of Infection

When considering the infectious disease problems of the transplant patient, the skin must be carefully and repeatedly evaluated for two reasons: (a) It can be an important portal for the entry of a variety of microbial pathogens causing both localized and disseminated infection; (b) it can be a site of spread of infection metastatic from another site, often providing the first indication of the presence of such disseminated infection. The patient's immunosuppressive therapy can greatly modify the appearance of infection invading the skin; thus, even trivial-appearing skin lesions that are unexplained merit biopsy for culture and pathological assessment.

The dermatologic manifestations of infection in this patient population may be divided into four categories:[1,136]

1. Infection originating in the skin and typical of that occurring in immunocompetent patients, although with the potential for more serious disease
2. Extensive involvement of the skin with organisms that usually produce localized or trivial infection in immunocompetent individuals
3. Infection originating in the skin caused by opportunistic organisms that rarely produce disease in immunocompetent patients but that may produce localized or disseminated infection in immunocompromised patients
4. Disseminated systemic infection metastatic to the skin from a noncutaneous portal of entry

There are two considerations regarding the first category. First, because of the attenuation of skin integrity associated with steroid use, minor trauma to the skin results in an increased incidence of typical cellulitis due to group A streptococci and *Staphylococcus aureus*. Second, the range of organisms causing a particular gross morphologic picture is much greater in this patient population than the other categories, and includes gram-negative bacilli and a variety of fungi such as *C. neoformans* and *Candida* species. On clinical grounds alone, cryptococcal cellulitis may be difficult to distinguish from a staphylococcal cellulitis; thus, biopsy is indicated in any patient slow to respond to adequate anti-staphylococcal therapy.

The major examples of infections in the second category are infection with papillomavirus (DNA viruses that cause human warts) and infection with a variety of "nonvirulent" skin fungi. In the case of papillomavirus infection, the number of warts may be so great as to be disfiguring, with the extent of such involvement being directly related to the intensity of the immunosuppressive therapy administered. In addition, human papillomavirus DNA has been demonstrated in the skin cancers of these patients, and it is likely that such cancers arise as a result of the combined effects of the virus, immunosuppression, and ultraviolet irradiation.

Examples of localized infections of the third type include those caused by such atypical mycobacteria as *Mycobacterium marinum,* the fungus *Paecilomyces,* and the alga *Prototheca wickerhamii.* Of far greater concern are those patients who develop systemic infection following primary skin invasion with *Aspergillus, Candida,* or *Rhizopus* species. The pathogenesis of these cases of disseminated fungal infection originating in the skin is similar: trauma to the skin due to maceration by occlusive dressing or tape, followed by invasion of the damaged skin and subsequent systemic dissemination.

In the fourth category, cutaneous lesions may be the first clinical sign of disseminated life-threatening infection in the compromised host. This is particularly important with such opportunistic organisms as *N. asteroides, C. neoformans, Aspergillus* species, and *Candida* species. Approximately 20% to 30% of patients with cryptococcal infection have skin lesions weeks to months before the development of CNS disease, and 10% to 15% of patients with disseminated candidal infection have skin lesions early in their course. It is far easier to treat such patients early in their disease, on the basis of the skin findings, than after the CNS and other metastatic sites become involved.

PRINCIPLES OF ANTIMICROBIAL THERAPY IN LIVER TRANSPLANTATION

Antimicrobial therapy can be administered to the transplant patient in three modes: (a) therapeutic, in which the antimicrobial agent is administered to treat established clinical infection; (b) prophylactic, in which antimicrobial therapy is administered to an entire population before an event in order to prevent the occurrence of infection common enough or important enough to justify such an intervention; and (c) preemptive, in which antimicrobial therapy is administered before clinical disease to a subgroup of patients determined on the basis of a laboratory marker or a clinical or epidemiologic characteristic to be at particularly high risk for a given infection.[1,2,9]

Because of the importance of preventing infection in this patient population, there is a particular emphasis on prophylactic and preemptive antimicrobial strategies. By far the most successful prophylactic strategy is low-dose trimethoprim-sulfamethoxazole therapy (1 single-strength tablet daily), which has essentially eradicated *Pneumocystis, Listeria, Nocardia,* and, perhaps, *Toxoplasma* infection in these patients. Preemptive strategies include the following: intravenous ganciclovir for patients with asymptomatic CMV viremia, intravenous followed by oral ganciclovir for CMV-seropositive patients being treated with antilymphocyte antibody therapy, fluconazole therapy for patients with *Candida* in the biliary tree or urine in order to prevent obstructing fungal balls, and amphotericin therapy in patients whose respiratory tract is colonized with *Aspergillus fumigatus* (subsequent risk of infection of 50% to 75%).[1,2,9]

The final area of antimicrobial therapy in liver transplant patients that merits comment is that of drug interactions. The key step in the metabolism of both cyclosporine and tacrolimus is via hepatic cytochrome P-450–linked enzymes. There are two forms of metabolic interaction between the calcineurin inhibitors and antimicrobial agents:[1,2,9]

1. Drug-induced upregulation of cyclosporine and tacrolimus metabolism, resulting in decreased drug levels and the possibility of too little immunosuppression, resulting in rejection. The antimicrobial agents most commonly causing this effect are rifampin, isoniazid, and nafcillin.
2. Drug-induced downregulation of cyclosporine and tacrolimus metabolism, resulting in increased cyclosporine levels, an increased incidence of nephrotoxicity, and the possibility of overimmunosuppression, resulting in an added risk of infection. The antimicrobial agents most commonly causing this effect are the macrolides (erythromycin, clarithromycin, and azithromycin, in that order) and the azole antifungal agents (ketoconazole, itraconazole and voriconazole, and fluconazole, in that order).

These effects can be well managed by prospectively monitoring cyclosporine and tacrolimus blood levels and making appropriate adjustments. More problematic are interactions that are not related to drug metabolism, but rather are due to synergistic nephrotoxicity. Thus, the administration of amphotericin, the aminoglycosides, high-dose trimethoprim-sulfamethoxazole, and vancomycin in the face of therapeutic levels of cyclosporine and tacrolimus can result in severe nephrotoxicity. As a consequence, every effort should be made to avoid these drugs in the management of transplant patients.

SUMMARY AND CONCLUSIONS

Table 17.4 summarizes the different categories of infection observed in liver transplant patients. Great progress has been made and will continue to be made in the prevention and treatment of the infectious complications, technical problems, and excessive environmental hazards that occur within the hospital. At present, the emergence of antimicrobial-resistant infection with vancomycin-resistant enterococci, methicillin-resistant staphylococci, highly resistant gram-negative bacilli,

TABLE 17.4. *Classification of infections of major importance in organ transplant recipients*

Infections related to technical complications[a]
Transplantation of a contaminated allograft
Anastomotic leaks or stenoses
Wound hematoma
Intravenous line contamination
Urinary or biliary catheter contamination
Iatrogenic damage to the skin
Infections related to excessive nosocomial hazard
Aspergillus species
Legionella species
Pseudomonas aeruginosa and other gram-negative bacilli
Nocardia asteroides
Infections related to particular exposure within the community
Systemic mycotic infections in certain geographic areas
   Histoplasma capsulatum
   Coccidiodes immitis
   Blastomyces dermatitidis
Community-acquired opportunistic infection due to ubiquitous saprophytes in the environment[b]
   Cryptococcus neoformans
   Aspergillus species
   N. asteroides
   Pneumocystis carinii
Mycobacterium tuberculosis
Strongyloides stercoralis
Respiratory infections circulating in the community
   Influenza
   Streptococcus pneumoniae
Infections acquired by the ingestion of contaminated food or water
   Salmonella species
   Listeria monocytogenes
Viral infections of particular importance in the transplant patient
Herpes group viruses
Hepatitis viruses
Papovavirus
Human immunodeficiency virus
Adenoviruses

[a]All lead to infection with gram-negative bacilli, *Staphylococcus* species, and/or *Candida* species.
[b]The incidence and severity of these infections and, to a lesser extent, of the other infections listed are directly related to the state of immunosuppression present in the particular patient.
Modified from Rubin RH. Infection in renal and liver transplant recipients. In: Rubin RH, Young LS, eds. *Clinical approach in the compromised host,* 2nd ed. New York: Plenum Publishing, 1988:567–621.

and azole-resistant candidal species constitutes a major new challenge for these susceptible patients. Viral infections, including community-acquired respiratory viruses, remain a continuing issue, but new antiviral agents hold great promise in controlling these traditional scourges of transplantation.

As the clinician approaches the infectious disease problems of the liver transplant patient, he or she should be aware of the challenges ahead. The chronic requirement for immunosuppression to prevent allograft rejection not only increases the incidence and severity of acute infections but also results in chronic progressive disease from microbial agents unlikely to have such effects in immunologically intact individuals. The prevention of infection is the primary aim in this patient population, because every episode of clinical infection requiring treatment carries the potential for lethal consequences. Thus, the therapeutic prescription for the transplant patient has two components: the immunosuppressive program to treat and prevent rejection, and the antimicrobial strategy to make the immunosuppressive program safe.

The prompt recognition of and aggressive therapy of those infections that do occur are the critical factors in the successful treatment of this patient population. This may be a particularly difficult problem because the suppressed inflammatory reaction that is present often blunts the signs and symptoms of infection, necessitating great skill on the part of the clinician in interpreting the significance of subtle findings.

Although one must recognize the challenges inherent in caring for these patients, the rewards are great in terms of the promise and potential success of liver transplantation being brought to an increasing number of patients.

REFERENCES

1. Rubin RH. Infection in the organ transplant recipient. In: Rubin RH, Young LS, eds. *Clinical approach to infection in the compromised host,* 4th ed. New York: Plenum Publishing, 2000 *(in press).*
2. Fishman JA, Rubin RH. Infection in organ-transplant recipients. *N Engl J Med* 1998;338:1741–1751.
3. Lebeau G, Yanaga K, Marsh JW, et al. Analysis of surgical complications after 397 hepatic transplantations. *Surg Gynecol Obstet* 1990; 170:317–322.
4. George DL, Arnow PM, Fox AS, et al. Bacterial infection as a complication of liver transplantation: epidemiology and risk factors. *Rev Infect Dis* 1991;13:387–396.
5. Barkholt L, Ericzon BG, Tollemar J, et al. Infections in human liver recipients: different patterns early and later after transplantation. *Transpl Int* 1993;6:77–84.
6. Garcia S, Rogue J, Ruza F, et al. Infection and associated risk factors in the immediate postoperative period of pediatric liver transplantation: a study of 176 transplants. *Clin Transplant* 1998;12:190–197.
7. Arnow PM, Zachary KC, Thistlewaite JR, et al. Pathogenesis of early operative site infections after orthotopic liver transplantation. *Transplantation* 1998;65:1500–1503.
8. Gayowski T, Marino IR, Singh N, et al. Orthotopic liver transplantation in high-risk patients: risk factors associated with mortality and infectious morbidity. *Transplantation* 1998;65:499–504.
9. Rubin RH, Tolkoff-Rubin NE. Antimicrobial strategies in the care of organ transplant recipients. *Antimicrob Agents Chemother* 1993; 37(4):619–624.
10. Scowden EB, Schaffner W, Stone WJ. Overwhelming strongyloidiasis: an unappreciated opportunistic infection. *Medicine (Baltimore)* 1978;57:527–544.
11. Morgan JS, Schaffner W, Stone WJ. Opportunistic strongyloidiasis in renal transplant recipients. *Transplantation* 1986;42:518–524.
12. Purtilo DT, Meyers WN, Connor DH. Fatal strongyloidiasis in immunosuppressed patients. *Am J Med* 1974;54:488–493.
13. White JV, Garvey C, Hardy MA. Fatal strongyloidiasis after renal transplantation: a complication of immunosuppression. *Ann Surg* 1982;48:39–41.
14. Fowler CA, Lindsay I, Lewin J, et al. Recurrent hyperinfestation with *Strongyloides stercoralis* in a renal allograft recipient. *Br Med J* 1982;285:1394.
15. DeVault GA, Brown St, Montoya SP, et al. Disseminated strongyloidiasis complicating acute renal allograft rejection. Prolonged thiabenda-

zole administration and successful retransplantation. *Transplantation* 1982;34:220–221.

16. Schad GA. Cyclosporine may eliminate the threat of overwhelming strongyloidiasis in immunosuppressed patients. *J Infect Dis* 1986;153:178.

17. Jones CA. Clinical studies in human strongyloidiasis. *Gastroenterology* 1950;16:743–746.

18. Pohl C, Green M, Wald ER, et al. Respiratory syncytial virus infection in pediatric liver transplant recipients. *J Infect Dis* 1992;165:166–169.

19. Panuska JR, Hertz MI, Taraf H, et al. Respiratory syncytial virus infection of alveolar macrophages in adult transplant recipients. *Am Rev Respir Dis* 1992;145:934–939.

20. Whimbey EE, Englund JA. Community respiratory virus infections in transplant recipients. In: Bowden RA, Ljungman P, Paya CV, eds. *Transplant infections*. Philadelphia: Lippincott-Raven Publishers, 1998:295–308.

21. Rubin RH. The compromised host as sentinel chicken. *N Engl J Med* 1987;317:1151–1153.

22. Pananicolau GA, Meyers BR, Meyers J, et al. Nosocomial infections with vancomycin-resistant *Enterococcus faecium* in liver transplant recipients: risk factors for acquisition and mortality. *Clin Infect Dis* 1996;23:760–766.

23. Fortun J, Lopez-San Roman A, Velasco JJ, et al. Selection of *Candida glabrata* strains with reduced susceptibility to azoles in four liver transplant patients with invasive candidiasis. *Eur J Clin Microbiol Infect Dis* 1997;16:314–318.

24. Orloff SL, Busch AM, Olyaei AJ, et al. Vancomycin-resistant enterococci in liver transplant patients. *Am J Surg* 1999;177:418–422.

25. Hopkins C, Weber DJ, Rubin RH. Invasive aspergillus infection: possible non-ward common source within the hospital environment. *J Hosp Infect* 1989;12:19–25.

26. Allo MD, Miller J, Townsend T, et al. Primary cutaneous aspergillosis associated with Hickman intravenous catheters. *N Engl J Med* 1987;317:1105–1008.

27. Ettinger NA, Trulock EP. Pulmonary considerations of organ transplantation. *Am Rev Respir Dis* 1991;143:1386–1405, 144:213–223, 144:433–451.

28. Rubin RH, Wolfson JS, Cosimi AB, et al. Infection in the renal transplant recipient. *Am J Med* 1981;70:405–411.

29. Nelson PW, Delmonico FL, Tolkoff-Rubin NE, et al. Unsuspected donor *Pseudomonas* infection causing arterial disruption after renal transplantation. *Transplantation* 1984;37:313–314.

30. Rubin Rh, Fishman JA. A consideration of potential donors with active infection—is this a way to expand the donor pool? *Transpl Int* 1998;11:333–335.

31. Busuttil RW, Goldstein LI, Danovitch G, et al. Liver transplantation today. *Ann Intern Med* 1986;104:377–389.

32. Starzl TE, Iwatsuki S, Van Thiel DH, et al. Evolution of liver transplantation. *Hepatology* 1982;2:614–636.

33. Wozney P, Zajko AB, Bron KM, et al. Vascular complications after liver transplantation: a 5-year experience. *AJR Am J Roentgenol* 1986;147:657–663.

34. Tzakis BG, Gordon RD, Shaw BW Jr, et al. Clinical presentation of hepatic artery thrombosis after liver transplantation in the cyclosporine era. *Transplantation* 1985;40:667–671.

35. Segel MC, Zajko AB, Bowen A, et al. Hepatic artery thrombosis after liver transplantation: radiologic evaluation. *AJR Am J Roentgenol* 1986;146:137–141.

36. Starzl TE, Demetris AJ. *Liver transplantation: a 31 year perspective*. Chicago: Year Book Medical Publishers, 1990.

37. Annunziata GM, Blackstone M, Hart J, et al. Candida (*Torulopsis glabrata*) liver abscesses eight years after orthotopic liver transplantation. *J Clin Gastroenterol* 1997;24:176–179.

38. Bubak ME, Porayko MK, Krom RA, et al. Complications of liver biopsy in liver transplant patients: increased sepsis associated with choledochojejunostomy. *Hepatology* 1991;14:1063–1065.

39. Castaldo P, Strata RJ, Wood RP, et al. Clinical spectrum of fungal infections after orthotopic liver transplantation. *Arch Surg* 1991;126:149–156.

40. Colonna JO II, Winston DJ, Brill JE, et al. Infectious complications in liver transplantation. *Arch Surg* 1988;123:360–364.

41. Kusne S, Dummer JS, Singh N, et al. Infections after liver transplantation: an analysis of 101 consecutive cases. *Medicine (Baltimore)* 1988;67:132–143.

42. Cuervas-Mons V, Barrios C, Garrido A, et al. Bacterial infections in liver transplant patients under selective decontamination with norfloxacin. *Transplant Proc* 1989;21:3558.

43. Wajsczak CP, Dummer JS, Ho M, et al. Fungal infections in liver transplant recipients. *Transplantation* 1985;40:347–353.

44. Rosman C, Klompkmaker IJ, Bousel GJ, et al. The efficacy of selective bowel decontamination as infection prevention after liver transplantation. *Transplant Proc* 1990;22:1554–1555.

45. van Zeijl JH, Kroes ACM, Metselaar HJ, et al. Infections after auxiliary partial liver transplantation. Experiences in the first ten patients. *Infection* 1990;18:146–151.

46. Wiesner RH, Hermans PE, Rakela J, et al. Selective bowel decontamination to decrease gram negative aerobic bacterial and candidal colonization and prevent infection after orthotopic liver transplantation. *Transplantation* 1988;45:570–574.

47. Wiesner RH. Selective decontamination for infection prophylaxis in liver transplantation patients. *Transplant Proc* 1991;23:1927–1928.

48. Arnow PM, Furmaga K, Flaherty JP, et al. Microbiological efficacy and pharmacokinetics of prophylactic antibiotics in liver transplant patients. *Antimicrob Agents Chemother* 1992;36:2125–2130.

49. Steffen R, Reinhartz O, Blumhardt G, et al. Bacterial and fungal colonization and infection using oral selective bowel decontamination in orthotopic liver transplantation. *Transpl Int* 1994;7:101–108.

50. Arnow PM, Carandang GC, Zabner R, et al. Randomized controlled trial of selective bowel decontamination for prevention of infections following liver transplantation. *Clin Infect Dis* 1996;22:997–1003.

51. Arnow PM. Prevention of bacterial infection in the transplant recipient. The role of selective bowel decontamination. *Infect Dis Clin North Am* 1995;9:849–862.

52. Krowka MJ, Cortese DA. Pulmonary aspects of chronic liver disease and liver transplantation. *Mayo Clin Proc* 1985;60:407–413.

53. Jensen WA, Rose RM, Hammer SM, et al. Pulmonary complications of orthotopic liver transplantation. *Transplantation* 1986;42:484–490.

54. Singh N, Gayowski T, Wagener MM, et al. Pulmonary infiltrates in liver transplant recipients in the intensive care unit. *Transplantation* 1999;67:1138–1144.

55. Koskinen PK, Kallio EA, Tikkanen JM, et al. Cytomegalovirus infection and cardiac allograft vasculopathy. *Transplant Infect Dis* 1999;1:115–126.

56. Rubin RH. Infectious disease complications of renal transplantation. *Kidney Int* 1993;44:221–236.

57. Rubin RH. Impact of cytomegalovirus infection on organ transplant recipients. *Rev Infect Dis* 1990;12(suppl 7):S754–S766.

58. Reinke P, Prösch S, Kern F, et al. Mechanism of human cytomegalovirus (HCMV) reactivation and its impact on organ transplant patients. *Transplant Infect Dis* 1999;1:157–164.

59. Fietze E, Prösch S, Reinke P, et al. Cytomegalovirus infection in transplant patients: role of tumor necrosis factor-alpha. *Transplantation* 1994;58:675–680.

60. Docke WB, Prösch S, Fietze E, et al. Cytomegalovirus reactivation and tumor necrosis factor-alpha. *Lancet* 1994;343:268–269.

61. Prösch S, Staak K, Stein J, et al. Stimulation of the human cytomegalovirus IE enhancer/promoter in HL-60 cells by TNF-alpha is mediated via induction of NFκB. *Virology* 1995;208:107–116.

62. Preiksaitis JK, Cockfield SM. Epstein-Barr virus and lymphoproliferative disorders after transplantation. In: Bowden RA, Ljungman P, Paya CV, eds. *Transplant infections*. Philadelphia: Lippincott-Raven Publishers, 1998:245–263.

63. Cathomas G, Tamm M, McGandy CE, et al. Transplantation-associated malignancies: restriction of human herpesvirus 8 to Kaposi's sarcoma. *Transplantation* 1997;64:175–178.

64. Kedda MA, Margolius L, Kew MC, et al. Kaposi's sarcoma-associated herpesvirus in Kaposi's sarcoma occurring in immunosuppressed renal transplant recipients. *Clin Transplant* 1996;10:429–431.

65. Alkan S, Karcher DS, Ortiz A, et al. Human herpesvirus 8/Kaposi's sarcoma-associated herpesvirus in organ transplant patients with immunosuppression. *Br J Haematol* 1997;96:412–414.

66. Rezeig MA, Fashir BM. Kaposi's sarcoma in liver transplant recipients on FK506: two case reports. *Transplantation* 1997;63:1520–1521.

67. Basgoz N, Preiksaitis J. Post-transplant lymphoproliferative disease. *Infect Dis Clin North Am* 1995;9:901–923.

68. Ho M, Miller G, Atchison RW, et al. Epstein-Barr virus infections and DNA hybridization studies in posttransplantation lymphoma and lymphoproliferative lesions: the role of primary infection. *J Infect Dis* 1985;152:876–886.

69. Snydman DR, Werner BG, Dougherty NN, et al. A randomized, double-blind, placebo-controlled trial of cytomegalovirus immune globulin prophylaxis in liver transplantation. *Ann Intern Med* 1993;119:984–991.

70. Hibberd PL, Tolkoff-Rubin ME, Cosimi AB, et al. Symptomatic cytomegalovirus disease in the cytomegalovirus antibody seropositive renal transplant recipient treated with OKT3. *Transplantation* 1992;53:68–72.

71. Hibberd PL, Tolkoff-Rubin NE, Conti D, et al. Preemptive ganciclovir therapy to prevent cytomegalovirus disease in cytomegalovirus antibody-positive renal transplant recipients: a randomized controlled trial. *Ann Intern Med* 1995;123:18–26.

72. Savage LJ, Gonwa TA, Goldstein RM, et al. Cytomegalovirus infection in orthotopic liver transplantation. *Transpl Int* 1989;2:96–101.

73. Kanj SS, Sahara AI, Clavein PA, et al. Cytomegalovirus infection following liver transplantation: review of the literature. *Clin Infect Dis* 1996;22:537–549.

74. Stratta RJ, Shaefer MS, Markin RS, et al. Clinical patterns of cytomegalovirus disease after liver transplantation. *Arch Surg* 1989;124;1443–1450.

75. Paya CV, Herman PE, Wiesner RH, et al. Cytomegalovirus hepatitis in liver transplantation: prospective analysis of 93 consecutive orthotopic liver transplantations. *J Infect Dis* 1989;160:752–758.

76. Alessiani M, Kusne S, Fung JJ, et al. CMV infection in liver transplantation under cyclosporine or FK506 immunosuppression. *Transplant Proc* 1991;23:3035–3037.

77. Alexander JA, Cueller RE, Fadden RJ, et al. Cytomegalovirus infections of the upper gastrointestinal tract before and after liver transplantation. *Transplantation* 1988;46:378–382.

78. Escudero-Fabre A, Cummings O, Kirklin JK, et al. Cytomegalovirus colitis presenting as hematochezia and requiring resection. *Arch Surg* 1992;127:102–104.

79. Mayoral JL, Loeffler CM, Fasola CG, et al. Diagnosis and treatment of cytomegalovirus disease in transplant patients based on gastrointestinal tract manifestations. *Arch Surg* 1991;126:202–206.

80. Van Thiel DH, Gavaler JS, Schade RR, et al. Cytomegalovirus infection and gastric emptying. *Transplantation* 1992;54:70–73.

81. Sakr M, Hassanein T, Gavaler J, et al. Cytomegalovirus infection of the upper gastrointestinal tract following liver transplantation—incidence, location, and severity of cyclosporine- and FK506-treated patients. *Transplantation* 1992;53:786–791.

82. Sinzger C, Plachter B, Stenglein S, et al. Immunohistochemical detection of viral antigens in smooth muscle, stromal, and epithelial cells from acute human cytomegalovirus gastritis. *J Infect Dis* 1993;167:1427–1432.

83. Tilsed JVT, Morgan JDT, Veitch PS, et al. Reactivation of duodenal cytomegalovirus infection mimicking a transplant lymphoma. *Transplantation* 1992;54:945–946.

84. Shutze WP, Kirklin JK, Cummings OW, et al. Cytomegalovirus hemorrhoiditis in cardiac allograft recipients. *Transplantation* 1991;51:918–920.

85. Chou S. Newer methods for diagnosis of cytomegalovirus infection. *Rev Infect Dis* 1990;12(suppl 7):S727–S736.

86. Patel R, Paya CV. Cytomegalovirus infection and disease in solid organ transplant recipients. In: Bowden RA, Ljungman P, Paya CV, eds. *Transplant infections.* Philadelphia: Lippinocott-Raven Publishers, 1998:229–244.

87. Lowance D, Neumayer H-H, Legendre CM, et al. Valacyclovir for the prevention of cytomegalovirus disease after renal transplantation. *N Engl J Med* 1999;340:1462–1470.

88. Turgeon N, Fishman JA, Basgoz N, et al. Effect of oral acyclovir or ganciclovir therapy after preemptive intravenous ganciclovir therapy to prevent cytomegalovirus disease in cytomegalovirus seropositive renal and liver transplant recipients of antilymphocyte antibody therapy. *Transplantation* 1998;66:1780–1786.

89. Straus SE, Cohen JI, Tosato G, et al. Epstein-Barr virus infections: biology, pathogenesis, and management. *Ann Intern Med* 1993;118:45–58.

90. Preiksaitis JK, Diaz-Mitoma F, Mirzayans F, et al. Quantitative oropharyngeal Epstein-Barr virus shedding in renal and cardiac transplant recipients: relationship to immunosuppressive therapy, serologic responses, and the risk of post-transplant lymphoproliferative disorder. *J Infect Dis* 1992;166:986–994.

91. Pagano JS. Epstein-Barr virus: culprit or consort? *N Engl J Med* 1992;327:1750–1752.

92. Salt A, Sutehall G, Sargaison M, et al. Viral and *Toxoplasma gondii* infections in children after liver transplantation. *J Clin Pathol* 1990;43:63–67.

93. Randhawa PS, Markin RS, Starzl TE, et al. Epstein-Barr virus-associated syndromes in immunosuppressed liver transplant recipients. Clinical profile and recognition on routine allograft biopsy. *Am J Surg Pathol* 1990;14:538–547.

94. Stephaman E, Gruber SA, Dunn DL, et al. Post-transplant lymphoproliferative disorders. *Transplant Rev* 1991;5:120–129.

95. Malatack JJ, Gartner JC Jr, Urbach AH, et al. Orthotopic liver transplantation, Epstein-Barr virus, cyclosporine, and lymphoproliferative disease: a growing concern. *J Pediatr* 1991;118:667–675.

96. Leach CT, Sumaya CV, Brown NA. Human herpesvirus-6: clinical implications of a recently discovered, ubiquitous agent. *J Pediatr* 1992;121:173–181.

97. Lusso P, Malnati M, DeMaria A, et al. Productive infection of CD4+ and CD8+ mature human T cell populations and clones by human herpesvirus 6. Transcriptional down-regulation of CD3. *J Immunol* 1991;147:685–691.

98. Flamand L, Gosselin J, Stefanescu I, et al. Immunosuppressive effect of human herpesvirus 6 on T-cell function: suppression of interleukin-2 synthesis and cell proliferation. *Blood* 1995;85:1263–1271.

99. Dockrell DH, Prada J, Jones MF, et al. Seroconversion to human herpesvirus 6 following liver transplantation is a marker of cytomegalovirus disease. *J Infect Dis* 1997;176:1135–1140.

100. Singh N, Carrigan DR, Gayowski T, et al. Variant B human herpesvirus-6 associated febrile dermatosis with thrombocytopenia and encephalopathy in a liver transplant recipient. *Transplantation* 1995;60:1355–1357.

101. Singh N, Carrigan DR, Gayowski T, et al. Human herpesvirus-6 infection in liver transplant recipients: documentation of pathogenicity. *Transplantation* 1997;64:674–678.

102. Chang FY, Singh N, Gayowski T, et al. Fever in liver transplant recipients: changing spectrum of etiologic agents. *Clin Infect Dis* 1998;26:59–65.

103. Rubin RH, Tolkoff-Rubin NE. The problem of human immunodeficiency virus (HIV) infection and transplantation. *Transpl Int* 1988;26:59–65.

104. Tzakis AG, Cooper MH, Dummer JS. Transplantation in HIV+ patients. *Transplantation* 1990;49:354–358.

105. Erice A, Rhame FS, Heussner RC, et al. Human immunodeficiency virus infection in patients with solid organ transplant: report of five cases and a review. *Rev Infect Dis* 1991;13:537–547.

106. Patijn GA, Strengers PFW, Harvey M, et al. Prevention of transmission of HIV by organ and tissue transplantation. *Transpl Int* 1993;6:165–172.

107. Rubin RH, Jenkins RL, Shaw BW Jr, et al. The acquired immunodeficiency syndrome and transplantation. *Transplantation* 1987;44:1–4.

108. Simonds RJ, Holmberg SD, Hurwitz RL, et al. Transmission of human immunodeficiency virus type 1 from a seronegative organ and tissue donor. *N Engl J Med* 1992;326:726–732.

109. Bzowej NH, Wright TL. Viral hepatitis in the transplant patient. In: Bowden RA, Ljungman P, Paya CV, eds. *Transplant infections.* Philadelphia: Lippincott-Raven Publishers, 1998:309–324.

110. Todo S, Demetris A, Van Thiel D, et al. Orthotopic liver transplantation for patients with hepatitis B virus-related liver disease. *Hepatology* 1991;13:619–626.

111. Samuel D, Muller R, Alexander G, et al. Liver transplantation in European patients with the hepatitis B surface antigen. *N Engl J Med* 1993;329:1842–1847.

112. Marcellin P, Samuel D, Areias J, et al. Pretransplantation interferon treatment and recurrence of hepatitis B virus infection after liver transplantation for hepatitis B-related end-stage liver disease. *Hepatology* 1994;19:6–12.

113. Rakela J, Wooten R, Batts K, et al. Failure of interferon to prevent recurrent hepatitis B infection in hepatic allograft. *Mayo Clin Proc* 1989;64:429–432.

114. Grellier L, Brown D, McPhilips P, et al. Lamivudine prophylaxis: new strategy for prevention of reinfection in liver transplantation for hepatitis B DNA positive cirrhosis. *Hepatology* 1995;22:224A.

115. Ling R, Mutimer D, Ahmed M, et al. Selection of mutations in the hepatitis B virus polymerase during therapy of transplant recipients with lamivudine. *Hepatology* 1996;24:711–713.

116. Tipples G, Ma M, Fischer K, et al. Mutations in HBV RNA-dependent DNA polymerase confer resistance to lamivudine *in vivo. Hepatology* 1996;24:714–717.

117. Samuel D, Bismuth A, Mathieu D, et al. Passive immunoprophylaxis after liver transplantation in HbsAg-positive patients. *Lancet* 1991;337:813–815.

118. Terrault N, Zhou S, Combs C, et al. Prophylaxis in liver transplant recipients using schedule of hepatitis B immunoglobulin. *Hepatology* 1996;24:1327–1333.
119. McGory R, Ishitani M, Oliveira W, et al. Improved outcome of orthotopic liver transplantation for chronic hepatitis B cirrhosis with aggressive passive immunization. *Transplantation* 1996;61:1358–1365.
120. Perrillo R, Rakela J, Martin P, et al. Long term lamivudine therapy of patients with recurrent hepatitis B post liver transplantation. *Hepatology* 1997;26:177A.
121. Dickson RC, Everhart JE, Lake JR, et al. Transmission of hepatitis B by transplantation of livers from donors positive for antibody to hepatitis B core antigen. The National Institute of Diabetes and Digestive and Kidney Diseases. *Gastroenterology* 1997;133:1668–1674.
122. Uemoto S, Sugiyama K, Marusawa H, et al. Transmission of hepatitis B virus from hepatitis B core antibody-positive donors in living related liver transplants. *Transplantation* 1998;65:494–499.
123. Feray C, Gigou M, Samuel D, et al. Influence of the genotypes of hepatitis C virus on the severity of recurrent liver disease after liver transplantation. *Gastroenterology* 1995;108:1088–1096.
124. Martin P, Munoz S, Di Bisceglie A, et al. Recurrence of hepatitis C virus infection following orthotopic liver transplantation. *Hepatology* 1991;13:719–721.
125. Wright TL, Donegan E, Hsu H, et al. Recurrent and acquired hepatitis C viral infection in liver transplant recipients. *Gastroenterology* 1992;103:317–322.
126. Detre K. Liver transplantation for chronic viral hepatitis. Presented at the American Association for the Study of Liver Diseases Single Topic Conference, Reston, VA, 1995.
127. Chemello L, Bernardineelo E, Guido M, et al. The effect of interferon alpha and ribavirin combination therapy in naive patients with chronic hepatitis C. *Hepatology* 1995;23(suppl 2):8–12.
128. Brillanti S, Miglioli M, Barbara L. Combination antiviral therapy with ribavirin and interferon alpha in interferon alpha relapsers and nonresponders: Italian experience. *J Hepatol* 1995;23(suppl 2):13–16.
129. Schvarcz R, Ando Y, Sonnerborg A, et al. Combination treatment with interferon alpha-2b and ribavirin for chronic hepatitis C in patients who have failed to achieve sustained response to interferon alone: Swedish experience. *J Hepatol* 1995;23(suppl 2):17–21.
130. Lai M, Yang P, Wang JT, et al. Long-term efficacy of ribavirin plus interferon alpha in the treatment of chronic hepatitis C. *Gastroenterology* 1996;111:1307–1312.
131. Pereira B, Wright T, Schmid C, et al. Screening and confirmatory testing of cadaver organ donors for hepatitis C virus infection: a US national collaborative study. *Kidney Int* 1994;46:886–892.
132. Pereira B, Milford E, Kirkman R, Levey A. Transmission of hepatitis C virus by organ transplantation. *N Engl J Med* 1991;325:454–460.
133. Pereira B, Milford E, Kirkman R, et al. Prevalence of hepatitis C virus RNA in organ donors positive for hepatitis C antibody and in the recipients of their organs. *N Engl J Med* 1992;327:910–915.
134. Pereira B, Wright TL, Schmid C. A controlled study of hepatitis C transmission by organ transplantation. The New England Organ Bank Hepatitis C Study Group. *Lancet* 1995;345:484–487.
135. Tolkoff-Rubin NE, Hoving GK, Rubin RH. Central nervous system infections. In: Wijdicks EFM, ed. *Neurologic complications in organ transplant recipients.* (*Blue books of practical neurology,* vol 21.) Boston, MA: Butterworth Heinemann, 1999:141–168.
136. Wolfson JS, Sober AJ, Rubin RH. Dermatologic manifestations of infection in immunocompromised patients. *Medicine (Baltimore)* 1985;64:115–124.

Transplantation of the Liver, edited by Willis C. Maddrey, Eugene R. Schiff, and Michael F. Sorrell. Lippincott Williams & Wilkins, Philadelphia © 2001.

CHAPTER 18

Neurologic Complications of Liver Transplantation

Zbigniew K. Wszolek and Jimmy R. Fulgham

Since the first orthotopic liver transplantation (OLT) was performed in 1963,[1] improved patient selection, the emergence of specialized transplantation centers, and better immunosuppression have all had an impact on patient survival. Despite advances, complications occur. Neurologic complications are responsible for significant mortality and morbidity: 8.3% to 47% in clinical series.[1-4] Neuropathologic studies of fatalities after OLT demonstrated neurologic abnormalities in most cases.[5-8] Complications may affect the central nervous system, peripheral nervous system, or both, and patients may present with diffuse neurologic dysfunction or focal abnormalities. The signs and symptoms frequently do not indicate the cause, and often the clinical features do not predict the underlying neuropathologic changes.[6] To find the underlying cause of the neurologic dysfunction and to prevent permanent impairment or death require timely evaluation, diagnostic acuity, and a multidisciplinary approach to these patients.

Neurologic syndromes that occur after OLT include seizures, changes in the level of consciousness, focal deficits, and peripheral nervous system involvement. Frequently, central and peripheral dysfunction occur simultaneously; however, the central abnormalities often obscure the peripheral nervous system deficits. This chapter discusses the signs, symptoms, and diagnostic evaluation of patients presenting with neurologic complications after liver transplantation and the underlying causes of the complications.

Z. K. Wszolek: Senior Associate Consultant, Department of Neurology, Mayo Clinic, Jacksonville, Jacksonville, Florida; Associate Professor of Neurology, Mayo Medical School, Rochester, Minnesota 55905. J. R. Fulgham: Consultant, Department of Neurology, Mayo Clinic and Mayo Foundation; Assistant Professor of Neurology, Mayo Medical School; Rochester, Minnesota 55905.

CENTRAL NERVOUS SYSTEM COMPLICATIONS

There are various signs and symptoms of central nervous system abnormalities in OLT patients (Table 18.1). Seizures will be discussed first and in considerable detail. They are common neurologic events, and the causes of seizures exemplify the range of disorders that may affect OLT patients.

Seizures

Ictal events are among the most frequently observed neurologic complications after OLT in clinical series.[2,4,8,9] In clinical consecutive series, the incidence of seizures varied from 2.8% to 42%.[10] Seizures tended to occur in a bimodal distribution, with the highest frequency in the first week after OLT and then between 5 weeks and 16 weeks after transplantation (Fig. 18.1).[4,10-12] In an analysis of deaths occurring after liver transplantation, seizures were present in up to 36% of adult autopsied cases studied.[7]

TABLE 18.1. *Neurologic complications after orthotopic liver transplantation*

Seizures
Encephalopathy or confusion
Infection
Meningitis
Encephalitis
Abscess
Cerebrovascular complications
Anoxic or hypoxic changes
Infarction
Hemorrhage
Focal motor deficits (pyramidal, extrapyramidal, cerebellar)
Other
Headaches
Delusions or hallucinations
Movement disorders

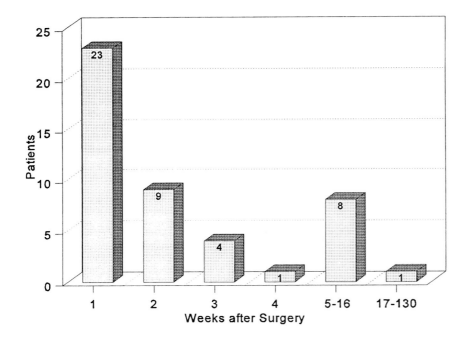

FIG. 18.1. Bimodal distribution of seizures after liver transplantation. Data are from a review of consecutive series of published reports of liver transplant recipients. (From Wszolek ZK, Steg RE. Seizures after orthotopic liver transplantation. *Seizure* 1997; 6:31–39, with permission from the British Epilepsy Association.)

Seizures may be focal or generalized, or the patient may present with status epilepticus (Table 18.2). Vogt et al.[9] found generalized seizures to be the most common but also reported focal motor seizures as well as a patient with generalized tonic-clonic seizures and myoclonus. Multiple or recurrent seizures are frequent. For patients in whom status epilepticus develops, the mortality is high and often associated with severe neuropathologic abnormalities.[1,9,11,13]

The precise cause of seizures in these patients is often difficult to establish. Liver transplant recipients are critically ill, and multiple abnormalities may be present that could cause seizures either alone or in combination (Table 18.3). A detailed analysis of 11 OLT patients with epileptiform abnormalities on their electroencephalograms (EEGs) was described previously.[13] Electrolyte (sodium, calcium, and magnesium) disturbances after OLT are common. Hypocalcemia can produce encephalopathy, obtundation, and seizures. Increased or decreased serum sodium concentration disturbs intracerebral water balance and can result in seizures. In addition, rapid correction of a low serum sodium value has been associated with central pontine and extrapontine myelinolysis.[14,15] Hypomagnesemia in conjunction with cyclosporine therapy has been associated with seizures; however, this association is not absolute, and a low serum magnesium level has been found in some cases of seizures associated with cyclosporine and not in others.[4,11]

The hyperglycemic nonketotic state has been shown to result in seizures and coma in OLT patients. This phenomenon is attributed to water flux secondary to hyperosmolality caused by disturbed glucose homeostasis during liver transplantation. Glucose infusion during operation may exacerbate this situation, resulting in coma, seizures, and death.[16,17]

Cerebrovascular complications were the cause of seizures in 18 (86%) of 21 patients who died after OLT.[11] The pathologic features identified were cerebral infarction, intracerebral hemorrhage, arteriovenous malformation, and subarachnoid hemorrhage. The most frequent histologic finding was ischemic neuronal changes, with or without cortical laminar necrosis. The latter finding may reflect acute, global cerebral ischemia associated with hy-

TABLE 18.2. *Practical seizure classification paradigm*

Generalized tonic-clonic seizure
  Primary
  Secondary
Partial seizures
  Simple partial seizures
  Complex partial seizures
Status epilepticus
  Convulsive status epilepticus
  Nonconvulsive status epilepticus

TABLE 18.3. *Recognized causes of seizures after liver transplantation*

Electrolyte disturbances
  Hyponatremia
  Hypocalcemia
  Hypomagnesemia
Hyperglycemic nonketotic state
Cerebral infarction
Anoxic or hypoxic encephalopathy
Intracerebral hemorrhage
Infection
Cyclosporine
Tacrolimus
OKT3
Coexisting seizure disorder

potension or cardiac arrest during operation or in the post-operative period.

Sepsis is a frequent systemic complication after OLT and may be due to bacteremia, fungemia, or viremia. In addition, there may be infection with multiple organisms, and several different microbial classes may be involved. Meningitis or encephalitis[9] has been identified at autopsy in patients with sepsis, and seizures were often the first manifestation of cerebral involvement. Pathogens identified in OLT patients who experience seizures include *Klebsiella pneumoniae, Listeria monocytogenes, Cryptococcus neoformans, Mycobacterium tuberculosis, Candida* species, *Aspergillus* species, and cytomegalovirus.[2,5,18–20] Frequently, there are structural or metabolic abnormalities to which the seizures are attributed, and the possibility of central nervous system involvement in the infectious process may be overlooked. In OLT patients, as in other transplant recipients, immunosuppression may predispose to infection with unusual pathogens.[21,22]

Various medications can cause seizures (Table 18.4); in liver transplant recipients, however, the drug cited most often is cyclosporine.[23–29] Cyclosporine has been implicated even when drug levels are in the therapeutic range, and seizures have also occurred at subtherapeutic levels. Often seizure activity resolves when the dose of cyclosporine is decreased or the drug is discontinued. Concomitant factors implicated in cyclosporine-induced seizures include hypocholesterolemia, hypomagnesemia, and corticosteroid infusion.[4,29,30] A striking change has been demonstrated in the cerebral white matter of patients receiving cyclosporine, whether seizures occurred or not.[29] This change is associated with a florid reactive astrocytosis affecting predominantly white matter, but it may also involve the cortex. These changes may provide the substrate for seizure initiation.

Tacrolimus (FK506) and orthoclone (OKT3) are newer immunosuppressive agents, with the former now being used as a primary immunosuppressive agent in some patients after OLT.[31,32] Both have been associated with seizures in transplant recipients, and seizures may resolve after lowering the dose or discontinuing the medication.[31,32] Interestingly, tacrolimus has been associated with a posterior leukoencephalopathy, as seen with cyclosporine toxicity.[31] Other medications that may cause seizures in OLT patients or other critically ill patients are listed in Table 18.4.

In patients with a preexisting seizure disorder, control of seizures may become difficult and may require a change in the antiepileptic medication or a change in dosage (personal observation). It is possible that an underlying structural abnormality (for example, a remote contusion) may become actively epileptogenic after OLT.[11] In the patient who has had liver transplantation for alcoholic liver disease, a late seizure after OLT should make one consider an alcohol withdrawal seizure.

Clinical observation and examination are of paramount importance for any patient with a seizure disorder. The observer should look for evidence of focal onset, such as jacksonian motor seizure or posturing of an extremity. Patients should be tested for evidence of dominant or nondominant hemisphere involvement, such as aphasia. Postictal Todd's paralysis also may have significance for localization. Tremor, asterixis, and segmental myoclonus all can be seen in liver transplant recipients and may be mistaken for seizures. Conversely, seizures may not be associated with tonic-clonic activity or other motor manifestations. Rather, mental clouding, confusion, or obtundation may be the only clinical sign of seizure activity.

Because confusion and mental status changes occur frequently in liver transplant recipients, EEG is extremely useful for diagnosis and follow-up. With the evolution of digitalized EEG equipment, continuous EEG monitoring in the intensive care unit is feasible. Monitoring during the first few days after operation, when associated with deterioration in mental status or a change in the level of neurologic functioning, can greatly facilitate the diagnosis of seizures and the subsequent care and management of these patients. Figures 18.2 and 18.3 are EEGs and case summaries of patients after liver transplantation.

Computed tomography (CT) and magnetic resonance imaging (MRI) of the head have well-established value in the assessment of patients with neurologic disease. When confronted with new-onset seizures in the posttransplantation patient, one of these modalities should be used promptly. This will exclude most of the structural abnormalities discussed previously. CT scanning should be performed with contrast enhancement if possible; however, a study that does not use contrast material will demonstrate mass effect and hemorrhage localization as well as a scan with contrast material. MRI has the advantage of superb anatomic detail, multiple imaging sequences, and multiplanar views. However, logistically it is more difficult to perform in the critically ill patient. MRI with gadolinium often demonstrates subtle meningeal enhancement that is not apparent with CT scanning.

Conventional cerebral angiography and MRI with angiographic sequences may occasionally be used if a vascular abnormality is suspected as the cause of seizures. Stereotaxic brain biopsy is a procedure that can be performed with acceptable risk and should be considered if an unknown

TABLE 18.4. *Medications that can precipitate seizure in liver transplant recipients*

Lidocaine
Theophylline
Tricyclic antidepressants
Antibiotics
   Aminoglycoside
   Penicillin
   Imipenem
   Vancomycin
   Isoniazid
Immunosuppressive agents
   Cyclosporine
   Tacrolimus
   Azathioprine
   Prednisone
   OKT3

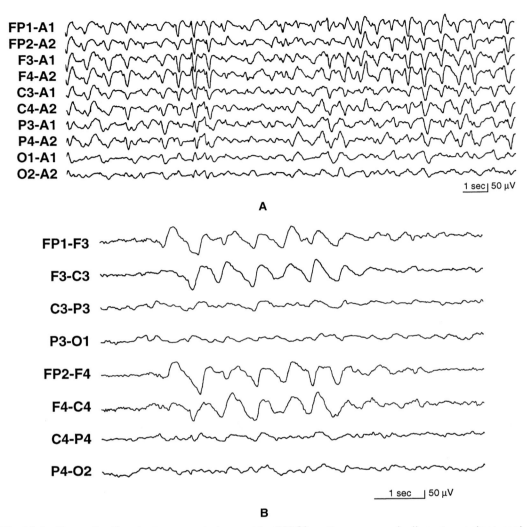

FIG. 18.2. Nonepileptic electroencephalographic (EEG) patterns seen in liver transplant recipients. **A:** A 51-year-old woman with end-stage liver disease caused by cryptogenic cirrhosis was found confused. An EEG demonstrated typical triphasic waves that can be seen before or after liver transplantation and are consistent with hepatic encephalopathy. **B:** A 43-year-old patient was confused 2 days after orthotopic liver transplantation (OLT). An EEG demonstrated bifrontal intermittent rhythmic delta activity, but no triphasic waves or seizure patterns were present. **C:** A 52-year-old man underwent liver transplantation for Laënnec's cirrhosis and had a history of alcohol and polysubstance abuse. He presented 263 days after OLT with delirium tremens following binge drinking. An EEG was performed to exclude partial complex status epilepticus and demonstrated excessive beta activity consistent with benzodiazepine administration, but no epileptiform activity. **D:** A 40-year-old woman complained of headache 1 month after OLT for hepatocellular carcinoma. The headache was transient, and a computed tomographic (CT) head scan at her initial visit was normal. The headache returned, and she rapidly became comatose. Repeat head CT scan demonstrated a right cerebellar hematoma (*inset*). The EEG showed a theta coma pattern, which is a poor prognostic indicator for neurologic recovery. **E:** A 61-year-old man developed post-transplantation movements of his jaw that were thought to be a seizure. The EEG clearly demonstrated movement artifact and muscle artifact but no potentially epileptiform activity. (**A, C,** and **D:** From Steg RE, Wszolek ZK. Electroencephalographic abnormalities in liver transplant recipients: practical considerations and review. *J Clin Neurophysiol* 1996;13:60–68, with permission from the American Clinical Neurophysiology Society. **E:** From Wszolek ZK, Steg RE. Seizures after orthotopic liver transplantation. *Seizure* 1997;6:31–39, with permission from the British Epilepsy Association.)

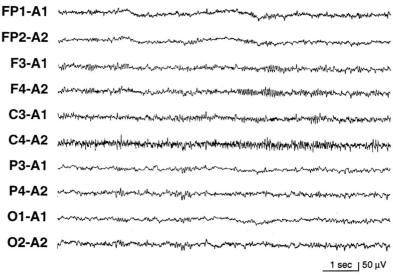

C

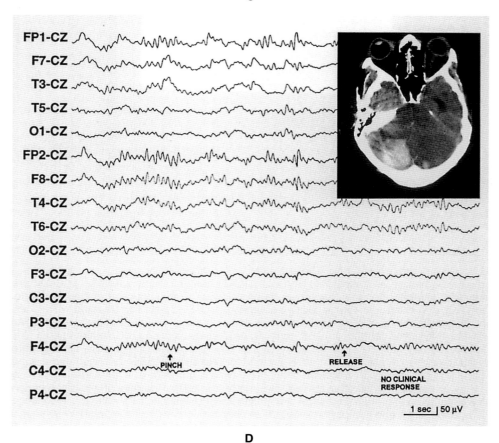

FIG. 18.2. Continued

structural abnormality is demonstrated on neuroimaging studies. It is used not only for diagnostic purposes but also to guide therapy. One potential problem in the OLT patient is the presence of a preexisting coagulopathy, which would preclude such an invasive procedure.

Laboratory investigations are important in the evaluation of patients with seizures after OLT. Serum electrolytes; blood glucose, cyclosporine, and tacrolimus levels; and blood clotting parameters should be checked immediately. A complete blood cell count, including platelets, should be performed.

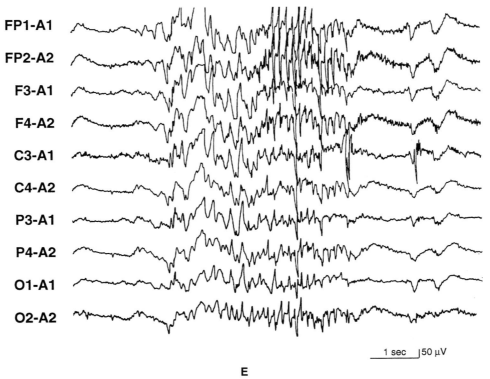

FP1-A1

FP2-A2

F3-A1

F4-A2

C3-A1

C4-A2

P3-A1

P4-A2

O1-A1

O2-A2

1 sec ⌐50 µV

E

FIG. 18.2. Continued

Patients who have taken antiepileptic medications should have the levels measured, and cardiorespiratory status should be ascertained from chest radiograph, electrocardiogram, and arterial blood gases. Measuring the liver enzymes and ammonia can assess the status of the liver graft.

Because involvement of the central nervous system by an infectious process may be heralded by the onset of seizures, an examination of the cerebrospinal fluid is essential. This may require correction of a coagulopathy with fresh frozen plasma, platelets, or cryoprecipitate. The

FIG. 18.3. Electroencephalographic (EEG) epileptiform patterns in liver transplant recipients. **A:** A 4-year-old girl who had an orthotopic liver transplant (OLT) at age 3 months for biliary atresia presented with peritonitis, and after treatment underwent a second OLT. One day postoperation, rhythmic jerking of the arm, leg, and head, and eye deviation were noted. An EEG revealed spike-and-wave activity over the right temporal lobe, and magnetic resonance imaging demonstrated biparieto-occipital and right temporal lobe infarctions (*bottom left* and *right*). **B:** A 57-year-old male OLT recipient had a respiratory arrest followed a day later by bilateral facial jerking. The EEG shows myogenic potentials intermixed with polyspike-and-wave activity (*left*). After 2 mg of lorazepam, the EEG demonstrated a suppressed background that coincided with cessation of the facial twitching (*right*). **C:** A 40-year-old patient suffered a respiratory arrest 18 months after an OLT. Despite resuscitation, the patient was unresponsive. The EEG shows continuous generalized spike and polyspike-and-wave activity without clinical accompaniment. The patient died, and autopsy revealed diffuse anoxic ischemic brain injury. **D:** A 56-year-old man developed necrotizing bronchopneumonia after his second OLT. Nine days postoperation he developed tonic-clonic seizure activity. The EEG demonstrated diffuse spike and polyspike-and-wave activity similar to **(C);** however, the electrographic changes were accompanied by clinical seizures. **E:** A 67-year-old man developed seizures after OLT and, despite fosphenytoin and lorazepam, seizures continued. Gabapentin was added to his treatment, and seizures were controlled. The EEG demonstrates midline repetitive sharp waves without clinical accompaniment. (**A** and **E:** From Wszolek ZK, Steg RE, Wijdicks EFM. Seizures. In: Wijdicks EFM, ed. *Blue books of practical neurology: neurologic complications in organ transplant recipients.* Boston: Butterworth-Heinemann, 1999:107–125, with permission from the Mayo Foundation. **B left** and **C:** From Steg RE, Wszolek ZK. Electroencephalographic abnormalities in liver transplant recipients: practical considerations and review. *J Clin Neurophysiol* 1996; 13:60–68, with permission from the American Clinical Neurophysiology Society. **D:** From Wszolek ZK, Steg RE. Seizures after orthotopic liver transplantation. *Seizure* 1997;6:31–39, with permission of the British Epilepsy Association.)

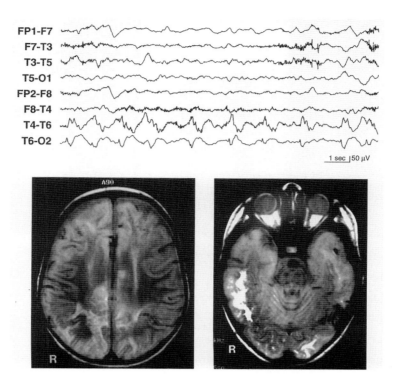

A

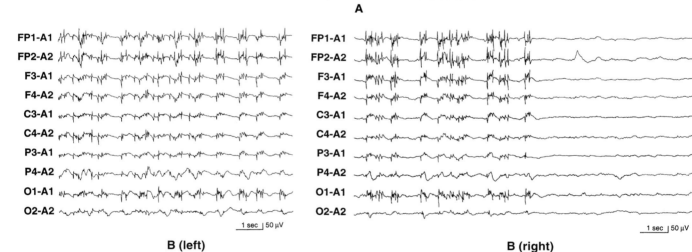

B (left)   **B (right)**

C

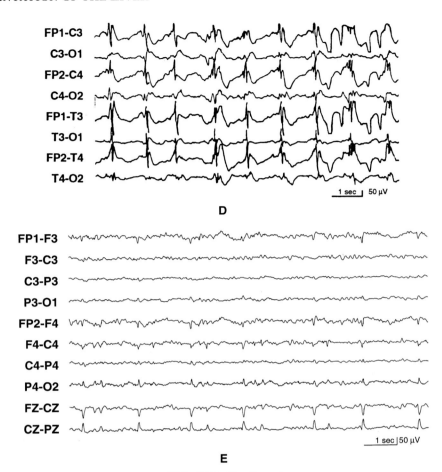

FIG. 18.3. *Continued*

lumbar puncture may be technically difficult; if problems are anticipated, the procedure can be performed with fluoroscopic guidance.

The two agents we consider as primary for the treatment of seizures in our patients are phenytoin and phenobarbital. Both have the advantages of intravenous administration, established efficacy, and predictable pharmacokinetics and side effect profiles. In status epilepticus, diazepam or lorazepam may be used initially, but they are not a substitute for starting a maintenance anticonvulsant such as phenytoin or phenobarbital. Although there are no studies that particularly indicate an advantage of phenytoin over phenobarbital, our personal choice is to initiate therapy with phenytoin. Phenytoin will precipitate out in solutions containing glucose; thus, it should be administered with normal saline or half-normal saline. Lines previously used with a solution containing glucose should be flushed before use. Intravenously administered phenytoin can be locally irritating, causing phlebitis; if a central venous line is available, it should be used. A better option for parenteral administration is fosphenytoin. This medication is administered in phenytoin equivalents, has fewer side effects, and can be given intramuscularly.

Anticonvulsant drug levels should be monitored. For phenytoin both the total and free drug levels should be measured initially, and then, if different, the free drug levels should be followed. In a retrospective analysis of total and free phenytoin levels in OLT patients, Bennett and Murrin[33] found several biochemical abnormalities in the transplant patient that may decrease phenytoin binding and, therefore, total phenytoin levels. Increased values for total bilirubin, creatinine, and blood urea nitrogen and decreased serum albumin concentration correlated with therapeutic free phenytoin levels when total levels were subtherapeutic.

Gabapentin, lamotrigine, and topiramate are new antiepileptic medications. There are no published reports on the use of these in the OLT patient. Gabapentin, however, is an attractive agent to consider in liver transplantation because it is eliminated by renal excretion and not appreciably metabolized by the liver. We have on several occasions used gabapentin with benefit for seizure control and without any untoward side effects.

Carbamazepine is not an attractive agent for patients experiencing seizures after OLT. Patients with preexisting epilepsy satisfactorily managed with carbamazepine should continue on this medication. Valproic acid, which is avail-

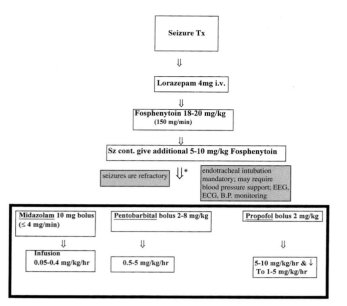

*At the point of seizures being refractory anesthetic doses of medications are
  required. The choice is a matter of preference.

*Phenobarbital can be given at this point. Bolus of 18-20 mg/kg
  @ 100 mg/ min. If seizure activity continues the dosage can be increased
  in 10 mg/kg increments to a maximum of 60 mg/kg or burst suppression
  pattern on the EEG.

FIG. 18.4. Protocol for the management of status epilepticus
in liver transplant recipients. B.P., blood pressure; ECG, electrocardiogram; EEG, electroencephalogram; Sz, seizure; Tx,
therapy.

able in a parenteral form, in our view should not be used for
management of seizures in the liver transplant recipient.

In patients who develop status epilepticus, a protocol should
be in place to aggressively manage this life-threatening situation (Fig. 18.4).

Disturbed Level of Consciousness

Liver failure leading to coma was first described in the
nineteenth century. Of the numerous changes in blood composition produced by hepatic failure, change in ammonia
has gained the most attention as causing altered cerebral
function. Other substances implicated include branched-chain amino acids, mercaptans, and short-chain fatty acids.
The syndrome produced is hepatic encephalopathy, and it
has a characteristic but nonspecific EEG pattern. The main
features are periodic triphasic waves having a duration of
300 to 500 ms and a repetition rate of 1.5 to 2.5 Hz. They
are bilaterally synchronous and symmetric but often with
frontal predominance. A phase lag, usually frontal to occipital, is common (Fig. 18.2A).

Before liver transplantation almost all patients have some
degree of hepatic encephalopathy. After OLT, levels of consciousness may vary from clouding of the sensorium to
fluctuating levels of awareness to frank coma (Fig. 18.2).
The liver functions measured by serum enzymes may be in-

creased, suggesting graft dysfunction. This condition is more
appropriately termed *transplantation encephalopathy*[7] and is
often difficult to distinguish from hepatic encephalopathy.
Neurologic signs such as asterixis, gagenhalten, and extensor
plantar responses may be present in either situation. However, other causes of altered mentation may be present (Table
18.5). Therefore, it is important to proceed with diagnostic
studies to exclude infection, structural abnormalities, or seizures as the cause of altered mental status.

Meticulous recording of all laboratory measurements
and diagnostic evaluations is helpful to follow moment-to-moment and day-to-day trends. Even with these measures,
it has been our experience that it is often necessary to proceed to repeat neuroimaging studies, electrophysiologic
testing, and perhaps cerebrospinal fluid examinations to exclude the multiple causes of transplantation encephalopathy. Despite these efforts, a significant number of patients
have encephalopathy of indeterminate origin.

Other causes of encephalopathy after OLT include Wernicke's encephalopathy, akinetic mutism, and effects from
medication. As in all patients in the intensive care unit or
after a major surgical procedure, hypnosedatives and other
medications may have a profound and often prolonged effect on alertness.

Specific treatment of mental status changes depends on
their cause. All efforts should be made to correct electrolyte
abnormalities, maintain adequate oxygenation, and maintain cerebral perfusion. Monitoring intracerebral pressure is
of value in posttransplantation patients.[34–36] Fiber-optic intracerebral pressure monitors provide an accurate and relatively safe method to measure intracerebral pressure, from
which the cerebral perfusion pressure can be obtained.
Seizures should be treated aggressively. Sepsis and meningitis are excluded by appropriate cultures, including blood,

TABLE 18.5. *Causes of disturbed
levels of consciousness in orthotopic
liver transplant recipients*

Infection
  Sepsis
  Meningitis
  Encephalitis
  Abscess
Seizures
Postictal confusion
Nonconvulsive status epilepticus
Hyperosmolality
Cerebral edema
Cerebral ischemia
  Global
  Focal
Graft failure or rejection
Medications
  Cyclosporine
  Tacrolimus
Central pontine myelinolyis
Undetermined

sputum, cerebrospinal fluid, and urine. Empiric use of antibiotics may be started in some cases while the culture results and sensitivities are pending. Structural abnormalities or mass lesions require the appropriate neuroimaging studies and may require neurosurgical consultation. If graft failure is the cause of the encephalopathy, then retransplantation is appropriate.

Cerebrovascular Complications

Cerebrovascular complications after OLT may be the result of a focal process such as infarction or hemorrhage or may be multifocal or global (Table 18.6). The latter type is often the result of anoxia following cardiorespiratory failure or systemic hypotension.

Hemorrhages may involve any of the intracranial spaces and can be intraparenchymal, subdural, or subarachnoid (Figs. 18.2D, 18.5, and 18.6). In the cases presented by Ferreiro et al.,[6] 17% of the patients had intracerebral hemorrhages, of which four were large intracerebral or cerebellar hematomas, three were subdural hematomas, and two were subarachnoid hemorrhages. In combined data from the University of Nebraska and the Mayo Clinic,[13] 19 (53%) of 36 patients who had an EEG and underwent neuropathologic examination after death had intracranial hemorrhages. This series included intraparenchymal, subdural, and subarachnoid hemorrhages. The group in Pittsburgh[7,37,38] reported similar hemorrhagic complications.

TABLE 18.6. *Cerebrovascular complications in patients after liver transplantation*

Cerebral ischemia or infarction
  Global
    Hypotension
    Hemodynamic instability
  Focal or multifocal
    Embolic
    Vasculitis
    Hypercoagulable state
Hemorrhage
  Subdural hematoma
  Intraparenchymal hematoma
    Lobar
    Hypertensive
    Bleeding diathesis (coagulopathy)
  Subarachnoid hemorrhage
Venous sinus thrombosis

The cause of hemorrhages is often secondary to a hemorrhagic diathesis, with thrombocytopenia or prolongation of the prothrombin or partial thromboplastin times.[37] In addition, some cases may be secondary to infections. Fungi, in particular *Aspergillus* and *Candida,* may result in mycotic aneurysms and subarachnoid or intraparenchymal hemorrhages.[18,37,39,40] Other bacterial infections may result in mycotic hemorrhages, but *Aspergillus* has a propensity for vascular invasion. Hypertension, either essential or medication

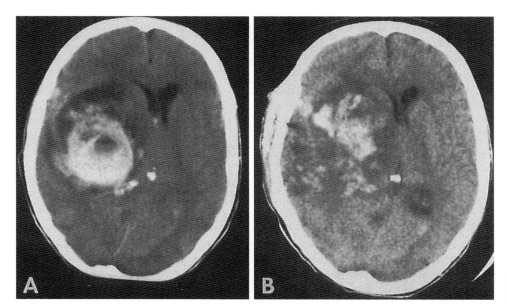

FIG. 18.5. A 51-year-old woman with primary biliary cirrhosis had an orthotopic liver transplant for endstage liver disease and did well until day 25, when an acute right hemiplegia developed and her level of consciousness deteriorated into coma. **A:** Computed tomographic scan of the head demonstrated a massive intracerebral hemorrhage with mass effect causing midline shift. A craniotomy led to partial evacuation of the hematoma and improvement of the right hemisphere mass effect. **B:** Despite these efforts, the patient died on day 31 from progressive herniation. At autopsy, there was no evidence of an arteriovenous malformation or other structural abnormality to account for the hemorrhage.

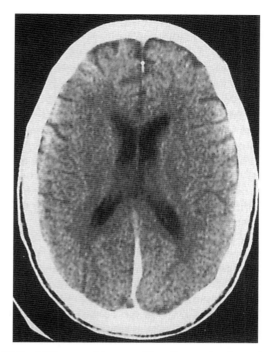

FIG. 18.6. A 33-year-old man with a diagnosis of cryptogenic cirrhosis and end-stage liver disease underwent orthotopic liver transplantation. Bleeding complicated his postoperative course, and he required 90 units of packed red blood cells and 50 units of fresh frozen plasma. On day 4, he lapsed into coma. A computed tomographic scan of the head revealed a small left parafalcine subdural hematoma that resolved. He remained unresponsive throughout the remainder of his hospital course and died on day 64 with *Staphylococcus aureus* sepsis. An asymptomatic parafalcine subdural hematoma that would not account for the patient's coma can be seen. Follow-up studies showed resolution of this hematoma. At autopsy, the patient demonstrated central pontine myelinolysis.

induced, can result in hypertensive hemorrhages. The location of hypertensive hemorrhages is usually in the basal ganglia, thalamus, and cerebellum. Lobar hemorrhages may also be secondary to hypertension.

Ischemic cerebral infarction (Fig. 18.3A), when present, is most often associated with global ischemia and decreased cerebral perfusion.[37] Pathologically, there is hippocampal neuronal ischemia, with or without laminar necrosis. Discrete cerebral infarcts are unusual in liver transplant recipients, and when present, the etiology is often unidentified.[6] Ischemic infarction has been associated with the presence of an anticardiolipin antibody and presumed hypercoagulable state.[41] Patients with the anticardiolipin antibody syndrome are prone to venous and arterial thrombosis. This is particularly true if venous and arterial thrombosis are associated with a lupus anticoagulant. Patients have presented with focal neurologic deficits after OLT with no other stroke mechanism identified other than the presence of anticardiolipin IgG antibody, and in those patients treatment with warfarin was initiated. The presence of an anticardi-

olipin antibody is not sufficient to warrant anticoagulation when there are no ischemic symptoms. Nor is there reason to screen patients routinely for the antibody. However, a patient presenting with focal neurologic symptoms does warrant investigation.

Another mechanism for ischemic stroke in the liver transplant recipient is vasculitis due to tacrolimus, resulting in multifocal cerebral infarcts.[42] Cyclosporine has also been implicated in causing reversible perfusion abnormalities; this abnormal perfusion may be the etiology of the posterior leukoencephalopathy seen with cyclosporine and perhaps other medications.[43,44] The perfusion abnormality is proposed to be due to reversible vasoconstriction caused by the release of endothelin, a potent vasoconstrictor.[44] It is possible that both cyclosporine and tacrolimus affect cerebral perfusion and that at times the effect is reversible whereas at other times it results in cerebral infarction.

Venous sinus thrombosis results in venous hypertension and may cause venous infarction. Thrombosis of the sinuses may be caused by infection or dehydration and may be seen in patients with a circulating procoagulant. Venous sinus thrombosis should be suspected in OLT patients presenting with bilateral, multifocal infarcts, especially if hemorrhagic. Treatment is anticoagulation.[45]

The hallmark of vascular events affecting the central nervous system is the temporal profile of the sudden onset of a neurologic deficit. Although this pattern is seen in OLT patients, it may be obscured. Encephalopathy from causes discussed earlier and generalized disability may make new focal findings difficult to recognize. Frequent neurologic assessment is mandatory in these patients so that subtle neurologic changes may be recognized early.

Neuroimaging studies, CT and MRI, play a central role in recognizing hemorrhages and ischemic complications after liver transplantation. In cases of global ischemia, patients may become progressively obtunded and have a "normal" CT scan. In those situations, there may be subtle obliteration of the gray-white interface and so-called normalization of the scan. New techniques using MRI with diffusion and perfusion studies may be useful in recognizing early ischemia. Angiographic MRI sequences can identify large vessel occlusions, and studies of the venous phase can diagnose venous sinus occlusions. EEG may provide valuable information, demonstrating periodic lateralizing epileptiform discharges associated with cortical laminar necrosis.[46] Cerebral angiography may be indicated in some cases. Cardiac monitoring for arrhythmias and echocardiography to investigate new murmurs should be done in all patients who suffer cerebral ischemic events.

Treatment is aimed at correction of any coagulopathy and identification of possible embolic sources, and it may include neurosurgical intervention. Fresh frozen plasma and platelet transfusions are helpful to correct the coagulopathy, especially if surgery is anticipated. Endocarditis should be assessed with echocardiography; transesophageal echocardiography is the modality of choice. Because of the frequency of *Aspergillus* infections in these patients, any hemorrhagic cerebral event should raise the suspicion of aspergillosis, and appropriate cultures should be performed.

Infections

In this patient population, sepsis is common and immunosuppression is the major predisposing factor. The pathogens involved are often opportunistic, and the infections are frequently polymicrobial. Involvement of the central nervous system can be indirect, such as in encephalopathy due to fever and septic shock. Direct involvement may be as meningitis, encephalitis, or cerebral abscess (Figs. 18.7 and 18.8), which may be multiple (Table 18.7) or as local mass effect (Fig. 18.9). As already discussed, intracerebral hemorrhage can be the presenting sign of central involvement with *Aspergillus*.

In the clinical series by Krom et al.,[2] a case of *Listeria* meningitis was reported, and Rowley et al.[47] reported a case of cytomegalovirus infection. In the series by Busuttil et al.,[8] infection occurred in 51% of patients after liver transplantation, and half of those who died had at least one infection identified. In neuropathologic series, infection involving the central nervous system is frequent. In the data from the Pittsburgh group and the group at the University of California at Los Angeles (UCLA),[7,8] infections were present in 26% and 47% of cases at autopsy, respectively. Pathogenic organisms include fungi, bacteria, and viruses. The incidence of fungal infection was the greatest, accounting for 15% and 25% in the Pittsburgh and UCLA data, respectively.[7,8] Autopsies reviewed at the University of Nebraska demonstrated similar findings.[20,39]

Viral encephalitis is often diagnosed indirectly by the presence of microglial nodules either on brain biopsy or at autopsy.[6] The polymerase chain reaction, *in situ* hybridization, and immunohistochemical techniques may also demonstrate a viral genome in spinal fluid or brain tissue of patients after OLT.[48–51] These techniques demonstrate a higher frequency of viral genomic material in patients after liver transplantation who come to autopsy compared with age-matched controls.[51]

Progressive multifocal leukoencephalopathy (PML) is a subacute demyelinating disorder that has been found in patients who are immunosuppressed, including liver transplant recipients.[52,53] This disorder is caused by infection

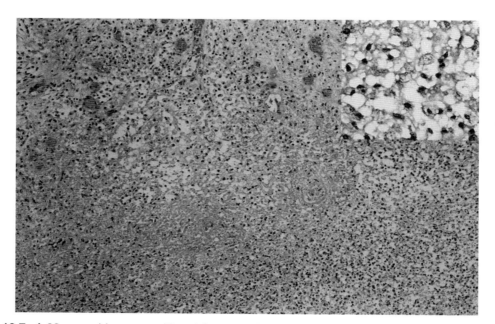

FIG. 18.7. A 23-year-old woman with autoimmune chronic active hepatitis since the age of 13 years underwent three orthotopic liver transplantations (OLTs), and each postoperative course was complicated. After her first operation, she became confused, with diminished strength and tone in all four extremities that improved over 3 days. A second OLT was performed 24 days later because of fulminant hepatic rejection, and a third OLT was performed 49 days after the first, also because of graft rejection. She was dismissed from the transplantation center with no focal neurologic deficits but returned 6 weeks later and was readmitted with intraabdominal infections; 80 days after the third OLT, she became comatose. She ultimately died of overwhelming multiple opportunistic infections 169 days after her first OLT. Neuropathologic evaluation showed central pontine and extrapontine myelinolysis and a small tuberculosis abscess in the right precentral area from the meninges through the cortex into the subcortical white matter. Microscopic sections of the abscess showed necrotic material in the center surrounded by neutrophils and granulation tissues. (Hematoxylin and eosin/Luxol fast blue stain, original magnification ×10.) The inset demonstrates intracellular acid fast bacilli. (Ziehl-Nielson stain, original magnficiation ×60.) This case was described in Wszolek et al.[59] as case 9. (Photographs courtesy of Dr. Rodney D. McComb and Dr. Grace Gilgenast.)

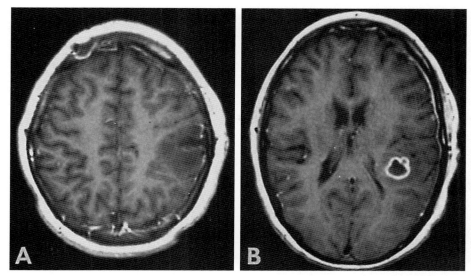

FIG. 18.8. In a 17-year-old woman with hepatic failure secondary to acute viral hepatitis, progressive hepatic encephalopathy developed. A left frontal epidural intracranial pressure (ICP) monitor was placed 1 day before orthotopic liver transplantation (OLT). OLT was performed uneventfully; however, 1 day later ICP increased to 52 mm Hg. The ICP improved with osmotic and barbiturate therapy so that by day 9 only intermittent agitation was noted. Twenty-seven days after OLT, the patient became unresponsive and had right-sided focal motor findings and anisocoria, with the left pupil larger than the right. Imaging studies of the head demonstrated a ring-enhancing left frontoparietal lesion, and a biopsy was performed on day 28 with drainage of an *Aspergillus* abscess. **A:** A T1-weighted magnetic resonance image (MRI) demonstrates the postoperative defect with considerable mass effect remaining. **B:** A ring-enhancing lesion in the deep parietal lobe consistent with a second abscess (T1-weighted MRI with gadolinium contrast). The patient died 36 days after OLT.

with the papovavirus JC. Antiviral therapy is reasonable, but PML is usually progressive and fatal. This disorder should be suspected in transplant recipients who become confused or obtunded, with or without focal findings.

Fungal species most commonly identified include *Aspergillus, Candida,* and *Cryptococcus.*[7,8,20,39,40,54] Other fungal species that usually do not cause deep infections in humans have been identified as a cause of intracerebral abscess after liver transplantation.[55]

A transmissible disorder related not to immunosuppression but to the allograft is Creutzfeldt-Jakob disease after OLT.[56] Patients may present with dementia, startle myoclonus, or

TABLE 18.7. *Infectious involvement of nervous system after liver transplantation*

Direct	Indirect	
Meningitis	Sepsis	
Encephalitis	Endotoxin	
Abscess	Shock	
Brain		
Paraspinal		
Organisms		
Bacterial	Viral	Fungal
Listeria species	Cytomegalovirus	*Aspergillus*
Klebsiella species	JC virus	*Candida*
Proteus species	Epstein-Barr virus	Cocci
Staphylococcus species	Herpes simplex virus	Other
Nocardia	Varicella-zoster virus	
Mycobacterium		
Pseudomonas species		
Parasitic		
Strongyloides		
Toxoplasma		
Other		
Creutzfeldt-Jakob or prion disease		

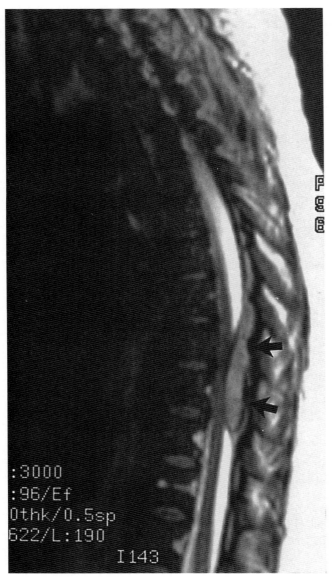

FIG. 18.9. A 40-year-old woman developed methicillin-resistant *Staphylococcus aureus* sepsis 2 years after OLT. She was treated with vancomycin. Six weeks later paraparesis and urinary retention developed. A magnetic resonance image demonstrated an epidural mass from T7 to T10 (arrows), and emergent decompression was performed. Cultures were positive for methicillin-resistant *S. aureus*. (From Wszolek ZK, McCashland TM, Witte RJ, et al. Spinal epidural abscess in a liver transplant recipient. *Transplant Proc* 1996;28:2978–2979, with permission from Appleton & Lange.)

ataxia. Diagnosis is supported by clinical features, the presence of periodic sharp waves on the EEG, and neuron-specific enolase elevation in the spinal fluid.

Patients who have central involvement by infection often present with subtle changes in the level of consciousness. Signs of meningeal irritation, such as nuchal rigidity, may

not be present because of immunosuppression. Similarly, the cerebrospinal fluid may not show pleocytosis despite the presence of an infection involving the central nervous system. Repeated cerebrospinal fluid examinations may be necessary to exclude an infectious process and to guide therapy.

Neuroimaging studies may be helpful in identifying focal abnormalities such as an abscess (Fig. 18.5), and MRI with gadolinium contrast may reveal meningeal enhancement when other studies have negative results. Cultures of body fluids, including cerebrospinal fluid, and brain biopsy specimens in appropriate cases may give a specific diagnosis and guide selection of therapy.

Treatment for specific infectious agents depends on laboratory studies, particularly species identification and sensitivity results. Fungal therapy is often delayed because of the time necessary to culture the organisms. Identification of fungal species by specific DNA probes allows more rapid identification than in the past. The effective treatment of infections requires a multidisciplinary approach in these immunosuppressed patients, who often have polymicrobial infections. For specific antimicrobial therapies, readers are referred to Chapter 17.

Central Pontine and Extrapontine Myelinolysis

Adams et al.[57] described an unusual clinicopathologic entity seen in alcoholic and malnourished patients for which they coined the term *central pontine myelinolysis* (CPM). The cause of this disorder has been thought to be secondary to the rapid correction of hyponatremia and a local myelinotoxic effect.[15] This phenomenon was first described in OLT patients by Starzl et al.[58] in 1978. Although the pathologic changes were first noted in the basis pontis (Fig. 18.10), it is now known that changes can occur elsewhere in the brain and there may be little change in the pons. Extrapontine myelinolysis (EPM) and CPM can occur in the same patient (Fig. 18.11).

Correction of the serum sodium concentration in OLT patients from a relative hyponatremia to normonatremia or hypernatremia is associated with CPM or EPM.[59,60] The perioperative period has been identified as a time of particular risk for rapid and wide changes in the serum sodium concentration. Wszolek et al.[59] reported four cases in which myelinolysis was demonstrated at autopsy. In all, a change in the serum sodium value of 20 mEq/L or more was identified in the perioperative period (Fig. 18.11), defined as the 5 days before and the 5 days after operation. In those cases, the maximum rate of change in the serum sodium concentration occurred on the operative day. There have been anecdotal reports of CPM associated with cyclosporine toxicity.[61]

Because the effects of CPM and EPM often produce quadriparesis, eye movement abnormalities, or death, we think prevention is of utmost importance. We suggest frequent monitoring of serum sodium concentration in the perioperative period and the avoidance of rapid correction or

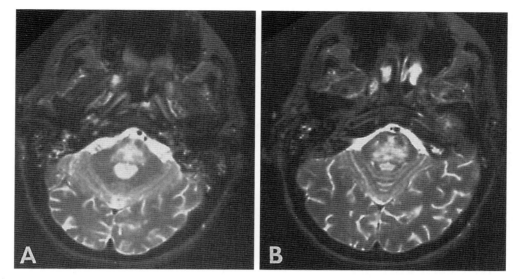

FIG. 18.10. A 54-year-old man with a 10-year history of chronic active hepatitis underwent orthotopic liver transplantation (OLT) and did well until day 2, when he experienced diffuse left-sided weakness and was increasingly unresponsive. He lapsed into coma by day 8 and remained comatose until his death 44 days after OLT. **A:** and **B:** Magnetic resonance images of the head showed areas of increased T2 signal in the basis pontis consistent with central pontine myelinolysis. This was confirmed at autopsy. A review of serum sodium values in the perioperative period (see text for definition) showed an increase of 22 mEq/L, from a low of 129 mEq/L to a maximum of 151 mEq/L.

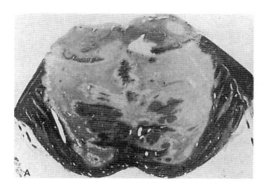 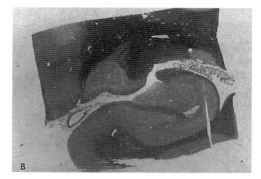

FIG. 18.11. A 53-year-old woman with end-stage liver disease secondary to non-A, non-B hepatitis who presented for orthotopic liver transplantation had no focal neurologic deficits but mild encephalopathy. Her first postoperative day was uneventful; however, by the fifth day, she became confused and seizures developed, and by the eighth postoperative day she was comatose with a left abducens nerve palsy. Fifteen days postoperatively, magnetic resonance imaging showed abnormal signal intensities in the pons and basal ganglia bilaterally. Acute pneumonia developed on the nineteenth postoperative day, and she died. Neuropathologic evaluation revealed widespread myelinolysis involving the pons **(A)**, caudate nucleus, putamen, thalamus, mamillary bodies, lateral geniculate bodies **(B)**, and other structures. Microscopically, there was relative neuronal preservation, with mild loss in the center of areas of demyelination and a varied amount of gliosis. **C:** Section from pons. (Hematoxylin and eosin/Luxol fast blue, original magnification ×100.) **D:** Section from lateral geniculate nucleus. (Hematoxylin and eosin/Luxol fast blue, original magnification ×25.) **E:** Serum sodium concentration increased from the severely hyponatremic level of 113 mEq/L preoperatively to 135 mEq/L during operation and remained relatively constant thereafter. (**E:** From Wszolek ZK, McComb RD, Pfeiffer RF, et al. Pontine and extrapontine myelinolysis following liver transplantation: relationship to serum sodium. *Transplantation* 1989;48:1006–1012, with permission from Williams & Wilkins Company.) The clinical description of this case was described in Wszolek et al.[59] as case 7; electroencephalographic findings were described in Wszolek et al.[13] as case 8. (Photographs of pathologic specimens courtesy of Dr. Rodney D. McComb.)

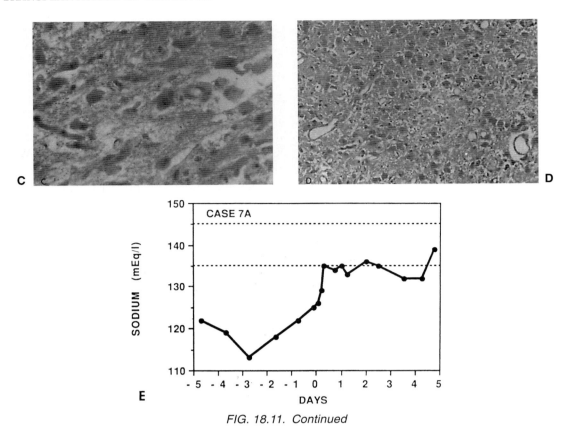

FIG. 18.11. Continued

changes in the serum sodium level of greater than 20 mEq/L. Although prevention of CPM and EPM is the main goal of management, patients do survive and can have a good recovery. Therefore, supportive care is essential. This may often mean admission to an intensive care unit.

IMMUNOSUPPRESSIVE DRUGS

The incidence of rejection after solid-organ transplantation has decreased substantially since the introduction of cyclosporine. Its use, however, has not been without associated neurotoxicity. In the liver transplant population, cyclosporine neurotoxicity has been reported in 10% to 25% of patients.[25,29] Syndromes include hypertension, headache, seizures, cortical blindness, akinetic mutism, and various motor abnormalities, including a spinocerebellar syndrome.[3,4,29,62–65]

The mechanism of neurotoxicity due to cyclosporine is unknown. Several investigators[24,26,66] suggested that there may be a perturbation in the blood-brain barrier. Analysis of cerebrospinal fluid after OLT demonstrated cyclosporine and its metabolites,[24] and high-dose corticosteroids have been thought to displace cyclosporine from central nervous system binding sites.[30,67] Both observations suggest a direct toxic effect of cyclosporine on neural tissue. Access to neural tissue may be gained via membrane toxicity of cyclosporine[26] or possibly indirectly through blood-brain barrier disruption associated with severe hepatic failure.[68]

Concomitant derangements in magnesium and cholesterol values have been implicated in the neurotoxic effects of cyclosporine.[4,29,69] These may be epiphenomena rather than directly related to cyclosporine neurotoxicity. Low magnesium levels may reflect cyclosporine nephrotoxicity,[69] and hypocholesterolemia may reflect decreased hepatocellular function.[29] In the latter instance, deGroen et al.[70] hypothesized that an episode of hepatic encephalopathy before transplantation increases the incidence of cyclosporine neurotoxicity. Hypocholesterolemia in these cases is a marker for decreased synthetic function of the liver, and the inverse relationship of cholesterol and the incidence of cyclosporine neurotoxicity reflects advanced liver failure.[70]

Seizures associated with cyclosporine have already been discussed. Hypomagnesemia alone has been associated with seizures and it is possible that together, cyclosporine and a low serum magnesium level may increase the likelihood of a seizure in some cases. White matter changes have been associated with cyclosporine neurotoxicity and have been found after OLT and after transplant of other solid organs (Fig. 18.12).[29,66] Stein et al.[3] described an unusual condition seen in OLT patients and associated with cyclosporine. In 4 of 40 patients, a cerebrocerebellar syndrome was found that led to partial recovery in 2 pa-

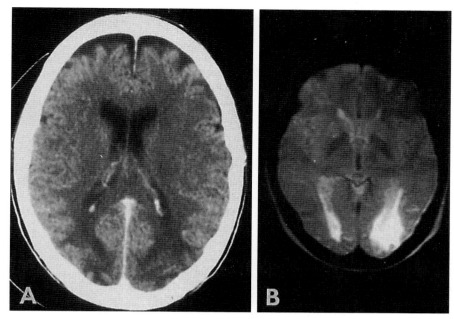

FIG. 18.12. A 47-year-old woman with cryptogenic cirrhosis had an orthotopic liver transplant (OLT) for impending liver failure. Seventeen days later, a second OLT was performed because of steroid-resistant allograft rejection. Four days after the first OLT, the patient was disoriented and complained of blindness; examination demonstrated right hemiparesis that progressed to spastic quadriparesis and cortical blindness. An initial computed tomographic (CT) scan of the head was normal; however, follow-up CT scan **(A)** and magnetic resonance imaging **(B)** demonstrated low-attenuation changes in the white matter **(A)** and increased T2 signal in the occipital lobes, with the left greater than the right **(B).** Initial immunosuppression consisted of cyclosporine, azathioprine, and prednisone. With discontinuation of cyclosporine, the patient's mental status improved to baseline. A second similar episode occurred, again associated with cyclosporine. During this second episode, there was also a clinical seizure, and electroencephalograms demonstrated nonspecific slowing, triphasic waves, and decreased amplitude over the left parieto-occipital region.

tients after discontinuation of cyclosporine, stabilization in 1 after stopping cyclosporine but worsening with rechallenge, and complete recovery in 1 patient.

The reversibility of signs and symptoms with decreasing dosage or discontinuation of cyclosporine is a major line of evidence linking this medication and neurotoxicity. Recurrence of the same syndrome when cyclosporine is presented again is further evidence. Why some patients are affected and not others, even when otherwise clinically similar, is unknown. Similarly, why some patients make a complete recovery and others an incomplete recovery is not known. Perhaps, as suggested by Boon et al.,[23] poor recovery signifies severe cyclosporine neurotoxicity and significant blood-brain barrier compromise. The oral form of cyclosporine, Neoral, has significantly reduced the major neurologic complications associated with intravenous cyclosporine.[71]

Because of the neurologic toxicity associated with cyclosporine, the drug tacrolimus has been used as a primary immunosuppressant in patients after liver transplantation. Although it has been demonstrated to be effective, it too has been associated with significant neurologic toxicity. Posterior leukoencephalopathy, seizures, vasculitis with infarc-

tion, headache, tremor, dysarthria, speech apraxia, and cortical blindness have all been reported.[32,72–78]

At present there does not appear to be an immunosuppressive agent, either alone or in combination, that has not been associated with some neurotoxicity. Detailed discussions of the immunosuppressive medications used in liver transplantation can be found in Chapter 13.

PERIPHERAL NERVOUS SYSTEM

Although less common, neurologic complications involving the peripheral nervous system have been reported (Fig. 18.13),[3,8,29,64,79–81] namely, plexopathy, polyneuropathy, and mononeuropathy. These complications are often masked or obscured by the critical illness of the patient or by the more prominent central nervous system manifestations.

Patients may have an antecedent peripheral neuropathy that becomes apparent only after OLT and not as a result of the transplantation. The peripheral nerves are particularly prone to injury during prolonged surgical procedures, either as a result of positioning or as a result of a specific procedure such as venovenous shunting or cross-clamping the vena cava.[3,79] A case of chronic inflammatory demyelinating polyneuropathy

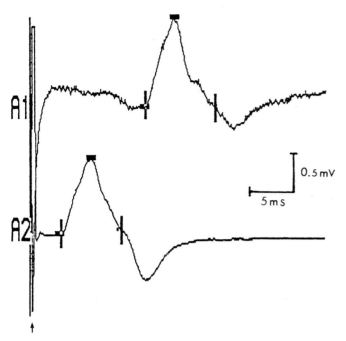

FIG. 18.13. A 71-year-old man with end-stage liver disease secondary to cirrhosis of unknown cause and chronic renal insufficiency developed right hand weakness, pain radiating from the axilla down to the fifth and fourth fingers, and paresthesias of these two fingers soon after orthotopic liver transplantation. Neurophysiologic assessment, including nerve conduction studies, concentric needle examination, and somatosensory evoked potentials, established the diagnosis of right brachial plexopathy predominantly involving the lower trunk. There was superimposed mild generalized sensorimotor axonal peripheral neuropathy. Motor nerve conduction studies performed in the right ulnar nerve 46 days after orthotopic liver transplantation are shown. Compound muscle action potentials recorded over the hypothenar muscle by surface electrodes were elicited with supermaximal stimulation at the elbow (trace *A1*) and at the wrist (trace *A2*). Distal latency measured from the shock artifact (*arrow*) to the onset of negative deflection (the first vertical marker, trace *A2*) was borderline (3.5 ms; normal value in our laboratory, <3.6 ms). Compound muscle action potential amplitude measured from the onset of the negative deflection to the peak of this deflection (horizontal markers, trace *A1*) was significantly decreased (1.1 mV; normal value, >6 mV). Filters: 2 Hz to 20 kHz.

has been reported after liver transplantation. The patient improved with plasma exchange followed by intravenous γ-globulin.[82] Somatosensory evoked potential monitoring during the operation may help eliminate these complications, especially in patients predisposed to neuropathies, such as those who have diabetes. Autonomic nervous system dysfunction has not been explored in these patients.

OTHER COMPLICATIONS

Headache

Headache is a common complaint in patients after OLT. When confronted with a patient complaining of a head-

ache, one must exclude infection, structural abnormalities such as hemorrhage or infarction, or medication side effect before concluding that the head pain is benign. Stein et al.[3] reported new-onset headache that heralded acute occipital hemorrhage in a patient with little else to suggest a focal lesion. The location, quality, and frequency of headache in these patients are often not helpful in predicting cause.

Well-controlled migraine headaches before transplantation can become difficult to control after OLT and often result in frequent visits to the emergency department for pain relief. One of the most common neurologic side effects of immunosuppressants, including tacrolimus and cyclosporine, is headache. Headache secondary to these medications often responds to decreasing the dose or stopping the medication. Unfortunately, headaches often return when the medication is restarted.

The investigation of patients with headache should include a CT scan of the head or another neuroimaging study. Cerebrospinal fluid examination may be necessary but must be individualized for each patient. Cyclosporine and tacrolimus blood levels should be measured. If pain appears to be coming from specific areas and would be more appropriately called facial pain, then specialty consultations may be in order (e.g., oral surgery or otolaryngology).

Specific treatment depends on the underlying cause of the headache. If no specific cause requiring specific intervention is found, then symptomatic therapy is appropriate. Nonnarcotic analgesics may be effective, but one should not withhold narcotics from these patients if these agents are necessary to manage their discomfort. Calcium channel blockers, β-adrenergic receptor blockers, or tricyclic antidepressants can be used for management of chronic headache. In the acute situation, high-flow oxygen may provide relief.

Movement Disorders

Abnormal movements such as myoclonus and tremor are not unusual in OLT patients (Fig. 18.2E). Asterixis is often present and may be mixed with a tremor, making a nosologic diagnosis difficult. Postural tremor is a common side effect associated with tacrolimus.[78] In many cases, decreasing the dosage of medication resulted in improvement, although a fine tremor may persist. Switching to cyclosporine was not associated with recurrence of tremor,[78] although tremor is also noted as a side effect of cyclosporine therapy.[83,84] There are anecdotal reports of other movement disorders in liver transplant recipients, including chorea, hemiballismus, and parkinsonism.[85–87] Multichannel surface electromyographic recordings and the EEG can help delineate the nature of the movement. Treatment is often difficult. Decreasing the dose of immunosuppressive medications may be helpful, and gabapentin has been shown to be beneficial in some patients with tremor. Clonazepam has been beneficial in the treatment of myoclonus in some patients and is worth trying.

Psychiatric Disturbances

Various psychiatric disturbances have been described in OLT patients, including anxiety, hallucinations, depression, adjustment disorders, delirium, and psychotic states.[88–90] The prevalence of short-term psychiatric morbidity ranges from 30% to 40% of patients. Symptoms may occur early, especially acute delirium. Acute delirium may be more common in patients with significant hepatic encephalopathy before OLT or in the alcoholic patient. Depression, psychosis, and late-onset delirium may present with subtle signs and may be difficult to recognize. Psychiatric consultation and support are important not only for the patient but also for family members. The psychiatrist's input before transplantation can be invaluable in preparing the patient and the family to understand and cope with these problems if they arise.

The psychiatrist is invaluable in assisting with the management of preexisting psychopathology. A full discussion of these issues is beyond the scope of this chapter.

INVESTIGATIONS

Laboratory investigations should not replace a thorough neurologic examination; however, this population of patients often presents with subtle and nonspecific findings. The complex issues that arise may require complete neurodiagnostic testing and may require repeated testing; the choice of diagnostic modalities should be individualized for each patient. The challenge is to recognize catastrophic neurologic compli-

TABLE 18.8. *Investigations in patients with neurologic signs and symptoms after orthotopic liver transplantation*

Imaging studies
  Computed tomography scan with or without contrast material
  MRI scan
  MRI scan with angiographic sequences
  Cerebral angiography
Electrophysiologic tests
  Electroencephalography
  Electromyography
  Evoked potentials
Laboratory tests
  Cerebrospinal fluid
  Complete blood cell count
  Coagulation measurements
  Ammonia
  Liver enzymes
  Electrolytes
  Osmolality
  Cultures for bacteria, viruses, and fungi
  Serologic tests
  Arterial blood gases
  Cyclosporine blood level
  Tacrolimus blood level
Ancillary investigations
  Brain biopsy
  Intracerebral pressure monitoring
  Echocardiography

MRI, magnetic resonance imaging.

cations early so that appropriate therapy can be initiated. Useful diagnostic tests are listed in Table 18.8.

SUMMARY

Neurologic complications are unfortunately common after OLT and involve the central and peripheral nervous systems either directly or indirectly. Seizures, disturbed levels of consciousness, and infections are the most frequent causes of significant morbidity and mortality. Although improved immunosuppression has increased survival in these patients, it has also contributed to the neurologic complications. Patients who survive are often left with little in the way of neurologic morbidity, but neurologic dysfunction contributes significantly to deaths in nonsurvivors. Modern diagnostic techniques help improve the response to neurologic catastrophe and improve survival with limited morbidity. Preventive techniques, such as electrophysiologic monitoring during operation or continuous EEG monitoring after operation, may further enhance the management of these patients. New developments in liver transplantation may eliminate some of the neurologic problems but may present the neurologist with new challenges.

REFERENCES

1. Starzl TE, Marchioro TL, Von Kaulla KN, et al. Homotransplantation of the liver in humans. *Surg Gynecol Obstet* 1963;117:659–676.
2. Krom RAF, Wiesner RH, Rettke SR, et al. The first 100 liver transplantations at the Mayo Clinic. *Mayo Clin Proc* 1989;64:84–94.
3. Stein DP, Lederman RJ, Vogt DP, et al. Neurological complications following liver transplantation. *Ann Neurol* 1992;31:644–649.
4. Adams DH, Ponsford S, Gunson B, et al. Neurological complications following liver transplantation. *Lancet* 1987;1:949–951.
5. Power C, Poland SD, Kassim KH, et al. Encephalopathy in liver transplantation: neuropathology and CMV infection. *Can J Neurol Sci* 1990;17:378–381.
6. Ferreiro JA, Robert MA, Townsend J, et al. Neuropathologic findings after liver transplantation. *Acta Neuropathol* 1992;84:1–14.
7. Martinez AJ, Estol C, Faris AA. Neurologic complications of liver transplantation. *Neurol Clin* 1988;6:327–348.
8. Busuttil RW, Colonna JO II, Hiatt JR, et al. The first 100 liver transplants at UCLA. *Ann Surg* 1987;206:387–399.
9. Vogt DP, Lederman RJ, Carey WD, et al. Neurologic complications of liver transplantation. *Transplantation* 1988;45:1057–1061.
10. Wszolek ZK, Steg RE. Seizures after orthotopic liver transplantation. *Seizure* 1997;6:31–39.
11. Estol CJ, Lopez O, Brenner RP, et al. Seizures after liver transplantation: a clinicopathologic study. *Neurology* 1989;39:1297–1301.
12. Wszolek ZK, Steg RE. Seizures after liver transplantation. *Liver Transplant Surg* 1995;1:334–339.
13. Wszolek ZK, Aksamit AJ, Ellingson RJ, et al. Epileptiform electroencephalographic abnormalities in liver transplant recipients. *Ann Neurol* 1991;30:37–41.
14. Burcar PJ, Norenberg MD, Yarnell PR. Hyponatremia and central pontine myelinolysis. *Neurology* 1977;27:223–226.
15. Norenberg MD. A hypothesis of osmotic endothelial injury: a pathogenetic mechanism in central pontine myelinolysis. *Arch Neurol* 1983;40:66–69.
16. Lampe EW II, Simmons RL, Najarian JS. Hyperglycemic nonketotic coma after liver transplantation. *Arch Surg* 1972;105:774–776.
17. Machado MCC, Monteiro da Cunha JE, Margarido NF, et al. Hyperosmolar coma associated with clinical liver transplantation. *Int Surg* 1976;61:368–369.
18. Boon AP, Adams DH, Buckels J, et al. Cerebral aspergillosis in liver transplantation. *J Clin Pathol* 1990;43:114–118.

19. Green M, Wald ER, Tzakis A, et al. Aspergillosis of the CNS in a pediatric liver transplant recipient: case report and review. *Rev Infect Dis* 1991;13:653–657.

20. Markin RS, Hollins S, Wood RP, et al. Main autopsy findings in liver transplant patients. *Mod Pathol* 1989;2:339–348.

21. Hall WA, Martinez AJ, Dummer JS. Progressive multifocal leukoencephalopathy after cardiac transplantation. *Neurology* 1988;38: 995–996.

22. Aldape KD, Fox HS, Roberts JP, et al. *Cladosporium trichoides* cerebral phaeohyphomycosis in a liver transplant recipient: report of a case. *Am J Clin Pathol* 1991;95:499–502.

23. Boon AP, Adams DH, Carey MP, et al. Cyclosporin-associated cerebral lesions in liver transplantation [Letter]. *Lancet* 1988;1:1457.

24. Gottrand F, Largillière C, Fairiaux J-P. Cyclosporine neurotoxicity [Letter]. *N Engl J Med* 1991;324:1744–1745.

25. Grant D, Wall W, Duff J, et al. Adverse effects of cyclosporine therapy following liver transplantation. *Transplant Proc* 1987;19:3463–3465.

26. Powell-Jackson PR, Carmichael FJL, Calne RY, et al. Adult respiratory distress syndrome and convulsions associated with the administration of cyclosporine in liver transplant recipients. *Transplantation* 1984; 38:341–343.

27. Deierhoi MH, Kalayoglu M, Sollinger HW, et al. Cyclosporine neurotoxicity in liver transplant recipients: a report of three cases. *Transplant Proc* 1988;20:116–118.

28. Polson RJ, Powell-Jackson PR, Williams R. Convulsions associated with cyclosporin A in transplant recipients [Letter]. *Br Med J* 1985; 290:1003.

29. de Groen PC, Aksamit AJ, Rakela J, et al. Central nervous system toxicity after liver transplantation: the role of cyclosporin and cholesterol. *N Engl J Med* 1987;317:861–866.

30. Durrant S, Chipping PM, Palmer S, et al. Cyclosporin A, methylprednisolone, and convulsions [Letter]. *Lancet* 1982;2:829–830.

31. Small SL, Fukui MB, Bramblett GT, et al. Immunosuppression-induced leukoencephalopathy from tacrolimus. *Ann Neurol* 1996;40: 575–580.

32. European FK506 Multicentre Liver Study Group. Randomised trial comparing tacrolimus (FK506) and cyclosporin in prevention of liver allograft rejection. *Lancet* 1994;344:423–428.

33. Bennett DR, Murrin C. Phenytoin binding in liver transplant patients [Abstract]. *Neurology* 1991;41(suppl 1):140.

34. Donovan JP, Shaw BW Jr, Langnas AN, et al. Brain water and acute liver failure: the emerging role of intracranial pressure monitoring. *Hepatology* 1992;16:267–268.

35. Lidofsky SD, Bass NM, Prager MC, et al. Intracranial pressure monitoring and liver transplantation for fulminant hepatic failure. *Hepatology* 1992;16:1–7.

36. Keays R, Potter D, O'Grady J, et al. Intracranial and cerebral perfusion pressure changes before, during and immediately after orthotopic liver transplantation for fulminant hepatic failure. *Q J Med* 1991;79: 425–433.

37. Estol CJ, Pessin MS, Martinez AJ. Cerebrovascular complications after orthotopic liver transplantation: a clinicopathologic study. *Neurology* 1991;41:815–819.

38. Cienfuegas JA, Martínez AJ, Van Thiel K, et al. Neuropathologic abnormalities in liver transplant patients. A study of 29 cases. *Med Clin (Barcelona)* 1985;84:169–175.

39. Boes B, Bashir R, McComb R, et al. CNS aspergillosis: review of twenty-six patients [Abstract]. *Neurology* 1992;42(suppl 3):458.

40. Wijdicks EF, de Groen PC, Wiesner RH, et al. Intracerebral hemorrhage in liver transplant recipients. *Mayo Clin Proc* 1995;70: 443–446.

41. Bronster DJ, Gousse R, Fassas A, et al. Anticardiolipin antibody-associated stroke after liver transplantation. *Transplantation* 1997;63: 908–909.

42. Pizzolato GP, Sztajzel R, Burkhardt K, et al. Cerebral vasculitis during FK 506 treatment in a liver transplant patient. *Neurology* 1998;50: 1154–1157.

43. Lorberboym M, Bronster DJ, Lidov M, et al. Reversible cerebral perfusion abnormalities associated with cyclosporine therapy in orthotopic liver transplantation. *J Nucl Med* 1996;37:467–469.

44. Truwit CL, Denaro CP, Lake JR, et al. MR imaging of reversible cyclosporin A-induced neurotoxicity. *AJNR Am J Neuroradiol* 1991;12: 651–659.

45. Einhaupl KM, Villringer A, Meister W, et al. Heparin treatment in sinus venous thrombosis. *Lancet* 1991;338:597–600.

46. Grabow J, Okazaki H. Generalized periodic complexes associated with laminar cortical necrosis in a case of hepatic encephalopathy and liver transplantation [Abstract]. *Electroencephalogr Clin Neurophysiol* 1990;76:34P.

47. Rowley HA, Kaku DA, Ascher NL, et al. Neurologic findings in 100 consecutive liver transplant recipients [Abstract]. *Neurology* 1990; 40(suppl 1):181.

48. Mutimer D. CMV infection of transplant recipients. *J Hepatol* 1996;25:259–269.

49. Samuel D, Dussaix E. Cytomegalovirus infection, fulminant hepatitis, and liver transplantation: the sides of the triangle [Editorial]. *Liver Transplant Surg* 1997;3:547–551.

50. Mutimer DJ, Shaw J, O'Donnell K, et al. Enhanced (cytomegalovirus) viral replication after transplantation for fulminant hepatic failure. *Liver Transplant Surg* 1997;3:506–512.

51. Power C, Poland SD, Kassim KH, et al. Encephalopathy in liver transplantation: neuropathology and CMV infection. *Can J Neurol Sci* 1990;17:378–381.

52. Aksamit AJ Jr, de Groen PC. Cyclosporine-related leukoencephalopathy and PML in a liver transplant recipient. *Transplantation* 1995;60: 874–876.

53. Worthmann F, Turker T, Muller AR, et al. Progressive multifocal leukoencephalopathy after orthotopic liver transplantation. *Transplantation* 1994;57:1268–1271.

54. Jabbour N, Reyes J, Kusne S, et al. Cryptococcal meningitis after liver transplantation. *Transplantation* 1996;61:146–149.

55. Patel R, Gustaferro CA, Krom RA, et al. Phaeohyphomycosis due to *Scopulariopsis brumptii* in a liver transplant recipient [Letter]. *Clin Infect Dis* 1994;19:198–200.

56. Creange A, Gray F, Cesaro P, et al. Creutzfeldt-Jakob disease after liver transplantation. *Ann Neurol* 1995;38:269–272.

57. Adams RD, Victor M, Mancall EL. Central pontine myelinolysis: a hitherto undescribed disease occurring in alcoholic and malnourished patients. *Arch Neurol Psychiatry* 1959;81:154–172.

58. Starzl TE, Schneck SA, Mazzoni G, et al. Acute neurological complications after liver transplantation with particular reference to intraoperative cerebral air embolus. *Ann Surg* 1978;187:236–240.

59. Wszolek ZK, McComb RD, Pfeiffer RF, et al. Pontine and extrapontine myelinolysis following liver transplantation: relationship to serum sodium. *Transplantation* 1989;48:1006–1012.

60. Estol CJ, Faris AA, Martinez AJ, et al. Central pontine myelinolysis after liver transplantation. *Neurology* 1989;39:493–498.

61. Fryer JP, Fortier MV, Metrakos P, et al. Central pontine myelinolysis and cyclosporine neurotoxicity following liver transplantation. *Transplantation* 1996;61:658–661.

62. Appleton RE, Farrell K, Teal P, et al. Complex partial status epilepticus associated with cyclosporin A therapy. *J Neurol Neurosurg Psychiatry* 1989;52:1068–1071.

63. Bird GLA, Meadows J, Goka J, et al. Cyclosporin-associated akinetic mutism and extrapyramidal syndrome after liver transplantation. *J Neurol Neurosurg Psychiatry* 1990;53:1068–1071.

64. Rubin AM, Kang H. Cerebral blindness and encephalopathy with cyclosporine A toxicity. *Neurology* 1987;37:1072–1076.

65. Casanova B, Prieto M, Deya E, et al. Persistent cortical blindness after cyclosporine leukoencephalopathy. *Liver Transplant Surg* 1997;3: 638–640.

66. Lane RJM, Roche SW, Leung AAW, et al. Cyclosporin neurotoxicity in cardiac transplant recipients. *J Neurol Neurosurg Psychiatry* 1988; 51:1434–1437.

67. Boogaerts MA, Zachee P, Verwilghen RL. Cyclosporine, methylprednisolone, and convulsions [Letter]. *Lancet* 1982;2:1216–1217.

68. Wacks I, Oster JR, Roth D, et al. Severe cerebral edema in a patient with anasarca and hypernatremia. *Clin Nephrol* 1992;37:19–22.

69. Thompson CB, June CH, Sullivan KM, et al. Association between cyclosporin neurotoxicity and hypomagnesaemia. *Lancet* 1984;2: 1116–1120.

70. deGroen PC, Wiesner RH, Krom RAF. Advanced liver failure predisposes to cyclosporine-induced central nervous system symptoms after liver transplantation. *Transplant Proc* 1989;21:2456.

71. Wijdicks EF, Dahlke LJ, Wiesner RH. Oral cyclosporine decreases severity of neurotoxicity in liver transplant recipients. *Neurology* 1999;52:1708–1710.

72. Lopez OL, Martinez AJ, Torre-Cisneros J. Neuropathologic findings in liver transplantation: a comparative study of cyclosporine and FK 506. *Transplant Proc* 1991;23:3181–3182.

73. Eidelman BH, Abu-Elmagd K, Wilson J, et al. Neurologic complications of FK 506. *Transplant Proc* 1991;23:3175–3178.
74. Neuhaus P, Langrehr JM, Williams R, et al. Tacrolimus-based immunosuppression after liver transplantation: a randomised study comparing dual versus triple low-dose oral regimens. *Transpl Int* 1997;10:253–261.
75. Nakamura M, Fuchinoue S, Sato S, et al. Clinical and radiological features of two cases of tacrolimus-related posterior leukoencephalopathy in living related liver transplantation. *Transplant Proc* 1998; 30:1477–1478.
76. Shutter LA, Green JP, Newman NJ, et al. Cortical blindness and white matter lesions in a patient receiving FK506 after liver transplantation. *Neurology* 1993;43:2417–2418.
77. Boeve BF, Kimmel DW, Aronson AE, et al. Dysarthria and apraxia of speech associated with FK-506 (tacrolimus). *Mayo Clin Proc* 1996; 71:969–972.
78. Wijdicks EF, Wiesner RH, Dahlke LJ, et al. FK506-induced neurotoxicity in liver transplantation. *Ann Neurol* 1994;35:498–501.
79. Veitch JE, McAllister V, Hutton L, et al. Phrenic nerve: diaphragm function following liver transplantation [Abstract]. *Muscle Nerve* 1992;15:1174.
80. Moreno E, Gomez SR, Gonzalez I, et al. Neurologic complications in liver transplantation. *Acta Neurol Scand* 1993;87:25–31.
81. Bronster DJ, Yonover P, Stein J, et al. Demyelinating sensorimotor polyneuropathy after administration of FK506. *Transplantation* 1995; 59:1066–1068.
82. Taylor BV, Wijdicks EF, Poterucha JJ, et al. Chronic inflammatory demyelinating polyneuropathy complicating liver transplantation. *Ann Neurol* 1995;38:828–831.
83. LeDoux MS, McGill LJ, Pulsinelli WA, et al. Severe bilateral tremor in a liver transplant recipient taking cyclosporine. *Mov Disord* 1998; 13:589–596.
84. Wijdicks EF, Wiesner RH, Krom RA. Neurotoxicity in liver transplant recipients with cyclosporine immunosuppression. *Neurology* 1995; 45:1962–1964.
85. Coelho JC, Wiederkehr JC, Cat R, et al. Extrapyramidal disorder secondary to cytomegalovirus infection and toxoplasmosis after liver transplantation. *Eur J Pediatr Surg* 1996;6:110–111.
86. Provenzale JM, Glass JP. MRI in hemiballismus due to subthalamic nucleus hemorrhage: an unusual complication of liver transplantation. *Neuroradiology* 1996;38(suppl 1):S75–S77.
87. Combarros O, Fabrega E, Polo JM, et al. Cyclosporine-induced chorea after liver transplantation for Wilson's disease. *Ann Neurol* 1993;33:108–109.
88. Gold LM, Kirkpatrick BS, Fricker FJ, et al. Psychosocial issues in pediatric organ transplantation: the parents' perspective. *Pediatrics* 1986;77:738–744.
89. Surman OS, Dienstag JL, Cosimi AB, et al. Liver transplantation: psychiatric considerations. *Psychosomatics* 1987;28:615–621.
90. Reich D, Rothstein K, Manzarbeitia C, et al. Common medical diseases after liver transplantation. *Semin Gastrointest Dis* 1998;9:110–125.

Transplantation of the Liver, edited by Willis C. Maddrey, Eugene R. Schiff, and Michael F. Sorrell. Lippincott Williams & Wilkins, Philadelphia © 2001.

CHAPTER 19

Liver Transplantation in the Alcoholic Patient

Michael R. Lucey

HISTORICAL BACKGROUND

Alcoholic patients rarely received liver transplantation between 1975 and 1985 for two reasons. First, it was thought that the outcome after liver transplantation for alcoholic liver disease was worse than for other diagnoses.[1] Second, many physicians were concerned that alcoholic patients would return to drinking after transplantation. Indeed, the authors of the influential National Institutes of Health (NIH) Consensus Conference on Liver Transplantation statement in 1983 acknowledged this anxiety. Their summary report stated that whereas patients with alcoholic liver disease "who are judged likely to abstain from alcohol and have established clinical indicators of fatal outcomes may be candidates for liver transplantation . . . only a small proportion of alcoholic patients with liver disease would be expected to meet the rigorous [selection] criteria."[2] The experience of the next 15 or more years has borne out neither the presumption of poor prognosis nor the prediction of a lack of suitable alcoholic candidates.

The first indication that alcoholic patients could achieve reasonable short-term survival after liver transplantation came from Starzl, who reported in 1988 that 41 alcoholic patients who underwent transplantation in Pittsburgh between 1980 and 1987 had a 1-year survival rate of 73.2%.[3] Furthermore, he recorded an unexpectedly infrequent relapse to alcohol use, leading him to coin the aphorism that "liver transplantation was the ultimate sobering experience." Since then, alcoholic liver disease has become one of the most common reasons for liver transplantation. In February 1998, 9,823 patients were on the waiting list for liver transplantation in the United States; alcoholic liver disease was the primary diagnosis in 1,736 (24%) of these patients, either alone or in conjunction with chronic hepatitis C infection.[4] In 1997, alcoholic cirrhosis was the underlying diagnosis in 777 (18.6%) of 4,167 liver transplanta-

tions in the United States. As this chapter documents, there have been numerous reports of alcoholic patients undergoing liver transplantation for whom 1- and 5-year survival rates were on the order of 70% and alcoholism relapse rates were between 30% and 50% in the first 5 years.

Whether these data are interpreted as indicating success or failure depends on one's perspective.[5] It is clear that the general public retains considerable ambivalence about providing liver transplants to alcoholic patients.[6] Even among medical professionals, the reactions of transplant physicians and surgeons to alcoholic relapse among their transplant recipients are different from those of specialists in addiction medicine. This dichotomy between transplant medicine and addiction medicine led to a watershed conference on liver transplantation and the alcoholic patient held under the auspices of the National Institutes of Health in 1997.[7] This conference showed that liver transplantation provides a good outcome for most alcoholic patients who receive a transplant. It showed also that the challenges ahead include trying to understand the mechanisms that lead some patients to relapse, and adapting patient management to limit the risks of relapse and graft loss.

EFFICACY OF LIVER TRANSPLANTATION IN ALCOHOLIC LIVER DISEASE

Patients with alcoholic liver disease who are selected for and undergo liver transplantation have an acceptable initial survival. Table 19.1 shows data from the United Network for Organ Sharing (UNOS) database for 1- and 5- year patient survival for patients with seven common diagnoses.[4] The survival rate for patients with alcoholic liver disease is similar to that for patients with chronic viral hepatitis, somewhat inferior to that for chronic cholestatic disorders, but substantially better than that for malignant liver disease. Belle and co-workers analyzed the UNOS database further in 1997.[8] They found that the causes for and frequency of graft dysfunction and loss were alike in alcoholic and nonalcoholic

M. R. Lucey: Department of Medicine, Hospital of the University of Pennsylvania, Philadelphia, Pennsylvania 19104.

TABLE 19.1. *Survival after liver transplantation*

	1-year survival		5-year survival	
	Percentage	No. of patients	Percentage	No. of patients
Acute hepatic necrosis	72.0	1,403	65.4	7,105
Alcoholic liver disease	81.9	3,063	67.6	1,561
Autoimmune hepatitis	83.5	907	77.2	386
Chronic viral hepatitis	80.3	4,267	65.3	2,102
Hepatoma	68.1	521	34.5	355
PBC	85.8	1,726	79.4	860
PSC	87.0	1,601	76.2	776
All diagnoses	81.3	14,771	68.4	7,141

Data are from the United Network for Organ Sharing database.
PBC, primary biliary cirrhosis; PSC, primary sclerosing cholangitis.

transplant recipients. The strength of this database lies in its size and duration; the weaknesses arise from the inexact data recording and retrospective analysis.

A more complex picture emerges from prospectively gathered data from the NIH's liver transplant database, in which 139 alcoholic patients were among the 625 patients receiving primary grafts for chronic liver disease and followed for 7 years.[9] Patients with fulminant hepatic failure, hepatitis B infection, or hepatocellular carcinoma were excluded from the control group. In this study, 3-year patient survival was significantly less in the alcoholic group (73%) compared with the nonalcoholic recipients (86%). This occurred in the setting of more severe liver failure at transplantation among the alcoholic cohort. The difference in graft, as opposed to patient, survival between the alcoholic and nonalcoholic cohorts was less striking (71% versus 78%). Furthermore, the frequency of retransplantation was less among alcoholic recipients: 3% of the alcoholic cohort required retransplantation at 4 years compared with 9% of the nonalcoholic cohort. These data were interpreted to show that the initial response to transplantation was similar in both alcoholic and nonalcoholic patients, but that there was a reluctance to perform retransplantations in alcoholic recipients, resulting in a disproportionate decline in patient survival over time among alcoholic recipients.

There are no controlled trials to demonstrate that liver transplantation is more efficacious than other forms of treatment for patients with alcoholic liver disease. Nevertheless, a strong case can be made that liver transplantation is the best available therapy for *some* patients with alcoholic liver disease. In 1992, Lucey et al. showed that among a cohort of alcoholic patients considered for liver transplantation, the survival at 12 months of 45 patients selected for the procedure was 78% compared with 50% in 54 patients who were not selected for transplantation.[10] Subsequently, Poynard et al. used a mathematical model to demonstrate that survival among alcoholic patients with life-threatening liver disease was improved by liver transplantation compared with the predicted outcome with medical management.[11] However, these investigators were not able to show a benefit in less severely affected patients with alcoholic cirrhosis. Although these data suggest that liver transplantation is the best treatment for at least some alcoholic patients, it is more difficult to show efficacy in less urgently ill alcoholic patients because of the capacity of patients with acute alcoholic hepatitis to recover when alcohol is withheld.

ETHICAL ISSUES

In the past few years the debate on the appropriateness of placing alcoholic patients on the transplantation waiting list has centered on the question of whether such patients should be given equal or reduced access to donor organs on account of the "voluntary" nature of alcoholism. (See reference 12 for my review of the topic.) The sheer numbers of alcoholic patients receiving liver transplants might suggest that there is little opposition to performing transplantations in alcoholic patients. That observation ignores the (unknown) denominator of alcoholic individuals with liver disease in the community and the possibility of unrecognized discrimination. A recent opinion poll in Great Britain showed that both the general population and family physicians believed that alcoholic patients should receive a lesser priority compared with other candidates for scarce donor organs, even when the alternative recipients had a lesser chance of a successful outcome from transplantation.[6]

Nevertheless, in the idealistic realm of "best practice," there is little support for discrimination against alcoholic patients when rationing donor livers. For example, Krom concluded for an international consensus-gathering exercise that "medical selection criteria should be the same for all patients with end-stage liver disease."[13] This view also informed the discussion on determining minimal criteria for placement on the liver transplantation waiting list in the United States.[14]

PREDICTING PROGNOSIS IN ALCOHOLIC LIVER DISEASE

The syndrome of acute alcoholic hepatitis, which presents as acute hepatic injury following recent excessive drinking, complicates the assessment of prognosis in alcoholic patients with liver failure, because of the propensity for patients with this syndrome to recover with abstinence from alcohol.[15] At the most severe end of the spectrum, Maddrey and co-workers have described a discriminant function based on prothrombin time and serum bilirubin level that stratifies those patients at greatest risk of early death.[16] The revised discriminant function is derived as follows:

$$[4.6 \times (\text{prothrombin time in seconds} > \text{control time})] + \text{serum bilirubin (mg/dL)}$$

Values greater than 32 indicate a high risk of early mortality. The development of acute renal failure in the setting of acute alcoholic hepatitis is an antemortem event.[17]

The current consensus in the United States is that patients with acute alcoholic hepatitis should not receive liver transplantation. This is a difficult rule to apply in some cases, especially when acute hepatic failure results unexpectedly from a combination of alcohol use and acetaminophen intake.[18] This situation shows that even with fixed rules, a case-by-case assessment should be made.

The Child-Pugh scoring system has become the most widely used instrument to estimate prognosis in alcoholic and other forms of cirrhosis.[19] As shown in Table 19.2, it is a scoring system based on clinical features of portal hypertension and liver failure. It is used to determine minimal criteria for placement on the transplantation waiting list in the United States.[14] The limitations of the Child-Pugh system are that it is less predictive in acute (or acute on chronic) liver failure and chronic cholestatic disease. Consequently, the Child-Pugh score is a poor prognostic instrument in acute alcoholic hepatitis or for acute toxic hepatic injury in an alcoholic individual. In addition, although the Child-Pugh score is a useful, albeit empirical, method to stratify cirrhotic patients into high- or low-risk groups, it is unhelpful in predicting the risks of mortality with or without transplantation in individual patients.

MEDICAL ASSESSMENT OF THE ALCOHOLIC CANDIDATE

A second element of the pretransplantation evaluation is the assessment of the general health of the patient, focusing on conditions that might limit the potential for successful transplantation, such as end-organ damage to the heart, pancreas, kidneys, or CNS or poor general nutritional status.[15] This component of the evaluation is also directed to assessing the presence and consequence of comorbid disorders, including chronic viral hepatitis, malignancy, metabolic disorders, and chronic bacterial infection.

Alcoholic candidates need careful assessment for the cardiovascular risks of surgery and recovery after surgery. Curiously, alcoholic cardiomyopathy is rarely a reason for refusal to transplant.[20] This is probably because the greatest myopathic effects are observed during active drinking, and patients who are currently drinking are screened out by the referring physicians or during the evaluation process. However, cardiomyopathy may evade recognition even during extensive pretransplantation assessment, because of low peripheral resistance in patients with advanced cirrhosis, portal hypertension, and ascites. Peripheral resistance recovers almost immediately in a successful liver transplantation. Consequently, liver transplant recipients, alcoholic and nonalcoholic alike, occasionally experience acute cardiac failure immediately on completion of transplantation, when a previously unrecognized myopathic heart has to function with a restored afterload.

The choice of cardiac test depends on local preference. Noninvasive methods, including dobutamine echocardiography and 12-lead stress electrocardiographic testing, are commonly used. Many alcoholic patients have a history of cigarette smoking or hypertension, or both. Formal cardiac catheterization is advisable in any patient in whom there is concern regarding undetected or suspected coronary artery disease.

Acute or chronic pancreatitis is rarely if ever a reason to refuse transplantation to an alcoholic candidate.

Assessment of CNS function in alcoholic candidates with end-stage liver failure is confounded by the difficulty of distinguishing hepatic encephalopthy, which is reversible upon restoration of hepatic function, from an organic fixed brain syndrome consequent on alcoholism. We generally rely on a brain imaging study (CT or MR), and in the absence of a structural lesion give the patient the benefit of the doubt.

Many alcoholic patients with end-stage liver disease are malnourished. Although there are few data to show that restoration of nutritional status in anticipation of transplantation has a salutary effect, it stands to reason that the better nourished patient is in better shape to overcome major surgery. In particular, we should not withhold protein merely on account of a history of encephalopathy. Kearns et al.

TABLE 19.2. *Child-Pugh classification*

	Points		
	1	2	3
Encephalopathy grade	None	1, 2	3, 4
Ascites	Absent	Slight	Moderate
Bilirubin level (mg/dL)	1–2	2–3	>3
Albumin level (g/dL)	>3.5	2.8–3.5	<2.8
Prothrombin time			
(secs prolonged)	1–4	4–6	>6
Prothrombin time (INR)	<1.7	1.8–2.3	>2.3
PBC or PSC			
Bilirubin level (mg/dL)	1–4	4–10	>10

Grading (total score): Class A, 1–6 points; class B, 7–9; class C, 10–15.

PBC, primary biliary cirrhosis; PSC, primary sclerosing cholangitis.

Adapted from Pugh RNH, Murray-Lyon IM, Dawson JL, et al. Transection of the esophagus for bleeding esophageal varices. *Br J Surg* 1973;60:649–654.

have shown that patients with alcoholic cirrhosis benefit from a daily diet containing 1.5 g protein per kg ideal body weight.[21]

Chronic hepatitis C infection is present in many patients with presumed alcoholic liver disease and may exacerbate the injury process.[22,23] Similarly, markers for chronic hepatitis B infection should be sought in any putative alcoholic individual presenting for liver transplantation. Primary hepatocellular carcinoma (hepatoma) may complicate alcoholic cirrhosis. This risk is greatest in alcoholic men with chronic viral hepatitis.[24] All alcoholic patients undergoing evaluation should receive an imaging study (sonogram, CT, or MR) and measurement of serum α-fetoprotein. The role of liver transplantation in patients with hepatoma is considered elsewhere. Tuberculosis is a risk for any alcoholic patient, and all candidates being evaluated for liver transplantation should have skin testing for reactivity to purified protein derivative (PPD).[25]

PSYCHOLOGICAL ASSESSMENT OF THE ALCOHOLIC CANDIDATE

Everhart and Beresford studied the use of assessment of psychological stability and the potential for sobriety. They received mailed questionnaires from 69 programs in the United States, representing 90% of the programs performing more than five adult liver transplantations in 1995.[26] Their data, presented as percentage of centers with positive replies, showed that 93% of centers thought that psychiatric evaluation was very important in making the diagnosis of alcoholic liver disease in liver transplant candidates. In 83% of the centers, a psychiatrist or other expert in addiction medicine routinely sees each case of alcoholic liver disease, and in 74% of centers this expert actively participates in the decision to list the patient for transplantation. Social or family support, duration of abstinence, a history of other substance abuse, and a history of other psychiatric disorders were most frequently considered very important in making a decision to offer or withhold listing a patient with alcoholic liver disease. In contrast, less than half of the programs cited willingness to sign a rehabilitation contract as very important. These data indicate that assessment by an addiction specialist has become an integral part of transplantation evaluation for alcoholic patients in the United States.

The attitudes of transplant psychiatrists or psychologists toward alcoholic candidates for liver transplantation were surveyed in 1992 in 14 U.S. liver transplant programs. Each respondent was asked to react to five brief clinical scenarios.[27] There was little consensus, except that respondents preferred to advocate that patients with continuing alcohol use receive addiction therapy rather than be refused transplantation outright. This suggests that psychiatrists working in liver transplant evaluation programs are reluctant to make absolute judgments that have irrevocable negative consequences.

The Michigan Alcoholism Prediction Score (MAPS), devised by Beresford from longitudinal studies of alcoholic individuals, is an instrument to assist in the prediction of sobriety after transplantation.[10] It emphasizes insight into alcoholism, family support, and social stability as predictors of maintaining durable abstinence, and has been influential in establishing these factors in the psychological assessment of the alcoholic candidate. Unfortunately, the accuracy of the actual score as a predictor of future behavior is limited. As a result of selection practices among referring physicians, and perhaps also because of barriers to primary care for alcoholic individuals, the great majority of alcoholic candidates who were evaluated by Beresford had high (i.e., good) prognostic scores.[28] When pretransplantation MAPS scores were reviewed against subsequent drinking behavior up to 5 years after liver transplantation, there was no difference between drinkers and abstainers.[29]

The most widely discussed issue regarding the prediction of future abstinence in liver transplant candidates is the so-called 6-month abstinence rule, which states that an alcoholic patient should be abstinent for 6 months before receiving a liver transplant. As shown in Table 19.3, few of the published series have applied the 6-month rule. There is little evidence in the general literature on alcoholism to support the rule's utility as a predictor of future abstinence. This topic is reviewed by Vaillant, who pointed out that in many treatment studies and in longitudinal natural history cohorts, a majority of patients who continue to abuse alcohol achieve 6 months of abstinence at some time in their drinking career.[30]

The data from liver transplant studies regarding the value of 6 months' abstinence are mixed and controversial, although some authors have concluded that the 6-month rule is a useful guide to sobriety. For example, Osorio et al. found that patients with less than 6 months' abstinence were more likely to relapse.[31] However, their study is one of the few that used 6 months' abstinence as a requirement for transplantation, and the identification of patients who had less than 6 months' abstinence was made after the transplantation, when patients were reinterviewed. These data highlight the problem of misleading drinking histories rather than confirm the value of the rule itself.

A fundamental caveat relates to the discriminant power of the 6-month rule to distinguish future drinkers from nondrinkers. Most proponents of the rule have concentrated on documented relapse after transplantation. Even here the data are confusing, with as many studies showing no relation to future drinking as those showing an apparent association. Fewer authors have considered the possibility that application of a strict 6-months' abstinence criterion might unfairly penalize some patients who are prevented from receiving a transplant on its account. Yates and co-workers have shown in a mathematical model that strict application of the 6-month rule would exclude from transplantation

TABLE 19.3. *Alcoholic relapse data in 17 published studies*

Location	Ref.	Year	Patients	Lost to follow-up	Abstinence criteria	Follow-up (mo)	Relapse (%)	Methods
Pittsburgh	43	1990	52	21	No	NS	12	Telephone interview
Kings, London	44	1990	18	6	No	4 mo–7 yrs	17	Retrospective chart review
Madison	45	1992	32	9	No	NS	13	Psychiatric interview
Cal/Pacific	46	1995	29	0	No	24	21	Prospective follow-up
UCSF	32	1996	43	0	6 mo	21	19	Mail survey
Vienna	47	1994	44	38	No	78	32	Retrospective chart review
Michigan	21	1997	50	9	No	63	34	Combination survey, review
Kings, London	48	1994	20	20	NS	34	95	Psychiatric interview
Dallas	49	1996	41	26	No	NS	49	Telephone interview
Baltimore	50	1996	29	13	No	NS	7	Retrospective chart review
Italy	51	1997	18		6 mo	NS	27	Retrospective chart review
Spain	52	1998	44	NS	NS	39.5	18	Urinary ethanol
Pittsburgh	53	1996	58	45	No	NS	21	Retrospective chart review
Chicago	54	1997	63	21	No	49	22	Combination survey, review
Birmingham, UK	38	1998	56	14	No	NS	50	Patient interview
Birmingham, UK	55	1997	39	NS	No	25	13	Retrospective chart review
Colorado	41	1997	42	26	No	NS	17	Telephone interview

NS, not stated; UCSF, University of California at San Francisco.

many alcoholic patients who are in need of transplantation but who are at no greater risk of relapse.[32]

Finally, the psychological evaluation includes an educational component to allow the patient to make well-informed decisions about sobriety, liver transplantation, and the management of alcoholism.

SELECTION FOR LIVER TRANSPLANTATION

The process of selection for liver transplantation requires the patient to negotiate many steps even before reaching the transplant center. These include obtaining access to medical care, overcoming limitations from financial or insurance provisions, and overcoming the biases about referral to tertiary care centers among primary care providers. There are few data to indicate how these influences affect alcoholic patients with significant liver disease in the United States.

It is evident in Great Britain that alcoholic patients may be discriminated against prior to referral to liver transplant centers.[33] In addition, Neuberger and his colleagues have recently reported the results of a survey of the general public, family physicians, and gastroenterologists.[6] The respondents were asked to allocate four donor livers among eight hypothetical recipients, who epitomized the difficult choices involved. Although there was disagreement among the three groups of respondents regarding the relative importance of some recipient characteristics, such as age and the likelihood of success of the transplant, all three groups gave low priority to the alcoholic candidate. These data suggest that there is continuing ambivalence (at least in Great Britain) regarding the medical model of alcoholism. Whether such ambivalence about performing transplanta-

tions in alcoholic patients is common in the United States remains uncertain.

MORBIDITY AFTER LIVER TRANSPLANTATION FOR ALCOHOLIC LIVER DISEASE

There are only subtle differences in patient survival, graft survival, adherence to medication regimens, or other measures of health between alcoholic recipients and the remainder of liver transplant recipients. On the other hand, there are many striking anecdotes involving alcoholic liver recipients regarding alcohol use, poor compliance with medical care, graft injury, and patient death.

Wiesner and co-workers demonstrated in their analysis of the NIH liver transplant database that alcoholic patients did not spend more time in the hospital either in the initial transplant admission or in the first year posttransplantation compared with nonalcoholic recipients.[9] These data confirm earlier reports that alcoholic patients do not consume a disproportionate amount of resources when undergoing liver transplantation, nor do alcoholic patients demonstrate greater early morbidity.[34]

Alcoholic recipients do not appear to miss medication doses more frequently than nonalcoholic recipients.[9,35] Indeed, an unexpected observation by a number of transplant groups is that alcoholic liver transplant recipients experience less frequent episodes of acute cellular rejection than patients who undergo transplantation for other reasons.[9,36,37] These data may reflect a state of partially suppressed cellular immunity in alcoholic patients with end-stage liver failure. It is unlikely that this is a direct effect of alcohol on the cellular immune system, since most of the recipients in these three studies were abstinent for 6 months or more at the time of transplantation. Whether alcoholic patients who relapse into abusive drinking are more prone to miss doses of immunosuppressants than abstinent recipients is not known, although individuals for whom this appears to have been the case have been described.[29,38] Both our group and that in Birmingham have noted that the alcoholic recipients relapsing into significant alcohol use after liver transplantation appear to have an increased frequency of nonhepatic problems, such as pancreatitis and pneumonia, in addition to acute intoxication, that may require admission to hospital.[29,30]

The psychological health of alcoholic recipients after liver transplantation has been studied in a number of ways. Beresford et al. compared the psychological health of 22 alcoholic liver transplant recipients with that of 39 nonalcoholic recipients in a telephone survey conducted at least 6 months after transplantation and found no differences in frequency of return to work, incidence of depression, or episodes of missed medications.[35] Wiesner et al. used a prospectively gathered quality-of-life questionnaire to assess patient perception of well-being before and after transplantation.[9] Their data show that four measures of well-being (general health perception, well-being, affect, and stress) all improve substantially 1 year after liver transplantation compared with pretransplantation assessments in both alcoholic and nonalcoholic recipients alike. After transplantation, there are small but significant differences between the two groups for each of the scores, with worse scores being recorded for alcoholic recipients. These differences in psychological health between nonalcoholic and alcoholic recipients appeared to increase by years 2 and 3 posttransplantation.

Ability to return to work is a more concrete measure of psychological health. In Wiesner's study, a significantly greater proportion of alcoholic patients were out of work prior to their transplant procedure compared with nonalcoholic patients (80% versus 63%).[9] However, these differences had become insignificant by 1 year after transplantation (42% versus 38%). Adams et al. found that frequency of return to work was comparable in alcoholic and nonalcoholic recipients, and that the duration of pretransplantation lack of employment was the most important predictor of the likelihood of returning to work.[39]

Alcoholic relapse is the aspect of psychological health after liver transplantation that has received the most attention. The NIH-sponsored workshop on liver transplantation in alcoholic liver disease revealed a clash of cultures between addiction specialists and liver transplant specialists that encompassed goals of therapy and definitions of success or failure. This culture clash is well illustrated by the notion of a "slip" versus "recidivism." The perspective of the addiction or liaison psychiatrist distinguishes between alcohol use of an occasional and minor degree (a slip), and addictive or harmful drinking. This view is illustrated by Fuller, who stated that "although a slip is an unwelcome event, if it occurs and does not progress to a relapse it is unlikely to cause harm and should not be treated punitively.

A slip often provides an opportunity for the patient to reexamine his or her life and renew the commitment to abstinence."[40] Fuller argues that the term "recidivism" should be avoided because of its implications of culpability.[40]

In contrast, most descriptions of transplantation in alcoholic patients are written by liver transplant physicians and surgeons, who define any use of alcohol by the transplant recipient as an alcoholic failure, often termed "recidivism." Such behavior is judged to warrant severe consequences, often including withholding retransplantation where it might otherwise be deemed medically necessary. The low retransplantation rates for alcoholic patients recorded by Wiesner support this conclusion.[9] Further adding to the uncertainty about alcohol relapse after transplantation is the inherent conflict of interest about the accuracy of data documenting alcohol use when the provider of the information (the patient) has many reasons to conceal his or her drinking.

Many studies of posttransplantation alcohol use have now been published, and are summarized in Table 19.3. Relapse is defined as *any* alcohol use in every study. Most published studies are retrospective, relatively short term, and compromised by missing patients. All have the inherent problem of determining the accuracy of data about drinking. Few of the studies cover a period beyond the first 5 years posttransplantation. The 17 studies in Table 19.3 therefore probably underestimate actual drinking. Nevertheless, taken together these studies reveal some coherent messages. First, Starzl's initial observation that relapses were less common than might have been expected is holding up. Probably one-third to one-half of alcoholic recipients admit to or are discovered to have consumed some alcohol in the first 5 years. Viewed from the other way about, probably half of the patients maintain strict abstinence, which is remarkable given the natural history of alcoholism. Vaillant has written that "under conventional treatment for alcoholism, a 2 year relapse rate of 60% to 80% is common."[30] The prevalence of alcohol use increases as the interval after transplantation progresses through the first 5 years. It is not known whether it plateaus then or continues to rise.

Many of the episodes of alcohol use included in the relapse data referred to earlier are individual drinking events, after which the patient reestablishes abstinence (see reference 30 for a description of one such cohort). Sustained or abusive drinking is much less common, affecting about 10% or fewer alcoholic recipients. Both Everson et al.[41] and Tang et al.[38] suggest that the interval from transplantation to resumption of abusive drinking is short, often less than 1 year. Since this is the period during which the recipient is under greatest scrutiny by the transplant center, it is likely that these drinking episodes will come to attention. Individual patients have been described who have died after transplantation and whose death could be attributed in whole or in part to abusive drinking, sometimes linked with depression and refusal to take immunosuppressants, although this appears to be an exceptional event (such patients are included in references 3, 9, 10, and 29, among others). Furthermore, as mentioned previously, relapse to alcohol use may lead to significant morbidity, including pneumonia, pancreatitis, and acute alcoholic hepatitis, that may require admission to the hospital.[28,39]

ALCOHOLISM TREATMENT AFTER LIVER TRANSPLANTATION

There are no published studies of the application of a formal treatment program for alcoholism after liver transplantation. Weinrieb has undertaken a randomized pilot study, sponsored by the National Institute on Alcohol Abuse and Alcoholism, in which three treatment programs are evaluated: a combination of pharmacotherapy with naltrexone and motivational enhancement therapy (MET), placebo plus MET, or standard posttransplantation therapy in 60 patients surviving the immediate postoperative period.[42] The main observation from the study so far is that specific impediments are encountered when trying to conduct a study such as this in the complex setting of care after liver transplantation. To date, the majority of potential candidates for the study have declined to enter. Three reasons are given: fear of hepatotoxicity due to naltrexone, lack of interest because the patient's current management regimen is so taxing, and finally the perception that alcoholism is no longer a problem.

These observations indicate that future treatment studies should be tailored to address the factors that foster relapse in alcoholic liver transplant recipients. Because we understand only poorly what leads an alcoholic person to resume drinking, this is a challenge. Future studies must also be compatible with the health concerns of the posttransplantation patient and recognize the already complex demands placed on such patients.

REFERENCES

1. Scharschmidt BF. Human liver transplantation: an analysis of 540 patients from 4 centers. *Hepatology* 1984;4:95S–111S.
2. National Institutes of Health consensus development conference statement: liver transplantation. *Hepatology* 1984;4:107S–110S.
3. Starzl TE, Van Thiel D, Tzakis AG, et al. Orthotopic liver transplantation for alcoholic cirrhosis. *JAMA* 1988;260:2542–2544.
4. The U.S. Scientific Registry for Transplant Recipients and the Organ Procurement and Transplantation Network—transplant data. Richmond, VA: UNOS; Rockville, MD: Division of Transplantation, Office of Special Programs, Health Resources and Services Administration, U.S. Department of Health and Human Services.
5. Lucey MR, Weinrieb R. Liver transplantation and alcoholics: is the glass half full or half empty? *Gut* 1999 *(in press)*.
6. Neuberger J, Adams D, MacMaster P, et al. Assessing priorities for allocation of donor liver grafts: survey of public and clinicians. *Br Med J* 1998;317:172–175.
7. Hoofnagle JH, Kresina T, Fuller RK, et al. Liver transplantation for alcoholic liver disease: executive statement and recommendations. *Liver Transplant Surg* 1997;3:347–350.
8. Belle SH, Beringer KC, Detre KM. Liver transplantation for alcoholic liver disease in the United States: 1988 to 1995. *Liver Transplant Surg* 1997;3:212–219.
9. Wiesner RH, Lombardero M, Lake JR, et al. Liver transplantation for end-stage alcoholic liver disease: an assessment of outcomes. *Liver Transplant Surg* 1997;3:231–239.
10. Lucey MR, Merion RM, Henley KS, et al. Selection for and outcome of liver transplantation in alcoholic liver disease. *Gastroenterology* 1992;102:1736–1741.
11. Poynard T, Barthelemy P, Fratte S, et al. Evaluation of efficacy of liver transplantation in alcoholic cirrhosis by a case control study and simulated controls. *Lancet* 1994;344:502–507.
12. Lucey MR, Beresford TP. Ethical considerations regarding orthotopic liver transplantation for alcoholic patients. In: Shelton WN, Edwards RB, eds. *Values, ethics and alcoholism.* (*Advances in bioethics.*) Greenwich, CT: JAI Press, 1998.
13. Krom RAF. Liver transplantation and alcohol: who should get transplants? *Hepatology* 1994;20:28S–32S.
14. Lucey MR, Brown KA, Everson GT, et al. Minimal criteria for placement of adults on the liver transplant waiting list: a report of a national conference organized by the American Society of Transplant Physicians and the American Association for the Study of Liver Diseases. Conference proceedings. *Liver Transplant Surg* 1997;3:628–637.
15. Lucey MR. Medical assessment of alcoholic candidates for liver transplantation. In: Lucey MR, Merion RM, Beresford TP. *Liver transplantation and the alcoholic patient.* Cambridge, UK: Cambridge University Press, 1994:50–79.
16. Carithers RL, Herlong HR, Diehl AM, et al. Methylprednisolone therapy in patients with severe alcoholic hepatitis. *Ann Intern Med* 1989;110:685–690.
17. Mutimer DJ, Burra P, Neuberger JM, et al. Managing severe alcoholic hepatitis complicated by renal failure. *Q J Med* 1993;86:649–656.
18. Schiodt FV, Rochling FA, Casey DL, et al. Acetaminophen toxicity in an urban county hospital. *N Engl J Med* 1997;337:1485–1492.
19. Pugh RNH, Murray-lyon IM, Dawson JL, et al. Transection of the esophagus for bleeding esophageal varices. *Br J Surg* 1973;60:649–654.
20. Donovan CL, Marcovitz PA, Punch JD, et al. Two-dimensional and dobutamine stress echocardiography in the preoperative assessment of patients with end stage liver disease prior to orthotopic liver transplantation. *Transplantation* 1996;61:1180–1188.
21. Kearns PJ, Young H, Garcia G, et al. Accelerated improvement of alcoholic liver disease with enteral nutrition. *Gastroenterology* 1992;102:200–205.
22. Corrao G, Arico S. Independent and combined action of hepatitis C virus infection and alcohol consumption on the risk of symptomatic liver cirrhosis. *Hepatology* 1998;27:914–949.
23. Ostapowicz G, Watson KJR, Locarnini SA, et al. Role of alcohol in the progression of liver disease caused by hepatitis C virus infection. *Hepatology* 1998;27:1730–1735.
24. Schafer DF, Sorrell MF. Hepatocellular carcinoma. *Lancet* 1999;353:1253–1257.
25. Friedman LN, Sullivan GM, Bevilaqua RP, et al. Tuberculosis screening in alcoholics and drug addicts. *Am Rev Resp Dis* 1987;136:1188–1192.
26. Everhart JE, Beresford TP. Liver transplantation for alcoholic liver disease: a survey of transplantation programs in the United States. *Liver Transplant Surg* 1997;3:220–226.
27. Snyder SL, Drooker M, Strain JJ. A survey estimate of academic liver transplant teams' selection practices for alcohol-dependent applicants. *Psychosomatics* 1996;37:432–437.
28. Beresford TP. Psychiatric assessment of alcoholic candidates for liver transplantation. In: Lucey MR, Merion RM, Beresford TP. *Liver transplantation and the alcoholic patient.* Cambridge, UK: Cambridge University Press, 1994:29–49.
29. Lucey MR, Carr K, Beresford TP, et al. Alcohol use after liver transplantation in alcoholics—a clinical-cohort follow-up study. *Hepatology* 1997;25:1223–1227.
30. Vaillant GE. The natural history of alcoholism and its relationship to liver transplantation. *Liver Transplant Surg* 1997;3:304–310.
31. Osorio RW, Ascher NL, Avery M, et al. Predicting recidivism after orthotopic liver transplantation for alcoholic liver disease. *Hepatology* 1996;20:105–110.
32. Yates WR, Martin M, LaBrecque D, et al. A model to examine the validity of the 6-month abstinence criterion for liver transplantation. *Alcohol Clin Exp Res* 1998;22:513–517.
33. Davies MH, Langman MJS, Elias E, et al. Liver disease in a district hospital remote from a transplant center: a study of admissions and death. *Gut* 1992;33:1397–1399.
34. McCurry KR, Baliga P, Merion RM, et al. Resource utilization and outcome of liver transplantation for alcoholic cirrhosis: a case-control study. *Arch Surg* 1992;127:772–777.

35. Beresford TP, Schwartz J, Wilson D, et al. The short-term psychological health of alcoholic and non-alcoholic liver transplant recipients. *Alcohol Clin Exp Res* 1992;16:996–1000.

36. Berlakovich GA, Rockenschaub S, Taucher S, et al. Underlying disease as a predictor for rejection after liver transplantation. *Arch Surg* 1998;133:167–172.

37. Farges O, Saliba F, Farhamant H, et al. Incidence of rejection and infection after liver transplantation as a function of the primary disease: possible influence of alcohol and polyclonal immunoglobulins. *Hepatology* 1996;23:240–248.

38. Tang H, Boulton R, Gunson B, et al. Patterns of alcohol consumption after liver transplantation. *Gut* 1998;43:140–145.

39. Adams P, Ghent C, Grant D, et al. Employment after liver transplantation. *Hepatology* 1995;21:140–144.

40. Fuller RK. Definition and diagnosis of relapse to drinking. *Liver Transplant Surg* 1997;3:258–262.

41. Everson G, Bharadhwaj G, House R, et al. Long-term follow-up of patients with alcoholic liver disease who underwent hepatic transplantation. *Liver Transplant Surg* 1997;3:263–274.

42. Weinrieb RM, O'Brien CP. Current research in the treatment of alcoholism in liver transplant recipients. *Liver Transplant Surg* 1997;3:328–336.

43. Kumar S, Stauber RE, Gavaler JS, et. al. Orthotopic liver transplantation for alcoholic liver disease. *Hepatology* 1990;11:159–164.

44. Bird DLA, O'Grady JG, Harvey FAH, et al. Liver transplantation in patients with alcoholic cirrhosis: selection criteria and rates of survival and relapse. *Br Med J* 1990;301:15–17.

45. Knechtle SJ, Fleming MF, Barry KL, et al. Liver transplantation for alcoholic liver disease. *Surgery* 1992;112:694–703.

46. Gish RG, Lee AH, Keeffe EB, et al. Liver transplantation for patients with alcoholism and end-stage liver disease. *Am J Gastroenterol* 1993; 88:1337–1342.

47. Berlakovich GA, Steininger R, Herbst F, et al. Efficacy of liver transplantation for alcoholic cirrhosis with respect to recidivism and compliance. *Transplantation* 1994;58:560–565.

48. Howard LM, Fahy T, Wong P, et al Psychiatric outcome in alcoholic liver transplant patients. *Q J Med* 1994;87:731–773.

49. Gerhardt TC, Goldstein RM, Urschel HC, et al. Alcohol use following liver transplantation for alcoholic cirrhosis. *Transplantation* 1996;62: 1060–1063.

50. Zibari GB, Edwin D, Wall L, et al. Liver transplantation for alcoholic liver disease. *Clin Transplant* 1996;10:676–679.

51. Stefanini GF, Biselli M, Grazi GL, et al. Orthotopic liver transplantation for alcoholic liver disease: rates of survival, complications and relapse. *Hepatogastroenterology* 1997;44:1356–1360.

52. Fabrega E, Crespo J, Casafont F, et al. Alcoholic recidivism after liver transplantation for alcoholic cirrhosis. *J Clin Gastroenterol* 1998;26: 204–206.

53. Tringali RA, Trzepacz PT, DiMartini A, et al. Assessment and follow-up of alcohol-dependent liver transplantation patients. A clinical cohort. *Gen Hosp Psychiatry* 1996;18:70S–77S.

54. Foster PF, Fabrega F, Karademir S, et al. Prediction of abstinence from ethanol in alcoholic recipients following liver transplantation. *Hepatology* 1997;25:1469–1477.

55. Anand AC, Ferraz-Neto B, Nightengale P, et al. Liver transplantation for alcoholic liver disease: evaluation of a selection protocol. *Hepatology* 1997;25:1478–1484.

Transplantation of the Liver, edited by Willis C. Maddrey, Eugene R. Schiff, and Michael F. Sorrell. Lippincott Williams & Wilkins, Philadelphia © 2001.

CHAPTER 20

Liver Transplantation in Patients with Chronic Hepatitis B and C

Hugo R. Rosen and Paul Martin

LIVER TRANSPLANTATION AND HEPATITIS B INFECTION

By the late 1980s orthotopic liver transplantation (OLT) for patients infected with the hepatitis B virus (HBV) had been identified as having important limitations regarding graft and patient outcomes because of reinfection of the allograft by HBV following otherwise technically successful transplantation.[1] As a result, enthusiasm for offering OLT to HBV-infected patients waned, and the percentage of transplantations performed in the United States for this indication declined through the early 1990s.[2,3] However, a number of important clinical observations, most notably the recognition of the prognostic significance of active HBV replication pretransplantation, and advances such as the protective effect of high-dose hepatitis B immune globulin (HBIG) helped in the development of strategies to help prevent graft reinfection by HBV.[4] More recently, the introduction of nucleoside analogues with efficacy against HBV has further diminished the burden of recurrent hepatitis posttransplantation.[5]

Important issues that remain to be resolved include the prevention of mutant forms of HBV, which have been recognized with monotherapy with either nucleoside analogues[6] or HBIG,[7,8] as well as how to provide adequate protection against recurrent HBV without the prohibitively high cost of high-dose HBIG. Despite these concerns, the management of HBV in the OLT candidate has improved substantially in the last decade; it is now possible to anticipate an excellent outcome with a low likelihood of serious graft reinfection for the OLT candidate with HBV. Although universal vaccination against HBV will ultimately reduce the burden of HBV-related cirrhosis and hepatocellular carcinoma (HCC), as has already been achieved in Taiwan,[9] it will be at least several more decades before HBV disappears as an important indication for OLT given that 300 million individuals worldwide are already chronically infected.

Course and Mechanisms of Recurrent Hepatitis B

Prior to the introduction of effective immunoprophylaxis, a series of papers described the course of graft infection by HBV[1,10,11] (Fig. 20.1). Serial graft biopsies identified the progression of recurrent HBV from initial acute hepatitis to chronic hepatitis and frequently to cirrhosis, although some patients did have more indolent recurrent HBV. The initial postoperative course is clinically indistinguishable from that of patients who undergo transplantation for other indications.[1] Hepatitis B surface antigen (HBsAg) may or may not disappear from serum in the first few weeks, but within 2 to 5 weeks after OLT, immunoperoxidase staining on liver biopsy can identify cytoplasmic expression of hepatitis B core antigen (HBcAg), typically without histologic features of hepatitis.[1] In the subsequent several weeks, biochemical evidence of graft dysfunction is accompanied by biopsy features of acute viral hepatitis, although the inflammatory response may be somewhat attenuated, presumably because of immunosuppression. Within several months of OLT, features of chronic hepatitis emerge, with accelerated progression to cirrhosis and graft failure within an average of 2.5 years postoperatively. However, the tempo of graft injury can be even more rapid, with graft cirrhosis developing within 1 year of OLT.

A particular form of HBV recurrence, fibrosing cholestatic hepatitis (FCH), is associated with profound hepatic dysfunction and rapid graft failure.[12] The biopsy features

H. R. Rosen: Department of Medicine, Molecular Microbiology, and Immunology; Director, Research Development; Division of Gastroenterology/Hepatology, Medical Director, Liver Transplantation Program; Portland Veterans Administration Medical Center and Oregon Health Sciences University, Portland, Oregon 97207.

P. Martin: Department of Medicine, Dumont-UCLA Transplant Program, Center for Health Sciences, University of California at Los Angeles, Los Angeles, California 90095.

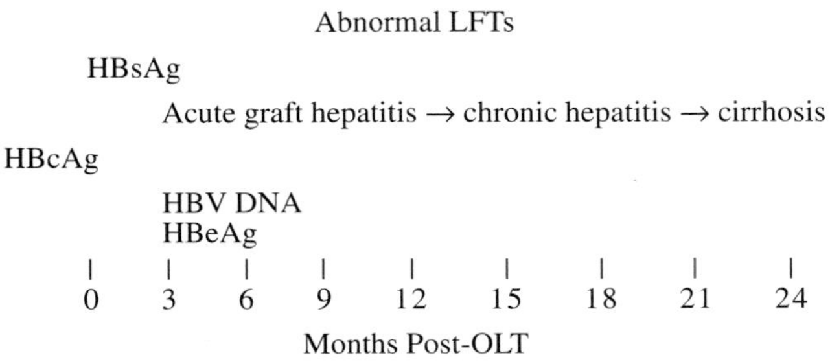

Abnormal LFTs

HBsAg

Acute graft hepatitis → chronic hepatitis → cirrhosis

HBcAg

HBV DNA
HBeAg

```
  |     |     |     |     |     |     |     |     |
  0     3     6     9    12    15    18    21    24
```
Months Post-OLT

FIG. 20.1. Course of recurrent hepatitis B virus infection after orthotopic liver transplantation. HBsAg, hepatitis B surface antigen (serum); HBcAg, hepatitis B core antigen (hepatocyte); HBeAg, hepatitis B e antigen (serum); HBV DNA, hepatitis B viral DNA (serum); LFTs, liver function tests; OLT, orthotopic liver transplantation.

of FCH are notable for relatively little inflammation, with periportal fibrosis and ballooning of pericentral hepatocytes, in addition to cholestasis and fibrosis.[13] Immunohistochemical studies have shown abundant expression of HBsAg and HBcAg, which, in conjunction with the modest degree of inflammation, has led to the hypothesis that this form of graft injury is due to a direct cytopathic effect of HBV. Experimental proof for this hypothesis is provided by a transgenic mouse model of excessive surface antigen production and accumulation in the hepatocytes in which liver injury similar to FCH occurs,[14] as well as by the demonstration in patients with FCH of increased transcription of HBV.[15] HBV recurrence can also rapidly progress to acute hepatocellular failure,[2] reminiscent of fulminant hepatic failure.

Rapid graft reinfection despite the removal of the major source of HBV replication (i.e., the infected native liver) reflects the presence of viable virions in extrahepatic reservoirs and bone marrow[16] (Table 20.1). Colonization of the graft leads to the establishment of replicating hepatic HBV. The more aggressive course of post-OLT HBV infection probably results from a number of factors, including enhanced viral replication and attenuated host response. In the absence of some form of antiviral prophylaxis, there is a logarithmic increase in serum HBV DNA levels as well as appearance of hepatitis B e antigen (HBeAg) even if this antigen was absent pretransplantation.[17]

Therapeutic immunosuppression is implicated in the enhanced viral replication by a series of observations. For example, the HBV genome contains a steroid-sensitive receptor with *in vitro* data from a hepatoma cell line of increased HBV DNA production upon exposure to steroids or azathioprine.[18] In the woodchuck model of HBV, protracted treatment with cyclosporine in acute infection increased viral replication, as reflected in increased serum DNA levels and hepatocyte core antigen expression.[19] In an *in vitro* study in hepatocytes from patients with chronic HBV, acute tacrolimus (FK506) administration did not increase HBV replication, in contrast to

TABLE 20.1. *Mechanism of recurrence of hepatitis B infection after orthotopic liver transplantation*

Extrahepatic reservoirs
Permissive effect of immunosuppressive agents
Glucocorticoid-responsive receptor on HBV genome

HBV, hepatitis B virus.

methylprednisolone in the same system.[20] However, it is conceivable that longer tacrolimus administration might affect HBV replication in a manner analogous to cyclosporine in acute infection.[2]

Immunopathogenesis

Immunologic mechanisms have also been invoked to explain the aggressive course of HBV recurrence post-OLT. In the immunocompetent (non-OLT) patient, elimination of HBV-infected hepatocytes is mediated by cytotoxic CD8+ cells that recognize HBV determinants processed by the host's cells expressed in association with HLA class I antigens on the hepatocyte surface.[21] Therefore, in acute HBV infection, a cytolytic response can aid in resolution of viral infection at the cost of liver cell injury.

Typically, OLT recipients are not HLA class I matched, suggesting that the mechanisms of hepatocyte injury are likely to be independent of classic HLA restriction, although one report did suggest that when HLA class I matching occurred, recurrent hepatitis was more clinically severe.[22] HLA class II molecules also present viral peptides to CD4+ cells at the hepatocyte surface, and recipient CD4+ cells that repopulate the graft are HLA mismatched with the donor (target) organ.[23] An alternative mechanism involves activation of T lymphocytes leading to cytokine release [e.g., tumor necrosis factor α (TNF-α)] and cell injury.[2,23]

Natural History

The burden of recurrent HBV is graphically illustrated in a report from the University of Pittsburgh from the early 1990s, before the introduction of effective immunoprophylaxis.[1] HBV recurrence was observed in over 80% of patients surviving more than 2 months post-OLT and was implicated in 73% of all post-OLT deaths beyond the first 60 days. A more recent retrospective multicenter U.S. experience has again highlighted the poorer outcome for HBV-infected patients in the absence of adequate prophylaxis when compared with patients who undergo transplantation for causes other than viral hepatitis.[11] The 1- and 5-year survival rates were significantly diminished (72% and 51%, respectively) for patients receiving transplantations for HBV compared with the control group (84% and 74%, respectively). The difference in survival rates was predominantly related to HBV recurrence.

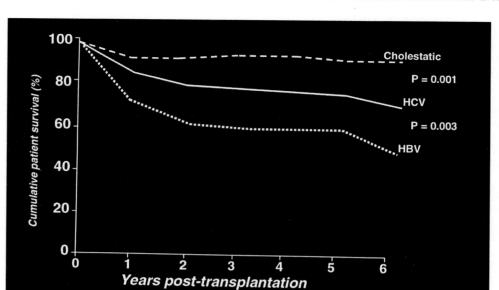

FIG. 20.2. Poor survival for patients with hepatitis B virus infection after orthotopic liver transplantation. Data are from the National Institute of Diabetes and Digestive and Kidney Diseases liver transplant database, 1990–1994. (From Charlton M, Seaberg E, Wiesner R, et al. Predictors of patient and graft survival following liver transplantation for hepatitis C. *Hepatology* 1998;28:823–830, with permission.)

Charlton and colleagues[24] have also provided recent information from the prospectively collected National Institute of Diabetes and Digestive and Kidney Diseases (NIDDK) liver transplantation database on the outcome of patients undergoing transplantation in the United States from the three major participating programs between 1990 and 1994. Although the focus of this paper was hepatitis C virus (HCV) recurrence following OLT, patients who underwent transplantation for HBV had a significantly poor survival compared with the HCV-infected group ($P = 0.003$). The survival rate for the HCV-infected patients was in turn poorer ($P = 0.001$) than the benchmark cholestatic cirrhosis group (Fig. 20.2).

Predictors of Hepatitis B Virus Recurrence

The importance of HBV replicative status pre-OLT as a predictor of HBV recurrence was demonstrated in a large multicenter European study of over 300 patients.[4] The highest risk of recurrence, 83% actuarial rate at 3 years, was observed in recipients who had HBeAg in serum and HBV DNA detectable by molecular hybridization pre-OLT. The lowest HBV recurrence rate (16%) occurred in patients who underwent transplantation for fulminant HBV, in which spontaneous clearance of HBV is frequent, although severe liver injury may have already resulted. Patients with chronic HBV without markers of active replication had an intermediate rate of HBV recurrence (58%). Coinfection with hepatitis D virus (HDV) resulted in a lower rate of HBV recurrence (32%). By multivariate analysis, HDV coinfection and acute rather than chronic HBV infection were significant predictors of nonrecurrence, as was administration of high-dose HBIG for more than 6 months post-OLT. A high level of HBV replication pre-OLT reflects a larger circulating population of virus in the bloodstream that has the potential to rapidly recolonize the allograft, with accentuation of replication caused by the immunosuppressive regimen.

Asian race with presumed infancy or childhood acquisition of HBV was initially reported as a predictor of a poor outcome due to aggressive recurrence of HBV post-OLT,[25] although a more recent experience suggested that this apparent association may be due to more advanced liver disease at the time of OLT rather than any unique effect of race.[26] A recent update has indicated no adverse effect on HBV recurrence due to race[27] (Table 20.2).

A subset of patients with a particularly poor outlook has been those patients who undergo retransplantation following initial graft failure due to HBV recurrence.[28] The FCH pattern of recurrence showed an even more accelerated course of recurrence in the second graft. However, this observation is now probably moot because of the advent of effective prophylactic strategies to prevent HBV recurrence; a recent multicenter experience reported survival of 6 (86%) of 7 patients following retransplantation using high-dose HBIG.[29] Similarly good results have also been reported from Europe with the use of a variety of antiviral agents in combination with HBIG[30] (see Chapter 21).

Precore mutant forms of HBV that fail to secrete HBeAg have been implicated in severe liver disease in nontransplantation patients,[31] and some reports have also implicated

TABLE 20.2. *Predicting hepatitis B infection recurrence after orthotopic liver transplantation*

Positive predictors
High replication (HBeAg, HBV DNA)
Absence of viral coinfection (HCV, HDV)
OLT for cirrhosis
Negative predictors
Administration of high-dose HBIG
Lamivudine therapy
OLT for fulminant hepatic failure
Unproven predictors
Ethnicity
Concomitant hepatocellular carcinoma

HBeAg, hepatitis B e antigen; HBV DNA, hepatitis B viral DNA; HCV, hepatitis C virus; HDV, hepatitis D virus; OLT, orthotopic liver transplantation; HBIG, hepatitis B immune globulin.

analogous mutations in severe recurrent HBV post-OLT.[32] Again, in the era of effective prophylaxis against HBV recurrence, the presence of a precore mutant does not per se increase the likelihood of reinfection or graft failure, whereas pre-OLT viral load does, according to Naumann and colleagues, who studied a large cohort of HBV patients who received high-dose HBIG post-OLT and many of whom had this mutant.[33]

Hepatitis B Recurrence and Coinfection with Other Hepatotropic Viruses

Coinfection with other hepatotropic viruses attenuates HBV recurrence post-OLT. This has been best characterized with HDV coinfection,[34] but there is also evidence that hepatitis C virus coinfection may similarly reduce the impact of HBV recurrence.[35] Because all three viruses are parenterally spread, coinfection is not infrequent in OLT candidates, although HDV has a lower background prevalence in North America than in Western Europe both in the transplant and nontransplant setting. Thus, in a recent multicenter U.S. study, HDV coinfection was identified in only 6.2% of HBV-infected OLT candidates[36] compared with an earlier European experience reported by Samuel et al. in which one-third of HBV-positive recipients had HDV coinfection that reduced the risk of HBV recurrence.[4]

HDV coinfection typically results in interference with HBV replication, which in turn diminishes the risk of HBV recurrence post-OLT. Even if HBV does recur, HDV coinfection is associated with a more indolent course of infection than is typically observed in its absence.[4] In a more recent report of long-term HBIG prophylaxis in HDV-coinfected OLT recipients, Samuel and co-workers not only observed a low overall rate of HBV recurrence of 10.3% but also an absence of cirrhosis in patients with HBV recurrence in a follow-up extending over a mean of 3 years, implying that HDV offered some protection even in the face of HBV recurrence.[37]

Some observations had suggested that HDV could recur in the graft in the absence of HBV. In one study, HDV antigen was present in hepatocytes, and HDV RNA reappeared in serum without detection of routine HBV markers of reinfection such as serum HBV DNA or HBV core antigen in hepatocytes.[34] A recent study has revisited this issue and has detected evidence of HBV replication, albeit low grade, by molecular techniques.[38] The difficulty of detecting HBV replication in these circumstances may be due in part to the administration of HBIG. If HBV surface antigen does not reappear, isolated HDV markers are not durable, reflecting the inability of HDV to persist without established HBV reinfection.

A complex relationship also exists between HBV and HCV in the transplant and nontransplant setting. Coinfection has been implicated in more severe clinical liver disease in the latter situation, although a suppressive effect of HCV on HBV replication has also been demonstrated.[39] A report from Huang and colleagues from San Francisco described improved survival in OLT recipients with recurrent HBV who had HCV coinfection compared with those with HBV infection alone.[35] A more recent European report suggests that coinfected patients given HBIG before anti-HCV screening was available had a greater reduction in HCV recurrence than those who underwent transplantation after anti-HCV–positive lots were no longer used, implying that the passively acquired antibodies offered some protection against HCV recurrence.[40]

De Novo Hepatitis B Virus Infection Posttransplantation

Although most cases of HBV in OLT recipients are clearly related to recurrence of infection, a number of reports have implicated the allograft as a source of HBV infection. Donor markers typical of remote resolved HBV infection with IgG antibody to HBcAg (anti-HBc) seropositivity, with or without the presence of antibody to HBsAg (anti-HBs), have been convincingly associated with the subsequent development of graft dysfunction and the appearance of serum HBsAg positivity in the recipient following OLT from both cadaveric[41] and living-related donors.[42] The putative mechanism is amplification of minute amounts of viable virions in the graft by therapeutic immunosuppression following OLT.[43] This postulate is further supported by a recent report of a high prevalence of HBV DNA detectable by polymerase chain reaction (PCR) in patients with chronic HCV who had anti-HBc positivity but were negative for HBsAg.[44] The course of HBV acquired peritransplantation had initially appeared more indolent than that due to reinfection, although poor graft and patient outcomes can also be seen with HBV infection acquired in this manner.[45,46]

According to data from the NIDDK database, allografts from donors with anti-HBc seropositivity and absent HBsAg are highly likely to transmit HBV infection to HBV-naive recipients. Dickson and colleagues[41] reviewed the outcome of hepatitis B–naive transplant recipients at four American centers who had received allografts from donors seropositive for anti-HBc but not HBsAg. Eighteen (78%) of 23 such recipients developed HBV infection, in contrast to only 3 (0.5%) of 651 recipients of anti-HBc–negative grafts ($p < 0.0001$). Survival was also affected in recipients who had acquired HBV from the allograft; such patients had a diminished 4-year survival rate compared with patients who remained uninfected. In contrast, use of such donor grafts in OLT recipients with preexisting HBV infection who receive adequate prophylaxis against HBV recurrence does not appear to increase the risk of allograft infection by HBV (S. Han, personal communication, 2000). In addition, markers of prior resolved HBV infection, notably anti-HBc seropositivity with or without anti-HBs seropositivity in the recipient, may offer protection against graft HBV infection.[47]

Hepatitis B and Hepatocellular Carcinoma

Hepatocellular carcinoma (HCC) is a frequent complication of chronic HBV infection, especially if cirrhosis has developed. OLT is potentially curative in a subset of patients with HCC with a small tumor burden. The generally accepted criteria for a positive outcome are a tumor diameter less than 5 cm if the lesion is solitary or, if there are (less than 3) lesions, a tumor diameter less than 3 cm; and a negative metastatic workup.[48] However, the experience with OLT in the patient with both HCC and HBV infection had not been very encouraging until recently because of HBV recurrence rather than metastatic spread.[49] The confounding effects of adjuvant chemotherapy as well as absence of adequate immunoprophylaxis against HBV may have been important factors in the poor results.

More recently a large multicenter European experience has shown that only pre-OLT replicative activity and post-OLT immunoprophylaxis were significant predictors of HBV recurrence, and that HCC per se does not increase the likelihood of HBV recurrence.[50] Thus, the current assessment of the OLT candidate with HCC and HBV should focus initially on the likelihood of cure of the tumor by OLT using the criteria described previously and then on providing adequate prophylaxis against HBV recurrence.

CHRONIC HEPATITIS C INFECTION

Since its molecular characterization in 1989, hepatitis C virus has been implicated as the main cause of posttransfusion and sporadic non-A, non-B hepatitis.[51] An estimated 300 million people worldwide are infected with HCV, which has now replaced HBV infection as the leading cause of cirrhosis and hepatocellular carcinoma in the Western world.[52] Moreover, HCV is an important cofactor in the natural history of other primary liver diseases, including alcoholic liver disease,[53] acute hepatitis A,[54] and hepatitis B.[55] Not surprisingly, as of 1993, HCV had become the single leading indication for orthotopic liver transplantation worldwide, surpassing alcoholic liver disease. Moreover, human liver transplantation repre-

sents the only available model system for studying this common disease because a suitable animal model (the endangered chimpanzee model has significant limitations) or tissue culture system for HCV propagation does not exist.

Epidemiology

Blood transfusion, which accounted for a substantial proportion of HCV infections acquired more than 10 years ago, accounts for a minimal fraction of recently acquired infections.[56] In fact, by 1995, the risk of transfusion-associated HCV infection was so low that the Centers for Disease Control and Prevention's sentinel surveillance system was unable to detect any cases.[57] In contrast, intravenous drug use is an attributable risk factor for recent acquisition of HCV infection in 60% of cases. Although HCV is most efficiently transmitted by large or repeated percutaneous exposures to blood, cases of sexual transmission,[58] perinatal transmission,[59] and acquisition from mucous membrane exposure[60] have been described.

Molecular Virology and Immunopathogenesis

HCV is a single-stranded RNA virus within the *Flaviviridae* family. The structural proteins [i.e., nucleocapsid protein and envelope glycoprotein (E1 and E2)] are encoded at the 5′ end, followed by the nonstructural proteins (NS2 to NS5B) with various functions, including a helicase/protease (NS3) and an RNA polymerase (NS5).[61] Like many positive-stranded RNA viruses, HCV expresses its genetic information in the form of a single large "polyprotein" of approximately 3,000 amino acid residues encoded by a single open reading frame.

Different isolates of HCV display substantial nucleotide sequence variability distributed throughout the viral genome. Furthermore, genotype-specific changes in one region of the HCV genome of an isolate are highly predictive of type-specific changes in other regions. For example, genotype 1b–specific changes in the capsid region of HCV are associated with type-specific changes in the 5′ untranslated region, and either region can be used to assign genotype. HCV genotypes have been reported to affect the natural history of liver disease, the risk of neoplastic transformation, and response to therapy; it also appears that specific genotypes are associated with longer duration of infection.[62]

The low fidelity of the RNA-dependent RNA polymerase is responsible for genetic heterogeneity, leading to the evolution of *quasispecies,* a complex population of closely related virions in a given host. The biologic consequences of quasispecies include the development of escape mutants, variable cell tropism (e.g., lymphotropic versus hepatotropic), vaccine failure, and rapid development of drug resistance.[63] For example, it has been demonstrated that the emergence of HCV variants with altered peptide ligands as T-cell receptor antagonists provides a mechanism for HCV chronicity.[64] The estimated frequency of spontaneous nucleotide substitutions is very high, namely, about 10^{-2} to 10^{-3} substitutions per nucleotide per year.[65]

Despite significant advances in our understanding of the epidemiology and molecular biology of HCV, the mechanisms responsible for hepatocellular injury in chronic HCV infection remain poorly understood. Although the contribution of a direct cytopathic effect of HCV is still controversial, several lines of evidence indicate that immune-mediated mechanisms are likely to play an important role in the pathogenesis of HCV. A number of studies have demonstrated the presence of CD4+ and CD8+ T cells that recognize structural and nonstructural HCV antigens within the liver as well as the peripheral blood of patients with chronic HCV infection.[66,67] However, the fundamental question why HCV persists in the presence of a specific immune response remains unanswered.

Natural History Prior to Transplantation

Acute HCV infection is notable for its propensity to develop chronicity, with approximately 85% of individuals demonstrating evidence of infection 6 months following acute infection.[68] Data suggest that the immune response at the time of acute infection is crucial in determining the outcome of infection. In a study by Missale et al.,[69] the 12 patients with self-limited infection who subsequently became HCV RNA negative had more frequently detectable and significantly stronger T-cell responses to HCV antigens compared with the 9 patients who developed persistent viremia and biochemical evidence of chronic liver injury.

Factors predictive of progression include the age of exposure (older age at acquisition is associated with a greater risk of cirrhosis),[70] duration of infection, route of transmission (blood transfusion is associated with a greater risk of cirrhosis than intravenous drug use),[71] HCV genotype,[72,73] coexistent alcoholism,[74] and the degree of damage seen on initial liver biopsy.[75] In patients with established cirrhosis related to HCV infection, the 5-year risk of hepatic decompensation (ascites, jaundice, hepatic encephalopathy, or variceal bleeding) is 18%, and that of hepatocellular carcinoma is 7%.[76] It is estimated that the number of deaths attributable to HCV-related chronic liver disease, including hepatocellular carcinoma, will increase substantially during the next two decades. The potential economic and clinical burden related to HCV is staggering.

Outcome following Liver Transplantation

HCV reinfection after OLT occurs universally in patients with pretransplantation viremia, and 50% to 70% of these patients develop graft hepatitis.[77–79] However, graft and patient survival for the first 10 years following OLT appear to be unaffected by the HCV serostatus of the recipient.[80] In some series, approximately one-third of patients undergoing OLT for HCV-related liver disease have HCC, and OLT in this setting is associated with reduced survival due to

CAUSES OF GRAFT LOSS FOLLOWING LIVER Tx

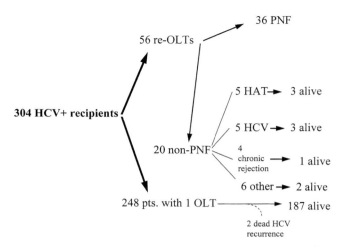

FIG. 20.3. Outcome of 304 HCV-positive liver transplant recipients. HCV, hepatitis C virus; HAT, hepatic artery thrombosis; PNF, primary nonfunction; CR, chronic rejection.

recurrence of tumors rather than recurrence of HCV.[52] An analysis of 304 HCV-seropositive liver transplant recipients from the University of California at Los Angeles (UCLA) showed that less than 5% develop graft failure due to recurrent HCV within the first 3 years (Fig. 20.3).[81]

The natural history of recurrent HCV infection was further described by the King's College group in London by comparing 1- and 5-year protocol biopsies from OLT recipients with and without HCV infection.[82] Almost 90% of the HCV-infected patients (n = 149) had chronic hepatitis by 5 years, compared with approximately 20% of the HCV-negative group (n = 623), in whom allograft hepatitis was predominantly related to HBV infection. Of concern, approximately 20% of the HCV-infected patients had evidence of allograft cirrhosis at the 5-year protocol biopsy (Fig. 20.4); there-

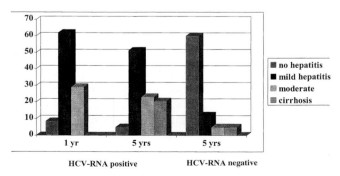

FIG. 20.4. Allograft biopsy findings at 1 and 5 years in patients positive for hepatitis C virus (HCV) and at 5 years in HCV-negative patients. (From Gane EJ, Portmann BC, Naoumouv NV, et al. Long-term outcome of hepatitis C infection after liver transplantation. *N Eng J Med* 1996;334:821–827, with permission.)

fore, the natural history of HCV infection appears to be accelerated in transplant recipients in comparison with immunocompetent individuals. Although studies with longer follow-up periods are required to determine the proportion of patients who will ultimately develop allograft cirrhosis related to HCV recurrence, it appears that fewer than 10% of patients with mild hepatitis at 1 year progress to allograft cirrhosis at 5 years. In contrast, two-thirds of patients with at least moderate HCV activity at 1 year progressed to cirrhosis by 5 years in the King's College series.

A number of studies have confirmed that findings at the onset of histologic recurrence[83] and at 1 year[84] appear to be predictive of long-term HCV-related graft injury. Rosen and colleagues reported that transient hyperbilirubinemia (attributable solely to HCV recurrence) and hepatocyte ballooning on allograft biopsy were predictive of progressive allograft injury.[83] In addition, as previously described in recurrent HBV infection, a severe progressive cholestatic syndrome due to HCV recurrence has been reported by a number of centers. The frequency of this syndrome appears to be 2% to 10%. The syndrome is associated with extremely high circulating and intrahepatic levels of HCV RNA, suggesting a direct cytopathic effect.[85,86]

Mechanisms of Allograft Injury Related to Hepatitis C Infection

Liver transplantation for HCV is analogous to acute HCV infection in that a naive uninfected liver is placed into a viremic host, and the allograft is invariably infected. As such, the human liver transplantation model offers an opportunity to study viral kinetics and immunopathogenic mechanisms of both acute and chronic HCV-related liver disease. The spectrum of allograft injury related to HCV recurrence ranges from no evidence of biochemical or histologic injury to mild abnormalities to graft failure that requires retransplantation in a subset of patients. Several interrelated viral and host factors have been proposed to explain the variable outcomes, including HCV viral load, genotype and quasispecies, and rejection and immunosuppression (Fig. 20.5).

Viral Load

The influence of the level of viremia on the severity of histologic recurrence at different time points has been assessed by a number of investigators. Chazouilleres et al. quantified serum HCV RNA levels of 100 patients who were HCV RNA positive before liver transplantation and reported that most developed high-titer viremia, with a mean 10- to 20-fold increase following liver transplantation.[87] However, the levels of HCV RNA did not correlate with serum alanine transaminase changes or histologic findings, and indeed, the patient with the highest circulating HCV RNA did not demonstrate any evidence of histologic recurrence. These early findings suggested that HCV per se probably

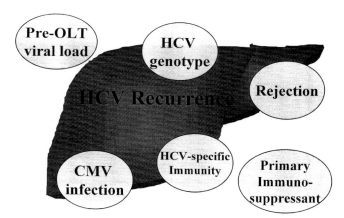

FIG. 20.5. A number of host and viral factors have been postulated to explain the variable severity of hepatitis C virus recurrence following liver transplantation.

does not have a direct cytopathic effect, supporting the hypothesis that immune-mediated mechanisms may play a central role in the pathogenesis of HCV infection. However, a subsequent study by Gretch and colleagues demonstrated that serum HCV RNA levels in the first 2 weeks following OLT were significantly higher in patients who subsequently developed chronic active hepatitis within their allografts than in those patients who did not.[88]

A longitudinal analysis by Gane and colleagues[78] found that the onset of acute allograft hepatitis was associated with peak circulating levels of HCV RNA, which in the majority of patients decreased over time. Moreover, an analysis of the NIDDK liver transplantation database showed the predictive value of pretransplantation viral levels: patients with circulating HCV RNA levels of 1×10^6 Eq/mL or higher just prior to OLT had significantly diminished graft and patient survival (Fig. 20.6),[24] suggesting that the size of the viral innoculum is crucial and providing a rationale for preemptive therapeutic regimens (see Chapter 21).

In theory, direct hepatocellular damage may occur only above a critical threshold of intracellular virus accumulation, and this level may be reached in a larger proportion of hepatocytes in recipients with a higher viral load. Alternatively, the greater viral innoculum may overwhelm the immune system's capacity to contain the virus. These findings are remininscent of those suggesting that acquisition of HCV from a blood transfusion is more likely to lead to cirrhosis than acquisition of infection related to intravenous drug use.

Viral Heterogeneity

The relative importance of different HCV genotypes following transplantation remains the subject of considerable debate. Several European groups have suggested that infection with HCV genotype 1b is associated with a higher prevalence of histologic recurrence[89] and more severe allograft

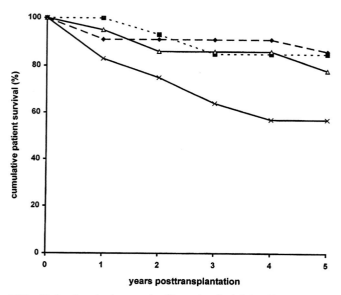

FIG. 20.6. Survival was significantly diminished in patients undergoing orthotopic liver transplantation if their pretransplantation viral load was greater than 1×10^6 Eq/mL. Data are from the National Institute of Diabetes and Digestive and Kidney Diseases liver transplant database (see ref. 24).

hepatitis.[82] However, most series from major transplant centers in the United States have not confirmed this finding,[90,91] whereas others have found that genotype 1a, which shares 85% homology at the amino acid level with genotype 1b, is associated with higher histologic severity scores than non-1 genotypes.[92] These discrepant results with respect to HCV genotype and recurrent disease may be related to the use of different histologic criteria and varying length of follow-up to assess severity, use of different genotyping technologies,[93] or to the interplay of genotype with other unmeasured factors (i.e., genotype may only represent a relative risk factor). Recently, a series from Spain of homogeneous HCV-1b OLT recipients demonstrated a correlation between cumulative steroids and an accelerated natural history of recurrent hepatitis.[94] The authors concluded that unequivocal histologic evidence of rejection needs to be present to treat HCV-1b patients with steroids. This study reflects the difficulty of assigning the relative importance of the multiple factors involved in HCV recurrence.

Work by Gretch and colleagues has demonstrated that HCV genetic divergence post-OLT correlates with outcome.[95] In patients who develop severe HCV recurrence following liver transplantation, the major quasispecies variants are efficiently propagated, whereas patients without any evidence of significant histologic recurrence show emergence of new quasispecies variants by posttransplantation day 30, and consensus sequences of the quasispecies major variants present in pretransplantation serum are not detectable at any time after liver transplantation.[96] From a mechanistic standpoint, these data are in accord with the findings (described below) of an impaired HCV-specific immune response in patients with severe recurrence; that is, a lack of immunologic selection allows efficient propagation of a dominant quasispecies.

Immunosuppression and Rejection

The majority of retrospective data indicate that the 3-year patient and graft survival rates for HCV-seropositive OLT recipients are not affected by the choice of induction immunosuppression, that is, cyclosporine versus tacrolimus.[24,82,97,98] Although use of tacrolimus did confer a 5-year patient survival advantage in HCV-positive recipients registered in the United States FK506 Study Group,[99] this difference may have been a reflection of the significantly lower rates of rejection in the tacrolimus group (68% versus 76% for cyclosporine-treated recipients within the first year). Moreover, an ongoing, prospective, randomized trial at UCLA (using lower doses of tacrolimus than the initial trials) has failed to show any difference in the prevalence or severity of HCV recurrence or on survival according to which calcineurin inhibitor is used.[100] There are limited data concerning the impact of newer immunosuppressive agents (e.g., mycophenolate mofetil, rapamycin, interleukin 2 antibodies) on the natural history of HCV post-OLT.

Patients undergoing OLT for HCV-related liver failure appear to experience frequencies of acute cellular rejection (ACR) and steroid-resistant rejection that are comparable with those of patients undergoing OLT for other indications. Undoubtedly, the most difficult challenge facing the transplant physician caring for the HCV-positive liver transplant recipient is the differentiation between ACR and HCV recurrence, which can have considerable histologic overlap (Table 20.3).[101] Our current approach in a patient with equivocal findings of rejection—namely, to hold off on presumptive treatment, repeat daily laboratory tests, and repeat an allograft biopsy several days later—is predicated on the reported increase in mortality in HCV-infected recipients (relative risk 2.9) treated for ACR.[102] In contrast, a single episode of ACR in the non-HCV-infected OLT recipient appears to confer a survival advantage.[102] It seems intuitive that in patients with progressive HCV-related allograft injury, the level of immunosuppression should be reduced, particularly in light of recent data showing the safety of steroid withdrawal; however, no study to date has specifically addressed this important question.

Sheiner and colleagues from Mt. Sinai in New York have demonstrated that the incidence of histologic recurrence is directly correlated with the degree of post-OLT immunosuppression, approaching 72% in patients treated for multiple or steroid-resistant rejection as compared with 18% in patients never treated for rejection.[103] In a case control study from UCLA, Rosen and colleagues reported that patients receiving OKT3 had earlier and more severe recurrence compared with a contemporary cohort matched for key variables.[104] Five (26.3%) of 19 patients who received OKT3 ultimately developed allograft cirrhosis, versus 2 (6%) of 33 patients treated for steroid-responsive rejection

TABLE 20.3. *Histologic features of recurrent hepatitis C infection versus acute cellular rejection*

	Recurrent hepatitis C infection	Rejection
Time posttransplantation	Anytime; onset usually within first year	Usually in first 2 months
Portal inflammation	Most cases	Always
Lymphocytes	Bland, uniform	Activated
Aggregates	Usually	Occasionally
Follicles	50% of cases	Very rarely
Eosinophils	Inconspicuous	Almost always
Steatosis	Often	Never
Acidophilic bodies	Common	Uncommon
Duct damage	About 50% of cases	Very common
Atypical features	Cholestasis, ballooning degeneration without significant inflammation, marked ductular proliferation mimicking obstruction, granulomas	Prominent periportal and lobular necroinflammatory activity without subendothelial venular inflammation

From Rosen HR, Martin P. Liver transplantation. In: Schiff ER, Sorrell MF, Maddrey WC, eds. *Schiff's disorders of liver disease,* 8th ed. Philadelphia: Lippincott-Raven Publishers, 1999:1589–1615, with permission.

($p < 0.03$). A subsequent analysis combining data from both centers demonstrated that HCV-positive patients receiving OKT3 experienced a 10-fold increase in graft loss.[105]

Cellular Immune Response

In addition to the association of OKT3 with augmented severity of HCV recurrence, several lines of indirect evidence suggest that deficient cell-mediated immunity plays a contributory role in the pathogenesis of HCV-related liver injury following transplantation. Coinfection with cytomegalovirus (CMV), which has been shown to induce cell-mediated immune defects and consequently a higher risk of opportunistic infections following transplantation, has been associated with a higher risk of HCV-related allograft cirrhosis.[106] A

follow-up study from the NIDDK database confirmed the independent association of CMV infection with allograft cirrhosis and mortality.[107]

A failure to mount an efficient immune response to HCV antigens, either because of selective defects in the host immune system or because of viral interference with the normal function of the immune cells, could account for the inability of the large proportion of HCV-infected transplant recipients to eradicate HCV. A recent analysis has shown that approximately 40% of patients with minimal or self-limited recurrent HCV demonstrate proliferative responses to HCV antigens, whereas none of the patients with severe recurrence do so (Fig. 20.7).[108] These emerging data suggest that the inability to generate adequate virus-specific T-cell responses plays at least a contributory role in the

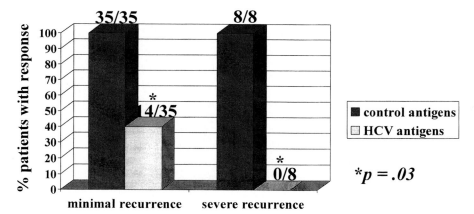

FIG. 20.7. Proliferative responses of peripheral blood T-helper cells to control non–hepatitis C virus (HCV) antigens (either tetanus toxoid or cytomegalovirus) were detectable in all liver transplant patients. However, whereas 40% of the patients with minimal recurrence responded to at least one of the HCV antigens, none of the patients with severe histologic recurrence demonstrated any significant proliferation to the HCV proteins. A stimulation index of 3 or above was considered significant. (From Rosen HR, Hinrichs DJ, Gretch DR, et al. Association of multispecific CD4+ response to hepatitis C and severity of recurrence after liver transplantation. *Gastroenterology* 1999;117:926–932.)

pathogenesis of progressive HCV-related graft injury following OLT. It is hoped that the characterization of the immunoregulatory mechanisms involved in this setting will lead to the development of highly specific therapeutic strategies. The roles of nonspecific (bystander) T-cell activation within the allograft, of cytokines, and of nitric oxide production also remain to be defined.

An immunohistochemical analysis demonstrated that patients with severe recurrence show marked and aberrant intrahepatic expression of molecules involved in lymphocyte

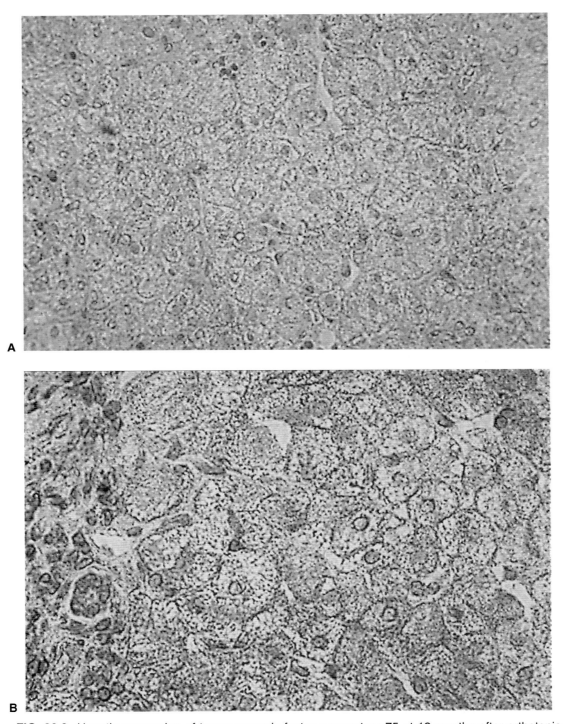

FIG. 20.8. Hepatic expression of tumor necrosis factor α receptor p75 at 12 months after orthotopic liver transplantation in **(A)** a patient with minimal histologic changes and in **(B)** a patient with progressive allograft damage. (Courtesy of Ed Gane.)

activation and antigen presentation, as well as intercellular and vascular adhesion.[109] In another study, a strong correlation was shown between expression of hepatic and soluble TNF-α receptor p75 and histologic activity of allograft hepatitis[110] (Fig. 20.8). An analysis of TNF-α polymorphisms has shown that recipients of a donor liver expressing an allele associated with higher constitutive and inducible expression of TNF-α are more susceptible to severe HCV recurrence (Fig. 20.9).[111]

In summary, the cellular immune response appears to play a central role in the pathogenesis of HCV following OLT. The converse also appears to be true; that is, recurrent HCV disease induces defects in the cellular immune response, as suggested by the University of Pittsburgh series showing a higher incidence of major and late infections in OLT patients with recurrent HCV (27% versus 6% in HCV-negative recipients).[112]

The Humoral Immune Response

Negro et al. found that anti-HCV core IgM antibodies were persistently undetectable more often in patients who did not develop any evidence of recurrent hepatitis after liver transplantation.[113] Another study from Spain of 25 OLT recipients confirmed these findings, demonstrating a significant correlation between the presence of anti-HCV core IgM before OLT and at 15 days, 90 days, and 1 year post-OLT with the presence of recurrent hepatitis.[114] A more recent analysis using recombinant immunoblot assays found that patients with minimal recurrence had significantly lower titers of antibody reactivity to NS4 and NS5.[115] However, the HCV-related humoral immune response likely does not play an important direct role in the pathogenesis of graft injury.

Approximately one-third of HCV-infected individuals have detectable cryoglobulins following OLT, and a possible association between immune complex deposition and more severe allograft hepatitis as well as late hepatic artery thrombosis has been suggested.[52,116] Moreover, HCV-related membranoproliferative glomerulonephritis may account for significant renal impairment in an unknown proportion of HCV-positive patients before and after OLT. In one experience, 6 (21%) of 28 patients awaiting OLT had histologically confirmed glomerulonephritis and significant proteinuria.[117]

Use of Grafts Infected with Hepatitis C Virus

In a preliminary analysis of the United Network for Organ Sharing (UNOS) database,[118] use of HCV-positive donor livers in HCV-positive recipients (n = 71) was associated with graft and patient survival rates comparable with those achieved with use of HCV-negative donor livers (n = 2,257), suggesting that such a policy might be a feasible means of expanding the donor organ pool. Furthermore, Vargas et al.[119] observed that the histologic outcome in HCV-positive liver recipients was usually better when they received an HCV-positive versus an HCV-negative graft.

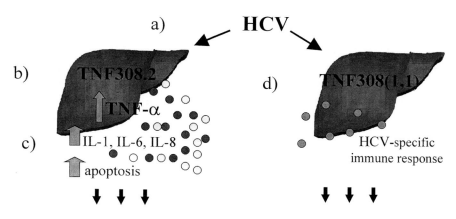

Early and severe recurrence   **Minimal recurrence**

FIG. 20.9. A conceptual paradigm for the role of specific tumor necrosis factor α (TNF-α) polymorphisms within the donor as a contributing factor for the variable severity of hepatitis C virus (HCV) recurrence following orthotopic liver transplantation. **A:** Following liver transplantation for HCV, acute HCV infection of the allograft invariably occurs. **B:** The patient who receives a donor liver with a TNF308.2 allele inherits an increased susceptibility for TNF-α production. **C:** TNF-α is an important early mediator of the cytokine cascade, generating production of interleukins 1, 6, and 8. This leads to recruitment and activation of nonspecific lymphocytes and effector cells. What ensues is an immunopathologic response that is ultimately ineffective in containing the virus. In addition, TNF-α has been shown to be an important mediator of hepatocyte apoptosis. **D:** In contrast, the majority of patients will receive a donor liver homozygous for the 308.1 allele. In this setting, acute infection of the allograft is followed by induction of an HCV-specific immune response. Recent work has demonstrated a correlation between a vigorous HCV-specific immune response and self-limited or minimal recurrence.

Whenever genotypes 1a or 1b were present in the donor/recipient pair, they eventually became the prevalent genotype, suggesting a possibly replicative advantage for these strains.

Retransplantation

The prevalence of HCV infection in patients undergoing liver retransplantation has increased significantly, from 6.5% in 1990 to 38.4% in 1995 ($p < 0.0001$; Fig. 20.10).[120] Although this rising prevalence likely represents the increase in HCV-related liver failure as a primary indication for OLT and more accurate testing for HCV infection, it does raise concern about the relative contribution of HCV to graft failure.

Data have suggested that survival following retransplantation is particularly poor in patients with recurrent HCV, even in those with other causes of graft failure. For example, an analysis of 27 HCV-positive patients undergoing retransplantation at the University of Pittsburgh demonstrated a mortality rate of 67% at a median follow-up of 120 days.[121] Twelve of these patients had concurrent chronic rejection, and 3 had vascular thrombosis. A study by Feray et al. of 119 French patients undergoing liver retransplantation demonstrated a significantly diminished 1-year graft survival (40%) in the subset of 20 patients who had developed allograft cirrhosis due to recurrent HCV, even when compared with patients retransplanted for hepatitis B–related graft failure.[122] Of note, all 20 patients developed evidence of histologic recurrence in their second grafts, leading to recurrent graft failure in 3 patients. Moreover, 15 (28%) of the 54 patients who underwent retransplantation for chronic rejection had histologic evidence of HCV infection. In a more recent study from UCLA, retransplantation in 20 patients with HCV infection was associated with a 4-fold increase in mortality compared with primary transplantation for HCV-related liver failure, irrespective of the etiology of graft failure (i.e., chronic rejection versus re-

current HCV).[81] These reports have led to the impassioned plea by some transplant physicians that retransplantation for recurrent HCV be abandoned.[123]

Analysis of the UNOS database demonstrated significantly diminished patient survival in the HCV-positive group: 57%, 55%, and 54% at 1, 3, and 5 years, respectively, compared with 65%, 63%, and 61%, respectively, in the HCV-negative group ($p = 0.008$, log-rank test).[120] The subgroup of HCV-positive patients undergoing retransplantation for causes other than primary nonfunction who had serum bilirubin levels of 10 mg/dL or higher and creatinine concentration of 2 mg/dL or higher had particularly poor outcomes. We conclude that acceptable results following liver retransplantation for severe recurrent HCV are attainable in highly selected patients, that is, those without severe hyperbilirubinemia and renal failure, and that retransplantation remains the only viable option for patients whose allografts fail because of recurrent disease.

CONCLUDING PERSPECTIVES

The evolution of our understanding and management of HBV and HCV infection in the OLT recipient has been rapid in the last decade. Although there remain important limitations to currently available antiviral strategies (see Chapter 21), it is now possible to offer OLT to the virally infected patient in the expectation that recurrent virus will not limit graft or patient outcomes.

ACKNOWLEDGMENTS

H.R. Rosen is supported in part by research funding from the American Society of Transplant Physicians, the American Digestive Health Foundation, and a Merit Review Grant, Washington, DC.

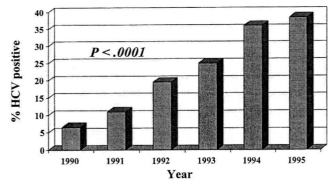

FIG. 20.10. The relative prevalence of hepatitis C virus infection in patients undergoing liver retransplantation has dramatically increased since 1990. (From Rosen HR, Martin P. Hepatitis C infection in patients undergoing liver retransplantation. *Transplantation* 1998;66:1612–1616, with permission.)

REFERENCES

1. Todo S, Demetris A, Van Thiel D, et al. Orthotopic liver transplantation for patients with hepatitis B virus-related liver disease. *Hepatology* 1991;13:619–626.
2. Terrault NA. Hepatitis B virus and liver transplantation. *Clin Liver Dis* 1999;2:389–415.
3. Huang EJ, Wright TL, Lake JR, et al. Hepatitis B and C coinfections and persistent hepatitis B infections: clinical outcome and liver pathology after transplantation. *Hepatology* 1996;3:396–404.
4. Samuel D, Muller R, Alexander G, et al. Liver transplantation in European patients with the hepatitis B surface antigen. *N Engl J Med* 1993;329:1842–1847.
5. Perrillo R, Rakela J, Martin P, et al. Lamivudine for suppression and/or prevention of hepatitis B when given pre/post transplantation [Abstract]. *Hepatology* 1997;26:260A.
6. Tipples G, Ma M, Fischer K, et al. Mutations in HBV RNA-dependent DNA polymerase confers resistance to lamivudine *in vitro*. *Hepatology* 1996;24:714–717.
7. Terrault N, Zhou S, McCory RW, et al. Incidence and clinical consequences of surface and polymerase gene mutations in liver transplant recipients on hepatitis B immunoglobulin. *Hepatology* 1998,28:555–561.

8. Ghany M, Ayola B, Villamil F, et al. Hepatitis B virus S mutants in liver transplant recipients who were reinfected despite hepatitis B immune globulin prophylaxis. *Hepatology* 1998;27:213–222.
9. Chang M-H, Chen C-J, Lai M-S, et al. Universal hepatitis B vaccination in Taiwan and the incidence of hepatocellular carcinoma in children. *N Engl J Med* 1997;1855.
10. Lucey M, Graham D, Martin P, et al. Recurrence of hepatitis B and delta hepatitis after orthotopic liver transplantation. *Gut* 1992;33:1390.
11. Terrault N, Pessoa M, Singleton S, et al. Improved survival of hepatitis B patients undergoing liver transplantation: effects independent of therapeutic interventions [Abstract]. *Hepatology* 1997;26:177A.
12. Davies SF, Portmann BC, O'Grady JG, et al. Hepatic histological findings after transplantation for chronic hepatitis B virus infection, including a unique pattern of fibrosing cholestatic hepatitis. *Hepatology* 1991;13:150–157.
13. Benner K, Lee R, Keeffe E, et al. Fibrosing cytolytic liver failure secondary to recurrent hepatitis B after liver transplantation. *Gastroenterology* 1992;103:1307–1312.
14. Chisari F, Klopchin K, Moriyama T, et al. Molecular pathogenesis of hepatocellular carcinoma in hepatitis B virus transgenic mice. *Cell* 1989;59:1145.
15. Mason AL, Wick M, White HM, et al. Increased hepatocyte expression of hepatitis B virus transcription in patients with features of fibrosing cholestatic hepatitis. *Gastroenterology* 1993;4:1269–1270.
16. Ilan Y, Galun E, Nagler A, et al. Sanctuary of hepatitis B virus in bone-marrow cells of patients undergoing liver transplantation. *Liver Transplant Surg* 1996;3:206–210.
17. O'Grady J, Smith H, Davies S, et al. Hepatitis B virus reinfection after orthotopic liver transplantation. Serological and clinical implications. *J Hepatol* 1992;1:104–111.
18. McMillan J, Shaw T, Angus P, et al. Effect of immunosuppressive and antiviral agents on hepatitis B virus replication *in vitro. Hepatology* 1995;9:36–43.
19. Cote P, Korba B, Steinberg H, et al. Cyclosporin A modulates the course of woodchuck hepatitis virus infection and induces chronicity. *J Immunol* 1991;146:3138–3144.
20. Wong PY, Marinos G, Peakman M, et al. FK506 in liver transplantation for chronic hepatitis B: *in vitro* studies on lymphocyte activation and virus replication. *Liver Transplant Surg* 1995;6:362–370.
21. Chang KM, Chisari FV. Immunopathogenesis of hepatitis B virus infection. *Clin Liver Dis* 1999;3:221–239.
22. Calmus Y, Hannoun L, Dousset B, et al. HLA class I matching is responsible for the hepatic lesions in recurrent viral hepatitis B after liver transplantation. *Transplant Proc* 1990;5:2311–2313.
23. Missale G, Brems J, Takiff H, et al. Human leukocyte antigen class I-independent pathways may contribute to hepatitis B virus-induced liver disease after liver transplantation. *Hepatology* 1993;3:491–496.
24. Charlton M, Seaberg E, Wiesner R, et al. Predictors of patient and graft survival following liver transplantation for hepatitis C. *Hepatology* 1998;28:823–830.
25. Jurim O, Martin P, Shaked A, et al. Liver transplantation for chronic hepatitis B in Asians. *Transplantation* 1994;9:1393–1395.
26. Ho BM, So SK, Esquivel CO, et al. Liver transplantation in Asian patients with chronic hepatitis B. *Hepatology* 1997;1:223–225.
27. So SK, Esquivel CO, Imperial JC, et al. Does Asian race affect hepatitis B virus recurrence or survival following liver transplantation for hepatitis B cirrhosis? *J Gastroenterol Hepatol* 1999;(suppl):S48–S52.
28. Crippin J, Foster B, Carlen S, et al. Retransplantation for hepatitis B—a multicenter experience. *Transplantation* 1994;6:823–826.
29. Ishitani M, McGory R, Dickson R, et al. Retransplantation of patients with severe posttransplant hepatitis B in the first allograft. *Transplantation* 1997;3:410–414.
30. Roche B, Samuel D, Feray C, et al. Retransplantation of the liver for recurrent hepatitis B virus infection: the Paul Brousse experience. *Liver Transplant Surg* 1999;3:166–174.
31. Omata M, Ehata T, Yokosuka O, et al. Mutations in the precore region of hepatitis B virus DNA in patients with fulminant and severe hepatitis. *N Engl J Med* 1991;324:1699.
32. Belle S, Beringer K, Detre K. Long-term outcome of liver transplant recipients in the US. *Clin Transpl* 1995;19–31.
33. Naumann U, Protzer-Knolle U, Berg T, et al. A pretransplant infection with precore mutants of hepatitis B virus does not influence the outcome of orthotopic liver transplantation in patients on high dose anti-hepatitis B virus surface antigen immunoprophylaxis. *Hepatology* 1997;2:478–484.
34. Ottobrelli A, Marzano A, Smedile A, et al. Patterns of hepatitis delta virus reinfection and disease in liver transplantation. *Gastroenterology* 1991;101:1649.
35. Huang EJ, Wright TL, Lake JR, et al. Hepatitis B and C coinfections and persistent hepatitis B infections: clinical outcome and liver pathology after transplantation. *Hepatology* 1996;3:396–404.
36. Pessoa M, Kim E, Martin P, et al. Dual effects of hepatitis B (HBV) infection and hepatitis B immunoglobulin in reducing the incidence of acute rejection post transplantation [Abstract]. *Gastroenterology* 1998;114:A1322.
37. Samuel D, Zignego A, Reynes M, et al. Long-term clinical and virological outcome after liver transplantation for cirrhosis caused by chronic delta hepatitis. *Hepatology* 1995;21:333.
38. Smedile A, Casey JL, Cote PJ, et al. Hepatitis D viremia following orthotopic liver transplantation involves a typical HDV virion with a hepatitis B surface antigen envelope. *Hepatology* 1998;6:1723–1729.
39. Alberti A, Pontisso P, Chemello L, et al. The interaction between hepatitis B and hepatitis C virus in acute and chronic liver disease. *J Hepatol* 1995;2(suppl):38–41.
40. Feray C, Gigou M, Samuel D, et al. Incidence of hepatitis C in patients receiving different preparations of hepatitis B immunoglobulins after liver transplantation. *Ann Intern Med* 1998;10:810–816.
41. Dickson RC, Everhart JE, Lake JR, et al. Transmission of hepatitis B by transplantation of livers from donors positive for antibody to hepatitis B core antigen. *Gastroenterology* 1997;5:1668–1674.
42. Uemoto S, Sugiyama K, Marusawa H, et al. Transmission of hepatitis B virus from hepatitis B core antibody-positive donors in living related liver transplants. *Transplantation* 1998;4:494–499.
43. Chazouilleres O, Mamish D, Kim M, et al. "Occult" hepatitis B virus as source of infection in liver transplant recipients. *Lancet* 1994;8890:677–678.
44. Cacciola I, Pollicino T, Squadrito G, et al. Occult hepatitis B virus infection in patients with chronic hepatitis C liver disease. *N Engl J Med* 1999;341:22–26.
45. Douglas DD, Rakela J, Wright TL, et al. The clinical course of transplantation-associated *de novo* hepatitis B infection in the liver transplant recipient. *Liver Transplant Surg* 1997;2:105–11t.
46. Crespo J, Fabrega E, Casafont F, et al. Severe clinical course of *de novo* hepatitis B infection after liver transplantation. *Liver Transplant Surg* 1999;3:175–183.
47. Dodson SF, Issa S, Araya V, et al. Infectivity of hepatic allografts with antibodies to hepatitis B virus. *Transplantation* 1997;11:1582–1584.
48. Mazzaferro V, Regalia E, Doci R, et al. Liver transplantation for the treatment of small hepatocellular carcinomas in patients with cirrhosis. *N Engl J Med* 1996;11:693–699.
49. Wong PY, McPeake JR, Portmann B, et al. Clinical course and survival after liver transplantation for hepatitis B virus infection complicated by hepatocellular carcinoma. *Am J Gastroenterol* 1995;1:29–34.
50. Mazzaferro V, Regalia E, Montalto F, et al. Risk of HBV reinfection after liver transplantation in HBsAg-positive cirrhosis. Primary hepatocellular carcinoma is not a predictor for HBV recurrence. *Liver* 1996;2:117–122.
51. Alter MJ. The detection, transmission, and outcome of hepatitis C virus infection. *Infect Agents Dis* 1993;2:55–66.
52. Gane E. Hepatitis C virus infection following liver transplantation. *Viral Hepatitis Rev* 1998;4:97–125.
53. Brechot C, Nalpas B, Feitelson MA. Interactions between alcohol and hepatitis viruses in the liver. *Clin Lab Med* 1996;16:273–287.
54. Vento S, Garofano T, Renzini C, et al. Fulminant hepatitis associated with hepatitis A virus superinfection in patients with chronic hepatitis C. *N Engl J Med* 1998;338:286–290.
55. Cacciola I, Pollicino T, Squadrito G, et al. Occult hepatitis B virus infection in patients with chronic hepatitis C liver disease. *N Engl J Med* 1999;341:22–26.
56. Alter MJ. The epidemiology of acute and chronic hepatitis C. *Clin Liver Dis* 1997;1:559–568.
57. Rosen HR. Primer on hepatitis C for the hospital epidemiologist. *Infect Control Hosp Epidemiol* 2000;21:229–234.
58. Alter MJ, Coleman PJ, Alexander WJ, et al. Importance of heterosexual activity in the transmission of hepatitis B and non-A, non-B hepatitis. *JAMA* 1989;262:1201–1205.
59. Lam JP, McOmish F, Burns SM, et al. Infrequent vertical transmission of hepatitis C virus. *J Infect Dis* 1993;167:572–576.
60. Rosen HR. Acquisition of hepatitis C by a conjunctival splash. *Am J Infect Control* 1997;25:2427.

61. Rosen HR, Gretch DR. Hepatitis C virus: molecular aspects and implications for future therapy. *Molec Med Today* 1999;5:393–399.

62. Rosen HR, Chou S, Sasaki AS, et al. Molecular epidemiology of hepatitis C infection in U.S. veteran liver transplant recipients: evidence for decreasing relative prevalence of genotype 1b. *Am J Gastroenterol* 1999;94:3013–3019.

63. Bukh J, Miller RH, Purcell RH. Genetic heterogeneity of hepatitis C virus: quasispecies and genotypes. *Semin Liver Dis* 1995;15:41–63.

64. Tsai S-L, et al. Hepatitis C virus variants circumventing cytotoxic T lymphocyte activity as a mechanism of chronicity. *Gastroenterology* 1998;115:954–966.

65. Fang JWS, Chow V, Lau JYN. Virology of hepatitis C virus. *Clin Liver Dis* 1997;1:493–514.

66. Koziel MJ, Dudley D, Afdhal N, et al. Hepatitis virus-specific cytotoxic T lymphocytes recognize epitopes in the core and envelope proteins of HCV. *J Virol* 1993;67:7522–7532.

67. Ferrari C, Valli A, Galati L, et al. T-cell response to structural and nonstructural hepatitis C virus antigens in persistent and self-limited hepatitis C virus infections. *Hepatology* 1994;19:286–295.

68. Tong MJ, El-Farra NA, Reikes AR, et al. Clinical outcomes after transfusion-associated hepatitis C. *N Engl J Med* 1995;332:1463–1466.

69. Missale G, et al. Different clinical behaviors of acute hepatitis C virus infection are associated with different vigor of the anti-viral cell-mediated immune response. *J Clin Invest* 1996;98:706–714.

70. Poynard T, Bedossa P, Opolon P, et al. Natural history of liver fibrosis progression in patients with chronic hepatitis C. *Lancet* 1997;349:825–832.

71. Gordon SC, Bayati N, Silverman AL. Clinical outcome of hepatitis C as a function of mode of transmission. *Hepatology* 1998;28:562–567.

72. Marrone A, Sallie R. Genetic heterogeneity of hepatitis C virus: the clinical significance of genotypes and quasispecies behavior. *Clin Lab Med* 1996;16:429–449.

73. Simmonds P. Variability of hepatitis C virus. *Hepatology* 1995;21:570–583.

74. Brechot C, Nalpas B, Feitelson MA. Interactions between alcohol and hepatitis viruses in the liver. *Clin Lab Med* 1996;16:273–287.

75. Yano M, et al. The long-term pathological evolution of chronic hepatitis C. *Hepatology* 1996;23:1334–1340.

76. Fattovich G, Giustina G, Degos F, et al. Morbidity and mortality in compensated cirrhosis type C: a retrospective follow-up study of 384 patients. *Gastroenterology* 1997;112:463–472.

77. Ferrell LD, et al. Hepatitis C viral infection in liver transplant recipients. *Hepatology* 1992;16:865–876.

78. Gane EJ, Naoumov NV, Qian K-P, et al. A longitudinal analysis of hepatitis C virus replication following liver transplantation. *Gastroenterology* 1996;110:167–177.

79. Fukumoto T, Berg T, Ku Y, et al. Viral dynamics of hepatitis C early after orthotopic liver transplantation: evidence for rapid turnover of serum virions. *Hepatology* 1996;24:1351–1354.

80. Boker K, Dalley G, Bahr M, et al. Long-term outcome of hepatitis C virus infection after liver transplantation. *Hepatology* 1997;25:203–210.

81. Rosen HR, O'Reilly PM, Shackleton CR, et al. Graft loss following liver transplantation in patients with chronic hepatitis C. *Transplantation* 1996;62:1773–1776.

82. Gane EJ, Portmann BC, Naoumov NV, et al. Long-term outcome of hepatitis C infection after liver transplantation. *N Engl J Med* 1996;334:821–827.

83. Rosen HR, Gretch DR, Oehlke M, et al. Timing and severity of hepatitis C recurrence following liver transplantation as predictors of longterm allograft injury. *Transplantation* 1998;65:1178–1182.

84. Prieto M, Berenguer M, Rayon JM, et al. High incidence of allograft cirrhosis in hepatitis C virus genotype 1b infection following transplantation: relationship with rejection episodes. *Hepatology* 1999;29:250–256.

85. Dickson RC, Caldwell SH, Ishitani MB, et al. Clinical and histologic patterns in early graft failure due to recurrent hepatitis C infection after liver transplantation. *Transplantation* 1996;61:701–705.

86. Schluger LK, Sheiner PA, Thung SN, et al. Severe recurrent cholestatic hepatitis C following orthotopic liver transplantation. *Hepatology* 1996;23:971–976.

87. Chazouilleres O, Kim M, Combs C, et al. Quantitation of hepatitis C virus RNA in liver transplant recipients. *Gastroenterology* 1994;106:994–999.

88. Gretch DR, Bacchi CE, Corey L, et al. Persistent hepatitis C virus infection after liver transplantation: clinical and virological features. *Hepatology* 1995;22:1–9.

89. Feray C, Gigou M, Samuel D, et al. Influence of the genotypes of hepatitis C virus on the severity of recurrent liver disease after liver transplantation. *Gastroenterology* 1995;108:1088–1096.

90. Vargas HE, Laskus T, Wang LF, et al. The influence of hepatitis C virus genotype on the outcome of liver transplantation. *Liver Transplant Surg* 1997;4:22–27.

91. Zhou S, Terrault NA, Ferrell L, et al. Severity of liver disease in liver transplantation recipients with hepatitis C virus infection: relationship to genotype and level of viremia. *Hepatology* 1996;24:1041–1046.

92. Shuhart MC, Bronner MP, Gretch DR, et al. Histological and clinical outcome after liver transplantation for hepatitis C. *Hepatology* 1997;26:1646–1652.

93. Gonzalez-Peralta R, Lau JYN. Do viral genotypes and HLA matching influence the outcome of recurrent hepatitis C virus infection after liver transplantation? *Liver Transplant Surg* 1998;4:104–108.

94. Berenguer M, Prieto M, Cordoba J, et al. Early development of chronic active hepatitis in recurrent hepatitis C virus infection after liver transplantation: association with treatment of rejection. *J Hepatol* 1998;28:756–763.

95. Gretch DR, Polyak SJ, Wilson JJ, et al. Tracking hepatitis C virus quasispecies major and minor variants in symptomatic and asymptomatic liver transplant recipients. *J Virol* 1996;70:7622–7631.

96. Sullivan DG, Wilson JJ, Carithers RL, et al. Multigene tracking of hepatitis C virus quasispecies after liver transplantation: correlation of genetic diversification in the envelope region with asymptomatic or mild disease patterns. *J Virol* 1998;72:10036–10043.

97. Ghobrial RM, Colquhoun S, Rosen HR, et al. Tacrolimus versus cyclosporine immunosuppression in liver transplantation for hepatitis C [Abstract]. *Hepatology* 1998;28:261A.

98. Zervos XA, Weppler D, Fragulidis GP, et al. Comparison of tacrolimus with microemulsion cyclosporine as primary immunosuppression in hepatitis C patients after liver transplantation. *Transplantation* 1998;65:1044–1046.

99. Wiesner RH for the United States FK506 Study Group. A long-term comparison of tacrolimus (FK506) versus cyclosporine in liver transplantation. *Transplantation* 1998;66:493–499.

100. Martin P, Goldstein RM, Goss J, et al. A prospective controlled trial of tacrolimus vs. cyclosporine in orthotopic liver transplant recipients with hepatitis C virus: lack of effect on recurrent hepatitis [Abstract]. *Hepatology* 1998;28:313A.

101. Rosen HR, Martin P. Liver transplantation. In: Schiff ER, Sorrell MF, Maddrey WC, eds. *Schiff's disorders of liver disease,* 8th ed. Philadelphia: Lippincott-Raven Publishers, 1999:1589–1615.

102. Charlton M, Seaberg E. Impact of immunosuppression and acute rejection on recurrence of hepatitis C: results of NIDDK liver transplantation database. *Liver Transplant Surg* 1999;5:S107–S114.

103. Sheiner PA, Schwartz ME, Mor E, et al. Severe or multiple rejection episodes are associated with early recurrence of hepatitis C after orthotopic liver transplantation. *Hepatology* 1995;21:30–34.

104. Rosen HR, Martin P, Shackleton CR, et al. Use of OKT3 (monoclonal antibody) associated with early and severe hepatitis C recurrence following liver transplantation. *Am J Gastroenterol* 1997;92:1453–1456; comments, 1416–1417.

105. Rosen HR, Martin P. OKT3 and hepatitis C: defining the risks. *Transplantation* 1997;63:171–172.

106. Rosen HR, Chou S, Gretch DR, et al. Cytomegalovirus viremia: risk factor for allograft cirrhosis following liver transplantation for hepatitis C. *Transplantation* 1997;64:721–726.

107. Charlton M, Seaberg EC, Wiesner RH, et al. Increased mortality following CMV infection in patients transplanted for HCV: results of the NIDDK liver transplantation database [Abstract]. *Hepatology* 1998;4:345A.

108. Rosen HR, Hinrichs DJ, Gretch DR, et al. Association of multispecific CD4+ response to hepatitis C and severity of recurrence after liver transplantation. *Gastroenterology* 1999;117:926–932 (with comments, 1012–1014).

109. Asanza C, Garcia-Monzon C, Clemente G, et al. Immunohistochemical evidence of immunopathogenetic mechanisms in chronic hepatitis C recurrence after liver transplantation. *Hepatology* 1997;26:755–763.

110. Gane E, Williams R, Naoumov N, et al. The role of TNF-alpha in HCV recurrence following liver transplantation. *(Submitted).*

111. Rosen HR, Lentz JJ, Rose SL, et al. Donor polymorphism of tumor necrosis factor gene associated with variable severity of hepatitis C

recurrence following liver transplantation. *Transplantation* 1999;68: 1898–1902.

112. Singh N, Gayowski T, Wagener MM, et al. Increased infections in liver transplant recipients with recurrent hepatitis C virus hepatitis. *Transplantation* 1996;61:402–406.

113. Negro F, Gijostra E, Rubbia-Brandt L, et al. IgM anti-hepatitis C virus core antibodies as marker of recurrent hepatitis C after liver transplantation. *J Med Virol* 1998;56:224–229.

114. Crespo J, Carte B, Lozano JL, et al. Hepatitis C virus recurrence after liver transplantation: relationship to anti-HCV core IgM, genotype, and level of viremia. *Am J Gastroenterol* 1997;9: 1458–1462.

115. Rosen HR, Gretch DR, Kaufman E, et al. The humoral immune response to hepatitis C following liver transplantation: assessment of a new immunoblot assay. *Am J Gastroenterol (in press).*

116. Ishitani M, McGory R, Dickson R, et al. Late hepatic artery thrombosis: a potential complication of viral hepatitis [Abstract]. *Hepatology* 1996;24:293A.

117. Altraif IH, Abdulla AS, al Sebayel MI, et al. Hepatitis C associated glomerulonephritis. *Am J Nephrol* 1995;15:407–410.

118. Johnson LB, Edwards E, Rustgi VK, et al. Impact of donor hepatitis C infection on recipient outcome following liver transplantation in the hepatitis C positive recipient: an analysis of the UNOS data [Abstract]. *Hepatology* 1998;28:388A.

119. Vargas HE, Laskus T, Wang L-F, et al. Outcome of liver transplantation in hepatitis C virus-infected grafts. *Gastroenterology* 1999;117: 149–155.

120. Rosen HR, Martin P. Hepatitis C infection in patients undergoing liver retransplantation. *Transplantation* 1998;66:1612–1616.

121. Casavilla FA, Lee R, Lim J, et al. Outcome of liver retransplantation for recurrent hepatitis C infection [Abstract]. *Hepatology* 1995;22:153A.

122. Feray C, Habsanne A, Samuel D, et al. Poor prognosis of patients retransplanted for recurrent liver disease due to hepatitis C virus [Abstract]. *Hepatology* 1995;22:135A.

123. Carithers RL. Recurrent hepatitis C after liver transplantation. *Liver Transplant Surg* 1997;3:S16–S17.

Transplantation of the Liver, edited by Willis C.
Maddrey, Eugene R. Schiff, and Michael F.
Sorrell. Lippincott Williams & Wilkins,
Philadelphia © 2001.

CHAPTER 21

Antiviral Therapy before and after Transplantation

Marina Berenguer and Teresa L. Wright

Liver disease due to hepatitis viruses B (HBV) and C (HCV) is the major cause for liver transplantation in the majority of transplant centers. Unfortunately, in the absence of prophylactic measures, viral recurrence following transplantation is almost universal. Graft injury from viral reinfection may result in significant morbidity, with graft failure and the need for retransplantation, and even mortality.

Generally, there are four main approaches to the patient with HBV, hepatitis D virus (HDV) or HCV infection undergoing liver transplantation (Fig. 21.1): (a) prevention of progressive liver disease prior to transplantation so that the need for liver transplantation is obviated; (b) prevention of recurrent infection after transplantation by administration of agents prior to, at the time of, or following transplantation, or during all these periods; (c) treatment of disease when and if it occurs; and (d) prevention of serious disease following transplantation through several interventions such as patient selection and modification of immunosuppression. These strategies can be implemented prior to transplantation when the patient is awaiting the availability of an organ donor (e.g., with the use of nucleoside analogues for HBV), at the time of transplantation (e.g., with the use of hepatitis B immmune globulin, or HBIG), and/or following transplantation (e.g., with the use of nucleoside analogues or HBIG, or both, for HBV, and of a combination of interferon and ribavirin for HCV).

Although the untreated natural history of posttransplantation HCV infection is more benign than that of posttransplantation HBV infection, the recent availability of several treatment options for HBV-infected patients, such as nucleoside analogues, has greatly improved the outcome of

the latter group, with a subsequent increased interest in transplantation for HBV.

This chapter reviews the spectrum of therapeutic strategies in patients undergoing liver transplantation for HBV (with or without HDV-) or HCV-related liver disease, with particular emphasis on recent antiviral agents such as nucleoside analogues or the combination of interferon and ribavirin.

HEPATITIS B VIRUS INFECTION

Natural History

Early experience with liver transplantation for hepatitis B–infected patients was discouraging,[1] with reinfection rates of approximately 80%, frequently resulting in graft loss.[1,2] One-year patient survival was significantly reduced in patients positive for hepatitis B surface antigen (HBsAg) compared with those who were HBsAg negative (45% versus 62%, respectively),[1] with a significant variability in outcome depending on the serologic and virologic status of the patient.[1,2] Patients with low indices of replication, such as those with fulminant hepatitis, those coinfected with HDV, and those with cirrhosis without detectable hepatitis B e antigen (HBeAg) or HBV DNA pretransplantation, have a lower rate of reinfection than patients with indices of active replication.[2]

Thinking has evolved over the past 5 years so that patients with HBV infection are currently considered good candidates for liver transplantation. This change in clinical practice has resulted from improved outcomes with specific interventions, mainly the use of hepatitis B immune globulin and, more recently, the use of nucleoside analogues. The debate on transplantation for HBV has thus evolved from whether HBV-infected patients should receive transplants to how we should manage these patients before and after transplantation. Several questions need to be addressed:

M. Berenguer: Servicio de Hepato-Gastroenterología, Hospital Universitari La FE, Valencia 46009, Spain.

T. L. Wright: Veterans Administration Medical Center, San Francisco, California 94121.

A. Preemptive therapy

1. Pretransplantation antiviral therapy

   - To eradicate pretransplantation infection
   - To reduce the risk and severity of posttransplantation recurrence by decreasing levels of viremia pretransplantation
   - To delay or obviate the need for transplantation

2. Early posttransplantation antiviral therapy

   - To reduce the rate of recurrent infection
   - To reduce the risk and severity of recurrent disease

3. Posttransplantation prophylactic therapy

   - To reduce the rate of recurrent infection

B. Treatment of recurrent disease

   - To treat acute hepatitis in order to eradicate infection and/or reduce the risk of progression
   - To treat chronic hepatitis in order to eradicate infection and/or improve histologic disease severity

C. Management of immunosuppression

   Selection of
   - Tacrolimus versus cyclosporine
   - Use of mycophenolate
   - Treatment of rejection

D. Retransplantation (early versus late)

FIG. 21.1. Therapeutic strategies for patients undergoing liver transplantation who are infected with hepatitis B or hepatitis C virus.

1. Should HBIG remain the standard of care for these patients?
2. Can passive immunoprophylaxis be stopped in the long term?
3. Should antiviral agents be used preemptively or only as therapeutic agents?
4. Should antiviral agents be used alone or in combination?
5. Should patients undergoing transplantation for HBV receive a specific immunosuppressive regimen?
6. Is retransplantation an option for patients with recurrent HBV-related graft failure?

Prevention of Graft Reinfection with Hepatitis B Virus

Hepatitis B Immune Globulin

The standard of care in most liver transplantation programs is the use of lifelong passive immunization with high-dose HBIG (Table 21.1).[2-8] HBIG consists of polyclonal antibodies directed against the viral envelope, and was originally derived from donors positive for antibody to HBsAg (anti-HBs). The presumed mechanism of action of this antibody is to neutralize circulating virus by binding to the viral envelope, preventing infection of the transplanted liver.

In early studies, the administration of HBIG during the anhepatic phase and in the short term posttransplantation did not effectively reduce the incidence of recurrent HBV infection. In contrast, long-term administration of HBIG for more than 6 months was shown to reduce the rate of HBV recurrence dramatically to a median rate of 20% after 2 years.[2-8] In the largest European multicenter study, involving 17 countries, the recurrence rate was 75% in patients receiving no or short-term HBIG versus 33% in those receiving long-term HBIG ($p < 0.001$).[2] Long-term administration of HBIG reduced the rate of recurrence to less than 10% in patients with fulminant HBV hepatitis, to between 10% and 15% in HDV-coinfected patients, and to less than 30% in HBV DNA–negative cirrhotic patients. However, it did not reduce the rate of recurrence in patients with HBV DNA–positive HBV cirrhosis.[2] More recent reports using higher doses of HBIG with maintenance titers over 500 IU/L have shown positive results even among those patients who were HBV DNA positive prior to transplantation.[7,8] In summary, the protocol of HBIG administration appears to have an effect on the rate of recurrence,[2-8] with lower recurrence rates seen in patients achieving titers of anti-HBs higher than 500 IU/L compared with studies in which the end point is 100 IU/L.

Various regimens have been described, with most including the administration of 10,000 IU HBIG intravenously during the anhepatic phase and 10,000 IU HBIG daily for the first week posttransplantation. The subsequent dosing is

TABLE 21.1. *Experience with long-term hepatitis B immune globulin prophylaxis in the liver transplant setting*

Author and year (Reference)	Number of patients	Duration of therapy (mo)	Anti-HBs* titers (IU/L)	Recurrence rate
Muller et al. 1991 (3)	23	6–12	≥100	25% at 1 year
Samuel et al. 1991 (4)	110	Indefinite	≥ 100	59% at 2 years
Samuel et al. 1993 (2)	209	≥ 6	Variable	35% at 3 years
Devlin et al. 1994 (6)	27	Indefinite	≥ 100	48% at 1 year
Konig et al. 1994 (5)	44	Indefinite	≥ 100	39% at 1 year
McGory et al. 1996 (7)	27	Indefinite	≥ 500[a]	11% at 2 years
Terrault et al. 1996 (8)	24	Indefinite	≥ 500[b]	19% at 2 years

*anti-HBs, antibody to hepatitis B surface antigen.
[a]Targeted trough anti-HBs levels varied with time posttransplantation: ≥ 500 IU/L during the first 7 days, ≥ 250 IU/L until the end of the third month, and ≥ 100 IU/L afterward.
[b]Mean titers obtained by hybridization assay: 1,275 IU/L.

given on a monthly basis,[8] with the tapering schedule being weekly to monthly[7] or based on anti-HBs titers.[4–7] With the fixed monthly schedule,[8] the majority of patients will achieve trough anti-HBs titers in serum of at least 500 IU/mL, with median titers of 1,250 IU/mL.

Although to this date, passive long-term immunoprophylaxis is the best way of preventing HBV recurrence, there are several limitations to its long-term use (Table 21.2). The first limitation is its lack of efficacy in approximately 20% of patients, who will become HBsAg positive despite high doses of HBIG. The causes of breakthrough are probably multifactorial and include inadequate anti-HBs titers following transplantation, mutations in the region of the surface gene of the HBV genome that encodes the a determinant region, and high levels of viremia. A second limitation of HBIG is the reduced availability of this drug and the subsequent effect on

TABLE 21.2. *Prophylaxis with long-term hepatitis B immune globulin: disadvantages and reasons against discontinuation*

Disadvantages
HBV recurrence (overall rate of 15% to 20% at 2 years)
Limited availability
High cost
Side effects
Heavy surveillance
Reasons against discontinuation
Persistence of HBV DNA in PBMC, liver, and/or serum of HBsAg-negative recipients
Only HBIG has demonstrated improved survival to date
Recurrence described in patients discontinuing HBIG prophylaxis years following transplantation

HBV, hepatitis B virus; PBMC, peripheral blood mononuclear cells; HBsAg, hepatitis B surface antigen; HBIG, hepatitis B immune globulin.

drug cost, which has tripled in the period from 1995 to 1998. A single dose of 10,000 IU costs between $3,000 and $4,700 in 1998 depending on the product used.

The need for parenteral administration, with variable patient tolerance and the development of side effects in a substantial proportion of patients, represents an additional problem. Major side effects include back or chest pain, which occurs in the majority of treated patients (90%), headaches (20%), and flushing (5%), requiring a slow infusion rate and treatment with antihistamines, corticosteroids and narcotics.[7–9] Although elevated mercury levels have been documented, only one report has suggested mercury toxicity from the mercurial thimoseral used to preserve the drug.[10]

The final limitation is the difficulty in discontinuing this product in the long term. Recurrent infection has been documented in patients stopping prophylaxis with HBIG after 1 year.[11] Furthermore, HBV DNA has been detected by highly sensitive molecular techniques in the serum, liver, and peripheral blood mononuclear cells of HBsAg-negative patients on HBIG prophylaxis, suggesting that indefinite treatment is required.[8,12,13]

To reduce the cost of HBIG administration, low-dose subcutaneous administration has been advocated by some.[14] This approach has been associated with a high rate of recurrence when used as monotherapy.[14] However, low-dose HBIG should be revisited in the era of combination therapy. Three recent reports have described their initial experience with the combination of lamivudine with low doses of intramuscular HBIG used prophylactically from the time of transplantation, with promising results.[15–17] Of a total of 26 patients receiving this regimen and followed for a mean of 16 months, only 1 has developed allograft reinfection at 6 months posttransplantation.[15–17] Interestingly, this protocol was effective in patients who were either HBV DNA positive or negative at the time of transplantation, and in patients with precore mutants.[17] Besides the potential to offer synergy or decrease resistance to HBIG, the economic implications of this approach are notable.[15]

Some of the limitations of HBIG may be reduced with a new intravenous formulation (IVHBIG; NABI, Rockville, Maryland). In a preliminary clinical trial, this new HBIG preparation has been shown to induce longer-lasting levels of circulating antibodies to HBsAg compared with previous experience with conventional HBIG preparations. Furthermore, the new HBIG was well tolerated, and no adverse effects were observed.[18] This profile, in particular the prolonged elimination half-life, may reduce the cost of administration by approximately 30% and improve the quality of life of patients by extending the interval between repeated immune globulin injections.

Mutations in the region of the surface gene that encodes the A determinant, believed to be the immunodominant epitope of the surface gene and the putative region for antibody binding, have been associated with treatment failure and disease recurrence, and thus are termed *escape mutants*.[19–25] In patients with these mutations, serum HBsAg becomes detectable, generally accompanied by an increase in levels of HBV DNA and positivity of HBeAg and by signs of histologic disease.

In patients failing HBIG therapy, graft loss is common. However, treatment with nucleoside analogues has shown promising results, with a decrease in HBV replication and improvement in liver enzymes and histologic disease severity.[25,26] Surface gene mutations have been described in approximately half of the patients failing HBIG prophylaxis, with the most common mutation being a substitution of glycine for arginine at amino acid position 145.[21,23–25] Discontinuation of HBIG results in reversion of the mutations to the wild type virus in the majority of patients (78%).[23] The remaining 50% of patients failing HBIG have no surface gene mutations. It is likely that several factors may have contributed to the failure, such as the level of HBV replication prior to transplantation, the amount and dosing of HBIG, and the type and amount of immunosuppression.[25] Debate still exists as to whether HBV escape mutants are selected by treatment from preexisting populations, or whether they emerge under therapy.[21,24,25,27] In the absence of antiviral treatment with nucleoside analogues, graft failure is more frequently seen in patients with escape mutants than in those without them.[24]

Alternatives

Given the previously mentioned disadvantages of HBIG, several alternatives have being proposed, including preemptive therapy with nucleoside analogues, the combination of HBIG with one or more nucleoside analogues, and HBV vaccination of transplant recipients receiving HBIG prophylaxis. However, whether these options will improve the outcome in HBV-infected patients undergoing liver transplantation (mainly in the subset of patients with pretransplantation

active replication) or decrease the incidence of viral surface gene mutations remains to be seen.

Antiviral Therapy

Antiviral Agents

Several agents have been used to treat hepatitis B in the transplant setting. Of these, lamivudine appears the most promising agent.

Interferon

Interferon alfa is an effective antiviral and immunomodulatory agent that has been extensively used for the treatment of chronic hepatitis B. Complete response, defined as the disappearance of HBV DNA and the loss of HBeAg, has been achieved in approximately one-third of treated patients. Patients with chronic HBV appear to obtain long-term benefit from interferon therapy, with improved survival and reduced complications. The patients included in most clinical trials of interferon represent a highly select group of chronic HBV carriers. In particular, patients with decompensated liver disease have been excluded. Although low-dose interferon is tolerated in patients with hepatic decompensation and may even result in improvement in synthetic function, the risk of worsening hepatic decompensation limits its use in this setting.[28]

Nucleoside Analogues

Several agents that specifically inhibit HBV replication are in clinical development for the treatment of chronic hepatitis B infection.[29] Nucleoside analogues (Table 21.3) have been shown to inhibit viral replication and improve liver enzymes and histology in infected individuals.[30,31] After being incorporated into the growing DNA chain, they terminate replication by inhibiting the reverse transcription process. Unfortunately, they are only capable of blocking replication of the intermediates; they have limited efficacy at eliminating the source of replication. As a consequence, rises in liver enzymes have been observed following cessation of treatment.[32–35] The clinical significance of these "hepatic flares" is under investigation. Thus, the need for long-term therapy appears likely, although there is concern that prolonged treatment will result in the development of viral resistance with DNA breakthrough in a large proportion of patients.[27,36–39] This resistance is associated with specific mutations in the YMDD locus, the same region of the viral polymerase that has been associated with resistance to lamivudine in the therapy of infection with the human immunodeficiency virus (HIV).[40,41]

Lamivudine. The negative enantiomer of 2′-deoxy-3′thiacytidine, lamivudine is a cytosine analogue that inhibits the reverse transcriptase of HBV by interfering with the synthesis of the proviral DNA chain from pregenomic viral messenger RNA. It has good oral bioavailability and is well tolerated.[30] There are extensive data on the safety of lamivudine for both HIV and HBV patients.

TABLE 21.3. *Nucleoside analogues for the prevention and treatment of hepatitis B infection following liver transplantation*

Drug	Mechanism of action	Pharmacokinetics	Adverse effects	Other viruses affected
Ganciclovir	Inhibition of viral DNA polymerase	Oral bioavailability, 10%; plasma half-life, 2.5 h	Bone marrow suppression (common), renal insufficiency, fever, headache (uncommon)	CMV, HSV, VZV, Epstein-Barr
Famciclovir	Inhibition of viral DNA polymerase	Oral bioavailability, 75%; plasma half-life, 2 h	Headache, nausea, diarrhea (uncommon)	HSV, VZV
Lamivudine	Inhibition of viral DNA polymerase and reverse transcriptase	Oral bioavailability, 85%; plasma half-life, 5–7 h	Mild paresthesias (uncommon); asymptomatic elevations in serum amylase, lipase, and creatine phosphokinase levels (uncommon)	HIV-1
Adefovir	Inhibition of viral DNA polymerase and reverse transcriptase	Oral bioavailability, 85%	Asymptomatic elevations in serum amylase, lipase, and creatine phosphokinase levels (uncommon); transaminase elevations during and after therapy	HIV-1, CMV, HSV

CMV, cytomegalovirus; HSV, herpes simplex virus; VZV, varicella-zoster virus; HIV, human immunodeficiency virus.

In the case of HBV infection, lamivudine has proven to be extremely safe in a variety of patient groups, including those with stable HBV,[32–34] those with hepatic decompensation awaiting transplantation,[42,43] and those with recurrent HBV following transplantation.[44] The only side effects reported have been asymptomatic elevations in serum amylase, lipase, and creatine phosphokinase levels and mild paresthesias, which usually resolve despite continuation of therapy.[32–34,45] More severe side effects included a severalfold increase of serum alanine aminotransferase (ALT), which may simply represent reactivation of HBV and is usually seen before seroconversion to anti-HBe. Besides its high safety profile, lamivudine has potent anti-HBV activity. In the three groups of patients mentioned earlier, lamivudine is universally effective at suppressing HBV replication to levels below detection of the abbott liquid hybridization assay (approximately 3 logs).

Famciclovir and Ganciclovir. Ganciclovir, famciclovir, and penciclovir are a family of related guanosine analogues that inhibit viral DNA and protein synthesis. These drugs differ in their oral bioavailability and anti-HBV potency.[30] Ganciclovir was the first agent to be used in the treatment of recurrent hepatitis B following transplantation, with promising results.[46] Unfortunately, this drug has several drawbacks that limit its use in this setttting, including its modest anti-HBV activity in comparison with second-generation nucleoside analogues and the need for intravenous administration given its poor oral bioavailability.

Famciclovir, the oral form of penciclovir, is a guanosine analogue with good oral bioavailability and is well tolerated both in immunocompetent and immunocompromised patients.[29] In contrast to other nucleoside analogues, no evidence of hepatic decompensation or ALT flare has been described with famciclovir.[47] Treatment with famciclovir leads to a rapid dose-dependent reduction of both HBV DNA levels and transaminases, with the greatest activity seen with 500 mg three times daily.[35] Although there has been no direct comparison between lamivudine and famciclovir, the antiviral effect of the former agent appears to be greater than that of the latter drug.

Other Agents. Other nucleotide and nucleoside analogues with anti-HBV activity include adefovir and lobucavir. More data are available for the former than the latter. Adefovir dipivoxil is an oral prodrug of the adenine nucleotide analogue adefovir that has anti-HBV activity.[30] Unlike nucleoside analogues with antiviral activity, adefovir does not require the nucleoside kinase enzyme for initial phosphorylation.[48] Since nucleoside kinase may be absent in 1% to 2% of hepatocytes, adefovir could potentially have antiviral activity in a broader range of cells than lamivudine or famciclovir. Dose-finding studies have shown that a single daily dose of 30 mg is well tolerated and has a potent antiviral activity.[48] As with nucleoside analogues, adefovir is well tolerated, with similar side effects. Liver enzyme elevations that required dose modification or interruption have been described during both treatment and follow-up. Final analysis of the safety profile of this agent is awaited. Adefovir may have an advantage over other drugs in the treatment of lamivudine-resistant infection prior to and following liver transplantation, because this agent has demonstrated activity *in vitro* against HBV strains with genetic resistance to lamivudine.[49]

Lobucavir is a guanosine analogue with potent anti-HBV activity. However, data from preclinical animal studies have suggested toxicities that have halted further clinical development.

Preemptive Antiviral Therapy

Several antiviral agents have been used in the pretransplantation setting, the rationale being that by decreasing HBV replication to undetectable levels, the rate of recurrent infection will be reduced posttransplantation. Additional and more difficult end points to reach are the stabilization of liver disease and the postponement or even obviation of the need for transplantation. To date, however, no drug has yet been proven in a controlled trial to reduce clinical progression of decompensated liver disease or reduce the need for transplantation.

Traditionally, the only available option for clearing HBV DNA from serum prior to transplantation was interferon. However, candidates for transplantation are generally a subgroup of patients difficult to treat with interferon because of its severe side effects and the possibility of precipitating further deterioration of liver function. Therapy with low doses of interferon (0.5 MU per day to 3 MU three times a week) adjusted according to tolerability is an option for these patients. Although the benefit of treating such patients is not established, limited studies involving patients with decompensated disease suggest that interferon therapy may be of minor benefit and may produce sustained inhibition of viral replication and clinical stabilization.[28] In a recent study, prolonged interferon therapy (3 to 48 months) given at low doses (3 MU) resulted in a sustained loss of serum HBV DNA associated with biochemical response in 10 (66%) of the 15 treated patients with decompensated HBV cirrhosis.[50] During follow-up, 7 of these 10 patients showed marked clinical improvement. Unfortunately, interferon alfa prophylaxis appeared to be of little use in preventing reinfection in patients undergoing transplantation. In a study in which 22 HBV-infected patients awaiting transplantation were treated prophylactically with interferon at low doses, recurrence was similar in HBV DNA–positive and HBV DNA–negative patients treated with interferon therapy compared with untreated patients (80% vs. 91%, and 31% vs. 33%, respectively).[51]

More promising results have been described with nucleoside analogues such as lamivudine and famciclovir. Most of the experience published to date is with lamivudine. An early report showed that lamivudine was able to clear HBV DNA from serum in cirrhotic patients awaiting transplantation.[43] In this report, lamivudine was maintained for 1 year after transplantation with a low rate of HBV reinfection. Only 1 patient of 10 developed recurrent HBV at 24 weeks, associated with a mutation in the polymerase gene.[43] In a larger open-label study that included 10 centers across the United States and Canada, lamivudine was administered at a dose of 100 mg daily prior to transplantation and for 12 months following transplantation.[52] With this approach, HBV DNA levels were undetectable by the Abbott assay in all patients in the early posttransplantation period, 83% of patients lost HBsAg at the end of posttransplantation follow-up, and disappearance of HBeAg occurred in approximately one-third of individuals initially positive for this marker. The major drawback of this approach is the development of resistance to lamivudine, with HBV DNA reappearance, during both the pre- and posttransplantation period (see "Emergence of Nucleoside Analogue Resistance," later in this chapter).

Famciclovir has also been tried as preemptive therapy in patients undergoing liver transplantation. In a pilot study, eight HBsAg-positive patients were treated with famciclovir for 6 months.[53] Although an initial decline in HBV DNA titers occurred in all patients, only two (25%) of the patients became HBV DNA negative before transplantation and underwent liver transplantation. Seroconversion to anti-HBs (and anti-HBe in the HBeAg-positive patient) was demonstrated at the conclusion of famciclovir therapy in the patients who underwent transplantation. Both patients remained HBV DNA negative at nearly 2 years of follow-up after transplantation. Treatment was well tolerated, and no side effects attributable to famciclovir were observed. Several studies are currently evaluating this approach, but no results have been published to date. As with lamivudine, there are concerns regarding the development of famciclovir-resistant variants, which may in turn demonstrate cross-resistance to lamivudine.

Because treatment failures occur at a rate of approximately 20% after 1 to 2 years of treatment with either HBIG or lamivudine when given as single prophylactic agents, some alternatives have been proposed. In a recent study, Markowitz et al. demonstrated that lamivudine in combination with high doses of HBIG is safe and highly effective in preventing HBV recurrence following liver transplantation.[54] In this study, 13 patients were treated prophylactically with lamivudine (150 mg daily) and high-dose HBIG, starting with 10,000 IU during the anhepatic phase. No treatment failures were observed after 1 year of treatment, and 1-year patient survival reached 92%. Whether the frequency of viral resistance will increase with more prolonged follow-up periods is still unknown.[54] Preliminary data on combination prophylaxis with low doses of intramuscular HBIG and lamivudine have also shown this regimen to be effective and potentially cost saving.[15]

Lamivudine has recently been compared with HBIG as a prophylactic agent against HBV recurrence. Twenty-four liver transplant recipients who underwent transplantation for HBsAg-positive cirrhosis and who had received HBIG for at least 6 months with no evidence of HBV recurrence were randomized to lamivudine (100 mg daily, n = 12) or standard HBIG (n = 12) for 52 weeks. Of 21 patients who completed the study, all remained HBsAg negative with undetectable HBV DNA (by Abbott assay) in serum and undetectable HBsAg and HBcAg in the liver graft. HBV DNA was detected by polymerase chain reaction (PCR) initially in 8 patients (4 in the lamivudine group and 4 in the HBIG group). At the end of the 52 weeks of treatment, the same number of patients had detectable HBV DNA by PCR in serum (6 in the lamivudine group, 2 in the HBIG group). HBV recurrence occurred in 3 patients: 1 in the HBIG group and 2 in the lamivudine group. Although this study suggests that, given their similar efficacy profile, lamivudine may be a more attractive approach than HBIG for the prevention of HBV recurrence, the follow-up period is too short to draw definite conclusions.[55] Resistance will likely become an issue with longer follow-up.

Famciclovir in association with HBIG has also been tried in a preliminary study in patients with indices of active replication, suggesting that this approach can also achieve a reduction in HBV recurrence. Several studies are currently underway to assess the efficacy of both drugs given either alone or in combination with HBIG as a means of preventing HBV recurrence.

Treatment of Hepatitis B Disease of the Graft

Treatment of HBV-related liver disease in transplant patients is difficult for several reasons, including the high levels of HBV replication and the ongoing immunosuppressive treatment. Interferon has been used in this setting without major efficacy. New nucleoside analogues are promising in this setting because of their potent antiviral effect and their lack of side effects, particularly regarding the risk of rejection. Resistance, however, is an issue.

Interferon has been used to treat recurrent hepatitis B with discouraging results, despite a low risk of rejection.[56,57] Some benefit was observed in one study in which 14 patients with recurrent hepatitis B, all with active viral replication, were treated with interferon alfa, 3 MU thrice weekly for a mean period of 23 weeks. Loss of HBV DNA was seen in 4, loss of HBeAg in 2, and loss of HBsAg in 1 patient after therapy. No effect was seen on aminotransferase levels, however, and 1 patient developed graft rejection with subsequent graft loss, highlighting the potential adverse effect of this drug.[58] In another recent case report, two patients who had failed HBIG were treated with interferon alfa; normalization of ALT and loss of HBeAg, HBV DNA, and HBsAg were seen in both. One patient was coinfected with HDV, and the other was treated with high and prolonged doses of interferon (6 MU three times a week for 6 months, then lower doses for 22 months).[59] The recent advent of potent antiviral agents such as nucleoside analogues has limited the role of interferon as a prophylactic or therapeutic agent. However, if resistance to nucleoside analogues becomes an increasingly important problem, the interest in interferon alone or in combination with nucleoside analogues may increase.

Lamivudine is the most widely used nucleoside analogue.[26,38,44,60] In most studies, liver transplant recipients with documented HBV recurrence (elevated serum ALT levels, HBsAg positivity, and detectable HBV DNA) have been treated with lamivudine (100 mg daily) with good tolerance and rapid loss of HBV DNA in serum.[26,38,44,60] Good response has been achieved not only in patients with chronic hepatitis B following transplantation but also in the setting of acute hepatitis B of the graft[61] and in the most severe cases of fibrosing cholestatic hepatitis.[62] In the largest series, 52 patients with recurrent HBV hepatitis (histologic evidence of damage, with HBsAg seropositivity and detectable HBV DNA) were treated with lamivudine (100 mg daily) for 52 weeks. After treatment, 31 (60%) had undetectable HBV DNA by solution hybridization, 14 (31%) of the 45 initially HBeAg-positive patients lost HBeAg, 3 (6%) became HBsAg negative, and 37 (71%) normalized the serum alanine aminotransferase levels. Although fibrosis remained

unaffected in the majority, portal and lobular inflammation and periportal necrosis improved significantly.[44] The downside of this agent is the need for continuous treatment because relapse is the rule once the drug is discontinued. Prolonged therapy is associated with the potential development of breakthrough due to the emergence of HBV escape mutants, which occurred in 14 (27%) of these patients.

Famciclovir has also been used to treat liver transplant recipients with HBV recurrence. In a pilot study, 12 liver recipients who had initially failed HBIG were treated with famciclovir (500 mg thrice daily) for a mean duration of 13.5 months (range, 3–30 months). After 12 months of therapy, a 95% reduction in HBV DNA was detected in 9 patients, which was associated with a decrease in serum aminotransferase levels and clinical improvement.[63] Several case reports have published similar data.[64,65] A large multicenter study of 107 patients has been initiated with treatment periods of up to 4 years.[66] After 6 months of treatment with famciclovir (500 mg thrice daily, with dosing adjusted to renal function), a median reduction in ALT levels was observed in 45 (42%) of the patients, with a reduction in HBV DNA in 86 (80%).[66] However in the long term, most of the patients treated with famciclovir relapse.[67]

Emergence of Nucleoside Analogue Resistance

Monotherapy with both lamivudine and famciclovir has resulted in the emergence of HBV mutants that are resistant to these compounds. This resistance generally occurs after prolonged therapy (more than 6 months).[36–42,44] In both instances, the appearance of resistant mutants is associated with a rise in serum HBV DNA and ALT levels, indicating a breakthrough infection. Molecular analysis of these mutations has shown that they are located in the viral DNA polymerase gene.[27] Because of the overlapping nature of the HBV open reading frames, nucleotide changes in the polymerase may result in amino acid changes not only in the polymerase protein but also in the surface protein, which could in turn theoretically alter binding of HBIG.[27] Thus, long pretransplantation treatment with nucleoside analogues could select changes within the polymerase protein, which in turn could result in immunologically relevant alterations to the viral envelope that have the potential to produce HBsAg variants not neutralized by HBIG at the time of transplantation.[27]

Resistance to lamivudine is associated with changes in both the B and C domains of the polymerase, whereas changes associated with famciclovir occur mainly in the B domain. In the case of lamivudine, mutations are located within the tyrosine-methionine-aspartate-aspartate (YMDD) amino acid motif, which is involved in the nucleotide binding in the catalytic domain of the polymerase.[40] The most common mutations described are the mutation of the methionine at amino acid position 550 to either isoleucine or valine, with the latter often seen in combination with a leucine-to-methionine change in the B domain of the polymerase at position 526.[36,40,68] These mutations have been shown to confer reduced sensitivity to lamivudine *in vitro* and in the duck model. When lamivudine is stopped, the wild variant reemerges as the dominant viral population, but retreatment is again associated with the development of resistant mutants at an accelerated rate.[41,68,69]

In contrast, mutations generated by famciclovir are not located within the YMDD motif, but in a region upstream from it.[39] The most common mutations are the valine-to-leucine change at amino acid position 519 and a leucine-to-methionine change at position 526. Since the YMDD motif is located in the C domain of the polymerase, lamivudine-resistant mutants associated only with changes in this motif should theoretically remain sensitive to famciclovir. However, lamivudine-induced mutations can also occur in the B domain of the polymerase, where changes have also been described with famciclovir. Thus famciclovir-resistant virus may not be sensitive to lamivudine, a situation recently described in several patients.[27,70]

The long-term rate of emergence of drug-resistant mutants and their implications for the natural history of HBV infection are still unknown. Although some cases of histologic and clinical deterioration have been reported when drug-resistant mutants develop,[70,71] these changes are not consistently associated with hepatic disease progression.[44] It is possible that differences in the replicative competence or "fitness" of the mutants may account for these differences in outcome.[72] *In vitro* studies with adefovir have shown that although cross-resistance occurs between lamivudine and famciclovir, variants resistant to both these drugs remain sensitive to adefovir, suggesting that adefovir dipivoxil may be very important in the treatment of HBV with or without resistance to other oral agents.[73,74]

An understanding of the viral dynamics in HBV infection is essential for achieving antiviral treatment success. Studies suggest that no single agent is able to clear the virus effectively without resistant mutants emerging.[75,76] Synergistic combination regimens with one or more nucleoside or nucleotide analogues and immune stimulants such as interferon or therapeutic vaccines are likely to be the best strategy for maximizing antiviral activity and preventing the development of resistant HBV variants. As in the HIV field, combination therapy is inevitable. Our goal should be to select the most potent synergistic drugs for which (a) development of resistance requires multiple viral mutations, (b) the viral mutations conferring resistance do not overlap, and (c) development of mutations can reinstate sensitivity to a drug to which the virus had previously become resistant. The ultimate decision on the choice of drugs for combination therapy awaits the results of ongoing phase III trials on long-term monotherapy with lamivudine and famciclovir and on combination therapy with lamivudine and interferon alfa, and phase III trials with adefovir.

In conclusion, there are limitations to all current practices (Tables 21.2 and 21.4) for preventing HBV recurrence. Treatment with nucleoside analogues prior to transplantation is limited by the possible development of drug-resistant

TABLE 21.4. *Advantages and disadvantages of nucleoside analogues for the prevention and treatment of hepatitis B infection following liver transplantation*

Advantages
High bioavailability by the oral route
Relative lack of adverse effects
Lack of effect on the immune system
Possible capability of blocking the supercoiled HBV-DN Accc (famciclovir, adefovir)
Effective against other viruses
Disadvantages
Need for prolonged therapy
Development of drug-resistant viral mutants

HBV-DNAccc, circular covalently closed DNA.

mutants that in turn may impair the ability of HBIG to prevent HBV recurrence. Deciding the optimal time to begin therapy is unclear because long waiting times would place patients at risk for development of resistance if treatment were initiated too early. In contrast, if treatment is begun when patients are profoundly decompensated, then an opportunity to stabilize the liver disease and postpone or even eliminate the need for transplantation may be missed. Limitations of prolonged HBIG therapy mainly include the cost and side effects. If lamivudine is to be used in combination with HBIG, the dose and duration of HBIG treatment remains uncertain, and the efficacy of long-term lamivudine therapy may be impaired by the development of drug-resistant mutants.

Alternative Approaches

Prevention of serious disease following transplantation may be attempted through several interventions, such as patient selection and modification of immunosuppression.

Patient Selection

Until the introduction of nucleoside analogues, the presence of HBV replication was considered by some centers as a contraindication to transplantation because the rate of recurrence is higher in these patients than in those who are HBV DNA and HBeAg negative prior to transplantation.[2] The availability of new and effective treatments, mainly nucleoside analogues, that can reduce the level of viral replication prior to transplantation may obviate the need for selection on this basis.

HBV-infected patients are at high risk for developing hepatocellular carcinoma, a circumstance that is not uncommon in the transplant setting. Although the rate of cancer recurrence was very high in early series, more promising results have been obtained with an accurate staging of tumors and improved patient selection.[77,78] The criteria for selecting these patients are tumors without evidence of macroscopic vascular invasion, less than 3 lesions, and no single lesion greater than 5 centimeters in diameter.

Patient Management: Modification of Immunosuppression

Studies performed both *in vitro* and *in vivo* in immunocompetent patients have shown a detrimental effect of steroids on HBV replication. Although azathioprine also increases viral replication in *in vitro* models, it does so at concentrations not likely to be achieved in liver transplantation patients.[79,80] These effects have been reproduced in patients with chronic hepatitis B, in whom treatment with prednisolone and azathioprine led to an increase in both staining intensity and number of cells with hepatitis B core antigen, hepatitis e antigen, and HBV DNA.[81] Reactivation of quiescent infection, with rapid progression of liver disease in some cases, has been described after immunosuppression is initiated, supporting the deleterious effect of immunosuppression.[82] The mechanism by which steroids increase HBV replication is through the activation of a corticosteroid-responsive promoter region in the HBV genome.[83] These studies and observations have led to the common practice of rapidly lowering the dose of prednisone in patients undergoing transplantation for HBV-related end-stage liver disease. Although this practice seems relatively safe, its efficacy is yet to be proven.

The effect of other immunosuppressive agents, such as cyclosporine and tacrolimus (FK506), is uncertain. Neither cyclosporine nor tacrolimus given alone has an effect on HBV replication *in vitro*.[80,84] These *in vitro* studies were performed with short-term drug exposure, however, and thus may not correlate to the liver transplant situation, where long-term exposure is typical. In woodchucks with acute woodchuck hepatitis virus infection (WHV), 4 weeks of cyclosporine had no effect on viral replication, whereas longer treatment led to an increase in serum WHV DNA and enhanced hepatic expression of virus core antigen.[85] There are no studies directly comparing tacrolimus- and cyclosporine-based regimens in HBV-infected transplant recipients. As with patient selection, the introduction of highly effective prophylactic therapies may limit the importance of the type and dose of immunosuppression in determining the risk of recurrence.

Retransplantation

The initial results of retransplantation for patients with graft failure due to recurrent hepatitis B were discouraging because of high rates of HBV reinfection and even more aggressive disease in the second graft.[86] Improved outcomes have been achieved with specific interventions, mainly with the use of aggressive immunoprophylaxis to prevent HBV reinfection.[87,88]

De Novo Hepatitis B Infection

Donors who are positive for anti-HBc have been shown to transmit HBV infection despite negativity of the serum HBsAg in the donor.[89–92] Variable rates have been described, depending on the geographical prevalence of anti-HBc positivity in the general population. Variables associated with transmission include the anti-HBc status and the functional status of the recipient, and the age of the donor.[92] Several policies have been adopted, including use of these organs only for recipients already infected with HBV, and utilization of these organs only in cases of emergency or borderline indications. In the latter situations, HBIG alone or in combination with lamivudine is administered to prevent transmission, with good results, at least in the short term.[90,93]

Alternatively, because many of the patients undergoing transplantation have never been exposed to hepatitis B, it has been recommended that patients be vaccinated prior to transplantation, generally at the time of listing. An accelerated vaccination regimen has been adopted, with vaccine given at 0, 1, and 2 months and a follow-up vaccine at 6 months. However, as with other immunosuppressed populations, the results of vaccination in these patients have been disappointing.[94] Efficacy may improve with the use of new pre-S vaccines and DNA-based vaccines that promote high levels of HBV antigen expression and antigen presentation by major histocompatibility complex (MHC) molecules.[95]

HEPATITIS C VIRUS INFECTION

Natural History

HCV-related liver disease, alone or in combination with alcoholic liver disease, has become the leading indication for liver transplantation among adults, accounting for approximately half of transplantations in many centers. There is real concern that the number of patients in need of transplantation will increase in coming years given the prevalence of infection in the general population (1.8%), the 3-fold greater prevalence in those who are 30 to 50 years old as compared with older age groups, the eventual progression to cirrhosis in approximately one-fifth of those infected, and the lack of consistently effective antiviral therapy.

Recurrent infection after liver transplantation, defined as the presence of virus in serum, is universal.[96] Although histologic evidence of liver injury will develop in the majority within the first year posttransplantation, severe graft dysfunction is rare in the short term.[97] With longer periods of follow-up, a significant proportion of patients progress to cirrhosis (8% to 30% after a median of 5 to 7 years),[98,99] yet both patient and graft survival rates are comparable with that observed in patients undergoing transplantation for other nonmalignant indications.[98–101]

Several factors complicate the assessment of the long-term outcome of recurrent HCV infection. These include the insufficient number of patients or duration of follow-up in the majority of studies, the uncertainty about the most appropriate control group, the presence of pretransplantation or posttransplantation confounding or unidentified variables that may alter the outcome, and the end points chosen. Typical end points used, such as mortality, are unlikely to develop frequently within short and medium durations of follow-up. As a consequence, studies measuring the full effect of HCV infection on posttransplantation outcome will likely require long duration of follow-up and large numbers of cases and controls. Intermediate end points, such as histologic disease progression, have been recently applied in a large cohort of transplant patients. The rate of fibrosis progression per year was reported to be higher than that reported in the nontransplant population, suggesting that the duration required to develop signficant HCV-related liver damage will be shorter in immunosuppressed patients than in those who are immunocompetent.[102] Studies in which strict histologic follow-up is performed also suggest a more rapid progression to end-stage liver disease in these patients compared with those who are immunocompetent.[99] It is thus likely that the full effect of recurrent HCV infection will become apparent only with time. Although short-term survival is sufficiently good to warrant continued transplantation of this group of patients, the potential seriousness of this disease has led to therapeutic trials of antiviral agents for this indication.

Currently, several important questions are as yet unanswered:

1. What is the real effect of antiviral therapy in the natural history of HCV infection posttransplantation?
2. Can the patients most likely to benefit from therapy be identified?
3. Can treatment regimens be modified to improve the long-term response rate?
4. Should patients undergoing liver transplantation for HCV disease receive unique immunosuppression?
5. Is retransplantation an option for liver transplant recipients with HCV-related graft failure?
6. Should some HCV-infected patients be denied transplantation?

Prophylactic Therapy

In contrast to HBV infection, for which HBIG has been shown to be beneficial, there is currently no available intervention to prevent recurrence of HCV infection. In one study, polyclonal immunoglobulins containing anti-HCV were shown to decrease the incidence of recurrent HCV viremia measured 1 year posttransplantation.[103] However, given the humoral immune failure in providing adequate and long-lasting neutralizing immunity against HCV, one would predict that additional approaches will be necessary.

Preemptive Antiviral Therapy

Pretransplantation

Preemptive therapy may be initiated while awaiting liver transplantation in order to (a) stabilize or improve the hepatic function so that the need for liver transplantation may be delayed or even obviated, and (b) suppress viral replication so that the risk of posttransplantation HCV recurrence or aggressive recurrent HCV disease is reduced.

Studies of the kinetics of HCV have suggested that the effect of interferon, at least in genotype 1 infection, is dose dependent and directly antiviral, with a rapid HCV decline starting the first day of therapy.[104] These data suggest that therapy with interferon early before transplantation can theoretically become a way of improving long-term survival of these patients. There have been anecdotal case reports of the use of interferon in decompensated HCV cirrhotic patients, since these patients have typically been excluded from randomized trials. Interferon is poorly tolerated in this setting and could potentially precipitate worsening hepatic function. Modified regimens or combinations with ribavirin may be considered in these patients.

Although also scarce, more data are available on the efficacy of interferon with or without ribavirin in compensated cirrhotic patients. Results from several trials on interferon monotherapy have consistently shown a lower biochemical and virologic sustained response rate in cirrhotic patients (9% to 16%) compared with noncirrhotic patients (17% to 34%). This may not be true with combination therapy, however. Additional benefits from antiviral therapy may be reduction in the risk of developing hepatocellular carcinoma and in the risk of decompensation of hepatic function. Indeed, data are emerging that suggest that the incidence of hepatocellular carcinoma, hepatic decompensation, and the need for transplantation are reduced among compensated cirrhotic patients treated with interferon.[105-107] Cirrhotic patients should thus be included in studies evaluating the benefits of antiviral therapy, particularly combination therapy, in preventing the development of complications and ultimately in reducing the need for transplantation.

Posttransplantation

Another preemptive approach recently described is the use of either interferon alone[108,109] or in combination with ribavirin[110] early after liver transplantation in an attempt to prevent HCV disease recurrence or diminish the risk of aggressive histologic progression (Table 21.5). In one study,[108] 86 transplant recipients were randomized within 2 weeks of transplantation to receive either interferon alone (n = 38) or placebo (n = 48) for 1 year. Although patient and graft survival rates at 2 years did not differ between the groups, and the rate of persistence of HCV was not affected by treatment, histologic disease recurrence was observed less frequently in interferon-treated patients (8 of 30 who were evaluable at 1 year) than in those who were not treated (22 of 41; $p = 0.01$). In a second controlled trial,[109] 24 transplant recipients were randomized at 2 weeks posttransplantation to receive interferon or placebo for 6 months. Both the incidence of histologic recurrence and its severity did not differ between groups. However, interferon treatment delayed the development

TABLE 21.5. *Preemptive posttransplantation therapy for recurrent hepatitis C infection*

Reference (No. of patients)	Study type	Time from OLT to treatment (wk)	Type, dose, and duration of treatment	Histologic hepatitis C recurrence (treated vs untreated)	Differences in survival	Rejection rate (treated vs untreated)
109 (n = 24)	C, R	2	IFN-α_{2b}, 3 MU thrice weekly for 6 mo	50% vs. 42%	No	50% vs. 42%
108 (n = 38)	C, R	2	IFN-α_{2b}, 3 MU thrice weekly for 12 mo	25% vs. 53%	Yes	56% vs. 56%
110 (n = 21)	UC	3	Ribavirin (10 mg/kg/day) plus IFN-α_{2b} (216 MU) for 12 mo	57%[a]	NA	No rejection; hemolytic anemia, 38%

OLT, liver transplantation; C, controlled; R, randomized; UC, uncontrolled; NA, not available or not applicable; IFN-α_{2b}, interferon alfa 2b.

[a]Only 4.7% of patients developed significant histologic disease.

of HCV hepatitis, which occurred at a median of 408 days after transplantation in the treated group versus 193 days in the untreated group ($p = 0.05$). No differences in graft or patient survival were observed.

In a case series,[110] 21 recipients (19 of whom were infected with HCV genotype 1b) were treated with interferon alfa 2b and ribavirin starting the third week posttransplantation. After a median follow-up period of 12 months, 4 patients (19%) had developed acute recurrent hepatitis C, but only 1 (5%) had evolved to chronic active hepatitis, despite the presence of viremia in 12 (59%) of the patients. Common side effects included hemolytic anemia and asthenia, which were well controlled with dose reduction. No follow-up data were provided. Well-designed controlled randomized studies are needed to confirm these encouraging findings.

Treatment of Graft Disease Related to Hepatitis C

Treatment of recurrent HCV disease with interferon has thus far been disappointing, but initial results from combination therapy with interferon and ribavirin are encouraging (Table 21.6).

Interferon

The experience with interferon alone has been limited, and its efficacy appears to be moderate and transient. Interferon at doses of 3 MU, thrice weekly for 6 months, has failed to clear serum HCV RNA despite normalization of ALT values in a subset of patients treated (0% to 28%).[111,112] Relapse after discontinuing treatment is almost the rule, and posttreatment improvement in liver damage is not common. The potential reasons for the poor antiviral effect of interferon in the transplant setting are many, and likely relate to

high levels of HCV RNA during the posttransplantation period and to the high rate of infection by genotype 1, both of which have been associated with poor response to interferon in immunocompetent patients. Moreover, there has been concern about using interferon in solid-organ transplant recipients because it can upregulate the expression of HLA class I and II, which may in turn increase the risk of allograft rejection. In contrast to the renal transplant experience, interferon-induced rejection appears to be uncommon in the setting of liver transplantation.

Identification of variables associated with a sustained response could be useful for selecting patients most likely to benefit from interferon therapy. Unfortunately, because of the small number of studies evaluating this strategy as well as the low rates of sustained response, there are almost no data on predictive variables of response in this population. In general, low pretreatment levels of HCV RNA are associated with better initial responses to interferon therapy than high levels.[111]

In order, to improve on the rate of response, strategies such as optimization of the dose and duration of interferon or fine tuning the timing of initiation of therapy have been attempted. Prolonged interferon therapy has been described in one uncontrolled small study,[113] in which patients were treated for a mean of 21 months with an apparent enhanced response rate, which unfortunately was assessed by biochemical but not virologic end points. Two small case series have reported preliminary data on the use of interferon in the setting of acute hepatitis posttransplantation with the aim of decreasing the persistence of infection and the progression of disease.[114,115] Although this strategy was clearly ineffective in the first trial and was associated with a high rate of graft rejection, longer therapy appeared beneficial in the second study. Well-designed prospective trials are needed to assess this approach.

TABLE 21.6. *Therapy of recurrent hepatitis C infection with interferon or ribavirin or a combined regimen*

Reference (No. of patients)	Study type	Time from OLT to treatment (mo)	Type, total dose, and duration of treatment	Biochemical or virologic response at end of treatment*	Biochemical or virologic response after follow-up*	Histologic improvement after follow-up*	Rejection rate
111 (n = 18)	UC	15 ± 2 (4–38)	IFN-α_{2b}, 205 MU (mean), 5.7 ± 0.1 mo (4–6 mo)	BR: 5 (28%) VR: 1 (0.05%)	BR: 4 (22%) VR: 0	5 (28%)	0.05%
112 (n = 46)	C (n = 32), NR	31 ± 19 (7–60)	IFN-α_{2b}, 180 MU (mean), 5 ± 1.8 mo (1–6 mo)	BR: 2/9 (22%)[a] VR: 2/9 (22%)	BR: 1/9 (11%) VR: 1/9 (11%) Control: 0%	22% vs. 0%	35% vs. 3%
113 (n = 18)	UC	6.4 (1–37)	IFN-α, 108 MU (n = 10), 216 MU (n = 5), or 360 MU (n = 3); 6 mo (n = 7) and 11–36 mo (n = 11)	BR: 5 (28%)	BR: 11 (61%); 8/11 (73%) with maintenance IFN; 3/7 (43%) with 6-month course	75% vs. 0%	Acute rejection, 6% vs. 11%; chronic rejection, 0%
114 (n = 14)	C (n = 7), NR	2–3 mo	IFN-α_{2b}, 216 MU, 6 mo	BR: 0% vs. 0% VR: 0% vs. 0%	NA	Treated group, 0%; control group, NA	Acute rejection, 28% vs. 14%; chronic rejection, 28% vs. 0%
118 (n = 9)	UC	5 ± 3, 7	Ribavirin, 1,000–1,200 mg vo, 3 mo	BR: 4 (44%) VR: 0	BR: 0 VR: 0	25%	No rejection; symptomatic reversible hemolytic anemia in 3
119 (n = 30)	C, R	6–7	IFN (3 MU 3 times weekly) vs. ribavirin (1,200 mg/day), 6 mo	BR: 43% vs. 85% VR: 46% vs. 0%	NA	No improvement in fibrosis or HAI	2 patients withdrawn due to severe hemolysis
120 (n = 21)	UC	9 (3–24)	Ribavirin + IFN-α_{2b} (ribavirin, 1,000–1200 mg vo[b]; IFN, 216 MU), 6 mo	BR: 21 (100%) VR: 10 (48%)	During ribavirin maintenance: BR: 17/18 (94%) VR: 5/18 (28%)	94%	No rejection; symptomatic reversible hemolytic anemia in 3

OLT, orthotopic liver transplantation; C, controlled; UC, uncontrolled; R, randomized; NR, nonrandomized; IFN-α_{2b}, interferon alfa 2b; BR, biochemical response; VR, virologic response; NA, not available or not applicable; HAI, hepatic activity index.

*treated vs untreated

[a]Five patients developed chronic rejection; thus, analysis of response rate was performed on the remaining 9 patients.

[b]vo = oral route of administration

Ribavirin

Ribavirin is another agent that has been recently evaluated in small case series in the transplant population. This guanosine analogue inhibits the replication of a wide range of RNA and DNA viruses, but has been tested in immunocompetent patients with limited efficacy when administered alone. When administered in combination with interferon, efficacy is clearly increased.[116] In liver transplant recipients, ribavirin monotherapy was associated with biochemical improvement in many patients, but virologic clearance in none.[117–119] Biochemical relapse was universal after cessation of therapy, and no histologic improvement was observed. The main side effect was hemolysis, which resolved after the cessation of therapy. In one randomized trial,[119] 31 liver transplant recipients with chronic hepatitis C in the graft were randomized to receive either interferon or ribavirin for 24 weeks. After 12 months of therapy, ribavirin was superior to interferon in achieving normalization of serum aspartate aminotransferase levels (85% versus 43%, $p < 0.05$) and in reducing lobular inflammation (64% versus 21%, $p = 0.05$), but not in reducing the fibrosis stage or the total histologic activity index. In contrast, patients receiving interferon alone had reduction in HCV RNA but not complete elimination of viremia.

Combination Therapy

Combination therapy is an approach with initial promising results.[120–122] In a nonrandomized pilot study, Bizollon et al. assessed the safety and efficacy of combination therapy with ribavirin and interferon for the treatment of recurrent hepatitis C.[120] Twenty-one patients with early documented recurrent HCV hepatitis were treated with interferon alfa 2b (3 MU thrice weekly) and ribavirin (1,000 mg per day) for 6 months and then maintained on ribavirin monotherapy until the end of the study. All patients normalized ALT, and 11 (50%) cleared HCV RNA from serum at the end of the treatment period. The remaining patients, although viremic, experienced a 50% reduction in viral load. Only one patient had a biochemical relapse during the 6-months period on ribavirin alone, despite reappearance of serum HCV RNA in 50% who had initially cleared HCV RNA. Most important, all but one patient who tolerated the drug showed an improvement in liver histology. Safety and tolerability were satisfactory, with reversible hemolytic anemia being the most common side effect. No patient experienced graft rejection.[120] This favorable outcome is noteworthy because all patients had high HCV RNA levels (mean value of 125 mEq/mL), and 92% were infected with HCV genotype 1, features classically associated with lack of response to therapy. Early intervention with combined therapy at a stage when patients had not progressed to severe forms of liver injury may explain the good results obtained. Off-treatment response rates were not provided in this initial report, but maintenance therapy with ribavirin is probably important to avoid relapse, since all 3 patients who stopped ribavirin be-

cause of adverse events had a biochemical relapse associated with histologic deterioration.

The same authors have recently reported on the 12-month follow-up of 11 treated patients who cleared HCV RNA from serum and liver after the 12 months of ribavirin monotherapy. Ten (90%) of the patients maintained a sustained biochemical and virologic response, without significant histologic changes compared with the end-of-treatment biopsies.[121] These preliminary data suggest that maintenance therapy may be discontinued in patients who have responded virologically.

In another recent nonrandomized Italian multicenter study,[122] 122 liver transplant recipients with histologic evidence of recurrent hepatitis C were treated with interferon (3 MU thrice weekly) and ribavirin (600–1000 mg daily) for 6 to 12 months. Virologic response did not differ in patients treated for 6 months compared with those treated for 12 months (50% versus 50%). The cumulative probabilities of developing biochemical and virologic responses at the end of treatment were 72% and 35%, respectively. Of 78 patients with at least 6 months of follow-up, relapse was common, with 41 (53%) patients experiencing a biochemical relapse and 39 (50%) having detectable HCV RNA again in serum. These studies are encouraging, but the duration of follow-up once therapy is discontinued is still too short to draw valid conclusions. Randomized controlled trials, currently underway, are needed to define the true efficacy of this approach.

Alternative Approaches

In contrast to treatment of HBV infection, where important advances have been made, treatment of HCV infection continues to be based on interferon, either alone or in combination with ribavirin. In that sense, patient selection and patient management probably remain an important step in improving the long-term outcome of HCV-infected patients undergoing liver transplantation.

Patient Selection

Predictors of disease progression have been identified that could potentially be used to target treatment to patients with a high likelihood of progressive disease. HCV RNA levels prior to transplantation or in the early posttransplantation period (or both),[100,102] severe and early acute hepatitis,[99,123] and strong immunosuppression[124–126] currently appear as the three variables most consistently associated with poor outcome, but further analysis is required to confirm these findings. To this point, however, no single variable or combination of variables is capable of accurately predicting which individual will develop serious disease posttransplantation and which individual will not, thus preventing the precise selection of patients for early intervention or for transplant denial.

Coexistent hepatocellular carcinoma is increasingly common in patients with HCV infection. The criteria for selecting patients with HCV and localized hepatocellular carcinoma are no different from other indications, that is, tumors without evidence of macroscopic vascular invasion, less than 3 lesions, and no single lesion greater than 5 centimeters in diameter. With these selection criteria, survival rates do not differ from those achieved by HCV-infected patients without hepatocellular carcinoma.[77,78]

Patient Management

Identification of variables associated with worse outcome may help in the selection of HCV-infected liver transplant recipients who will benefit from therapy. In particular, since pretransplantation and early posttransplantation serum HCV RNA levels have been associated with the outcome following transplantation,[98,100,102] specific interventions prior to transplantation in order to decrease viral load may ultimately affect the posttransplantation course. The main limitation of this approach, however, is the tolerability and safety of interferon in patients with decompensated liver disease (see previous discussion).

The use of a specific immunosuppressive regimen less deleterious to HCV-infected patients is another approach that could theoretically improve the outcome. The optimal immunosuppressive regimen for HCV-infected patients is still unknown, however. The majority of studies have found no differences in patient or graft survival in recipients treated with cyclosporine-based versus tacrolimus-based induction regimens.[98,100] However, accurate assessment of the precise role played by specific immunosuppressive drugs in the progression of HCV-related liver disease may be impaired by the development of several new agents, with the subsequent multiplicity of combination regimens and the difficulty in quantifying the potency of new drugs. Studies of the role of immunosuppression in disease progression are problematic.

Because evidence is accumulating that the intensity of the immunosuppression (i.e., the number of grams of methylprednisolone, cumulative steroids, or OKT3 used) is related to the aggressiveness of HCV-related disease posttransplantation,[99,102,124–126] caution should be applied when deciding treatment for rejection. Currently, in many centers, mild rejection episodes are no longer treated, moderate episodes either remain untreated or are treated with low doses of methylprednisolone (1–3 g), and severe episodes continue to be treated with methylprednisolone boluses or by switching the immunosuppressive regimen.

Differentiating rejection episodes from recurrent hepatitis C may be difficult.[97] Histologic findings of marked ductal injury and venulitis, although occasionally seen in patients with recurrent hepatitis C, are also seen in episodes of rejection. Features suggestive of HCV infection include lymphoid aggregates, fatty changes, presence of acidophilic bodies, and sinusoidal dilatation, whereas those suggestive of rejection include endotheliitis, bile duct necrosis, and a mixed portal inflammatory infiltrate (eosinophils and neutrophils as well as mononuclear cells). Knowledge of the date of transplantation may also facilitate the interpretation of liver histology because rejection episodes typically occur earlier than recurrent hepatitis C, which is rarely observed in the first month after transplantation. If doubts persist, serial biopsies should be performed. A therapeutic trial with a short course of steroids, although previously proposed as a means to differentiate these entities, may be detrimental in the long term and thus is not currently recommended. If data exist that support the presence of both entities, treatment with corticosteroids may be initiated. Although rapid reduction in the doses of corticosteroids is becoming common practice in these patients, the efficacy of this approach is unproven.

Additional factors that have been implicated in the severity of HCV disease include necroinflammatory activity and fibrosis staging on the initial liver biopsy or first-year biopsy.[99,102,123] These data suggest that management should include early biopsies to identify patients for whom antiviral therapy will be beneficial or for whom high doses of immunosuppression will be detrimental.

Retransplantation

Because of the progressive nature of recurrent HCV disease, it is likely that in the next decade there will be a marked increase in the number of HCV-infected recipients in need of retransplantation. Indeed, the prevalence of HCV infection in patients undergoing retransplantation has increased significantly, from 6.5% in 1990 to 38.4% in 1995.[127] It has thus become imperative to determine whether all patients with graft failure due to recurrent HCV disease are candidates for further transplantation. This is a difficult issue to resolve currently because very few studies have focused on this problem, with early reports suggesting poor outcome;[128] also, there is an increasing shortage of organ donors, and doubts exist about retransplantation because of the incidence of recurrent severe HCV disease in the second graft.

Initial data have suggested that survival following retransplantation is particularly poor in patients with recurrent HCV.[127,128] Analysis of the United Network for Organ Sharing (UNOS) database demonstrated significantly diminished patient survival in HCV-infected patients undergoing retransplantation compared with uninfected patients (57%, 55%, and 54% at 1, 3, and 5 years, respectively, versus 65%, 63%, and 61%; $p = 0.0038$, log-rank test).[127] However, other factors, such as creatinine concentration, bilirubin level, and UNOS status, appear to have greater predictive value than HCV status in patients undergoing retransplantation.[129,130] Indeed, more recent data have suggested improved outcome, particularly when retransplantation is performed before severe hyperbilirubinemia and development of renal complications occur.[129,130]

In a recent study, Rosen et al. have developed and validated a survival model based on five readily available "bedside" variables—age, bilirubin level, creatinine concentration, UNOS status, and cause of graft failure—that accurately predicts survival after retransplantation. Although two models identified HCV seropositivity as significant, this variable was not included in the final model because it did not add to the estimation of prognosis.[130] This study suggests that application of retransplantation in low-risk patients, independent of HCV status, is a reasonable option because outcomes are comparable with primary transplantation. Whether retransplantation is justifiable in patients with high risk scores needs to be carefully evaluated.

The severity of recurrent HCV disease in the first graft does not seem to predict that observed in the second graft. Larger studies are needed to address this issue in more detail, however. The combination of an increasing shortage of organ donors and a growing number of patients in need of first transplantation will likely determine the candidacy of patients being considered for retransplantation.

CONCLUSION

In the absence of specific therapeutic interventions, viral reinfection with HBV or HCV is the rule. Although prophylactic therapy with HBIG has proved to be highly beneficial for HBV infection, there are currently no similar approaches for HCV infection. Despite the efficacy of HBIG, there are serious limitations to this approach, such as cost, side effects, and a 20% failure rate, that have focused interest on well-tolerated and effective nucleoside analogues. Although their evaluation is still underway, there are limitations to their use as monotherapy in the transplant setting; drug resistance in particular remains an issue. Defining the actual role of HBIG and nucleoside analogues in the transplant setting will likely be a difficult task to solve during the next several years.

Despite uncertainties regarding rates of posttransplantation disease progression, there is a consensus emerging that recurrent HCV infection results in liver failure in a significant although currently unmeasured proportion of patients and that the time course over which this progression occurs is shorter than in the immunocompetent population. As the disease process moves into its second decade, it can be anticipated that future morbidity and liver-related mortality will increase. Strategies to prevent or to reduce the effect of HCV infection after liver transplantation are therefore essential. Our ability to intervene in this disease is currently limited. The main obstacles are the difficulty in predicting the outcome in the individual patient and the lack of effective therapy. Neither interferon nor ribavirin, when administered as single agents, result in sustained viral clearance. However, administration of both drugs given in combination either to prevent disease or to treat recurrence when it occurs appears promising.

The inability of currently available antiviral therapies to eliminate HCV or HBV in the setting of liver transplantation suggests that indefinite treatment designed to suppress viral replication will be necessary. The feasibility of such an approach will depend on development of drugs that re-duce the histologic activity of hepatitis, improve graft and patient survival, have acceptable side effect profiles, and have an acceptable cost.

REFERENCES

1. Todo S, Demetris A, Van Thiel D, et al. Orthotopic liver transplantation for patients with hepatitis B virus-related liver disease. *Hepatology* 1991;13:619–626.
2. Samuel D, Muller R, Alexander G, et al. Liver transplantation in European patients with the hepatitis B surface antigen. *N Engl J Med* 1993;329:1842–1847.
3. Muller R, Gubernatis G, Farle M, et al. Liver transplantation in HBs antigen (HBsAg) carriers: prevention of hepatitis B virus (HBV) recurrence by passive immunization. *J Hepatol* 1991;13:90–96.
4. Samuel D, Bismuth A, Mathieu D, et al. Passive immunoprophylaxis after liver transplantation in HBsAg-positive patients. *Lancet* 1991; 337:813–815.
5. Konig V, Hopf U, Neuhaus P, et al. Long-term follow up of hepatitis B virus-infected recipients after orthotopic liver transplantation. *Transplantation* 1994;58:553–559.
6. Devlin J, Smith H, O'Grady J, et al. Impact of immunoprophylaxis and patient selection on outcome of transplantation for HBsAg-positive liver recipients. *J Hepatol* 1994;21:204–210.
7. McGory RW, Ishitani MB, Oliveira WM, et al. Improved outcome of orthotopic liver transplantation for chronic hepatitis B cirrhosis with aggressive passive immunization. *Transplantation* 1996;61:1358–1364.
8. Terrault N, Zhou S, Combs C, et al. Prophylaxis in liver transplant recipients using a fixed dosing schedule of hepatitis B immunoglobulin. *Hepatology* 1996;24:1327–1333.
9. Al-Hemsi B, McGory R, Shepard B, et al. Liver transplantation for hepatitis B cirrhosis: clinical sequelae of passive immunization. *Clin Transpl* 1996;10:668–675.
10. Lowell JA, Burgess S, Shenoy S, et al. Mercury poisoning associated with high-dose hepatitis-B immune globulin administration after liver transplantation for chronic hepatitis B. *Liver Transplant Surg* 1996; 2:475–478.
11. Muller R, Samuel D, Fassati L, et al. "EUROHEP" consensus report on the management of liver transplantation for hepatitis B virus infection. *J Hepatol* 1994;21:1140–1143.
12. Feray C, Zignego A, Samuel D, et al. Persistent hepatitis B virus infection of mononuclear blood cells without concomitant liver infection. *Transplantation* 1990;49:1155–1158.
13. Brind A, Jiang J, Samuel D, et al. Evidence for selection of hepatitis B mutants after liver transplantation through peripheral blood mononuclear cell infection. *J Hepatol* 1997;26:228–235.
14. Villamil E, Kuhn M, Makowka L, et al. Quantitative anti-HBs titers during intramuscular (IM) hepatitis B immunoglobulin (HBIG) administration post-liver transplantation (LT) for hepatitis B [Abstract]. *Hepatology* 1992;16:49A.
15. Yao FY, Osorio RW, Roberts JP, et al. Intramuscular hepatitis B immune globulin combined with lamivudine for prophylaxis against hepatitis B recurrence after liver transplantation. *Liver Transplant Surg* 1999;5:491–496.
16. Yoshida EM, Erb SR, Partovi N, et al. Liver transplantation for chronic hepatitis B infection with the use of combination lamivudine and low-dose hepatitis B immune globulin. *Liver Transplant Surg* 1999;5:520–525.
17. McCaughan GW, Spencer J, Koorey D, et al. Lamivudine therapy in patients undergoing liver transplantation for hepatitis B virus precore mutant-associated infection: high resistance rates in treatment of recurrence but universal prevention if used as prophylaxis with very low dose hepatitis B immune globulin. *Liver Transplant Surg* 1999;5:512–519.
18. Adler R, Safadi R, Caraco Y, et al. Comparison of immune reactivity and pharmacokinetics of two hepatitis B immune globulins in patients after liver transplantation. *Hepatology* 1999;29:1299–1305.
19. Cariani E, Ravaggi A, Tanzi E, et al. Emergence of hepatitis B virus S gene mutant in a liver transplant recipient. *J Med Virol* 1995;47: 410–415.
20. Trautwein C, Schrem H, Tillmann HL, et al. Hepatitis B virus mutations in the pre-S genome before and after liver transplantation. *Hepatology* 1996;24:482–488.

21. Carman WF, Trautwein C, van Deursen FJ, et al. Hepatitis B virus envelope variation after transplantation with and without hepatitis B immune globulin prophylaxis. *Hepatology* 1996;24:489–493.
22. Hawkins AE, Gilson RJ, Gilbert N, et al. Hepatitis B virus surface mutations associated with infection after liver transplantation. *J Hepatol* 1996;24:8–14.
23. Ghany MG, Ayola B, Villamil FG, et al. Hepatitis B virus S mutants in liver transplant recipients who were reinfected despite hepatitis B immune globulin prophylaxis. *Hepatology* 1998;27:213–222.
24. Protzer-Knolle U, Naumann U, Bartenschlager R, et al. Hepatitis B virus with antigenically altered hepatitis B surface antigen is selected by high-dose hepatitis B immune globulin after liver transplantation. *Hepatology* 1998;27:254–263.
25. Terrault NA, Zhou S, McCory RW, et al. Incidence and clinical consequences of surface and polymerase gene mutations in liver transplant recipients on hepatitis B immunoglobulin. *Hepatology* 1998;28:555–561.
26. Nery JR, Weppler D, Rodriguez M, et al. Efficacy of lamivudine in controlling hepatitis B virus recurrence after liver transplantation. *Transplantation* 1998;65:1615–1621.
27. Locarnini S. Hepatitis B virus surface antigen and polymerase gene variants: potential virological and clinical significance. *Hepatology* 1998;27:294–297.
28. Perrillo R, Tamburro C, Regenstein F, et al. Low-dose, titratable interferon alfa in decompensated liver disease caused by chronic infection with hepatitis B virus. *Gastroenterology* 1995;109:908–916.
29. Balfour HH. Antiviral drugs. *N Engl J Med* 1999;340:1255–1268.
30. Berenguer M, Wright TL. Hepatitis B and C viruses: molecular identification and targeted antiviral therapies. *Proc Assoc Am Physicians* 1998;110:98–112.
31. Zoulim F, Trepo C. Drug therapy for chronic hepatitis B: antiviral efficacy and influence of hepatitis B virus polymerase mutations on the outcome of therapy. *J Hepatol* 1998;29:151–168.
32. Dienstag JL, Perrillo RP, Schiff ER, et al. A preliminary trial of lamivudine for chronic hepatitis B infection. *N Engl J Med* 1995;333:1657–1661.
33. Lai CL, Ching CK, Tung AK, et al. Lamivudine is effective in suppressing hepatitis B virus DNA in Chinese hepatitis B surface antigen carriers: a placebo-controlled trial. *Hepatology* 1997;25:241–244.
34. Lai CL, Chien RN, Leung NW, et al. A one-year trial of lamivudine for chronic hepatitis B. Asia Hepatitis Lamivudine Study Group. *N Engl J Med* 1998;339:61–68.
35. Main J, Brown JL, Howells C, et al. A double blind, placebo-controlled study to assess the effect of famciclovir on virus replication in patients with chronic hepatitis B virus infection. *J Viral Hepat* 1996;3:211–215.
36. Ling R, Mutimer D, Ahmed M, et al. Selection of mutations in the hepatitis B virus polymerase during therapy of transplant recipients with lamivudine. *Hepatology* 1996;24:711–713.
37. Tipples GA, Ma MM, Fischer KP, et al. Mutation in HBV RNA-dependent DNA polymerase confers resistance to lamivudine *in vivo*. *Hepatology* 1996;24:714–717.
38. Bartholomew MM, Jansen RW, Jeffers LJ, et al. Hepatitis-B-virus resistance to lamivudine given for recurrent infection after orthotopic liver transplantation. *Lancet* 1997;349:20–22.
39. Aye TT, Bartholomeusz A, Shaw T, et al. Hepatitis B virus polymerase mutations during antiviral therapy in a patient following liver transplantation. *J Hepatol* 1997;26:1148–1153.
40. Allen M, Deslauriers M, Andrews C, et al. Identification and characterization of mutations in hepatitis B virus resistant to lamivudine. *Hepatology* 1998;27:1670–1677.
41. Chayama K, Suzuki Y, Kobayashi M, et al. Emergence and takeover of YMDD motif mutant hepatitis B virus during long-term lamivudine therapy and re-takeover by wild type after cessation of therapy. *Hepatology* 1998;27:1711–1716.
42. Bain VG, Kneteman NM, Ma MM, et al. Efficacy of lamivudine in chronic hepatitis B patients with active viral replication and decompensated cirrhosis undergoing liver transplantation. *Transplantation* 1996;62:1456–1462.
43. Grellier L, Mutimer D, Ahmed M, et al. Lamivudine prophylaxis against reinfection in liver transplantation for hepatitis B cirrhosis. *Lancet* 1996;348:1212–1215.
44. Perrillo R, Rakela J, Dienstag J, et al. Multicenter study of lamivudine therapy for hepatitis B after liver transplantation. *Hepatology* 1999;29:1581–1586.

45. Nevens F, Main J, Honkoop P, et al. Lamivudine therapy for chronic hepatitis B: a six-month randomized dose-ranging study. *Gastroenterology* 1997;113:1258–1263.
46. Gish RG, Lau JY, Brooks L, et al. Ganciclovir treatment of hepatitis B virus infection in liver transplant recipients. *Hepatology* 1996;23:1–7.
47. Cirelli R, Herne K, McCrary M, et al. Famciclovir: review of clinical efficacy and safety. *Antiviral Res* 1996;29:141–151.
48. Cundy KC. Clinical pharmacokinetics of the antiviral nucleotide analogues cidofovir and adefovir. *Clin Pharmacokinet* 1999;36:127–143.
49. Xiong X, Flores C, Yang H, et al. Mutations in hepatitis B DNA polymerase associated with resistance to lamivudine do not confer resistance to adefovir *in vitro*. *Hepatology* 1998;28:1669–1673.
50. Marcellin P, Giuily N, Loriot MA, et al. Prolonged interferon-alpha therapy of hepatitis B virus-related decompensated cirrhosis. *J Viral Hepat* 1997;4(suppl 1):21–26.
51. Marcellin P, Samuel D, Areias J, et al. Pretransplantation interferon treatment and recurrence of hepatitis B virus infection after liver transplantation for hepatitis B-related end-stage liver disease. *Hepatology* 1994;19:6–12.
52. Perrillo R, Rakela J, Martin P, et al. Lamivudine for suppression and/or prevention of hepatitis B when given pre/post transplantation [Abstract]. *Hepatology* 1997;26:260A.
53. Singh N, Gayowski T, Wannstedt CF, et al. Pretransplant famciclovir as prophylaxis for hepatitis B virus recurrence after liver transplantation. *Transplantation* 1997;63:1415–1419.
54. Markowitz JS, Martin P, Conrad AJ, et al. Prophylaxis against hepatitis B recurrence following liver transplantation using combination lamivudine and hepatitis B immune globulin. *Hepatology* 1998;28:585–589.
55. Naoumov NV, Lopes R, Crepaldi G, et al. Randomized trial of lamivudine (LAM) versus hepatitis B immunoglobulin (HBIG) for prophylaxis of HBV recurrence after liver transplantation [Abstract]. *J Hepatol* 1999;30(suppl 1):51.
56. Wright HI, Gavaler JS, Van Theil DH. Preliminary experience with alpha-2b-interferon therapy of viral hepatitis in liver allograft recipients. *Transplantation* 1992;53:121–124.
57. Hopf U, Neuhaus P, Lobeck H, et al. Follow-up of recurrent hepatitis B and D infection in liver allograft recipients after treatment with recombinant interferon-alpha. *J Hepatol* 1991;13:339–346.
58. Terrault NA, Holland CC, Ferrell L, et al. Interferon alfa for recurrent hepatitis B infection after liver transplantation. *Liver Transplant Surg* 1996;2:132–138.
59. Ben-Ari Z, Shmueli D, Shapira Z, et al. Loss of serum HBsAg after interferon-A therapy in liver transplant patients with recurrent hepatitis-B infection. *Liver Transplant Surg* 1997;3:394–397.
60. Ben-Ari Z, Shmueli D, Mor E, et al. Beneficial effect of lamivudine in recurrent hepatitis B after liver transplantation. *Transplantation* 1997;63:393–396.
61. Andreone P, Caraceni P, Grazi GL, et al. Lamivudine treatment for acute hepatitis B after liver transplantation. *J Hepatol* 1998;29:985–989.
62. Al Faraidy K, Yoshida EM, Davis JE, et al. Alteration of the dismal natural history of fibrosing cholestatic hepatitis secondary to hepatitis B virus with the use of lamivudine. *Transplantation* 1997;64:926–928.
63. Kruger M, Tillmann HL, Trautwein C, et al. Famciclovir treatment of hepatitis B virus recurrence after liver transplantation: a pilot study. *Liver Transplant Surg* 1996;2:253–262.
64. Klein M, Geoghegan J, Schmidt K, et al. Conversion of recurrent D-positive hepatitis B infection to seronegativity with famciclovir after liver transplantation. *Transplantation* 1997;64:162–163.
65. McCaughan G, Angus P, Bowden S, et al. Retransplantation for precore mutant-related chronic hepatitis B infection: prolonged survival in a patient receiving sequential ganciclovir/famciclovir therapy. *Liver Transplant Surg* 1996;2:472–474.
66. Neuhaus P, Manns M, Atkinson G for the FCV Liver Transplant Study Group. Safety and efficacy of famciclovir for the treatment of recurrent hepatitis B in liver transplant recipients [Abstract]. *Hepatology* 1997;26:260A.
67. Rayes N, Seehofer D, Bechstein WO, et al. Long-term results of famciclovir for recurrent or *de novo* hepatitis B virus infection after liver transplantation.

68. Niesters H, Honkoop P, Haagsma E, et al. Identification of more than one mutation in the hepatitis B virus polymerase gene arising during prolonged lamivudine treatment. *J Infect Dis* 1998;177: 1382–1385.

69. Marzano A, Debernardi-Venon W, Condreay L, et al. Efficacy of lamivudine re-treatment in a patient with hepatitis B virus (HBV) recurrence after liver transplantation and HBV-DNA breakthrough during the first treatment. *Transplantation* 1998;65:1499–1500.

70. de Man RA, Bartholomeusz AI, Niesters HG, et al. The sequential occurrence of viral mutations in a liver transplant recipient re-infected with hepatitis B: hepatitis B immune globulin escape, famciclovir non-response, followed by lamivudine resistance resulting in graft loss. *J Hepatol* 1998;29:669–675.

71. Ben-Ari Z, Pappo O, Zemel R, et al. Association of lamivudine resistance in recurrent hepatitis B after liver transplantation with advanced hepatic fibrosis. *Transplantation* 1999;68:232–236.

72. Melegari M, Scaglioni PP, Wands JR. Hepatitis B virus mutants associated with 3TC and famciclovir administration are replication defective. *Hepatology* 1998;27:628–633.

73. Gibbs CS, Westland CW, Yang H, et al. *In vitro* analysis of cross-resistance profiles of new antivirals for chronic HBV infection [Abstract]. *J Hepatol* 1999;30(suppl 1):62.

74. Xiong X, Yang H, Westland CE, et al. *In vitro* evaluation of hepatitis B virus polymerase mutations associated with famciclovir resistance. *Hepatology* 2000;31:219–224.

75. Nowak MA, Bonhoeffer S, Hill AM, et al. Viral dynamics in hepatitis B virus infection. *Proc Natl Acad Sci U S A* 1996;93:4398–4402.

76. Zeuzem S, de Man RA, Honkoop P, et al. Dynamics of hepatitis B virus infection *in vivo*. *J Hepatol* 1997;27:431–436.

77. Figueras J, Jaurrieta E, Valls C, et al. Survival after liver transplantation in cirrhotic patients with and without hepatocellular carcinoma: a comparative study. *Hepatology* 1997;25:1485–1489.

78. Mazzaferro V, Regalia E, Doci R, et al. Liver transplantation for the treatment of small hepatocellular carcinomas in patients with cirrhosis. *N Engl J Med* 1996;334:693–699.

79. Lau JY, Bain VG, Smith HM, et al. Modulation of hepatitis B viral antigen expression by immunosuppressive drugs in primary hepatocyte culture. *Transplantation* 1992;53:894–898.

80. McMillan JS, Shaw T, Angus PW, et al. Effect of immunosuppressive and antiviral agents on hepatitis B virus replication *in vitro*. *Hepatology* 1995;22:36–43.

81. Lau JY, Bird GL, Alexander GJ, et al. Effects of immunosuppressive therapy on hepatic expression of hepatitis B viral genome and gene products. *Clin Invest Med* 1993;16:226–236.

82. Lok A, Liang R, Chiu E, et al. Reactivation of hepatitis B virus replication in patients receiving cytotoxic therapy. *Gastroenterology* 1991; 100:182–188.

83. Tur-Kaspa R, Burk R, Shaul Y, et al. Hepatitis B virus DNA contains a glucocorticoid-responsive element. *Proc Natl Acad Sci U S A* 1986; 82:1627–1631.

84. Wong PY, Marinos G, Peakman M, et al. FK506 in liver transplantation for chronic hepatitis B: *in vitro* studies on lymphocyte activation and virus replication. *Liver Transplant Surg* 1995;1:362–370.

85. Cote PJ, Korba BE, Steinberg H, et al. Cyclosporin A modulates the course of woodchuck hepatitis virus infection and induces chronicity. *J Immunol* 1991;146:3138–3144.

86. Crippin J, Foster B, Carlen S, et al. Retransplantation for hepatitis B— a multicenter experience. *Transplantation* 1994;57:823–826.

87. Ishitani M, McGory R, Dickson R, et al. Retransplantation of patients with severe posttransplant hepatitis B in the first allograft. *Transplantation* 1997;64:410–414.

88. Roche B, Samuel D, Feray C, et al. Retransplantation of the liver for recurrent hepatitis B virus infection: the Paul Brousse experience. *Liver Transplant Surg* 1999;5:166–174.

89. Dickson RC, Everhart JE, Lake JR, et al. Transmission of hepatitis B by transplantation of livers from donors positive for antibody to hepatitis B core antigen. The National Institute of Diabetes and Digestive and Kidney Diseases liver transplantation database. *Gastroenterology* 1997;113:1668–1674.

90. Uemoto S, Sugiyama K, Marusawa H, et al. Transmission of hepatitis B virus from hepatitis B core antibody-positive donors in living related liver transplants. *Transplantation* 1998;65:494–499.

91. Van Thiel DH, De Maria N, Colantoni A, et al. Can hepatitis B core antibody positive livers be used safely for transplantation? Hepatitis B

92. Prieto M, García A, Gómez MD, et al. *De novo* hepatitis B virus infection after liver transplantation (OLT) from anti-HBc positive donors. *Transplantation* 1999;67:S17.

93. Dodson SF, Bonham CA, Geller DA, et al. Prevention of *de novo* hepatitis B infection in recipients of hepatic allografts from anti-HBc positive donors. *Transplantation* 1999;68:1058–1061.

94. Chalasani N, Smallwood G, Halcomb J, et al. Is vaccination against hepatitis B infection indicated in patients waiting for or after orthotopic liver transplantation? *Liver Transplant Surg* 1998; 4:128–132.

95. Rollier C, Sunyach C, Barraud L, et al. Protective and therapeutic effect of DNA-based immunization against hepadnavirus large envelope protein. *Gastroenterology* 1999;116:658–665.

96. Wright T, Donegan E, Hsu H, et al. Recurrent and acquired hepatitis C viral infection in liver transplant recipients. *Gastroenterology* 1992; 103:317–322.

97. Ferrell L, Wright T, Roberts J, et al. Hepatitis C viral infection in liver transplant recipients. *Hepatology* 1992;16:865–876.

98. Gane E, Portmann B, Naoumov N, et al. Long-term outcome of hepatitis C infection after liver transplantation. *N Engl J Med* 1996;334: 815–820.

99. Prieto M, Berenguer M, Rayón M, et al. High incidence of allograft cirrhosis in hepatitis C virus genotype 1b infection following transplantation: relationship with rejection episodes. *Hepatology* 1999;29:250–256.

100. Charlton M, Seaberg E, Wiesner R, et al. Predictors of patient and graft survival following liver transplantation for hepatitis C. *Hepatology* 1998;28:823–830.

101. Feray C, Caccamo L, Alexander GJM, et al. European collaborative study on factors influencing the outcome after liver transplantation for hepatitis C. *Gastroenterology* 1999;117:619–625.

102. Berenguer M, Ferrell L, Watson J, et al. HCV-related fibrosis progression following liver transplantation: increase in recent years. *J Hepatol* 2000 *(in press)*.

103. Feray C, Gigou M, Samuel D, et al. Incidence of hepatitis C in patients receiving different preparations of hepatitis B immunoglobulins after liver transplantation. *Ann Intern Med* 1998;128:810–816.

104. Neumann AU, Lam NP, Dahari H, et al. Hepatitis C viral dynamics *in vivo* and the antiviral efficacy of interferon-alpha therapy. *Science* 1998;282:103–107.

105. International Interferon-α Hepatocellular Carcinoma Study Group. Effect of interferon-α on progression of cirrhosis to hepatocellular carcinoma: a retrospective cohort study. *Lancet* 1998;351:1535–1539.

106. Kasahara A, Hayashi N, Mochizuki K, et al. Risk factors for hepatocellular carcinoma and its incidence after interferon treatment in patients with chronic hepatitis C. *Hepatology* 1998;27:1394–1402.

107. Serfarty L, Aumaître H, Chazouillères O, et al. Determinants of outcome of compensated hepatitis C virus-related cirrhosis. *Hepatology* 1998;27:1435–1440.

108. Sheiner P, Boros P, Klion FM, et al. The efficacy of prophylactic interferon alfa-2b in preventing recurrent hepatitis C after liver transplantation. *Hepatology* 1998;28:831–838.

109. Singh N, Gayowski T, Wannstedt C, et al. Interferon-α for prophylaxis of recurrent viral hepatitis C in liver transplant recipients. *Transplantation* 1998;65:82–86.

110. Mazzaferro V, Regalia E, Pulvirenti A, et al. Prophylaxis against HCV recurrence after liver transplantation. Effect of interferon and ribavirin combination. *Transplant Proc* 1997;29:519–521.

111. Wright TL, Combs C, Kim M, et al. Interferon alpha therapy for hepatitis C virus infection following liver transplantation. *Hepatology* 1994;20:773–779.

112. Feray C, Samuel D, Gigou M, et al. An open trial of interferon alfa recombinant for hepatitis C after liver transplantation: antiviral effects and risk of rejection. *Hepatology* 1995;22:1084–1089.

113. Singh N, Gayowski T, Wannstedt CF, et al. Interferon-alpha therapy for hepatitis C virus recurrence after liver transplantation: long-term response with maintenance therapy. *Clin Transplant* 1996;10:348–351.

114. Vargas V, Charco R, Castells L, et al. Alpha-interferon for acute hepatitis C in liver transplant patients. *Transplant Proc* 1995;27:1222–1223.

115. Boillot O, Berger F, Rasolofo E, et al. Effects of early interferon alfa therapy for hepatitis C virus infection recurrence after liver transplantation. *Transplant Proc* 1995;27:2501.

116. Liang TJ. Combination therapy for hepatitis C infection. *N Engl J Med* 1998;339:1549–1550.

117. Gane EJ, Tibbs CJ, Ramage JK, et al. Ribavirin therapy for hepatitis C infection following liver transplantation. *Transpl Int* 1995;8:61–64.

118. Cattral MS, Hemming AW, Wanless IR, et al. Outcome of long-term ribavirin therapy for recurrent hepatitis C after liver transplantation. *Transplantation* 1999;67:1277–1280.

119. Gane EJ, Lo SK, Riordan SM, et al. A randomized study comparing ribavirin and interferon alfa monotherapy for hepatitis C recurrence after liver transplantation. *Hepatology* 1998;27:1403–1407.

120. Bizollon T, Palazzo U, Ducerf C, et al. Pilot study of the combination of interferon alfa and ribavirin as therapy of recurrent hepatitis C after liver transplantation. *Hepatology* 1997;26:500–504.

121. Bizollon T, Ducerf C, Chevallier M, et al. Long-term efficacy of ribavirin plus IFN in the treatment of HCV recurrence after liver transplantation. Presented at the eleventh Congress of the European Society for Organ Transplantation, Oslo, June 1999. Abstract 20.

122. Bellatti G, Alberti AB, Belli LS, et al. Therapy of chronic hepatitis C after liver transplantation: multicenter italian experience [Abstract]. *J Hepatol* 1999;30(suppl 1):51.

123. Rosen HR, Gretch DR, Oehlke M, et al. Timing and severity of initial hepatitis C recurrence as predictors of long-term liver allograft injury. *Transplantation* 1998;65:1178–1182.

124. Sheiner PA, Schwartz ME, Mor E, et al. Severe or multiple rejection episodes are associated with early recurrence of hepatitis C after orthotopic liver transplantation. *Hepatology* 1995;21:30–34.

125. Berenguer M, Prieto M, Córdoba J, et al. Early development of chronic active hepatitis in recurrent hepatitis C virus infection after liver transplantation: association with treatment of rejection. *J Hepatol* 1998;28:756–763.

126. Rosen HR, Shackleton CR, Higa L, et al. Use of OKT3 is associated with early and severe recurrence of hepatitis C after liver transplantation. *Am J Gastroenterol* 1997;92:1453–1457.

127. Rosen HR, Martin P. Hepatitis C infection in patients undergoing liver retransplantation. *Transplantation* 1998;66:1612–1616.

128. Sheiner PA, Schluger LK, Emre S, et al. Retransplantation for recurrent hepatitis C. *Liver Transplant Surg* 1997;3:130–136.

129. Rosen H, O'Reilly P, Shackleton C, et al. Graft loss following liver transplantation in patients with chronic hepatitis C. *Transplantation* 1997;62:1773–1776.

130. Rosen HR, Madden JP, Martin P. A model to predict survival following liver retransplantation. *Hepatology* 1999;29:365–370.

Transplantation of the Liver, edited by Willis C. Maddrey, Eugene R. Schiff, and Michael F. Sorrell. Lippincott Williams & Wilkins, Philadelphia © 2001.

CHAPTER **22**

Liver Transplantation in Patients with Fulminant Hepatitis

Didier Samuel and Henri Bismuth

The field of liver transplantation has changed dramatically in the last 15 years. Liver transplantation was initially established as a treatment for patients with end-stage chronic liver disease; transplantation for acute liver failure was proposed later. Before 1986, few cases of liver transplantation for fulminant hepatitis had been reported, with only some successful cases.[1-3] The reasons for the low success rate were multiple: (a) The criteria for the indications of liver transplantation as well as for the timing of transplantation were not clearly defined, (b) the national organizations of organ sharing were not well organized for emergency liver allocation, and (c) there were technical limits to the ability to correct coagulation defects or to perform transplantation in patients with multiple organ failure (associated anuria, sepsis, etc.). In our center, a program of emergency liver transplantation for fulminant and subfulminant hepatitis was begun in January 1986; our experience was previously reported.[4,5]

In the last few years, there has been a dramatic increase in the number of liver transplantations performed worldwide for fulminant or subfulminant hepatitis. These conditions represented 10% of the indications for liver transplantation in the European Liver Transplant Registry in 1996 (Fig. 22.1).[6]

DEFINITION

Three main definitions have been given for fulminant hepatitis. Trey and Davidson have defined fulminant hepatitis as acute hepatitis complicated by acute liver failure, with hepatic encephalopathy occurring less than 8 weeks

after the onset of jaundice.[7] Bernuau and colleagues have defined fulminant hepatitis as acute hepatitis complicated by acute liver failure, with hepatic encephalopathy occurring less than 2 weeks after the onset of jaundice; and subfulminant hepatitis as acute hepatitis complicated by acute liver failure, with hepatic encephalopathy occurring 2 weeks to 3 months after the onset of jaundice.[8] The group at King's College have defined three categories: hyperacute liver failure, with a delayed onset of jaundice and encephalopathy of 7 days; acute liver failure, with a delayed onset of jaundice and encephalopathy of less than 28 days; and subacute liver failure, with a delayed onset of jaundice and encephalopathy of less than 3 months.[9] The common points of these definitions are the occurrence of encephalopathy during the course of acute hepatitis in a patient without known previous liver diseases, and the spontaneous poor prognosis (an 85% mortality rate). This chapter uses Bernuau and colleagues' definitions of fulminant and subfulminant hepatitis.

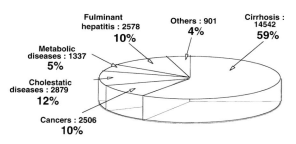

FIG. 22.1. Indications for liver transplantation in Europe from January 1988 to June 1998 in 24,743 patients. (Adapted from the European Liver Transplant Registry held at Hopital Paul Brousse, Villejuif, France; property of the European Liver Transplant Association.)

D. Samuel and H. Bismuth: Centre HépatoBiliaire, Faculté de Médecine Paris Sud, Hopital Paul Bousse, 94800, Villejuif, France.

Hepatic encephalopathy is classified into four stages according to the definition of Trey and Davidson:[7]

Stage 1: Slow consciousness
Stage 2: Accentuation of stage 1 and presence of asterixis
Stage 3: Presence of deep confusion or only reactive to vocal stimuli
Stage 4: Presence of deep coma assessed by at least the absence of reactions to vocal stimuli

In stage 3 and 4 encephalopathy, the presence of coma is classified into four grades:

Grade 1: Reactivity to vocal stimuli
Grade 2: Absence of reactivity to vocal stimuli, with coordinate response to nociceptive stimuli
Grade 3: Absence of reactivity to vocal stimuli, with incoordinate response to nociceptive stimuli
Grade 4: Brain death

Intracranial hypertension can be suspected on the occurrence of the following clinical symptoms: marked hyperventilation, opisthotonos, hyperpronation-adduction of the arms, cardiac arrhythmia, myoclonias, seizures, and poorly reactive pupils.

CAUSES OF FULMINANT AND SUBFULMINANT HEPATITIS

In France, acute viral hepatitis is the major cause of fulminant and subfulminant hepatitis. In our series of 150 patients admitted for fulminant or subfulminant hepatitis, 48% were affected with acute viral hepatitis: hepatitis B virus (HBV) either alone or together with hepatitis D virus (HDV) in 33.5% and 7%, respectively; hepatitis A virus (HAV) in 5%; non-A, non-B, non-C hepatitis in 2%; and herpesviruses in 0.5%. The other causes were drug-induced hepatitis in 21%, toxic ingestion (e.g., *Amanita phalloides* ingestion, massive acetaminophen ingestion) in 3%, various causes in 4%, and indeterminate causes in 24%. Hepatitis C virus (HCV) infection by itself is almost never responsible for the occurrence of fulminant hepatitis.[10,11] In contrast to France, acetaminophen overdose was the main cause of fulminant hepatitis in Great Britain. In a British series of 342 patients admitted from 1993 to 1994, the cause of the hepatitis was acetaminophen overdose in 250 (73%), HAV infection in 8 (2%), HBV infection in 8 (2%), non A–E hepatitis in 28 (8%), drug-induced hepatitis in 9 (3%), and other causes in 39 (12%).[12]

Rare causes of fulminant liver disease are a fulminant course of Wilson's disease, Budd-Chiari syndrome, Reye syndrome, massive malignant infiltration of the liver (liver metastasis, leukemia, lymphoma), hypoxic hepatitis due to cardiac failure, heatstroke, fatty infiltration of the liver, and HELLP syndrome (hemolysis, elevated liver function, and low platelets).

FULMINANT OR SUBFULMINANT HEPATITIS BEFORE THE ADVENT OF LIVER TRANSPLANTATION

Patient Outcome

Before the advent of liver transplantation, the overall mortality rate in patients with fulminant and subfulminant hepatitis was around 80%.[8] The main cause of death was cerebral edema complicated by brain herniation.[13] In viral hepatitis, one characteristic feature was the complete recovery of patients who survived without evolution to chronicity. The survival rate was partially dependent on the etiology: The mortality rate was between 75% and 80% for patients with HBV or HBV-HDV fulminant hepatitis, and between 80% and 95% in those with drug-induced fulminant hepatitis, such as from halothane fulminant hepatitis due to halothane ingestion, fulminant hepatitis of indeterminate cause, and so-called non-A, non-B fulminant hepatitis. The survival rate was higher for patients with fulminant hepatitis A, reaching 55%, and was between 50% and 60% for those with acetaminophen overdose.[12]

Medical Treatments

Before the advent of liver transplantation, many treatments were attempted without any improvement in survival, such as exchange blood transfusion, cross-circulation with a human or an animal donor,[7] corticosteroid therapy,[14–16] intravenous infusion of mannitol,[15,16] hemodialysis and continuous hemofiltration on polyacrylonitrile membranes,[17,18] and charcoal hemoperfusion.[19–21] A beneficial effect of a continuous intravenous infusion of prostaglandin E_1 on survival was reported in a nonrandomized series of 17 patients,[22] but these encouraging results were not confirmed in a randomized study from the same group.[23]

Although some of these treatments did not show any effect on the survival rate, other favorable effects were observed. Mannitol infusion seems useful to decrease brain edema at least transiently. In patients treated with continuous venovenous hemofiltration or hemodialysis, the main causes of death were sepsis or bleeding rather than brain death, suggesting a favorable effect of these therapies on brain edema. The aim of all of these treatments was to wait until liver regeneration occurred. The causes of failure of these treatments were probably multifactorial: (a) They were not able to replace the synthetic functions of the liver, and (b) liver regeneration is probably not a constant event after fulminant hepatitis and, when it occurs, may be insufficient, as is observed in patients with subacute hepatitis who develop poorly efficient nodules of regeneration.

LIVER TRANSPLANTATION FOR FULMINANT OR SUBFULMINANT HEPATITIS

Criteria for Patient Selection

Because 15% to 20% of patients with fulminant or subfulminant hepatitis will improve spontaneously, it is necessary to determine the subset of patients who will die without transplantation. Thus, it is necessary to have reliable criteria for the indications for liver transplantation. In addition, these criteria are needed early in the course of the hepatitis so that there is time to find a donor if transplantation is required. When transplantation is decided on for a patient, the delay to find a donor can be extreme, depending on organ availability and the geographic locality of the transplant team; in addition, the procedure itself can take as long as 12 hours.

In our common experience with the Clichy's group, the appearance of confusion or coma along with a marked decrease in factor V level to less than 30% of normal in a patient older than 30 years or to less than 20% of normal in a patient 30 years or younger was associated with a spontaneous mortality rate of more than 90% independent of the etiology.[4,24,25] Criteria for liver transplantation differ among transplant centers. Table 22.1 summarizes the different criteria reported in the literature.

The King's College group considers the etiology of the hepatitis as the most important prognostic factor: they use different criteria in patients with and without acetaminophen toxicity. In the nonacetaminophen group they consider the etiologies of non-A, non-B virus infection and drug-induced hepatitis as indications per se for liver transplantation independent of other factors.[26] One of the difficulties of comparing the criteria for liver transplantation among centers is the use of factor V level expressed in percentage of normal in the French groups and of prothrombin time expressed in prolonged seconds in comparison to normal in the British group.[27] A correlation between prothrombin time in seconds and factor V percentage has been reported using the international normalized ratio (INR). The Paul Brousse–Clichy criteria described previously are used in all centers in France and in several countries, whereas the criteria developed by the King's College group are used in the United Kingdom and in many other countries, including the United States. A standardization of these criteria should be attempted in the future.

Other centers have defined still other criteria for liver transplantation. Liver biopsy, mainly by the transjugular route, is of great help in determining the etiology of liver failure, particularly in the absence of classic viral markers or of evident etiology (e.g., acetaminophen overdose). For example, cases of fulminant Budd-Chiari syndrome, hypoxic hepatitis secondary to cardiac failure, malignant infiltration of the liver, and herpes hepatitis can be identified in this manner.

The role of liver biopsy as a prognostic indicator is a matter of debate, however. The extent of necrosis can be very heterogenous, and great changes can occur in a few days. In some cases little necrosis is present but hepatocytes can be nonfunctioning, and the extent of and capacity for liver regeneration is difficult to evaluate even with immunohistochemical markers. Liver biopsy may be of help in intermediate cases when the decision to proceed to transplantation is difficult; however, in the end, decisions must be based on clinical and biochemical grounds. The clinician is thus in a delicate situation. It is difficult to know a posteriori if transplantation is not indicated; in contrast, if transplantation is not carried out and the patient dies, the wrong approach is clearly underscored. In conclusion, this area remains controversial.

Using our criteria defined earlier, of 177 patients meeting these criteria for liver transplantation, 25 died before a donor could be found, 2 recovered spontaneously and were removed from the waiting list, and the other 150 underwent transplantation. The fact that only 2 patients survived among the 27 who did not receive a transplant supports the accuracy of our selection criteria.

Contraindications to Liver Transplantation

In our experience, the contraindications to emergency liver transplantation for patients with fulminant hepatitis are related to inability to support the operative procedure, namely, age older than 70 years, and severe cardiac, lung, or multiple organ failure. These contraindications have to be discussed case by case and are related to the experience of each center. Some centers are reluctant to perform liver transplantation

TABLE 22.1. *Criteria for liver transplantation in French centers and in King's College*

Clichy and Paul Brousse[5,24,25]	King's College[26]	
	Acetaminophen toxicity	Non–acetaminophen toxicity
Factor V < 30% if age > 30 yr or Factor V < 20% if age < 30 yr and Confusion or coma (encephalopathy stage 3 or 4)	Arterial ph < 7.3 or 3 of the following criteria: PT > 100 sec (INR > 7) Creatinine > 300 μmol/L Encephalopathy stage 3 or 4	PT > 100 sec (INR > 7) or 3 of the following criteria: Etiology: non-A, non-B hepatitis; or halothane- or drug-induced hepatitis Delay in onset of jaundice and encephalopathy > 7 days PT > 50 sec (INR > 3.5) Bilirubin > 300 μmol/L Age < 10 yr or > 40 yr

PT, prothrombin time; INR, international normalized ratio.

in the high-risk patient (i.e., with deep coma and hemo-dynamic instability), considering that these patients have a poorer expectancy of survival after liver transplantation and that the graft should be given to less risky recipients. We consider this to be a debate in ethics.

We have observed full neurologic recovery in some of our patients with very severe coma (i.e., seizures, low cerebral perfusion pressure, asymmetric dilated pupils) and hemody-namic instability requiring high doses of adrenaline or nora-drenaline. Thus, in our opinion, the neurologic limit to trans-plantation before death is never known. We consider that the neurologic contraindication for liver transplantation is the occurrence of brain death, defined, in a patient who has re-ceived no barbiturates, as the presence of bilateral nonre-active pupils, lack of spontaneous ventilation, and two con-secutive flat electroencephalograms. However, patients with fixed pupils with persistence of spontaneous ventilation, pa-tients with stage 4 encephalopathy and grade 3 coma with cerebral perfusion pressure below 40 mm Hg for more than 1 hour, and with seizures have a high risk of postoperative brain death or survival with neurologic sequelae.[5]

Should patients with sepsis prior to transplantation receive a transplant? Sepsis is a frequent event in patients with fulmi-nant liver failure.[28–30] We do not consider the presence of pos-itive blood cultures prior to transplantation a contraindication per se to liver transplantation. However, the presence of a se-vere pneumonia or of uncontrolled septic shock prior to trans-plantation is a contraindication to liver transplantation.

MANAGEMENT OF PATIENTS WITH FULMINANT OR SUBFULMINANT HEPATITIS

Pretransplantation Management

Except in cases of acetaminophen overdose and herpetic hep-atitis, there is no specific medical treatment for fulminant hep-atitis. For acetaminophen overdose, N-acetylcysteine should be administered as soon as possible even if the patient is referred late. For herpetic hepatitis, intravenous acyclovir should be administered as soon as possible. As soon as liver transplantation is indicated, the search for a liver donor should be initiated. In France, there is a national superemergency procedure conducted by the national organ-sharing agency (Etablissement Francais des greffes) that gives absolute prior-ity to patients with fulminant or subfulminant hepatitis for any donor liver in the country. The mean waiting time is around 1.4 days (0.5–4.0 days). Most of the organ-sharing organiza-tions in Europe use the same procedure for these patients. In the United States, patients are listed in United Network for Organ Sharing (UNOS) category 1 (i.e., fulminant liver fail-ure, patients in the intensive care unit).

Patients should be monitored for glucose level because they are exposed to hypoglycemia, which can cause cere-bral function to deteriorate. It is necessary to maintain the glucose level by the administration of a minimal daily dose of 200 g carbohydrates.

Infection should be searched for routinely by performing blood, urine, and sputum cultures. Patients with acute liver failure are susceptible to bacteremia, septic shock, and fungal complications, especially when liver failure is prolonged over several days.[28–30] In our series and in the series from King's College in London, 26% of the patients developed bac-teremia. In the series from King's College in London, 32% of the patients with fulminant liver failure developed fungal in-fections. The prophylactic use of antimicrobial treatments in patients with fulminant hepatitis has been suggested by some authors. We routinely administer antimicrobial treatments against gram-negative bacteria as soon as patients are placed on mechanical ventilation. When liver failure persists over several days, we add antifungal prophylactic therapy with in-travenous amphotericin B.

Clinical neurologic examinations should be performed to classify encephalopathy and to survey the appearance or degree of intracranial hypertension. When signs of cerebral edema are present, intravenous mannitol (0.5 g to 1 g/kg body weight every 4 hours) can be used as a first-line ther-apy. When renal failure is present, mannitol can be delete-rious. We use continuous venovenous hemofiltration or he-modialysis with polyacrylonitrile membranes when mannitol is contraindicated. Continuous venovenous hemofiltration can be used during the surgical procedure. Thiopental has been suggested in patients refractory to mannitol, but re-mains difficult to manage.[31]

Monitoring of the intracranial pressure by using an intra-cranial sensor remains controversial.[32,33] For several teams, its use seems beneficial for controlling the intracranial pres-sure and the cerebral perfusion pressure (the difference be-tween the mean arterial pressure and the intracerebral pres-sure) during the preoperative and perioperative transplant phase.[5,34] Some authors consider the cerebral perfusion pres-sure an aid in the decision of whether to transplant.[35] They believe that liver transplantation is contraindicated if the cerebral perfusion pressure is less than 40 mm Hg for several hours.[34] In our experience, monitoring of the intracranial pressure was not used in the decision to transplant but was useful for several reasons in patients with deep coma. First, there are some discrepancies between the clinical symptoms and the degree of intracranial pressure.[36] Second, during the surgical procedure under anesthesia, there are no reliable clinical symptoms, and the intracranial pressure can vary during the various phases of the procedure.[36] Finally, after transplantation, brain death can occur due to the persistence of high intracranial pressure, and careful monitoring until the patient awakens seems necessary.[4,5]

There are some difficulties in the use of intracerebral monitoring. It is an invasive method, and there is a risk of bleeding complications in patients with major coagulation disorders. The morbidity rate and the mortality rate with these sensors are 10% and 2%, respectively, in our experi-ence. It is not certain whether these sensors are completely reliable, and the more reliable sensors (i.e., those placed in subdural or intraventricular positions) are more dangerous.[37] We consider intracranial pressure monitoring to be useful, and we currently use this monitoring as soon as the patient is placed on mechanical ventilation. However, insertion of the sensor should be done cautiously because of the risk of bleeding. We recommend that coagulation defects be corrected prior to insertion of the sensor, and that hemostasis be adequately controlled at the insertion point. In agreement with Blei et al.,[37] we recommend that sensors be placed in extradural positions rather than an intracerebral position.

Sedative drugs must be avoided in these patients prior to transplantation in order to avoid modifying neurologic status and therefore the criteria indicating the need for liver transplantation. We restrict the use of sedatives to patients who require mechanical ventilation. Ventilation is indicated only in case of respiratory failure or deep coma. We believe that fresh frozen plasma and other plasma substitutes should be avoided in these patients prior to transplantation so that the levels of coagulation factors are not altered, since these factors remain one of the main criteria in the decision to transplant. In addition, the risk of spontaneous bleeding is lower in acute liver failure. Thus, we administer fresh frozen plasma only before insertion of an intracerebral sensor or at the beginning of the transplant procedure. In general, all therapies that increase the degree of liver failure should be avoided, in particular, the administration of acetaminophen, commonly prescribed before the advent of encephalopathy. For this reason some advocate the systematic use of N-acetylcysteine in all cases of fulminant hepatitis. The group at King's College have reported some improvement after administration of N-acetylcysteine even in non-acetaminophen-induced hepatitis.

When a liver donor is available, liver transplantation has to be performed as soon as possible. Our center used to accept the first liver graft available for the most seriously ill patients, even if the graft demonstrated fatty infiltration or was ABO incompatible. However, because of a high rate of graft failure, leading to retransplantation or death, some organ-sharing organizations and many centers are reluctant to use ABO-incompatible liver grafts. This should be balanced with the risk of death of the patient during the wait for another opportunity to obtain a donor organ.

Some patients with fulminant or subfulminant hepatitis referred for transplantation die before transplantation can be performed. This occurred in 15% to 30% of our cases in which transplantation had been decided upon. This rate of death varies from country to country depending on the opportunity for obtaining grafts in emergencies.[5,38]

Most of the patients (70%) who die before transplantation die of brain death. The other main causes of death are sepsis, hemodynamic instability, multiple organ failure, and gastrointestinal bleeding. A few patients improve before transplantation and can be removed from the waiting list. In our experience, this occurred in 2 (1%) of 177 patients for whom the decision to transplant had been made. This event can always occur because the predictive factors of spontaneous death are not 100% accurate. Thus, it is necessary to reevalu-

ate the patient at the time of the offer of a graft in order to decide if the transplantation is still indicated.

The clinical condition of the fulminant liver failure patient at the time of transplantation is different from that of patients with chronic liver disease. Most of the liver failure patients are in a coma at the time of transplantation, have signs of intracranial hypertension, and are on mechanical ventilation. Renal failure is a common event, and sometimes hemodialysis or continuous hemofiltration has to be performed before or during the surgical procedure. Positive blood cultures can be present. Some patients are in septic shock or have severe pneumonia, and there is a question whether these patients can undergo operation. There are no general rules; each team must decide for each patient if transplantation is feasible or not. One can attempt to control sepsis and to delay the transplantation for several days if possible.

Hemodynamic instability may require the use of pressor drugs such as adrenaline or noradrenaline. The cause of this hemodynamic instability is frequently a profound vasodilatation, which can be the consequence of an unrecognized sepsis or of the liver failure itself. There is a relationship between the severity of vasodilatation and the severity of the liver failure. Transplantation can be performed because hemodynamic instability does not represent an absolute contraindication; however, the risk of perioperative or postoperative death is probably higher. Some teams have proposed performing an emergency total hepatectomy along with a portacaval anastomosis in these cases to reverse the hemodynamic shock.[39] The rationale for such an approach is that the necrotic liver is responsible for the delivery of toxins that cause the hemodynamic shock. The patient is then placed in the intensive care unit again to wait for a liver graft. This approach has been carried out mainly in patients with necrotic livers rather than in patients with fulminant hepatitis. Some cases of hemodynamic improvement have been described; however, the postoperative mortality was high.[39] The risk of postoperative death was related to the length of waiting time for the liver graft. The risk of such a procedure is that the patient will die before a graft can be found. For this reason, the procedure remains controversial.

Perioperative Management

To correct coagulation defects, fresh frozen plasma is administered at the beginning of the procedure. It is necessary to maintain a balance between fluid restriction to avoid the increase of brain edema and maintenance of a satisfactory cerebral perfusion pressure. The total clamping of the inferior vena cava (IVC) and of the portal vein is poorly tolerated. Two techniques are used: transplantation using a venovenous bypass with a venous return in the axillary vein rather than in the jugular vein; and transplantation with conservation of the IVC[40] and lateral clamping of the IVC, associated with temporary portacaval anastomosis. In patients with renal failure or high intracranial pressure, or both, perioperative venovenous hemofiltration can be performed.

The surgical procedure itself is generally technically easy: the coagulation defects can be corrected with infusion of fresh frozen plasma and platelets. The hepatectomy is facilitated because of the presence of an atrophic liver and the absence of severe portal hypertension. However, sometimes the transplantation can be difficult. When the liver graft is of poor quality there is a risk of immediate graft nonfunction after revascularization, with diffuse abdominal bleeding. When there is a size mismatch between donor and recipient, the size of the graft needs to be reduced.[41] The combination of several factors, such as graft reduction and massive steatosis, may increase the risk of diffuse abdominal bleeding.

Postoperative Management

Irreversible brain damage can be observed even during the first hours after transplantation;[4,5] thus, it remains necessary to perform neurologic assessments until the patient is completely awake.

RESULTS OF LIVER TRANSPLANTATION FOR FULMINANT AND SUBFULMINANT HEPATITIS

The survival rate after transplantation for fulminant hepatitis ranges between 50% and 75% in different series in the literature (Fig. 22.2).[4,5,42–46] The actuarial 1- and 5-year survival rates of 150 patients who received transplants between January 1986 and January 1996 at our center were 68% and 61%, respectively (Fig. 22.3). As observed in other series, the postoperative mortality was high. In our experience, most of the deaths occurred in the first 3 postoperative months.

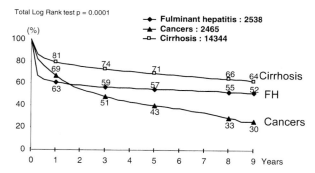

FIG. 22.2. Survival after liver transplantation in Europe in relation to the initial liver disease. Note the higher posttransplantation mortality in patients who undergo transplantation for fulminant hepatitis, with a low decline in survival after 1 year. This reflects the critical clinical condition of the patients at the time of transplantation and the poor quality of grafts used in some patients due to the context of emergency. (Adapted from the European Liver Transplant Registry held at Hopital Paul Brousse, Villejuif, France; property of the European Liver Transplant Association.)

LIVER TRANSPLANTATION FOR FH AND SFH

HOPITAL PAUL BROUSSE 1986 - 1996

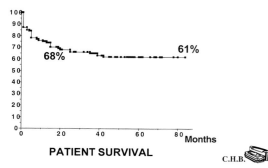

PATIENT SURVIVAL

FIG. 22.3. Survival after liver transplantation in patients with fulminant (7H) and subfulminant hepatitis (CSFH) at the Centre HépatoBiliare at Paul Brousse. The 1- and 5-year survival rates were 68% and 61%, respectively.

The main causes of death during and after transplantation were brain death and sepsis. Brain death can occur during the surgical procedure and sometimes in the immediate postoperative period; thus, the risk of brain death is not eliminated as soon as the new liver is in place. We and others have observed some cases of brain death occurring several hours or days following transplantation.[4,5] Intracranial sensors have shown that the intracranial pressure can increase during the surgical procedure.[36] During the dissection phase, the intracranial pressure seems to increase; during the anhepatic phase, the London group showed a decline in the intracranial pressure values, which, however, remained higher than the pretransplantation values.[36] In a study from San Francisco, there was no decrease noted in the intracranial pressure. During the reperfusion phase, the intracranial pressure rose again in the London study and decreased slightly in the San Francisco study. In both studies, the intracranial pressure values were higher at the end of the procedure than prior to transplantation.[34,36] Thus, it is necessary to remain cautious until the patient is fully awake.

Sepsis is another major cause of death, for several reasons. First, as described earlier, sepsis is common in patients with fulminant hepatitis. Second, patients in a coma before transplantation may remain on mechanical ventilation after transplantation for several days, increasing the risk of sepsis. Finally, patients receiving ABO-incompatible grafts receive aggressive antirejection therapy, which increases the risk of sepsis.

Morbidity

Neurologic sequelae can be observed after transplantation. This was rarely described in patients with fulminant hepatitis who survived spontaneously before the era of liver trans-

TABLE 22.2. *Outcome of 150 patients who received transplants at Hospital Paul Brousse from 1986 to 1996 in relation to the grade of coma at time of transplantation*

Encephalopathy stage[a]	Grade of coma	Number of patients	Survival (%)	Pre- or posttransplantation brain deaths	Neurologic sequelae
3	0[b]	8	87	0	0
3	1	21	67	0	0
4	2	41	78	3	1
4	3	80	56[c]	12	6

Note the relationship between the severity of coma pretransplantation and the survival rate, risk of occurrence of brain death, and rate of occurrence of neurological sequelae among survivors.

[a]Trey's classification.
[b]Marked confusion.
[c]$P < 0.01$.

plantation. Neurologic sequelae can be minor, such as memory defects, or major, such as hemiplegia or severe mental deterioration. The neurologic complications can be the direct consequences of the severity of the pretransplantation coma or the consequence of cerebral bleeding related to the intracranial pressure monitor.[37]

Sepsis is a frequent complication after liver transplantation for fulminant hepatitis; see the previous section.

Retransplantation

The rate of retransplantation in our series was much higher than in the elective series (13% versus 7%). The main causes of retransplantation were acute rejection, primary graft nonfunction, and intrahepatic biliary strictures. This high rate of retransplantation was related mostly to the condition of the patient prior to transplantation. The use of ABO-incompatible grafts was responsible for a high rate of severe acute rejection episodes and the occurrence of biliary strictures in the graft.[47,48] The use of steatotic grafts may be responsible for a high rate of primary graft nonfunction.[49]

Many complications are related to the quality of the graft or to graft compatibility. In theory, these severely ill patients need a very good graft in order to recover from their liver failure as quickly as possible; however, due to the emergency situation, they receive the first liver available, which could be of poor quality or ABO blood group incompatible. It is the responsibility of the team to decide if ABO-incompatible grafts should be used in an emergency. However, in order to conserve grafts, most organ-sharing organizations do not offer ABO-incompatible grafts even in the emergency setting (Fig. 22.4).

Viral Hepatitis B Recurrence after Liver Transplantation for Fulminant Hepatitis B

HBV can recur after transplantation for fulminant hepatitis B, but the rate of recurrence is much lower than for patients

who undergo transplantation for chronic liver disease caused by HBV. Recurrence is rare (less than 10% of cases) if patients receive long-term posttransplantation passive immunoprophylaxis.[50,51] In addition, when HBV recurred in the graft, it seemed less severe than in patients with HBV recurrence after transplantation for chronic HBV liver disease.

The rate of HBV recurrence was 25% in patients who underwent transplantation because of fulminant hepatitis due to HBV and HDV and who received long-term passive immunoprophylaxis with antibody to hepatitis B surface antigen.

Quality of Life and Long-term Survival

The quality of life of the survivors is generally good and seems similar to that of patients who undergo transplantation for chronic liver disease. The great majority of young patients will return to a normal social life and to work. However, psychological troubles can be observed in the early postoperative period and are explained mainly by the pretransplantation

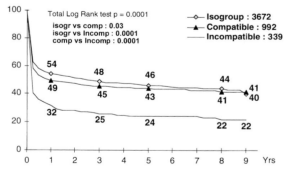

FIG. 22.4. Graft survival after emergency liver transplantation using ABO-identical, ABO-compatible, or ABO-incompatible grafts. There is a significantly lower graft survival rate in ABO-incompatible transplantation. (Adapted from the European Liver Transplant Registry held at Hopital Paul Brousse, Villejuif, France; property of the European Liver Transplant Association.)

encephalopathy and by the fact that these patients were not prepared psychologically for transplantation, in contrast to patients receiving transplants for chronic liver disease.

Long-term survival is generally good. There are few deaths after 1 year, due in part to the low rate of HBV recurrence in fulminant hepatitis B and to the absence of recurrence in other causes of fulminant hepatitis. There are no reports on the long-term outcome of these patients; however, in our own series the 1-year survival rate was 72% and the 5-year actuarial survival rate was 65%.

NEW TRENDS IN LIVER TRANSPLANTATION FOR FULMINANT HEPATITIS

New therapeutic strategies based on the concept of liver regeneration in fulminant hepatitis have been devised.

Auxiliary Liver Transplantation

Auxiliary orthotopic transplantation,[52] a procedure that requires partial left or right hepatectomy of the original liver and leaves in place part of the native liver, has been proposed for the treatment of patients with fulminant or subfulminant hepatitis. It is postulated that the native liver will regenerate, with the graft placed in orthotopic position acting as a temporary support. A number of reports of successful auxiliary liver transplantation have been published. In a multicenter European study, the overall survival rate was 63%. Sixty-eight percent of the survivors (i.e., 43% of all patients) permanently stopped immunosuppressive therapy with full recovery of the native liver.[53]

The key issue is the characterization of criteria by which native liver regeneration can be predicted. Complete regeneration was frequent in patients younger than 40 years, in those in whom the cause of fulminant hepatitis was viral hepatitis or acetaminophen overdose, and in those in whom fulminant hepatitis followed a hyperacute course.

Auxiliary partial liver transplantation may have some drawbacks: (a) The native liver does not always regenerate correctly, especially in patients with subfulminant hepatitis; (b) when hepatitis is due to hepatitis viruses, there is a risk of chronic viral persistence because of the immunosuppressive drugs; (c) there is only moderate portal hypertension in these patients, and because part of the portal flow must be diverted to the graft, the loss of flow could negatively affect the regeneration of the native liver; and (d) there is a competition between the two livers, such that the venous blood flow may favor the native liver or the graft, depending on events such as rejection. The main disadvantage of auxiliary orthotopic liver transplantion is that it is technically more difficult and may delay the development of satisfactory graft function, whereas most patients require a functional liver as soon as possible; this delay may be deleterious in more severely ill patients. Thus, the exact place of auxiliary liver transplantation in the armamentarium of liver

transplantation and the indications for this surgical technique remain ill defined.[54,55]

When auxiliary transplantation is performed, the extent of native liver regeneration can be assessed by the combined use of biochemical liver test results, analysis of biopsies of the two livers, appreciation of the volumes of both livers by computed tomographic scan, and dimethyl iminodiacetic acid (HIDA) scanning. This latter examination is the most useful in determining the function of each liver.

When the native liver has regenerated, the question arises as to the best way to deal with the graft. One option is to taper the immunosuppression to provoke a controlled rejection of the donor liver, thereby leaving it to atrophy. The theoretical disadvantage of this approach is the risk of causing a severe graft rejection that would require its prompt surgical removal, which can be a difficult procedure in an inflamed organ. The other option is to take out the graft electively without discontinuing the immunosuppression. The procedure of surgical removal of the graft may be difficult, however. In the absence of regeneration of the native liver, the question is whether to remove the native liver or not. There may be a long-term risk involved in leaving in place a native liver, particularly in the case of viral hepatitis B, where there may be an oncogenic risk.

Liver Supports

Bioartificial supports have been developed recently for the treatment of patients with fulminant hepatitis. Their current aim is more to increase the length of time a patient can survive while waiting for a graft than to replace liver transplantation.

Ex Vivo Liver Perfusion

Ex vivo liver perfusion had been attempted before the era of liver transplantation; the animals used included baboons, chimpanzees, and pigs. The results were disappointing in terms of survival. Recently, *ex vivo* pig liver perfusion has again been attempted in a few patients.[56] The results were not compelling, and several problems appeared. The duration of perfusion was limited to a mean of 6 hours because of the deterioration of the function of the pig liver. Hyperacute and acute rejection phenomena occurred within the pig liver and could not be prevented by a filter for xenogenic antibodies placed on the circuit. There was also a sharp decrease in the platelet count. This technique cannot be used widely in the future, because the pig liver is harvested emergently, which raises a concern regarding the risk of pathogen transmission.

Hepatocyte Transplantation

Hepatocyte transplantation is still experimental and has been used in humans mainly for treating metabolic disorders[57] and not for acute liver failure. To be effective experimentally it must be performed before the onset of liver failure.

Extracorporeal Bioartificial Liver Supports

The development of bioartificial livers utilizing extracorporeal circuits has been reported. Three systems have been applied experimentally in humans. One system uses hepatocytes from a human hepatoblastoma cell line.[58] This system is an extracorporeal circuit in which the whole blood of the patient is passed through a hollow fiber cartridge in which the hepatocytes are placed in the extracapillary part of the capillary fibers. Despite the presence of several security levels, the main concern is that malignant hepatocytes may pass into the patient's circulation. A recent report of its use in patients with fulminant liver failure in a randomized trial has shown mixed results, with some improvement in the neurologic condition of the patients but no clear improvement in survival.[59] All other systems currently developed use porcine hepatocytes placed in a cartridge in an extracorporeal circuit. The type of cartridge, the number of cells, and the arrangement of the cells differ from one system to another. The tridimensional system developed by Gerlach is in evaluation in humans.[60]

The system developed by Demetriou and Circe Biomedical was evaluated at Cedars Sinai, the University of California at Los Angeles, and our center and is used during the waiting time for transplantation. This system is an extracorporeal circuit that carries out plasmapheresis. The plasma of the patient is then passed through a charcoal filter and a hollow fiber cartridge, in which 5 billion hepatocytes on dextran microcarriers are placed in the extracapillary part of the cartridge. Exchange is carried out between the plasma and the hepatocytes through the capillary semipermeable membranes.[61,62] At our center, 10 patients with fulminant hepatitis listed for emergency liver transplantation have been treated with one to three courses of 6 hours on the bioartificial liver apparatus; all have undergone transplantation, and 8 survived. The main clinical outcome was neurologic improvement. One of the promising features of this system is that the porcine hepatocytes are kept cryopreserved and are unfrozen only when a patient is available. The advantage is that the hepatocytes can be shipped in the cryopreserved state, and the harvesting of porcine hepatocytes and all procedures for isolation and preservation of the hepatocytes are performed under strict regulatory conditions to avoid any transmission of pathogenic agents from pigs to humans. The use of porcine hepatocytes is a matter of concern because of the risk of xenoreactions and particularly of the risk of transmission from pigs to humans of a pig endogenous retrovirus (PERV) present in the germ line of the pigs.[63] Although no case of transmission has been described,[64,65] a virologic survey is warranted.

These bioartificial livers are at a first stage. Future developments are anticipated, particularly in increasing the number of cells in these systems and in using normal human hepatocytes rather than xenohepatocytes.

CONCLUSIONS

Liver transplantation represents a breakthrough in the treatment of patients with fulminant or subfulminant hepatitis. Patients with fulminant hepatitis should be referred as early as possible to a specialized center with a liver transplant unit. Liver transplantation, if necessary, should be performed early, before the advent of irreversible brain damage. Reliable criteria for the indication for transplantation have been developed, and the creation of a superemergency waiting list has increased the feasibility of transplantation. However, brain edema remains difficult to control medically and is the main cause of death before and after transplantation, which explains in part the higher mortality rate in these patients. Auxiliary orthotopic liver transplantation is a very interesting option but should be reserved for young patients, those with a high probability of liver regeneration, and those without a severe grade of coma. Therapies such as extracorporeal bioartificial liver support have to be evaluated as possible therapies for the prevention of fulminant hepatitis or for prolonging the waiting time for a graft.

REFERENCES

1. Iwatsuki S, Esquivel CO, Gordon RD, et al. Liver transplantation for fulminant hepatic failure. *Semin Liver Dis* 1985;5:325–328.
2. Ringe B, Pichlmayr R, Lauchart W, et al. Indications and results of liver transplantation in acute hepatic failure. *Transplant Proc* 1986;18:86–88.
3. Williams R, Gimson AE. An assessment of orthotopic liver transplantation in acute liver failure. *Hepatology* 1984;4:22S–24S.
4. Bismuth H, Samuel D, Gugenheim J, et al. Emergency liver transplantation for fulminant hepatitis. *Ann Intern Med* 1987;107:337–341.
5. Bismuth H, Samuel D, Castaing D, et al. Orthotopic liver transplantation in fulminant and subfulminant hepatitis. The Paul Brousse experience. *Ann Surg* 1995;222:109–119.
6. Bismuth H, Samuel D, Castaing D, et al. Liver transplantation for patients with acute liver failure. *Semin Liver Dis* 1996;16:415–425.
7. Trey C, Davidson CS. In: Popper H, Shaffner F, eds. *Progress in liver diseases: the management of fulminant hepatic failure,* vol. 3. New York: Grune and Stratton; London: Heinemann, 1970:282–298.
8. Bernuau J, Rueff B, Benhamou JP. Fulminant and subfulminant liver failure: definition and causes. *Semin Liver Dis* 1986;6:97–106.
9. O'Grady JG, Shalm SW, Williams R. Acute liver failure: redefining the syndromes. *Lancet* 1993;342:273–275.
10. Feray C, Gigou M, Samuel D, et al. Hepatitis C virus RNA and hepatitis B virus DNA in serum and liver of patients with fulminant hepatitis. *Gastroenterology* 1993;104:549–555.
11. Wright TL, Hsu H, Donegan E, et al. Hepatitis C virus not found in fulminant non-A non B hepatitis. *Ann Intern Med* 1991;115:111–112.
12. Williams R. Classification, etiology and considerations of outcome in acute liver failure. *Semin Liver Dis* 1996;16:343–348.
13. Ware AJ, D'Agostinho A, Combes B. Cerebral edema: a major complication of massive hepatic necrosis. *Gastroenterology* 1971;61:877–884.
14. EASL Trial Committee. Randomized trial of steroid therapy in acute liver failure. *Gut* 1979;20:620–623.
15. Canalese J, Gimson AES, Davis C, et al. Controlled trial of dexamethasone and mannitol for the cerebral edema of fulminant hepatic failure. *Gut* 1982;23:625–629.
16. Ede RJ, Williams R. Occurrence and management of cerebral edema in liver failure. In: Williams R, ed. *Clinics in critical care medicine: liver failure.* Edinburgh: Churchill Livingstone, 1986:26–46.

17. Denis J, Opolon P, Nusinovici V, et al. Treatment of encephalopathy during fulminant hepatic failure by haemodialysis with high permeability membrane. *Gut* 1978;19:787–793.

18. Denis J, Opolon P. Traitement de l'encephalopathie aigüe au cours des hépatites par hemofiltration continue. Résultats d'une étude controllée. In: Gauthier A, ed. *Soins intensifs en hepato-gastro-enterologie.* Paris: Masson, 1983:5–12.

19. O'Grady J, Gimson AES, O'Brien CJ, et al. Controlled trials of charcoal hemoperfusion and prognostic factors in fulminant hepatic failure. *Gastroenterology* 1988;94:1186–1192.

20. Gazzard BG, Portmann B, Weston MJ, et al. Charcoal haemoperfusion in the treatment of fulminant hepatic failure. *Lancet* 1974; 1:1301–1307.

21. Gimson AES, Braude SE, Mellon PJ, et al. Earlier charcoal haemoperfusion in fulminant hepatic failure. *Lancet* 1982;2:681–683.

22. Sinclair SB, Greig PD, Blendis LM, et al. Biochemical and clinical response of fulminant viral hepatitis to administration of prostaglandin E. A preliminary report. *J Clin Invest* 1989;84:1063–1069.

23. Sheiner P, Sinclair S, Greig PD, et al. A randomized control trial of PGE2 in the treatment of fulminant hepatic failure [Abstract]. *Hepatology* 1992;16:88A.

24. Bernuau J, Goudeau A, Poynard T, et al. Multivariate analysis of prognostic factors in fulminant hepatitis B. *Hepatology* 1986;6:648–651.

25. Bernuau J, Samuel D, Durand F, et al. Criteria for emergency liver transplantation in patients with acute viral hepatitis and factor V below 50% of normal: a prospective study [Abstract]. *Hepatology* 1991;14:49A.

26. O'Grady JG, Alexander GJM, Hayllar KM, et al. Early indicators of prognosis in fulminant hepatic failure. *Gastroenterology* 1989;97: 439–445.

27. O'Grady JG, Hambley H, Williams R. Prothrombin time in fulminant hepatic failure. *Gastroenterology* 1991;100:1480–1481.

28. Rolando N, Harvey F, Brahm J, et al. Prospective study of bacterial infection in acute liver failure: an analysis of fifty patients. *Hepatology* 1990;11:49–53.

29. Rolando N, Harvey F, Brahm J, et al. Fungal infections: a common, unrecognised complication of acute liver failure. *J Hepatol* 1991;12: 1–9.

30. Rolando N, Philpott-Howard J, Williams R. Bacterial and fungal infection in acute liver failure. *Semin Liver Dis* 1996;16:389–402.

31. Forbes A, Alexander GJM, O'Grady JG, et al. Thiopental infusion in the treatment of intracranial hypertension complicating fulminant hepatic failure. *Hepatology* 1989;10:306–310.

32. Schafer DF, Shaw BW. Fulminant hepatic failure and orthotopic liver transplantation. *Semin Liver Dis* 1989;9:189–194.

33. Blei AT. Cerebral edema and intracranial hypertension in acute liver failure: distinct aspects of the same problem. *Hepatology* 1991;13:376–379.

34. Lidofski SD, Bass NM, Prager MC, et al. Intracranial pressure monitoring and liver transplantation for fulminant hepatic failure. *Hepatology* 1992;16:1–7.

35. Donovan JP, Shaw BW, Langnas AN, et al. Brain water and acute liver failure: the emerging role of intracranial pressure monitoring. *Hepatology* 1992;16:267–268.

36. Keays R, Potter D, O'Gray J, et al. Intracranial and cerebral perfusion pressure changes before, during and immediately after orthotopic liver transplantation for fulminant hepatic failure. *Q J Med* 1991;289: 425–433.

37. Blei AT, Olafson S, Webster S, et al. Complications of intracranial pressure monitoring in fulminant hepatic failure. *Lancet* 1993;341:157–158.

38. Castells A, Salmeron JM, Navasa M, et al. Liver transplantation for acute liver failure: analysis of applicability. *Gastroenterology* 1993; 105:532–538.

39. Ringe B, Lubbe N, Kuse E, et al. Total hepatectomy and liver transplantation as a two-stage procedure. *Ann Surg* 1993;218:3–9.

40. Cherqui D, Lauzet JY, Rotman N, et al. Orthotopic liver transplantation with preservation of the caval and portal flows. Technique and results in 62 cases. *Transplantation* 1994;58:793–796.

41. Bismuth H, Houssin D. Reduced-sized orthotopic liver grafts in hepatic transplantation in children. *Surgery* 1984;95:367–370.

42. Brems JJ, Hiatt JR, Ramming KP, et al. Fulminant hepatic failure: the role of liver transplantation as primary therapy. *Am J Surg* 1987;154: 137–141.

43. Peleman RR, Gavaler JS, Van Thiel DH, et al. Orthotopic liver transplantation for acute or subacute hepatic failure in adults. *Hepatology* 1987;7:484–489.

44. Vickers C, Neuberger J, Buckels J, et al. Transplantation of the liver in adults and children with fulminant hepatic failure. *J Hepatol* 1988;7: 143–150.

45. O'Grady JG, Alexander GJM, Thick M, et al. Outcome of orthotopic liver transplantation in the aetiological and clinical variants of acute liver failure. *Q J Med* 1988;69:817–824.

46. DeVictor D, Desplanques L, Debray D, et al. Emergency liver transplantation for fulminant liver failure in infants and children. *Hepatology* 1992;16:1156–1162.

47. Gugenheim J, Samuel D, Reynes M, et al. Liver transplantation across ABO blood group barrier. *Lancet* 1990;336:519–523.

48. Farges O, Kalil A, Samuel D, et al. The use of ABO incompatible grafts in liver transplantation: a life saving procedure in highly selected patients. *Transplantation* 1995;59:1124–1133.

49. Adam R, Reynes M, Johann M, et al. The outcome of steatotic grafts in liver transplantation. *Transplant Proc* 1991;23:1538–1540.

50. Samuel D, Bismuth A, Mathieu D, et al. Passive immunoprophylaxis after liver transplantation in HBsAg positive patients. *Lancet* 1991; 337:813–815.

51. Samuel D, Muller R, Alexander G, et al. and EUROHEP. Liver transplantation in European patients with the hepatitis B surface antigen. *N Engl J Med* 1993;329:1842–1847.

52. Boudjema K, Cherqui D, Jaeck D, et al. Auxiliary liver transplantation for fulminant and subfulminant hepatic failure. *Transplantation* 1995; 59:218–223.

53. Chenard-Neu MP, Boudjema K, Bernuau J, et al. Auxiliary liver transplantation: regeneration of the native liver and outcome in 30 patients with fulminat hepatic failure. A multicenter study. *Hepatology* 1996; 23:1119–1127.

54. Bismuth H, Azoulay D, Samuel D, et al. Auxiliary partial orthotopic liver transplantation for fulminant hepatitis. The Paul Brousse experience. *Ann Surg* 1996;224:712–726.

55. Pereira SP, McCarthy M, Ellis AJ, et al. Auxiliary partial orthotopic liver transplantation for acute liver failure. *J Hepatol* 1997;26:1010–1017.

56. Chari RS, Collins BH, Mage EJC, et al. Treatment of hepatic failure with *ex-vivo* pig-liver perfusion followed by liver transplantation. *N Engl J Med* 1994;331:234–237.

57. Fox IJ, Chowdhury JR, Kaufman SS, et al. Treatment of the Crigler-Najjar syndrome type I with hepatocyte transplantation. *N Engl J Med* 1998;338:1422–1426.

58. Sussman NL, Chong MG, Koussayer T, et al. Reversal of fulminant hepatic failure using an extracorporeal liver assist device. *Hepatology* 1992;16:60–65.

59. Ellis AJ, Hughes RD, Wendon J, et al. Pilot controlled trial of the extracorporeal liver assist device in acute liver failure. *Hepatology* 1996;24:1446–1451.

60. Gerlach JC. Development of a hybrid liver support system: a review. *Int J Artif Organs* 1996;19:645–654.

61. Rozga J, Williams F, Ro MS, et al. Development of a bioartificial liver: properties and function of a hollow-fiber module inoculated with liver cells. *Hepatology* 1993;17:258–265.

62. Watanabe FD, Mullon CJP, Hewitt WR, et al. Clinical experience with a bioartificial liver in the treatment of severe liver failure. A phase 1 clinical trial. *Ann Surg* 1997;225:484–494.

63. Patience C, Patton GS, Takeuchi Y, et al. No evidence of pig DNA or retroviral infection in patients with short-term extracoporeal connection to pig kidneys. *Lancet* 1998;352:699–701.

64. Heneine W, Tibell A, Switzer WM, et al. No evidence of infection with porcine endogenous retrovirus in recipients of porcine islet-cell xenografts. *Lancet* 1998;352:695–699.

65. Paradis K, Langford G, Long Z, et al. for the Xen 111 Study Group. Search for cross species transmission of porcine endogenous retrovirus in patients treated with living pig tissue. *Science* 1999;285:1236–1241.

Transplantation of the Liver, edited by Willis C. Maddrey, Eugene R. Schiff, and Michael F. Sorrell. Lippincott Williams & Wilkins, Philadelphia © 2001.

CHAPTER 23

Recurrent Disease of Presumed Autoimmune Origin

Thomas W. Faust

Liver transplantation is the treatment of choice for patients with end-stage liver disease resulting from a variety of disorders. Viral hepatitis and malignancy are known to recur after transplantation, but whether diseases of presumed autoimmune origin, including primary biliary cirrhosis (PBC), primary sclerosing cholangitis (PSC), and autoimmune hepatitis, recur after transplantation is controversial. As the organ donor shortage continues and waiting times and mortality rates for potential recipients increase, the issue of recurrent disease after transplantation leading to the need for retransplantation becomes increasingly important. With improvements in surgical techniques, medical management, and immunosuppression, long-term survival is expected, and physicians assuming responsibility for the care of allograft recipients must be cognizant that disease recurrence is possible.

After transplantation, most patients with suspected recurrence are asymptomatic, abnormalities in standard liver function test results are nonspecific, and autoimmune markers frequently persist or recur, making a clinical diagnosis of recurrent disease difficult. Posttransplantation biliary strictures are not specific for PSC, but may be seen with ischemic or preservation injury, ABO incompatibility, and chronic rejection. Likewise, inflammatory infiltrates on liver biopsy are not specific for recurrent PBC or autoimmune hepatitis; acute rejection, graft versus host disease, viral infections, drug toxicity, and biliary ductal obstruction produce similar findings. Immunosuppression may modify expression of autoimmune diseases and delay recurrence for diseases known to evolve slowly within the native liver before transplantation. HLA disparity between donor and recipient may also influence disease expression. Consequently, the clinician should exercise caution when making a diagnosis of recurrent disease. Over the intermediate term, recurrent disease appears to be of little

clinical significance, but long-term studies will be required to assess the impact of recurrence on patient and graft survival.

PRIMARY BILIARY CIRRHOSIS

Primary biliary cirrhosis is thought to be a disease of disordered immune regulation.[1] Antimitochondrial antibodies (AMA) are present in 95% of patients. A family of antibodies exist to different mitochondrial antigens. Over 90% of patients with PBC have anti-M2 antibodies against the E2 subunits of pyruvate dehydrogenase, branched-chain α-oxoacid dehydrogenase, and oxoglutarate dehydrogenase complexes; however, other antibodies (anti-M4, M8, and M9) are also present. The relationship between AMA and bile duct injury is unclear, but immune attack of aberrantly expressed antigenic molecules on biliary epithelial cells with similarities to the E2 subunit is possible. Through molecular mimicry, certain microbial proteins are antigenically similar to the E2 subunit.[2] Pathophysiologically, an immune response may be generated to an unidentified microbe, followed by immune attack on biliary epithelial cells expressing similar antigens.

Lymphocytic destruction of medium-size bile ducts expressing increased amounts of class I and II antigens is characteristic.[1] Four stages of PBC are known.[3,4] Stage 1 is associated with segmental and patchy granulomatous destruction of interlobular and septal bile ducts with chronic mononuclear inflammatory cells (the florid duct lesion). Bile duct loss associated with ductular proliferation and portal tract expansion with chronic inflammatory cells represents stage 2, whereas stage 3 is identified with a reduction in portal inflammation followed by septal fibrosis, bile duct loss, and cholestasis. Cirrhosis represents stage 4. Granulomatous destruction of bile ducts is considered pathognomonic, whereas other features (breaks in the biliary epithelial basement membrane, loss of biliary epithelial cells, portal and periportal inflammatory infiltrates, lymphocytic bile duct destruction,

T. W. Faust: Department of Medicine, The University of Chicago Hospitals and Clinics, Chicago, Illinois 60637.

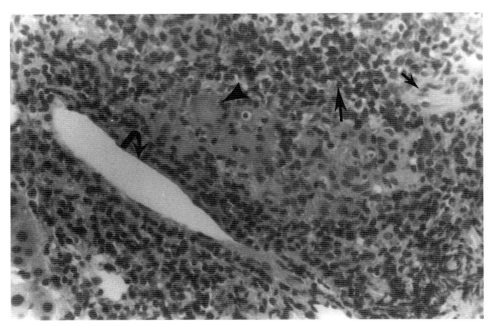

FIG. 23.1. Periportal granulomatous inflammation suggestive of recurrent primary biliary cirrhosis. The portal vein (*curved arrow*) and hepatic artery (*small arrow*) are surrounded by a dense infiltrate of mononuclear cells (*large arrow*). A granuloma is apparent (*arrowhead*). The intrahepatic bile duct is destroyed by the inflammatory reaction. (Courtesy of David L. Watkins, Baylor Medical Center, Dallas, Texas.)

ductopenia, noncaseating granulomas) are suggestive, but not diagnostic (Fig. 23.1). Staging of PBC is subject to sampling error with biopsy because different stages may be present within different hepatic segments.

Evidence for Recurrence

Studies offering evidence for the recurrence of PBC are summarized in Table 23.1. Neuberger et al. were the first to suspect recurrent PBC.[5] Three patients who received transplants for PBC were followed for 3.5 to 4.5 years. Three years after transplantation, all patients experienced elevations of bilirubin and alkaline phosphatase; persistence of the sicca syndrome was seen in one patient, development of pruritus in two, and hypothyroidism in one. Titers of AMA fell to undetectable levels in all recipients, followed by values similar to or higher than before transplantation. Immunoglobulin M (IgM) was also increased in one recipient. Biopsies revealed portal inflammation, bile duct injury, ductopenia, lymphoid aggregates, granulomas, and increased copper-binding protein. The histologic findings were not suggestive of chronic rejection. Five controls who received transplants for other conditions did not exhibit the clinical, biochemical, serologic, or histologic abnormalities described earlier. The authors concluded that PBC recurred after transplantation.

In a follow-up paper from the same group, 23 patients with PBC surviving longer than 1 year after transplantation were studied, 10 of whom underwent biopsy.[6] One hundred and two controls underwent transplantation for conditions other than PBC, 50 of whom also underwent biopsy. All patients who underwent transplantation for PBC exhibited significant improvement in clinical symptoms and liver function test results; however, 5 recipients experienced recurrence of pruritus, and several patients developed *de novo* Raynaud's phe-

TABLE 23.1. *Incidence of recurrent primary biliary cirrhosis after transplantation*

Author (Ref.)	Length of follow-up (yr)	Incidence by biopsy (%)
Neuberger et al. (5)	3.5–4.5	NA
Polson et al. (6)	>1	90
Dietze and Margreiter (7)	1.0–3.5	33
Hubscher et al. (8)	1.0–8.3	16
Balan et al. (9)	>1	8
Sebagh et al. (10)	>1	9
Van De Water et al. (11)	>0.3	21
Kim et al. (12)	0.2–7.5	11
Wong et al. (13)	0.9–1.0	NA
Dmitrewski et al. (14)	>1	30
Mazariegos et al. (15)	0.6–2.0	15
Slapak et al. (16)	>5	24
Haagsma et al. (17)	>1	0
Klein et al. (18)	>1	0
Demetris et al. (19)	>0.5	0
Esquivel et al. (20)	1.0–6.5	0
Buist et al. (21)	>0.25	0
Samuel et al. (22)	0.25–4.8	0
Gouw et al. (23)	1–11	0
Dubel et al. (24)	>4	0

NA, not applicable.

nomenon, sicca syndrome, and sclerodactyly. As in the initial study, AMA titers and IgM fell in most recipients immediately after transplantion, followed by elevated values over time. Nine (90%) of 10 biopsied patients had histologic features consistent with early recurrent disease: ductular proliferation, breaks in the bile duct membrane, lymphocytic aggregates within portal tracts, granulomas, and deposition of copper-associated protein. There was no correlation between histologic recurrence and liver function test results in patients who received transplants for PBC. Bile duct proliferation was seen in 12 (24%) of 50 biopsied controls, but ductal obstruction and chronic rejection accounted for the findings. The authors concluded that PBC recurs; however, several potential flaws of the study exist. Biopsies of PBC and control patients were not blinded, matching of PBC recipients and controls was not clearly discussed, and testing for hepatitis C was not available. The florid duct lesion was not present in any sample, making a diagnosis of recurrent disease tenuous, and follow-up biopsies of patients with suspected recurrence revealed nonspecific changes.

Six patients who underwent transplantation for PBC were followed for 14 to 43 months by Dietze and Margreiter.[7] As with previous studies, a similar pattern of AMA fluctuation was apparent. Protocol biopsies were obtained at discharge; 1 month, 6 months, and 12 months after transplantation; yearly; and whenever indicated. Two recipients displayed granulomatous destruction of bile ducts suggesting recurrent disease without evidence of rejection or infection. The authors concluded that most patients had a stable clinical course and that disease expression may be attenuated by immunosuppression; however, determining the impact of recurrent disease on patient and graft survival would require prolonged follow-up.

Hubscher et al. studied 172 biopsies from 83 patients whose indication for transplantation was PBC and 181 biopsies from 105 non-PBC controls.[8] Biopsies were obtained from 12 to 100 months after transplantation in conjunction with clinical, biochemical, and serologic data. Thirteen (16%) of 83 patients who underwent transplantation for PBC experienced recurrence. Two biopsies revealed granulomatous duct destruction, whereas in other samples, mononuclear infiltrates, lymphoid aggregates, epithelioid granulomas, ductular proliferation, ductopenia, and portal fibrosis were suggestive but not diagnostic of recurrent PBC. Most biopsies were consistent with early patchy involvement (stage 1 or 2). No lesions suggesting PBC were apparent in the controls. Twelve of 13 PBC were asymptomatic, with normal liver biochemistry 13 to 51 months posttransplantation; 8 of 11 and 9 of 11 recipients had positive AMA and elevated IgM, respectively. There was no correlation between AMA titer, IgM, and histologic recurrence. The authors stressed that viral hepatitis, biliary obstruction, and chronic rejection should be excluded prior to diagnosing PBC recurrence.

In a similar investigation, 60 patients whose indication for transplantation was PBC and 156 non-PBC controls with at least 1 year of follow-up were studied.[9] Liver function tests, AMA, and IgM were assessed. Patients underwent protocol liver biopsy at 1 and 3 weeks posttransplantation, 4 months, yearly, and as needed. Granulomatous destruction of interlobular and septal bile ducts suggested recurrence. Most PBC patients experienced symptomatic improvement in association with normal biochemistry and a fall in AMA and IgM titers. Florid duct lesions were seen in 5 (8%) of 60 PBC patients 2 to 6 years after transplantation, whereas granulomatous destruction was not present in the control group. Because there was no correlation among clinical symptoms, liver function test findings, AMA titers, IgM, and histologic recurrence, a clinical diagnosis of recurrent PBC could not be made. Balan et al. concluded that an unequivocal diagnosis of recurrence could be made if the florid duct lesion was found; careful exclusion of other disorders as described previously is mandatory. As with other studies, the short-term prognosis for recurrent PBC was excellent, but prolonged follow-up would be required to address the impact of recurrent disease and immunosuppression on patient and graft survival.

Sebagh et al. examined 69 patients who underwent transplantation for PBC and 53 controls.[10] Biopsies were obtained per protocol and when indicated. Six (8.7%) PBC patients exhibited nonsuppurative destructive cholangitis, portal inflammatory infiltrates, and ductopenia suggestive of mildly recurrent disease. The authors suggested that periportal plasma cell infiltrates were highly sensitive and specific for PBC recurrence. Other causes for graft dysfunction were excluded.

Advances in immunohistochemistry lend further support for PBC recurrence after transplantation. Van De Water et al. studied 38 patients who received transplants for PBC and 29 non-PBC controls with a minimum of 4 months follow-up.[11] Recurrent disease was assessed using murine monoclonal antibodies (C355.1) to the E2 subunit of pyruvate dehydrogenase complex, which are known to react with apical biliary epithelial antigens of PBC patients. Twenty-eight (74%) of the 38 PBC patients exhibited intense apical staining with C355.1 compared with none of the controls; 8 (28%) of 28 patients positive for C355.1 also demonstrated histologic evidence of recurrent PBC. None of the subjects with histologic recurrence was negative for C355.1. Nonspecific portal infiltrates, idiopathic hepatitis, acute and chronic rejection, and normal histology accounted for the remainder positive for C355.1. Fifty percent of PBC patients with recurrent disease also displayed cholestatic indices. The authors concluded that PBC recurred after transplantation and that apical staining with C355.1 may be the earliest marker for disease recurrence.

In a subsequent study, 6 patients who received transplants because of autoimmune cholangiopathy (AMA-negative PBC) were compared with 12 AMA-positive controls.[12] One of 6 AMA-negative and 1 of 12 AMA-positive recipients manifested histologic evidence of recurrence. As with previous studies, the authors concluded that patient and graft survival were not compromised over the short term.

The Role of Immunosuppression

Recurrent PBC may be influenced by the immunosuppressive regimen and the method of weaning patients from immunosuppression.[13–16] Wong et al. reported recurrent disease within 1 year of transplantation in two patients receiving tacrolimus (FK506).[13] Both patients demonstrated granulomatous bile duct destruction with cholestasis, pruritus, and the sicca syndrome. The authors suggested that cyclosporine may be preferable to tacrolimus in patients whose indication for transplantation was PBC.

In a similar paper, 27 PBC patients with graft survival over 1 year were studied; 11 patients received cyclosporine and 16 patients received tacrolimus.[14] Protocol biopsies were obtained at 1 and 2 years after transplantation. The definition of recurrence was based on characteristic portal and periportal pathology. After the first year, 5 (31%) of 16 patients receiving tacrolimus developed hepatic granulomas, whereas none was present in patients receiving cyclosporine. After 2 years, lesions suggestive of PBC recurrence were present in 7 (44%) of 16 patients receiving tacrolimus, and 1 (9%) of 11 patients receiving cyclosporine. The authors concluded that PBC recurred more frequently and sooner in patients receiving tacrolimus, but that graft survival was not compromised in the medium term; however, details regarding exclusion of other causes for granulomas were not provided.

Previous studies have suggested that rapid weaning of immunosuppression in PBC patients may be harmful.[15,16] Two (15%) of 13 patients exhibited histologic evidence of recurrence 7 and 24 months after being weaned from a cyclosporine-based regimen in the study by Mazariegos et al.[15] Slapak et al. examined 33 patients who underwent transplantation for PBC, 8 of whom developed portal-based granulomas and inflammatory infiltrates consistent with recurrent disease.[16] As with previous studies, the authors advised caution in weaning patients with autoimmune diseases from immunosuppression. The effect of rapid corticosteroid withdrawal on the rate of PBC recurrence is not known and will require additional studies.

Evidence against Recurrence

Even though many studies support recurrent PBC after transplantation, others have challenged this concept (Table 23.1). Haagsma et al. studied 15 PBC and 16 control patients with at least 1 year of posttransplantation follow-up.[17] Titers of M2, M4, and M8 antibodies, liver function tests, and biopsies were obtained routinely. AMA titers fell 1 month after transplantation, M2 antibodies were present in low titer, and M4 and M8 antibodies became undetectable with prolonged follow-up. Liver function test results were similar between groups, and histologic evidence of PBC recurrence was not present even though one sample revealed nonsuppurative destructive cholangitis (attributable to rejection). The study concluded that AMA titers fell after transplantation secondary to the effects of immunosuppression, that no correla-

tion existed between AMA titer before transplantation and biochemical and histologic abnormalities afterward, and that histologic recurrence could not be demonstrated in patients receiving transplants for PBC; however, mention was made that longer follow-up would be required to assess the recurrence of disease in patients who underwent transplantation for PBC. In a similar investigation, Klein et al. studied M2, M4, M8, and M9 antibodies in 23 patients who underwent transplantation for PBC and survived for at least 1 year.[18] Sixteen (69.5%) of 23 patients remained anti-M2 positive at low titer, whereas other antibodies became undetectable in the majority. With 13 years of follow-up, histologic evidence of recurrent disease was not seen despite the presence of M2 antibodies.

Demetris et al. performed a retrospective study of 106 PBC patients and 288 non-PBC controls.[19] Titers of AMA fell slightly after transplantation or remained the same. Even though there was an insignificant increase in the incidence of chronic rejection in PBC transplant patients, no evidence of recurrent disease could be found. Graft dysfunction did not correlate with AMA titers, and patient and graft survival were similar between groups. The authors concluded that recurrent disease could not be diagnosed with certainty and that the effects of immunosuppression may modify disease expression within the graft; however, the lack of long-term histologic follow-up in patients who underwent transplantation for PBC was a major drawback to the study.

In a subsequent paper, Esquivel's group examined biochemical and histologic data on 76 patients receiving transplants for PBC, with follow-up between 1 and 6.5 years.[20] As with prior investigations, AMA titers fell or remained the same in the majority. Thirteen (17%) of 76 patients demonstrated evidence of hepatic dysfunction secondary to acute or chronic rejection, but none of the subjects was found to have recurrent disease; however, biopsies were taken within the first few months after transplantation, 5 of 13 patients did not undergo liver biopsy, and the mean follow-up period was short. Even though nonsuppurative cholangitis was present, the histology was most compatible with rejection.

Buist et al. performed a prospective study of 30 patients who underwent transplantation for PBC with at least 3 months of follow-up.[21] As with previous investigations, clinical, biochemical, serologic, and histologic variables were analyzed. Abnormal liver function test results were present in 10 recipients either due to "transient causes" or chronic rejection, and AMA and IgM fell or became undetectable in most, followed by a subsequent rise. Fifteen PBC patients and 9 non-PBC controls underwent biopsy; no difference in histology was seen between the groups. Granulomas were present in 1 PBC patient, but no details regarding etiology were provided.

Similarly, PBC recurrence was assessed in 44 patients with a mean survival of 25 months.[22] Raynaud's phenomena, sicca syndrome, pulmonary hypertension, and scleroderma reappeared in 6 recipients (14%). The authors suggested that PBC does not recur after transplantation; however, details of posttransplantation liver biopsies were not provided.

Gouw et al. studied 19 PBC patients and 14 non-PBC controls with a median follow-up of 5 years; biochemical, serologic, and histologic parameters were assessed.[23] Protocol liver biopsies were obtained annually. There were no differences in liver function test results and biopsies between groups; however, granulomas were present 3 years after transplantation in 2 patients with PBC. Details regarding exclusion of other causes for hepatic granulomas were not given.

Other studies have assessed the relationship between autoantibodies and PBC recurrence.[24–26] Dubel et al. evaluated 16 PBC patients for M2 antibodies with a minimum of 4 years of follow-up.[24] Liver function tests and biopsies were performed monthly and yearly, respectively. As with aforementioned studies, AMA titer fell or became normal in the majority, but no histologic evidence of recurrent disease was apparent. Antibodies against nuclear components (gp210 and Sp100) have been observed in patients with PBC.[25,26] In a study by Dubel's group, 76 PBC transplant patients were assessed for anti-gp210 and antinuclear dot antibodies.[25] Antibody titers fell in the majority, but only 1 patient experienced recurrent PBC. The authors concluded that there was no correlation between antibodies to nuclear components and recurrent disease within the graft. Luettig et al. studied PBC-specific antinuclear (Sp100 and gp210) and antimitochondrial antibodies in 42 patients who underwent transplantation for PBC compared with 93 controls.[26] Even though antibody titers fell after transplantation, the qualitative pattern remained the same. There was no correlation among antinuclear and antimitochondrial antibody titers, liver function test results, and histologic recurrence.

Conclusions

The recurrence of PBC after transplantation is controversial. Differences in study design, numbers of patients, immunosuppressive regimens, lengths of follow-up, and criteria for recurrence account for discrepant results. AMA are present in the majority of recipients, but there is no correlation between a positive titer and clinical, biochemical, or histologic recurrence.

Because most patients with suspected recurrence are asymptomatic and liver function test results are nonspecific, liver biopsy remains the gold standard for diagnosis. Well-defined histologic criteria for PBC must be used, and granulomatous destructive cholangitis should be present. Lymphocytic cholangitis, ductular proliferation, ductopenia, and portal mononuclear infiltrates are not specific for PBC, and florid duct lesions on occasion may be found in patients with hepatitis C and ischemic cholangitis. Exclusion of other conditions mimicking PBC (acute and chronic rejection, graft versus host disease, biliary obstruction, viral hepatitis, drug effects) is paramount prior to making a diagnosis of PBC recurrence. Numerous infectious and noninfectious etiologies

account for hepatic granulomas after transplantation.[27] Cytomegalovirus (CMV) infection, hepatitis B and C, tuberculosis, acute rejection, preservation injury, and foreign-body reactions should be considered. Acute rejection and preservation injury or hepatitis account for early portal-based and parenchymal granulomas, respectively, whereas late portal-based granulomas are possibly caused by recurrent disease. The effects of immunosuppression may delay or modify disease expression within the graft.

If PBC recurs, intermediate-term patient and graft survival rates are excellent, but long-term studies will be required to assess disease recurrence and its impact on the allograft. Advances in immunohistochemistry may provide additional insight about recurrent PBC. What effect will newer immunosuppressive agents or rapid steroid withdrawal protocols have on the incidence and severity of recurrent disease? Should PBC transplant patients receive ursodeoxycholic acid as preventive therapy for recurrence? Supplementary studies will be necessary to answer these questions.

PRIMARY SCLEROSING CHOLANGITIS

Primary sclerosing cholangitis is a progressive cholestatic disease of unknown etiology associated with insidious inflammation and fibrosis of intrahepatic or extrahepatic bile ducts, or both. Disordered immune regulation may play a role. A diagnosis of PSC is based on clinical, biochemical, cholangiographic, and histologic criteria. Cholestatic liver indices and perinuclear antineutrophil cytoplasmic antibodies are characteristic. Irregular ductal strictures, beading, diverticular outpouchings, and pruning are seen on cholangiography, whereas biopsy reveals concentric rings of fibrous tissue with edema and inflammatory cells around interlobular bile ducts (fibrous cholangitis), and replacement of ducts with fibrous scars (fibroobliterative lesions). Fibroobliterative lesions are infrequently found on biopsy (fewer than 50% of samples), and other ischemic, infectious, obstructive, and iatrogenic causes may account for similar histopathology. As with PBC, PSC is associated with four histologic stages.[28] Portal hepatitis and edema without extension beyond the limiting plate define stage 1, whereas periportal inflammation with fibrosis and piecemeal necrosis constitutes stage 2. Stage 3 is linked to septal fibrosis with or without bridging necrosis, and stage 4 is associated with cirrhosis. Cholangiectases and cholangitic abscesses may be present in combination with these histologic findings.

The recurrence of PSC after transplantation is controversial. Careful exclusion of other conditions identified with intrahepatic and extrahepatic biliary strictures is mandatory.[29] Ischemic strictures resulting from hepatic arterial occlusion and preservation injury have similar cholangiographic and histologic appearances to that of PSC. Chronic rejection, ABO incompatibility between donor and recipient, viral and bacterial infections, and technical misadventures can mimic the cholangiographic features associated with PSC.

Evidence for Recurrence

Table 23.2 summarizes the studies presenting evidence concerning the recurrence of primary sclerosing cholangitis. Figures 23.2 through 23.4 illustrate the histologic and cholangiographic findings suggestive of recurrent PSC.

McDonald et al. evaluated 20 biliary strictures (6 anastomotic, 8 central hilar, and 6 peripheral nonanastomotic) in patients who underwent transplantation for different diseases.[30] Hepatic arterial patency, acute and chronic rejection, and ischemia times were assessed in all recipients. Among the 6 patients who developed peripheral strictures, 3 patients had PSC prior to transplantation. Hepatic arterial occlusion was not present in any PSC transplant recipient who developed strictures. Mean cold ischemia times were longer in patients who developed peripheral lesions; however, the authors failed to clearly state whether prolonged ischemia times were present in patients who underwent transplantation for PSC. Chronic rejection was more prevalent in recipients with peripheral strictures. The study concluded that PSC may recur, but that careful exclusion of other causes for nonanastomotic strictures was warranted.

Biliary obstruction, fibrous cholangitis, and fibroobliterative lesions were assessed in patients who underwent transplantation for PSC with a minimum of 6 months follow-up.[31] Twenty-two PSC transplant patients with Roux-en-Y anastomoses were matched with 185 non-PSC controls and 22 non-PSC Roux-en-Y controls; the Roux-en-Y controls were used to evaluate the effect of Roux-en-Y loops on subsequent development of fibrosis. Seven (32%) of 22 PSC patients, 19 (10%) of 185 non-PSC controls, and 3 (14%) of 22 Roux-en-Y controls developed biliary obstruction on biopsy, whereas 6 (27%) of 22 PSC patients, 4 (2%) of 185 non-PSC controls, and 1 (5%) of 22 Roux-en-Y controls developed fibrous cholangitis. Fibroobliterative lesions were seen in 3 (14%) of 22 patients who underwent transplantation for PSC but in none of the controls. The Birmingham study concluded that fibrous cholangitis was more common in patients who underwent transplantation for PSC, that fibroobliterative lesions were only seen in patients with PSC, and that patient

and graft survival were not affected over the intermediate term. Fibroobliterative lesions could not be explained by the creation of Roux-en-Y anastomoses. Data on cold ischemia times, hepatic arterial patency, and cholangiography were not provided.

Sheng et al. studied the prevalence of intrahepatic, extrahepatic nonanastomotic, and choledochojejunal anastomotic strictures in 100 patients (112 grafts) who underwent transplantation for PSC compared with 543 non-PSC controls (575 grafts).[32] Hepatic arterial patency was evaluated with Doppler sonography and angiography, and cold ischemia times were assessed for all subjects. Thirty (27%) of 112 grafts from PSC patients and 75 (13%) of 575 grafts from the control group displayed intrahepatic strictures by cholangiography, whereas 7 (6%) of 112 grafts from PSC patients and 10 (2%) of 575 grafts from the control group exhibited nonanastomotic extrahepatic biliary strictures. Intrahepatic and nonanastomotic extrahepatic strictures were significantly more frequent in patients who received transplants for PSC. Diverticulum-like outpouchings were seen in conjunction with intrahepatic strictures in several PSC patients. There were no significant differences in the frequency of anastomotic strictures or the prevalence of hepatic arterial occlusion and cold ischemia times between PSC and control groups. The authors concluded that nonanastomotic intrahepatic and extrahepatic lesions were more common in patients who underwent transplantation for PSC, whereas anastomotic strictures most likely resulted from technical errors; however, histopathology, ABO compatibility between donor and recipient, and chronic rejection were not discussed.

In a subsequent investigation, 130 grafts with intrahepatic strictures and 130 grafts without strictures were studied. Both groups were matched as to the type of anastomosis—either choledochojejunostomy or choledochocholedochostomy.[33] Hepatic arterial patency, cold ischemia times, preservation solution, and ABO compatibility were assessed for both groups. An original diagnosis of PSC was seen in 32 (24.6%) of 130 grafts with intrahepatic strictures and in 11 (8.5%) of 130 grafts without intrahepatic strictures; however, intrahepatic strictures were significantly more common with choledochojejunostomy, hepatic arterial occlusion, and grafts preserved in Euro-Collins solution. Liver biopsies were reviewed in 101 and 109 grafts with and without strictures, respectively. Even though cholangitis was significantly more common in patients with strictures, there were no significant differences in the incidences of ischemia, chronic rejection, preservation injury, acute rejection, and CMV infection between groups. The authors concluded that technical factors accounted for most anastomotic strictures, whereas recurrent PSC, hepatic arterial occlusion, prolonged cold ischemia times, chronic rejection, and ABO incompatibility were responsible for the majority of intrahepatic lesions.

The cholangiographic appearances of 32 allografts from patients who underwent transplantation for PSC were compared with those of 32 grafts from non-PSC controls.[34] Both groups were matched for choledochojejunostomy, time elapsed between transplantation, and the diagnosis

TABLE 23.2. *Incidence of recurrent primary sclerosing cholangitis after transplantation*

Author (Ref.)	Length of follow-up (yr)	Incidence by cholangiography or biopsy (%)
Harrison et al. (31)	>0.5	41
Sheng et al. (32)	0.01–3.9	33
Sheng et al. (34)	0.01–9.0	25
Narumi et al. (35)	0.6–3.8	12
Goss et al. (37)	>0.5	9
Jeyarajah et al. (38)	>1	15
Graziadei et al. (39)	>0.25	20
Marsh et al. (40)	0.3–3.8	Not defined
Letourneau et al. (41)	>0.1	Not defined
Lerut et al. (42)	0.3	Not defined
Haagsma et al. (44)	0.25–4.0	0

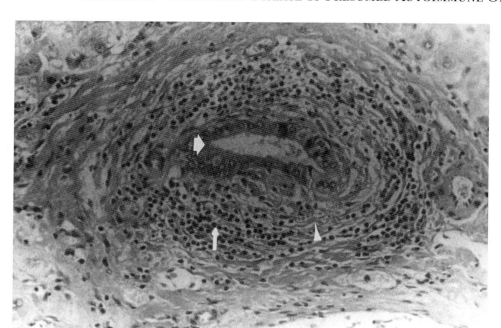

FIG. 23.2. Mononuclear cells (*arrow*) and lamellar fibrosis (*thin arrowhead*) surround an intrahepatic bile duct (*thick arrowhead*). Fibrous cholangitis is suggestive of recurrent primary sclerosing cholangitis. (Courtesy of George E. Bridges and G. Weldon Tillery, Baylor Medical Center, Dallas, Texas.)

of nonanastomotic strictures. Single or multiple strictures, length, focal dilation, mural irregularity, and diverticulum-like outpouchings were analyzed in both groups. Mural irregularity was present in 15 (47%) of 32 grafts from patients whose indication for transplantation was PSC and in 4 (13%) of 32 grafts from the control group, whereas diverticulum-like outpouchings were seen in 6 (19%) of 32 grafts from PSC patients and 1 (3%) of 32 grafts from controls. There were no significant differences in the frequency, number, and length of biliary strictures between th

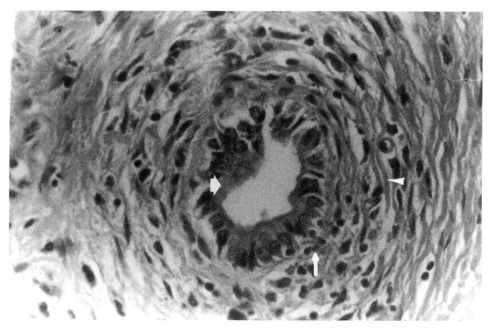

FIG. 23.3. Fibrous cholangitis consistent with recurrent primary sclerosing cholangitis is present at higher magnification. A damaged intrahepatic bile duct (*thick arrowhead*) is surrounded by mononuclear cells (*arrow*) and lamellar fibrosis (*thin arrowhead*). (Courtesy of George E. Bridges and G. Weldon Tillery, Baylor Medical Center, Dallas, Texas.)

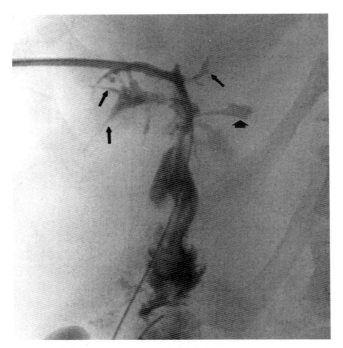

FIG. 23.4. Transhepatic cholangiogram demonstrating features suggestive of recurrent primary sclerosing cholangitis. Multiple intrahepatic strictures (*arrows*) and diverticulum-like outpouchings (*arrowhead*) are characteristic. (Courtesy of Jeffery A. Leef, The University of Chicago Hospitals and Clinics, The University of Chicago, Chicago, Illinois.)

experimental and control groups. The incidence of hepatic arterial occlusion and the use of Euro-Collins preservation solution were no more frequent in patients who acquired nonanastomotic strictures. Sheng et al. concluded that mural irregularities and diverticulum-like outpouchings suggested PSC recurrence; however, histology was not available to strengthen their case. In addition, the authors failed to provide information about matching PSC and non-PSC patients for ABO compatibility, cold ischemia times, acute and chronic rejection, or CMV infection. The majority of strictures attributed to PSC were diagnosed early after transplantation, raising concern about indicting recurrent PSC, a disease that is normally slow to evolve.

Narumi et al. studied 33 patients who underwent transplantation for PSC, with a mean follow-up of 37 months.[35] Diagnosis of recurrence was based on biochemical, cholangiographic, and histologic criteria in the absence of other known causes for biliary strictures. Four (12%) of 33 patients experienced recurrence based on periportal fibrosis and pericholangitis in conjunction with multiple nonanastomotic strictures between 7 and 45 months after transplantation. Ischemia times were not prolonged, ABO-identical grafts were used, and CMV infection was not significant.

Further data suggesting PSC recurrence was provided in a study by Fuller et al.[36] Twenty patients with biliary strictures were compared with 32 controls. Sixteen (80%) of

20 patients and 4 (20%) of 20 acquired nonanastomotic and anastomotic strictures, respectively. Five (31%) of 16 patients with nonanastomotic lesions had undergone transplantation for PSC. There were no differences between the groups regarding cold ischemia times, ABO incompatibility, rates of hepatic arterial occlusion, or rejection.

In a follow-up study, recurrent disease was assessed in 127 patients who underwent transplantation for PSC.[37] Eleven (8.6%) of 127 patients exhibited cholangiographic and histologic evidence of recurrence with a median follow-up of 3 years. The definition of recurrence was based on clinical symptoms and signs of cholestasis, nonanastomotic strictures within intrahepatic and extrahepatic bile ducts, and periductal inflammation with fibrosis at least 6 months after transplantation. There were no significant differences in patient or graft survival between PSC recipients and controls, although follow-up was short. Even though hepatic arterial patency was assessed, information about cold ischemia times and ABO matching was not provided. Postoperative viral infections were mentioned, but details regarding the types of infection and their relevance to biliary strictures after transplantation were not provided.

Distinguishing recurrent PSC from chronic rejection is difficult. Clinical, histologic, and cholangiographic data from patients with suspected PSC recurrence and chronic rejection were analyzed.[38] One hundred patients who received transplants for PSC with a minimum of 12 months follow-up were divided into one of three groups: group A (recurrent PSC), group B (PSC history with chronic rejection), and group C (PSC history without disease recurrence or chronic rejection). Cholangiographic and histologic data were obtained for each group. PSC recurrence and chronic rejection were apparent in 15% and 13% of patients, and the mean times to recurrent PSC and chronic rejection were 21 and 5 months, respectively. Intrahepatic strictures without biliary sludge and casts were seen in patients with suspected recurrence but not in those with chronic rejection. Ductal scarring, concentric periductal lamellar fibrosis, and obliterative arteriopathy were equally prevalent in groups A and B. There were no significant differences between groups regarding hepatic arterial occlusion, ABO incompatibility, and cold ischemia times; however, CMV infection was more common in patients with recurrent PSC. Patient and graft survival rates were significantly lower and transplantation rates significantly higher in patients with chronic rejection. Several potential flaws of the study exist. How can we be sure that recurrent disease was present in the PSC patients with obliterative arteriopathy (classically found in chronic rejection) or that chronic rejection was present in the subjects with lamellar fibrosis (characteristic of PSC)? What role did CMV play in stricture development in the group with suspected recurrent PSC?

In a recent paper, Graziadei et al. provide compelling evidence for PSC recurrence.[39] One hundred and twenty patients who underwent transplantation for PSC were compared with a group of 415 non-PSC controls after applying careful exclusion criteria (hepatic artery stenosis or thrombosis, chronic rejection, ABO incompatibility, anastomotic strictures, and nonanastomotic strictures developing less than 90 days after transplantation). Recurrence of disease was based on cholangiographic or histologic data, or both. Nonanastomotic strictures of intrahepatic or extrahepatic bile ducts developing more than 90 days after transplantation defined cholangiographic recurrence, whereas fibroobliterative lesions and fibrous cholangitis with or without ductopenia and cirrhosis were consistent with histologic recurrence. Twenty-two (18.3%) of 120 PSC patients and 5 (1.2%) of 415 non-PSC controls developed nonanastomotic strictures. Biliary strictures developed significantly later in patients who underwent transplantation for PSC. Nine patients with cholangiographic findings consistent with recurrent disease were also found to have compatible histology; however, 2 recipients who underwent transplantation for PSC developed fibrosis and ductopenia that suggested recurrence but had no cholangiographic findings. There were no significant differences in cold ischemia times, preservation solutions, CMV infections, and positive lymphocytotoxic crossmatches between patients who developed recurrence and those who did not; however, inflammatory bowel disease was more prevalent in patients who developed recurrent PSC. Five-year patient and graft survival rates were similar between PSC patients with recurrent disease and those without.

Evidence against Recurrence

Marsh et al. studied 55 patients who underwent transplantation for PSC with a mean follow-up of 19 months.[40] One of 55 patients developed biliary strictures; however, similar lesions were seen in 4 patients who underwent transplantation for other indications. In the patient with PSC, the authors failed to provide information regarding histology, ABO compatibility, cold ischemia time, and past or current viral infections. There was no conclusive evidence that PSC recurred.

In a follow-up study, biliary complications were analyzed in 9 patients who underwent transplantation for PSC and in 30 non-PSC controls.[41] Choledochojejunostomy and choledochocholedochostomy were performed in PSC and control patients, respectively. Six (67%) of 9 PSC patients developed biliary strictures. Strictures at the anastomosis were present in each recipient, whereas 2 patients developed intrahepatic lesions. Only 3 (10%) of 30 controls experienced biliary problems consisting of strictures or leaks. Letourneau et al. concluded that biliary complications were significantly more common in patients who underwent transplantation for PSC, and that the choledochojejunostomy may be a predisposing factor; however, the authors did not conclusively state that PSC recurred.

Lerut et al. evaluated 55 patients who received transplants for PSC, 1 of whom developed intrahepatic strictures.[42] Biopsy demonstrated features indicative of biliary obstruction. Cold and warm ischemia times were satisfactory, the donor and recipient were ABO identical, and hepatic arterial patency was confirmed. Even though the authors suggested that PSC may recur, the effects of choledochojejunostomy and the possibility of chronic rejection could not be discounted.

Hilar biliary strictures were examined in 152 patients undergoing transplantation for different etiologies.[43] Sixteen (10.5%) of 152 patients developed hilar strictures; most strictures were seen within the first 3 months. Ductal mucosal casts suggestive of ischemia were frequently present in patients who developed strictures. Strictures were no more frequent in patients who underwent transplantation for PSC than in patients who underwent transplantation for other indications. In the 5 patients with PSC who developed hilar strictures, hepatic arterial occlusion was present in 2, chronic rejection in 3, and CMV infection in 2. The Mayo study concluded that biliary strictures were frequent after transplantation, that strictures were no more common in patients who underwent transplantation for PSC than in other transplant recipients, and that other factors may account for their development.

In a subsequent paper, Haagsma et al. studied the relationship between perinuclear antineutrophil cytoplasmic antibodies (p-ANCA) and PSC after transplantation.[44] Nine patients receiving grafts for PSC were compared with 10 non-PSC controls. Biopsies and p-ANCA titers were obtained at scheduled intervals. As with PBC, autoantibody titers fell immediately after transplantation, followed by an increase over time. No patient positive for p-ANCA experienced histologic recurrence. The authors concluded that the role of p-ANCA in PSC recurrence was not clear, that immunosuppression may influence autoantibody titer, and that a correlation between p-ANCA titer and disease recurrence did not exist. Even though biopsy did not support disease recurrence in this study, cholangiographic data were not provided for any patient.

Conclusions

Because of a lack of a gold standard for diagnosis, the recurrence of PSC remains controversial. Clinical parameters and routine liver function tests are not specific for recurrent disease. Most patients with suspected recurrence are asymptomatic. Autoantibodies (p-ANCA) are ubiquitous before and after transplantation and do not correlate with histology. Differences in study design, methods of diagnosis, number of patients, and lengths of follow-up account for discrepancies between studies. To accurately diagnose PSC recurrence, well-defined cholangiographic and histologic criteria will be needed. Exclusion of other disorders (preservation injury, ABO incompatibility, chronic rejection, hepatic arterial occlusion, viral infections) that produce similar lesions is essential. Three to 5 years after transplantation, nonanastomotic intrahepatic and extrahepatic strictures are seen in 20% to 25% of PSC patients.

As with PBC, the effects of immunosuppression may modify or delay disease expression within the graft. Although recurrent disease may be more prevalent in patients receiving cyclosporine than in those receiving tacrolimus, additional studies with a larger number of patients will be required.[38] Studies will be essential to resolve the issue of recurrent PSC and the effects of different immunosuppressants and corticosteroid withdrawal on recurrence rates. Patient and graft survival do not appear to be affected in the medium term. Therapeutic options for posttransplantation biliary strictures include balloon dilation with or without placement of stents, surgical revision, or retransplantation.[30,33,41,43,45]

AUTOIMMUNE HEPATITIS

As with PBC and PSC, autoimmune hepatitis is thought to be a disease of disordered immune regulation.[46] Aberrant display of HLA class II antigens or enhanced presentation of normal elements on hepatocytes followed by activation and proliferation of cytotoxic T lymphocytes may be important. Sensitized T cells release proinflammatory cytokines, leading to hepatocellular necrosis. Criteria for diagnosis include periportal hepatitis with or without lobular inflammation in association with biochemical and serologic aberrations. Abnormalities in serum transaminases; hypergammaglobulinemia; and autoantibodies to nuclear antigen (ANA), smooth muscle (SMA), or liver-kidney microsome 1 (LKM-1) are characteristic. Chronic liver diseases caused by viral hepatitis, Wilson's disease, hemochromatosis, α_1-antitrypsin deficiency, and steatohepatitis require exclusion prior to diagnosing autoimmune hepatitis. Corticosteroids, with or without azathioprine, and transplantation are accepted therapies.

As with other disorders of immune regulation, the existence of recurrent autoimmune hepatitis is controversial. Diagnosis of recurrence is based on clinical, biochemical, serologic, and histologic criteria. Exclusion of acute rejection, viral hepatitis, drug effects, and biliary obstruction is imperative.

Evidence for Recurrence

Studies presenting evidence for the recurrence of autoimmune hepatitis are summarized in Table 23.3. Figure 23.5 shows histologic findings suggestive of recurrence.

Neuberger et al. reported a case of a 26-year-old HLA-B8-DR3–positive woman with autoimmune hepatitis who received an HLA-B8-DR3–negative graft.[47] Normal liver function test results and loss of autoantibodies were documented 6 months after transplantation; however, by 18 months the patient experienced recrudescence of clinical disease in combination with abnormal transaminase levels and serologies. There was no evidence of hepatitis A or B, CMV infection, or toxoplasmosis. Serologic and polymerase chain reaction (PCR) tests for hepatitis C were not available at the time of the study. Biopsy revealed a mononuclear cell infiltrate in association with piecemeal necrosis and bridging collapse. The patient improved with an increase in immunosuppres-

TABLE 23.3. *Incidence of recurrent autoimmune hepatitis after transplantation*

Author (Ref.)	Length of follow-up (yr)	Incidence by biopsy (%)
Neuberger et al. (47)	1.5	NA
Wright et al. (48)	>0.8	26
Birnbaum et al. (49)	0.2–1.7	83
Sempoux et al. (50)	0.3	NA
Ahmed et al. (51)	>0.5	61
Prados et al. (52)	0.7–4.4	33
Kerkar et al. (53)	0.5–3.8	4
Sanchez-Urdazpal et al. (54)	0.04–6.0	0

NA, not applicable.

sion. The authors concluded that recurrent autoimmune hepatitis was present based on clinical, serologic, and histologic criteria and that abnormal histology could not be explained by viral infection, acute or chronic rejection, or drug toxicity; however, hepatitis C could not be excluded.

In a subsequent paper, Wright et al. studied the relationship between HLA-B8-DR3 status and disease recurrence.[48] Forty-three patients underwent transplantation for autoimmune hepatitis, with a minimum of 10 months of follow-up. Autoimmune markers were present and serologic markers for viral hepatitis were absent in all patients; however, testing for hepatitis C RNA was not performed. Liver biopsies were obtained only when clinically indicated. Eleven (25.6%) of 43 recipients exhibited evidence of recurrent disease manifested by dense mononuclear portal infiltrates and piecemeal necrosis in association with persistence of autoantibodies and hyperglobulinemia. All cases of recurrent disease were in patients who received HLA-DR3–negative grafts. Nine (45%) of 20 HLA-DR3–positive recipients and 2 (12%) of 17 HLA-DR3–negative recipients experienced disease recurrence. Similar trends with HLA-B8–positive recipients were present but were not statistically significant. The authors concluded that HLA-DR3–positive recipients of HLA-DR3–negative grafts were at risk for recurrent autoimmune hepatitis. Recurrent disease was not present in recipients of HLA-DR3–positive grafts, and HLA-B8 status did not influence disease recurrence. Recurrence was not confused with rejection or biliary obstruction. Information was not provided regarding histologic criteria or timing of recurrence, dosage of immunosuppression at the time of recurrence, and the effects of increased immunosuppression on recurrent disease.

Six children underwent transplantation for autoimmune hepatitis, 5 (83%) of whom developed recurrence with a mean follow-up of 11 months.[49] The definition of recurrence was based on histology, autoantibodies, and hyperglobulinemia. Rejection was frequent but not confused with recurrent disease. Other causes (ischemic, obstructive, viral) for hepatic dysfunction were excluded, but exclusion of hepatitis C by PCR was not performed. Three of 5 patients with recurrent autoimmune hepatitis required a second graft within 1 year. Unfortunately, recurrent disease developed in all pa-

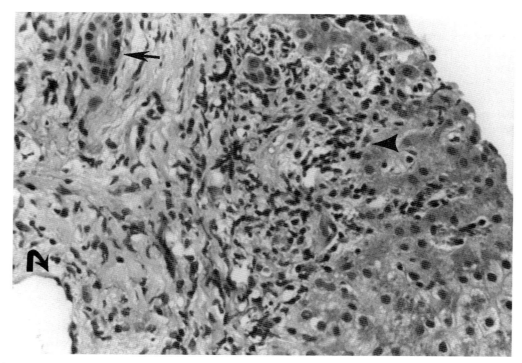

FIG. 23.5. Mononuclear cells invade the hepatic lobule in conjunction with piecemeal necrosis suggestive of recurrent autoimmune hepatitis (*arrowhead*). A normal intrahepatic bile duct (*arrow*) and portal vein (*curved arrow*) are present. (Courtesy of Georges J. Netto, Baylor Medical Center, Dallas, Texas.)

tients after retransplantation. The Mount Sinai study concluded that autoimmune hepatitis recurred frequently in the pediatric population, that recurrence was associated with aggressive disease requiring retransplantation, and that efforts to develop an immunosuppressive regimen to prevent recurrence should continue.

Sempoux et al. suggested that acute lobular hepatitis may be an early manifestation of recurrent disease after transplantation.[50] Portal mononuclear infiltrates with associated piecemeal and lobular necrosis were present in a 43-year-old man 4 months after transplantation. Viral infection was excluded by appropriate serology and nucleic acid analysis. Clinical and biochemical remission was obtained with increased immunosuppression; however, repeat liver biopsy was not performed. The authors concluded that lobular inflammation may be the first indication of recurrent autoimmune hepatitis, that immunosuppression may modify disease expression, and that caution should be exercised when weaning patients from immunosuppression.

In a subsequent study, 53 patients underwent transplantation for autoimmune hepatitis.[51] Twenty (61%) of 33 subjects followed for more than 6 months developed chronic hepatitis. Autoantibodies persisted in most, but information regarding histologic evidence of recurrence or data excluding other causes of inflammation were not provided. The authors concluded that chronic inflammation within the graft may represent disease recurrence in patients who underwent transplantation for autoimmune hepatitis.

In a recent study, the incidence of recurrent autoimmune hepatitis, associated risk factors, response to treatment, and patient and graft survival after recurrence were assessed by Prados et al.[52] Recurrent disease was defined by sustained elevation of transaminases of at least 1 month's duration and consistent histopathology. Positive autoimmune markers (ANA, SMA, LKM) with or without elevated IgG or γ-globulin were also required. Recipients with a history of viral hepatitis, alcohol abuse, suspected drug toxicity, or bile duct problems were not considered to have recurrent disease. Twenty-seven patients with a mean follow-up of 3.7 years met inclusion criteria, 9 (33%) of whom exhibited recurrent autoimmune hepatitis at a mean of 2.6 years. The risk of recurrence was 8% for the first year, 20% by the third year, and 68% after 5 years. Recurrent disease was more frequent in HLA-DR3–positive recipients on less immunosuppression with longer follow-up. Asymptomatic recurrences were associated with abnormal liver function test results, autoantibodies, and elevated globulins. Histopathology consisted of periportal and lobular hepatitis with lymphoplasmocytic infiltrates, plasma cells, piecemeal necrosis, and bridging fibrosis. Recipients with LKM antibodies did not develop recurrent disease. Biochemical parameters improved with increased immunosuppression, but hepatic inflammation did not improve or worsened in the majority. With a mean follow-up of 2.4 years, there was no significant difference in patient or graft survival between recipients who developed recurrence and those who did not. The authors concluded that recurrent autoimmune hepatitis was frequent, that the risk of recurrence increased over time with reduced immunosuppression, and that longer follow-up was required to assess the impact of recurrent disease on patient and graft survival.

Kerkar et al. proposed that autoimmune hepatitis may occur *de novo* after transplantation.[53] Seven (4%) of 180 children who underwent transplantation for conditions other than autoimmune hepatitis developed graft dysfunction after a median follow-up of 24 months. Viral infections, hepatic arterial patency, acute or chronic rejection, and bile duct abnormalities were assessed. Transplant recipients with suspected recurrence developed abnormalities in transaminases, autoantibodies, and IgG. Biopsy revealed a mixed lymphocytic and plasma cell infiltrate with piecemeal necrosis and bridging fibrosis. With increased immunosuppression, 6 of 7 patients displayed improvement in biochemical and histologic indices. The authors concluded that the abnormalities in liver function test findings, serology, and histology were consistent with *de novo* occurrence of autoimmune hepatitis, but that additional studies were necessary to rule out other causes for these abnormalities.

Evidence against Recurrence

Serial liver function test results, ANA, SMA, and γ-globulins were assessed in 24 patients who underwent transplantation for autoimmune hepatitis; 22 of these patients also underwent protocol liver biopsy.[54] Recurrence was defined by the presence of autoantibodies in association with periportal hepatitis in the absence of viral infection or rejection. ANA or SMA, or both, and γ-globulins decreased and ultimately became negative in all patients. There was no histologic evidence of recurrence in any patient with a mean follow-up of 39 months. The Mayo group concluded that autoimmune hepatitis did not recur after transplantation; however, recipients routinely received triple immunosuppression, which may have accounted for the negative results (Table 23.3).

Conclusions

Recurrent autoimmune hepatitis after transplantation is supported by most studies. The existence of disease recurrence is based on well-defined clinical, biochemical, serologic, and histologic criteria. As with patients who receive transplants for PBC and PSC, differences in study design, immunosuppressive regimens, and length of follow-up periods influence the recurrence rates seen. Rejection, viral infections, drug effects, and biliary obstruction require exclusion prior to making a diagnosis of recurrence. Most transplant recipients respond to an increase in corticosteroids and azathioprine, but the prognosis for pediatric patients appears to be inferior to that of adults. The value of using tacrolimus rather than cyclosporine for the prevention of recurrent disease is unclear. Weaning of immunosuppression should be approached with caution in patients who undergo transplantation for autoimmune hepatitis. Longer follow-up will be necessary to assess the consequences of recurrent disease on patient and graft survival, and future studies addressing the effects of novel immunosuppressants on disease recurrence are warranted.

SUMMARY

The reappearance of PBC after transplantation remains controversial. There is no correlation between titer of AMA and clinical, biochemical, or histologic recurrence. Granulomatous destructive cholangitis should be present, and exclusion of other disorders (acute or chronic rejection, graft versus host disease, biliary obstruction, viral hepatitis, drug effects) is mandatory prior to making a diagnosis of recurrent disease. Therapeutic strategies for the prevention and treatment of recurrent PBC remain to be defined. Patient and graft survival do not appear to be affected over the intermediate term.

The existence of recurrent PSC is even more controversial because of lack of a diagnostic gold standard. Well-defined cholangiographic and histologic criteria are requisite for diagnosis, and preservation injury, ABO incompatibility, chronic rejection, hepatic arterial occlusion, and viral infections require exclusion. Balloon dilation with or without biliary stents, surgical revision, and retransplantation are therapeutic options. Patient and graft survival are excellent over the medium term.

Most studies support the existence of recurrent autoimmune hepatitis based on clinical, biochemical, serologic, and histologic criteria. As with PBC and PSC, other disorders (rejection, viral infections, drug effects, biliary obstruction) require exclusion. The majority of adults respond well to increased immunosuppression, whereas the prognosis for pediatric patients is not as favorable.

Differences in study designs, numbers of patients, immunosuppressive regimens, lengths of follow-up, and criteria for recurrence account for discrepancies in the results among studies in patients who undergo transplantation for autoimmune disorders. Longer follow-up periods will be essential to assess the impact of recurrent disease on patient and graft survival. Additional investigations should concentrate on preventive and therapeutic strategies for recurrent autoimmune diseases after transplantation.

REFERENCES

1. Lee Y-M, Kaplan MM. Primary biliary cirrhosis. In: Friedman LS, Keefe EB, eds. *Handbook of liver disease.* Edinburgh: Churchill Livingstone, 1998:197–214.
2. Van de Water J, Turchany J, Leung PSL, et al. Molecular mimicry in primary biliary cirrhosis. Evidence for biliary epithelial expression of a molecule cross-reactive with pyruvate dehydrogenase complex-E2. *J Clin Invest* 1993;91:2653–2664.
3. Scheuer PJ, Lefkowitch JH. Primary biliary cirrhosis. In: Scheuer PJ, Lefkowitch JH, eds. *Liver biopsy interpretation,* vol. 31. London: WB Saunders Company, 1994:51–58.

4. Batts KP, Wang X. Recurrence of primary biliary cirrhosis, autoimmune cholangitis and primary sclerosing cholangitis after liver transplantation. *Clin Liver Dis* 1998;2:421–435.

5. Neuberger J, Portmann B, Macdougall BRD, et al. Recurrence of primary biliary cirrhosis after liver transplantation. *N Engl J Med* 1982;306:1–4.

6. Polson RJ, Portmann B, Neuberger J, et al. Evidence for disease recurrence after liver transplantation for primary biliary cirrhosis. Clinical and histologic follow-up studies. *Gastroenterology* 1989;97:715–725.

7. Dietze O, Margreiter R. Primary biliary cirrhosis (PBC) after liver transplantation. *Transplant Proc* 1990;22:1501–1502.

8. Hubscher SG, Elias E, Buckels JAC, et al. Primary biliary cirrhosis. Histological evidence of disease recurrence after liver transplantation. *J Hepatol* 1993;18:173–184.

9. Balan V, Batts KP, Porayko MK, et al. Histological evidence for recurrence of primary biliary cirrhosis after liver transplantation. *Hepatology* 1993;18:1392–1398.

10. Sebagh M, Farges O, Dubel L, et al. Histological features predictive of recurrence of primary biliary cirrhosis after liver transplantation. *Transplantation* 1998;65:1328–1333.

11. Van De Water J, Gerson LB, Ferrell LD, et al. Immunohistochemical evidence of disease recurrence after liver transplantation for primary biliary cirrhosis. *Hepatology* 1996;24:1079–1084.

12. Kim WR, Poterucha JJ, Jorgensen RA, et al. Does antimitochondrial antibody status affect response to treatment in patients with primary biliary cirrhosis? Outcomes of ursodeoxycholic acid therapy and liver transplantation. *Hepatology* 1997;26:22–26.

13. Wong PYN, Portmann B, O'Grady JG, et al. Recurrence of primary biliary cirrhosis after liver transplantation following FK506-based immunosuppression. *J Hepatol* 1993;17:284–287.

14. Dmitrewski J, Hubscher SG, Mayer AD, et al. Recurrence of primary biliary cirrhosis in the liver allograft: the effect of immunosuppression. *J Hepatol* 1996;24:253–257.

15. Mazariegos GV, Reyes J, Marino IR, et al. Weaning of immunosuppression in liver transplant recipients. *Transplantation* 1997;63:243–249.

16. Slapak GI, Saxena R, Portmann B, et al. Graft and systemic disease in long term survivors of liver transplantation. *Hepatology* 1997;25:195–202.

17. Haagsma EB, Manns M, Klein R, et al. Subtypes of antimitochondrial antibodies in primary biliary cirrhosis before and after orthotopic liver transplantation. *Hepatology* 1987;7:129–133.

18. Klein R, Huizenga JR, Gips CH, et al. Antimitochondrial antibody profiles in patients with primary biliary cirrhosis before orthotopic liver transplantation and titres of antimitochondrial antibody-subtypes after transplantation. *J Hepatol* 1994;20:181–189.

19. Demetris AJ, Markus BH, Esquivel C, et al. Pathologic analysis of liver transplantation for primary biliary cirrhosis. *Hepatology* 1988;8:939–947.

20. Esquivel CO, Van Thiel DH, Demetris AJ, et al. Transplantation for primary biliary cirrhosis. *Gastroenterology* 1988;94:1207–1216.

21. Buist LJ, Hubscher SG, Vickers C, et al. Does liver transplantation cure primary biliary cirrhosis? *Transplant Proc* 1989;21:2402.

22. Samuel D, Gugenheim J, Mentha G, et al. Liver transplantation for primary biliary cirrhosis. *Transplant Proc* 1990;22:1497–1498.

23. Gouw ASH, Haagsma EB, Manns M, et al. Is there recurrence of primary biliary cirrhosis after transplantation? A clinicopathologic study in long-term survivors. *J Hepatol* 1994;20:500–507.

24. Dubel L, Farges O, Bismuth H, et al. Kinetics of anti-M2 antibodies after liver transplantation for primary biliary cirrhosis. *J Hepatol* 1995;23:674–680.

25. Dubel L, Farges O, Courvalin J-C, et al. Persistence of gp210 and multiple nuclear dots antibodies does not correlate with recurrence of primary biliary cirrhosis 6 years after liver transplantation. *J Hepatol* 1998;28:169–170.

26. Luettig B, Boeker KHW, Schoessler W, et al. The antinuclear antibodies Sp100 and gp210 persist after orthotopic liver transplantation in patients with primary biliary cirrhosis. *J Hepatol* 1998;28:824–828.

27. Ferrell LD, Lee R, Brixko C, et al. Hepatic granulomas following liver transplantation. *Transplantation* 1995;60:926–933.

28. Wiesner RH. Primary sclerosing cholangitis. In: Friedman LS, Keeffe EB, eds. *Handbook of liver disease.* Edinburgh: Churchill Livingstone, 1998:215–225.

29. Sebagh M, Farges O, Kalil A, et al. Sclerosing cholangitis following human orthotopic liver transplantation. *Am J Surg Pathol* 1995;19:81–90.

30. McDonald V, Matalon TAS, Patel S, et al. Biliary strictures in hepatic transplantation. *J Vasc Interv Radiol* 1991;2:533–538.

31. Harrison RF, Davies MH, Neuberger JM, et al. Fibrous and obliterative cholangitis in liver allografts: evidence of recurrent primary sclerosing cholangitis? *Hepatology* 1994;20:356–361.

32. Sheng R, Zajko AB, Campbell WL, et al. Biliary strictures in hepatic transplants: prevalence and types in patients with primary sclerosing cholangitis vs those with other liver diseases. *AJR Am J Roentgenol* 1993;161:297–300.

33. Campbell WL, Sheng R, Zajko AB, et al. Intrahepatic biliary strictures after liver transplantation. *Radiology* 1994;191:735–740.

34. Sheng R, Campbell WL, Zajko AB, et al. Cholangiographic features of biliary strictures after liver transplantation for primary sclerosing cholangitis: evidence of recurrent disease. *AJR Am J Roentgenol* 1996;166:1109–1113.

35. Narumi S, Roberts JP, Emond JC, et al. Liver transplantation for sclerosing cholangitis. *Hepatology* 1995;22:451–457.

36. Feller RB, Waugh RC, Selby WS, et al. Biliary strictures after liver transplantation: clinical picture, correlates and outcomes. *J Gastroenterol Hepatol* 1996;11:21–25.

37. Goss JA, Shackleton CR, Farmer DG, et al. Orthotopic liver transplantation for primary sclerosing cholangitis. A 12-year single center experience. *Ann Surg* 1997;225:472–483.

38. Jeyarajah DR, Netto GJ, Lee SP, et al. Recurrent primary sclerosing cholangitis after orthotopic liver transplantation. *Transplantation* 1998;66:1300–1306.

39. Graziadei IW, Wiesner RH, Batts KP, et al. Recurrence of primary sclerosing cholangitis following liver transplantation. *Hepatology* 1999;29:1050–1056.

40. Marsh JW, Iwatsuki S, Makowka L, et al. Orthotopic liver transplantation for primary sclerosing cholangitis. *Ann Surg* 1988;207:21–25.

41. Letourneau JG, Day DL, Hunter DW, et al. Biliary complications after liver transplantation in patients with preexisting sclerosing cholangitis. *Radiology* 1988;167:349–351.

42. Lerut J, Demetris AJ, Stieber AC, et al. Intrahepatic bile duct strictures after human orthotopic liver transplantation. *Transpl Int* 1988;1:127–130.

43. Ward EM, Kiely MJ, Maus TP, et al. Hilar biliary strictures after liver transplantation: cholangiography and percutaneous treatment. *Radiology* 1990;177:259–263.

44. Haagsma EB, Mulder AHL, Gouw ASH, et al. Neutrophil cytoplasmic autoantibodies after liver transplantation in patients with primary sclerosing cholangitis. *J Hepatol* 1993;19:8–14.

45. Davern TJ, Lake JR. Recurrent disease after liver transplantation. *Semin Gastrointest Dis* 1998;9:86–109.

46. Czaja A. Autoimmune hepatitis. In: Friedman LS, Keefe EB, eds. *Handbook of liver disease.* Edinburgh: Churchill Livingstone, 1998:63–83.

47. Neuberger J, Portmann B, Calne R, et al. Recurrence of autoimmune chronic active hepatitis following orthotopic liver grafting. *Transplantation* 1984;37:363–365.

48. Wright HL, Bou-Abboud CF, Hassanein T, et al. Disease recurrence and rejection following transplantation for autoimmune chronic active liver disease. *Transplantation* 1992;53:136–139.

49. Birnbaum AH, Benkov KJ, Pittman NS, et al. Recurrence of autoimmune hepatitis in children after liver transplantation. *J Pediatr Gastroenterol Nutr* 1997;25:20–25.

50. Sempoux C, Horsmans Y, Lerut J, et al. Acute lobular hepatitis as the first manifestation of recurrent autoimmune hepatitis after orthotopic liver transplantation. *Liver* 1997;17:311–315.

51. Ahmed M, Mutimer D, Hathway M, et al. Liver transplantation for autoimmune hepatitis: a 12 year experience. *Transplant Proc* 1997;29:496.

52. Prados E, Cuervas-Mons V, De La Mata M, et al. Outcome of autoimmune hepatitis after liver transplantation. *Transplantation* 1998;66:1645–1650.

53. Kerkar N, Hadzic N, Davies ET, et al. De-novo autoimmune hepatitis after liver transplantation. *Lancet* 1998;351:409–413.

54. Sanchez-Urdazpal L, Czaja AJ, van Hoek B, et al. Prognostic features and role of liver transplantation in severe corticosteroid-treated autoimmune chronic active hepatitis. *Hepatology* 1992;15:215–221.

CHAPTER 24

Critical Care of Liver Transplant Recipients

Selected Topics

Jeffrey A. Lowell and Byers W. Shaw, Jr.

A comprehensive discussion of the intensive care of patients who have undergone liver transplantation is beyond the intended scope of this chapter. What we have attempted to do is explore several unique aspects of this care in a simplified manner. Our fears that we risk oversimplification are assuaged to some degree by presuming our audience to be the clinician who has a working knowledge of the care of liver transplant recipients but who needs a brief refresher course in some of the more basic aspects of intensive care. Our use of a model for reviewing the various physiologic factors affecting oxygen transport, for instance, may seem too elementary for most practicing intensive care specialists. But it has proved useful to students and residents who spend a few months on the service and for whom management of critically ill patients is not yet second nature.

We have neglected to include any discussion of numerous important aspects of the care of the patient in the intensive care unit (ICU). These include, but are not limited to, the role of infection prophylaxis, protocols for cardiopulmonary resuscitation, management of acute liver failure, and withdrawal of care when hope for recovery recedes. The astute clinician will also recognize the need to carefully tailor the use of immunosuppressive medications, antibiotics, and other medications when caring for critically ill patients, matters that we skillfully skirt in this chapter.

Perhaps most glaring is our failure to mention what is undoubtedly the most important problem encountered in patients requiring prolonged care in an ICU, namely, sepsis. Sepsis is the most common reason for readmission to the ICU after surgery as well as for delayed discharge or death. Affected patients simply will not leave the ICU alive unless

one can identify and treat the cause of sepsis. All of the ventilator management skill in the world will fail if what a patient really needs is surgical drainage of an abscess or the addition of appropriate antibiotics. Because these matters are discussed elsewhere in this book, our efforts have concentrated on topics for which having a working knowledge serves as a basic foundation for understanding the more comprehensive care of these difficult patients.

NUTRITION

Pretransplantation nutritional assessment in the patient with end-stage liver disease is problematic. Peripheral edema, ascites accumulation, and fluid retention make changes in body weight or anthropometric measurements unreliable. Serum levels of albumin, transferrin, prealbumin, and retinal-binding globulin are all depressed in patients with end-stage liver disease, and are also affected by hydration, renal function, and iron stores. Development of the hepatorenal syndrome will make calculations of the creatinine/height index unreliable.[1–9] Using a system that provides a "global assessment" of a patient's nutritional status, more than 80% of transplant candidates demonstrate moderate to severe malnutrition.[7,10] Perhaps the best predictors of the severity of malnutrition are the cause of the patient's liver disease and the pace at which it progresses. For example, a patient with rapid development of acute hepatic failure will have a much higher nutritional reserve than a patient with long-standing sclerosing cholangitis with active cholangitis and significant portal hypertension.[11]

In contrast to the difficulties in precisely quantitating the amount of protein and calories remaining in the nutritional reserve of the pretransplantation patient, vitamin, mineral, and trace element levels are all easily obtainable. As might

Transplantation of the Liver, edited by Willis C. Maddrey, Eugene R. Schiff, and Michael F. Sorrell. Lippincott Williams & Wilkins, Philadelphia © 2001.

J. A. Lowell and B. W. Shaw, Jr.: Department of Surgery, University of Nebraska College of Medicine, Omaha, Nebraska 68198.

be expected, patients with end-stage liver disease have significantly lower levels of fat-soluble vitamins (A, D, E, and K). Serum copper and magnesium levels are frequently elevated, whereas zinc levels are depressed.[5]

Posttransplantation allograft function is the main determinant of metabolic stress and nutritional needs. In a patient with excellent early allograft function, the period of postoperative hypermetabolism is short, and patients usually can achieve their nutritional goals, as calculated by resting energy expenditure (REE), with a normal enteral diet. The rapid return to enteral diet, whether it is taken entirely by mouth or with the aid of nasoenteric tube feedings, is desirable for several reasons.[12–19] The immediate posttransplantation period is commonly associated with liver function test derangements related to several causes, including allograft rejection, infection, drug toxicity, or bile duct obstruction. In patients who receive parenteral nutrition (PN), a nonspecific cholestasis may occur, especially in those patients who receive caloric intake in excess of requirements.[20,21] This cholestasis may confound the interpretation of posttransplantation liver function test abnormalities. In addition, higher rates of visceral protein synthesis occur in patients who receive enteral alimentation. Enterocyte stimulation leads to the release of trophic factors and aids in the maintenance of the small bowel mucosa and in the prevention of bacterial translocation.[13,14,16]

In contradistinction to the patient with good early allograft function, those with delayed function are typically volume overloaded and intolerant of enteral feedings. Virtually all of these patients require PN with a goal of providing adequate calories and protein, correcting metabolic abnormalities and vitamin and trace element deficiencies, and minimizing sodium and water accumulation.[4] With the current group of commercially available nutrient stock solutions, it is common for these patients to receive less than their calculated energy requirements because of volume constraints. The development of more concentrated nutrient solutions will eventually eliminate this problem.

To assess the efficacy of nutritional support after liver transplantation, Reilly et al. performed a randomized prospective study.[6] In this investigation, 28 liver transplant patients were divided into three groups: one group received no specific nutritional therapy; the second received "standard" PN, with 35 kcal/kg per day of nonprotein calories and 1.5 g/kg per day of protein; and the third group received PN with a branched-chain-enriched amino acid solution. At the end of 7 days, the PN groups had better nitrogen balance and no worsening of encephalopathy or elevations in serum ammonia concentration. The PN groups required a shorter period of posttransplantation mechanical ventilation and had shorter ICU stays. The total hospital charges were in fact greatest in the group that received no nutritional support. No benefit of a branched-chain-enriched amino acid solution over the standard amino acid solution was identified. It is unfortunate that this well-designed study did not include a treatment arm that used enteral nutrition. As discussed previously, enteral nutri-

tion is preferred in the posttransplantation patient for many reasons, not least of which is that it can be delivered at a fraction of the cost of PN.

The posttransplantation caloric and protein requirements of the liver transplant recipient may be difficult to estimate. Nutritional requirements should be tailored to the individual patient's needs. The Harris-Benedict equation, which is one of the most common tools to predict basal energy expenditure (BEE), uses body weight as one of the variables:[22]

$$BEE \text{ for males} = 66 + 13.7w + 5h - 6.8a$$

$$BEE \text{ for females} = 655 + 9.6w + 1.7h - 4.7a$$

In these equations, a is age in years, w is weight in kilograms, and h is height in centimeters. A patient's weight before and after transplantation poorly reflects true lean body mass because of an increase in total body water. Ascites and anasarca due to diminished protein stores pretransplantation, and volume overload posttransplantation, make caloric expenditure predictions based on weight inaccurate.

The metabolic cost of overfeeding (that is, providing more calories than are being consumed) translates into a respiratory quotient (R) that is greater than 1.0, which means that more carbon dioxide is being produced than oxygen consumed. More ventilatory work is thus needed to eliminate the extra carbon dioxide. A posttransplantation patient is frequently hypoventilatory for several reasons. Upper abdominal incisions, abdominal distention due to large amounts of ascites or ileus, and metabolic alkalosis all lead to posttransplantation hypoventilation. This state, coupled with additional carbon dioxide production due to overfeeding, may precipitate respiratory failure in the patient with a tenuous pulmonary reserve.

Cholestasis is also common in the posttransplantation patient and may be significantly worsened by hypercaloric PN feeding. For this reason, it is safest to measure the actual REE with a metabolic cart, an instrument that uses the principle of indirect calorimetry. This is easy to perform, gives an accurate assessment of caloric needs, and allows for a direct measurement of R. If a metabolic cart is not available, REE can be approximated from measurements of oxygen consumption ($\dot{V}O_2$) in a patient with a pulmonary artery catheter, using a modification of the Fick equation:

$$\text{Metabolic rate (kcal/hr)} = \dot{V}O_2 \text{ (mL/min)} \times 60 \text{ min/h} \times 4.83 \text{ kcal/L} \times 1 \text{ L/1000 mL}$$

$$\dot{V}O_2 \text{ (mL/min)} = 13.9 \times \text{hemoglobin} \times \text{cardiac output} \times (SaO_2 - S\bar{v}O_2)$$

SaO_2 is arterial oxygen saturation, and $S\bar{v}O_2$ is mixed venous oxygen saturation.

The REE of most posttransplantation patients will calculate to be about 30 kcal/kg per day.[23] In a study by Shanbhogue and colleagues, the mean REE of 11 consecutive, nonseptic liver transplant recipients over the first three postoperative days was 920 ± 190 kcal/m[2] per day.[11] Surprisingly, this was not significantly different from their pretransplantation REE. Thus, the immediate pretransplantation period in a patient with end-stage liver disease is an extremely hypermetabolic one. The similarities in the caloric demands before and after surgery speak to the major metabolic stresses of the patient with end-stage liver disease.

Protein requirements also increase significantly after transplantation. Metabolism of muscle to generate free amino acids for gluconeogenesis occurs at an accelerated rate. This catabolic response to surgery is enhanced by the administration of high-dose corticosteroids. Clinically, the increase in catabolism is measured by a rise in the excretion of urinary urea nitrogen (UUN) posttransplantation.[5,11] Typically, nitrogen balance (protein intake minus urinary, fecal, and insensible nitrogen losses) is negative for 7 to 14 days posttransplantation regardless of the amount of protein provided.

$$N_2 \text{ balance (g)} = \text{protein (g)}/6.25 \text{ (g)} - \text{UUN (g)} + 4$$

Protein provided in excess of 1.5 to 1.75 g/kg daily in the postoperative period does not serve to lessen the negative nitrogen balance, but only contributes to an elevation in the serum urea nitrogen level. Some investigators have used growth hormone in an effort to improve protein utilization in the postoperative period, with some early favorable results.[14,15,24]

The nonprotein calories of the nutrient admixture are made up of carbohydrates and fats. Excess administration of either of these is associated with potential complications in the posttransplantation period. Optimum glucose utilization occurs at a rate of 4.5 mg/kg per minute. Glucose infusion at a rate greater than 7 mg/kg per minute will lead to lipogenesis in the liver.[12,25] The use of lipids as a caloric source has several advantages. At 9 kcal/g, lipids supply nearly 3 times the calories per volume as glucose (3.4 kcal/g). However, no more than 40% of calories should be given as lipids. Triglyceride levels should be monitored during lipid infusion to avoid levels over 500 mg/dL. The rapid infusion of lipids is associated with a flooding of the reticuloendothelial system and fixed tissue macrophages (e.g., Kupffer cells) and impairs bacterial clearance. This obviously should be avoided in the heavily immunosuppressed patient in the early posttransplantation period. However, the continuous delivery of less than 1 g/kg per day does not adversely affect the reticuloendothelial system. In a typical patient this is accomplished by giving 250 cc of a 20% Intralipid solution daily.

The addition of vitamins and trace elements to the daily nutritional formula should not be overlooked. In addition to providing the recommended daily allowance of water-soluble and fat-soluble vitamins, supplemental vitamin K is frequently given, especially in patients receiving antibiotics that may alter gut flora and thus endogenous reabsorption. Iron and zinc are the two trace elements that are most commonly deficient in the postoperative patient. Iron is required for hematopoiesis, and zinc as a cofactor for protein synthesis.

Drugs are frequently added to PN admixtures. The continuous infusion of certain drugs has several pharmacokinetic, therapeutic, and cost advantages over intermittent bolus administration. Medications commonly added to PN solutions

include albumin, aminophylline, cimetidine or ranitidine, heparin, hydrochloric acid, and insulin.[26]

Monitoring nutritional therapy is extremely important in the critically ill patient because many metabolic complications associated with parenteral nutrition are possible.[26] Daily assessment of electrolyte, calcium, phosphate, and magnesium levels is necessary because these may change rapidly. Frequent blood glucose measurements are also necessary in patients receiving hypertonic dextrose solutions, especially when they are receiving high-dose corticosteroids. Insulin should be added to the PN solution and supplemented with a sliding scale of subcutaneous or intravenous insulin to keep blood glucose levels lower than 210 mg/dL. Blood glucose levels above this value are associated with a higher incidence of postoperative sepsis.[27] Accurate daily weights and fluid balances are important in the postoperative period. Frequent alterations in PN volume and electrolytes are common in the first several days after transplantation.

Our approach to nutritional support in the posttransplantation patient is typified by the following example. A 42-year-old woman underwent a complicated retransplantation for chronic allograft rejection. She was quite ill before surgery and was receiving enteral tube feedings to supplement her oral diet. She had evidence of mild malnutrition preoperatively. After retransplantation, she has gained 12 kg from her preoperative weight of 70 kg (without any significant ascites present). By postoperative day 2, it is clear that she will require several days of ventilatory support, and her gastrointestinal function has not yet returned. This patient is clearly total body volume overloaded, and in such a patient we restrict intravenous fluid to a maximum of 1,500 cc per day. Caloric and protein requirements are determined using the preoperative weight. If a metabolic cart is available, REE is measured or calculated using the modified Fick equation if a pulmonary artery catheter is in place. Otherwise, caloric needs are estimated to be 25 kcal/kg, or about 1,750 kcal/day in this patient. Protein requirements are 1.5 kcal/kg or about 105 g/day. This amount of protein (4 kcal/g) provides 420 kcal/day, leaving 1,330 kcal to be supplied from dextrose and lipids. No more than 40% of nonprotein calories should be from lipid sources. Fifty grams of lipid will give 450 kcal/day, leaving 980 kcal from dextrose, or approximately 280 g. Commercially available nutrient stock solutions are 70% dextrose, 15% amino acids, and 20% lipids.[28] Thus, the PN formulation for this patient provides 400 cc of 70% dextrose, 700 cc of 15% amino acids, and 250 cc of 20% lipids.

As the patient recovers and gastrointestinal function returns, an enteral diet is begun. During the transition, daily total calories and protein are maintained as the amount of enteral nutrition is increased and PN decreased. During the recovery phase, nitrogen balances are checked weekly, and if the patient is behind more than 4 g daily, protein intake is increased.

Central amino acid clearance is a measure of the ability of the liver to use amino acids. The clearance through the liver of free amino acids has been used experimentally to predict the quality of allograft function after liver transplantation. To date, this test has not had wide clinical application but continues to be used on an investigational basis in some centers.[29]

FLUID, ELECTROLYTE, AND ACID-BASE STATUS

Patients who have undergone orthotopic liver transplantation have many similarities with regard to fluid, electrolyte, and acid-base status in the early phase of their ICU stay. The majority of patients with end-stage liver disease have significant increases in total body sodium and water content, primarily due to a state of hyperaldosteronism. Following liver transplantation, total body sodium and water content may be further increased, and intravascular volume can be quite variable. As is discussed in the section "Hemodynamic Monitoring," the determination of intravascular volume status should be guided by pulmonary artery catheter pressures, mixed venous oxygen saturation, and calculations of oxygen delivery and consumption as well as by measures of end-organ function such as urine output.

Patients with end-stage liver disease frequently have some element of renal dysfunction before transplantation. In addition, they usually receive high-dose corticosteroids during the procedure as well as large amounts of crystalloids and blood products. These elements all have predictable outcomes and allow the physician to anticipate the need for various metabolic interventions.

Although not consistent with our experience, some authors have stated that most patients have a mild metabolic acidosis upon arrival in the ICU.[30,31] They attribute this phenomenon to the production and accumulation of lactic acid due to decreased tissue perfusion during the anhepatic phase of the transplant procedure and to allograft reperfusion effects. These effects may be lessened with the use of systemic and portal venous bypass. Massive blood transfusion may also contribute to a metabolic acidosis because during storage, blood pH falls as red cells use dextrose for metabolism and produce lactate and pyruvate.[32,33]

After a transient period of acidosis most patients will develop a metabolic alkalosis.[30,31] This alkalosis occurs for many reasons. Sodium bicarbonate is commonly given during the anhepatic phase in anticipation of allograft reperfusion. Patients receive high doses of corticosteroids in the early days after transplantation, which, when combined with diuretics, leads to the development of a hypochloremic, hypokalemic alkalosis. High volumes of nasogastric hydrogen losses and extracellular volume contraction will also worsen a developing alkalosis. The use of large amounts of citrate-containing blood products may contribute to a postoperative metabolic alkalosis.[34–38] Citrate is used as an anticoagulant by acting as a calcium chelator. Citrate dissociation generates 3 mol of bicarbonate. Arterial pH is the rate-limiting step in citrate metabolism. Patients who receive massive transfusions during the transplant procedure develop a huge citrate debt that leads to the gradual development of an alkalosis. This debt may be worsened by the administration of large volumes of crystalloid solutions containing lactate or acetate.[39] The effects of diuretics and steroids will also contribute to the acid-base derangement. The ability to clear citrate is dependent on hepatocellular function, and the delayed development of metabolic alkalosis may be an indirect indication of poor allograft function. Treatment of metabolic alkalosis is important for several reasons. Most enzyme systems function better at a slightly acid pH. In the allograft that is attempting to recover from a period of cold and warm ischemia, the metabolic environment should be optimal. Perhaps more important, however, is the effect that metabolic alkalosis has on ventilatory status. Hypoventilation posttransplantation is common for many reasons, such as incisional pain, abdominal distention from ascites or ileus, a large donor liver that makes abdominal wall closure difficult, intraabdominal sepsis, or phrenic nerve dysfunction.[37] Hypercarbia is the appropriate respiratory compensation for a severe metabolic alkalosis. This decrease in minute ventilation may be enough to either make weaning from mechanical ventilation unsafe or make reintubation and continued ventilatory support necessary. In such cases, active correction of the metabolic alkalosis is warranted.

In most patients, mild metabolic alkalosis is not a significant problem. Once the liver allograft demonstrates satisfactory function, one can begin to replace potassium stores. With improved intraoperative anesthetic management, most patients return from the operating room nearly euvolemic. This obviates the need for the use of large doses of diuretics postoperatively. Also, with refinements in surgical technique, massive transfusion during the transplant procedure is uncommon, limiting the citrate burden postoperatively. In most patients gastrointestinal function returns quickly and the gastric volume losses are minimal. Histamine-2 (H_2) blockade is effective in reducing the hydrogen ion loss in the patient who requires gastric decompression. However, H_2 blockers contribute to hyponatremia because sodium ion is lost in place of hydrogen ion.

In patients who develop a significant metabolic alkalosis (pH greater than 7.60), several treatment options exist. These include restoration of extracellular volume, elimination of gastric hydrogen losses, and replacement of serum potassium losses. In addition, one can use acetazolamide, a carbonic anhydrase inhibitor that blocks urinary losses of hydrogen ion while leading to increased renal excretion of bicarbonate. However, care must be taken in the use of this drug in patients with poor initial allograft function because of the potential for ammonia accumulation when less hydrogen ion is available for tubular conversion of ammonia to ammonium.

In hypochloremic patients, chloride ion can be replaced with the use of potassium chloride, calcium chloride, or magnesium chloride. Hydrogen chloride can also be used safely to correct a metabolic alkalosis. Fifty to 150 mL of a 0.1 N solution is delivered through a central venous catheter over a 24-hour period.[40] In patients receiving parenteral nutrition, hydrogen chloride can be added as long as the PN admixture does not contain lipids that may deemulsify. Caution should be used if hydrogen chloride and acetazolamide are used together, because this may lead to overcorrection of serum pH.[40]

The most common electrolyte abnormalities posttransplantation are hyponatremia and hypokalemia. Many patients have hyponatremia pretransplantation, and despite isotonic fluid resuscitation the decreased serum sodium concentration may persist after surgery. Caution should be used prior to transplantation for patients who have severe hyponatremia with serum sodium levels less than 120 mEq/dL, because rapid correction may lead to an acute neurologic decompensation due to central pontine myelinolysis. After transplantation, many patients still are total body salt and water overloaded, and correction of both occurs slowly over the first days as hepatic allograft and renal function improve and sodium stores are mobilized.

Hyponatremia posttransplantation rarely requires major intervention, aside from diuresis. Sodium-containing intravenous solutions should be avoided. Hyponatremia secondary to hypoglycemia may occur in the diabetic patient (or newly diagnosed diabetic patient) who receives high-dose corticosteroids in the early posttransplantation period. This is treated with a continuous infusion of regular insulin until blood glucose levels have normalized.

Hypokalemia is extremely common posttransplantation. During transplantation, serum potassium levels are purposefully kept low to prevent the cardiac complications associated with abrupt rises immediately after revascularization of the liver allograft. In general, hypokalemia is well tolerated postoperatively, and potassium replacements should be given judiciously until it is ensured that the hepatic allograft is functioning and that renal function is also satisfactory.

Hyperkalemia is a more significant problem. Causes include primary graft nonfunction and fulminant hepatic necrosis or, more commonly, renal dysfunction due to either tubular necrosis or cyclosporine toxicity. Cyclosporine toxicity may also induce a type 4 renal tubular acidosis leading to bicarbonate wasting and potassium retention. Hyperkalemia posttransplantation is treated in a standard fashion with intravenous administration of calcium and insulin, the use of oral or rectal potassium binding resin (Kayexelate), systemic alkalinization, and, in severe cases, hemodialysis.

Other frequently encountered electrolyte abnormalities include those of calcium, phosphate, and magnesium. Hypocalcemia may result from hypoalbuminemia, chelation from a large citrate load, or hepatocyte injury that leads to an intracellular shift of calcium. These effects may exacerbate a pretransplantation deficiency due to an impaired metabolism of vitamin D and parathormone.[37] Hypercalcemia in the posttransplantation period occurs from excess replacement. Elevated serum phosphate levels posttransplantation are due to renal insufficiency and are treated with phosphate binders. When present, hypophosphatemia should be corrected be-

cause phosphate is necessary for adenosine triphosphate (ATP) production. Magnesium is a cofactor for many enzyme systems. Many patients with end-stage liver disease have hypomagnesemia, which can be exacerbated in the early posttransplantation period by the effects of cyclosporine on the renal tubule. Amphotericin B can also cause significant magnesium wasting. High levels of magnesium are uncommon and are most likely due to large doses of magnesium-containing antacids.

RENAL CONSIDERATIONS

Oliguria is extremely common in the early recovery phase following liver transplantation. The most common form manifests itself within 12 to 18 hours of completion of the operation and occurs regardless of whether cyclosporine or tacrolimus (FK506) has been given. Oliguria in this early phase is not usually responsive to fluid administration and does not appear to be related to hypovolemia. The exact mechanisms are not well understood, although the effect is most likely due to fluid shifts and abnormalities of intrarenal perfusion. However, in the absence of other factors (such as mentioned below), the uncomplicated case of oliguria usually resolves within 24 hours and rarely progresses to overt renal failure.

Many recognizable factors may lead to overt renal dysfunction after orthotopic liver transplantation. These include pretransplantation renal insufficiency, intravascular volume status, allograft function, the presence of systemic sepsis, cyclosporine and tacrolimus use, use of nephrotoxic antibiotics or antiviral and antifungal agents, and the use of other nephrotoxic medications.

Many patients who undergo liver transplantation have abnormal renal function preoperatively. Not uncommonly, patients will have a component of prerenal azotemia due to diuretic use, hypoalbuminemia, and frequent paracentesis. In addition, there may be a component of acute tubular necrosis due to hypotension from sepsis or blood loss, or from the use of nephrotoxic medications.

One of the most ominous pretransplantation phenomena is the development of hepatorenal syndrome, which is defined clinically by the following: end-stage liver disease, no history of renal disease prior to the onset of liver failure, normal renal sediment, absence of proteinuria, marked oliguria, urine sodium concentration less than 10 mEq/L, fractional excretion of Na (FE_{Na}) less than 1%, progressive rise in the serum urea nitrogen to creatinine ratio in spite of adequate blood pressures and volumes, and lack of response to volume expansion.[41–43] Hepatorenal syndrome is an acute functional disturbance in renal function in the patient with end-stage liver disease. Spontaneous recovery from hepatorenal syndrome is extremely uncommon. The kidneys in patients with hepatorenal syndrome are normal and have been used successfully as donor organs when transplanted into noncirrhotic patients.[44] Recovery of normal renal function occurs after liver transplantation when hepatic allograft function is satisfactory. Patients with hepatorenal syndrome have been shown to have an intense renal vasoconstriction that may be improved with the administration of prostaglandin E_1.[43] Hepatorenal syndrome does not seem to predispose patients to posttransplantation tubular necrosis.[42]

Cyclosporine and tacrolimus are both nephrotoxic, particularly when administered intravenously. Oral preparations of both are given as soon as possible because these preparations have significantly less nephrotoxicity. When given intravenously, the drugs are administered either as a continuous infusion or over a period of 6 to 8 hours. In patients with adequate left heart filling pressures, the acute onset of oliguria is the first sign of cyclosporine or tacrolimus toxicity. If patients have significant pretransplantation renal impairment or show evidence of cyclosporine or tacrolimus intolerance, induction immunosuppression with OKT3 is utilized. Caution must be used in the volume-overloaded patient because of the possibility of cytokine-mediated acute pulmonary edema after the administration of OKT3. If necessary, hemodialysis, continuous arteriovenous hemofiltration, or slow continuous ultrafiltration may be necessary to remove excess extracellular volume. We also commonly use a low-dose dopamine infusion (2–5 μg/kg per minute) in the early postoperative period in an attempt to improve renal perfusion.[45]

The nephrotoxic effects of cyclosporine or tacrolimus may be recognized by a disproportionate rise in the serum urea nitrogen concentration compared with the serum creatinine concentration. This may be due to alterations in intrarenal blood flow caused by cyclosporine-induced thromboxane A_2 production.[46] Furosemide, although primarily used posttransplantation as a potent loop diuretic, has also been shown to increase renal blood flow.[47] Low-dose furosemide may counteract the cyclosporine nephrotoxicity by increasing renal prostaglandin levels, some of which are vasodilatory, in the cortical microcirculation of the kidney.[48] However, aggressive diuretic use will lead to intravascular volume contraction and contribute to cyclosporine nephrotoxicity.

Many medications that prove necessary in the management of patients after liver transplantation are nephrotoxic. In addition, serum creatinine levels or direct measurements of creatinine clearance frequently lead to overestimation of renal function in patients receiving cyclosporine.[42] Therefore, when choosing doses of drugs that depend on renal elimination, one must rely on frequent measurements of blood levels. The same concerns must be addressed in the use of drugs that require hepatic metabolism for elimination. The use of common antibiotics such as vancomycin and aminoglycosides requires close monitoring of peak and trough serum levels. Ganciclovir and acyclovir are used for both prophylaxis and treatment of cytomegalovirus infection. Dosing of both of these antiviral agents requires adjustments based on creatinine clearance. Amphotericin B is also nephrotoxic, and its use leads to a predictable series of metabolic sequelae. Virtually all patients will develop a renal tubular acidosis and have significant sodium and magnesium losses.

Our approach to the patient who develops oliguria after liver transplantation is first to ensure that left-sided filling pressures (pulmonary artery diastolic or pulmonary capillary wedge pressures) are at least 15 mm Hg. In the patient who develops oliguria during cyclosporine or tacrolimus parenteral infusion, that dose is held and the amount of the next scheduled dose is decreased. Renal-dose dopamine is liberally utilized. Consideration is also given to postrenal causes, and the Foley catheter is irrigated and abdominal ultrasonography may be performed to rule out hydronephrosis. If return of gastrointestinal function allows for predictable absorption of oral cyclosporine or tacrolimus, these agents should be given enterally. If oliguria persists and creatinine concentration rises, OKT3 (5.0 mg IV for adults and 2.5 mg for children under 30 kg) may be used and cyclosporine or tacrolimus discontinued. Induction with OKT3 is used routinely in patients with significant pretransplantation renal dysfunction.

In patients without an obvious etiology for posttransplantation renal failure, occult sources of sepsis should be carefully searched for. Renal dysfunction that is attributable to poor liver allograft function is similar to that caused by pretransplantation hepatorenal syndrome in that the renal dysfunction will persist until graft recovery or retransplantation is accomplished.

Polyuria after orthotopic liver transplantation is uncommon. Causes include a postacute tubular necrosis diuresis or hypoglycemia. Adequate intravascular volume should be maintained during a period of significant diuresis.

HEMODYNAMIC MONITORING

Having dealt in the foregoing discussion with some of the general concerns associated with managing renal function and fluid and electrolyte balance in patients recovering from liver transplant surgery, we can consider the special challenges these patients present in the routine use of hemodynamic monitors and ventilator support. In large part, much of what makes the proper care of these patients different from that needed by the usual postsurgical patient is the extremely hyperdynamic circulatory status. Hyperdynamic circulation makes both the interpretation and response to standard measures of hemodynamic status hazardous for the uninitiated physician. Unfortunately, the available literature does not adequately address the peculiar responses of patients with chronic liver disease to acute stress, such as that associated with major surgery. Much of the discussion that follows is, in fact, based more on the authors' experience than on well-controlled clinical or laboratory studies. Delineation of the neural and hormonal causes of the hyperdynamic state associated with chronic liver disease would go a long way toward allowing a more erudite discussion of this matter.

TABLE 24.1. *Classification of liver transplant recipients*

Group	Hyperdynamic circulation	Abnormal sodium metabolism	Malnutrition	Pulmonary hypertension	Cardiac dysfunction
I	—	—	—	—	—
II	+	±	±	—	—
III	++	++	++	—	—
IV	++	++	++	+	+

To better understand the management of patients after liver transplantation, we find it convenient to assign a patient to one of several possible groups as depicted in Table 24.1. Group I represents patients with little or no evidence of the hyperdynamic circulation associated with chronic liver disease. This group includes patients with primary hepatic malignancies but without underlying liver disease. It might also include some patients with acute liver failure, although these patients will develop hyperdynamic circulation in the advanced stages of liver failure even in the acute setting.

Group I patients normally tolerate the stress of surgery much as would any patient without liver disease who undergoes major surgery. These patients are more likely to be able to withstand the anhepatic phase of the transplant surgery without the need for venous bypass. Blood loss in these patients should be minimal, as should the need for volume resuscitation, leading to minimal fluid shifts in the immediate postoperative period.

In the early management of group I patients, adequate vascular volume must be maintained. Even in the absence of large-volume fluid or blood losses during the transplant operation, fluid sequestration will occur in the abdomen because of the extensive raw surface areas and intestinal ileus. Group I patients are most likely to be able to maintain adequate arterial blood pressure even in the face of progressive dehydration and volume contraction. The use of a pulmonary artery pressure catheter will yield information much as it does in other postsurgical patients. Inadequate vascular volume will be reflected by a fall in cardiac output and an increase in systemic vascular resistance associated with low filling pressures, such as central venous pressure or pulmonary artery wedge pressure (PAWP). In the setting of hypovolemia, group I patients will demonstrate an increase in the difference between arterial and venous blood oxygen content ($\Delta Ca\text{-}\bar{v}o_2$) as oxygen delivery decreases. This is associated with decreased cardiac output without a concomitant fall in oxygen consumption. With further volume depletion, compensatory mechanisms eventually will lead to a decrease in oxygen consumption in association with increased anaerobic metabolism. Low oxygen saturation in mixed venous blood samples along with increasing concentration of blood lactate levels are associated with the most severe manifestations of hypovolemic shock.

Group I patients respond to fluid infusion much as do so-called healthy patients (those without advanced liver disease). Low urine output in association with low filling pressures will usually respond promptly to fluid administration that is titrated to achieve a PAWP in the 12 to 15 mm Hg range. In those patients in whom a satisfactory response (manifested by restoration of urine output) is not seen, a search for other causes of low urine output should be repeated (as discussed previously).

Group II patients are those with chronic liver disease who have hyperdynamic circulation but who have maintained normal or near-normal levels of serum albumin and have normal or near-normal sodium metabolism. The major difference from group I patients is the high cardiac output and relatively low arterial-venous oxygen content difference ($\Delta Ca\text{-}\bar{v}o_2$) manifested by group II patients. In the immediate period following surgery, this may lead to confusion if one relies on these measurements to judge the adequacy of fluid resuscitation. Group II patients with low urine output may manifest both normal cardiac output and satisfactory mixed venous blood oxygen saturation ($S\bar{v}o_2$) and $\Delta Ca\text{-}\bar{v}o_2$ and yet still require fluid administration. In such cases, it is helpful to review the values of hemodynamic parameters maintained during surgery. By doing so, one can usually discover which values were associated with the best evidence of end-organ function (e.g., urine output) during surgery. These values can then serve as targets during the early postoperative phase should the patient experience a fall in urine output below 25 to 30 mL per minute or 0.5 to 1.0 mL/kg per minute.

Both group I and group II patients can suffer dramatic falls in serum levels of albumin in the immediate period after transplantation. The cause may be iatrogenic as a result of large-volume losses of body fluids with high protein content and replacement with crystalloid. It may also stem from inadequate replacement of protein losses from ascites in the operative and immediate postoperative phases. In mild cases of hypoalbuminemia and with good liver graft function, these patients usually do not need supplementation with exogenous albumin. Nevertheless, some authors have suggested that maintenance of serum albumin levels above 3.0 to 3.2 g/dL is beneficial and reduces the incidence of oliguria.[49] Our bias is to avoid exogenous albumin unless oliguria presents in the face of both hypovolemia and a serum albumin level that is less than 3.0 g/dL.

Group I and II patients who have experienced uncomplicated intraoperative courses with low blood losses and good fluid management will normally arrive in the intensive care unit in a euvolemic to slightly hypervolemic state. In these cases, administration of normal maintenance fluids, such as D5W normal saline at 100 to 150 mL/h in most adults, will suffice as a starting point for postoperative fluid orders. The regimen can be modified in the next several hours according to individual patient needs. For example, whereas a group I patient may have little or no ascites output from abdominal drains, a group II patient might lose several liters in the first few hours. The latter patient's losses of fluid, electrolytes, and protein will require more aggressive replacement than the former. Furthermore, unlike group III or IV patients, the group II patient may respond in an entirely appropriate manner to early fluid replacement. As liver allograft function improves and portal hypertension resolves, these patients may begin to behave much like group I patients.

Group III and IV patients represent difficult challenges, both during the transplant operation and in the immediate period afterward. These are patients with advanced liver disease who have extremely hyperdynamic circulation, severe hypoalbuminemia and associated severe malnutrition, abnormal sodium metabolism, and abnormal renal function. Such patients come to operation with massive ascites and some degree of hepatorenal syndrome, usually complicated by a degree of acute tubular necrosis or perhaps interstitial nephritis secondary to antibiotics or other medications. Group IV patients are distinguished from group III patients by having the added disadvantage of clinically significant cardiopulmonary dysfunction. Long-standing hyperdynamic circulation can be associated with severe cardiomyopathy or pulmonary hypertension. Although the causative mechanisms for either of these complications is not well understood, each can represent a prohibitive risk for the patient who requires liver transplantation. For those in whom the degree of either cardiac failure or pulmonary hypertension is not severe enough to warrant exclusion from transplantation, the early postoperative management will be complicated nonetheless.

Oliguria or hypotension in the early postoperative period requires a more careful approach in group III and IV patients than in group I or II patients. Exuberant use of albumin or plasma fractions may result in overcorrection of hyponatremia, with the attendant risk of central pontine myelinolysis. Overuse of hypotonic crystalloid solutions will only worsen hyponatremia while leading to further accumulation of total body water. One must keep in mind that the intravascular life span of most intravenously administered crystalloid solutions is likely to be quite short in these patients. Thus, for the most part, the use of large boluses of colloid solutions is reserved for those instances when rapid restoration of intravascular volume is required. If hyponatremia is already present, care must be taken to avoid the use of rapid infusions of isotonic solutions. Instead, the judicious use of a mixture of isotonic and hypotonic solutions will be less likely to result in the kind of rapid fluxes in serum sodium levels that are associated with central pontine myelinolysis (namely, a change of 23 mEq/L or more in less than 48 hours).

The fluid of choice to use for maintenance purposes in group III and IV patients is somewhat controversial. One option is to use large volumes (150–250 mL) of 25% albumin infused over several hours. Proportionate to the amount of albumin administered, the amount of sodium and water given will be much less than with an oncotically equivalent amount of 5% albumin or other plasma fractions. However, this technique is extremely expensive and will result in only temporary improvements in serum albumin levels because these patients will lose much of the exogenously administered protein via ascites. Our preference is to use moderate amounts of 25% albumin in an attempt to raise serum albumin levels to the 3.0 g/dL range in patients in whom some correction of hypovolemia is required.

In reality, until normal liver function succeeds in restoring sodium metabolism, protein synthesis, and whatever else is responsible for correction of hyperdynamic circulation and portal hypertension, some degree of relative hypovolemia will need to be tolerated in these patients. The trick is to avoid excessive volume contraction. Once again, a review of the intraoperative course may provide useful guidelines. In contrast to group I or II patients, however, group III and IV patients will not benefit in the long run by overzealous attention to maintaining adequate filling pressures. Such an approach will always result in a self-sustaining spiral of more fluid causing more ascites, which, when removed through the abdominal drains, leads to further volume contraction followed by further fluid administration and more ascites formation. (The alternative of allowing ascites to accumulate has other undesirable effects, including the risk of peritonitis, alteration of renal hemodynamics, and ventilatory compromise from increased intraabdominal pressure.) Although a fluid bolus will result in a temporary improvement—perhaps even a brief episode of increased urine output—eventual interruption of this cycle will require an acceptance of the abnormal physiology and maintenance of the delicate balance between too little and too much intravascular expansion. This balance is almost never well identified by the usual measures of filling pressures or cardiac output, but rather by the combination of these values that yields acceptable renal function and tolerable ascites production.

If urine output falls below 20 to 30 mL per hour for adults or 0.5 mL/kg per hour for children, and in the face of filling pressures that are less than optimal (PAWP above 15 to 18 mm Hg), a single 250 mL bolus of 5% albumin is administered over 20 to 30 minutes and hemodynamic pressures measured again. If urine output remains low and filling pressures remain below a PAWP of 10 to 12 mm Hg, a second bolus is given. If, in response, filling pressures have risen to a PAWP of between 12 and 15 mm Hg and urine output has not improved, further boluses are unlikely to be

TABLE 24.2. *Vasoactive drugs and their specific actions*

Class	Drug	BP	SVR	Cardiac output	HR	Inotropic low dose	Inotropic high dose	Renal blood flow	Coronary blood flow	$S\bar{v}O_2$
α only	Phenylephrine	↑↑↑	↑↑↑↑	↓↓↓	↓↓↓	±	±	↓↓↓↓	±↑↑	↑
α and β	Norepinephrine	↑↑	↑↑↑	↓↓	↓↓±	↑	↑	↓↓↓↓	↑↑	↑↑
α and β	Epinephrine	↑±	↑±	↑↑	↑↑↑	↑↑	↑↑↑	↓±	↑↑	↑↑↑
β only	Isoproterenol	↑±	↓↓	↑↑↑↑	↑↑↑↑	↑↑↑	↑↑↑↑	±	↑↑↑	↑↑↑↑
β only	Dobutamine	↓↓	↓↓↓	↑↑↑	↑↑	↑↑↑	↑↑↑	±	↑↑↑	↑↑↑↑
α and β	Dopamine	↑↑	↑↑	↑↑	↑	±	↑↑	↑↑↑	↑↑	↑↑
β-Blocker	Propranolol	±↓	±	↓↓↓	↓↓↓↓	↓↓	↓↓↓	↓	↓↓	↓↓↓
β-Blocker	Metoprolol	↓↓↓	↓	↓↓	↓↓↓	↓↓	↓↓↓	±	↓↓	↓↓
Other	Nitroglycerine	±↓	↓↓	↑↑	±	±	±	±↑	↓	↓↓↓
Other	Hydralazine	↓↓↓	↓↓↓	↑↑	↑↑	±	±	±↑	↓	↓↓
Other	Prazosin	↓↓↓	↓↓	↑↑	±	±	±	±↑	↓	↓↓
Other	Nitroprusside	↓↓	↓↓↓	↑↑↑	±↑	±	±	↑↑	±	↓↓

BP, blood pressure; SVR, systemic vascular resistance; HR, heart rate; $S\bar{v}O_2$, mixed venous oxygen saturation.

Table courtesy of T.P. Clemmer, Director, Shock and Trauma ICU, LDS Hospital, Salt Lake City, Utah, 1979.

of further benefit. This is the point where considerable personal preference, sometimes immodestly referred to as the art of medicine, is inclined to rule the day. We will discuss a few of our favorite courses of action.

Most of our colleagues are fond of using "renal-dose" dopamine at 2 to 3 μg/kg per minute. Some authors have provided anecdotal evidence to suggest that in this setting, low-dose dopamine has a beneficial effect on renal function.[45] However, in view of a lack of specific scientific data and an inconsistent personal experience, we remain skeptical of the benefits of this approach. Of course, lack of data rarely serves as a worthy adversary to faith. So it is that we too often start low-dose dopamine at an early stage in the management of these patients, once we are convinced that volume status is not severely contracted. One must keep in mind, however, that the use of this agent only makes the task of maintaining adequate filling pressures all the more important. The unwary clinician may return to the bedside at a later hour to find that volume contraction has led to hypotension and that hypotension has resulted in an insidious upward creep in the dose of dopamine. Of course, this caveat only serves to point out the more general need for all active members of the care team to understand the goals and imposed limits on the use of all medications, especially powerful vasoactive agents.

Another favorite technique, often following soon after the dopamine has been discovered to be lacking in restorative powers, is the "albumin cocktail with Lasix chaser." The proponents of this remedy administer 50 to 100 mL of 25% albumin over 20 to 30 minutes and follow it with an intravenous bolus of furosemide (20–80 mg, per taste). If this results in a noticeable response in the urine output, it may be repeated every 4 to 8 hours, apparently dependent more on how anxious the physician is about the low urine output than on any more mundane issues (such as cost or effectiveness).

Traditionally, one approaches the hypoperfused patient with three basic questions: Is intravascular volume adequate? Is cardiac contractility optimal? Would afterload reduction improve cardiac function? One does not traditionally believe that an increase in afterload can improve oxygen delivery, except perhaps for a brief period in emergency situations when one is attempting to maintain brain and myocardial perfusion.

Table 24.2 lists the more common vasoactive drugs and their effects on various physiological parameters. These drugs may be used alone or in combination, depending on the specific needs of the patient. For example, a patient with low cardiac output in the face of adequate filling pressures and high systemic vascular resistance may respond to low-dose epinephrine (inotropic effect and afterload reduction from vasodilatory β-agonist effect), amniodorone and related compounds, or a combination of inotrope and peripheral vasodilator (e.g., dopamine in the 10–15 μg/kg range and nitroprusside). In the following section, we discuss some unique problems that may attend the management of the group of patients we have categorized as group IV.

PROBLEMS OF GROUP IV PATIENTS

Pulmonary Hypertension

Pulmonary hypertension is a complication of chronic liver disease. When severe, it must be viewed as a contraindication to liver transplantation. In our experience, patients with resting mean pulmonary artery pressures above 45 to 50 mm Hg have a prohibitive risk of mortality with liver transplantation. Although some authors have suggested that pulmonary hypertension does not resolve after liver transplantation,[50] others have had reasonable success in this setting.[51,52] The difficulties that have been encountered with such patients occur in the intraoperative and postoperative course and appear to arise chiefly as the result of such patients' intolerance to fluid overload, pulmonary atelectasis, the effects of positive pressure ventilation, or significant increases in systemic vascular resistance that also lead to critical increases in pulmonary vascular resistance.

Measures that may be of value in keeping pulmonary vascular resistance within an acceptable range include vigorous pulmonary toilet; early extubation; avoidance of fluid overload; the use of hemofiltration in the event that an effective diuresis cannot be accomplished; and the administration of aerosolized or intravenous bronchodilators and a variety of vasoactive substances intended to dilate pulmonary vascular beds, including isoproterenol, priscoline, prostaglandin E_1, aminophylline, and nitroprusside. However, all of these measures may fail and the patient succumb to right-sided cardiac failure. The use of a right ventricular assist device, although not yet reported in the literature, may be of value as a means of providing temporary support for such patients. Pulmonary hypertension can be expected to resolve gradually during the first 3 to 6 months posttransplantation provided the patient has sustained normal liver function.[53]

Pulmonary Shunting

Intrapulmonary shunting, in the absence of pulmonary hypertension, is a recognized complication of advanced liver disease.[54] The shunting is caused by the formation of abnormal communicating channels, presumably between pulmonary arterioles and venules, that result in right-to-left shunting of blood. Nuclear scanning techniques and angiography often reveal that they are most severe in the lung bases.[55] In severe cases, the calculated degree of shunting may be as high as 75%. The specific stimulation for the development of these arteriovenous malformations is not known. In response to a verbal report from the University of Pittsburgh hailing the effectiveness of somatostatin analogue (octreotide) in reversing shunts prior to liver transplantation, we and others undertook empirical treatment of small groups of patients. However, using the same protocol as well as higher doses of somatostatin analogue, we were not able to confirm any beneficial effect in five patients with severe shunting who were awaiting liver transplantation. Krowka et al. from the Mayo Clinic reported a similar failure of somatostatin to alter the degree of shunting in patients with the hepatopulmonary syndrome.[56] Fortunately, as reported by several investigators, shunting begins to resolve within several months of successful liver transplantation.[57,58]

The perioperative management of such patients may be extremely difficult. As with pulmonary hypertension, multiple changes in a patient's condition that are normal events after liver transplantation can have a profound negative effect on pulmonary shunts. Atelectasis is perhaps the most common problem. Normally, alveolar collapse results in some increased pulmonary vascular resistance in atelectatic segments as a reflex response intended to decrease shunting by not perfusing those pulmonary capillary beds associated with unventilated alveoli. However, because the abnormal vascular shunts do not respond to hormonal or neurogenic control mechanisms, this reflex response causes a greater proportion of pulmonary arterial blood to flow through the shunts.

As in the management of pulmonary hypertension, vasoactive drugs that dilate normal pulmonary vascular beds may have a critical role in maintaining adequate oxygen delivery in patients with severe hypoxia secondary to intrapulmonary shunting. Isoproterenol, nitroglycerin, prostaglandin E_1, and priscoline are four agents that we have found to be of variable assistance in these patients. In all cases, one should be more concerned with assessing the evidence of adequate oxygen transport to the tissues than with concentrating solely on the arterial Po_2. In most cases, these patients have developed remarkable adaptive mechanisms for dealing with severely depressed levels of arterial oxygen content. Nevertheless, they do not develop the capacity of surviving on anaerobic metabolism. Agitation, air hunger, and tachypnea are physical signs that should alert the clinician to the possibility of inadequate oxygenation. Lactic acidosis is a late sign of ongoing anaerobic metabolism and mandates aggressive measures to improve oxygen transport.

OXYGEN DELIVERY AND TRANSPORT

In approaching the hemodynamic and ventilatory management of the critically ill patient, including one who has undergone liver transplantation, we find it useful to focus on the goals of that management. The most basic need of the patient is delivery of adequate oxygen to mitochondria. The most important mitochondria are those in the brain and myocardium. The organs supported by those mitochondria are among the least tolerant tissues to hypoxia because they are not capable either of sustained suspension of metabolic activity or of metabolizing lactate, the product of anaerobic metabolism. In addition, loss of even small amounts of tissue in these organs to hypoxic death can have devastating results, in contrast to similar tissue destruction in other organ systems. Nevertheless, during any resuscitative efforts, we eventually have to provide the rest of the organism's mitochondria with oxygen as well. The earlier we accomplish that goal in stabilizing the critical patient, the less organ damage the patient will sustain.

Shunting and Ventilation-Perfusion Mismatch

In practice, the usual first clue of possible problems with oxygen delivery is a fall in arterial Po_2 (Pao_2). When this happens, it is important to distinguish whether the fall in Pao_2 is significant. To do so, calculate the actual content of oxygen in arterial blood (Cao_2 = Sao_2 × 1.34 × hemoglobin + Po_2 × 0.003). (Table 24.3 defines pulmonary-respiratory symbols that are used in the following discussion. Table 24.4 lists important equations.) At the levels of Pao_2 normally found in postoperative patients, the contribution of dissolved oxygen to the total oxygen content of blood is negligible. Thus the

TABLE 24.3. *Common symbols used in discussion of oxygen transport*

Symbol	Meaning
Po_2	Partial pressure of oxygen
Pao_2	Arterial partial pressure of oxygen
PAo_2	Partial pressure of oxygen in the alveoli
$P\bar{v}o_2$	Venous partial pressure of oxygen
$P(A\text{-}a)o_2$	Alveolar-arterial difference in partial pressure of oxygen
P_B	Barometric pressure
Cao_2	Arterial oxygen content
$Cc'o_2$	Pulmonary capillary oxygen content
$C\bar{v}o_2$	Mixed venous oxygen content
$Ca\text{-}\bar{v}o_2\Delta$	Difference between arterial and venous oxygen content
Fio_2	Fraction of inspired gas that is oxygen
R	Respiratory quotient
Sao_2	Arterial hemoglobin oxygen saturation
$S\bar{v}o_2$	Mixed venous hemoglobin oxygen saturation
Qs/Qt	Pulmonary shunt fraction
$\dot{V}/\dot{Q}$	Ventilation to perfusion ratio

Sao_2 is a much more important indication of the amount of oxygen contained in blood. Because of the wide variation in the affinity of hemoglobin (Hgb) for oxygen often found in critically ill patients, one should be certain that the value of Sao_2 that one uses is *measured* and not calculated from the Pao_2 using a standard nomogram.

It is also important to distinguish whether the observed fall in Pao_2 is related to pulmonary disease processes rather than alveolar hypoventilation. This is done by calculating the alveolar-arterial oxygen gradient [$P(A\text{-}a)o_2$]. A few simple examples using the formulas in Table 24.4 will suffice to show the importance of this distinction.

An anxious 45-year-old man with deep venous thrombosis following living-related liver donation develops atypical

TABLE 24.4. *Equations used in evaluating oxygen transport*

$Cao_2 = Sao_2 \times 1.39 \times Hgb + Pao_2 \times 0.0031$
$C\bar{v}o_2 = S\bar{v}o_2 \times 1.39 \times Hgb + P\bar{v}o_2 \times 0.0031$
$Cc'o_2 = Hgb \times 1.39 + PAo_2 \times 0.0031$
$Ca\text{-}\bar{v}o_2 = Cao_2 - C\bar{v}o_2$
$PAo_2 = (P_B - 47) \times Fio_2 - Pco_2[Fio_2 + (1 - Fio_2)/R]$[a]
$PAo_2 = (P_B - 47) - Pco_2$ when $Fio_2 = 1.00$
$P(A-a)o_2 = PAo_2 - Pao_2$
$Qs/Qt = (Cc'o_2 - Cao_2)/(Cc'o_2 - C\bar{v}o_2)$
Fick equation: $\dot{V}o_2 = $ Cardiac output $\times (Cao_2 - C\bar{v}o_2) \times 10$[b]

Hgb, hemoglobin. See Table 23.3 for definitions of the respiratory symbols.

[a]R is usually assumed to be 0.75.

[b]Oxygen consumption (in mL/min) equals cardiac output (in L/min) times the difference between the arterial and mixed venous oxygen content (in mL/dL) times 10 dl/L. This equation can be simplified to the following: $\dot{V}o_2 = $ Cardiac output $\times 13.9 \times Hgb \times (Sao_2 - S\bar{v}o_2)$.

chest pain and tachypnea on the third postoperative day and is found to have the following arterial blood gases:

pH	7.48
$Paco_2$	23
Hco_3	15
Pao_2	93
Sao_2	96
Hgb	14.2
Fio_2	0.21

Does this patient have a problem with oxygen transport or delivery that should cause concern and lead to further investigations? Using the equations in Table 24.4, we can calculate the $P(A\text{-}a)o_2$, which in this patient is 27.7 mm Hg. The alveolar-arterial gradient increases with age, but a rough rule of thumb is that it should be about one-third of the patient's age, in this case 15 mm Hg. Therefore, this patient has an abnormal $P(A\text{-}a)o_2$. Our clinical suspicion that he has suffered a pulmonary embolism is supported by the blood gases. In this case, the Pao_2 and Sao_2 both appear satisfactory. However, the patient has been hyperventilating, with a resultant decrease in alveolar (and hence arterial) Pco_2. The calculations reveal the abnormality in oxygen delivery in the form of an elevated $P(A\text{-}a)o_2$.

The second example patient is a 59-year-old woman who underwent liver transplantation 12 hours earlier and has been extubated for 2 hours. She is described by the nurse as sleepy but arousable. Her spontaneous respiratory rate is 6 breaths per minute. Cutaneous oximetry reveals a Sao_2 of 80%. The following arterial blood gases are obtained:

pH	7.40
$Paco_2$	59
Pao_2	45
Sao_2	80
Hgb	14.2
Fio_2	0.21

Calculation of the $P(A\text{-}a)o_2$ shows that it is about 16 mm Hg, within the normal range for this patient. The low Pao_2 is not related to primary pulmonary pathology, but rather to alveolar hypoventilation. The patient needs ventilator support, not an increased Fio_2. The elevation in $Paco_2$ is responsible for an elevated $PAco_2$, which, because of the law of partial pressures of gases, leads to the reduction in PAo_2. The hypoventilation may be in response to a severe metabolic alkalosis, since the pH is normal. This is not an unusual set of circumstances early after liver transplantation, especially if the patient has developed citrate overload, as described previously.

If we determine that the fall in Pao_2 is not related to alveolar hypoventilation, we must next determine whether the abnormal process in the lungs is caused by an increase in the amount of blood that is shunted through the lungs without the benefit of gas exchange with ventilated alveoli (dead space) or by an increase in the number of alveoli that are ventilated but not perfused (ventilation-perfusion mismatch). Although extremely rare after liver transplantation, pulmonary embolism is the most common cause of increased dead space in other surgical patients. Atelectasis, on the other hand, is the most common cause of increased shunting. In addition, as discussed previously, advanced liver disease may be attended by severe anatomical shunting.

One immediate clinical distinction between shunting and ventilation-perfusion ($\dot{V}/\dot{Q}$) mismatch is that correction of a lower Pa_{O_2} in patients with increased dead space usually can be accomplished with small increases in Fi_{O_2} (an exception would be a massive pulmonary embolism). This is in contrast to the situation when dealing with shunts. Figures 24.1 and 24.2 show why this is the case. Figure 24.1A shows the profound effect that a shunt has on the Pa_{O_2} in a patient breathing room air with a PA_{O_2} of 150 mm Hg. Figure 24.1B demonstrates why supplemental oxygen may have little effect toward improving oxygenation in a patient with severe shunting. Even though the PA_{O_2} has been increased to 713 mm Hg in the ventilated alveoli, the mixing of blood that has perfused unventilated alveoli (shunted blood) effectively dilutes the increased oxygen content obtained with supplemental oxygen.

In contrast, Figure 24.2 shows how little effect a $\dot{V}/\dot{Q}$ mismatch caused by a pulmonary embolus has on Pa_{O_2}. The cause of hypoxia associated with a pulmonary embolus is, in most cases, related to reflex bronchoconstriction in the area of the occluded blood vessel. This leads to a lower rate of diffusion of oxygen into the nonoccluded capillaries perfusing affected alveoli. Figure 24.3 demonstrates how a relatively small increase in the Fi_{O_2} will lead to normalization of arterial oxygen saturation.

In practice, problems of $\dot{V}/\dot{Q}$ mismatch are less common than problems with shunting after liver transplantation. However, we should keep in mind some unique problems that these patients may have, some of which lead to increased shunting but are still readily corrected.

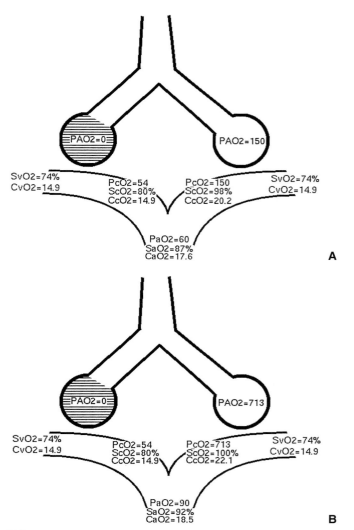

FIG. 24.1. A: The effect of a shunt in a patient breathing room air. Note the effect on Pa_{O_2} of mixing shunted blood with non-shunted blood. **B:** The relatively minor effect of increased fraction of inspired oxygen on Pa_{O_2} in a patient with a shunt. (Adapted from Clemmer TP, Director, Shock and Trauma Unit, LDS Hospital, Salt Lake City, Utah.)

Pleural Effusions

Patients with chronic liver disease may develop significant pleural effusions. The amount of pleural fluid that accumulates is dependent on the type and size of communicating channels between the peritoneal and pleural cavities as well as the pressure differential between these cavities. For instance, some patients with massive ascites may accumulate only small amounts of fluid in the chest because of the small size of the channels. At the other extreme, patients may present with massive pleural effusions with no evidence of significant ascites owing to large communicating channels combined with a substantial pressure gradient favoring movement of ascites into the chest. In any case, the reaccumulation of ascites during the first few days or weeks after liver transplantation may be associated with the development of clinically significant pleural effusions. In fact,

because removal of the native liver involves dissection into the bare area of the abdominal surface of the diaphragm, the threat of pleural effusion may be greater after transplantation than before.

Pleural effusions usually result in increased shunting as accumulating fluid causes alveolar or airway collapse, usually without a proportionate alteration in perfusion. Lung volumes may also be compromised by limitations in diaphragmatic excursion imposed by reaccumulation of fluid in the abdomen independent of the development of pleural effusions. In fact, these considerations are the main reason that drains are placed in the abdomen prior to abdominal wall closure during the transplant procedure. These drains can provide an important tool in the management of fluid accumulation in the early postoperative period. This may

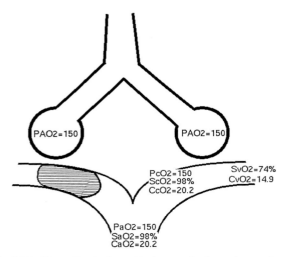

FIG. 24.2. The effect of ventilation-perfusion mismatch secondary to pulmonary embolism on Pao_2. (Adapted from Clemmer TP, Director, Shock and Trauma Unit, LDS Hospital, Salt Lake City, Utah.)

prove of critical importance in those patients with marginal pulmonary function.

Some investigators have claimed that patients with chronic liver disease have abnormally low airway closure pressures.[56] This may lead to an increased risk of atelectasis in these patients, particularly after major surgery. Combined with the observed tendency toward fluid accumulation in the chest cavity, liver transplant patients may exhibit an increased risk of respiratory failure following early extubation. This is of major importance in the early postoperative management of group III or IV patients. This translates to the need to be certain that these patients are fully awake and that one has reasonable control of the fluid dynamics prior to extubation. Removal from positive pressure ventilation may be associated with rapid accumulation of pleural fluid or, more frequently, widespread atelectasis. Reintubation should not be delayed in the event a patient shows early signs of tiring out or becoming hypoxic after extubation.

A Model for Understanding Oxygen Transport

The essential point of the foregoing discussion has been to emphasize the critical need to define exactly what problem the patient is having. Let us assume that at this point, we have examined the patient and found clinical evidence of inadequate oxygenation. Furthermore, we have measured the Pao_2 and calculated the alveolar-arterial gradient and found it to be abnormal, suggesting that alveolar hypoventilation is *not* the primary problem. Further, we have documented that the patient does not have evidence of either massive ascites or pleural effusion compromising ventilatory status. Likewise, a chest x-ray does not reveal any evidence either of pneumothorax or of major segmental collapse that might benefit from therapeutic bronchoscopy. We do not suspect pulmonary embolism both because it is exceedingly uncommon after liver transplantation and because a moderate increase in Fio_2 has not improved the patient's Pao_2. At this point, we are left to deal with a patient who requires more aggressive maneuvers to improve the transport of adequate oxygen to tissues. To aid in understanding how various measures interact with the physiological mechanisms of oxygen delivery, it is useful to review a simple model.

One can think of the entire process of oxygen delivery as analogous to the series of tasks necessary to supply a busy factory with raw materials. For our purposes here, we will consider a coal-burning power plant that is supplied by a coal train. The train is filled with chunks of coal at the coal mine and travels to the coal factory, where the coal is unloaded while the train remains in motion. The train moves in a continuous circle between the coal factory and the power plant. Depending on the demand on the plant for power, the train can be ordered to increase or decrease the speed at which it delivers coal. In addition, the amount of coal loaded into each train car can vary, as can the number of cars on the train. However, the carrying capacity of each car is limited, meaning that they cannot be more than 100% filled. To some degree, the size of the opening through which the coal can be loaded into the cart (and through

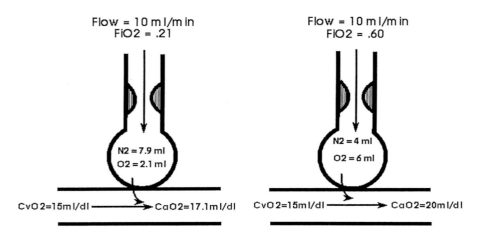

FIG. 24.3. The effect of increased fraction of inspired oxygen on ventilation-perfusion mismatch related to regional bronchospasm in pulmonary embolism. Note the relatively greater benefit of supplemental oxygen compared with Fig. 24.1B, depicting a shunt. (Adapted from Clemmer TP, Director, Shock and Trauma Unit, LDS Hospital, Salt Lake City, Utah.)

TABLE 24.5. *Physiological equivalents to the coal train and power plant model*

Physiology	Model
Cardiac output	Speed of the train
Arterial oxygen content (Cao_2)	Total amount of coal per train
Arterial oxygen saturation (Sao_2)	Percent filling of cars with coal at the coal mine
Mixed venous oxygen saturation ($S\bar{v}o_2$)	Percentage of car occupied by coal when train returns to be reloaded
Hemoglobin	Number of cars on train
Oxygen-hemoglobin dissociation (P_{50})	Size of cars
Dissolved oxygen ($Po_2 \times 0.003$)	Coal dust
Arterial partial pressure of oxygen (Pao_2)	Filling pressure at coal mine
Arterial-venous oxygen content difference ($Ca-\bar{v}o_2$)	Difference in amount of coal leaving mine from that returning in cars from power plant

which the coal is unloaded at the power plant) can be varied. Table 24.5 shows the physiological equivalents in this coal mine–power plant model. The chunks of coal are equivalent to oxygen molecules carried by hemoglobin; each individual car can be thought of as a discrete amount of hemoglobin, such as that contained in a red blood cell. The number of cars in the train is equivalent to blood hemoglobin concentration, and the speed of the train is equivalent to cardiac output.

A student once asked where dissolved oxygen fits into this model. After some discussion, we decided that the arterial Po_2 is represented in the model by the force with which coal comes down the chute and into the coal cars. If this force is high, cars are filled rapidly and efficiently. The dissolved oxygen is perhaps best thought of as the coal dust that inevitably accompanies the loading of great chunks of coal. Higher loading force probably yields more coal dust within the cars. Coal dust is certainly unloaded at the plant and it is undoubtedly used, but it is normally a relatively unimportant amount of coal compared with the amount represented by the large chunks loaded into the cars. This relatively minute quantity of coal is analogous to the small quantity of oxygen transported as dissolved gas in blood.

To carry the analogy further, we should recognize that at normal operating forces, the cars are over 90% filled with chunks of coal. Nevertheless, one can also understand that as the loading force decreases (analogous to a falling arterial Po_2), at some point the filling of the cars will become inefficient enough that cars leave the coal mine severely underfilled. The relationship between the loading forces and the degree of filling of the cars is represented by the oxygen-hemoglobin dissociation curve. In our model, the shape and position of this curve is perhaps most analogous to the size of the train cars. Hence, a shift in the curve to the right that results in a lower affinity of hemoglobin for oxygen means that a higher Po_2 is required to achieve the same degree of hemoglobin saturation. This is analogous to saying that it takes a higher loading pressure to get a larger car as full when the speed of the train is held constant. But, this also means that more coal is available at the power plant per car on the train for the same degree of car filling, just as a higher

Po_2 will be achieved at the capillary level for a given Sao_2 when the oxygen-hemoglobin dissociation curve shifts to the right. Of course, the size of our cars is not unlimited. In addition, too large a car results in inadequate filling at the achievable filling pressure levels. (I think this means that the cars are emptied at the power plant through the top and when the cars are not very full, not very much coal is retrieved, regardless of how big the cars are.)

One of the problems with management of our power plant is the fact that we have not yet found the key to unlock the door and allow us to walk inside, view the gauges, and make direct determinations about whether the plant is receiving enough coal in proportion to the demand for power. Instead, we have to make certain assumptions about the relative proportions of the amount of coal going into the plant and the amount of coal left behind in the coal cars when they leave the plant. If the coal cars come out of the plant empty, then we have no way of knowing whether we have supplied enough coal to meet the demands. However, if the cars exit the power plant with a substantial amount of coal still in them, we can have some confidence that we have supplied enough coal. Through past experience, we have learned that if the coal cars return to the mine approximately 70% to 75% full, we can be fairly certain that we have met the demands of the power plant.

Continuing the analogy, when we begin to see evidence that the power plant is not receiving enough coal (in the physiologic case, by end-organ dysfunction and lactic acidosis), we should examine how we might better supply coal. One option is to speed up the train, which in the patient means increasing cardiac output. Cardiac output can be enhanced by ensuring that the intravascular volume is adequate, that cardiac contractility is satisfactory, and that afterload is not so high that it causes cardiac dysfunction. Second, we can increase the number of cars on the train by transfusing the patient with red blood cells. Similarly, we should be concerned about how full the cars are when they leave the mine and recognize that only when the force with which the coal is loaded into the cars falls below a certain level will there be a noticeable decline in the percentage of filling in the cars. This is equivalent to saying that only below a certain partial pressure of oxygen in arterial blood do we begin to see clinically significant oxygen desaturation of hemoglobin. However, once we do fall below that level (typically an arterial Po_2 of 50 to 65 mm Hg), the oxygen saturation can fall dramatically as we enter the steep part of the oxygen-hemoglobin dissociation curve (Fig. 24.4).

The difference between the amount of coal being delivered to the power plant and the quantity arriving back at the mine is equivalent to the arterial-venous oxygen content difference. As this difference widens, we need to be concerned about the efficiency of coal delivery. We also need to recognize that under certain abnormal conditions, the difference between the amount of coal entering and the amount of coal coming out of the power plant may be within the satisfactory range but the coal may not actually be accessible or properly used within the power plant. This is equivalent to the type of physiological shunting that occurs in association with septic shock or, in relevance to our current discussions, in advanced liver disease.

This model is useful when approaching the management of the patient with problems of either gas exchange or hemodynamic instability. The first chore in approaching a patient with hypotension, low urine output, or hypoxemia involves assessment of the entire process of oxygen delivery. Before initiating therapy, one has to define the problem. We start by obtaining a set of standard hemodynamic parameters and laboratory blood tests. Because we cannot go into the power plant, we must look directly at the amount of coal left in the cars as the train returns to the coal mine for reloading. This means measuring the oxygen saturation of mixed venous blood from the distal port of the pulmonary artery catheter. We can use this, along with a measurement of the hemoglobin concentration and the $P\bar{v}o_2$, to calculate the total oxygen content of venous blood. If this amount of oxygen is within the acceptable range ($P\bar{v}o_2$ greater than 30 mm Hg, and $S\bar{v}o_2$ greater than 70% to 75%) and the patient still appears to be in shock (i.e., has evidence of low tissue perfusion), then the value of the $P\bar{v}o_2$ (or $S\bar{v}o_2$) measurements depreciates dramatically. This suggests a situation involving extensive peripheral shunting. Blood is circulating to tissues, but oxygen extraction is not taking place. Therefore, the "normal" $P\bar{v}o_2$ is not indicative of normal tissue perfusion. Our assumption that inspecting the coal cars as they return to the coal mine will tell us whether the plant is receiving enough coal is wrong. Something is wrong inside the plant, and coal is going in but is not being used. In fact, in this situation, we often find that the amount of coal still in the cars as they return to be reloaded is surprisingly high, yielding a difference with the amount loaded that is lower than expected. In effect, this is a case of decreased oxygen consumption.

If the $P\bar{v}o_2$ is low, it confirms our clinical impression that oxygen delivery is inadequate. But why? And, more important, what can we do about it? It is useful to recall what factors influence the amount of coal left in the cars when they return to be reloaded. One major factor is the amount loaded into them in the first place, that is, the Cao_2. If we find that the Cao_2 is below the normal value of 20 mL/dL, then we know that this is one factor that we should try to correct in order to supply more oxygen. We can do this by increasing the pressure head of coal loading, that is, by increasing the Fio_2 of the inspired gas. However, the relationship between this pressure and the degree to which the train cars are filled is represented by a sigmoid-shaped curve. We find that unless we are dealing with very low pressures (i.e., those below 60–70 mm Hg, where we enter the steep portion of the oxygen-hemoglobin dissociation curve), even fairly large increases in pressure yield minuscule increases in oxygen content because the cars are already nearly full. Therefore, we need to try something else. Often, the best idea is to add more cars to the train. Hemoglobin concentrations should be optimized to 13 to 15 g/dL by judicious transfusion of packed red blood cells. This is the most effective way to increase Cao_2.

However, if the Pao_2 is indeed low enough to yield a Sao_2 below 85% to 90%, increasing the Pao_2 may lead to substantial improvements in Cao_2. An increase in Sao_2 of 1% will only yield an increase in Cao_2 of 0.0134 mL per every gram of hemoglobin, or 0.201 for a hemoglobin level of 15 g/dL. On the other hand, an increase of 10% to 15% in Sao_2 under these circumstances yields 2 to 3 additional mL of oxygen per mL of blood.

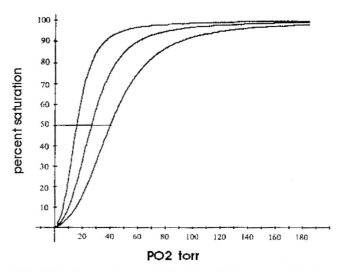

FIG. 24.4. Oxygen-hemoglobin dissociation curve showing three different P_{50} relationships: 16 mm Hg (torr), 26.6 mm Hg (the normal P_{50}), and 40 mm Hg. The latter represents a shift to the right.

Positive End Expiratory Pressure

When Cao_2 is low because of a low Sao_2, we need to consider how to increase the filling of the coal car. Obviously, we can increase the Fio_2. But this may not yield satisfactory results; in addition, when FiO_2 remains above 50% for more than 48 hours, we will begin to dramatically increase the risk of oxygen-induced lung damage. Another option is the use of positive end expiratory pressure (PEEP). PEEP results in higher mean airway pressure-time multiples, which then lead to better alveolar ventilation of collapsed or atelectatic airways. The idea is to recruit more of the damaged alveoli to the task of oxygen delivery to the pulmonary capillary beds, thereby decreasing the intrapulmonary shunting that occurs when blood traverses the capillary bed but is not exposed to ventilated alveoli. Contrary to the opinion all too often expressed by trainees during good-natured grilling on ICU rounds, PEEP does not result in increased oxygen delivery by increasing the diffusion pressure gradient across edematous alveolar-capillary interstitial space. Oxygen diffusion is rarely a problem; keeping the airways open when the normal protective mechanisms of the lung have been subverted is. Oxygen cannot diffuse into the blood stream if the blood passes by alveoli that are not being ventilated.

Once PEEP has been added to the support of a patient, the next question should be: How much? One can answer this question in one of several ways, although the most popular among housestaff often seems to be, "use the level of PEEP that yields the best PaO_2, but not more than about 15 to 20 cm because PEEP will blow out the lungs if it's too high!" The fact that this answer, though hardly erudite, often suffices for the management of most patients does not mean it is correct. Optimization of PEEP is a relatively simple process and can be very important in providing the best care to the most critically ill patients.

One definition of "best PEEP" is that level of PEEP that yields the best lung compliance. One starts by measuring static lung compliance. This can be done by measuring the airway pressure in the patient at the completion of the inspiratory cycle. In older models of the popular Puritan-Bennett MA1 ventilator, one pinched the pressure tube to the expiratory valve just at the end of the inspiratory cycle, preventing the expiratory escape of the delivered volume. The value of the plateau pressure obtained at that moment was divided into the expiratory volume to obtain the value of static lung compliance. Most modern ventilators have an expiratory hold button that will allow one to obtain the plateau pressure associated with the tidal volume of a breath. One then adds a certain trial level of PEEP (e.g., 5 cm) and remeasures static lung compliance after 15 to 20 minutes. In theory, if more alveoli have been recruited, lung compliance will improve. More PEEP is added and compliance remeasured until one sees either a leveling off or a decrease in lung compliance. At the point of leveling off, one most likely has reached the point of maximum expansion of the available alveoli, and any further pressure increases may result in overdistention manifested by decreased lung compliance. The major advantage of this method is its simplicity. One can very rapidly obtain the maximum improvement in lung compliance at the bedside. The major disadvantage of this method is that it does not actually measure the success of PEEP in reducing pulmonary shunting. The point of maximum compliance may not be the point of optimum oxygen delivery.

For a more direct method of estimating best PEEP, one can use serial measurements of cardiac output and both mixed venous and arterial oxygen contents to calculate the shunt fraction using the Fick equation. Once again, one starts with a trial level of 5 cm PEEP, then performs the measurements necessary to calculate shunt fraction. PEEP is then increased by 2 to 5 cm H_2O and the measurements and calculations repeated. In this manner, one can see at which point the additional benefit of improved arterial Po_2 is outweighed by the decrements in cardiac output attending higher levels of PEEP. This may be very important in patients with poor cardiac reserve in whom the best lung compliance may initially be obtained at a level of PEEP that reduces cardiac output to a degree sufficient to actually reduce oxygen transport. An understanding of these principles is even more important when faced with managing poor oxygen transport problems in those patients that we have previously classified as group IV.

Other ways of increasing CaO_2 with an eye toward improving $C\bar{v}O_2$ are mostly indirect. Decreasing total lung water in an effort to improve alveolar ventilation by forced diuresis may be of benefit in those with evidence of adequate or increased intravascular volume. High-frequency ventilation techniques may serve to provide better alveolar ventilation with less barotrauma and less effect on cardiac output than conventional ventilation. Differential lung ventilation may allow optimal management of lungs with different degrees of injury. In general, these techniques are reserved for situations of severe pulmonary failure, such as adult respiratory distress syndrome (ARDS) associated with sepsis. They rarely prove necessary in the short-term management of most patients immediately after liver transplantation.

Perhaps the most important variable affecting $C\bar{v}O_2$ is cardiac output. Slow the train down and, in the face of unchanged demand for coal, the amount of coal consumed from each car will increase, resulting in a measurable reduction in the amount left in the cars upon return to the loading point. As mentioned earlier, cardiac output can be enhanced by optimizing preload, afterload, and cardiac contractility. Improving these variables will often allow further optimization of PEEP in those instances when both $C\bar{v}O_2$ and CaO_2 are decreased in the face of a widening $Ca\text{-}\bar{v}O_2\Delta$. This is most likely to be the case in those patients with enough cardiac dysfunction to prevent achievement of optimum PEEP levels.

The third variable that one must consider when examining the causes of reduced $P\bar{v}O_2$ is oxygen consumption. Increased oxygen consumption can result from increased metabolic needs associated with the stress of surgery or infection, patient agitation resulting in straining against restraints or resistance to ventilator assistance, overfeeding, hyperthyroidism, corticosteroid use, or fever. If CaO_2 and cardiac output have both been addressed and the patient is still showing signs of inadequate oxygen transport, then reduction of the demand for oxygen may be necessary. Possible measures include sedation, neuromuscular blockade, and reduction of body temperature.

Finally, one should also consider the effect of the oxygen-hemoglobin dissociation curve on $P\bar{v}o_2$. The P_{50} is the level of Po_2 at which hemoglobin is 50% saturated. Normal P_{50} is 26.6 mm Hg, but it can vary from 16 to 40 mm Hg in critically ill patients. We often talk of factors that shift the curve to the right or left. A shift to the right results in a higher P_{50}, meaning that it requires a higher Po_2 to achieve the same degree of hemoglobin saturation. It also means that oxygen is unloaded more readily in the peripheral tissues since the same degree of saturation yields a higher Po_2 within the capillary bed. The opposite applies to leftward shifts of the curve. As long as Cao_2 is sufficient to allow compensation for more peripheral oxygen unloading, a shift of the curve to the right will result in an increase in the $P\bar{v}o_2$, assuming oxygen consumption does not increase. Factors that result in a shift of the curve to the right include acidosis, hypercapnia, increased temperature, corticosteroids, β-blockers (particularly propranolol), and phosphates (increased 2,3-diphosphoglycerate). Decreased temperature, alkalosis, and hypocapnia all shift the curve to the left, increasing the affinity of hemoglobin for oxygen and thereby decreasing peripheral availability of hemoglobin-associated oxygen.

In practice, we seldom manipulate these variables in an effort to increase oxygen availability. However, it is important to keep these relationships in mind because one may be dealing with a patient who has developed hypothermia, alkalosis, and hypocapnia from other causes. Correction of these abnormalities, if not harmful in other ways, might result in improved oxygen transport.

In summary, our management of critically ill patients, including those who have undergone liver transplantation, should include careful consideration of oxygen delivery and transport. Based on our preceding discussion, our primary goal is the provision of adequate oxygen to the mitochondria. Because we have no method of directly measuring the happiness of these organelles, we must look for indirect evidence. The accumulation in the blood of the products of anaerobic metabolism, such as lactate, is a sign that we are failing to achieve our stated goal. But, even prior to the development of significant anaerobic metabolism, we should be able to gain some clues about the effectiveness of our management. The oxygen content of mixed venous blood is a useful approximation of the amount of oxygen still left in the blood after peripheral tissues have had the opportunity to extract their fair share. If $P\bar{v}o_2$ falls below 20 mm Hg, we can be fairly certain that the peripheral tissues have not received enough. On the other hand, if the $P\bar{v}o_2$ is satisfactory (above 30 mm Hg), or, more often, higher than normal, all may not be well out there in the peripheral tissues. There may be some sort of process (shunting) going on that prevents the mitochondria from using oxygen. This is often the case in sepsis.

Assuming that the $P\bar{v}o_2$ is a useful measurement in our patient, and that Cao_2 remains constant, maneuvers that lessen the difference between the amount of oxygen contained in arterial blood and that in mixed venous blood can be presumed to improve oxygen transport, whereas those that increase the gap may do harm. We can also use our various measurements to calculate the shunt fraction, oxygen delivery, and oxygen consumption. We want to improve oxygen consumption by improving oxygen transport, not by increasing the demand in peripheral tissues for oxygen. Thus, comparisons of oxygen consumption are of value when we are careful to maintain a constant and reasonably normal demand for oxygen by avoiding fever, agitation, or excess work of breathing.

Ventilator Management Made Simple

When placing a patient on ventilator support, one will need to specify initial machine settings. At a minimum these include ventilator mode, tidal volume, ventilator rate in breaths per minute (bpm), PEEP, and Fio_2. We will discuss each of these variables independently.

The modes available on most modern ventilators include controlled ventilation (CV), assisted controlled ventilation (ACV), intermittent mandatory ventilation (IMV), and continuous positive airway pressure (CPAP). Under CV, whatever rate is specified will be delivered to the patient regardless of respiratory effort. Additional breaths that the patient might initiate are not supported by ventilator cycling. Under ACV, in addition to supplying a minimum number of breaths as specified, the ventilator will cycle in response to patient effort. In general, the ventilator is set to respond to negative pressure generated by the patient of -1 to -2 mm Hg. Thus, the rate specified will be a minimum rate and the patient may generate additional assisted breaths. This is distinct from IMV, where the rate specified is the maximum number of ventilator-assisted breaths that will be supplied. As with CV, the patient can spontaneously breathe at a higher rate. The major difference between simple CV and IMV is that the IMV breaths are coordinated with patient effort. (This mode is also referred to as synchronized IMV, or SIMV).

Simple controlled ventilation is appropriate for use in the patient without spontaneous respiratory effort. If the patient is capable of spontaneous breathing, a better choice will be to use IMV. This is particularly true in confused, combative, or sleepy patients with uncoordinated breathing in whom CV may not be adequate or may result in stacking of breaths as the ventilator struggles to deliver the specified rate in the face of erratic breathing. In circumstances in which weaning from the ventilator is not an immediate goal, the use of ACV may be most appropriate because it will deliver a full breath each time the patient initiates sufficient negative pressure.

For purposes of weaning patients from ventilator support, gradual reduction of IMV rates is routine. One may find the use of pressure support useful in the weaning of those patients who have required prolonged ventilator support. Pressure support provides additional pressure during the inspiratory phase of the nonmandatory or spontaneous breaths, thus increasing the volume of these breaths. In fact, a minimum of 5 to 10 mm Hg of pressure support is recommended in patients who are placed on IMV support, mainly to overcome airway resistance within the apparatus.

The appropriate tidal volume can be estimated in one of several ways. The most common is to use 10 to 15 mL per kg of body weight. Hence, a 70 kg patient would have a tidal volume of 700 to 1,000 mL. This is probably a reasonable starting point, but should be monitored and quickly modified if found inappropriate. For specifying initial settings when the patient arrives in the ICU after surgery, a review of the settings used in the operating room will be very helpful. The major adverse effect of inappropriately low tidal volumes, independent of minute ventilation, is atelectasis. Too much tidal volume may result in barotrauma from overdistension of airways. Physical examination, including the chest rise, auscultation of breath sounds, and monitoring of peak inspiratory pressure (PIP), must be performed immediately after placing a patient on mechanical ventilator support and again at several later times to be sure a proper volume has been chosen.

Tidal volume multiplied by rate yields minute ventilation. An initial ventilator rate that will yield approximately 100 to 150 mL/kg minute ventilation is a reasonable starting point. Once again, a review of the minute ventilation used in the operating room may be of assistance. One may also wish to specify both the inspiratory time and the inspiratory flow rate to be used with the specified rate. Normally, inspiratory times of 1.0 to 1.5 seconds with rates of 6 to 12 bpm will yield an inspiratory to expiratory time ratio (I/E) of 1:2 or more. Flow rates of 40 L/min or slower will yield good gas exchange, with slower flow rates allowing better intrapulmonary gas exchange but yielding higher PIPs when lung compliance is abnormally low. Thus, our 70 kg patient will start out with a tidal volume of 700 mL, a rate of 10 bpm, a flow rate of 30 L/min for an inspiratory (I) time of 1.4 sec, and an I/E ratio of 1:3.3.

We have already discussed the use of PEEP and how to select the best PEEP. In our initial ventilator settings, we usually choose to place the patient on PEEP equivalent to the physiological level normally generated in the nonintubated patient by the upper airway. This "physiological PEEP" is about 3 cm H_2O.

The choice of a starting FiO_2 is best guided by an understanding of why the patient needs ventilator support. The patient who develops ARDS in association with sepsis and is found to be profoundly hypoxic prior to intubation will have distinctly different oxygen requirements when first placed on ventilator support than will the patient who has just arrived in the ICU after a liver transplant. In the support of hypoxic patients, we start with the highest practical levels of FiO_2, avoiding 100% oxygen because of the associated risk of absorption atelectasis. One can then wean

the FiO_2 as rapidly as appropriate for the patient. Cutaneous oximetry is extremely useful in accomplishing this rapidly, although care must be taken in deeply jaundiced patients because hyperbilirubinemia results in false elevation of oxygen saturation readings with oximeters employing infrared spectrometry. Once again, for the patient fresh from the operating room, a review of the anesthesia record will serve as a guide to a starting point for the FiO_2. As mentioned previously, one should avoid prolonged use of FiO_2 greater than 0.50 for more than 48 hours.

Weaning from Ventilation

Table 24.6 lists the physiological criteria for weaning patients from mechanical ventilation. It is important to distinguish the methodology of weaning the healthy patient who is just awakening from major surgery from that involved in removing a patient from long-term support. In routine recovery from liver transplantation, as from any major surgery, the use of stepwise reduction in IMV rate will suffice. Weaning parameters can be obtained from the patient as soon as the patient is alert enough to cooperate or just before planned extubation to confirm the success of the weaning procedure. However, simple examination of the patient may suffice. If the patient is awake and responsive and has an acceptable minute ventilation on an IMV of 2 to 4 bpm, adequate oximetric saturation, and can cough and breathe deeply with gusto, the patient can be extubated. In the absence of large blood losses or preexisting pulmonary disease, most patients can be extubated 2 to 12 hours after liver transplantation.

The patient who has required prolonged ventilator support (more than 1 week) presents a different set of problems. These patients often require a careful stepwise approach, usually with forward and backward progress as they gain strength and their injured lungs recover. The specific approach that one takes is dependent on the reason for prolonged intubation. Those whose problem was mostly increased shunting and hypoxia may have been maintained on IMV rates low enough to allow preservation of some strength. On the other hand, prolonged use of neuromuscular blockade or sedation in the support of the patient with severe ARDS usually results in a devastating degree of weakness from which the patient may require many days or weeks to recover.

Before launching a program of weaning from the ventilator, one should obtain physiologic parameters from the patient at least daily and, if practical, before and after specific

TABLE 24.6. *Physiological criteria for weaning patients from mechanical ventilation*

$PaO_2 > 70$ mm Hg on FiO_2 40%
Maximum inspiratory force (MIF) > 20 cm of water
Tidal volume (V_T) = 5–8 mL/kg
Vital capacity (VC) = 10–15 mL/kg
Minute volume (MV) < 10 L/min

weaning maneuvers. These parameters include spontaneous tidal volume (V_T), vital capacity (VC), minute ventilation, and maximum inspiratory force (MIF). Patients too lethargic to cooperate with these tests are not candidates for weaning. In addition, those patients who, for one reason or another, have minute ventilation requirements in excess of 10 L/min are not likely to be able to support themselves, and weaning efforts should be forestalled until these requirements are reduced. More specifically, one can use the minute ventilation and V_T to calculate a projected rate for the patient, then estimate whether it is reasonable to expect the patient to sustain this degree of respiratory effort. A patient with a V_T of 300 mL and a minute volume of 12 L/min will need to breathe at a rate of 40 bpm continuously, compared with a rate of 12 bpm for a patient with a spontaneous V_T of 500 mL and a minute volume of 6 L/min. On the other hand, VC and MIF are effort-dependent parameters that may improve rapidly as the patient gains strength with one of the weaning programs described below. If minute volumes are consistently less than 10 L/min and the patient is alert and cooperative, one can start a weaning program that is designed to improve breathing performance as rapidly as possible without risking setbacks caused by overworking, atelectasis, hypoxia, and hypercapnea.

We have seldom found that simple weaning of IMV rates suffices for those patients who have lost considerable strength. In such cases, we resort to one of two approaches, often combining these techniques on alternate days if necessary. The first technique is called "wind sprints" and involves placing the patient on short periods of low IMV rates or CPAP alone and gradually increasing the duration and frequency of these trials over a period of days. Some patients will not tolerate this technique because they develop atelectasis very rapidly on the CPAP or low IMV settings, sometimes with disastrous results.

An alternative is to use a relatively high level of pressure support and wean the patient over time. The initial level of support should be sufficient to provide tidal volumes during spontaneous breaths equivalent to those generated during mandatory breaths. This provides a mode of support that is similar to ACV, but with volume cycling during mandatory breaths and pressure cycling during spontaneous breaths. This maneuver is initiated when the patient has been weaned to an IMV rate of less than 20 bpm but does not tolerate further weaning. With the addition of pressure support, one can reduce the IMV rate by 25% to 50%, and then daily or every other day reduce the level of pressure support by 3 to 5 cm H_2O. For each reduction in pressure of 10 cm, one can attempt a reduction in IMV of 2 to 4 bpm on alternate days. Signs of failure include the usual: increased respiratory rate, air hunger, atelectasis, hypercapnea, and in severe cases, hypoxia.

One should recall that the chief disadvantage of pressure cycled ventilation is the potential inconsistency of tidal volumes delivered. This can be a serious problem in the patient who begins to struggle against the ventilator in the face of inadequate support, setting up a potential vicious cycle.

One can establish proper alarm limits for low mandatory volumes on the ventilator, but we feel that a safer option is to always maintain some level of IMV.

The development of ARDS is associated with a decreased lung compliance. The resulting need for increased pressure to deliver adequate lung volumes leads ultimately to barotrauma. In those patients in whom levels of peak expiratory pressure greater than 10 to 15 cm H_2O are found necessary, one will need to pay close attention to both the peak inspiratory pressure and mean airway pressures to avoid serious barotrauma. It is often useful to lower tidal volume and raise ventilator rate to achieve the same minute volume at a lower mean airway pressure and with lower PIP. A recent multicenter trial revealed the efficacy of ultrahigh frequency (greater than 3 Hz) jet ventilation in improving Pao_2 and lowering PIP in patients with severe lung injury.[59] Although we have very little experience with this technique, in extreme cases of ARDS after liver transplantation it may be an option worth considering.

SUMMARY

We have discussed some of the more basic as well as a few unique issues associated with the care of patients who have undergone liver transplantation. In many cases, the problems these patients have and the approaches to their management are not substantially different from those experienced by other patients after major surgery. At the same time, the preexisting severe liver disease and the need for immunosuppression introduce a degree of complexity that is not often addressed in the mainstream critical care literature. The solutions to some of these problems await the development of a better understanding of the causes of the various physiological aberrations attending chronic liver disease.

REFERENCES

1. Hehir DJ, Jenkins RL, Bistrian BR, et al. Nutrition in patients undergoing orthotopic liver transplantation. *JPEN J Parenter Enteral Nutr* 1985;9:695–700.
2. Shronts EP, Teasley KM, Thoele SL, et al. Nutrition support of the adult liver transplant candidate. *J Am Diet Assoc* 1987;87:441–451.
3. Goulet OJ, de Goyet J, Otte JB, et al. Preoperative nutritional evaluation and support for liver transplantation in children. *Transplant Proc* 1987;19:3249–3255.
4. Porayko MK, DiCecco S, O'Keefe SJD. Impact of malnutrition and its therapy on liver transplantation. *Semin Liver Dis* 1991;11:305–314.
5. DiCecco SR, Plevak DJ, Wiesner RH, et al. Do we accurately estimate caloric and nitrogen requirements in the liver transplant patient? *Gastroenterology* 1991;100:A520.
6. Reilly J, Mehta R, Teperman L, et al. Nutritional support after liver transplantation: a randomized prospective study. *JPEN J Parenter Enteral Nutr* 1990;14:386–391.
7. Hasse JM. Nutritional implications of liver transplantation. *Henry Ford Hosp Med J* 1990;38:235–240.
8. Oellerich M, Burdelski M, Lautz HU, et al. Assessment of pretransplant prognosis in patients with cirrhosis. *Transplantation* 1991;51:801–806.
9. Chin SE, Shepherd RW, Cleghorn GJ, et al. Pre-operative nutritional support in children with end-stage liver disease accepted for liver transplantation: an approach to management. *J Gastroenterol Hepatol* 1990;5:566–572.

10. Moukarzel AA, Najm I, Vargas J, et al. Effect of nutritional status on outcome of orthotopic liver transplantation in pediatric patients. *Transplant Proc* 1990;22:1560–1563.

11. Shanbhogue RL, Bistrian BR, Jenkins RL, et al. Increased protein catabolism without hypermetabolism after human orthotopic liver transplantation. *Surgery* 1987;101:146–149.

12. Shanbhogue RL, Nompleggi D, Bell SJ, et al. Nutritional support in surgery of the liver. In: McDermott WV, ed. *Surgery of the liver.* Boston: Blackwell Scientific Publications, 1989:497–510.

13. Daly JM, Lieberman MD, Goldfine J, et al. Enteral nutrition with supplemental arginine, RNA, and omega-3 fatty acids in patients after operation: immunologic, metabolic and clinical outcomes. *Surgery* 1992;112:56–67.

14. Wilmore DW, Moylan JA Jr, Brslow BF, et al. Anabolic effects of human growth hormone and high caloric feedings following thermal injury. *Surg Gynecol Obstet* 1991;138:875–884.

15. Wilmore DW. Hormonal responses and their effects on metabolism. *Surg Clin North Am* 1976;56:999–1018.

16. Moore F, Moore E, Jones TN, et al. TEN versus TPN following major abdominal trauma: reduced septic morbidity. *J Trauma* 1989;29:916–922.

17. Wade JE, Echenique M, Blackburn GL. Enteral feeding in liver failure. In: Johnston IDA, ed. *Advances in clinical nutrition.* Boston: MTP Press, 1982:149–162.

18. Bothe A, Wade JE, Blackburn GL. Enteral nutrition; an overview. In: Hill GL, ed. *Nutrition and the surgical patient.* Edinburgh: Churchill Livingstone, 1981:76–103.

19. Alverdy J, Sang H, Sheldon GF. The effect of parenteral nutrition on gastrointestinal immunity. The importance of enteral stimulation. *Ann Surg* 1985;202:681–684.

20. Shanbhogue RLK, Chawls WJ, Weintranb M, et al. Parenteral nutrition in the surgical patient. *Br J Surg* 1987;4:172–180.

21. Roy CC, Belli DC. Hepatobiliary complications associated with TPN: an enigma. *J Am Coll Nutr* 1985;4:655–660.

22. Harris JA, Benedict FG. *A biometric study of basal metabolism in man.* Washington, DC: Carnegie Institute of Washington, 1919:279.

23. Bower RH. Nutrition for critically ill patients. In: Cameron JL, ed. *Current surgical therapy,* 4th ed. St. Louis: BC Decker, 1992:1051–1056.

24. Ziegler TR, Young LS, Ferrari-Baliviera E, et al. Use of human growth hormone combined with nutritional support in a critical care unit. *JPEN J Parenter Enteral Nutr* 1990;14:574–581.

25. Driscoll DF, Blackburn GR. Total parenteral nutrition 1990. A review of its current status in hospitalized patients and the need for patient-specific feeding. *Drugs* 1990;40:343–363.

26. Driscoll DF, Baptista RJ, Mitrano FP, et al. Parenteral nutrition admixtures as drug vehicles: theory and practice in the critical care setting. *DICP Ann Pharmacother* 1991;25:276–283.

27. Bagdade JD, Koot RK, Bulger RJ. Impaired leukocyte function in patients with poorly controlled diabetes. *Diabetes* 1974;23:9–15.

28. Driscoll DF, Bistrian BR, Baptista RJ, et al. Base solution limitations and patient-specific TPN admixtures. *Nutr Clin Prac* 1987;2:160–163.

29. Pearl RH, Clowes GHA, Loda M, et al. Hepatocyte function measured by central plasma clearance of amino acids: a method of patient selection and postoperative management in human liver transplantation. *Transplant Proc* 1985;17:276–278.

30. Driscoll DF, Bistrian BR, Jenkins RL, et al. Development of metabolic alkalosis after massive transfusion during orthotopic liver transplantation. *Crit Care Med* 1987;15:905–908.

31. Plevak DJ, Southorn PA, Narr BJ, et al. Intensive care unit experience in the Mayo liver transplantation program: the first 100 cases. *Mayo Clin Proc* 1989;64:433–445.

32. Bunker JP. Metabolic effects of blood transfusion. *Anesthesiology* 1966;27:446–455.

33. Povey MJC, Wales MB. pH changes during exchange transfusion. *Lancet* 1964;2:339–340.

34. Wilson RF, Gibons D, Percinel AK, et al. Severe alkalosis in critically ill surgical patients. *Arch Surg* 1972;105:197–203.

35. Miller RD, Tong MJ, Robbins TO. Effects of massive transfusion of blood on acid-base balance. *JAMA* 1972;216:1762–1765.

36. Schweitzer O, Howland WS. The effect of citrated bank blood on acid-base balance. *Surg Gynecol Obstet* 1962;114:90–96.

37. Thompson AE. Aspects of pediatric intensive care after liver transplantation. *Transplant Proc* 1987;19:34–39.

38. Bunker JP, Stetson JB, Coc RC, et al. Citric acid intoxication. *JAMA* 1955;157:1361–1367.

39. Griffel MI, Kaufman BS. Pharmacology of colloids and crystalloids. *Crit Care Clin* 1992;8:235–253.

40. Brimioulle S, Berre J, Vincent JL, et al. Hydrochloric acid infusion for treatment of metabolic alkalosis associated with respiratory alkalosis. *Crit Care Med* 1989;17:232–236.

41. Gonwa TA, Poplawski S, Paulsen W, et al. Pathogenesis and outcome of hepatorenal syndrome in patients undergoing orthotopic liver transplant. *Transplantation* 1989;47:395–397.

42. Ellis D, Avner ED, Starzl TE. Renal failure in children with hepatic failure undergoing liver transplantation. *J Pediatr* 1986;108:393–398.

43. Fevery J, Cutsem EV, Nevens F, et al. Reversal of hepatorenal syndrome by peroral misoprostol (prostaglandin E$_1$ analogue) and albumin administration. *J Hepatol* 1990;11:153–158.

44. Koppel MH, Coburn JW, Mims MM, et al. Transplantation of cadaveric kidneys from patients with hepatorenal syndrome: evidence for the functional nature of renal failure in advanced liver disease. *N Engl J Med* 1969;280:1367–1371.

45. Polson RJ, Park GR, Lindop MJ, et al. The prevention of renal impairment in patients undergoing orthotopic liver grafting by infusion of low dose dopamine. *Anesthesia* 1987;42:15–19.

46. Murray BM, Paller MS, Ferris TF. Effect of cyclosprine administration on renal hemodynamics in conscious rats. *Kidney Int* 1985;28:767–774.

47. Gerber JG. Role of prostaglandins in the hemodynamic and tubular effects of furosemide. *Fed Proc* 1983;42:1707–1710.

48. Driscoll DF, Pinson CW, Jenkins RL, et al. Potential protective effects of furosemide against early renal injury in liver transplant patients receiving cyclosporine. *Crit Care Med* 1989;17:1341–1343.

49. Dawidson IJ, Sandor ZF, Coorpender L, et al. Intraoperative albumin administration affects the outcome of cadaver renal transplantation. *Transplantation* 1992;53:774–782.

50. Prager MC, Cauldwell Ca, Ascher Nl, et al. Pulmonary hypertension associated with liver disease is not reversible after liver transplantation. *Anesthesiology* 1992;77:375–378.

51. Plevak D, Krowka M, Rettke S, et al. Successful liver transplantation on inpatients with mild to moderate pulmonary hypertension. *Transplant Proc* 1993;25:1840.

52. De Wolf Am, Scott VL, Easior T, et al. Pulmonary hypertension and liver transplantation. *Anesthesiology* 1993;78:2134.

53. Scott V, Miro A, Kang Y, et al. Reversibility of the hepatopulmonary syndrome by orthotopic liver transplantation. *Transplant Proc* 1993;25:1787–1788.

54. George J, Mellemgaard K, Tysthop N, et al. Venoarterial shunts in cirrhosis of the liver. *Lancet* 1960;1:852–854.

55. Wolfe JD, Tashkih DD, Holly FE, et al. Hypoxemia of cirrhosis: detection of abnormal small pulmonary vascular channels by quantitive radio imaging methods. *Am J Med* 1977;63:746–754.

56. Krowka MJ, Dickson ER, Cortese DA. Hepatopulmonary syndrome. Clinical observations and lack of therapeutic response to somatostatin analogue. *Chest* 1993;104:515–521.

57. Eriksson LS, Soderman C, Ericzon BG, et al. Normalization of ventilation/perfusion relationship after liver transplantation in patients with decompensated cirrhosis: evidence for hepatopulmonary syndrome. *Hepatology* 1990;12:135–157.

58. Stoller JK, Moodie D, Schiavonewa, et al. Reduction of intrapulmonary shunt and resolution of digital clubbing associated with primary biliary cirrhosis after liver transplantation. *Hepatology* 1990;11:54–58.

59. Gluck E, Heard S, Patel C, et al. Use of ultrahigh frequency ventilation in patients with ARDS. A preliminary report. *Chest* 1993;103:1313–1314.

Transplantation of the Liver, edited by Willis C. Maddrey, Eugene R. Schiff, and Michael F. Sorrell. Lippincott Williams & Wilkins, Philadelphia © 2001.

CHAPTER 25

Hepatopulmonary Syndromes

Michael J. Krowka

The relationship between the liver and the lungs has been receiving increased attention, in part because of the clinical experiences associated with orthotopic liver transplantation (OLT) in adults and children.[1] Experiences have ranged from the resolution of severe arterial hypoxemia following successful OLT in patients with hepatopulmonary syndrome to intraoperative death directly related to the effects of portopulmonary hypertension.

The spectrum of pulmonary dysfunction that complicates chronic liver disease has been recently reviewed.[1,2] This chapter emphasizes pulmonary consequences that have particular importance for the liver transplant candidate (Table 25.1). Topics addressed include pre-OLT pulmonary diagnostic approaches, clinically important pre-OLT pulmonary consequences of advanced liver disease, the effect of OLT on hepatopulmonary syndromes, and the current pulmonary indications and contraindications for OLT.

PRETRANSPLANTATION PULMONARY DIAGNOSTIC APPROACHES

Appropriate pulmonary diagnostic testing and experience with specific liver-lung syndromes continue to evolve as pre- and post-OLT experience accumulates.

Because post-OLT morbidity and mortality associated with pulmonary vascular consequences of liver disease are not uncommon, essential pre-OLT pulmonary screening includes assessment of arterial oxygenation, chest radiography, and Doppler echocardiography.[1,2] Only highly selected patients require additional routine pulmonary function testing (i.e., measurement of lung volumes, expiratory airflow, and diffusing capacity).

M. J. Krowka: Department of Medicine, Mayo Medical School, Mayo Clinic and Mayo Foundation, Rochester, Minnesota 55905.

Arterial Oxygenation

Arterial hypoxemia is defined by a Pao_2 of less than 70 mm Hg, an alveolar-arterial oxygen (A-a o_2) gradient greater than 20 mm Hg, or a hemoglobin oxygen saturation less than 92% by oximetry and is not uncommon in patients with liver disease. The major pulmonary mechanisms for arterial hypoxemia are shown in Fig. 25.1. The prevalence of hypoxemia ranges from 14% to 22% in the most recent series published.[3,4] Patients with encephalopathy and Child's class C severity of liver disease are most likely to be hypoxemic. The arterial oxygenation abnormality may be worse in the standing position compared with supine measurements, especially in patients with hepatopulmonary syndrome.[2] Arterial blood

TABLE 25.1. *Hepatopulmonary syndromes with implications for liver transplantation*

Syndrome	Potential reversibility with OLT
Pleural effusions (hepatic hydrothorax)	Yes
Hepatopulmonary syndrome	
Type I	Yes
Type II	No
Pulmonary hypertension	
Portopulmonary hypertension	Yes
Mild	Yes
Moderate	Yes?
Severe	No?
Hyperdynamic circulation/high-flow state	Yes
Volume excess	Yes
Specific pulmonary consequences of selected liver diseases	
α_1-Antitrypsin deficiency (emphysema)	No
Primary biliary cirrhosis (lung infiltrates)	
Lymphocytic	Yes?
Fibrotic	No?

OLT, orthotopic liver transplantation.

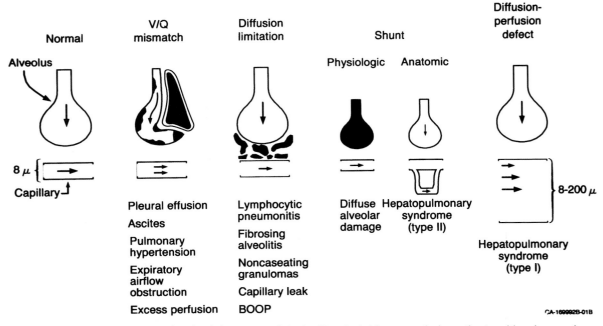

FIG. 25.1. Pulmonary pathophysiology associated with arterial hypoxemia in patients with advanced liver disease. Note the two types of physiology associated with hepatopulmonary syndrome. Severe pulmonary hypertension may be associated with severe hypoxemia due to intracardiac right-to-left shunting at the atrial level. (From Krowka MJ. Pulmonary manifestations of chronic liver disease. In: Schiff ER, Sorrell MF, Maddrey WC, eds. *Schiff's diseases of the liver,* 8th ed. Philadelphia: Lippincott Williams and Wilkins, 1999, pp. 489–502, with permission.)

gases (usually obtained from a single stick of the radial artery) are generally safe to obtain, even in patients with coagulopathy (increased prothrombin time) and thrombocytopenia.

Severe hypoxemia (PaO_2 less than 50 mm Hg) suggests the existence of hepatopulmonary syndrome or severe portopulmonary hypertension with intracardiac shunting.[1,2] In patients with significant fatigue that appears to be out of proportion to the degree of liver dysfunction, overnight oximetry may detect clinically important obstructive sleep apnea causing nighttime hemoglobin desaturations.[1]

Chest Radiography

Pre-OLT chest x-rays provide a baseline from which subsequent comparisons can be made. In addition, asymptomatic abnormalities (i.e., neoplasm or infection) that could affect the success of OLT may be detected and, therefore, require pre-OLT intervention. Significant pulmonary hypertension may be first suggested by the finding of enlarged central pulmonary arteries and cardiomegaly (Fig. 25.2). In patients with progressive dyspnea, the extent of clinically significant hepatic hydrothorax can be demonstrated and may be associated with additional reasons for hypoxemia (Fig. 25.3).

Doppler Echocardiography

Pre-OLT screening for clinically important pulmonary hypertension can be accomplished with the use of transthoracic

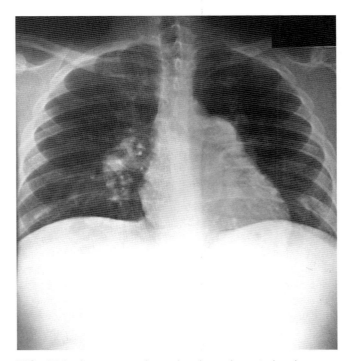

FIG. 25.2. Asymptomatic and enlarged central pulmonary vessels and cardiomegaly associated with portopulmonary hypertension (mean pulmonary artery pressure, 55 mm Hg; pulmonary vascular resistance, 430 dynes•s•cm^{-5}) can be seen in a 44-year-old man with hepatitis C liver disease. The patient was denied liver transplantation because of the severity of portopulmonary hypertension.

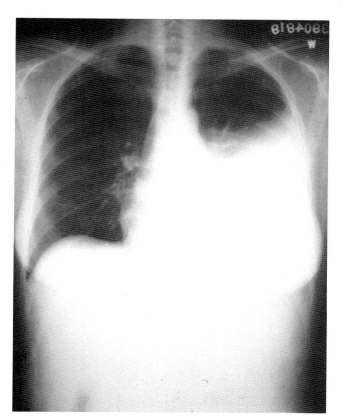

FIG. 25.3. Chest radiograph of a 57-year-old woman with stage IV primary biliary cirrhosis. The large left hepatic hydrothorax was associated with a PaO_2 of less than 48 mm Hg. Hypoxemia did not improve following therapeutic thoracentesis, and the patient was found to have moderate hepatopulmonary syndrome in addition to the pleural effusion.

Doppler echocardiography.[1,2] Approximately 12% to 15% of liver transplant candidates will demonstrate clinically significant increases in right ventricular systolic pressure, which in turn suggests increased pulmonary artery systolic pressure.[5,6] This technique estimates tricuspid valve peak regurgitant flow and provides a pressure estimate of the gradient between the right atrium and ventricle. It can be performed during a standard echocardiographic examination that also assesses valvular and left ventricular function.[5]

Preliminary data suggest a strong correlation ($r = 0.78$; $p < 0.01$) between pulmonary artery systolic pressures determined by Doppler echocardiography and right heart catheterization in 74 liver transplant candidates with mild to moderate portopulmonary hypertension (pulmonary artery systolic pressure less than 50 by Doppler echocardiography).[6] Contrast-enhanced echocardiography (transthoracic or transesophageal) is extremely useful to screen for pulmonary vascular dilatations associated with hepatopulmonary syndrome or intracardiac shunts, but this technique is not clinically necessary unless significant hypoxemia (PaO_2 below 70 mm Hg) exists.[1,2]

Pulmonary Function Tests

Routine pulmonary function testing in each liver transplant candidate is probably unnecessary.[1,7] Patients with progressive dyspnea should be studied with assessments of expiratory airflow, as measured by the ratio of forced expiratory volume in 1 second (FEV_1) to the forced vital capacity (FVC) (normal value is greater than 75%); lung volumes (total lung capacity and residual volume); and lung diffusing capacity for carbon monoxide (DLCO).[1] Although DLCO (which measures the efficiency of respiratory gas exchange) is reduced in approximately 50% of OLT candidates, the clinical importance of this finding in OLT patients is unclear.[7] Liver transplant candidates who are symptomatic smokers or have α_1-antitrypsin deficiency should undergo pretransplantation pulmonary function tests.

Exhaled nitric oxide has been recently reported to be an additional pulmonary function test that may have useful pre- and post-OLT correlations with arterial oxygenation and the hyperdynamic circulatory state associated with liver disease. Posttransplantation exhaled nitric oxide concentrations have been shown to decrease significantly (compared with abnormally increased pre-OLT values) in association with improvement in the A-a O_2 gradient.[8] Such measurements should be considered investigational at this time.

PULMONARY CONSEQUENCES OF ADVANCED LIVER DISEASE

Because of hepatic dysfunction, clinically significant abnormalities affect the pleural space, pulmonary vasculature, and lung parenchyma (airways and interstitium). Although these pulmonary problems are uncommon, respiratory symptoms in OLT candidates may overshadow the usual clinical problems encountered in such patients.[1]

Hepatic Hydrothorax

Pleural effusions occur in approximately 5% of patients as a direct consequence of portal hypertension.[9] These effusions (known as hepatic hydrothorax) are predominantly right-sided (70%), but may be bilateral (15%) or left-sided (15%). The classic chemistry of the pleural fluid is that of a transudate (fluid to serum total protein ratio less than 0.5 and fluid to serum lactate dehydrogenase ratio less than 0.6), similar to the characteristics of the ascitic fluid from which it originates. Rarely, chylous fluid comprises the hepatic hydrothorax;[10] that diagnosis is established by pleural fluid triglyceride levels above 110 mg/dL and a fluid to serum triglyceride ratio greater than 1. The pleural fluid accumulation occurs due to diaphragmatic defects that allow fluid to traverse through the hemidiaphragms. Negative pleural pressure generated with inspiration can result in effusions in the absence of clinical ascites.[9]

Hepatic hydrothorax may cause dyspnea due to lung compression. Severe hypoxemia (PaO_2 less than 50 mm Hg) is usually *not* characteristic of hepatic hydrothorax, and other causes should be explored (Fig. 25.3). Symptoms from these pleural effusions may be temporarily relieved by thoracentesis; however, unless the reasons for ascitic fluid accumulation are treated, the pleural effusions can be expected to rapidly recur.[11] Attempted pleural space obliteration with sclerosing agents such as talc or chemotherapeutic agents placed via chest tubes frequently fails. Although video thoracoscopy has been successful in identifying and closing the diaphragmatic defects, worsening ascites may result.[1,11] The placement of transjugular intrahepatic portosystemic shunts (TIPS) can dramatically reduce the degree of hepatic hydrothorax and the need for repeat thoracenteses.[12]

Pleural effusions associated with fever or chest pain, especially in OLT candidates, should be studied diagnostically by thoracentesis to rule out either infection of the fluid (spontaneous bacterial empyema) or metastatic malignancy such as hepatocellular carcinoma.[9]

Hepatopulmonary Syndrome

Most investigators agree that chronic liver disease (usually portal hypertension with or without cirrhosis) associated with arterial hypoxemia caused by pulmonary vascular dilatations characterizes the entity known as hepatopulmonary syndrome (HPS), which is considered a gas exchange problem.[1,2,13] Specific diagnostic criteria are summarized in Table 25.2.

Pulmonary vascular dilatations are inferred by noninvasive studies such as contrast-enhanced transthoracic echocardiography[14] and lung perfusion scanning with [99m]tech-

netium-labeled macroaggregated albumin ([99m]TcMAA).[15] The delayed appearance of microbubbles in the left atrium (after three cardiac cycles following opacification in right heart chambers) following peripheral injection of hand-agitated saline is considered positive for the existence of intrapulmonary vascular dilatations (Fig. 25.4). Normally the microbubbles (formed by agitated saline and further enhanced by agents such as indocyanine green dye) do not pass through the pulmonary vascular bed. Vascular dilatations greater than 10 μm in diameter, however, allow passage and subsequent detection in the pulmonary veins and left atrium.[14] In a similar manner, peripherally injected [99m]TcMAA passes through the dilated vasculature (diameter 10–90 μm) and can be quantitatively measured over the

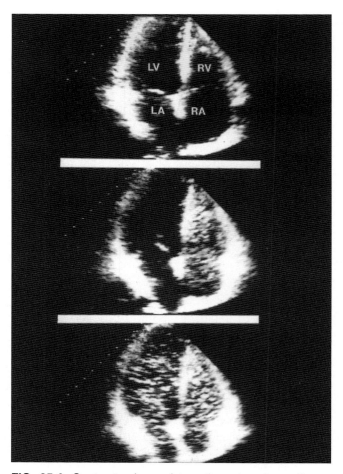

FIG. 25.4. Contrast-enhanced transthoracic echocardiography demonstrating the abnormal intrapulmonary passage of microbubbles induced by hand-agitated saline injection. **Top:** Normal cardiac chambers. **Middle:** Expected opacification of right heart chambers following peripheral injection of saline. **Bottom:** Abnormal opacification in left heart chambers six cardiac cycles after middle panel images. (From Krowka MJ, Tajik AJ, Dickson ER, et al. Intrapulmonary pulmonary vascular dilatations (IVPD) in liver transplant candidates: screening by two-dimensional contrast-enhanced echocardiography. *Chest* 1990;97:1165–1170, with permission.)

TABLE 25.2. *Diagnostic criteria for pulmonary vascular consequences of advanced liver disease*

Hepatopulmonary syndrome
Chronic liver disease (portal hypertension with or without cirrhosis)
Arterial hypoxemia
    $Pao_2 < 70$ mm Hg *or*
    Alveolar-arterial oxygen gradient > 20 mm Hg
Intrapulmonary vascular dilatation
    Positive delayed contrast-enhanced echocardiography[a] *or*
    Abnormal extrapulmonary uptake (>5%) following
    [99m]TcMAA lung perfusion scanning
Portopulmonary hypertension
Mean pulmonary artery pressure (MPAP) > 25 mm Hg
Pulmonary capillary wedge pressure (PCWP) < 15 mm Hg
Pulmonary vascular resistance[b] (PVR) > 120 dynes•s•cm^{-5}

[99m]TcMAA, [99m]technetium-labeled macroaggregated albumin.

[a]A positive scan is defined by the appearance of microbubbles in the left atrium three cardiac cycles after opacification in the right heart chambers following peripheral injection of hand-agitated saline.

[b]Some investigators (including this author) require the PVR criteria because increased cardiac output (CO) alone can cause increased MPAP without clinically significant pulmonary vascular histopathology. PVR = [(MPAP − PCWP) × 80]/CO.

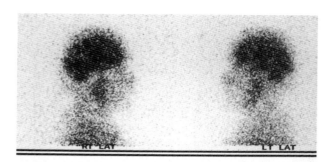

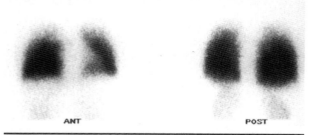

Geometric mean counts			
	Ant	Post	Geometric Mean
Lung	255244	368446	306665
	Left Lat	Rt Lat	
Brain	15333	14876	15103
	Shunt Index % =		27.47
	Normal shunt index < 5%		

FIG. 25.5. A 47-year-old man with Child-Turcotte-Pugh class C alcoholic cirrhosis demonstrated abnormal extrapulmonary (brain) uptake following 99mTcMAA lung perfusion scanning because of pulmonary vascular dilatations in hepatopulmonary syndrome. The Pao$_2$ was 46 mm Hg breathing room air, and 302 mm Hg breathing 100% oxygen.

brain and kidneys (Fig. 25.5).[15] Although contrast echocardiography is more sensitive in identifying pulmonary vascular dilatations, the 99mTcMAA method allows quantitation, which may be especially helpful in OLT patients to distinguish nonreversible reasons for hypoxemia (pulmonary fibrosis or emphysema) from potentially reversible hypoxemia caused by HPS.[16]

HPS is uncommon. Although positive contrast-enhanced echocardiograms associated with chronic liver disease are not infrequent (ranging from 13% to 47%), the occurrence of arterial hypoxemia in such patients only ranges from 5% to 13%.[2] The natural history of HPS is not well characterized. Retrospective data suggest a 40% mortality at 2.5 years following the diagnosis.[1,2] Subclinical expressions of this syndrome probably exist (vascular dilatations without hypoxemia), which, over time, will progress with worsening oxygenation.

The exact pathophysiology that causes this syndrome is unknown, but arterial hypoxemia results from a combination of excess perfusion for a given ventilation, diffusion limitation for oxygen across the alveolar-capillary interface, and anatomic right-to-left shunting between pulmonary arteries and veins (which bypass the alveolar-capillary unit).[2,17] Increased levels of exhaled nitric oxide can distinguish patients with HPS from those with cirrhosis and normal arterial oxygenation.[8] An animal model of this syndrome has been developed.[18]

The pulmonary vascular dilatations may be microscopic and diffuse (type I) or macroscopic and discrete (type II) (Fig. 25.6). Type I lesions, which are the most common, may be associated with normal pulmonary angiography, severe hypoxemia, and variable response to 100% inspired oxygen.[1] This pathophysiology is reversible in that OLT can result in resolution of hypoxemia. Type II lesions, which can be demonstrated with computed tomographic (CT) chest scanning or pulmonary angiography, have been associated with severe hypoxemia and very poor response to 100% inspired oxygen (Pao$_2$ below 300 mm Hg).[1,2] These lesions have been treated with coil embolotherapy, with dramatic improvement in oxygenation.[2] Very limited OLT experience in type II lesions has not demonstrated the consistent resolution of hypoxemia experienced with type I lesions.

Portopulmonary Hypertension

A spectrum of pulmonary hemodynamic abnormalities occurs in advanced liver disease[19] (Table 25.3). Although pulmonary hypertension occurs in up to 20% of patients with advanced liver disease, portopulmonary hypertension represents an uncommon subset (2% to 4%) of such patients as defined by the hemodynamic criteria obtained via right heart catheterization.[20] Unlike patients with primary pulmonary hypertension, patients with portopulmonary hypertension have a marked hyperdynamic circulatory state characterized by greater cardiac outputs than those measured in primary pulmonary hypertension.[21]

The clinical course of patients with portopulmonary hypertension has not been favorable. In a review of 78 patients with portopulmonary hypertension (mean pulmonary artery pressure of 59 mm Hg), the treatment was primarily palliative, with mean survival times of 15 months (median, 6 months) following the diagnosis of pulmonary hypertension.[22] Treatment of portopulmonary hypertension with intravenous epoprostenol, a potent pulmonary and systemic vasodilator, has been reported to dramatically improve pulmonary hemodynamics.[23,24]

The pathology of portopulmonary hypertension is characterized by a vasoconstrictive process that ranges from medial and intimal hypertrophy (potentially reversible) to vascular obliteration due to endothelial proliferation with recannulization (plexogenic arteriopathy, which may be irreversible). Also, thrombotic-fibrotic vascular obliteration (possibly irreversible) has been described in patients with portal hypertension.[25] Specific circulating causative factors have yet to be identified.

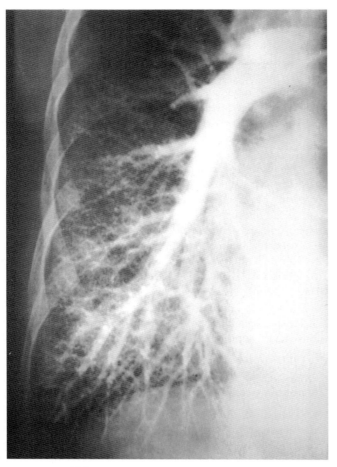
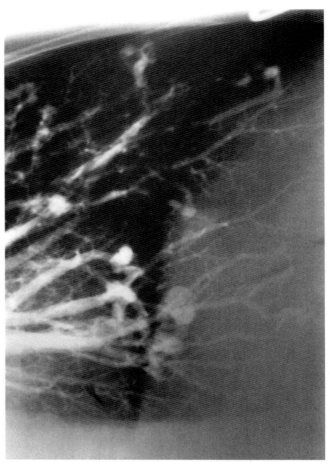

FIG. 25.6. Pulmonary angiograms demonstrating diffuse (type I) pulmonary vascular dilatations and discrete (type II) arteriovenous communications. Both patients had severe hypoxemia (Pao_2 below 50 mm Hg) due to hepatopulmonary syndrome. (From *Hepatology* 1995;21:96–100, with permission.)

Screening for portopulmonary hypertension can be accomplished with chest x-rays and Doppler echocardiography (which estimates the right ventricular systolic pressure), but the definitive diagnosis is established by pulmonary artery measurements obtained via right heart catheterization.[1,6]

In short, the two major pulmonary vascular consequences of advanced liver disease (hepatopulmonary syndrome and portopulmonary hypertension) represent distinct pulmonary pathophysiologies that occur as a consequence of factors (incompletely identified to date) associated with cirrhotic and noncirrhotic causes of portal hypertension.[19]

α_1-Antitrypsin Deficiency

The α_1-antitrypsin protein, a proteinase inhibitor (Pi), is predominantly synthesized by hepatocytes and, from a pul-

TABLE 25.3. *Pulmonary hemodynamic patterns in patients with advanced liver disease*

Hemodynamic patterns	MPAP	CO	PCWP	PVR
High-flow or hyperdynamic circulation (characteristic in hepatopulmonary syndrome)	N or ↑ (mild)	↑↑↑	↓	↓
Excess central volume	↑	↑	↑	↓↑
Vasoconstriction or obliteration (characteristic in portopulmonary hypertension)	↑↑↑	↑↓	↓	↑↑↑

MPAP, mean pulmonary artery pressure; CO, cardiac output; PCWP, pulmonary capillary wedge pressure; PVR, pulmonary vascular resistance: (MPAP − PCWP)/CO; N, normal (MPAP < 25 mm Hg); ↑, increased; ↓, decreased.

monary perspective, serves to oppose the powerful effects of leukocyte-derived neutrophil elastase.[26] Codominant, single–amino acid mutations on chromosome 14 (over 90 different alleles exist) can result in abnormal protein synthesis and folding within hepatocytes. Abnormal hepatocyte accumulation and impaired secretion of the resultant α_1 protein into the venous circulation follows and causes a deficiency that can be assessed by serum measurements. In a minority of patients, the hepatic accumulation and altered degradation can lead to cirrhosis. The degree of the deficiency is a function of the specific combination of abnormal alleles or phenotypes, which can be assessed by α_1 protein migration determined by serum isoelectric focusing methods. The normal phenotype is designated PiMM, whereas the most severe deficiencies associated with cirrhotic liver disease are documented in the PiSZ and PiZZ phenotypes.[26,27]

Emphysema due to severe serum deficiency of the α_1 protein (less than 80 mg/dL; normal range, 120–220 mg/dL) is the major pulmonary manifestation of this hepatic disorder.[27] Such patients classically have α_1 protein serum levels of less than 30 mg/dL and have the PiZZ phenotype. Severe expiratory airflow obstruction (FEV$_1$ less than 30% predicted) and hyperinflation of the chest (residual volume greater than 120% predicted) can occur as the elastic supporting structures of the alveoli are destroyed by unopposed effects of neutrophil elastase within the lung interstitium (Fig. 25.7). It is uncommon for patients with phenotypes such as PiMZ to have significant pulmonary dysfunction because they rarely have serum α_1 protein levels below the assumed protective threshold of 80 mg/dL. Children with the PiZZ phenotype and clinical liver disease rarely have significant expiratory airflow obstruction, but may demonstrate pulmonary function changes of mild hyperinflation.[27]

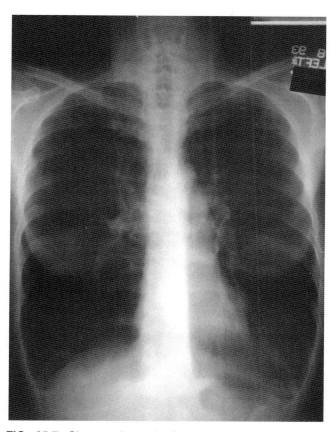

FIG. 25.7. Chest radiograph demonstrates advanced emphysema (hyperinflation of the chest with lower lobe bullae) with severe expiratory airflow obstruction (FEV$_1$ less than 30% predicted) due to PiZZ α_1-antitrypsin deficiency. This degree of pulmonary dysfunction would be a contraindication to liver transplantation.

Primary Biliary Cirrhosis

Of all the hepatic disorders that eventually result in OLT, primary biliary cirrhosis (PBC) is unique in its spectrum of potential pulmonary dysfunction.[27] In addition to the development of hepatic hydrothorax, hepatopulmonary syndrome, and portopulmonary hypertension, patients with PBC can present with interstitial lung disease in the form of lymphocytic pneumonitis, bronchiolitis obliterans with organizing pneumonitis, intrapulmonary granulomas, and fibrosing alveolitis (Fig. 25.8). These interstitial lung problems most likely relate to the immunologic aspects of PBC. Only the fibrosing alveolitis appears to be irreversible, with potentially severe restrictive pulmonary physiology and hypoxemia. Subclinical alveolitis has been described, and PBC patients (never-smokers) have abnormal DLCO measurements that appear more frequent in those with PBC of a more advanced pathologic stage.[27] Other hepatic disorders such as hepatitis C disease may have reversible, biopsy-proven interstitial lung disease associations, but these reports are quite rare to date.[27]

EFFECT OF LIVER TRANSPLANTATION ON HEPATOPULMONARY SYNDROMES

The results of orthotopic liver transplantation in patients with pulmonary consequences of advanced liver disease appear to be a function of the potential reversibility versus irreversibility of the pulmonary pathophysiology (Table 25.1), the predominant hepatic disorder, and post-OLT clinical management.

General Considerations

Changes in pulmonary function following OLT have been varied. Two observations should be stressed.[5] First, unlike other organ transplant procedures (such as bone marrow, heart-lung, or lung transplantation), the development of obliterative bronchiolitis (progressive small airway narrowing and expiratory airflow obstruction as measured by the FEV$_1$/FVC ratio, caused by graft versus host disease) has *not* been documented in liver transplant recipients. Second, abnormal pre-transplantation DLCO values, which measure the gas exchange efficiency of the lungs, do not always normalize following a

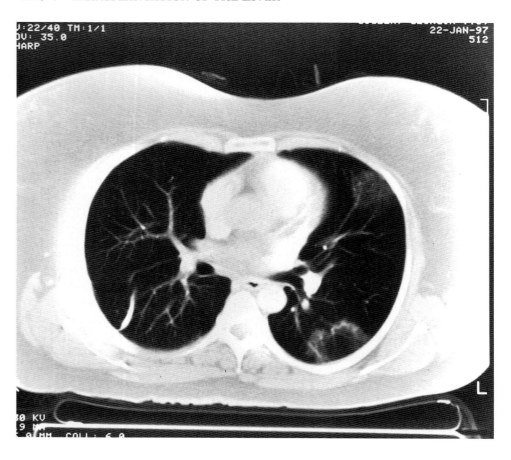

FIG. 25.8. Computed tomographic scan of the chest shows ring-like lesions due to biopsy-proven bronchiolitis obliterans with organizing pneumonitis in a 45-year-old woman with stage III-IV primary biliary cirrhosis. Pulmonary infiltrates resolved within 2 months following prednisone therapy.

successful OLT.[7] This phenomenon remains unexplained but does not appear to have a significant clinical correlate.

The resolution of pre-OLT arterial blood gas abnormalities (such as respiratory alkalosis and abnormal arterial oxygenation) following liver transplantation has been well documented. Although the exact mechanism causing respiratory alkalosis associated with chronic liver disease is unclear, normalization of hypocarbia and the alkalotic pH commonly occurs within months of OLT.[7,28]

Abnormal arterial oxygenation pre-OLT is of particular interest because of the multiple etiologies for hypoxemia (Fig. 25.1) and the potential for PaO_2 normalization post-OLT. Oxygenation abnormalities due to hepatic hydrothorax, physiologic shunting, diffusion-perfusion defects, selected ventilation-perfusion mismatches, and inflammatory interstitial lung disorders are potentially reversible (to varying degrees) with OLT. However, arterial hypoxemia due to anatomic shunting, fibrotic interstitial lung disease, bronchiectasis, or advanced emphysema (especially in the setting of α_1-antitrypsin deficiency) will most likely be unaffected by OLT; one should not expect normalization of PaO_2 abnormalities in such situations even with successful OLT.

Hepatopulmonary Syndrome

The first complete clinical description that documented the resolution of this syndrome following OLT was published in 1990.[29] A subsequent literature review of 73 HPS cases and 8 additional patients from the Mayo Clinic who underwent OLT has shown that 82% of patients (pediatric and adult) experience normalization of the oxygenation abnormality; attaining normal oxygenation may take up to 9 to 15 months posttransplantation.[30] Prolonged stay in the intensive care unit (with intubation and mechanical ventilation) was necessary in 22% of cases. Resolution of the hypoxemia was associated with normalization of the contrast echocardiograms and lung perfusion scans. Rarely, HPS can recur post-OLT.[31]

However, OLT in patients with HPS is not without risk. An overall postoperative mortality of 16% to 21% has been reported.[30,32] The most common associations with mortality include portal vein thrombosis, intracerebral hemorrhage, and refractory hypoxemia in the setting of multiorgan failure.[30,32] The only published risk factor associated with increased mortality is a pre-OLT PaO_2 of less than 50 mm Hg. A 30% mortality within 90 days of OLT was documented in such patients.[30] Other factors that may be related to increased post-OLT morbidity and mortality include a poor PaO_2 response to 100% inspired oxygen (PaO_2 less than 300 mm Hg), and the increased extrapulmonary (brain) uptake of [99m]TcMAA (greater than 30%; normal value, less than 5%) following lung perfusion scanning.[19,32] Published outcomes following OLT in patients with HPS are summarized in Table 25.4.

TABLE 25.4. *Hepatopulmonary syndrome and effects of orthotopic liver transplantation*

Syndrome resolution following OLT reported in 62% to 82% of cases,[30,32] but may require months of supplemental oxygen
Post-OLT mortality
  16% within 90 days of transplantation (n = 81)[30]
  30% by day 90 if pre-OLT Pao_2 < 50 mm Hg[30]
  32% at 1 year (n = 21)[32]
Greater pre-OLT extrapulmonary (brain) uptake of [99m]TcMAA associated with decreasing post-OLT survival[32]
Post-OLT nonresolution of HPS uncommon (2%)[30]
Post-OLT recurrence of HPS extremely rare[31]
HPS considered an indication for pediatric OLT[57]

HPS, hepatopulmonary syndrome; OLT, orthotopic liver transplantation; [99m]TcMAA, [99m]technetium-labeled macroaggregated albumin.

TABLE 25.5. *Posttransplantation clinical courses in 24 patients with pulmonary hypertension*

Intraoperative death[35]
Postoperative death (during hospitalization for transplantation)[36–40]
Postoperative death (after hospitalization for transplantation)[36]
Postoperative pulmonary hypertension unchanged[41,42]
Postoperative resolution or improvement in pulmonary hypertension[23,43–51]
Postoperative worsening of pulmonary hypertension[36]
Postoperative *de novo* occurrence of pulmonary hypertension[52,53]

Some patients in these studies were treated with intravenous epoprostenol before and after orthotopic liver transplantation.

Advances in perioperative management and careful patient selection have contributed to the favorable transplant outcomes in patients with HPS. Specifically, the use of inhaled nitric oxide (up to 40 ppm) to favorably alter postoperative ventilation-perfusion relationships and improve oxygenation has been reported.[33] Patients with significant comorbid conditions, such as cardiac dysfunction or concomitant pulmonary abnormalities such as pulmonary fibrosis or severe expiratory airflow obstruction due to emphysema, should be cautiously considered for OLT, because the hypoxemia caused by those conditions and the underlying pulmonary pathology would not be expected to improve post-OLT.[34]

Portopulmonary Hypertension

Unlike the frequent post-OLT resolution of hypoxemia associated with hepatopulmonary syndrome, the hemodynamic abnormalities associated with portopulmonary hypertension remain an intraoperative and post-OLT challenge.[19]

Mild to moderate pulmonary hypertension associated with chronic liver disease (high flow states, excess volume, or portopulmonary hypertension) does not appear to be associated with increased in-hospital mortality, especially if the calculated pulmonary vascular resistance (PVR) is less than 250 dynes•s•cm^{-5} and cardiac reserve is satisfactory.[20] However, patients with moderate to severe portopulmonary hypertension are problematic.[19,35] Such patients are defined by a mean pulmonary artery pressure (MPAP) higher than 35 mm Hg, a pulmonary capillary wedge pressure (PCWP) below 15 mm Hg, and a PVR greater than 250 dynes•s•cm^{-5} as determined during right heart catheterization.[19,35] Cardiac reserve is most likely a significant factor, and patients who did not demonstrate high cardiac outputs appeared to have poorer outcomes.[35]

The post-OLT outcomes in 43 patients with significant portopulmonary hypertension reported in the literature are summarized in Table 25.5. It is of interest that resolution or improvement in portopulmonary hypertension has been reported in highly selected cases. Reversibility of the pulmonary vasoconstrictive events may occur, up to a threshold that has yet to be determined and characterized. From the 18 published retrospective outcomes summarized in Table 25.5, the reported hemodynamic data associated with mortality and survival are summarized in Table 25.6. Although these data are incomplete and were collected from multiple institutions, they have provided a reference point for many transplant centers.[19,35,36] There are no guidelines concerning portopulmonary hypertension that have been embraced by the United Network for Organ Sharing (UNOS) to date.

TABLE 25.6. *Pulmonary hypertension: posttransplantation mortality and relationship with pretransplantation hemodynamics*

	No. of patients tested	Survivors	Cardiopulmonary Mortality	P
I. MPAP ≥ 35 mm Hg	29	15 (52%)	14 (48%)	.005
MPAP < 35 mm Hg	14	14 (100%)	0	
II. CO ≤ 8.0 L/min	31	20 (65%)	11 (35%)	.52
CO > 8.0 L/min	7	6 (86%)	1 (14%)	
III. PVR ≥ 250 dynes•s•cm^{-5}	20	9 (47%)	11 (55%)	.003
PVR < 250 dynes•s•cm^{-5}	18	17 (94%)	1 (6%)	

MPAP, mean pulmonary artery pressure; CO, cardiac output; PVR, pulmonary vascular resistance. All patients (N = 43) had MPAP measured; not all patients had CO and PVR determinations.

The preliminary effects of vasodilators such as intravenous epoprostenol on portopulmonary hypertensive patients considered for OLT are encouraging.[23,24] Epoprostenol may have additional anti–platelet-aggregating actions and vascular remodeling effects.[23] Although adverse events may occur, such as worsening thrombocytopenia with progressive splenomegaly,[54] the short-term use of epoprostenol to facilitate successful OLT in patients who otherwise would have been denied transplantation because of abnormal pulmonary hemodynamics has been reported.[23,48,51]

α₁-Antitrypsin Deficiency

Preliminary data from the Mayo Clinic suggest that progressive pre-OLT expiratory airflow obstruction and hyperinflation due to emphysema in adult patients with cirrhosis due to PiZZ phenotype may be associated with increased early mortality post-OLT.

Favorable long-term pulmonary function (12 to 82 months post-OLT) in patients who have undergone transplantation for PiZZ and PiMZ phenotypes has been reported in a single-institution series.[55] Theoretically, OLT should preclude further deterioration in pulmonary dysfunction caused by severe α₁-antitrypsin deficiency, but that hypothesis is yet to be tested.[27,56]

PULMONARY INDICATIONS AND CONTRAINDICATIONS FOR ORTHOTOPIC LIVER TRANSPLANTATION

Based on the evolving OLT experience in patients with concomitant pulmonary problems, consensus has developed concerning pulmonary indications and contraindications for OLT. Observations have translated into specific UNOS liver transplantation criteria, especially for the pediatric age group.

Severe and persistent hepatic hydrothorax, unresponsive to medical management or TIPS, is considered to be an indication for OLT in the pediatric and adult age groups if the Child-Turcotte-Pugh score is 7 or greater.[57]

Hepatopulmonary syndrome with progressive hypoxemia is reversible following OLT.[23] Several investigators view HPS as a reason to proceed with liver transplantation, regardless of the degree of hypoxemia in highly selected cases.[30,58,59] In addition, UNOS recognizes HPS as an indication for OLT in the pediatric age group (no specific PaO₂ criteria stated).[57] No formal guidelines concerning adults have been published. Severe HPS (PaO₂ below 50 mm Hg), especially when associated with comorbid conditions, may be a relative contraindication to OLT depending on individual transplant center experiences.

Increased pulmonary artery pressure caused by the hyperdynamic or high-flow circulatory state or increased central blood volume has not been associated with increased in-hospital mortality per se and should not be considered a contraindication to OLT.[20] These patients usually have only mild to moderate pulmonary hypertension and normal or slightly increased pulmonary vascular resistance.[20] However, pulmonary hypertension, regardless of the predominant physiology, has not been considered an indication for OLT to date.

Portopulmonary hypertension, with the potential for moderate to severe increases in pulmonary artery pressure (MPAP above 35 mm Hg), markedly increased pulmonary vascular resistance (greater than 250 dynes•s•cm⁻⁵), and detrimental effect on right heart function, remains a dilemma when contemplating potential liver transplantation.[19,60] Recent treatment advances with intravenous epoprostenol may allow successful OLT with favorable long-term outcomes.[23,48,51] Additional prospective experience with effective pulmonary vasodilators such as epoprostenol will be necessary to provide transplant centers with specific pulmonary hemodynamic criteria associated with not only a successful transplantation but also favorable long-term results. In short, moderate to severe portopulmonary hypertension as defined previously (untreated or refractory to treatment) remains a relative contraindication to OLT in most centers.

Severe α₁-antitrypsin deficiency associated with clinically significant emphysema (usually PiZZ or PiSZ phenotypes) poses a relative contraindication to OLT. Even with normalization of the α₁ protein serum level and conversion to the donor phenotype post-OLT, there are no data (or sound physiologic arguments) that suggest the pulmonary abnormality (panlobular emphysema) will resolve or improve. Patients with PiZZ α₁-antitrypsin deficiency can have hypoxemia due to hepatopulmonary syndrome, which does normalize post-OLT.[30,56] There are no published data addressing pulmonary function criteria that may preclude successful OLT. Intuitively, patients with severe expiratory airflow obstruction (FEV₁ less than 30% predicted) would likely have the greatest risk for post-OLT complications.

SUMMARY

There is reasonable consensus that several hepatopulmonary syndromes (pulmonary abnormalities that occur as a direct consequence of liver disease) can resolve with successful OLT. These pulmonary abnormalities include hepatic hydrothorax, type I hepatopulmonary syndrome, pulmonary hypertension due to the high-flow state or excess central volume, and mild to moderate portopulmonary hypertension in highly selected patients. Current data suggest that post-transplantation resolution of type II hepatopulmonary syndrome, severe portopulmonary hypertension (untreated), or advanced emphysema caused by α₁-antitrypsin deficiency is unlikely. Significant mortality is associated with hepatopulmonary syndromes, especially those with pulmonary vascular consequences of advanced liver disease.

REFERENCES

1. Krowka MJ. Pulmonary manifestations of chronic liver disease. In: Schiff ER, Sorrell MF, Maddrey WC, eds. *Schiff's diseases of the liver*, 8th ed. Philadelphia: Lippincott Williams and Wilkins, 1999:489–502.

2. Herve P, Lebrec D, Brenot, et al. Pulmonary vascular disorders in portal hypertension. *Eur Respir J* 1998;11:1153–1166.

3. Vachiery F, Moreau R, Hadengue A, et al. Hypoxemia in patients with cirrhosis: relationship with liver failure and hemodynamic alterations. *J Hepatol* 1997;27:492–495.

4. Moller S, Hillingso J, Christensen E, et al. Arterial hypoxemia in cirrhosis: fact or fiction? *Gut* 1998;42:868–874.

5. Donovan CL, Marcovitz PA, Punch JD, et al. Two-dimensional and dobutamine stress echocardiography in the preoperative assessment of patients with end-stage liver disease prior to orthotopic liver transplantation. *Transplantation* 1996;61:1180–1188.

6. Kim WR, Krowka MJ, Plevak DJ, et al. Accuracy of Doppler echocardiography in assessment of pulmonary hypertension in liver transplant candidates. *Liver Transpl* 2000;6:453–458.

7. Krowka MJ, Dickson ER, Wiesner RH, et al. A prospective study of pulmonary function and gas exchange in patients undergoing liver transplantation. *Chest* 1992;102:1161–1168.

8. Rolla G, Brussino L, Colagrande P, et al. Exhaled nitric oxide and impaired oxygenation in cirrhotic patients before and after liver transplantation. *Ann Intern Med* 1998;129:375–378.

9. Lazaradis KN, Kamath P, Krowka MJ. Hepatic hydrothorax. *Am J Med* 1999;107:262–267.

10. Romero S, Martin C, Hernandez L, et al. Chylothorax in cirrhosis of the liver. *Chest* 1998;114:154–159.

11. Mouroux J, Perrin C, Venissac N, et al. Management of pleural effusion of cirrhotic origin. *Chest* 1996;109:1093–1096.

12. Jeffries MA, Kazanjian S, Wilson M, et al. Transjugular intrahepatic portosystemic shunts and liver transplantation in patients with refractory hepatic hydrothorax. *Liver Transplant Surg* 1998;4:416–423.

13. Scott VL, Dodson SF, Kang Y. The hepatopulmonary syndrome. *Surg Clin North Am* 1999;79:23–41.

14. Krowka MJ, Tajik AJ, Dickson ER, et al. Intrapulmonary pulmonary vascular dilatations (IVPD) in liver transplant candidates: screening by two-dimensional contrast-enhanced echocardiography. *Chest* 1990;97:1165–1170.

15. Abrams GA, Nanda NC, Dubovsky EV, et al. Use of macroaggregated albumin lung perfusion scan to diagnose hepatopulmonary syndrome: a new approach. *Gastroenterology* 1998;114:305–310.

16. Abrams GA, Jaffe CC, Hoffer PB, et al. Diagnostic utility of contrast echocardiography and lung perfusion scan in patients with hepatopulmonary syndrome. *Gastroenterology* 1995;109:1283–1288.

17. Whyte MKB, Hughes JMB, Peters AM, et al. Analysis of intrapulmonary right to left shunt in hepatopulmonary syndrome. *J Hepatol* 1998;29:85–93.

18. Luo B, Abrams GA, Fallon MB. Endothelin-I in the rat bile duct ligation model of hepatopulmonary syndrome: correlation with pulmonary dysfunction. *J Hepatol* 1998;29:571–578.

19. Krowka MJ. Hepatopulmonary syndrome versus portopulmonary hypertension: distinctions and dilemmas. *Hepatology* 1997;25:1282–1284.

20. Castro M, Krowka MJ, Schroeder DR, et al. Frequency and clinical implications of increased pulmonary artery pressures in liver transplant patients. *Mayo Clin Proc* 1996;71:543–551.

21. Kuo PC, Plotkin JS, Johnson LB, et al. Distinctive features of portopulmonary hypertension. *Chest* 1997;112:980–986.

22. Robalino BD, Moodie DS. Association between primary pulmonary hypertension and portal hypertension: analysis of its pathophysiology and clinical, laboratory and hemodynamic manifestations. *J Am Coll Cardiol* 1991;17:492–498.

23. Krowka MJ, Frantz RF, McGoon MD, et al. Improvement in pulmonary hemodynamics during intravenous epoprostenol (prostacyclin): a study of 15 patients with moderate to severe portopulmonary hypertension. *Hepatology* 1999;30:641–648.

24. Kuo PC, Johnson LB, Plotkin JS, et al. Continuous intravenous infusion of epoprostenol for the treatment of portopulmonary hypertension. *Transplantation* 1997;63:604–616.

25. Edwards BS, Weir EK, Edwards WD, et al. Coexistent pulmonary and portal hypertension: morphologic and clinical features. *J Am Coll Cardiol* 1987;10:1233–1238.

26. Mahadeva R, Lomas DA. Alpha$_1$-antitrypsin deficiency, cirrhosis and emphysema. *Thorax* 1998;53:501–505.

27. Krowka MJ. Recent pulmonary observations in alpha$_1$-antitrypsin deficiency, primary biliary cirrhosis, chronic hepatitis C, and other hepatic problems. *Clin Chest Med* 1996;17:67–82.

28. Battaglia SE, Pretto JJ, Irving LB, et al. Resolution of gas exchange abnormalities and intrapulmonary shunting following liver transplantation. *Hepatology* 1997;25:1228–1232.

29. Stoller JK, Moodie D, Schiavone WA, et al. Reduction of intrapulmonary shunt and resolution of digital clubbing associated with primary biliary cirrhosis after liver transplantation. *Hepatology* 1990;11:54–58.

30. Krowka MJ, Porayko MK, Plevak DJ, et al. Hepatopulmonary syndrome with progressive hypoxemia as an indication for liver transplantation: case reports and literature review. *Mayo Clin Proc* 1997;72:44–53.

31. Krowka MJ, Wiseman GA, Steers JF, et al. Late recurrence and rapid evolution of hepatopulmonary syndrome. *Liver Transplant Surg* 1999;5:451–453.

32. Egawa H, Kasahara M, Inomata Y, et al. Long-term outcome of living related liver transplantation for patients with intrapulmonary shunting and strategy for complications. *Transplantation* 1999;67:712–717.

33. Alexander J, Greenough A, Baker A, et al. Nitric oxide treatment of severe hypoxemia after liver transplantation in hepatopulmonary syndrome. *Liver Transplant Surg* 1997;3:54–55.

34. Martinez G, Barbera JA, Navasa M, et al. Hepatopulmonary syndrome associated with cardiorespiratory disease. *J Hepatol* 1999;30:882–889.

35. Krowka MJ, Plevak DJ, Findlay JF, et al. Pulmonary hemodynamics and perioperative cardiopulmonary mortality in patients with portopulmonary hypertension undergoing liver transplantation. *Liver Transpl* 2000;6:443–450.

36. Ramsey MAE, Simpson BR, Nguyen AT, et al. Severe pulmonary hypertension in liver transplant candidates. *Liver Transplant Surg* 1997;3:494–500.

37. De Wolf AM, Gasior T, Kang Y. Pulmonary hypertension in a patient undergoing liver transplantation. *Transplant Proc* 1991;23:2000–2001.

38. Cheng EY, Woehlck HJ. Pulmonary artery hypertension complicating anesthesia for liver transplantation. *Anesthesiology* 1992;77:389–392.

39. Gillies BS, Perkins JD, Cheney FW. Abdominal aortic compression to treat circulatory collapse caused by severe pulmonary hypertension during liver transplantation. *Anesthesiology* 1996;85:420–422.

40. Losay J, Piot D, Bougaran J, et al. Early liver transplantation is crucial in children with liver disease and pulmonary artery hypertension. *J Hepatol* 1998;28:337–344.

41. Prager MC, Cauldwell CA, Ascher NL, et al. Pulmonary hypertension associated with liver disease is not reversible after liver transplantation. *Anesthesiology* 1992;77:375–378.

42. Liu G, Knudsen KE, Secher NH. Orthotopic liver transplantation in a patient with primary pulmonary hypertension. *Anesth Intens Care* 1996;2:714–716.

43. Yoshida EM, Erb S, Pflugfelder PW, et al. Single-lung versus liver transplantation for the treatment of portopulmonary hypertension—a comparison of two patients. *Transplantation* 1992;55:688–690.

44. Scott V, De Wolf A, Kang Y, et al. Reversibility of pulmonary hypertension after liver transplantation. *Transplant Proc* 1993;25:1789–1790.

45. Koneru B, Ahmed S, Wiesse AB, et al. Resolution of pulmonary hypertension of cirrhosis after liver transplantation. *Transplantation* 1994;58:1133–1135.

46. Mandell SM, Duke J. Nitric oxide reduces pulmonary hypertension during hepatic transplantation. *Anesthesiology* 1994;81:1538–1542.

47. Levy MT, Torzillo P, Bookallil M, et al. Case report: delayed resolution of severe pulmonary hypertension after isolated liver transplantation in a patient with cirrhosis. *J Gastroenterol Hepatol* 1996;11:734–737.

48. Plotkin JS, Kuo PC, Rubin LJ, et al. Successful use of chronic epoprostenol as a bridge to liver transplantation in severe portopulmonary hypertension. *Transplantation* 1998;65:457–459.

49. Tarquino M, Geggel RL, Strauss RS, et al. Treatment of pulmonary hypertension with inhaled nitric oxide during hepatic transplantation in an adolescent: reversibility of pulmonary hypertension after transplantation. *Clin Pediatr* 1998;37:505–510.

50. Boillot O, Bianco F, Viale JP, et al. Liver transplantation resolves the hyperdynamic circulation in hereditary hemorrhagic telangiectasia with hepatic involvement. *Gastroenterology* 1999;116:187–192.

51. Ramsay MAE, Spikes C, East CA, et al. The perioperative management of portopulmonary hypertension with nitric oxide and epoprostenol. *Anesthesiology* 1999;90:299–301.

52. Mandell MS, Groves BM, Duke J. Progressive plexogenic pulmonary hypertension following liver transplantation. *Transplantation* 1995;59:1488–1490.

53. Kaspar MD, Ramsay MAE, Shuey CB, et al. Severe pulmonary hypertension and amelioration of hepatopulmonary syndrome after liver transplantation. *Liver Transplant Surg* 1998;4:177–179.

54. Findlay JF, Plevak DJ, Harrison BA, et al. Development of worsening splenomegaly and thrombocytopenia with IV epoprostenol in patients with portopulmonary hypertension. *Liver Transplant Surg* 1999;5:362–365.

55. Vennarecci G, Gunson BK, Ismail T, et al. Transplantation for end stage liver disease related to alpha$_1$-antitrypsin. *Transplantation* 1996; 61:1488–1495.

56. Filipponi F, Soubrane O, Labrousse F, et al. Liver transplantation for end-stage liver disease associated with alpha$_1$-antitrypsin deficiency in children: pretransplant natural history, timing, and results of transplantation. *J Hepatol* 1994;20:72–78.

57. Amended UNOS Policy 3.6 (Amended Appendix 3B, Indications for liver transplantation in children). Approved by the UNOS Board of Directors on June 25, 1998.

58. LaBerge JM, Brandt Ml, LeBeque P, et al. Reversal of cirrhosis-related pulmonary shunting in two children by orthotopic liver transplantation. *Transplantation* 1992;53:1135–1138.

59. Hobieka J, Houssin D, Bernard O, et al. Orthotopic liver transplantation in children with chronic liver disease and severe hypoxemia. *Transplantation* 1994;57:224–228.

60. Kuo PC, Plotkin JS, Gaine S, et al. Portopulmonary hypertension and the liver transplant candidate. *Transplantation* 1999;67:1087–1093.

Transplantation of the Liver, edited by Willis C.
Maddrey, Eugene R. Schiff, and Michael F.
Sorrell. Lippincott Williams & Wilkins,
Philadelphia © 2001.

CHAPTER 26

Liver Transplantation for Malignancy

William J. Wall

During the early, developmental years of clinical liver transplantation there was enthusiasm for the treatment of liver cancer by total hepatectomy and liver grafting. The radical nature of the surgery for otherwise unresectable malignancy was appealing from a tumor perspective, and the operation was appealing from a technical viewpoint because it was easier to perform than transplants in patients with end-stage cirrhosis, portal hypertension, and coagulopathy. The recipients, although they had cancer, were in better physical condition than patients with liver failure from cirrhosis and thus were more likely to survive the immediate postoperative period. In centers that were at the forefront of liver grafting, cancer was the indication for transplantation in as many as one of every three patients.[1-3] All types of primary liver cancer were included in the early series—hepatocellular carcinoma and its fibrolamellar variant; hepatoblastoma; cholangiocarcinoma; angiosarcoma; and hemangioendothelioma. The optimism even extended to cases of liver grafting for hepatic metastases from colon cancer and for metastatic melanoma.[4]

Although many recipients did well in the short term, accumulated experiences soon revealed that the vast majority of patients succumbed from recurrent cancer, usually within 2 years of transplantation.[5-7] In many patients, tumor growth seemed to be accelerated by immunosuppression, a suspicion that was later confirmed.[8] The enthusiasm for treating cancer by liver grafting was replaced by the realization that transplantation was a biologically inadequate therapy for most liver malignancies. The dutifully reported failures from many centers coincided with the impact that the introduction of cyclosporine had on liver transplantation and transplantation overall. The proliferation of transplant centers and the tremendous surge in transplant activity that resulted from superior immunosuppression marked

the beginning of the widening gap between the supply of donor organs and the demand for them. The argument that liver grafting, although not curative for most cancer recipients, was still good palliation could not be justified in the face of organ shortages and long-term posttransplantation survival rates that were nearly 50% higher in cirrhotic patients without malignancy. That combination of factors forced transplant specialists to become far more selective in accepting patients with cancer for liver grafting.

Today, only certain types of malignancy that are deemed to be at an early stage are selected for treatment by liver transplantation. The objective is cure, and unless it is possible to achieve survival rates that parallel those of patients who receive transplants for nonneoplastic disease, it is hard to defend the allocation of organs for cancer patients. Registry data from the United States, Europe, Canada, and Australia show that the percentage of liver transplants performed for malignant indications varies from 3% to 8%.[9-12] Several factors contribute to differences in national statistics, including philosophical attitudes toward the treatment of cancer, the prevalence of viral hepatitis in the population, and the application of screening methods to detect cancer in patients with stable cirrhosis.

HEPATOCELLULAR CANCER

Hepatocellular carcinoma (HCC), the most common primary hepatic malignancy, is the most common malignant indication for transplantation. In the Western world, it is most often seen in combination with cirrhosis, and its prevalence is far less than that seen in Asia and Africa. In 1991, Penn[13] reported registry data on 365 patients with HCC treated by transplantation over the preceding decade. The 5-year patient survival rate was only 18%; recurrent cancer was the main cause of death between 2 and 5 years. The registry included cancers that were as large as 26 cm in diameter. Those data, in addition to the disappointing experiences from single centers,[14-16] clearly identified the need to refine

W. J. Wall: Multi-Organ Transplant Program, London Health Sciences Centre—University Campus, London, Ontario N6A 5A5, Canada.

selection criteria for candidates with HCC. In the 1990s, liver transplantation for malignancy focused on early cancer detection, accurate tumor staging, and the use of adjuvant or neoadjuvant chemotherapy in an attempt to achieve the highest rates of tumor-free survival.

Early Cancer Detection

Patients with stable cirrhosis frequently enter screening programs or attend surveillance clinics with the objective of detecting HCC when it is still in an early, asymptomatic stage. The tests most commonly used are serum α-fetoprotein (AFP) level and abdominal ultrasonography. The AFP value lacks specificity in substantial numbers of patients because of persistent or intermittent increases outside the normal range in chronic viral hepatitis and increases during exacerbations of hepatic inflammation. In various surveillance studies, the sensitivity of AFP levels (20 ng/mL or above) for detecting HCC ranges from 39% to 64% and the specificity ranges from 76% to 91%.[17,18]

Ultrasound for screening or surveillance is used to complement the AFP level. HCCs are commonly hypoechoic, and as they get larger their echogenicity becomes more heterogeneous due to tumor necrosis. Although ultrasound sensitivity and specificity rates of 78% and 94% have been reported for HCC,[18] the specificity of ultrasound for nodules less than 2 cm in diameter in cirrhotic livers has recently been reported to be less than 50%.[19] Regenerative nodules, dysplastic nodules, and focal fatty change can have features indistinguishable from small HCCs. Thus, ultrasonographic findings may not reliably characterize small nodules in cirrhotic livers in a relatively high percentage of cases. In addition to the detection of liver nodules, other relevant ultrasound findings that may be helpful include evidence of venous invasion or venous thrombosis.

When HCC is suspected on the ultrasound examination, contrast-enhanced computed tomography (CT) is the most appropriate test for confirming the diagnosis radiographically.[20] CT and its variations can detect most HCCs because their blood supply is almost entirely arterial. The tumors therefore typically are hypervascular on the arterial phase images (Fig. 26.1). CT is more sensitive and accurate than ultrasound in detecting multicentricity. In a retrospective study of 30 patients with HCC who underwent liver grafting, the sensitivities of ultrasound, CT, and hepatic angiography in detecting tumor multicentricity were 16%, 58%, and 58%, respectively.[21] Hepatic angiography combined with CT (angio-CT) can identify small foci of HCC during the arterial phase of the exam before portal venous delivery of contrast enhances the liver parenchyma.[22] Magnetic resonance imaging has been reported to detect tumors less than 2 cm in diameter in 81% of cases.[23] The choice of investigations at any given center will be largely influenced by the interests of the radiologists and their confidence in specific imaging modalities.

CT with iodized oil (lipoidal CT) is based on the tumor's uptake and retention of iodinated oil after intraarterial injection, and it has become a popular method to detect small tumors and to deliver chemotherapeutic agents in the oil emulsion. Lipoidal CT has been reported to accurately detect

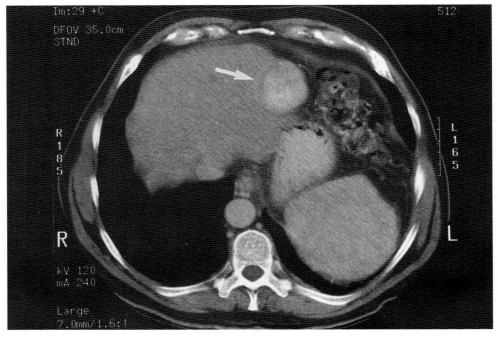

FIG. 26.1. Contrast-enhanced computed tomographic scan showing a 4.5 cm hypervascular hepatocellular carcinoma (*white arrow*) in the left lateral segment of an irregular, small, cirrhotic liver.

HCCs less than 1 cm in diameter in up to 83% of cases,[24] but other studies report much less favorable sensitivity rates.[25] Despite extensive radiographic investigations, confusion over the diagnosis of HCC or failure to identify small tumors occurs in 10% to 20% of cases. Multifocal lesions, satellite nodules, and vascular invasion are the findings that are most likely to be missed on preoperative imaging. Because the lungs are common sites of spread, a chest x-ray and CT of the chest should be performed as part of the workup of a patient with an HCC.

When a lesion that has typical features of an HCC is discovered radiographically, the use of needle biopsy to prove the diagnosis is controversial. Ultrasound or CT-guided needle biopsy may give false negative results, and there is the small but real risk of tumor seeding along the needle track. Percutaneous needle biopsy may have a more definite role in the diagnosis of indeterminate nodules that do not show characteristic radiographic features of HCC. If a hypervascular tumor that is not a hemangioma is visualized in a cirrhotic liver and the serum AFP level is greater than 100 ng/mL, the patient should be treated for HCC and a biopsy is not indicated. If a biopsy is deemed necessary, a core sample provides the pathologist with an appropriate specimen; fine-needle aspiration should be avoided.

Tumor Staging

For virtually all types of cancer, the size of the tumor, the existence of multiple foci, local invasion (vascular and lymphatic), and spread outside the organ of origin carry prognostic significance. In patients with HCC, large, multiple, and invasive cancers carry a worse prognosis.[26,27] The most detailed classification of tumor characteristics is the TNM system, which has been widely applied to all the common cancers. Several centers have found it useful in reporting their results of transplantation for HCC.[28,29] It is purely a pathological description of tumor variables and thus is different from the Okuda staging, which combines clinical variables (ascites, albumin and bilirubin levels) with the extent of liver involvement by the tumor.[30] In the TNM system, tumor characteristics are defined on the basis of the primary tumor (T) described by size, number, distribution in the liver, and the presence or absence of vascular invasion; the presence or absence of node (N) involvement; and the presence or absence of distant metastases (M). The TNM classification of HCC is described in Table 26.1,[31] and the Union Internationale Contre le Cancer (UICC) staging of the cancer is shown in Table 26.2.[32] At the University of Pittsburgh, 2-year patient survival rates of 75%, 75%, 56%, and 26% were reported after transplantation for stage I, II, III, and IVA HCC, respectively.[29]

The precision and detail of the TNM classification provides a useful system for comparing results and assessing the effect of various treatment regimens, but it has several important shortcomings that affect its practical application. With respect to tumor size, it is arguable whether 2 cm is

TABLE 26.1. *TNM classification of hepatocellular cancer*

T: Primary tumor

T1	Solitary, ≤ 2 cm without vascular invasion
T2	Solitary, ≤ 2 cm with vascular invasion
	Solitary, > 2 cm without vascular invasion
	Multiple, one lobe, ≤ 2 cm without vascular invasion
T3	Solitary, > 2 cm with vascular invasion
	Multiple, one lobe, ≤ 2 cm, with vascular invasion
	Multiple, one lobe, > 2 cm, with or without vascular invasion
T4	Multiple, more than one lobe
	Invasion of major branch of hepatic or portal veins
	Invasion of adjacent organs other than gallbladder
	Perforation of visceral peritoneum

N: Lymph nodes

N0	Nodes negative
N1	Nodes positive

M: Distant metastasis

M0	No distant metastasis
M1	Distant metastasis (e.g., lung, bone)

the most appropriate cut-off as opposed to 3 cm or even 5 cm, and there is no incremental weighting in the staging for tumors that are much larger than 2 cm. The analysis by McPeake et al.[33] found a significant impact of the size of HCC on outcome after transplantation when tumors of less than 4 cm, between 4 and 8 cm, and greater than 8 cm were compared (Fig. 26.2). Recent registry data compiled on 410 HCCs treated by transplantation showed a strong impact of tumor size on outcome.[34] Five-year actuarial patient survival rates were 59.9%, 48.7%, and 32.6% for tumors less than 3 cm, 3 to 5 cm, and greater than 5 cm, respectively.

The grouping of tumors with several different characteristics in the same stage is another criticism of the system, especially as it relates to tumors in the stage III category. Stage III is a heterogenous group into which tumors both with and without nodal involvement are assigned. When HCC involves lymph nodes, the prognosis is so poor that one has to seriously question the legitimacy of giving a node-positive tumor the same staging as a solitary 3 cm tumor with microscopic vascular invasion. A recent revision of the stage III category subclassifies node-negative and node-positive tumors into IIIA and IIIB, respectively,[32] which partially addresses this deficiency. Nonetheless, many would still argue that two small

TABLE 26.2. *Staging of hepatocellular cancer*

Stage I	T1	N0	M0
Stage II	T2	N0	M0
Stage IIIA	T3	N0	M0
Stage IIIB	T1	N1	M0
	T2	N1	M0
	T3	N1	M0
Stage IVA	T4	any N	M0
Stage IVB	any T	any N	M1

From Sobin LH, Wittekind C (International Union Against Cancer [UICC]), eds. *TNM classification of malignant tumours,* 5th ed. New York: John Wiley, 1997.

LIVER TRANSPLATATION FOR HCC

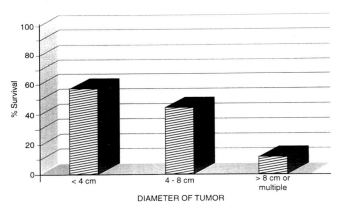

FIG. 26.2. Five-year actuarial survival after liver transplantation for hepatocellular carcinoma of different sizes. (Data are from McPeake, O'Grady JG, Azman S, et al. Liver transplantation for primary hepatocellular carcinoma: tumor size and number determine outcome. *J Hepatol* 1993;18:226–234.)

tumors in both lobes (i.e., stage IVA) carry a more favorable prognosis than a solitary IIIB tumor. Similarly, two 1 cm tumors in both lobes of the liver would be designated stage IVA, the same staging given to a 9 cm HCC invading the right hepatic vein. Finally, the TNM classification does not consider the degree of histologic differentiation of the tumor, which recently has been suggested to have prognostic significance in HCC treated by liver transplantation.[34]

These deficiencies of the TNM system are the likely explanation for why some recent series have failed to show a correlation between it and the outcome of HCC treated by transplantation.[35,36] Lack of an association between staging and survival is particularly relevant when reported series do not have comparable stratification of the tumor variables within the different stages, or when they have deliberately excluded tumors with certain characteristics, for example, node involvement or vascular invasion.[36] The TNM system as it applies to HCC will likely need modification if its full practical potential is to be realized.

Nevertheless, whenever transplantation is contemplated for the treatment of HCC, an attempt should be made to characterize the primary growth as accurately as possible and to detect or exclude extrahepatic spread. The presence of any demonstrable cancer outside the liver is the single most important contraindication to transplantation for HCC. There is no consensus on the size of an HCC that should be regarded as an absolute contraindication to transplantation, but many centers use an upper limit of 5 cm. Although rigid adherence to such a size limit will deny cure to an occasional patient with a larger tumor, patients with large cancers should not be accepted for transplantation unless they are participating in a specific protocol that has scientific merit. The experiences of many centers have identified those cancers that have better outcomes after transplantation, includ-

ing the futility of liver grafting for HCC in patients with hepatitis B cirrhosis without posttransplantation antiviral therapy.[37–40] If preoperative imaging suggests that a tumor is borderline, it is appropriate to have a backup recipient ready in the hospital if the transplant has to be abandoned because the operative findings reveal that the tumor is too advanced. Even with the most sophisticated preoperative imaging, pathological examination of the explanted liver will reveal understaging of the tumor in 25% to 43% of cases.[35,36]

Adjuvant and Neoadjuvant Chemotherapy

Recently there has been much interest in the use of adjuvant or neoadjuvant chemotherapy in combination with transplantation for HCC. The oncological argument for perioperative systemic chemotherapy is based on the observation that in the absence of any detectable tumor outside the liver, many patients develop seeding in the transplant and other sites (primarily lung) in the early postoperative period, indicating that either micrometastases are already present at the time of the transplant procedure or that tumor dissemination occurs during the surgery. It has been shown that HCC cells are recoverable from the right atrium and the portal vein during liver resection.[41,42] The risk of tumor emboli escaping into the circulation should be at least as great during hepatic transplantation. Thus, the administration of systemic perioperative chemotherapy with the intent of abolishing micrometastases is logical. The question is whether the logic of this approach is supported by clinical data.

In the early 1990s several pilot studies from different centers combined various chemotherapeutic protocols with transplantation for HCC.[43–47] It was the objective of the pilot studies to increase the curative benefit of transplantation for HCC by giving adjuvant treatment to patients with cancers that historically had poor survival rates with transplantation alone. The series, each with relatively small numbers of patients, are summarized in Table 26.3. Doxorubicin, cisplatin, and 5-fluorouracil were the most commonly used antineoplastic drugs, either alone or in combination. None of the chemotherapeutic regimens (agents, dosages, routes, timing, duration) is comparable in the various studies, nor are the mix of tumors (using the TNM classification). Notwithstanding these differences, the results showed 3-year actuarial survival rates of 46% to 64%, which were superior to previous reports of transplantation alone, at least for TNM stage III and stage IV HCC. However, there was deliberate exclusion of tumors with lymph node metastases or vascular invasion in some of the trials,[43–45] and therefore the studies are not really comparable with historical series of cancers of similar stage but with a different mix of tumor characteristics. The follow-up of patients in these trials was also quite short. In spite of these shortcomings, the results stimulated a great deal of interest in adjuvant chemotherapy in the transplant setting.

Since the latter part of the 1990s there has been more interest in the administration of transarterial chemoemboliza-

TABLE 26.3. *Liver transplantation and adjuvant chemotherapy for hepatocellular carcinoma*

Author (Ref.)	No. of patients	Treatment	TNM tumor stages (No. of patients)	Actuarial survival
Stone et al. 1993 (43)	20	Systemic chemotherapy (doxorubicin) pre-, intra-, and postoperatively	II (6), III (3), IVA (11)	59% (3 yr)
Carr et al. 1993 (44)	11	Monthly intraarterial chemotherapy pretransplantation (doxorubicin and cisplatin) and α-interferon	III (5), IVA (5), IVB (1)	91% (1 yr)
Cherqui et al. 1994 (45)	9	Preoperative TACE (lipoidal, doxorubicin, gelatin sponge) and radiotherapy; posttransplantation systemic chemotherapy (mitoxantrone)	II (1), III (1), IVA (9)	64% (3 yr)
Olthoff et al. 1995 (46)	25	Systemic chemotherapy posttransplantation (fluorouracil, doxorubicin, cisplatin) for 6 mo	II (6), III (8), IVA (10), IVB (1)	46% (3 yr)
Venook et al. 1995 (47)	17	TACE[a] (doxorubicin, cisplatin, mitomycin-c, gelfoam powder)	<5 cm, <4 tumors	Not stated

TACE, transarterial chemoembolization.
[a]Either tumor or whole-liver chemoembolization.

tion (TACE) using doxorubicin emulsified in iodized oil. When an HCC is identified and is suitable for treatment by transplantation, TACE has been advocated with the aim of causing necrosis of the primary tumor and diminishing the likelihood of further growth or metastasis between the time of treatment and the time of transplantation. The selective route minimizes systemic toxicity, delivers a high dose of the drug directly to the tumor, and maintains a high concentration of the drug within the tumor. Following infusion of the chemotherapy, gelatin sponge is used to embolize the tumor, leading to tumor infarction.[48]

Four reports deserve specific comment because each of them, by design, selected cirrhotic patients with what was believed to be early-stage HCC for treatment by transplantation.[35,36,49,50] Some of the patients received TACE and some did not. The four studies are summarized in Table 26.4. In each, the patients had underlying cirrhosis and superimposed hepatocellular carcinoma. Romani et al.[49] reported 27 cirrhotic patients who were found on screening to have a solitary HCC that was 5 cm or less in diameter. The discovery of the tumor was the indication for transplantation. Only a minority of patients received TACE prior to transplantation. Patients with lymph node metastases found preoperatively or intraoperatively were excluded. Patient survival at 3 years was 71%, and the cancer recurrence rate was only 7.4%.

TABLE 26.4. *Results of transplantation for early hepatocellular cancer*

Author (Ref.)	No. of patients	Selection criteria	Patients given neoadjuvant therapy	TNM staging (No. of patients)	Tumors understaged (%)	Recurrence rate (%)	Actuarial survival (%)
Romani et al. 1994 (49)	27	≤5 cm found on screening	3 TACE (doxorubicin), 1 ethanol injection	Not stated	20%	7.4%	71% (3 yr)
Mazzaferro et al. 1996 (35)	48	≤5 cm if single, ≤3 cm if multiple; no more than 4 lesions	26 TACE (14 doxorubicin, 12 mitoxantrone), 1 ethanol injection	I (15), II (18), III (13), IV (2)	27%	8%	75% (4 yr)
Figueras et al. 1997 (50)	38	<5 cm, localized	31 TACE (doxorubicin)	I (6), II (11), III (12), IVA (9)	12%	8%	79% (5 yr)
Llovet et al. 1998 (36)	58	≤5 cm, solitary, no vascular invasion	None	I (15), II (19), IIIA (11), IVA (13)	43%	3.5%	74% (5 yr)

TACE, transarterial chemoembolization.

Mazzaferro et al.[35] reported 48 cases of HCC that were smaller than 5 cm when single and smaller than 3 cm when multiple, with no more than three tumors. The tumors were not amenable to removal by partial hepatectomy because of their location or multifocality, or the severity of coexisting cirrhosis. If vascular or lymph node invasion was evident or suspected preoperatively, patients were excluded. Approximately half of the patients were given TACE at 6- to 8-week intervals prior to transplantation; the remaining patients did not receive neoadjuvant treatment because of insufficient hepatic reserve. The waiting time between tumor staging and transplantation was approximately 4 months. Two-thirds of the tumors were TNM stage I and II. The 4-year actuarial survival was 75%, and the tumor recurrence rate was 8% overall. Perhaps the most revealing observation in this study was the lack of a difference in overall or tumor-free survival between recipients who did and did not receive TACE. As shown in Fig. 26.3, preoperative chemoembolization did not increase tumor-free survival.

The study by Figueras et al.[50] involved 38 cases of localized HCC less than 5 cm in diameter. The main indication for transplantation was the presence of the HCC, irrespective of the degree of cirrhosis. Like the two previous studies, lymph node involvement was an exclusion criterion. Just over half of the tumors were stage III and stage IVA. Three-quarters of the patients received pretransplantation TACE. The recurrence rate was as low as in the other two series (8%), and the 5-year survival rate was 79%, which was not significantly different from the survival of a matched group of patients with cirrhosis undergoing liver transplantation during the same period. Tumors larger than 5 cm in diameter and those with vascular invasion had a worse prognosis.

The final and most recent study, by Llovet et al.,[36] reported 58 patients with HCC who were selected for transplantation because the tumors were solitary, less than 5 cm in diameter, and had no evidence of vascular invasion on preoperative imaging studies. Slightly less than half of the tumors were stage IIIA or IVA. In contrast to the other series, none of the patients received any chemotherapy or other antineoplastic treatment. The waiting time for transplantation averaged 2 months. The tumor recurrence rate was gratifyingly low at 3.5%, and the actuarial 5-year survival rate was 74%.

These studies show that excellent results can be obtained with transplantation in carefully selected patients with HCC. Unfortunately, they do not clarify the role of TACE as an adjunct to transplantation for tumors in the clinical stages that were represented in the series. None of the series provided proof that TACE improved cure rates, nor did they provide evidence that TACE made a significant difference for tumors that were of a more advanced stage, that is, stages III and IVA. Importantly, the effect of one of the most relevant variables—time—is unknown in the context of pretransplantation TACE. When the waiting time between tumor diagnosis and transplantation is only 1 or 2 months, TACE may have no role in management. On the other hand, if the waiting time to transplantation is many months, a valuable role for TACE could be found in early HCC by keeping the cancer in its earliest stage.

A recent analysis from Paris[51] provides further data but does not clarify the role of TACE. It reports a nonrandomized, retrospective study of 197 patients with HCC who underwent either liver transplantation or hepatic resection. TACE was given to approximately half of the patients prior to surgery. There was no significant increase in overall survival in those patients who had TACE, either in the resection or the transplantation group. Nevertheless, a subgroup of patients who had a 50% or more reduction in tumor size after TACE had an improved disease-free survival rate. That was true for patients who underwent either transplantation or resection. Without a randomized trial, it is impossible to claim a beneficial effect of TACE in patients with the earliest cancers (stages I and II), and whether TACE is effective for tumors of stage IIIA and stage IVA is yet to be proven.

The other undecided area is the place of postoperative chemotherapy for incidental cancers discovered by the surgeon at the time of transplantation or by the pathologist when the explanted liver is sectioned. From what is known, postoperative chemotherapy would not seem to be indicated for stage I or II cancers. It would be easier to justify the side effects and risks of systemic chemotherapy for a trial involving more advanced tumors, that is, larger, multiple tumors or those with vascular invasion.

All of the reported series differ to some degree in their selection criteria and treatment protocols, but they demonstrate that excellent survival rates are obtainable with very low rates of tumor recurrence. From the available informa-

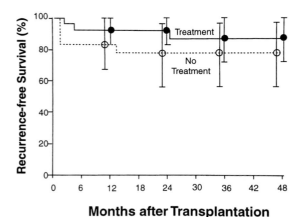

FIG. 26.3. Effect of treatment with transarterial chemoembolization before transplantation in 48 patients with cirrhosis and hepatocellular carcinoma. (From Mazzaferro, Regalia E, Doci R, et al. Liver transplantation for the treatment of small hepatocellular carcinomas in patients with cirrhosis. *N Engl J Med* 1996;334:693–699, with permission.)

tion, the following statements about the treatment of HCC by transplantation can be made:

1. The tumors with a more favorable prognosis are those that are less than 5 cm in diameter without gross vascular invasion. If multiple tumors are present, it is preferable that they be small (3 cm or less in diameter) and be three or fewer in number. It is impossible to say if multifocality confined to one lobe is more favorable than bilobar involvement when other tumor characteristics are excluded.

2. Perioperative chemotherapy, although theoretically appealing, is yet to be proven as necessary or beneficial for early-stage HCC when the waiting period between the time of diagnosis and the transplantation is short. It is not possible at this time to claim a beneficial effect of adjuvant therapy for specific tumor characteristics such as size, vascular invasion, or multiple nodules.

3. There is evidence that TACE causes tumor necrosis, and it may down-stage the primary cancer by size reduction; however, evidence is lacking that pretransplantation TACE results in improved cure rates. One could speculate that the greatest value of TACE in early HCC may be in preventing tumor growth and metastases when the waiting period between diagnosis and transplantation is substantial.

4. The shortcomings of the TNM classification, as they apply to HCC treated by liver grafting, need to be considered when results between centers or outcomes of different treatments are compared.

5. Preoperative imaging studies, as good as they are, frequently underestimate the true stage of HCCs. Small nodules and microscopic vascular invasion are pathological features that will continue to be difficult to document on imaging studies. Therefore, it seems certain that no matter what criteria are applied preoperatively, there will be a significant incidence of tumors that are more advanced than expected when the removed livers are examined.

Hepatic Resection versus Transplantation for Hepatocellular Carcinoma

The debate about partial liver resection versus transplantation for HCC will continue because there are no randomized trials that have addressed this controversy. Obviously, tumors that are anatomically unresectable because of their location or the severity of coexisting cirrhosis should be treated by transplantation when other transplantation criteria are satisfied. The debate relates mainly to patients whose tumors are anatomically resectable and whose underlying cirrhosis does not preclude partial hepatic resection with an acceptable perioperative mortality. The argument put forward for transplantation is that the underlying cirrhosis is treated as well as the tumor and that the neoplastic potential of the remaining cirrhotic liver is eliminated. Recurrent or new

primary cancers occur in a very high percentage of patients who undergo resection.[52] The advantages of transplantation have to be balanced against the higher perioperative mortality compared with resection and the risks and side effects of chronic immunosuppression.

Six different centers in Germany, France, Britain, and the United States have reported their retrospective experiences with resection and transplantation.[29,53–57] The selection criteria are different in each series and it is therefore not surprising that there is considerable variation in the results (Fig. 26.4). In three centers, patient survival rates after resection and transplantation were not significantly different; two centers' results favored resection; and one center favored transplantation. The outcomes undoubtedly reflect selection criteria and different approaches toward aggressive surgical management of liver cancer. For example, the 3-year patient survival after transplantation was more than twice as high in the Pittsburgh series compared with the Hanover series (39% versus 14%). But more than twice as many patients in the Hanover series had more advanced cancers, and nearly 20% of the patients had stage IVB tumors.[53] The apparently conflicting results are thus explained by the selection of different cancers for different treatment.

For tumors that are small (less than 3 cm) and situated in liver segments that are amenable to resection, our approach would be to resect them if coexistent cirrhosis is not severe. In patients with similar small tumors who have inadequate hepatic reserve or who have tumors that are more centrally located, transplantation would be offered. The argument that transplantation removes the risk of new primary tumors developing in the remaining lobe of a cirrhotic liver needs to be reassessed in the light of a recent case report of a *de novo* HCC developing in a transplanted liver in a patient with recurrent hepatitis C.[58] Universal reinfection with the hepatitis C virus after transplantation raises the specter of the carcinogenic effect of the virus on the transplanted organ and what it will mean over the long term to the thousands of patients who undergo transplantation for chronic hepatitis C.

Fibrolamellar Variant of Hepatocellular Carcinoma

The fibrolamellar variant of HCC is distinguished by its unique pathological characteristics and different clinical behavior from the much more common HCC. The patients tend to be younger, the majority of tumors occur in noncirrhotic livers, and the tumors typically grow much slower, with metastases occurring late.[59] Several series show that the natural history of nonsurgically treated fibrolamellar HCC is long and that patients can do well with both transplantation and nontransplantation-based treatment.[60–61] Even after incomplete removal by partial liver resection, long-term survival is possible. Fibrolamellar HCC is one of the rare liver primary cancers for which resection of local recurrences or nodal metastases is compatible with prolonged survival. So far there

RESECTION vs TRANSPLANTATION FOR HCC

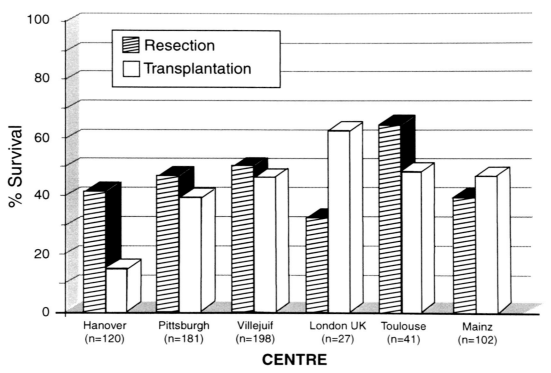

FIG. 26.4. Three-year patient survival rates after resection versus transplantation for hepatocellular carcinoma at six different centers (see references 29 and 53–57).

has been no beneficial effect demonstrated for perioperative chemotherapy for this neoplasm.

There is an association between tumor staging using the TNM system and cancer-free survival for fibrolamellar HCC. Nodal involvement and vascular invasion carry a worse prognosis. In the largest and most recent report of fibrolamellar HCC treated by either hepatic resection or transplantation at the University of Pittsburgh,[62] 10-year patient survival rates for 41 patients were better for resection than for transplantation (70% versus 28%, respectively). It should be stressed, however, that resection was the preferred procedure and that transplantation was resorted to when tumor extension precluded resection. Therefore, the circumstances for transplantation were distinctly unfavorable. Overall, 90% of the tumors were stage IVA or stage IVB. The fact that these tumors were so advanced at the time of surgery yet patients had overall survival rates of nearly 50% by 10 years is incontrovertible evidence that this distinctive histopathological tumor has a different biological behavior than nonfibrolamellar HCC.

OTHER PRIMARY LIVER CANCERS

Hepatoblastoma

Hepatoblastoma is a rare childhood tumor for which surgical resection has been the mainstay of treatment. It used to carry

a grim prognosis, but multimodal therapy has improved the outlook considerably for this cancer.[63–64] Combination chemotherapy preoperatively with doxorubicin and cisplatin can render previously unresectable tumors resectable, and metastatic disease in the lungs can respond dramatically to chemotherapy and surgery, with the prospect of long-term tumor-free survival. For hepatoblastomas that cannot be removed by partial hepatic resection because of their location or bilobar involvement, transplantation should be considered.[65] Systemic perioperative chemotherapy should be administered using the same regimen that would be used in combination with partial hepatectomy.

The tumor is so uncommon that the experience of single transplant centers is limited. In a review from several institutions in the United States, 6 of 12 children were alive with no evidence of malignancy from 2 to 6 years after transplantation.[66] Like the fibrolamellar variant of HCC, hepatoblastoma should not be excluded from consideration for treatment by transplantation because of the presence of extrahepatic disease.

Cholangiocarcinoma

In the historical series, cholangiocarcinoma had a miserably low cure rate with liver transplantation.[13,28] Experience showed the association between staging using the TNM system and the outcome for this malignancy.[28] The overwhelmingly lethal effect of tumor extension outside the liver was clearly shown, and the results were very poor even with apparently confined tumors. Early recurrences involved regional retroperitoneal lymph nodes and peritoneal surfaces. The dismal results led to the general view that cholangiocarcinoma should be an absolute contraindication to transplantation. The inability of radiation treatment or chemotherapy to cure these tumors is the reason that aggressive surgery and transplantation are still being explored as part of a multimodal approach to their management. In a series from Baylor Medical Center in Dallas, patients who received grafts for cholangiocarcinoma were given concurrent administration of 5-fluorouracil and radiotherapy to the porta hepatis and regional nodes 1 to 2 months after transplantation.[67] Tumors recurred in 11 of 14 recipients, and none of the patients who were tumor free at the time of the report had lived long enough to be assured of cure.

In the context of liver grafting, cholangiocarcinoma is usefully divided into three types. The first is cholangiocarcinoma arising from the biliary radicles within the liver, so-called intrahepatic or peripheral cholangiocarcinoma. Often it is multiple or diffuse, invades contiguous structures, spreads via perineural invasion, and metastasizes to local and regional nodes. Multicentricity and local invasion usually preclude removal by partial hepatectomy; hence, the consideration of transplantation arises. Unfortunately, the same pathological characteristics that preclude cure by partial liver resection defeat transplantation too. In the largest series reported to date, transplantation was unsuccessful in curing intrahepatic cholangiocarcinoma when there were multiple tumors, when nodes were involved, and when resection margins were positive.[68] Exenteration procedures of the upper abdomen and cluster transplants to obtain wider margins for this tumor have not received support. Transplantation cures intrahepatic cholangiocarcinoma so rarely that most transplant centers regard it as an absolute contraindication to transplantation even if imaging studies suggest the disease is confined to the liver.

The second type of bile duct cancer for which transplantation was initially hoped to be good treatment is the Klatskin carcinoma at the bifurcation of the common hepatic duct (Fig. 26.5). Sometimes referred to as hilar or central bile duct cancer, it is small and slow growing, but its location and propensity for local extension and lymphatic and perineural invasion prevent cure by radical surgery, including transplantation, with very few exceptions. Violation of the principles of cancer surgery by nonsurgical and surgical manipulation and mechanical intubation of the biliary tree prior to transplantation probably contributed to many early, fatal recurrences. But even when fresh cases are treated in the first instance by transplantation, recurrence is almost universal, although survivors can live for years before the cancer returns.

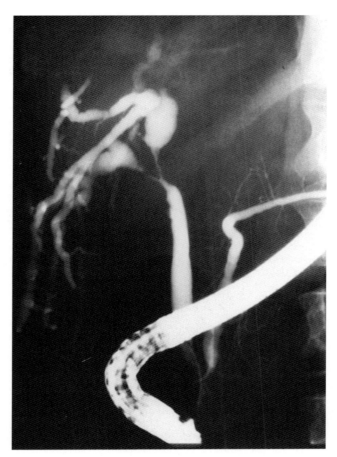

FIG. 26.5. Endoscopic retrograde cholangiopancreatogram showing a classic Klatskin carcinoma at the hepatic duct bifurcation.

Figure 26.6 shows the macroscopic appearance of a 2 cm Klatskin carcinoma on the coronal cut surface of a total hepatectomy specimen. Although the tumor is enticingly small, the histology in Fig. 26.7 shows cancer cells infiltrating through the wall of the duct onto the adventitia of the portal vein. The patient died of recurrent cancer 22 months after transplantation. Palliative bilioenteric bypass can achieve survival rates comparable with transplantation and thus is the treatment currently recommended at our center for Klatskin tumors.

The third type of cholangiocarcinoma relevant to transplantation is that which occurs in patients with primary sclerosing cholangitis. Cure is possible by transplantation when the tumors are found as incidental, *in situ* tumors when the indication for grafting is advanced primary sclerosing cholangitis.[69] The risk of developing cancer in primary sclerosing cholangitis is likely overstated, approximately 10% after 10 years, yet that alone has not been the leading indication for transplantation in this disease. When cholangiocarcinoma becomes clinically and grossly evident in patients with primary sclerosing cholangitis, transplantation is not appropriate because the chance of cure is remote. A few centers have investigated the role of high-dose

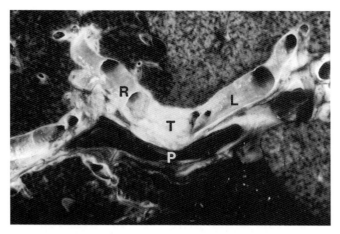

FIG. 26.6. Coronal section through the liver and Klatskin tumor shown in Fig. 26.5. T, tumor; R, right hepatic duct; L, left hepatic duct; P, portal vein bifurcation.

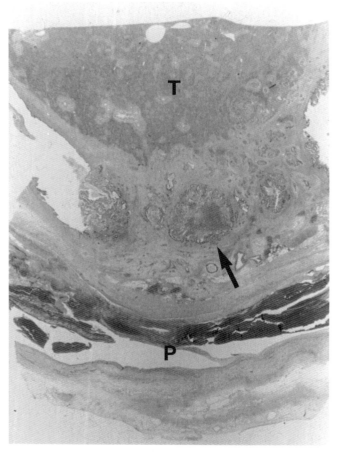

FIG. 26.7. Histologic section of the Klatskin tumor shown in Fig. 26.6. Arrow points to tumor invading the adventitia of the wall of the portal vein. T, tumor; P, portal vein.

intrabiliary radiotherapy with or without chemotherapy followed by liver transplantation for these cancers, but detailed reports have not been published.

Angiosarcoma and Hemangioendothelioma

Various sarcomas have been treated by hepatic transplantation. Angiosarcomas can originate in the liver, but they are aggressive cancers and spread early by hematogenous routes; thus, they should be regarded as a contraindication to transplantation. Epithelioid hemangioendothelioma, on the other hand, has a behavior that is quite variable. It is a rare cancer that tends to metastasize, but survival may be very prolonged.[28] Extrahepatic involvement at the time of transplantation is compatible with many years of survival.[70] Thus there is reason to continue to consider patients with this neoplasm for liver grafting.

METASTATIC TUMORS

Although liver grafting has been performed for many types of malignancy that have metastasized to the liver—including breast, kidney, colon, pancreas, and skin—the results are dismal for all except the neuroendocrine metastases. The liver is a frequent site of spread from neuroendocrine tumors originating in the gastrointestinal tract, pancreas, and other primary sites. They tend to be more indolent and slow growing than the other carcinomas of the gastrointestinal tract.

The treatment of choice for those secondary tumors is surgical resection when medical therapy cannot control the hormonal effects of the tumor. Prolonged survival can occur after removal of the majority of gross disease by partial hepatectomy or transplantation when there is bilobar liver involvement, but the results need to be interpreted in the context of survival rates without surgery. Five-year survival rates of up to 32% are reported for patients with unresected neuroendocrine liver secondary tumors, and thus the results of hepatic resection, whether partial or total, have to be assessed with that knowledge.[71] Although the intent in the past may have been cure, what is known about the biology of these tumors suggests that liver grafting should be regarded as palliation.

Since the first report of liver grafting for metastatic neuroendocrine tumors by Makowka and colleagues,[72] there have been a number of other reports that show long-term survival is possible.[73–76] In a review of the literature, the overall survival at 5 years was 24% in 103 patients after liver transplantation.[77] Recurrent cancer occurs frequently in the liver graft itself and in bone.

In a series of 31 patients collected from several transplant centers in France, the 5-year patient survival was much better for metastatic carcinoid tumors compared with the 4-year survival after transplantation for other neuroendocrine metastases (69% versus 8%, respectively).[78] Upper abdominal exenteration procedures have been performed to radically remove the primary growth, the liver secondaries, node-bearing tissue, and other visceral involvement.[79,80] The magnitude of the surgery and its morbidity, plus the comparable results for total hepatectomy and transplantation alone, make it difficult to recommend such radical surgery for palliation.

FUTURE CONSIDERATIONS

It seems certain that increasing numbers of patients with HCC will be candidates for liver transplantation over the next decade. The prevalence of liver disease, especially hepatitis C, and the application of screening and surveillance will result in more cases of HCC being referred for transplantation. Histologic studies of regenerative processes in cirrhotic livers and clonal analysis of regenerative nodules may aid in identifying those patients at greatest risk for the development of cancer.[81,82] The possibility of reducing the incidence of HCC in patients at risk by the administration of synthetic retinoids (polyprenoic acid) is intriguing,[83] but the ultimate solution will be the development of a vaccine for hepatititis C. Until that time, substantial numbers of the thousands of chronic carriers will develop HCC for which transplantation will offer the only hope of cure.

The effects of immunosuppression on the growth and spread of cancer suggest that patients who receive transplants for malignancy should be considered for specific tailoring of their immunosuppressive therapy. Centers that have reported the lowest HCC recurrence rates have withdrawn steroids 3 to 6 months after transplantation.[35,50] In a retrospective study from three Italian institutions, the relative risk of HCC recurrence increased almost four times when recipients received steroids indefinitely after grafting.[84] A recent experimental study in rodents examined the effect of immunosuppression on hepatoma recurrence in a syngeneic liver transplant model.[85] Cyclosporine administration significantly increased tumor recurrence in the lungs and other sites compared wtih nonimmunosuppressed animals. Rodent models of HCC and transplantation provide an excellent opportunity to study tumor variables and immunosuppression that should yield information that will guide clinicians in the selection of agents. Sirolimus (rapamycin), one of the newest drugs, has been shown to have antitumor effects and is an effective immunosuppressant in liver recipients.[86–88] Balancing the suppression of host immunity against the risk of accelerated tumor growth should be a paramount consideration in patients who receive grafts for malignancy. Recently the selective postoperative administration of iodine-131–labeled lipoidal reduced the recurrence rate of HCC and improved cancer-free survival in patients who underwent partial hepatic resection.[89] Because the transplanted liver is often the site of cancer recurrence, the treatment of the graft by this method in the immediate posttransplantation period has theoretical appeal.

It is not completely clear at this time what the true role of adjuvant and neoadjuvant chemotherapy is for HCC treated by liver grafting. It may be that chemotherapy truly benefits some patients, but the evidence for a definite effect as measured by cancer-free survival is largely circumstantial to date. The type of agents, their routes, their duration, and their dosages need to be investigated in randomized trials that stratify tumor characteristics by size, number of tumors, distribution in the liver, and vascular invasion. The trials will have to be multi-institutional in order to enroll the numbers of patients needed to provide conclusive data. Registry data are informative, but they cannot control for the many variables between participating centers.

REFERENCES

1. Starzl TE, Porter KA, Brettschneider L, et al. Clinical and pathological observations after orthotopic transplantation of the human liver. *Surg Gynecol Obstet* 1969;128:327–339.
2. Calne RY, Williams R. Orthotopic liver transplantation: the first 60 patients. *Br Med J* 1977;1:471–476.
3. Pichlmayr R, Brolsch C, Woniqeit K, et al. Experiences with liver transplantation in Hannover. *Hepatology* 1984;4:56S–60S.
4. Pichlmayr R. Is there a place for liver grafting for malignancy? *Transplant Proc* 1988;20(suppl 1):478–482.
5. Iwatsuki S, Klintmalm GBG, Starzl TE. Total hepatectomy and liver replacement (orthotopic liver transplantation) for primary hepatic malignancy. *World J Surg* 1982;6:81–85.
6. O'Grady JG, Polson RJ, Rolles K, et al. Liver transplantation for malignant disease: results in 93 consecutive patients. *Ann Surg* 1988;207:373–379.
7. Ringe B, Wittekind C, Bechstein WO, et al. The role of liver transplantation in hepatobiliary malignancy: a retrospective analysis of 95 patients with particular regard to tumor stage and recurrence. *Ann Surg* 1989;209:88–98.
8. Yokoyama I, Carr B, Saitsu H, et al. Accelerated growth of recurrent hepatocellular carcinoma after liver transplantation. *Cancer* 1991;68:2095–2100.
9. Annual report of the U.S. Scientific Registry for Organ Transplantation and the Organ Procurement and Transplantation Network, 1997. Richmond, VA: United Network for Organ Sharing; Bethesda, MD: Department of Health and Social Services.
10. Registry of the European Liver Transplant Association. Data analysis 1968–1997.
11. Annual report 1998, vol. 2: Organ donation and transplantation. Ottawa: Ontario: Canadian Organ Replacement Register, Canadian Institute for Health Information, June 1998.
12. Australian Liver Transplant Registry tenth report. Brisbane: Queensland Liver Transplant Service, 1998.
13. Penn I. Hepatic transplantation for primary and metastatic cancers of the liver. *Surgery* 1991;110:726–735.
14. Iwatsuki S, Gordon RD, Shaw BW Jr, et al. Role of liver transplantation in cancer therapy. *Ann Surg* 1985;202:401–407.
15. Iwatsuki S, Starzl TE, Todo S, et al. Experience in 1,000 liver transplants under cyclosporine-steroid therapy: a survival report. *Transplant Proc* 1988;20(suppl 1):498–504.
16. Bismuth H, Castaing D, Ericzon BGT, et al. Hepatic transplantation in Europe. First report of the European Liver Transplant Registry. *Lancet* 1987;2:674–676.
17. Oka H, Akihiro T, Kuroki T, et al. Prospective study of α-fetoprotein in cirrhotic patients monitored for development of hepatocellular carcinoma. *Hepatology* 1994;19:61–66.
18. Sherman M, Peltekian KM, Lee C. Screening for hepatocellular carcinoma in chronic carriers of hepatitis B virus: incidence and prevalence of hepatocellular carcinoma in a North American urban population. *Hepatology* 1995;22:432–438.
19. Kanematsu M, Hoshi H, Yamada T, et al. Small hepatic nodules in cirrhosis: ultrasonographic, CT, and MR imaging findings. *Abdom Imaging* 1999;24:47–55.

20. Miller WJ, Baron RL, Dodd GD, et al. Malignancies in patients with cirrhosis: CT sensitivity and specificity in 200 consecutive transplant patients. *Radiology* 1994;193:645–650.
21. Rizzi PM, Kane PA, Ryder SD, et al. Accuracy of radiology in detection of hepatocellular carcinoma before liver transplantation. *Gastroenterology* 1994;107:1425–1429.
22. Baron RL, Oliver JH, Dodd GD, et al. Hepatocellular carcinoma: evaluation with biphasic, contrast-enhanced, helical CT. *Radiology* 1996;199:505–511.
23. Hirai K, Aoki Y, Majiima Y, et al. Magnetic resonance imaging of small hepatocellular carcinoma. *Am J Gastroenterol* 1991;69:205–209.
24. Takayasu K, Moriyama N, Muramatsu Y, et al. The diagnosis of small hepatocellular carcinomas: efficacy of various imaging procedures in 100 patients. *Am J Radiol* 1990;155:49–54.
25. Spreafico C, Marchiano A, Mazzaferro V, et al. Hepatocellular carcinoma in patients who undergo liver transplantation: sensitivity of CT with iodized oil. *Radiology* 1997;203:457–460.
26. Fuster J, Garcia-Valdecassis JC, Grande L, et al. Hepatocellular carcinoma and cirrhosis: results of surgical treatment in a European series. *Ann Surg* 1996;223:297–302.
27. Okada S, Shimada K, Yamamoto J, et al. Predictive factors for postoperative recurrence of hepatocellular carcinoma. *Gastroenterology* 1994;106:1618–1624.
28. Pichlmayr R, Weimann A, Oldhafer KJ, et al. Role of liver transplantation in the treatment of unresectable liver cancer. *World J Surg* 1995;19:807–813.
29. Iwatsuki S, Starzl TE, Sheanan DG, et al. Hepatic resection versus transplantation for hepatocellular carcinoma. *Ann Surg* 1991;214:221–229.
30. Okuda K, Ohtsuki T, Obata H, et al. Natural history of hepatocellular carcinoma and progress in relation to treatment. *Cancer* 1985;56:918–928.
31. Hermanek P, Sobin LH. *TNM classification of malignant tumors.* Berlin: Springer-Verlag, 1987:53–55.
32. Sobin LH, Wittekind C (International Union Against Cancer [UICC]), eds. *TNM classification of malignant tumours,* 5th ed. New York: John Wiley, 1997:74–77.
33. McPeake JR, O'Grady JG, Azman S, et al. Liver transplantation for primary hepatocellular carcinoma: tumor size and number determine outcome. *J Hepatol* 1993;18:226–234.
34. Klintmalm GB. Liver transplantation for hepatocellular carcinoma. A registry report of the impact of tumor characteristics on outcome. *Ann Surg* 1998;228:479–490.
35. Mazzaferro V, Regalia E, Doci R, et al. Liver transplantation for the treatment of small hepatocellular carcinomas in patients with cirrhosis. *N Engl J Med* 1996;334:693–699.
36. Llovet JM, Bruix J, Fuster J, et al. Liver transplantation for small hepatocellular carcinoma: the tumor-node-metastases classification does not have prognostic power. *Hepatology* 1998;27:1572–1577.
37. Ismail T, Angrisani L, Gunson BK, et al. Primary hepatic malignancy: the role of liver transplantation. *Br J Surg* 1990;77:983–987.
38. Olthoff KM, Millis JM, Rosove MH, et al. Is liver transplantation justified for the treatment of hepatic malignancies? *Arch Surg* 1990;125:1261–1268.
39. Huag CE, Jenkins RL, Rohrer RJ, et al. Liver transplantation for primary hepatic cancer. *Transplantation* 1992;53:376–382.
40. Chung SW, Toth JL, Reziea M, et al. Liver transplantation for hepatocellular carcinoma. *Am J Surg* 1994;167:317–321.
41. Koo J, Fung K, Siu KF, et al. Recovery of malignant tumor cells from the right atrium during hepatic resection for hepatocellular carcinoma. *Cancer* 1983;52:1952–1956.
42. Yamanaka N, Okamoto E, Fujihara S, et al. Do the tumor cells of hepatocellular carcinomas dislodge into the portal venous stream during hepatic resection? *Cancer* 1992;70:2263–2267.
43. Stone MJ, Klintmalm GBG, Polter D, et al. Neoadjuvant chemotherapy and liver transplantation for hepatocellular carcinoma: a pilot study in 20 patients. *Gastroenterology* 1993;104:196–202.
44. Carr BI, Salby R, Madriaga J, et al. Prolonged survival after liver transplantation and cancer chemotherapy for advanced-stage hepatocellular carcinoma. *Transplant Proc* 1993;25:1128–1129.
45. Cherqui D, Piedbois P, Pierga J-Y, et al. Multinodal adjuvant treatment and liver transplantation for advanced hepatocellular carcinoma. *Cancer* 1994;73:2721–2726.
46. Olthoff KM, Rosove MH, Shackleton CR, et al. Adjuvant chemotherapy improves survival after liver transplantation for hepatocellular carcinoma. *Ann Surg* 1995;221:734–743.
47. Venook AP, Ferrell LD, Roberts JP, et al. Liver transplantation for hepatocellular carcinoma: results with preoperative chemoembolization. *Liver Transplant Surg* 1995;4:242–248.
48. Van Beers B, Roche A, Canguil P, et al. Transcatheter arterial chemotherapy using doxorubicin, iodized oil and gelfoam embolization in hepatocellular carcinoma. *Acta Radiologica* 1989;30:415–418.
49. Romani F, Belli LS, Rondinara GF, et al. The role of transplantation in small hepatocellular carcinoma complicating cirrhosis of the liver. *Surg Gynecol Obstet* 1994;178:379–384.
50. Figueras J, Juarieta E, Valls C, et al. Survival after liver transplantation in cirrhotic patients with and without hepatocellular carcinoma: a comparative study. *Hepatology* 1997;25:1485–1490.
51. Majno PE, Adam R, Bismuth H, et al. Influence of preoperative transarterial lipoidal chemoembolization on resection and transplantation for hepatocellular carcinoma in patients with cirrhosis. *Ann Surg* 1997;226:688–703.
52. Belghiti J, Paris Y, Farges O, et al. Intrahepatic recurrence after resection of hepatocellular carcinoma complicating cirrhosis. *Ann Surg* 1991;214:114–117.
53. Ringe B, Pichlmayr R, Witlekind C, et al. Surgical treatment of hepatocellular carcinoma: experience with liver resection and transplantation in 198 patients. *World J Surg* 1991;15:270–285.
54. Bismuth H, Chiche L, Adam R, et al. Liver resection versus transplantation for hepatocellular carcinoma in cirrhotic patients. *Ann Surg* 1993;218:145–151.
55. Tan KC, Rela M, Ryder SD, et al. Experience of orthotopic liver transplantation and hepatic resection for hepatocellular carcinoma of less than 8 cm in patients with cirrhosis. *Br J Surg* 1995;82:253–256.
56. Michel J, Suc B, Fourtainier G, et al. Recurrence of hepatocellular carcinoma in cirrhotic patients after liver resection or transplantation. *Transplant Proc* 1995;27:1799–1800.
57. Otto G, Heuschen U, Hoffman WJ, et al. Survival and recurrence after liver transplantation versus liver resection for hepatocellular carcinoma. *Ann Surg* 1998;227:424–432.
58. Saxena R, Ye MQ, Emre S, et al. *De novo* hepatocellular carcinoma in a hepatic allograft with recurrent hepatitis C cirrhosis. *Liver Transplant Surg* 1999;5:81–82.
59. Soreide O, Czerniak A, Bradpiece H, et al. Characteristics of fibrolamellar hepatocellular carcinoma. *Am J Surg* 1986;151:518–523.
60. Starzl TE, Iwatsuki S, Shaw BW Jr, et al. Treatment of fibrolamellar hepatoma with partial or total hepatectomy and transplantation of the liver. *Surg Gynecol Obstet* 1986;162:145–148.
61. Ringe B, Wittekind C, Weimann A, et al. Results of hepatic resection and transplantation for fibrolamellar carcinoma. *Surg Gynecol Obstet* 1992;175:299–305.
62. Pinna AD, Iwatsuki S, Lee RG, et al. Treatment of fibrolamellar hepatoma with subtotal hepatectomy or transplantation. *Hepatology* 1997;26:877–883.
63. Ortega JA, Krailo MD, Haas JE, et al. Effective treatment of unresectable or metastatic hepatoblastoma with cisplatin and continuous infusion Adriamycin chemotherapy: a report from the Children's Cancer Study Group. *J Clin Oncol* 1991;9:2167–2176.
64. Seo T, Ando H, Watanabe Y, et al. Treatment of hepatoblastoma: less extensive hepatectomy after effective preoperative chemotherapy with cisplatin and Adriamycin. *Surgery* 1998;123:407–414.
65. Tagge EP, Tagge DU, Reyes J, et al. Resection, including transplantation, for hepatoblastoma and hepatocellular carcinoma: impact on survival. *J Pediatr Surg* 1992;27:292–297.
66. Koneru B, Flye MW, Busuttil RW, et al. Liver transplantation for hepatoblastoma: the American experience. *Ann Surg* 1991;213:118–121.
67. Goldstein RM, Stone MJ, Tillery GW, et al. Is liver transplantation indicated for cholangiocarcinoma? *Am J Surg* 1993;166:768–772.
68. Casavilla FA, Marsh JW, Iwatsuki S, et al. Hepatic resection and transplantation for peripheral cholangiocarcinoma. *J Am Coll Surg* 1997;185:429–436.
69. Goss JA, Shackleton CR, Farmer DG, et al. Orthotopic liver transplantation for primary sclerosing cholangitis. A 12-year single center experience. *Ann Surg* 1997;225:472–481.
70. Marino IR, Todo S, Tzakis AG, et al. Treatment of epithelioid hemangioendothelioma with liver transplantation. *Cancer* 1998;62:2079–2084.
71. Delcore R, Friesen SR. Gastrointestinal neuroendocrine tumors. *J Am Coll Surg* 1994;178:188–211.
72. Makowka L, Tzakis AG, Mazzaferro V, et al. Transplantation of the liver for metastatic endocrine tumors of the intestine and pancreas. *Surg Gynecol Obstet* 1989;168:107–111.

73. Anthuber M, Karl-Walter J, Briegel J, et al. Results of liver transplantation for gastropancreatic tumor metastases. *World J Surg* 1996;20:73–76.

74. Dousset B, Houssin D, Soubrane O, et al. Metastatic endocrine tumors: is there a place for liver transplantation? *Liver Transplant Surg* 1995; 1:111–117.

75. Routley D, Ramage JK, McPeake J, et al. Orthotopic liver transplantation in the treatment of metastatic neuroendocrine tumors of the liver. *Liver Transplant Surg* 1995;1:118–121.

76. Lang H, Oldhafer KJ, Weimann A, et al. Liver transplantation for metastatic neuroendocrine tumors. *Ann Surg* 1997;225:347–354.

77. Lehnert T. Liver transplantation for metastatic neuroendocrine carcinoma. An analysis of 103 patients. *Transplantation* 1998;66:1307–1312.

78. LeTreut YP, Delpero JR, Dousset B, et al. Results of liver transplantation in the treatment of metastatic neuroendocrine tumors. *Ann Surg* 1997;225:355–362.

79. Alessiani M, Tzakis A, Todo S, et al. Assessment of five-year experience with abdominal organ cluster transplantation. *J Am Coll Surg* 1995;180:1–9.

80. Knechtle SJ, Kalayoglu M, D'Allesandro AM, et al. Should abdominal cluster transplantation be abandoned? *Transplant Proc* 1993;25: 1361–1363.

81. Shibata M, Morizane T, Uchida T, et al. Irregular regeneration of hepatocytes and risk of hepatocellular carcinoma in chronic hepatitis and cirrhosis with hepatitis-C-virus infection. *Lancet* 1998;351: 1773–1777.

82. Paradis V, Laurendeau I, Vidaud M, et al. Clonal analysis of macronodules in cirrhosis. *Hepatology* 1998;28:953–958.

83. Muto Y, Moriwaki H, Ninomiya M, et al. Prevention of second primary tumors by an acrylic retinoid, polyprenoic acid, in patients with hepatocellular carcinoma. *N Engl J Med* 1996;334:1561–1567.

84. Mazzaferro V, Rondinara GF, Rossi G, et al. Milan multicenter experience in liver transplantation for hepatocellular carcinoma. *Transplant Proc* 1994;26:3557–3560.

85. Freise CE, Ferrell L, Liu T, et al. Effect of systemic cyclosporine on tumor recurrence after liver transplantation in a model of hepatocellular carcinoma. *Transplantation* 1999;67:510–513.

86. Seghal S, Molnar-Kimber K, Ocain T, et al. Rapamycin: a novel macrolide. *Med Res Rev* 1994;14:1–22.

87. Price DJ, Grove JR, Calvo V, et al. Rapamycin-induced inhibition of the 70-kilodalton S6 protein kinase. *Science* 1992;257:973–977.

88. Watson CJE, Friend PJ, Jamieson NV, et al. Sirolimus: a potent new immunosuppressant for liver transplantation. *Transplantation* 1999; 67:505–509.

89. Lau WY, Leung TWT, Ho SKW, et al. Adjuvant intra-arterial iodine-131-labeled lipoidal for resectable hepatocellular carcinoma: a prospective randomized trial. *Lancet* 1999; 353:797–802.

Transplantation of the Liver, edited by Willis C. Maddrey, Eugene R. Schiff, and Michael F. Sorrell. Lippincott Williams & Wilkins, Philadelphia © 2001.

CHAPTER 27

Xenotransplantation

William E. Beschorner

The overriding limitation of liver transplantation today is the severe shortage of human organ donors. Most patients who could benefit from a liver transplant never receive one. Many patients experience significant deterioration of their clinical condition as they wait for a human liver. Approximately 4,000 liver transplants are performed annually in the United States. As of March 31, 1999, more than 62,000 high-priority patients in United States were on the United Network for Organ Sharing (UNOS) waiting list, including 12,600 patients waiting for a liver transplant. Because of the stringent criteria for the list, the actual number of patients who could benefit from transplantation is far greater. It has been estimated that 450,000 organ transplantations could be performed annually, including 52,000 liver transplantations, if the organs were available.[1]

The use of animals, particularly pigs, as an organ source presents a very attractive alternative to human organs. Animals can be bred and raised under very clean and controlled conditions. The anatomy and physiology of most organs is similar to the human counterparts. Sufficient organs can be provided for all recipient candidates. Xenografts provide specific advantages for liver recipients. The xenografts would be resistant to viral hepatitis. The transplant procedures could be performed in a timely manner, avoiding clinical deterioration. Liver damage by ischemia could also be avoided.

To a greater degree than with any other solid organ, clinical experience with liver xenografts already exists. On a short-term basis, pig livers have provided temporary support to recipients and to patients with acute liver failure. Some artificial liver devices use hepatocytes from nonhuman sources. Two baboon livers have been transplanted into human recipients. This experience gives us some insight into the potential utility and the potential problems associated with liver xenografts. In particular, these studies aid in the understanding of the physiology of liver xenografts.

Major issues still must be resolved before the transplantation of liver xenografts becomes widespread. The primary challenge, as with all organ xenografts, is severe rejection. Xenograft rejection is much more fulminant than allograft rejection and involves multiple mechanisms and antigens. The immunosuppression required to prevent xenograft rejection would leave the xenograft recipient much more immunodeficient than an allograft recipient, which leads to a related problem, namely, the risk of opportunistic and zoonotic infections.

CLINICAL EXPERIENCE WITH AND FUNCTION OF LIVER XENOGRAFTS

Compared with other organ xenografts, there is considerable clinical experience with liver xenotransplantation. These transplantations have proved useful in illustrating both the value and limitations of liver xenografts.

In 1992 and 1993, two orthotopic xenotransplantations were performed, placing baboon livers into patients with liver failure related to hepatitis B virus infection.[2,3] Multidrug therapy was administered to prevent cellular and antibody-mediated rejection. The patients survived 70 and 26 days. Rejection was not thought to be a serious problem, although the first patient died of invasive aspergillosis related to immunosuppression. This patient also had a history of infection with the human immunodeficiency virus (HIV) and a previous splenectomy. The liver xenografts appeared to provide at least partial function. The first patient recovered consciousness and did reasonably well during the early course. The liver xenograft demonstrated appropriate regeneration, growing from 600 g to an estimated 1.5 kg. There was no evidence of hepatitis B virus infection in the graft, although the posttransplantation interval was short.

The baboon liver xenografts were metabolically functional, producing multiple protein factors. The recipients' C3 and transferrin converted into baboon-derived proteins. Although the albumin and uric acid levels were abnormal for

W. E. Beschorner: Department of Surgery, University of Nebraska Medical Center; and Ximerex, Inc., Omaha, Nebraska 68198.

humans, they were in the normal range for baboons. The prothrombin time was normal, and complement function appeared normal.

On the other hand, the transplants raised several issues regarding xenograft function. Late in the course, the alkaline phosphatase and bilirubin levels rose. At autopsy both livers had severe bile sludging with denudation of the bile ducts. Both patients had renal failure, possibly related to hepatorenal syndrome. It is unknown if the abnormal levels of proteins such as albumin would cause long-term problems.

Serious questions have been raised about the risk of zoonotic infections from nonhuman primate donors. Indeed, retrospective analysis of the two baboon liver recipients identified such agents, although the viruses may have been related to the baboon chimerism present.[4] Because the risk of zoonotic infections is thought to be significantly less with pig donors than with primate donors, interest is now focused on pig liver xenografts.

If baboon livers proved to be moderately dysfunctional in human recipients, one would expect the problem to be even greater with pig liver xenografts. The major complement factors are only 70% homologous with human factors.[5] Pig and human albumin are only 65% homologous. Discrepancies between the pig and human factors would be amplified in cascade or regulatory systems. Some growth factors made in the liver, such as hematopoietic stem cell factor, are known to be species specific.

Possibly, "humanized" pigs could be produced through genetic engineering.[6] Considerable effort, however, would be required to identify all the significant discrepancies and to correct them with genetic insertions and deletions. Furthermore, the humanized liver would still need to support the life of the pig.

At this time, there have been no long-term pig-to-primate liver transplants to indicate whether pig livers can provide adequate function. Pig-to-baboon and pig-to-monkey liver xenografts cease functioning after only a few hours because of hyperacute rejection.[7]

Patients with acute liver failure have been supported for a few hours to days with extracorporeal liver perfusion (ECLP) while a human liver donor is sought.[8,9] Blood from the patient is perfused through the pig liver and returned. These procedures indicate that the pig liver is functional on a short-term basis. Patients typically show clinical improvement, with reduction of blood ammonia and lactic acid levels, conjugation and excretion of bilirubin, and stabilization of prothrombin time.[9,10] Often an overall improvement in mental status is observed. Indeed, for the short term, perfusion through pig livers appears to be as effective as short-term perfusion through human livers (I.J. Fox and A.N. Langnas, personal communication). Physiologic studies indicate good initial bile flow and excretion of cholesterol and phospholipids.[11]

As with the pig-to-primate liver xenografts, the porcine liver organs used in ECLP procedures stop functioning within a few hours because of hyperacute rejection. The issues of

function raised by the long-term baboon-to-human xenotransplantations cannot be answered given this short interval. The amount of protein synthesized in a few hours by the porcine liver would be very small compared with the factors subsequently produced by the human liver. Therefore any deficiency or competitive inhibition caused by the synthesis of incompatible porcine factors might not be recognized. These issues will require long-term pig-to-primate orthotopic liver xenotransplants. On the other hand, one would expect that significant amounts of pig liver factors would be released as the rejecting graft became necrotic. Complications related to circulating incompatible factors or to immune reactions to these factors have not been described.

REJECTION

Rejection has proved to be the most challenging and perplexing obstacle to widespread clinical use of organ xenografts. Initially, most of the focus centered on hyperacute rejection, which destroys the graft in a matter of hours. Now it appears that hyperacute rejection can be prevented by several different strategies. Acute xenograft rejection, occurring several days posttransplantation, has proved to be far more challenging. Strategies that worked well with allografts are ineffective with xenografts. Compared with the relatively simple phenomenon of allograft rejection, the complex and fulminant acute xenograft rejection involves more antigens and more immune mechanisms. In this review, the term *acute rejection* encompasses the phenomena of vascular rejection and cellular rejection. Most likely, chronic rejection will also occur in xenografts. At this time, however, there is very limited experience in discordant grafts. It is therefore unknown if chronic rejection will prove to be more or less serious than with allografts.

The reader should be cautioned that most of what we know of xenograft rejection is based on studies with heart and kidney xenografts. As was the case with allografts, most likely the story with the liver will be somewhat different. The liver is a very large organ with a dual source of circulation. Furthermore, the liver is a source of growth, coagulation, and complement factors. To the extent that these factors are species specific, the liver xenograft may influence the development of chimerism and rejection.

Hyperacute Rejection

For most combinations of species, the placement of a vascular graft into the recipient leads to destruction of the graft within minutes to hours of revascularization, a process termed hyperacute rejection (HAR). Complement binds to the endothelial cells throughout the graft and is activated, leading to adhesion of platelets, thrombosis, and ischemic necrosis of the tissue. In transplantation between many close species, such as monkey-to-baboon transplantation, HAR does not occur. Calne termed xenografts that typically undergo HAR, such as pig-to-primate transplants, *discordant*. Xenografts that do not undergo HAR, such as chimpanzee-to-human transplants, were termed *concordant*.[12]

Complement fixation can be by either the alternate or the classic pathway. When complement fixation is by the alternate pathway, such as with the guinea pig–to-rat model,[13] the endothelium shows deposition of properdin, C6, and membrane attack complex. C2 and C4 are not involved.

HAR of pig xenografts by Old World monkeys involves the immediate binding of circulating preformed antibodies to the endothelium and the classic complement pathway.[14–18] The binding of complement to the endothelial cells can then lead to loss of heparin sulfate, activation with change in shape, cell death and coagulation, and adhesion of neutrophils.[19] The widespread thrombosis of the vessels causes ischemic destruction of the xenograft.

In contrast to HAR of renal allografts due to sensitization, the responsible xenophyllic antibodies may involve IgM as well as IgG. The natural, preformed antibodies are primarily directed at a single epitope on the endothelial membrane, a glycoprotein with a terminal galactose α-1,3-galactose ("alpha gal") residue. This residue is expressed on most mammalian tissues. However, humans, apes, and Old World monkeys have a deficiency in the enzyme α-1,3-galactosyltransferase and therefore do not constituitively produce this epitope.[20] The oligosaccharide is generally expressed on intestinal bacteria, which most likely sensitizes hosts that do not constituitively produce it.

The expression of α-1,3-galactosyl residue is variable in different tissues.[21] Whereas it is extensively expressed on porcine endothelial cells, the expression is considerably less in fetal porcine pancreatic islets.[22] Thus, vascular grafts are more susceptible to HAR than pancreatic islets.

Though the alpha gal epitope is the primary target of natural antibodies involved in HAR, it is not the only epitope. When the antibodies to alpha gal were depleted, pig lungs still underwent HAR.[23] In transgenic knockout mice lacking the alpha gal antigen, pancreatic islets were rejected by antibodies to unrelated pig antigens.[24]

HAR of liver xenografts develops more slowly than HAR of heart and kidney xenografts. For example, pig livers are functional for several hours during an extracorporeal perfusion, whereas heart and kidney xenografts are destroyed within an hour in nonhuman primates. Alpha gal is expressed on the sinusoidal endothelium. *In vitro* studies indicate that the sinusoidal endothelium is capable of activating complement by either the classic or alternate pathways.[25] Most likely, the delay in dysfunction is related to the increased size of the perfused organ. Using intravital microscopy, HAR was shown in guinea pig livers to begin in the periportal sinusoids.[26] Furthermore, at any particular time, only a portion of the sinusoids were perfused.[27]

In addition to being a more diffuse target for natural antibodies, the liver may help prolong its survival by partially depleting natural antibodies from circulation. Indeed, extra-corporeal perfusion of pig livers has been used successfully to remove natural antibodies and prolong survival of subsequent vascular xenografts.

Acute Xenograft Rejection

Students of xenotransplantation were initially optimistic that once HAR could be prevented, the subsequent course would resemble that of an allograft transplant. They had hoped that acute xenograft rejection could be controlled with modest amounts of immunosuppression. Their optimism was based in part on experience with concordant xenotransplantation and in part on the weak *in vitro* cellular reaction of mouse lymphocytes to pig antigens. With pig xenografts, however, acute rejection has turned out to be far more challenging than either acute rejection of allografts or HAR of xenografts.

Acute xenograft rejection generally occurs between 2 and 8 days posttransplantation. At least three basic mechanisms are involved. These reactions have been called delayed hyperacute rejection, acute vascular rejection, and acute cellular rejection. While it is useful to study the mechanisms independently in the appropriate models, in reality these three mechanisms appear to be interrelated. One mechanism enhances the development of the next mechanism. A rejecting pig xenograft may progress seamlessly from one reaction into another, or components of all mechanisms might be present simultaneously. Any of these mechanisms would destroy the graft. Therefore, any successful strategy for xenotransplantation would need to prevent all these reactions.

Delayed Hyperacute Rejection and Acute Vascular Rejection

With delayed hyperacute rejection and acute vascular rejection, vascular grafts undergo rapid irreversible destruction in 2 to 8 days posttransplantation. Antibodies directed to endothelial cells bind to the cells, activate the endothelium, activate complement, and increase coagulation, leading to thrombosis and infarction of the graft. The histology of the rejected grafts shows vascular thrombosis and endothelial swelling. There is an infiltrate of large mononuclear cells, including macrophages and natural killer (NK) cells. Lymphocytes represent a minor population.[28] IgG is typically deposited on the endothelial cells, and complement may be detectable.

Delayed hyperacute rejection and acute vascular rejection represent closely related if not identical pathological processes.[29] The two terms imply different mechanisms leading to the final event. *Delayed hyperacute rejection* suggests that the causative elements were present in the recipient prior to transplantation. *Acute vascular rejection,* on the other hand, suggests that the causative elements or antibodies developed *de novo* following the transplantation. In most situations, both mechanisms contribute to graft rejection. This phenomenon is seen in models in which natural antibodies have been depleted or in which complement has been inhibited.[30] It is also observed in situations in which preformed natural antibodies would not be present, such as concordant grafts, xenografts into newborns, and allografts.[31,32]

The antibody specificity observed in acute vascular rejection differs from the IgM natural antibodies seen in HAR. The antibodies include IgG and are not directed against only the alpha gal epitope.[33] Because they are IgG, the reaction is most likely a secondary response to antigens seen previously. A study of sera from patients treated with extracorporeal perfusion of pig livers showed an early rise in IgG1 following the perfusion.[34]

In the guinea pig–to–rat model, acute vascular rejection does not appear to require T cells, since the reaction is also observed in nude rats.[35,36] If mature T cells were essential for xenograft rejection, then athymic (nude) mice or rats should accept xenografts. When guinea pig hearts were transplanted into nude rats treated with cobra venom factor to prevent HAR, the grafts were rejected as quickly as in normal rat recipients. Immunohistochemistry of the rejected graft showed a dense infiltrate of macrophages and NK cells but no B cells or T cells (T-cell receptor α or β).

Although this model appears to define a T-cell-independent process involved in the delayed destruction of xenografts, there is also compelling evidence supporting a T-cell response. The apparent discrepancy may relate to differences in the models. The guinea pig–to–rat model is known to differ from other models with respect to HAR. It may also differ from other models with respect to acute rejection. For example, whereas chemotherapy agents effective against T cells (cyclosporine, cyclophosphamide, etc.) can delay pig xenograft rejection in primates, they are relatively ineffective in the guinea pig-to-rat model.[37,38] Therefore, the contribution of T cells may be more important in primates. It is also possible that the few residual T cells remaining in the nude rats contribute to the rejection process.[39,40]

Acute Cellular Rejection

Concordant grafts between closely related species, such as transplants from Old World monkeys to baboons, are rejected in a manner similar to allografts. Heart xenografts are rejected in less than a week without immunosuppression. Although antibodies participate in the rejection, the predominant effector cells appear to be T cells. Several reports of long-term acceptance have been described. Using cyclosporine and steroids, heart xenografts survived for 77 and 94 days (mean graft survivals).[41,42] Transplanting monkey hearts into infant baboons and using suppression consisting of splenectomy, tacrolimus (FK506), methotrexate, and steroids, a mean survival of 127 days was achieved.[43] Adding total lymphoid irradiation to cyclosporine and azathioprine, Roslin attained a mean survival of 255 days.[44]

When HAR is prevented in discordant xenografts, the grafts are destroyed in a very narrow time frame, generally 3 to 8 days posttransplantation. This is consistent with a primary immune response. The severity of the rejection, however, appears to vary with the species combination and tissue involved.

In contrast to the primate-to-primate transplants, porcine organs transplanted into primates are rejected much more vigorously. This is evident by the immunosuppression required to block acute rejection and by the complications associated with the needed protocols. Immunosuppressive drugs, such as cyclosporine, that can provide for indefinite survival of allografts provide only limited survival of pig xenografts.[45] When HAR was prevented by splenectomy and plasmapheresis, pig kidneys functioned and survived within baboon recipients for up to 22 days.[46] The recipients received antithymocyte globulin, azathioprine, cyclosporine, and steroids. Of the five recipients, three developed irreversible vascular rejection, one died of pneumonia, and one was sacrificed with severe gastric dilatation.

In another series of pig-to-monkey kidney transplantations, HAR was prevented by *ex vivo* perfusion through either pig livers or an immunoadsorption column. Mixed chimerism was induced within the monkey to prevent acute rejection, using a nonmyeloablative protocol of wholebody and thymic irradiation and antibodies to lymphocytes or subsets. One recipient survived up to 15 days without rejection, but most of the kidneys were lost to vascular rejection during the second week.[47] The recipients that did not reject their grafts experienced complications such as severe anemia.[48]

The experience with pig-to-primate heart transplantation is similar. When sufficient immunosuppression is administered to prevent acute rejection, there is a high rate of complications involving infections or toxicity.[49,50] The difficulty is best illustrated in the experience with transgenic pigs that express human decay-accelerating factor.[51] Although HAR was not observed in these studies, the grafts were acutely rejected at 5.1 days without immunosuppression. Immunosuppression with cyclosporine, cyclophosphamide, and steroids was given in two other groups to prevent acute rejection. With an average daily dose of cyclophosphamide of 12 mg/kg per day, the median graft survival was prolonged only to 9 days. When the cyclophosphamide was increased to 21 mg/kg per day, the median survival was prolonged to 40 days. However, six of the ten animals had severe diarrhea or anemia requiring euthanasia.

The time of onset and the modest response to immunosuppression suggest that acute xenograft rejection is a primary immune response involving the sensitization of T and B cells. The experimental pathology studies reinforce that concept. When rats were given multiple doses of antithymocyte serum, human islet xenografts had significantly prolonged survival, suggesting that T cells were essential for xenograft survival.[52]

CD4+ cells were shown to be particularly important for xenograft rejection. With the depletion of CD4+ cells using monoclonal antibodies, fetal pig islets enjoyed prolonged survival.[53] The recipients were unable to mount antibody responses to pig cells. These studies indicated that CD4+ cells were important in at least the afferent limb of the immune response, particularly regarding the antibody response.[54] Although the studies emphasize CD4+ T cells, it is assumed that the antibodies also depleted CD4+ monocytes and macrophages as well.

Although the CD4+ cells certainly would contribute to the humoral response,[55] the CD4+ cells can destroy the target cells directly. Adoptive transfer studies of cell populations to SCID mice showed that the transfer of CD4+ cells without B cells led to rapid rejection of pig skin grafts.[56,57]

With allograft rejection, CD8+ cells are profoundly important in the tissue injury phase. With xenografts, however, these cells are less important. CD8+ cells are normally restricted to target cells expressing major histocompatibility (MHC) class I. Knockout mice deficient in β_2-microglobulin are deficient in class I antigen and therefore class I–restricted CD8+ T cells.[58] Mouse pancreatic islet allografts had prolonged survival within these hosts. However, rat islet xenografts were promptly rejected, suggesting that class I–restricted cytotoxicity is not essential for xenograft rejection.

A T-lymphocyte response is essential during the sensitization phase of the xenograft response. Treatment of mice with anti-CD2 antibodies (sheep red cell receptor) leads to prolonged acceptance of islet xenografts. If the treatment is delayed, however, no prolongation is observed.[59] When hamster hearts or livers are placed into rats, hematopoietic cells migrate to the spleen within 1 day, much like the migration from allografts.[60] The spleen shows a prompt response, with proliferation of IgM+ B cells and CD4+ T cells.

Thymus modification experiments also support the importance of a T-cell response.[61] The effect of intrathymic injection of splenocytes was assessed for either rat heart allografts or hamster heart xenografts. The injection induced indefinite survival of the allografts. When combined with a pulse of cyclophosphamide, intrathymic cell injection significantly prolonged survival as compared with the thymus and cyclophosphamide controls. By itself, however, the intrathymic injection had little effect on xenograft survival.

When fetal pig islets are transplanted into BALB/c nude mice, the grafts survived for over 28 days.[62] These nude mice had greater than 99% reduction in mature T cells. If normal mouse lymphocytes were adoptively transferred, the grafts were rejected within 7 days, indicating that the lymphocytes responsible for acute rejection of the pig islets were absent in the nude mouse. Transfer of CD4+ cells led to rapid rejection, whereas the transfer of CD8+ cells resulted in a delayed rejection. Because the nude mice had macrophages, the transfer most likely provided T cells that were missing. The responsible cells were also radiation sensitive. Xenografts were eventually rejected with the transfer of B cells and NK cells (i.e., CD4 and CD8 depleted). The findings support the proposal that xenografts can be rejected by at least two mechanisms: a T-cell process (particularly CD4+ T cells) and a non-T-cell process.

Similar results were achieved with the transfer of sensitized lymphocytes from a normal mouse rejecting a xenograft into a nude mouse containing the porcine islets.[63] Immunohistochemistry of the rejecting xenograft showed predominantly macrophages in the infiltrate, with a small number of CD3+ T cells at the periphery of the infiltrate. However, the macrophages were from the nude mouse. The study concluded that immunocompetent T cells were responsible for the activation and accumulation of macrophages.

T cells appear to be less important during the subsequent injury phase of xenograft rejection. Using the guinea pig–to-rat heart transplant model to focus on the effector arm of xenograft rejection, sensitized splenocytes were transferred into immunocompetent rats at the time of xenotransplantation. The sensitized cells accelerated the rejection process from the normal 4 days to less than 2 days.[64] The accelerated rejection was lost when either macrophages or B cells were depleted from the transferred suspension. Therefore, B cells and macrophages are important in the early tissue injury phase.

In vitro assays of cellular immunology have provided insights into the relative strength and mechanisms of allograft rejection. The mixed lymphocyte reaction with some discordant xenogeneic combinations was found to be weak.[65–67] It was widely believed at that time that cellular rejection of discordant xenografts would not present a major problem. Once HAR was resolved, cellular rejection could be controlled with immunosuppression, as was done with allografts. As discussed previously, that optimistic view is no longer appropriate. Acute cellular xenograft rejection is as strong or stronger than mismatched allograft rejection.[68] For the most relevant lymphocyte reactions—primate versus primate and human versus pig—the *in vitro* reaction is comparable in strength to human allogeneic reactions.[69,70]

Proliferative reactions of mouse lymphocytes to monkey, human, and pig stimulator cells were analyzed.[71] The weak *in vitro* reactions correlated with the weak direct interactions between the responder T-cell receptor and the stimulator MHC antigens. The adherence of accessory molecules to ligands, such as intercellular adhesion molecule 1 (ICAM-1) and lymphocyte function associated antigen 1 (LFA-1), was also weak. In contrast, the interaction was strong in closely related species, such as between mice and rats.[72,73] An *in vivo* test of this hypothesis with disparate xenografts, however, did not confirm this hypothesis. Pretransplantation coating of human islet xenografts with antibody to ICAM-1 delayed rejection in mouse hosts from 7 days to 21 days.[74] Similar results were observed with a rat-to-mouse islet model. Molecular binding studies indicated that the binding of LFA-1 to ICAM-1 was not species specific.

Effective sensitization requires the costimulation provided by the binding of CD28 on T lymphocytes to B7 on the antigen-presenting cells. Cytolytic T-lymphocyte antigen 4 (CTLA-4), a monoclonal antibody resembling CD28, blocks T-cell CD28 from binding to the antigen-presenting cells. Infusion of CTLA-4 blocks the rejection of human islets by recipient mice.[75]

Limiting dilution experiments can establish the relative number of lymphocytes reactive to xenogeneic stimulator cells.[76–78] The results with xenogeneic reactions are more complex than those observed with allogeneic cells. They suggest multiple mechanisms of T-cell sensitization, including direct and indirect antigen presentation.

With allogeneic reactions, the MHC antigens on allogeneic stimulator cells serve as both the antigen-presenting molecules and the antigenically distinct peptide. This is referred to as *direct antigen presentation*. Rather than a large number of cells with diverse peptides, all of the cells present the same antigen, leading to a much stronger reaction. The proliferation of human lymphocytes in response to pig stimulator cells has proved to involve direct antigen presentation that is at least as strong as the reaction to allogeneic human stimulator cells.[79,80] Porcine endothelial cells can directly stimulate human lymphocytes.[70,80] Similarly, porcine dendritic cells directly stimulate human T lymphocytes.[78] The reaction is against class II MHC antigen, specifically SLA-DR.

In a typical reaction to a foreign body, the foreign cells are engulfed and digested within the antigen-presenting cells. The digested peptides are then nestled on the surface within the class I or II MHC antigens. The responder cells recognize the MHC antigen and the associated peptide. This is referred to as *indirect antigen presentation*. Indirect xenoantigen presentation would utilize the recipient's T cells and antigen-presenting cells. It would not require compatibility between adhesion receptors and ligands in the donor and recipient. In the mixed lymphocyte reaction of human versus pig stimulator cells, the addition of purified human antigen-presenting cells (monocytes) enhances the proliferative response.[81]

Pig endothelial cells stimulate the proliferation of both purified CD4+ and CD8+ human lymphocytes.[70,80] Cytokine analysis of the mouse versus rat mixed lymphocyte reaction indicates that the CD4+ helper cells are those of T helper cell subtype 2 (T_H2), as compared with the usual T_H1 subtype seen with allogeneic reactions.[55] Whereas T_H1 cells participate in delayed-type hypersensitivity reactions, T_H2 cells typically contribute to the humoral response.

The immunopathological reviews of rejecting xenografts suggest that the mechanism of tissue injury differs from that seen with allografts. They emphasize the participation of bound immunoglobulins and NK cells. In contrast to rejecting allografts, T cells represent a minor population but may contribute to the tissue injury.

Most of the immunopathological surveys were performed using either the hamster-to-rat model or the guinea pig–to-rat model with cobra venom factor to prevent HAR.[82,83] The early pathology of the target organ shows vascular endothelial injury and thrombosis as well as tissue necrosis. The inflammation is limited, consisting primarily of macrophages and later eosinophils. The number of T and B lymphocytes is variable but is generally sparse. Immunoglobulin and fibrin are bound to the endothelium.

Immunoglobulins, particularly IgM and IgG2a, as well as C3, were shown to be bound to the endothelial cells following the transplantation of rat hearts into mice.[84] Depletion of CD4+ cells from the recipient blocked antibody production and acute xenograft rejection, suggesting that the CD4+ cells contributed to the humoral response.

The macrophages and NK cells are most likely recruited into the target tissue by the induced expression of monocyte chemoattractant protein (MCP-1).[85] The endothelial and vascular smooth muscle cells express MCP-1 within 12 hours of transplantation. It is believed that γ-interferon from NK cells induces the expression of MCP-1.

Most relevant to the clinical transplantation of porcine kidneys, the immunopathology of acute xenograft rejection of porcine xenografts transplanted into cynomolgus monkeys and baboons has been systematically described in grafts surviving 7 to 15 days.[86] Dying target cells were identified using the TUNEL (terminal deoxynucleotide transferase–mediated uridine nick-end labeling) assay for apoptosis; the mononuclear cell subtypes were identified with immunohistochemistry. Endothelial cells within the glomeruli and in the peritubular capillaries showed frequent apoptosis. Microangiopathic thrombi were present, with associated infarcts. Cellular infiltrates were identified around some arteries, consisting of granulocytes, T cells, and monocytes. Tubulitis was also seen, containing inflammatory cells and apoptotic epithelial cells.

Several immunopathological studies support a significant function for T cells in xenograft rejection. When human blood is perfused through a porcine kidney, the T cells and NK cells are removed from the blood. These cells were later identified attached to the vascular endothelial cells of the perfused graft.[87] T lymphocytes are more abundant with some nonvascular grafts, such as late in the rejection of corneas or in pancreatic islets.[53,88]

In vitro cell-mediated cell lysis assays suggest that T cells and NK cells collaborate in the destruction of pig endothelial cells. Human lymphocytes spontaneously lysed labeled pig endothelial cells.[89] The lysis was enhanced by interleukin 2 (IL-2) and inhibited by antibodies to CD2. Cell-mediated lysis has been correlated with acute rejection. Pig hearts transplanted into newborn baboons are not subject to HAR but are acutely rejected at 3.5 days. Immunopathological studies show the infiltrating cells to consist of mostly macrophages and NK cells (CD2+, CD16+). Only about 10% of the infiltrating cells were CD3+ T cells. Circulating peripheral blood mononuclear cells from the recipient baboons lysed cultured pig endothelial cells. IL-2 significantly enhanced the lysis. Antibodies against NK cells partially blocked the adhesion to pig endothelial cells.[90] Although the immunopathological studies favor an NK mechanism, the *in vitro* studies are consistent with a mixed cell reaction of T and NK cells. CD2 is expressed on peripheral T lymphocytes as well as NK cells. The binding of peripheral lymphocytes was only partially blocked by antibodies to

NK-associated integrin molecules. CD4+ T cells secrete IL-2. The activation of CD4+ cells therefore could enhance the NK or cytotoxic T-cell reaction.

A complementary study supports the involvement of human T cells, as well as non–T-cell mechanisms, in the lysis of pig endothelial cells.[79] The cell lysis was partially blocked by antibodies to CD3, which is expressed on mature T cells.

Chronic Rejection

In vascular allografts, chronic rejection is presently a major, unresolved problem. Months after the transplantation, the grafts undergo accelerated atherosclerosis, with diffuse intimal thickening and proliferation of the fibroblasts. In kidney allografts, there is an associated interstitial fibrosis and generalized loss of tubules.

Given the substantial barriers of HAR and vigorous acute rejection, there has been relatively little experience with long-term xenografts. Graft atherosclerosis has been observed in two baboon recipients of monkey hearts.[91] The recipients died at 74 and 502 days posttransplantation. The findings resembled accelerated arteriosclerosis seen with chronic allograft rejection. In the hamster-to-rat heart and aorta transplantation models, chronic vascular rejection has been described, also resembling chronic allograft rejection.[92–94]

In a systematic and quantitative study of hamster aorta xenografts, Scheringa demonstrated thickening and infiltration of the adventitia during the acute rejection (14 days).[92] This subsided and was followed during chronic rejection by a progressive thickening of the intima (at 56 days). Localized IgM deposits are seen in the arterial lesions.

Chronic xenograft rejection might prove to be more resistant to chemotherapy than is chronic allograft rejection.[95] Continuous cyclosporine or mycophenolate mofetil have been effective in reducing the intimal thickening seen in chronic xenograft rejection.[92,93,96]

Systemic Complications of Xenograft Rejection

Xenograft rejection could lead to complications well beyond the simple dysfunction of the organ xenograft. Fulminant rejection of an organ xenograft could lead to consumption of coagulation factors, activation of graft cells such as the endothelium, and release of xenogeneic proteins. Furthermore, the severe suppression required to prevent xenograft rejection would be associated with systemic complications from toxicity and infections.

Even after a conditioning regimen that included the removal of most xenoreactive natural antibodies and immunosuppression, three baboons fulminantly rejected porcine kidney xenografts.[97] Disseminated intravascular coagulation was observed in two of the recipients, with prolonged prothrombin and thromboplastin times and severe thrombocytopenia. Multiple mechanisms could have contributed to the

disseminated intravascular coagulation, including activation of complement, loss of endothelium and the corresponding anticoagulation factors, and the release of species-specific factors such as von Willebrand factor.

Recurrent or smoldering rejection with injury of xenograft cells might be expected to lead to immune complex disease, similar to that seen following repeated injections of horse serum.

With current technology, immunosuppression considerably greater than that used for allografts would be required to prevent xenograft rejection. As observed with primate recipients, the more aggressive immunosuppression would lead to greater toxicity and increased risk of opportunistic infections.

The basic dilemma of xenograft rejection is that the multiple xenogeneic antigens and multiple immune mechanisms involved make rejection very difficult to prevent. Immunosuppression would either be associated with partial rejection with organ dysfunction and systemic complications, or with severe immunodeficiency and associated infections. Not surprisingly, therefore, many now believe that specific immune tolerance is necessary for a viable xenotransplantation program.[47,98–100]

Summary

Compared with acute rejection of allografts, acute xenograft rejection is a complex phenomenon. When a transplant recipient "sees" an allograft, the immune system focuses on the polymorphic expression of major and minor histocompatibility antigens. The T cells interact directly with the tissue and the antigen-presenting cells from the donor. A humoral and cell-mediated response is mounted to rid the body of those few antigens.

When a recipient "sees" a xenograft, however, the immune system sees a foreign body in addition to an allograft. It mounts multiple defenses to rid the body of the complex object. When the two species are relatively closely related, such as with monkey-to-baboon transplants or pig-to-baboon transplants, the recipient can mount a direct antigen response. The recipient lymphocytes recognize the polymorphisms of the donor MHC as well as similarities. The accessory receptors bind to the corresponding ligands on the donor cells, and the immune response resembles the response to an allograft. When the two species are more disparate, this mechanism is less important.

However, the xenograft also brings with it numerous antigens not related to the histocompatibility antigens. These elicit a strong indirect response, wherein the xenogeneic cells are digested and the antigen presented through the recipient's antigen-presenting cells. Each of these antigens elicits a corresponding humoral or cellular response. In addition, the xenograft may elicit a primitive natural immune response.

For most xenotransplants, initial T-cell sensitization is essential. In particular, CD4+ T cells must be sensitized. If antibodies, drugs, or immune tolerance can block this initial step, the destruction of the xenografts will be postponed and possibly avoided.

The pathology of the rejected xenograft does not resemble the T-cell–mediated rejection of allografts, however. The grafts have bound immunoglobulins and complement and increased numbers of NK cells and macrophages. The T cells are variable and often sparse in number. Most of the injury is due to direct antibody response and complement fixation, antibody-dependent cell cytotoxicity by NK cells, and direct injury by NK cells. *In vitro* studies indicate that a minor population of T cells may also contribute to the tissue injury.

Efforts taken to reverse acute xenograft rejection should recognize the multiple effector cell mechanisms. For example, immunopathological studies of tissues at a later stage of rejection tend to emphasize the T-cell component.[86,87] If only one mechanism was prevented or reversed, another mechanism could still destroy the graft.

The different effector mechanisms could also be interacting to enhance the strength of the rejection. For example, early cell destruction could enhance the processing of cells and sensitization of additional effector cells. Cytokines produced by T cells, such as IL-2, may enhance the NK cell reaction. The activation of endothelium could lead to further adherence of T cells.

OPPORTUNISTIC AND ZOONOTIC INFECTIONS

The immunodeficient recipient is at significant risk for contracting infectious diseases from the organ donor. This has been demonstrated for allografts with the transmission of herpesviruses (including cytomegalovirus and Epstein-Barr virus), HIV, hepatitis, *Toxoplasma gondii,* and so forth. Precautions are now taken to minimize that risk. The risk of a human opportunistic infection would be minimized with animal donors. For example, even primates such as baboons are resistant to hepatitis B and human immunodeficiency virus.[2,101]

On the other hand, there is a potential risk of transmission of an infectious agent harbored by the animal donor. The zoonotic agents include exogenous infections as well as endogenous agents such as retroviruses. Although the exogenous agents can potentially be eliminated from the herd, endogenous retroviruses are coded in the genome.

The zoonotic agents may behave in a benign manner in the animal but act in an aggressive manner within the human host. For an individual patient, the benefit of a life-saving organ transplant would usually outweigh the risk of a possible infection. If the potential zoonotic infection were contagious, however, the public health risk must also be factored into the overall risk.

In comparing the potential use of swine and primate organs, the greatest concern has been expressed for the use of nonhuman primates as xenograft donors.[102,103] Whereas swine can be bred rapidly and can be raised under con-

trolled conditions, the conditions for primates cannot be as well controlled. There are several examples of viruses that are relatively benign in primates but have produced catastrophic results when they infect humans, such as the Marburg virus and the Ebola virus.[104,105] Although these viruses have a high mortality rate in humans, human hosts are unable to sustain the amplification for prolonged periods of time.[106] Proviral DNA for endogenous retroviruses is found in baboons and monkeys. When human cells are cocultured with baboon cells, the virus can be detected.[107]

Swine also pose a small risk for zoonotic infections, although most consider the risk to be much less than with nonhuman primates.[108] Multiple agents can potentially be passed from humans to pigs, which in turn could infect xenograft recipients. These include infections with bacteria such as *Salmonella, Campylobacter,* and *Yersinia,* parasites such as *Schistosoma,* and viruses such as influenza. Swine may also carry herpesviruses, including a swine cytomegalovirus.

High standards of animal husbandry have made these entities more theoretical than real. A thorough necropsy examination of ten pigs was performed, including 150 tests. The stool contained some parasites considered to be commensals; however, no agents pathogenic for humans were identified.[109]

Transformed porcine cell lines produce C-type endogenous retroviruses. When two such cell lines, PK-15 and MPK, were cocultured with human cell lines, porcine virus could be identified within the human cells.[110] The study raised the possibility that porcine retroviruses might infect humans. That, in turn, raises the risk that the virus may behave more aggressively in humans or transform into a more aggressive virus.

At this time, the concern is more theoretical than real. When porcine endothelial cells were transplanted into severely immunosuppressed baboons, there was no evidence of porcine endogenous retrovirus (PERV) in the blood or in multiple tissues.[111] Human recipients of porcine pancreatic islets were followed for up to 7 years posttransplantation. No evidence of PERV was found in the blood.[112] Neither PERV nor antibodies to PERV could be detected in patients after perfusion of their blood through porcine kidneys.[113]

The most reassuring study of the safety of pig tissues is a recently completed retrospective study of 160 patients exposed to viable pig tissues up to 12 years previously.[114] The specimens were analyzed in multiple laboratories, including the Centers for Disease Control and Prevention in Atlanta, Georgia. The analyses used a highly sensitive polymerase chain reaction (PCR) assay for PERV.[115] Because PERV is present in most pig cells, the analysis distinguished between the presence of PERV due to chimerism and true PERV infection. The patients included those treated with extracorporeal splenic perfusion, extracorporeal perfusion of whole liver and whole kidney, skin grafts, islet transplants, and treatment with artificial liver devices incorporating porcine hepatocytes. There was no evidence of PERV infection in any of the subjects, even though some demonstrated microchimerism up to 8.5 years after exposure. The failure to detect PERV infection after prolonged chimerism with porcine cells suggests that the lack of infection is more likely related to an unfavorable environment than to the lack of immune response.

In response to a proposal to treat a patient with acquired immunodeficiency syndrome (AIDS) with marrow transplanted from a baboon, the Food and Drug Administration held hearings and issued suggested guidelines related to the possibility of infectious diseases from xenotransplantation.[103] The suggestions include the formation of a registry for xenotransplantation, formation of institutional xenotransplant committees that include experts in infectious diseases, the surveillance of both animal donors and human recipients, the archiving of blood and tissues from donors and recipients, and the use of husbandry measures designed to provide pathogen-free animal donors.

THE PREVENTION OF XENOGRAFT REJECTION

Before xenotransplants can be performed routinely, it is imperative that xenograft rejection be prevented without seriously compromising the recipient's immunocompetence. Because xenografts express many more antigens than do allografts, they can be rejected by multiple immune mechanisms. A strategy that would inhibit all of the involved mechanisms would leave the recipient without any immune defenses.

Prevention of allograft rejection is, by comparison, relatively simple. The primary mechanism of rejection of allografts is by cytotoxic T cells and by direct antigen presentation. On the other hand, xenografts are rejected not only by cellular mechanisms, but also antibody-mediated mechanisms, NK cells, sensitized immune reactions and induced immune reactions. Sensitization is by indirect as well as direct antigen presentation.

The induction of immune tolerance is also a major challenge in xenotransplantation because of the numerous antigens expressed on xenografts. With allografts, the histocompatibility antigens are the primary targets. Therefore, the induction of tolerance to hematopoietic cells might also provide some protection against rejection of organ allografts. Xenografts, however, express many antigens not expressed on hematopoietic cells. Therefore, the induction of simple hematopoietic chimerism is probably insufficient to prevent rejection of xenografts. Most efforts at induction of tolerance to xenografts are only partially effective, preventing rejection by one mechanism but not by the other mechanisms.

Prevention of Hyperacute Rejection

Although HAR is a dramatic and nearly ubiquitous outcome of xenotransplantation, the problem has been defined and understood. For pig-to-primate xenotransplantations, the problem is simplified by the observations that natural antibodies are generally directed toward a single epitope and that complement is fixed by the classic pathway. Several successful strategies have been developed to prevent the immediate destruction of the xenograft.

Natural Antibodies

Four basic strategies have targeted HAR by natural antibodies: depletion from the serum, neutralization of antibodies, inhibition of complement, and development of specific immune tolerance.

Plasmapheresis has proved useful in preventing hyperacute rejection in ABO-mismatched recipients.[116] A similar removal of the natural xenogeneic antibodies by plasmapheresis was performed and showed a modest but significant prolongation compared with controls.[117] The shortcomings of plasmapheresis included incomplete removal of the antibodies and early return of the antibodies. With chronic plasmapheresis, coagulation factors were also depleted.

Better removal of antibodies was achieved using double-filtration plasmapheresis, with greater than 93% removal of the IgM natural antibody.[118,119] The prompt return of antibodies was delayed by either performing a splenectomy[46] or treating the patient with immune immunosuppressants such as cyclosporine.[120]

Because the alpha gal epitope is expressed on the endothelial cells, a more selective removal of antibodies could be achieved by perfusing the recipient's blood through a porcine liver. Indeed, the specific anti–alpha gal antibodies are undetectable immediately following the *ex vivo* perfusion.[27,121]

The antibodies can be depleted using immunoadsorption columns consisting of beads with bound antiimmunoglobulin antibodies[122] or bound antigen such as the alpha gal epitope.[28,123] The latter is the most specific method for antibody removal. With intermittent use of this column, pig graft survival of up to 3 weeks was achieved in discordant baboons. The IgM antibody returned within days of discontinuing the perfusions.

Neutralization with Soluble Oligosaccharides

Rather than removing the natural antibodies, soluble synthetic oligosaccharides with a terminal α-galactosyl residue could be infused into the recipient, effectively neutralizing the antibodies.[124] The soluble oligosaccharides prevented human serum from reacting with PK-15 pig tubular epithelial cells. Similarly, serum from baboons that were infused with the oligosaccharides showed decreased reactivity. Generally, larger oligosaccharides prove to be more effective than smaller oligosaccharides.[125] It is unknown if the prolonged circulation of immune complexes causes significant pathology. Immunoadsorption appears to be more effective than neutralization.

Xenotransplantation in Newborn Recipients

Natural antibodies to the alpha gal epitope are believed to be derived from a cross reaction against bacteria. One would therefore expect newborns to have a deficiency in these natural antibodies. Systematic studies found that newborn baboons and humans lack the IgM natural antibody, though many had the IgG anti–alpha gal antibody, presumably derived from the maternal blood.[126–128] Transplants from pigs to newborn baboons did not result in HAR, but were rejected in 3 to 4 days. Histology showed prominent mononuclear cell infiltrates consistent with acute rejection.[86,129]

The possibility was considered that newborn pigs do not express the alpha gal epitope. However, baboon serum was found to react equally with endothelial cells from newborn pigs and from mature pigs.[130]

Systemic Inhibitors of Complement

Early xenotransplantation models used cobra venom factor to block HAR. Cobra venom factor effectively blocked complement fixation by inactivating C'3c.[131] However, it was associated with significant toxicity. Less toxic inhibitors of complement have been tested for their ability to prevent HAR. Complement receptor 1 is normally expressed on red cells. It contributes to the clearance of immune complexes and blocks the terminal complement fixation for both the classic and alternate pathways. Recombinant soluble complement receptor (sCR1) was synthesized and has been tested for prevention of HAR.[38,132] With continuous administration, HAR was prevented in pig-to-monkey heart transplants. Recently a defective adenovirus vector containing sCR1 was developed.[133] Infected cells produced sCR1 and were protected from lysis by natural antibodies and complement.

Monoclonal antibodies against C5 and C8 have been produced.[134] They have blocked HAR in a perfusion model of pig heart xenografts.

Genetic Engineering

The natural antibodies responsible for hyperacute rejection of porcine xenografts are primarily directed at a single epitope, the galactose α-1-3-galactose epitope. The most obvious solution to this problem would be to genetically engineer a pig that fails to produce this oligosaccharide. A knockout mouse has been produced that fails to produce α-1,3-galactosyltransferase.[135] At this time, however, a similar knockout pig has yet to be produced.

Two other genetic engineering strategies have been taken to eliminate the problem of HAR of pig organs. First, genetic engineering can provide pigs with the human complement inhibitors that naturally protect human endothelium from complement-dependent lysis. Second, pigs can be produced that enzymatically remodel the α-galactosyl epitope into a harmless epitope such as seen on type O human red cells.

At least three groups have succeeded in producing transgenic pigs with human complement inhibitors. These inhibitors block the terminal sequence of complement activation and the development of the membrane attack complex that is responsible for cell lysis. The expression of human

CD59 or human CD59 and human decay-activating factor (DAF) significantly delayed rejection of pig hearts in monkeys up to 69 hours, as compared with about 1 hour in controls.[136,137]

In another study, hearts from pigs with human DAF and membrane cofactor protein (MCP) were transplanted into monkeys. HAR was effectively blocked and the grafts survived a median 5.1 days without any other measures taken to prevent HAR.[51] This group recognized that the tissue expression of human DAF was variable in different founder animals.[138] They selected and bred the founders expressing the product in the endothelial and smooth muscle cells.

In all these studies, the transgenic pigs have not shown any developmental or breeding abnormalities.[139]

Transgenic pig heart xenografts have been transplanted orthotopically into baboon recipients.[30] Combination chemotherapy (cyclophosphamide, cyclosporine, steroids) was given posttransplantation. Five of the ten grafts failed due to technical reasons. The remaining survived 4 to 9 days, at which point they were destroyed by vascular rejection.

Transgenic pigs have also been produced with altered antigen expression.[140] The enzymes α-1,3-galactosyltransferase and α-1,2-fucosyltransferase compete for the same substrate. Whereas the former produces the epitope for natural antibodies, the latter enzyme produces the H substance, as seen with blood group type O. By producing transgenic pigs expressing α-1,2-fucosyltransferase, the expression of the α-galactosyl epitope is significantly reduced. Cultured pig cells containing the fucosyltransferase enzyme are more resistant to lysis by natural antibody and complement.

Clinical studies have just started in several institutions using transgenic pig livers for extracorporeal perfusion of patients with acute liver failure. It is hoped that the transgenic livers will be functional for a longer term.

Organisms that produce the alpha gal epitope constitutively do not develop antibodies but rather specific tolerance to alpha gal. Humans and Old World monkeys fail to express alpha gal on their cells and therefore are not tolerant. Accordingly, it was thought that if the immune system were exposed to alpha gal during the development of tolerance, the animal would then fail to make specific antibodies.[141] This was tested with a knockout mouse that lacked the α-galactosyltransferase enzyme and accordingly made antibodies to alpha gal. Marrow was harvested and transduced with a gene for porcine α-galactosyltransferase. The altered marrow was infused into immunosuppressed mice. When the mice recovered, there was a marked reduction in antibody titers.

HAR, once considered the nemesis of xenotransplantation, can now be prevented by several strategies, with graft survival measured in days rather than minutes. The best strategy, however, will be determined based on long-term successes. The ideal strategy should not require repeated maneuvers for an indefinite period of time. If plasmapheresis or infusion of sCR1 or oligosaccharides were required indefinitely, the strategy would be expensive and inconvenient. The strategy should not chronically or severely suppress the host's immune response. If procedures to block complement fixation were combined with immunosuppression for preventing acute rejection, the host could end up with a severe combined immunodeficiency. The strategy should not adversely effect the graft function or contribute to acute or chronic rejection. Potential problems could arise from the persistent binding of immunoglobulins and early complement components or from a reaction to low-density expression of antigen.

Three potential outcomes could define a long-term solution for the prevention of HAR. First, the recipient could achieve accommodation, a phenomenon in which the immunoglobulins continue to circulate and bind to the tissue, but, through protective compensatory reactions by the host, the tissue is no longer injured. Second, the host could become specifically tolerant to the porcine endothelial antigens, such as alpha gal. Through negative selection, anergy, or suppression, the host stops making significant antibodies. Third, the responsible epitope could be permanently eliminated from the organ donor. Because humans have shown that tissue expression of alpha gal is not essential for life, the production of a knockout pig deficient in alpha gal remains an attractive goal.

Suppression of Acute Xenograft Rejection

Human allograft recipients are typically treated with long-term immunosuppression to prevent acute rejection. The drugs are relatively selective, and the recipient retains some ability to fight infections and neoplasms. The rejection of allografts differs in several respects from the immune destruction of xenografts. Rejection involves predominantly direct antigen presentation. Although antibodies contribute to the reaction, allograft rejection is predominantly a T-cell–dependent process.

The challenge to find a similarly selective immunosuppression protocol for xenografts will be considerably more difficult. Multiple mechanisms are involved, including indirect antigen presentation and antibody-mediated injury. NK cells are reactive with certain xenoantigens.

Many immunosuppressive drugs are being evaluated for their effectiveness with xenografts,[142] including cyclophosphamide,[38] cyclosporine,[38] tacrolimus,[143] leflunomide,[93] deoxyspergualin,[144,145] mycophenolate mofetil,[96,146] rapamycin (sirolimus),[147] brequinar,[148] and others. The humoral xenograft response appears to be the most resistant to suppression by chemotherapeutic agents.

It seems unlikely at this time that either a single agent or combination of agents can prevent xenograft rejection indefinitely without toxicity or severe deficiency. Additional strategies are required. Most likely, immunosuppression will be used in conjunction with other procedures intended to induce selective hyporesponsiveness to xenografts. Immunosuppression may be used to supplement these measures. For example, Sheffield and co-workers showed that injection of xenoanti-

gens into the thymus was ineffective in preventing rejection by itself.[61] However, the combination of intrathymic injection with temporary suppression with cyclophosphamide significantly prolonged xenograft survival. Similarly, Zhao et al. used temporary immune ablation to achieve immune tolerance to xenoantigens. After the chimeric mice achieved immunocompetence, pig skin grafts were accepted indefinitely without additional suppression.[149]

BASIC PREMISES FOR LONG-TERM XENOGRAFT ACCEPTANCE

For xenografts to achieve their potential, it will be necessary to preserve, at least partially, the immunocompetence of the recipient. Specific immune tolerance and accommodation to the xenograft can achieve that goal. Although the task is more formidable than with allografts, the opportunities are also greater. Porcine tissues can be modified in multiple ways that would be impractical for allografts. For example, herds can be produced with transgenic modifications.

With more opportunities for modification, a strategy needs to be devised. A successful approach would satisfy the following requirements. The recipient should be specifically unresponsive to all antigens expressed on the xenograft, including tissue-associated antigens. The recipient should remain immune responsive to all other antigens. The specific unresponsiveness should include all immune mechanisms: cellular, humoral, and natural. Tolerance should not develop against infectious organisms present in the donor or recipient. The recipient or donor animals should not be at increased risk for acquiring or activating an infection during the induction of immune unresponsiveness. The specific unresponsiveness should be permanent. If the recipient is chimeric, containing hematopoietic cells from the corresponding partner, the chimeric cells must be unresponsive to the recipient and not cause graft versus host disease (GVHD).

It is safe to say that no system exists today that satisfies all these goals. Particularly challenging is the need to induce tolerance to the xenograft without increasing the risk of infection. For example, systems that utilize immunosuppression during induction of tolerance not only increase the risk of developing an infection during the period of immunodeficiency but also increase the risk of inducing tolerance to those infectious organisms.

Development of the Universal Donor Animal?

Having demonstrated the insertion of human genes into pigs, it is naturally tempting to extrapolate these methods and propose the development either of a pig that is identical with the recipient or of a universal donor pig that humans cannot reject. Neither prospect seems plausible.

The task of deleting the numerous histocompatibility and xenogeneic antigens and then replacing them with the corresponding recipient antigens would be enormous, even with tomorrow's technology. Because most of the cell surface antigens have functions beyond immune recognition, it is highly unlikely that such a massive reengineering would result in a viable pig with a functional organ. A more believable proposal to achieve antigen identity would be to clone the recipient.[150] However, the ethical, legal, and serious logistical barriers make cloning impractical for transplantation.

Perhaps a universal donor pig could be engineered. Analogous to type O red cells, the recipient's immune system would simply fail to recognize the antigens. The level of difficulty, however, would be far greater than for red cells. There are numerous relevant antigens capable of triggering rejection. Most of the antigens have widely diverse polymorphisms. The cells and tissues are immunocompetent. If one were successful, a universal donor pig would pose two additional problems. First, if the pig had defective or absent antigen-presenting or accessory molecules, it would be severely immunodeficient. The pigs would need to be raised under gnotobiotic conditions. That would add greatly to the expense and make it much more difficult to satisfy the demand for organs. Of greater concern, however, are the consequences that follow the transplantation. First, if the transplanted organ became infected, the human immune system would not be able to react to it or defend it. Furthermore, the recipient might become tolerant to the infectious agent. Second, the recipient would experience severe GVHD if the pig lymphocytes were still capable of recognizing recipient antigen-presenting cells. The recipient would be incapable of rejecting the reactive pig lymphocytes.

A more achievable goal would be to produce xenogeneic donor cells that are partially identical with the recipient. The donor cells could express class I or II MHC antigens from the recipient or from the recipient species. This approach would need to be used in conjunction with other processes to establish accommodation or tolerance. By itself, the presence of recipient MHC antigen would make the donor cells more efficient as antigen-presenting cells. At the very least, these cells would enhance indirect antigen presentation. If the engineered cells had species-specific MHC but differed from the recipient, they would also enhance direct antigen presentation.

Genetic therapy can assist with the development of xenogeneic hematopoietic chimerism. Human class I antigen has been inserted into mouse hematopoietic cells using a retrovirus vector.[151] After lethal irradiation and bone marrow transplantation with the modified cells, stable chimerism with cells expressing the human antigen was observed. Furthermore, the chimeric animals developed a markedly reduced antibody response and a partially inhibited cellular response to immunization with this antigen, but retained a normal response to third-party antigens.[152,153]

An alternate approach would be to make the recipient's hematopoietic cells resemble the animal donor. Once tolerance is induced to the hybrid cell, tolerance should be established to the donor animal as well. Swine MHC class II antigen has been incorporated into murine and into baboon

CD34+ stem cells.[154,155] In two baboons receiving autologous stem cells transfected with swine antigen, prolonged survival of the cells was detected. Kidney xenografts from the corresponding swine were transplanted but promptly rejected. Because the hematopoietic chimerism persisted after rejection, it is assumed that the tolerance was incomplete. A humoral response reacted with other swine antigens.

Induction of Immune Tolerance

The mechanisms of immune tolerance have been thoroughly reviewed elsewhere.[156] Specific immune unresponsiveness requires both central tolerance and peripheral tolerance. Central tolerance develops in the thymus. Immature T cells rapidly proliferate within the cortex, and most of these cells become reactive to self antigens. Those T cells are eliminated (negatively selected) at the corticomedullary junction, an area rich in dendritic cells. The self-reactive T cells are greatly reduced in number by the time they enter the medulla and go into circulation. Peripheral tolerance includes mechanisms to protect the host from self-reactive cells. Some self-reactive cells escape negative selection. Furthermore, although the thymus undergoes marked involution with age and disease, the host is still capable of mounting a primary immune response to new antigens. Presumably, then, the host is still capable of producing naive T cells. Central tolerance is most important during development and immune reconstitution, deleting the bulk of self-reactive T cells. Peripheral tolerance is needed to enforce tolerance by those escaping the thymus during development and, later in life, to control T cells generated outside the thymus.

How does hematopoietic chimerism contribute to immune tolerance? The initial study by Medawar achieved at least partial tolerance through hematopoietic chimerism. The circulating cells can contribute in several ways. Antigen presentation of at least two signals can induce sensitization within naive lymphocytes, whereas presentation of only one antigen leads to anergy. In particular, B cells have been shown to be instrumental for induction of anergy. Dendritic cells are also instrumental in negative selection within the thymus. When the dendritic cells at the corticomedullary junction are permanently depleted through cyclosporine administration and mediastinal irradiation, self-reactive cells enter circulation and cause an autoimmune GVHD. The persistence of active suppressor cell mechanisms may also depend on chimerism. In a model of GVHD, when tolerant lymphocytes were deprived of tolerogenic strain leukocytes for a prolonged period, they lost their ability to suppress GVHD. With stimulation, however, the lymphocytes quickly regained their ability to suppress, in a manner similar to a secondary immune response.

Whether detectable chimerism is either necessary or sufficient for long-term organ graft acceptance, however, is still debated. Starzl et al. found evidence of microchimerism in patients with long-term allograft survival and in two human recipients of baboon liver grafts. Sykes et al. showed that donor cell chimerism was often lost long before the graft was rejected. Others have demonstrated donor cell chimerism in patients who have rejected their allografts. Even if a relationship between chimerism and organ graft acceptance were established, it would not necessarily indicate that the chimerism was responsible for the acceptance. Hematopoietic chimerism could simply be the result of immune tolerance.

A related issue is whether tolerance to hematopoietic cells is sufficient if tolerance to tissue- and species-associated antigens is also necessary. Initial studies of neonatal tolerance suggested that induction of tolerance to the donor's hematopoietic cells led to tolerance to peripheral tissues as well.[157] Medawar was surprised by this outcome, believing that the skin would have additional antigens not present on leukocytes. Further studies with different strains and with different sources of skin did, in fact, show rejection of skin grafts. Using different techniques and strains of animals, multiple tissue-associated antigens have since been identified. In spite of tolerance to the hematopoietic cells, these tissues are still rejected. Generally, rejection with a tissue-specific antigen mismatch is milder than with a major histocompatibility mismatch.

Triplett definitively demonstrated the importance of tissue-associated antigens in self-tolerance.[158] He removed the pituitary glands from developing tadpoles. When these glands were later transplanted back, they were promptly rejected. Similarly if the thyroid gland was totally removed from a fetal lamb and subsequently retransplanted into the mature sheep, it was rejected. On the other hand, if the thyroid was only partially removed, the sheep later accepted the thyroid autograft.[159] Tissue-associated antigens have been identified in multiple tissues, including skin, pituitary, thyroid, eye, and kidney in autograft and allograft transplants.[160] In some of these studies, recipients with donor cell hematopoietic chimerism rejected the tissue.

Although tissue-associated antigens have not been extensively studied in xenografts, they most likely represent a barrier, as they do with allografts. The best demonstration was made by Rice et al.[161] Human hematopoietic stem cells were infused into fetal lambs. Although the sheep demonstrated stable chimerism, the sheep still developed natural antibodies to human endothelium.

The ideal system for inducing immune tolerance to a xenograft must induce persistent tolerance to the xenograft, involving peripheral tolerance and probably central tolerance mechanisms. The tolerance must be antigen specific. The tolerance should be to tissue-associated and species-associated antigens as well as to the MHC. The tolerance must develop in a relatively immunodeficient state. The patient must be protected against opportunistic infections and against GVHD.

Accommodation

The body provides a fortuitous defensive mechanism against self-inflicted immune reactions, referred to as *accommoda-

tion* or *adaptation*. If tissues can survive the initial humoral or cellular reactions, with time the tissues become resistant to injury.

Accommodation has frequently been described with minor ABO-incompatible allografts. Passenger leukocytes produce IgG antibodies against the host's red cells. The IgG antibodies typically appear about 1 week posttransplantation and cause significant hemolysis. The reaction, however, is self-limiting. The hemolysis disappears in about 2 to 4 weeks, although the antibodies persist.[162,163]

A similar resolution of antibody-mediated rejection has been demonstrated for ABO-mismatched allografts and for discordant xenografts. Fischel et al. described a porcine cardiac xenograft surviving in a rhesus monkey for 8 days. Although circulating antibodies were bound to the endothelium, the graft had not undergone rejection.[164]

Hyperacute rejection was prevented in ABO-mismatched cardiac allografts in baboons by infusion of soluble trisaccharides of the A and B antigen to neutralize the antibodies. Although the circulating antibodies persisted after the oligosaccharides were discontinued, some grafts showed prolonged survival.[124]

Systemic and local effects may contribute to the protective effect of accommodation. Long-term (greater than 5 weeks) Lew rat recipients of hamster hearts have normal complement and circulating antihamster antibodies. Yet, a second fresh hamster heart graft is generally accepted.[165] Rat recipients of hamster hearts have circulating antibodies to hamster by 3 days posttransplantation. A second fresh hamster heart transplanted at that time is promptly rejected. The transplant of hamster hearts from rats undergoing accommodation, however, shows some protection.[166] When the accommodated tissue is transplanted into a naive rat, rejection is delayed.

The mechanism of accommodation is unknown. It is not caused by the depletion of antibodies or the replacement of donor endothelium with host endothelium within the graft. Immunohistochemistry of long-term cardiac xenografts (hamster to rat) shows deposition of IgG, IgM, C3, and C6 on the endothelium, but minimal fibrin formation. The possibility that accommodated endothelial cells lose their antigens was explored. Although some reduction in antigens such as alpha gal was observed with accommodation, it was not thought to be sufficient to protect the graft.[167]

Some have suggested that localized immunoregulation protects the graft. Within the myocardium are numerous CD4+ cells and macrophages. Many of the lymphocytes express IL-2 receptor (IL-2R). Cytokine stains reflect a T_H2 pattern (IL-4, IL-5) for the CD4+ cells rather than a T_H1 pattern.[168]

The regulatory cells infiltrating the tissues and the secreted cytokines probably provide some benefit by blocking the end stage of cell destruction. Terminal complement fixation does not occur. Natural killer cells and effector T lymphocytes are not recruited to the target tissues. Rosengard et al. observed that infiltrating lymphocytes extracted from tolerated allografts had suppressor cell activity with *in *vitro* assays.[169] Allografts retransplanted from tolerant recipients into naive recipients were protected from acute rejection.[170]

The induction of select protective genes might also provide protection. For example, these genes might inhibit apoptosis or produce nitric oxide and inhibit lymphocyte binding.[168,171]

PRELIMINARY STRATEGIES FOR PROLONGED XENOGRAFT ACCEPTANCE

Several novel systems have been proposed for establishing long-term xenograft survival with minimum toxicity from chemotherapy. These proposals and their supporting data, potential advantages, and disadvantages are briefly discussed in this section.

Transplantation into Immune Privileged Sites

Foreign antigens placed in certain anatomic locations (e.g., the brain, the testes, and the anterior chamber of the eye) are not rejected. These sites are known as *immune privileged sites*. It was originally believed that these sites were protected from infiltrating lymphocytes by tight junctions between vascular endothelial cells. That belief may prove to be simplistic, because activated lymphocytes can gain access to these sites. These sites have other properties that prevent normal immune sensitization. There are few antigen-presenting cells present and the sites do not have lymphatic drainage to regional lymph nodes.

Cultured human retinal pigment epithelial (RPE) cells have been transplanted into the retina space of rabbits without immunosuppression. The transplantation of RPE cells could potentially treat macular degeneration, a common cause of blindness. The transplanted cells became functional and showed prolonged acceptance. By 3 months, however, they showed evidence of early rejection.[172]

Dopaminergic neurons from a fetal pig were transplanted into the brain of a patient with Parkinson's disease.[173] The transplant significantly improved the clinical course of the patient. Seven months later, the fetal pig neurons were identified. They were intact and had extended their axons. The immune reaction was minimal.

Rat islet xenografts survived for a prolonged period in non-immunosuppressed mice when transplanted into the testes as opposed to the liver, spleen, or kidney capsule.[174] Similarly, islet allografts survive long term when transplanted into the brain.[175]

Although the cell grafts escape rejection in the immune privileged sites, the host does not develop tolerance to the graft. When donor strain skin grafts are placed on rats with long-term intracerebral islet grafts, the islets were rejected along with the skin grafts.[176]

The tissues of the immune privileged sites may be protected by local factors inhibiting inflammation. The brain,

eyes, and testes have increased expression of the Fas ligand.[177,178] When lymphocytes carrying the Fas receptor (CD95) encounter Fas ligand–containing cells, they undergo apoptosis, effectively depleting the tissue-reactive T cells.

When testicular tissue from a normal mouse was transplanted under the renal capsule of an allogeneic mouse, it survived. In contrast, testicular tissue from mice with a defective Fas ligand was promptly rejected.[179] The authors proposed that transgenic animals be produced in which the transplant tissue contains the Fas ligand. Donor tissue would then promptly induce tolerance to itself as the recipient's lymphocytes ligate the CD95R+ tissue.

Some studies have indicated, however, that the story might not be this straightforward. As expected, the lpr mouse, an autoimmune model of systemic lupus erythematosus, has a deficiency of CD95.[180] However, patients with lupus or rheumatoid arthritis actually have elevated levels of CD95.[181,182] Also contrary to expectation, rejecting allografts show induced expression of Fas on the infiltrating lymphocytes and expression of Fas ligand on the endothelial cells.[183]

CD95 can be modulated by various cytokines. For example, IL-4 downregulates the expression of CD95.[184] This is particularly troublesome for a recipient of discordant xenografts. IL-4 is increased in tissues demonstrating accommodation, because of numerous T_H2 type helper cells. Thus, accommodation could interfere with the induction of tolerance.

There is probably a good reason why CD95 is expressed in certain tissues at different stages and not expressed in other tissues. The immune privileged sites are relatively isolated and have limited risk of infection. If a mechanism for ready tolerance or evasion of immune response were present in other tissues, however, the host would be unable to destroy infectious agents or infected cells. A transgenic animal with widespread expression of Fas and Fas ligand would be effectively immunodeficient, making it difficult and expensive to produce. More important, infections acquired within the transplanted tissues, such as zoonotic viruses or host viruses, would escape the immune response and induce tolerance to the infectious organisms.

The strategy of exploiting immune privileged sites has limited application for liver xenotransplantation, because the liver is far larger than any of the proposed sites, with the possible exception of the brain. On the other hand, when the role of Fas and Fas ligand in apoptosis is fully understood, porcine hepatocytes could potentially be induced to express the appropriate Fas gene or ligand.[185]

Intrauterine Bone Marrow Transplantation

As a clinical application of the original Medawar model of developmental tolerance, some have proposed infusing marrow from the animal donor into preimmune human fetuses. After birth, the chimeric newborn should then accept an organ from the donor animal. In parallel, *in utero* marrow transplantation is being developed for the cure of congenital enzyme deficiencies.[186]

Harrison et al. established allogeneic chimerism in monkeys by infusing sex-mismatched rhesus monkey fetal liver cells.[187] As a preclinical model for transplanting xenografts into chimeric human newborns, Zanjani and Srour established chimerism between discordant species by injecting human stem cells into fetal lambs.[188,189] The human stem cells differentiated into erythroid, myeloid, and lymphoid cells. The lymphocytes differentiated into CD3+, CD4+, and CD8+ cells. Xenogeneic chimerism was stable for more than 2 years.

Human chimerism was established in fetal baboons when fetal liver cells were infused into first-trimester fetuses.[190] In general, donor cell chimerism has been limited in the recipient fetus. By purifying and injecting large numbers of stem cells, however, one baboon showed greater than 90% donor cell chimerism (K.J. Blakemore, personal communication).

The intrauterine transplantation of stem cells provides several major potential advantages. Even xenogeneic chimerism appears to be stable once established. The intrauterine environment is not only conducive to the induction of tolerance, but also is a protected and sterile environment. Thus, the risk of infectious complications during the period of immunodeficiency is minimal.

There are several limitations to *in utero* transplantation. The most obvious limitation is that it can be applied only to human fetuses with diagnosed congenital diseases. Second, the tolerance would only be against the hematopoietic cells transfused. Tissue-associated antigens in subsequent organ transplants would still be foreign to the chimeric patient. After inducing allogeneic chimerism in two fetal monkeys, kidney transplants from the donor monkey were performed 2 and 3 years after birth.[191] Mixed lymphocyte reactions between the chimeric recipients and the donors were markedly reduced, and the initial course of the graft was markedly better than in controls. Nonetheless, the grafts showed evidence of acute and chronic rejection. In the human-to-sheep chimeric model, antibody responses to the donor (human) endothelium was measured. In spite of persistent hematopoietic chimerism, the sheep developed normal titers of antibodies to the human endothelium.[161]

Third, there is a significant risk of developing lethal GVHD in the injected fetus. This system fully satisfies Billingham's requisites for GVHD. The preimmune fetus is antigenically distinct from the donor, the donor cells are immunocompetent, and the fetus is unable to reject the donor cells. Indeed, it is remarkable that not all chimeric fetuses develop GVHD. In looking at the role of T cells in allogeneic sheep-to-lamb *in utero* transplants, unfractionated marrow injected into fetal lambs invariably led to GVHD.[192] If the T cells were depleted, however, the resulting chimerism was very limited. When the mature T cells were reduced, good chimerism developed without evidence of GVHD. Apparently the fetus was able to

downregulate a limited number of mature reactive T cells and prevent GVHD.

Mixed Chimerism by Bone Marrow Transplantation

Since the vast majority of transplant recipients are beyond the fetal stage of development, an alternative approach would be to simulate the intrauterine environment within the recipient. As done with bone marrow transplants for the treatment of leukemia, irradiation and aggressive chemotherapy are used to eradicate the recipient's immune system. This allows engraftment and maturation of the subsequently infused marrow. As the immune system regenerates, the naive lymphocytes are in a fetuslike environment, that is, an environment of great antigen excess.

Bone marrow transplants with complete replacement of the recipient marrow with donor marrow can induce tolerance to the donor. The recipients, however, often develop lethal GVHD or are immunoincompetent.[193,194] To avoid these complications, Ildstad and Sachs proposed that the immunodeficient recipient be transplanted with *both* recipient and donor hematopoietic cells, establishing mixed chimerism.[195] Mixed chimerism would lead to tolerance to the donor antigens by the donor marrow and to immunocompetence of the recipient. The recipient marrow provides antigen-presenting cells. The T cells are depleted from both marrow populations in order to prevent lethal GVHD by the donor marrow and donor marrow rejection by the recipient's lymphocytes. The recipient is prepared with chemotherapy or irradiation.

As the two marrow populations reconstitute the recipient, the thymus is also regenerated with early thymocytes and dendritic cells from both partners. The differentiated lymphocytes are then negatively selected to deplete those lymphocytes reactive to donor or recipient hemopoietic cells. In the periphery donor or recipient, reactive lymphocytes become anergic and unreactive.

Mixed chimerism has proved successful in generating specific tolerance to the donor animal. In the rat-to-mouse transplantation model, it has led to very prolonged survival of rat skin grafts and pancreatic islet grafts in chimeric mice.[196] The reconstituted recipients are tolerant to the donor but remain fully responsive to third-party grafts.

Several significant improvements in the mixed chimerism system have been made to make it more practical for clinical transplants. A less toxic preparation of the recipient without ablating the myeloid elements still provides for good chimerism.[197] Antibodies to CD4 and CD8 given before and after the bone marrow transplantation lead to good engraftment of the thymus with donor cells, including dendritic cells, replacing the need for intense thymic irradiation. Finally, the graft can be placed at the time of the transplantation, rather than sequentially, following engraftment.

The mixed chimerism system is effective with pig allografts and has shown a partial effect with discordant pig-to-monkey xenograft transplantation.[47,48,198] Normal renal function without rejection was observed for up to 15 days. Low-level porcine chimerism was initially observed. Eventually, however, the monkeys either rejected the grafts or died of complications.

Xenogeneic chimerism was short lived compared with allogeneic chimerism.[198] The difference proved to be caused by the absence of species-specific hematopoietic growth factors and cytokines. When the monkey was administered recombinant porcine cytokines, IL-3, and stem cell factor, however, the survival of chimeric pig cells was markedly prolonged.[47]

Thymic Reeducation

The thymus is the principal provider of tolerant mature T cells. Prethymocytes from the bone marrow enter the thymus and proliferate without apparent restraint within the cortex. Thymocytes that react with self MHC as well as those that do not react with self are generated. Most of the autoreactive cells, however, are "filtered out" or clonally deleted at the corticomedullary junction.[193,199] Most of the cells migrating into the medulla and on to the peripheral lymph nodes are not reactive with self antigens.

Dendritic cells line the corticomedullary junction. These antigen-presenting cells define the antigen specificity of clonal deletion.[200,201] Cyclosporine combined with thymic irradiation depletes the corticomedullary dendritic cells and prevents their return. As the rodents recover from the immunosuppression, they develop an autoimmune disease resembling GVHD. Without the corticomedullary filter, the self-reactive cells migrated to the periphery and injured the tissues.

Three basic approaches have been proposed for thymic reeducation. The simplest approach is to inject these cells directly into the lobes of the thymus. Second, pharmacologic manipulation can be done to initially deplete the antigen-presenting cells from the thymus, followed by reexpansion of the thymus and recruitment of antigen-presenting cells. Third, a preimmune thymus from the fetal donor animal, already populated with donor antigen-presenting cells, can be transplanted into the recipient.

If thymic reeducation is done within a mature recipient with an established peripheral immune system, it will not be sufficient to prevent rejection. Other measures would need to be combined with it to prevent the peripheral T cells from reacting with the graft. With xenografts, additional measures would be needed for non–T-cell mechanisms of rejection.

Intrathymic Injection of Tolerogenic Antigen-Presenting Cells

Prolonged acceptance of pancreatic islet allografts was achieved when rats received a single dose of antilymphocyte serum (ALS) and islets were injected into the thymus.[202] Injection of islets under the renal capsule did not lead to prolonged acceptance. Those receiving intrathymic injections

were truly tolerant to the grafts. When islets were subsequently transplanted under the renal capsule, they were accepted for a prolonged period. In contrast, recipients who had received the initial islets in an immune privileged site (testicle) promptly rejected the secondary grafts. Many successful and unsuccessful studies have been performed with this basic technique.[203] The initial immunosuppression as provided by ALS appears to be critical. Some also suggest that the thymic inoculum must contain tissue-associated antigens.[204]

As with allografts, prolonged acceptance of rat xenografts in diabetic mice has been accomplished.[203,205] The same methods have not led to engraftment of mouse islets within rats, however. Sheffield found that in contrast to rat allografts, additional immunosuppression with cyclophosphamide was necessary to attain prolonged survival of hamster heart xenografts.[61] To the best of our knowledge, intrathymic injection has not yet been tested with large animal recipients of porcine xenografts.

By itself, however, intrathymic injection has several limitations. The need to severely suppress the peripheral immune system puts the recipient at risk for opportunistic infections. Intrathymic injection has not been as successful with larger animals as with rodents. Most significantly, this approach requires a sizeable thymus. It might be very difficult to inject recipients with thymic involution, such as those who are older or those with chronic illnesses.

Intrathymic Recruitment of Xenogeneic Dendritic Cells

Paradoxically, cyclosporine depletes the thymic dendritic cells needed for immune tolerance.[200,201] As discussed previously, a combination of cyclosporine and thymic irradiation leads to an autoimmune reaction resembling GVHD.[206] If the thymus is capable of regenerating, however, new dendritic cells can be recruited into the thymus and tolerance to new antigens is possible. Cyclosporine, therefore, serves the useful purpose of opening up space and allowing for the influx of new tolerogenic dendritic cells.[207,208]

The pharmacologic method of thymic reeducation offers significant advantages over the intrathymic injection method. Most notably, it can be used in situations with thymic involution. Growth hormones or select cytokines can be administered during the postcyclosporine period to enhance the reexpansion and repopulation of the thymus. The enhanced growth of the thymus could also lead to heightened immunocompetence while inducing specific tolerance. Because the method is systemic rather than local, recruitment may repopulate extrathymic sites of T-cell generation. At this time, pharmacologic thymic reeducation has not been tested in a xenogeneic system.

Transplantation of Fetal Porcine Thymus

Rather than repopulating the recipient thymus with donor antigen-presenting cells, the actual thymus from the donor animal can be placed in the recipient. Not only would the dendritic cells be of donor origin, but the thymic epithelium, which might be essential, would also be from the donor.[209] Transplants of allogeneic thymuses depleted of hematopoietic cells lead to tolerance as defined by the antigens on epithelium. Accordingly, Sykes et al. have proposed that in addition to performing a xenogeneic mixed chimerism bone marrow transplantation, the recipient also should be given a fetal thymus from the donor animal.[149] As the immature donor and host T cells repopulate and mature within the transplanted donor thymus, they would become tolerant to the donor animal.

Pig skin grafts have survived indefinitely on thymectomized mice reconstituted with mixed pig and mouse marrow and a fetal pig thymus. The tolerance is specific in that the mice reject third-party pig or mouse skin grafts. The mice are immunocompetent at the time of the skin transplant. This study constitutes a major milestone in establishing that permanent and specific tolerance can be established for grafts from a notably disparate xenogeneic donor. Besides providing porcine MHC antigen, the fetal pig thymus most likely provided an environment favorable to prolonged chimerism. Porcine class II–positive cells, probably dendritic cells, were evident 30 weeks posttransplantation. The V_β region of T-cell receptors was analyzed and demonstrated that clonal deletion was a major component of the induced tolerance. Initial studies in a baboon also demonstrated apparent prolongation of pig skin graft survival.[210]

Inhibition of T-Cell Costimulation

Effective T-cell activation requires multiple signals between the T cell and the antigen-presenting cell, in addition to the binding of the T-cell receptor to the corresponding antigen-presenting molecules. A major second signal is the CD28 receptor on the T cell.[211] When it binds to the corresponding B7-1 or B7-2 ligand expressed on the antigen-presenting cells, CD28 induces the production of interleukin 2. If the second signal fails to occur, the T cell becomes unresponsive or anergic.

CTLA-4 Ig is an immunoglobulin that binds to the B7-1 and B7-2 molecules, effectively blocking the needed stimulation of the T-cell CD28. Injecting CTLA-4 into xenograft recipients has led to prolonged acceptance of cardiac and pancreatic islet xenografts.[75,212] Graft survival was further prolonged when this was combined with antibodies to T-cell subsets. Eventually, however, the grafts were rejected by a humoral reaction. Although the CD28-B7 costimulation represents a primary second signal, it most likely is not the only second signal that could lead to sensitization.

The CD28 receptor on human T lymphocytes recognizes and binds to the corresponding B7-2 ligand on pig endothelial cells. Interruption of the costimulation with CTLA-4, therefore, could contribute to preventing porcine xenograft rejection. A recognized risk of inducing anergy within the recipient is that tolerance could inadvertently be induced to infectious agents as well.

Inhibition of costimulation would need to be supplemented with other therapies to prevent T-cell–independent reactions against the xenograft. If the recipient continues to produce new xenoreactive T cells, continuous therapy would be necessary to prevent later rejection.

Donor-Specific Transfusions

In reviewing the initial clinical trials of kidney allotransplants, it was unexpectedly discovered that transplant recipients with a history of multiple transfusions prior to transplantation experienced longer allograft survival rates than those without transfusions.[213,214] Consequently, until cyclosporine came into widespread use, candidates were intentionally transfused. The donor-specific transfusion phenomenon has been further studied in animal models.[215] Transfusions are typically performed in combination with temporary immunosuppression.

The transfusions probably induce multiple mechanisms of tolerance. As discussed elsewhere, the resulting chimerism participates in the two-way paradigm (graft vs. host and host vs. graft reactions) of transplant tolerance.[216] Two-way tolerance results with the resolution of these reactions. Chimerism also leads to repopulation of the tolerance-defining tissues such as the thymus (so-called reeducation of the thymus).[207] The donor dendritic cells at the corticomedullary junction effectively deplete many of the donor-reactive T cells produced by the thymus.

Modest prolongation of xenograft survival has been achieved when donor-specific transfusions are combined with chemotherapy or antibodies to T cells.[217,218] In comparison with allografts, however, xenogeneic transfusions are more likely to lead to sensitization than to tolerance.[219]

Surrogate Tolerogenesis

Applying the prevailing transplantation technology to prevention of xenograft rejection puts the recipient in a precarious position. Multiple immune mechanisms are capable of destroying the graft. Therefore, selective immunosuppression would not be effective. Induction of immune tolerance requires that the recipient endure a period of immunodepletion. Either of these approaches or a combination of these approaches would leave the recipient defenseless to combat opportunistic or zoonotic infections.

As an alternative to inducing immune unresponsiveness within the recipient, we propose instead to induce immune tolerance to the donor *within the xenograft donor* and adoptively transfer the tolerance back to the recipient. We have termed this process *surrogate tolerogenesis.*[220] The induction of tolerance within the donor animal provides considerably greater flexibility and opportunity. For example, with current approaches, developmental tolerance can only be applied to fetal or newborn patients. With surrogate tolerogenesis, however, developmental tolerance can be established within fetal donor animals and applied to recipients of any age. The preimmune fetal environment is not only conducive to the induction of immune tolerance but is also a naturally sterile environment.

The patient would be spared the need for eradication of the patient's immune system, because tolerance is induced outside the patient, within the immunodeficient fetal pig. Surrogate tolerogenesis utilizes not only clonal deletion and anergy, but also takes advantage of the active suppressor cell mechanisms that protect the fetus against differentiated maternal lymphocytes. The induction of antigen-specific suppressor cells outside the recipient allows the adoptive transfer of tolerance to the recipient without the need to destroy the patient's immune system. In contrast to tolerance induced with hematopoietic chimerism, tolerance would be established to all tissue-associated antigens as well as to the antigens on the hematopoietic cells.

Surrogate tolerogenesis provides the advantage of multiplicity. When tolerance is attempted in the transplant recipient, the outcome of the transplantation rests on the single attempt. If tolerance is induced within donor animals, however, multiple attempts can be made and the best chimeric animal can be chosen for transfer and transplantation into the recipient. If none of the transfused donor animals develops tolerance, the patient experiences only an irritating delay in the transplantation.

In surrogate tolerogenesis, bone marrow is aspirated from the intended xenograft recipient. The mature T cells are par-

tially reduced and the cells infused into fetal pigs (Fig. 27.1). After the birth of the litter, the best pig is selected. The splenocytes from the chimeric pig are harvested and infused back into the patient. If the chimeric cells provide immune tolerance to the chimeric pig, then a xenograft from the corresponding pig should be accepted.

Initial studies of surrogate tolerogenesis have demonstrated a specific inhibition in the immune response to pig antigens. Human lymphocytes infused into preimmune fetal pigs led to appropriate engraftment in the pig tissues, including thymus and spleen.[221] The chimeric lymphocytes specifically suppressed the mixed lymphocyte reaction of naive corresponding human lymphocytes to irradiated pig stimulator cells, even with a mixture of 1 lymphocyte per 100 responder cells.

Using a sheep xenograft model, the median survival of pig aorta xenografts was markedly prolonged compared with the appropriate controls (77 days versus 7 days, $P < 0.03$) without prolonged or severe immunosuppression.[222,223] The sheep received a single pretransplant injection of cyclophosphamide (35 mg/kg) and no posttransplant immunosuppression. The recipients remained immunocompetent throughout their course. No isolation precautions were required, and there were no significant infections. One of the experimental animals had an intact graft at 11 months posttransplantation, with only mild chronic rejection. Pig cell chimerism was demon-

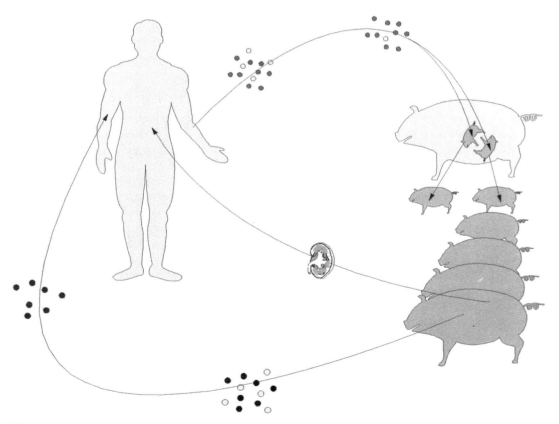

FIG. 27.1. Surrogate tolerogenesis.

strated in the spleen of this sheep by PCR. Surrogate tolerogenesis also markedly inhibited the induction of anti-pig antibodies in the recipients.

With the more stringent model of heterotopic pig heart xenografts, a partial success was observed with the initial transplants.[224] The control grafts were rejected at 3 to 4 days with classic vascular xenograft rejection. The experimental grafts were rejected at 4 to 6 days, which was not a significant prolongation in survival. Each of these grafts, however, developed cellular rather than vascular rejection.

If surrogate tolerogenesis in its current state of development could prevent vascular rejection, possibly it could be combined with selective immunosuppression to prevent cellular rejection as well. The sheep model was developed with daily administration of cyclosporine to the recipient, starting 2 days prior to transplantation. The level of immunosuppression was maintained at levels typical for heart allografts. As seen with other models, cyclosporine had little effect on the control animals, which rejected at 4 to 6 days. The first two experimental transplants lasted 9 and 25 days. The first recipient was euthanized due to a thrombus. The heart graft showed no evidence of rejection. The second graft developed an ischemic infarct due to a thromboembolus in the left main coronary artery. The uninvolved myocardium showed only mild, smoldering rejection, with scattered lymphocytes and minimal myocardial injury. Both sheep had normal lymphocyte and platelet counts throughout their course. The serum urea nitrogen and creatinine levels were normal. There was no evidence of significant infection.

How would preformed natural antibodies be managed with surrogate tolerogenesis? The technique could be combined with other technologies directed at HAR, such as antibody depletion, complement inhibitors, or transgenic pigs. Sheep do not produce antibodies to alpha gal because they express alpha gal constituitively. Transplant studies in nonhuman primates would be more appropriate for assessing the effect on antibodies to alpha gal.

Nonetheless, there is evidence that the induction of chimerism within the donor animal, as done with surrogate tolerogenesis, may have a beneficial effect on preformed antibodies.

The human marrow that was initially infused into preimmune fetal pigs was not depleted of B cells. Indeed, about 50% of the lymphocytes identified in the chimeric pigs were B cells. B cells committed to natural antibodies represent a large portion of the total population. Such B cells were most likely present in the chimeric pigs. The absence of any deleterious effect suggests that either the human cells were tolerant to the pig or that the pig tissues achieved accommodation.

Sheep normally have modest levels of noncytotoxic antibodies to pig cells. If sensitized, they develop high levels of cytotoxic antibodies. In the initial heart transplant studies, we were surprised to find that the levels of preformed antibodies to pig cells dropped precipitously after infusion of the chimeric pig splenocytes but not with infusion of nor-

mal control pig splenocytes. The mechanism is not understood at this time. The effect appears to be specific, because the levels of total IgG and IgM were unchanged.

Evidence of accommodation was observed with the experimental heart transplant recipients given cyclosporine. These sheep were found to be sensitized and had high levels of cytotoxic antibodies to pig cells as tested in a complement-dependent assay. Although the antibody levels did not drop after infusion, the grafts did not undergo vascular rejection as might be expected. When sensitized sheep received control pig heart xenografts and comparable treatment with cyclosporine, the grafts were rejected in 0.5 to 2 days.

Achieving accommodation in the donor pig prior to transplantation would greatly simplify the management of the xenograft recipient. The experimental retransplantation of grafts into recipients antigenically identical with the first recipient demonstrates that the accommodated graft carries some protection against rejection.[225] By achieving accommodation within the donor, as with surrogate tolerogenesis, this principle could potentially be utilized clinically.

Surrogate tolerogenesis provides several levels of protection against zoonotic infections. First, by using fetal surrogate and donor animals, surrogate tolerogenesis leads to immune tolerance within a sterile environment. Thus the risk of developing tolerance to infectious agents is minimized. Second, the coculture of human lymphocytes with porcine blood and tissues takes place prior to transplantation, outside the patient. The risk of activating a virus infection during lymphocyte activation is shifted to the pretransplantation period. Third, the chimeric donor, including the patient's lymphocytes, could be screened for zoonotic infection prior to transfusing the cells back to the patient. Finally, since the recipients do not undergo immune ablation, they could be vaccinated against any pathogen that might be present in pigs.

A potential drawback of surrogate tolerogenesis would be the need to wait for the xenograft. A patient requiring an emergency heart or liver transplantation would not benefit. Pigs have a short gestation period and grow rapidly after birth. Thus, the typical wait would be only 6 to 7 months for an adult-sized organ, which is less than the average wait for a human donor.

SUMMARY

The use of xenografts represents both a major opportunity and a major challenge. Animal donors, such as pigs, could be raised in sufficient numbers to totally resolve the shortage of organ donors. Transplants could be performed on an elective basis, eliminating the long waits, uncertainty, and clinical deterioration that often occurs with allotransplantation. The xenografts would be resistant to certain human infectious vectors such as hepatitis and HIV. Using state-of-the-art husbandry, xenograft donors such as pigs could be raised under very clean conditions and the risk of zoonotic infections minimized.

On the other hand, xenografts are subject to fulminant hyperacute and acute rejection. Technology that is effective with allografts will not prevent rejection of pig xenografts. Furthermore, the aggressive immunosuppression needed to prevent rejection would leave the recipient immunologically defenseless. Appropriate physiologic function has been demonstrated on a short-term basis, as with the extracorporeal perfusion of pig xenografts in patients with acute hepatic failure. The physiologic function of pig liver xenografts over the long term, however, remains to be proven. Some have postulated that endogenous viruses, coded in the genome of animal donors, represent a health risk. After considerable investigation, however, no evidence of disease has been identified and associated with these vectors in either patients or cohorts.

The opportunities and benefits of xenotransplantation clearly outweigh the risks and justify the innovative efforts required for meeting the challenges. The problems of xenotransplantation appear to be solvable. Although the issues are substantial and cannot be resolved with current technology, the use of xenografts provides for innovative approaches not available with allografts, such as modification of the xenograft by genetic engineering, immune modification, and stem cell therapy.

REFERENCES

1. Laing P. The unrecognized potential of xenotransplantation. Salomon Brothers report prepared for Sandoz, January 1996.
2. Starzl TE, Fung J, Tzakis A, et al. Baboon-to-human liver transplantation. *Lancet* 1993;34:65–71.
3. Starzl TE, Valdivia LA, Murase N, et al. The biological basis of and strategies for clinical xenotransplantation. *Immunol Rev* 1994;141: 213–244.
4. Allan JS, Broussard SR, Michaels MG, et al. Amplification of simian retroviral sequences from human recipients of baboon liver transplants. *AIDS Res Hum Retroviruses* 1998;14:821–824.
5. Hammer C. Physiological obstacles after xenotransplantation. *Ann N Y Acad Sci* 1998;862:19–27.
6. Starzl TE, Rao AS, Murase N, et al. Chimerism and xenotransplantation. New concepts. *Surg Clin North Am* 1999;79:191–205.
7. Luo Y, Kosanke S, Mieles L, et al. Comparative histopathology of hepatic allografts and xenografts in the nonhuman primate. *Xenotransplantation* 1998;5:197–206.
8. Chari RS, Collins BH, Magee JC, et al. Brief report: treatment of hepatic failure with *ex vivo* pig-liver perfusion followed by liver transplantation. *N Engl J Med* 1994;331:234–237.
9. Makowa L, Cramer DV, Hoffman A, et al. The use of a pig liver xenograft for temporary support of a patient with fulminant hepatic failure. *Transplantation* 1995;59:1654–1659.
10. Uesugi T, Ikai I, Yagi T, et al. Evaluation of ammonia and lidocaine clearance, and galactose elimination capacity of xenoperfused pig livers using a pharmacokinetic analysis. *Transplantation* 1999;68:209–214.
11. Foley DP, Vittimberga FJ, Quarfordt SH, et al. Biliary secretion of extracorporeal porcine livers with single and dual vessel perfusion. *Transplantation* 1999;68:362–368.
12. Calne RY. Organ transplantation between widely disparate species. *Transplant Proc* 1970;2:550.
13. Miyagawa S, Hirose H, Shirakura R, et al. The mechanism of discordant xenograft rejection. *Transplantation* 1988;46:825–830.
14. Gambiez L, Salame E, Chereau C, et al. The role of natural IgM in the hyperacute rejection of discordant heart xenografts. *Transplantation* 1992;54:577–583.
15. Platt JL, Turman MA, Noreen HJ, et al. An ELISA assay for xenoreactive natural antibodies. *Transplantation* 1990;49:1000–1001.
16. Platt JL, Lindman BJ, Chen H, et al. Endothelial cell antigens recognized by xenoreactive human natural antibodies. *Transplantation* 1990;50:817–822.
17. Platt JL, Vercellotti GM, Dalmasso AP, et al. Transplantation of discordant xenografts: a review of progress. *Immunol Today* 1990;11:450–456.
18. Dalmasso AP, Vercellotti GM, Fischel RJ, et al. Mechanism of complement activation in the hyperacute rejection of porcine organs transplanted into primate recipients. *Am J Pathol* 1992;140:1157–1166.
19. Platt JL. A perspective on xenograft rejection and accommodation. *Immunol Rev* 1994;141:127–149.
20. Galili U. Evolution and pathophysiology of the human natural anti-alpha galactosyl IgG (anti-Gal) antibody. *Springer Semin Immunopathol* 1993;15:155–171.
21. Oriol R, Ye Y, Koren E, et al. Carbohydrate antigens of pig tissues reacting with human natural antibodies as potential targets for hyperacute vascular rejection in pig-to-man organ xenotransplantation. *Transplantation* 1993;56:1433–1442.
22. Korsgren O, Jansson L, Moller E, et al. Pancreatic islet transplantation in the human. *Adv Nephrol Necker Hosp* 1993;22:371–386.
23. Macchiarini P, Oriol R, Azimzadeh A, et al. Evidence of human non-alpha galactosyl antibodies involved in the hyperacute rejection of pig lungs and their removal by pig organ perfusion. *J Thorac Cardiovasc Surg* 1998;116:831–843.
24. McKenzie IF, Koulmanda M, Mandel TE, et al. Pig islet xenografts are susceptible to "anti-pig" but not Gal-alpha(1,3)Gal antibody plus complement in Gal o/o mice. *J Immunol* 1998;161:5116–5119.
25. Tector AJ, Chen X, Soderland C, et al. Complement activation in discordant hepatic xenotransplantation. *Xenotransplantation* 1998;5:257–261.
26. Hammer C, Linke R, Seehofer D, et al. Xenogeneic rejection mechanisms shown by intravital microscopy. *Transplant Proc* 1998;30:4166–4167.
27. Sablinski T, Gianello PR, Bailin M, et al. Pig to monkey bone marrow and kidney xenotransplantation. *Surgery* 1997;121:381–391.
28. Bach FH, Winkler H, Ferran C, et al. Delayed xenograft rejection. *Immunol Today* 1996;17:379–384.
29. Saadi S, Platt JL. Immunology of xenotransplantation. *Life Sci* 1998;62:365–387.
30. Schmoeckel M, Bhatti FN, Zaidi A, et al. Orthotopic heart transplantation in a transgenic pig-to-primate model [published erratum appears in *Transplantation* 1998;66:943]. *Transplantation* 1998;65:1570–1577.
31. Xu H, Gundry SR, Hill AC, et al. Prolonged discordant cardiac xenograft survival in newborn recipients. *Circulation* 1997;96(suppl II):364–367.
32. Paul LC, Claas FH, van Es LA, et al. Accelerated rejection of a renal allograft associated with pretransplantation antibodies directed against donor antigens on endothelium and monocytes. *N Engl J Med* 1979;300:1258–1260.
33. Cooke SP, Hederer RA, Pearson JD, et al. Characterization of human IgG-binding xenoantigens expressed by porcine aortic endothelial cells. *Transplantation* 1995;60:1274–1284.
34. Yu PB, Parker W, Everett ML, et al. Immunochemical properties of anti-Gal alpha 1-3Gal antibodies after sensitization with xenogeneic tissues. *J Clin Immunol* 1999;19:116–126.
35. Candinas D, Belliveau S, Koyamada N, et al. T cell independence of macrophage and natural killer cell infiltration, cytokine production, and endothelial activation during delayed xenograft rejection. *Transplantation* 1996;62:1920–1927.
36. Candinas D, Koyamada N, Miyatake T, et al. Mononuclear cell infiltration, intragraft cytokine production and endothelial cell activation in delayed xenograft rejection are T cell-independent events. Presented at the Sixteenth International Congress of the Transplantation Society, 1996. Abstract Or422A.
37. Scheringa M, Schraa EO, Bouwman E, et al. Prolongation of survival of guinea pig heart grafts in cobra venom factor-treated rats by splenectomy. No additional effect of cyclosporine. *Transplantation* 1995;60:1350–1353.
38. Davis EA, Pruitt SK, Greene PS, et al. Inhibition of complement, evoked antibody, and cellular response prevents rejection of pig-to-primate cardiac xenografts. *Transplantation* 1996;62:1018–1023.
39. Hunig T, Bevan MJ. Ability of nude mice to generate alloreactive, xenoreactive and H-2-restricted cytotoxic T-lymphocyte responses. *Exp Cell Biol* 1984;52:7–11.
40. Vaessen LM, Broekhuizen R, Rozing J, et al. T-cell development during ageing in congenitally athymic (nude) rats. *Scand J Immunol* 1986;24:223–235.

41. Michler RE, McManus RP, Smith CR, et al. Prolongation of primate cardiac xenograft survival with cyclosporine. *Transplantation* 1987; 44:632–636.

42. McManus RP, Kinney T, Komorowski R, et al. Reversibility of cardiac xenograft rejection in primates. *J Heart Lung Transplant* 1991; 10:567–576.

43. Kawauchi M, Gundry SR, de Begona JA, et al. Prolonged survival of orthotopically transplanted heart xenograft in infant baboons. *J Thorac Cardiovasc Surg* 1993;106:779–786.

44. Roslin MS, Tranbaugh RE, Panza A, et al. One-year monkey heart xenograft survival in cyclosporine-treated baboons. Suppression of the xenoantibody response with total-lymphoid irradiation. *Transplantation* 1992;54:949–955.

45. Auchincloss H Jr. Xenogeneic transplantation. a review. *Transplantation* 1988;46:1–20.

46. Alexandre GPJ, Gianello P, Latinne D, et al. Plasmapheresis and splenectomy in experimental renal xenotransplantation. In: Hardy MA, ed. *Xenograft 25*. New York: Elsevier Science Publishers, 1989: 259–266.

47. Sachs DH. Pig-to-primate xenotransplantation: tolerance through mixed chimerism. *Xeno* 1995;3:52–55.

48. Latinne D, Gianello P, Smith CV, et al. Xenotransplantation from pig to cynomolgus monkey: approach toward tolerance induction. *Transplant Proc* 1993;25:336–338.

49. Pomerri F, Bressanin F, Muzzio PC. The kidney xenograft. An echographic assessment of the tissue parameters of the normal pig kidney [in Italian]. *Radiol Med (Torino)* 1994;87:107–110.

50. Kobayashi T, Taniguchi S, Ye Y, et al. Delayed xenograft rejection in C3-depleted discordant (pig-to-baboon) cardiac xenografts treated with cobra venom factor. *Transplant Proc* 1996;28:560.

51. Waterworth PD, Cozzi E, Tolan MJ, et al. Pig-to-primate cardiac xenotransplantation and cyclophosphamide therapy. *Transplant Proc* 1997;29:899–900.

52. Tze WJ, Tai J, Cheung S. Human islet xenograft survival in diabetic rats. A functional and immunohistological study. *Transplantation* 1990;49: 502–505.

53. Simeonovic CJ, Ceredig R, Wilson JD. Effect of GK1.5 monoclonal antibody dosage on survival of pig proislet xenografts in CD4+ T cell-depleted mice. *Transplantation* 1990;49:849–856.

54. Simeonovic CJ, Wilson JD, Ceredig R. Antibody-induced rejection of pig proislet xenografts in CD4+ T cell-depleted diabetic mice. *Transplantation* 1990;50:657–662.

55. Wren SM, Wang SC, Thai NL, et al. Evidence for early Th 2 T cell predominance in xenoreactivity. *Transplantation* 1993;56:905–911.

56. Wecker H, Winn HJ, Auchincloss H Jr. *Xenotransplantation* 1994;1: 8–16.

57. Friedman T, Shimizu A, Smith RN, et al. Human CD4+ T cells mediate rejection of porcine xenografts. *J Immunol* 1999;162:5256–5262.

58. Desai NM, Bassiri H, Kim J, et al. Islet allograft, islet xenograft, and skin allograft survival in CD8+ T lymphocyte-deficient mice. *Transplantation* 1993;55:718–722.

59. Chavin KD, Lau HT, Bromberg JS. Prolongation of allograft and xenograft survival in mice by anti-CD2 monoclonal antibodies. *Transplantation* 1992;54:286–291.

60. Langer A, Valdivia LA, Murase N, et al. Humoral and cellular immunopathology of hepatic and cardiac hamster-into-rat xenograft rejection. Marked stimulation of IgM++bright/IgD+dull splenic B cells. *Am J Pathol* 1993;143:85–98.

61. Sheffield CD, Hadley GA, Dirden BM, et al. Prolonged cardiac xenograft survival is induced by intrathymic splenocyte injection. *J Surg Res* 1994;57:55–59.

62. Mandel TE, Koulmanda M. Rejection of fetal allo and xenografts in nude mice reconstituted with defined cell populations. Presented at the Sixteenth International Congress of the Transplantation Society, 1996. Abstract Or457A.

63. Benda B, Korsgren O. Transfer of immunocompetent cells to athymic nude mice previously transplanted with fetal porcine islet-like cell clusters. *Transplant Proc* 1997;29:930.

64. Fryer JP, Leventhal JR, Dalmasso AP, et al. Beyond hyperacute rejection. Accelerated rejection in a discordant xenograft model by adoptive transfer of specific cell subsets. *Transplantation* 1995;59:171–176.

65. Woolnough JA, Misko IS, Lafferty KJ. Cytotoxic and proliferative lymphocyte responses to allogeneic and xenogeneic antigens *in vitro*. *Aust J Exp Biol Med Sci* 1979;57:467–477.

66. Swain SL, Dutton RW, Schwab R, et al. Xenogeneic human anti-mouse T cell responses are due to the activity of the same functional T cell subsets responsible for allospecific and major histocompatibility complex-restricted responses. *J Exp Med* 1983;157:720–729.

67. Yoshizawa K, Yano A. Mouse T lymphocyte proliferative responses specific for human MHC products in mouse anti-human xenogeneic MLR. *J Immunol* 1984;132:2820–2829.

68. Auchincloss H Jr. Why is cell-mediated xenograft rejection so strong? *Xeno* 1995;3:19–22.

69. Shah AS, Itescu S, O'Hair DP, et al. Importance of cell-mediated immune responses in rejection of concordant heart xenografts in primates. *Transplant Proc* 1996;28:775–776.

70. Bravery CA, Rose ML, Yacoub MH. Proliferative responses of highly purified human CD4+ T cells to porcine endothelial cells. *Transplant Proc* 1994;26:1157–1158.

71. Moses RD, Winn HJ, Auchincloss H Jr. Evidence that multiple defects in cell-surface molecule interactions across species differences are responsible for diminished xenogeneic T cell responses. *Transplantation* 1992;53:203–209.

72. Ohta Y, Gotoh M, Ohzato H, et al. Both donor and recipient adhesion molecules play a crucial role in inducing rejection of rat xenogeneic islets in mice. *Transplant Proc* 1997;29:953.

73. Wolf LA, Coulombe M, Gill RG. Donor antigen-presenting cell-independent rejection of islet xenografts. *Transplantation* 1995;60: 1164–1170.

74. Zeng Y, Torres MA, Thistelthwaite JR Jr, et al. Prolongation of human pancreatic islet xenografts by pretreatment of islets with anti-human ICAM-1 monoclonal antibody. *Transplant Proc* 1994;26:1120.

75. Lenschow DJ, Zeng Y, Thistlethwaite JR, et al. Long-term survival of xenogeneic pancreatic islet grafts induced by CTLA4lg. *Science* 1992;257:789–792.

76. Melchers I, Fey K, Eichmann K. Quantitative studies on T cell diversity. III. Limiting dilution analysis of precursor cells for T helper cells reactive to xenogeneic erythrocytes. *J Exp Med* 1982;156:1587–1603.

77. Cunningham AC, Butler TJ, Kirby JA. Demonstration of direct xenorecognition of porcine cells by human cytotoxic T lymphocytes. *Immunology* 1994;81:268–272.

78. Dorling A, Binns R, Lechler RI. Direct human T-cell anti-pig xenoresponses are vigorous but significantly weaker than direct alloresponses. *Transplant Proc* 1996;28:653.

79. Chan DV, Auchincloss H Jr. Human anti-pig cell-mediated cytotoxicity *in vitro* may have as many as three different components. Presented at the Third International Congress for Xenotransplantation, 1995.

80. Rollins SA, Kennedy SP, Chodera AJ, et al. Evidence that activation of human T cells by porcine endothelium involves direct recognition of porcine SLA and costimulation by porcine ligands for LFA-1 and CD2. *Transplantation* 1994;57:1709–1716.

81. Shishido S, Naziruddin B, Howard T, et al. Indirect recognition of porcine xenoantigens presented in the context of self HLA class II molecules by human CD4+ T cell clones. Presented at the sixteenth meeting of the American Society of Transplant Physicians, 1997. Abstract 630A.

82. Wallgren AC, Karlsson-Parra A, Korsgren O. The main infiltrating cell in xenograft rejection is a CD4+ macrophage and not a T lymphocyte. *Transplantation* 1995;60:594–601.

83. Marquet RL, van Overdam K, Boudesteijn EA, et al. Immunobiology of delayed xenograft rejection. *Transplant Proc* 1997;29:955–956.

84. Matsumiya G, Shirakura R, Miyagawa S, et al. Analysis of rejection mechanism in the rat to mouse cardiac xenotransplantation. Role and characteristics of anti-endothelial cell antibodies. *Transplantation* 1994;57:1653–1660.

85. Hancock WW, Bach FH. Monocyte chemoattractant protein (MCP-1) expression during xenograft rejection. Presented at the Third International Congress for Xenotransplantation, 1995. Abstract 285A.

86. Meehan SM, Kozlowski T, Sablinski T, et al. Delayed xenograft rejection in pig to primate renal xenografts: widespread endothelial apoptosis with little detectable antibody or inflammatory cell accumulation. Presented at the Sixteenth International Congress of the Transplantation Society, 1996. Abstract Or30A.

87. Khalfoun B, Janin P, Machet MC, et al. Discordant xenogeneic cellular interactions when hyperacute rejection is prevented: analysis using an *ex vivo* model of pig kidney perfused with human lymphocytes. *Transplant Proc* 1996;28:647.

88. Larkin DF, Takano T, Standfield SD, et al. Experimental orthotopic corneal xenotransplantation in the rat. Mechanisms of graft rejection. *Transplantation* 1995;60:491–497.
89. Itescu S, Kwiatkowski P, Wang SF, et al. Circulating human mononuclear cells exhibit augmented lysis of pig endothelium after activation with interleukin 2. *Transplantation* 1996;62:1927–1933.
90. Itescu S, Kwiatkowski PA, Artrip JH, et al. Role of natural killer cells and macrophages in delayed xenograft rejection of pig-to-primate cardiac transplantation. Presented at the meeting of the American Society of Transplant Physicians, 1997. Abstract 605A.
91. Fukushima N, Kawauchi M, Bouchart T, et al. Graft atherosclerosis in concordant cardiac transplantation. *Transplant Proc* 1994;26:1059–1060.
92. Scheringa M, Buchner B, Geerling RA, et al. Chronic rejection after concordant xenografting. *Transplant Proc* 1994;26:1346–1347.
93. Lin Y, Vandeputte M, Waer M. Effect of leflunomide and cyclosporine on the occurrence of chronic xenograft lesions. *Kidney Int* 1995; 52(suppl):S23–S28.
94. Xiao F, Shen J, Chong A, et al. Control and reversal of chronic xenograft rejection in hamster-to-rat cardiac transplantation. *Transplant Proc* 1996;28:691–692.
95. Dorling A, Riesbeck K, Warrens A, et al. Clinical xenotransplantation of solid organs. *Lancet* 1997;349:867–871.
96. O'Hair DP, McManus RP, Komorowski R. Inhibition of chronic vascular rejection in primate cardiac xenografts using mycophenolate mofetil. *Ann Thorac Surg* 1994;58:1311–1315.
97. Ierino FL, Kozlowski T, Siegel JB, et al. Disseminated intravascular coagulation in association with the delayed rejection of pig-to-baboon renal xenografts. *Transplantation* 1998;66:1439–1450.
98. Sachs DH, Sykes M, Greenstein JL, et al. Tolerance and xenograft survival. *Nat Med* 1995;1:969.
99. Dorling A, Lechler RI. T cell-mediated xenograft rejection: specific tolerance is probably required for long term xenograft survival. *Xenotransplantation* 1998;5:234–245.
100. Beschorner WE, Lomis TJ. Xenotransplantation: potential opportunity versus resistant challenge. In: Racusen LC, Solez K, Burdick JF, eds. *Kidney transplant rejection: diagnosis and treatment,* 3rd ed. New York: Marcel Dekker, 1998:201–250.
101. Gammie JS, Kaufman CL, Michaels MG, et al. Xenotransplantation: strategies to achieve donor-specific tolerance and immune reconstitution across species barriers through mixed bone marrow chimerism. *Mol Diagn* 1996;1:219–224.
102. Allan JS. Xenograft transplantation and the infectious disease conundrum. *Instit Lab Animal Resources J* 1995;37:37–48.
103. Shalala DE. Draft Public Health Service (PHS) guideline on infectious disease issues in xenotransplantation. *Federal Register* 1996;61:49920–49932.
104. Martini GA. Marburg agent disease in man. *Trans R Soc Trop Med Hyg* 1969;63:295–302.
105. Ebola haemorrhagic fever in Zaire, 1976. *Bull World Health Organ* 1978;56:271–293.
106. Chapman LE, Folks TM, Salomon DR, et al. Xenotransplantation and xenogeneic infections. *N Engl J Med* 1995;333:1498–1501.
107. Deinhardt F. Biology of primate retroviruses. In: Klein G, ed. *Viral oncology.* New York: Raven Press, 1980:357–398.
108. Michaels MG, Simmons RL. Xenotransplant-associated zoonoses. strategies for prevention. *Transplantation* 1994;57:1–7.
109. Ye Y, Niekrasz M, Kosanke S, et al. The pig as a potential organ donor for man. A study of potentially transferable disease from donor pig to recipient man. *Transplantation* 1994;57:694–703.
110. Patience C, Takeuchi Y, Weiss RA. Infection of human cells by an endogenous retrovirus of pigs. *Nat Med* 1997;3:282–286.
111. Martin U, Steinhoff G, Kiessig V, et al. Porcine endogenous retrovirus (PERV) was not transmitted from transplanted porcine endothelial cells to baboons *in vivo. Transpl Int* 1998;11:247–251.
112. Heneine W, Tibell A, Switzer WM, et al. No evidence of infection with porcine endogenous retrovirus in recipients of porcine islet-cell xenografts. *Lancet* 1998;352:695–699.
113. Patience C, Patton GS, Takeuchi Y, et al. No evidence of pig DNA or retroviral infection in patients with short-term extracorporeal connection to pig kidneys. *Lancet* 1998;352:699–701.
114. Paradis K, Langford G, Long Z, et al. Search for cross-species transmission of porcine endogenous retrovirus in patients treated with living pig tissue. *Science* 1999;285:1236–1241.
115. Switzer WM, Shanmugam V, Chapman L, et al. Polymerase chain reaction assays for the diagnosis of infection with the porcine endogenous retrovirus and the detection of pig cells in human and nonhuman recipients of pig xenografts. *Transplantation* 1999;68:183–188.
116. Alexandre GPJ, Squifflet JP, De Bruyere M, et al. Present experience in a series of 26 ABO-incompatible living donor renal allografts. *Transplant Proc* 1987;19:4538–4542.
117. Bier M, Beavers CD, Merriman WG, et al. Selective plasmapheresis in dogs for delay of heterograft response. *Trans Am Soc Artif Intern Organs* 1970;16:325–333.
118. Suga H, Ishida N, Kimikawa M, et al. Prolongation of cardiac xenograft function after reduction of natural antibodies using double filtration plasmapheresis. *ASAIO Trans* 1991;37:M433–M434.
119. Sato Y, Kimikawa M, Suga H, et al. Prolongation of cardiac xenograft survival by double filtration plasmapheresis and *ex vivo* immunoadsorption. *ASAIO J* 1992;38:M673–M675.
120. Van de Stadt J, Meriggi F, Vendeville B, et al. Prolongation of heart xenograft survival in the rat: effectiveness of cyclosporine in preventing early xenoantibody rebound after membrane plasmapheresis. *Transplant Proc* 1989;21:543–545.
121. Nair J, Fair JH, Burdick JF, et al. Role of naturally occurring xenoantibodies in hyperacute rejection strengthened by their avid binding to *ex vivo* pig to human liver xenografts and to isolated pig liver preparations. *Transplant Proc* 1994;26:1344–1345.
122. Kroshus TJ, Dalmasso AP, Leventhal JR, et al. Antibody removal by column immunoabsorption prevents tissue injury in an *ex vivo* model of pig-to-human xenograft hyperacute rejection. *J Surg Res* 1995;59:43–50.
123. Taniguchi S, Neethling FA, Korchagina EY, et al. *In vivo* immunoadsorption of antipig antibodies in baboons using a specific Gal(alpha)1-3Gal column. *Transplantation* 1996;62:1379–1384.
124. Cooper DK, Ye Y, Niekrasz M, et al. Specific intravenous carbohydrate therapy. A new concept in inhibiting antibody-mediated rejection—experience with ABO-incompatible cardiac allografting in the baboon. *Transplantation* 1993;56:769–777.
125. Li S, Neethling FA, Yeh JC, et al. Potent inhibition of human and baboon anti-alpha Gal antibodies by a subfraction of oligosaccharides derived from porcine stomach mucin. *Transplant Proc* 1996;8:558.
126. Xu H, Edwards NM, Chen JM, et al. Newborn baboon serum lacks natural anti-pig xenoantibody. *Transplantation* 1995;59:1189–1194.
127. Xu H, Edwards NM, Chen JM, et al. Natural antipig xenoantibody is absent in neonatal human serum. *J Heart Lung Transplant* 1995;14:749–754.
128. Minanov OP, Itescu S, Neethling FA, et al. Anti-GaL IgG antibodies in sera of newborn humans and baboons and its significance in pig xenotransplantation. *Transplantation* 1997;63:182–186.
129. Kaplon RJ, Michler RE, Xu H, et al. Absence of hyperacute rejection in newborn pig-to-baboon cardiac xenografts. *Transplantation* 1995;59:1–6.
130. Xu H, Oluwole S, Michler RE. Expression of newborn pig endothelial cell xenoantigens recognized by baboon natural xenoantibody. *Transplant Proc* 1996;28:627.
131. Snyder GB, Ballesteros E, Zarco RM, et al. Prolongation of renal xenografts by complement suppression. *Surg Forum* 1966;17:478–480.
132. Fearon DT. Anti-inflammatory and immunosuppressive effects of recombinant soluble complement receptors. *Clin Exp Immunol* 1991;86(suppl 1):43–46.
133. Tabei I, Elfeki SG, Nakamura J, et al. Construction, function and *in vivo* expression of a complement receptor type 1 containing recombinant adenovirus for use in xenotransplantation. *Transplant Proc* 1997;29:933–934.
134. Rollins SA, Matis LA, Springhorn JP, et al. Monoclonal antibodies directed against human C5 and C8 block complement-mediated damage of xenogeneic cells and organs. *Transplantation* 1995;60:1284–1292.
135. Tearle RG, Tange MJ, Zannettino ZL, et al. The alpha-1,3-galactosyltransferase knockout mouse. Implications for xenotransplantation. *Transplantation* 1996;61:13–19.
136. McCurry KR, Diamond LE, Kooyman DL, et al. Human complement regulatory proteins expressed in transgenic swine protect swine xenografts from humoral injury. *Transplant Proc* 1996;28:758.
137. Byrne GW, McCurry KR, Martin MJ, et al. Transgenic pigs expressing human CD59 and decay-accelerating factor produce an intrinsic barrier to complement-mediated damage. *Transplantation* 1997;63:149–155.

138. Rosengard AM, Cary NR, Langford GA, et al. Tissue expression of human complement inhibitor, decay-accelerating factor, in transgenic pigs. A potential approach for preventing xenograft rejection. *Transplantation* 1995;59:1325–1333.

139. White DJ, Cozzi E, Langford G, et al. The control of hyperacute rejection by genetic engineering of the donor species. *Eye* 1995;9:185–189.

140. Sandrin MS, Fodor WL, Mouhtouris E, et al. Enzymatic remodelling of the carbohydrate surface of a xenogenic cell substantially reduces human antibody binding and complement-mediated cytolysis. *Nat Med* 1995;1:1261–1267.

141. Bracy JL, Sachs DH, Iacomini J. Inhibition of xenoreactive natural antibody production by retroviral gene therapy. *Science* 1998;28: 1845–1847.

142. Nair RV, Morris RE. Immunosuppression in cardiac transplantation: a new era in immunopharmacology. *Curr Opin Cardiol* 1995;10: 207–217.

143. Starzl TE, Murase N, Demetris AJ, et al. Allograft and xenograft acceptance under FK-506 and other immunosuppressant treatment. *Ann N Y Acad Sci* 1993;685:46–51.

144. Valdivia LA, Monden M, Gotoh M, et al. Evidence that deoxyspergualin prevents sensitization and first-set cardiac xenograft rejection in rats by suppression of antibody formation. *Transplantation* 1990; 50:132–136.

145. Thomas F, Pittman K, Ljung T, et al. Deoxyspergualin is a unique immunosuppressive agent with selective utility in inducing tolerance to pancreas islet xenografts. *Transplant Proc* 1995;27:417–419.

146. Fujino Y, Kawamura T, Hullett DA, et al. Evaluation of cyclosporine, mycophenolate mofetil, and brequinar sodium combination therapy on hamster-to-rat cardiac xenotransplantation. *Transplantation* 1994;57:41–46.

147. Yatscoff RW, Wang S, Keenan R, et al. Efficacy of rapamycin, RS-61443 and cyclophosphamide in the prolongation of survival of discordant pig to rabbit cardiac xenografts. *Can J Cardiol* 1994;10: 711–716.

148. Cramer DV. Brequinar sodium. *Pediatr Nephrol* 1995;9:S52-S55.

149. Zhao Y, Swenson K, Sergio JJ, et al. Skin graft tolerance across a discordant xenogeneic barrier. *Nat Med* 1996;11:1211–1216.

150. Wilmut I, Schnleke AE, McWhir J, et al. Viable offspring derived from fetal and adult mammalian cells. *Nature* 1997;385:810–813.

151. Fox IJ, Athan E, Fisher J, et al. Use of gene therapy to induce human-mouse xenogeneic chimerism. *Surgery* 1993;114:174–181.

152. Schumacher I, Jeevarathnam S, Rubbocki R, et al. Use of gene therapy to induce antigen-specific immunologic unresponsiveness to class I xenogeneic major histocompatibility complex antigens. *Transplant Proc* 1995;27:313–314.

153. Schumacher IK, Newberg MH, Jackson JD, et al. Use of gene therapy to suppress the antigen-specific immune responses in mice to an HLA antigen. *Transplantation* 1996;62:831–836.

154. Shafer GW, Emery DW, Gustafsson K, et al. Expression of a swine class II gene in murine bone marrow hepatopoietic cells by retroviral-mediated gene transfer. *Proc Natl Acad Sci U S A* 1991;88:9760–9764.

155. Ierino FL, Banerjee PT, Gere J, et al. A genetic approach toward tolerance induction in a pig to baboon preclinical xenotransplantation model. Presented at the sixteenth annual meeting of the American Society of Transplant Physicians, 1997. Abstract 631A.

156. Schwartz RH. Immunological tolerance. In: Paul WE, ed. *Fundamental immunology*. New York: Raven Press, 1993:677–731.

157. Billingham R, Brent L, Medawar P. Quantitative studies on tissue transplantation immunity. III. Actively acquired tolerance. *Proc R Soc Lond Biol* 1956;238:357–415.

158. Triplett EL. On the mechanism of immunologic self recognition. *J Immunol* 1962;89:505–510.

159. McCullagh P. Interception of the development of self tolerance in fetal lambs. *Eur J Immunol* 1989;19:1387–1392.

160. Yard BA, Claas FH, Paape ME, et al. Recognition of a tissue-specific polymorphism by graft infiltrating T-cell clones isolated from a renal allograft with acute rejection. *Nephrol Dial Transplant* 1994;9: 805–810.

161. Rice HE, Flake AW, Hedrick MH, et al. Effect of xenogeneic chimerism in a human/sheep model on natural antibody. *J Surg Res* 1993;54:355–359.

162. Rios RP, Rodriguez PA, Ibanez GA, et al. Severe hemolytic anemia caused by anti-AB in renal transplantation with minor ABO incompatibility. *Sangre (Barcelona)* 1992;37:197–199.

163. Ramsey G. Red cell antibodies arising from solid organ transplants. *Transfusion* 1991;31:76–86.

164. Fischel RJ, Matas AJ, Platt JL, et al. Cardiac xenografting in the pig-to-rhesus monkey model: manipulation of anti-endothelial antibody prolongs survival. *J Heart Lung Transplant* 1992;11:965–973.

165. Hechenleitner P, Walter M, Candinas D, et al. Mechanisms of accommodation in hamster-to-rat cardiac xenografts: studies on second-set grafts. Presented at the Sixteenth International Congress of the Transplantation Society, 1996. Abstract 110or.

166. Vriens PW, Bouwman E, Scheringa M. Induction of accommodation prevents hyperacute rejection. *Transplant Proc* 1997;29:597–598.

167. Parker W, Holzknecht ZE, Song A, et al. Fate of antigen in xenotransplantation: implications for acute vascular rejection and accommodation. *Am J Pathol* 1998;152:829–839.

168. Bach FH, Ferran C, Hechenleitner P, et al. Accommodation of vascularized xenografts: expression of "protective genes" by donor endothelial cells in a host Th2 cytokine environment. *Nat Med* 1997;3: 196–204.

169. Rosengard BR, Kortz EO, Guzzetta PC, et al. Transplantation in miniature swine: analysis of graft-infiltrating lymphocytes provides evidence for local suppression. *Hum Immunol* 1990;28:153–158.

170. Rosengard BR, Fishbein JM, Gianello P, et al. Retransplantation in miniature swine. Lack of a requirement for graft adaptation for maintenance of specific renal allograft tolerance. *Transplantation* 1994; 57:794–799.

171. Dorling A, Delikouras A, Nohadani M, et al. *In vitro* accommodation of porcine endothelial cells by low dose human anti-pig antibody: reduced binding of human lymphocytes by accommodated cells associated with increased nitric oxide production. *Xenotransplantation* 1998;5:84–92.

172. He S, Wang HM, Ogden TE, et al. Transplantation of cultured human retinal pigment epithelium into rabbit subretina. *Graefes Arch Clin Exp Ophthalmol* 1993;231:737–742.

173. Deacon T, Schumacher J, Dinsmore J, et al. Histological evidence of fetal pig neural cell survival after transplantation into a patient with Parkinson's disease. *Nat Med* 1997;3:350–353.

174. Bobzien B, Yasunami Y, Majercik M, et al. Intratesticular transplants of islet xenografts (rat to mouse). *Diabetes* 1983;32:213–216.

175. Lee HC, Ahn KJ, Lim SK, et al. Allotransplantation of rat islets into the cisterna magma of streptozotocin-induced diabetic rats. *Transplantation* 1992;53:513–516.

176. Tze WJ, Tai J. Immunological studies in diabetic rat recipients with a pancreatic islet cell allograft in the brain. *Transplantation* 1989;47: 1053–1057.

177. French LE, Hahne M, Viard I, et al. Fas and Fas ligand in embryos and adult mice: ligand expression in several immune-privileged tissues and coexpression in adult tissues characterized by apoptotic cell turnover. *J Cell Biol* 1996;133:335–343.

178. Griffith TS, Yu X, Herndon JM, et al. CD95-induced apoptosis of lymphocytes in an immune privileged site induces immunological tolerance. *Immunity* 1996;5:7–16.

179. Bellgrau D, Gold D, Selawry H, et al. A role for CD95 ligand in preventing graft rejection. *Nature* 1995;377:630–632.

180. Rathmell JC, Cooke MP, Ho WY, et al. CD95 (Fas)-dependent elimination of self-reactive B cells upon interaction with CD4+ T cells. *Nature* 1995;376:181–184.

181. Knipping E, Krammer PH, Onel KB, et al. Levels of soluble Fas/APO-1/CD95 in systemic lupus erythematosus and juvenile rheumatoid arthritis. *Arthritis Rheum* 1995;38:1735–1737.

182. Amasaki Y, Kobayashi S, Takeda T, et al. Up-regulated expression of Fas antigen (CD95) by peripheral naive and memory T cell subsets in patients with systemic lupus erythematosus (SLE): a possible mechanism for lymphopenia. *Clin Exp Immunol* 1995;99:245–250.

183. Afford SC, Williams A, Fear J, et al. A potential role for Fas (CD95) and Fas ligand (CD95l) in liver allograft rejection following orthotopic liver transplantation. Presented at the Sixteenth International Congress of the Transplantation Society, 1996. Abstract Po153A.

184. Foote LC, Howard RG, Marshak-Rothstein A, et al. IL-4 induces Fas resistance in B cells. *J Immunol* 1996;157:2749–2753.

185. Krams SM, Fox CK, Beatty PR, et al. Human hepatocytes produce an isoform of FAS that inhibits apoptosis. *Transplantation* 1998;65: 713–721.

186. Cowan MJ, Golbus M. *In utero* hematopoietic stem cell transplants for inherited diseases. *Am J Pediatr Hematol Oncol* 1994;16:35–42.

187. Harrison MR, Slotnick RN, Crombleholme TM, et al. *In-utero* transplantation of fetal liver haemopoietic stem cells in monkeys. *Lancet* 1989;2:1425–1427.

188. Zanjani ED, Pallavicini MG, Ascensao JL, et al. Engraftment and long-term expression of human fetal hemopoietic stem cells in sheep following transplantation *in utero*. *J Clin Invest* 1992;89:1178–1188.

189. Srour EF, Zanjani ED, Brandt JE, et al. Sustained human hematopoiesis in sheep transplanted *in utero* during early gestation with fractionated adult human bone marrow cells. *Blood* 1992;79:1404–1412.

190. Shields LE, Bryant EM, Easterling TR, et al. Fetal liver cell transplantation for the creation of lymphohematopoietic chimerism in fetal baboons. *Am J Obstet Gynecol* 1995;173:1157–1160.

191. Mychaliska GB, Rice HE, Tarantal AF, et al. *In utero* hematopoietic stem cell transplants induce tolerance for postnatal kidney transplantation in monkeys. *Surg Forum* 1996;47:443–445.

192. Crombleholme TM, Harrison MR, Zanjani ED. *In utero* transplantation of hematopoietic stem cells in sheep: the role of T cells in engraftment and graft-versus-host disease. *J Pediatr Surg* 1990;25:885–892.

193. Marrack P, Lo D, Brinster R, et al. The effects of thymus environment on T cell development and tolerance. *Cell* 1988;53:627–634.

194. Sullivan KM. Graft-versus-host disease. In: Forman SJ, Blume KG, Thomas ED, eds. *Bone marrow transplantation.* Boston: Blackwell Scientific Publications, 1994:339–362.

195. Ildstad ST, Sachs DH. Reconstitution with syngeneic plus allogeneic or xenogeneic bone marrow leads to specific acceptance of allografts or xenografts. *Nature* 1984;307:168–170.

196. Sykes M, Lee LA, Sachs DH. Xenograft tolerance. *Immunol Rev* 1994;141:245–276.

197. Sharabi Y, Aksentijevich I, Sundt TM III, et al. Specific tolerance induction across a xenogeneic barrier: production of mixed rat/mouse lymphohematopoietic chimeras using a nonlethal preparative regimen. *J Exp Med* 1990;172:195–202.

198. Tanaka M, Latinne D, Gianello P, et al. Xenotransplantation from pig to monkey: the potential for overcoming xenograft rejection through induction of chimerism. *Transplant Proc* 1994;26:1326–1327.

199. Sprent J, Lo D, Gao E-K, et al. T cell selection in the thymus. *Immunol Rev* 1988;101:173–190.

200. Beschorner WE, Namnoum JD, Hess AD, et al. Cyclosporin A and the thymus. Immunopathology. *Am J Pathol* 1987;126:487–496.

201. Beschorner WE, Armas OA. Loss of medullary dendritic cells in the thymus after cyclosporine and irradiation. *Cell Immunol* 1991;132:505–514.

202. Posselt AM, Barker CF, Tamaszewski JE, et al. Induction of donor-specific unresponsiveness by intrathymic islet transplantation. *Science* 1990;249:1293–1295.

203. Markmann JF, Naji A, Barker CF. Acquired central immune tolerance following intrathymic inoculation. In: Alexander JW, Good RA, eds. *Transplantation tolerance induction.* Georgetown, TX: Landes Company, 1996:53–64.

204. Nakafusa Y, Goss JA, Mohanakumar T, et al. Induction of donor-specific tolerance to cardiac but not skin or renal allografts by intrathymic injection of splenocyte alloantigen. *Transplantation* 1993;55:877–882.

205. Zeng Y, Bluestone JA, Ildstad ST, et al. Long-term functional xenograft tolerance after intrathymic islet transplantation (Lewis rat-to-B6 mouse). *Transplant Proc* 1993;25:438–439.

206. Hess AD, Horwitz L, Beschorner WE, et al. Development of graft-vs-host disease-like syndrome in cyclosporine-treated rats after syngeneic bone marrow transplantation. *J Exp Med* 1985;16:718–730.

207. Beschorner WE, Yao X, Divic J. Recruitment of semiallogeneic dendritic cells to the thymus during post-cyclosporine thymic regeneration. *Transplantation* 1995;60:1326–1330.

208. Beschorner WE. Method for induction of antigen-specific immune tolerance. U.S. patent number 08/573,648, January 28, 1997.

209. Salaun J, et al. Thymic epithelium tolerizes for histocompatibility antigens. *Science* 1990;247:1471–1474.

210. Wu A, Yamada K, Awwad M, et al. Prolonged xenogeneic skin graft survival after porcine thymic transplantation in a nonhuman primate model. *Transplantation* 199;67:S419.

211. Harding FA, McArthur JG, Gross JA, et al. CD28-mediated signalling co-stimulates murine T cells and prevents induction of anergy of T-cell clones. *Nature* 1992;356:607–609.

212. Rehman A, Tu Y, Arima T, et al. Long-term survival of rat to mouse cardiac xenografts with prolonged blockade of CD28-B7 interaction combined with peritransplant T-cell depletion. *Surgery* 1996;120:205–212.

213. Morris PJ, Ting A, Stocker JW. Leucocyte antigens in renal transplantation. The paradox of blood transfusion in renal transplantation. *Med J Aust* 1968;2:1088–1090.

214. Opelz G, Senger DPS, Mickey MR, et al. Effect of blood transfusions on subsequent kidney transplants. *Transplant Proc* 1973;5:253–259.

215. Brunson ME, Tchervenkov JI, Alexandre JW. Enhancement of allograft survival by donor-specific transfusion one day prior to transplant. *Transplantation* 1991;52:545–549.

216. Rao AS, Starzl TE, Demetris AJ, et al. The two-way paradigm of transplantation immunology. *Clin Immunol Immunopathol* 1996;80:S46–S51.

217. Umesue M, Mayumi H, Nishimura Y, et al. Donor-specific prolongation of rat skin graft survival induced by rat-donor cells and cyclophosphamide under coadministration of monoclonal antibodies against T cell receptor alpha beta and natural killer cells in mice. *Transplantation* 1996;61:116–124.

218. Nardo B, Valdivia LA, Pan F, et al. Pretransplant xenogeneic blood transfusion combined with FK506 prolongs hamster-to-rat liver xenograft survival. *Transplant Proc* 1994;26:1208.

219. Valdivia LA, Monden M, Gotoh M, et al. Suppressor cells induced by donor-specific transfusion and deoxyspergualin in rat cardiac xenografts. *Transplantation* 1991;52:594–599.

220. Beschorner WE. Surrogate tolerogenesis for the development of tolerance to xenografts. Patent cooperation treaty serial number WO 94/27622, 1994.

221. Beschorner WE, Qian Z, Mattei P, et al. Induction of human chimerism and functional suppressor cells in fetal pigs: feasibility of surrogate tolerogenesis for xenotransplantation. *Transplant Proc* 1996;28:648–649.

222. Lomis TJ, Hess AD, Blakemore KJ, et al. Novel process for inducing specific immune tolerance to pig xenografts without severe immune suppression. *Surg Forum* 1996;47:411.

223. Beschorner WE, Lomis TJ, Hess AD, et al. Prolonged acceptance of pig xenografts without severe immune deficiency. Presented at the American Society of Transplant Physicians, Chicago, Illinois, 1997. Abstract 491.

224. Sudan DL, Radio SJ, Matamoros A Jr, et al. Effect of surrogate tolerogenesis on the vascular rejection of pig heart xenografts. *Transplantation (in press)*.

225. Miyatake T, Koyamada N, Hancock WW, et al. Survival of accommodated cardiac xenografts upon retransplantation into cyclosporine-treated recipients. *Transplantation* 1998;65:1563.

Transplantation of the Liver, edited by Willis C. Maddrey, Eugene R. Schiff, and Michael F. Sorrell. Lippincott Williams & Wilkins, Philadelphia © 2001.

CHAPTER 28

Hepatocyte Transplantation

Ira J. Fox and Jayanta Roy-Chowdhury

Liver transplantation has become the treatment of choice for liver failure and liver-based metabolic disorders. Improved survival following transplantation has led to a broader indication for its use. As a result, tremendous pressure has been placed on the supply of organs available for transplantation. Conceptually, hepatocyte transplantation could reduce the need for whole-organ transplantation. Numerous laboratory studies have shown that hepatocyte transplantation should be effective in the treatment of some forms of liver failure and metabolic disease. Livers not suitable for whole-organ transplantation could provide a source of hepatocytes for transplantation. Unlike whole livers, isolated hepatocytes can be cryopreserved for use when needed. In addition, laboratory studies have shown that hepatocytes can be modified, genetically or otherwise, to abrogate rejection.

Liver cell transplantation would require minimal intervention and would be unlikely to compromise native liver function. It has been considered particularly suitable for treating acute liver failure, in which the liver architecture remains normal and there is considerable restorative potential. Because the host liver and its vasculature remain intact, the consequences of graft loss would be relatively small. Hepatocyte transplantation could effectively replace whole-organ transplantation for the treatment of many inherited disorders of metabolism because transplantation of a relatively small number of liver cells, representing only a fraction of the liver mass, could be used to avoid removing an otherwise normally functioning native liver. Since only a fraction of normal protein activity will functionally correct many metabolic deficiencies, a single donor liver could potentially provide hepatocytes for more than one patient. The procedure would not interfere with subsequent liver trans-

plantation, should that become necessary, or liver-directed gene therapy, when it becomes available.

So far, human hepatocyte transplantation has been attempted in patients with acute liver failure, in chronic liver disease with cirrhosis, and in children with liver-based metabolic disease (Table 28.1). Although data concerning the efficacy of hepatocyte transplantation for liver failure in man have been difficult to interpret, at least one child with Crigler-Najjar syndrome type 1 has had unequivocal evidence of engraftment and function of transplanted allogeneic hepatocytes for more than a year. Unfortunately, many issues will need to be addressed before this technology can be applied to the great number of patients who could potentially benefit from it.

LABORATORY STUDIES

Hepatocyte Preparation

Hepatocytes are generally isolated by a variation of the *in situ* collagenase perfusion methods described by Berry, Friend, and Seglen.[1–3] The number of cells needed to treat liver failure or cure inherited disorders of metabolism, however, is variable for each condition and has yet to be determined. In most animal experiments, hepatocytes are transplanted fresh, but they can be used following cryopreservation as well. The ability to preserve and bank hepatocytes, either by cryopreservation or tissue culture, offers several theoretical advantages. These include donor-recipient tissue matching; possible immunologic modulation of donor cells; pooling of multiple donors, if needed, to increase cell numbers for transplantation; and allowing the transplant procedure to be performed semi-electively.

Although cryopreserved liver cells have been used in transplantation experiments, their ability to engraft as well as fresh hepatocytes has not been unequivocally established.[4] Unfortunately, human hepatocyte viability following cryopreservation is quite variable using present technology, and, despite

I. J. Fox: Department of Surgery, University of Nebraska Medical Center, Omaha, Nebraska 68198.

J. Roy-Chowdhury: Departments of Medicine and Molecular Genetics, Albert Einstein College of Medicine, Bronx, New York 10461.

TABLE 28.1. *Selected landmark developments in the research on liver cell transplantation*

Period	Development	Reference
1968	Isolation of primary hepatocytes	1
1970s	Early demonstration of bilirubin glucuronidation in Gunn rats	52
	Early studies on the treatment of acute liver failure	39
1980s	Hepatocyte engraftment at extrahepatic sites	15, 14, 45
	Treatment of acute liver failure in rats by hepatocyte transplantation	44
	Treatment of chronic liver failure in rats by hepatocyte transplantation	82
	Hepatocyte-based liver-directed gene therapy in an animal model	86
1990s	Demonstration of migration of intrasplenically transplanted hepatocytes to the liver	11
	Transplantation of conditionally immortalized hepatocytes for acute and chronic liver failure in animal models	46, 23
	Repopulation of the liver by transplanted primary hepatocytes in animal models	59, 61
	Hepatocyte-based *ex vivo* liver-directed gene therapy in humans	89
	Hepatocyte transplantation in humans for the treatment of liver failure	96
	Unequivocal demonstration of function of engrafted hepatocytes in a patient with Crigler-Najjar syndrome	97

recent advances that have made long-term maintenance of hepatocyte growth in culture possible, successful tissue culture often requires the use of biomatrices, which may adversely affect hepatocyte use for transplantation.[5–9]

Transplant Location

A number of ectopic sites have been examined for hepatocyte transplantation, but the vascular bed of the liver and the splenic pulp appear to be most appropriate for clinical application. Although not completely developed at this time, intraperitoneal transplantation of encapsulated cells may be possible in the future.

The liver appears to be the most accommodating site for engrafted hepatocytes, probably because of the availability of portal nutrients, contact with other hepatocytes and nonparenchymal cells, proximity to paracrine factors, and the ability to secrete into the biliary system. Hepatocytes can be seeded into the liver by intrasplenic injection, in which the spleen serves as a conduit for the distribution of cells into the liver parenchyma, or by intraportal injection. In the liver, transplanted hepatocytes retain normal architecture by light and electron microscopy and display all normal liver-specific characteristics; in rodents, the engrafted hepatocytes survive and function throughout the life of the recipient.[10,11]

Using standard histologic techniques, transplanted hepatocytes are difficult to identify in the host liver even a few days following transplantation.[12] As a result, early investigators were forced to examine hepatocyte engraftment in ectopic locations. These included the subcutaneous tissue, the dorsal fat pad, underneath the renal capsule, the lung, the peritoneal cavity, and the spleen. Identification of hepatocytes was facilitated by electron microscopy[13] and special histologic and immunohistochemical stains (glucose-6-phosphatase, albumin, and periodic acid-Schiff).[14–16]

The migration pattern of hepatocytes following transplantation was first determined by marking transplanted cells with fluorescent dyes such as DiI and carboxyfluorescein,[17–21] or with radioisotopes such as indium 111 or technetium 99m (^{99m}Tc). Use of molecularly marked hepatocytes, however, has permitted accumulation of far more detailed information regarding hepatocyte trafficking and integration. By transplanting hepatocytes transgenic for the hepatitis B virus surface antigen or human α_1-antitrypsin, confirmation of long-term engraftment has been accomplished by measuring transgene products in the blood or by localization of donor cells in the liver by *in situ* mRNA hybridization.[22] More recently, other techniques have been employed. Transplanting cells transduced to express the β-galactosidase gene allows localization by enzyme histochemistry,[23] using male donors in female recipients allows localization using fluorescence *in situ* DNA hybridization,[24] and using congenic rodents whose hepatocytes are dipeptidyl peptidase IV (DPPIV) deficient has allowed localization using enzyme histochemistry (Fig. 28.1).[25]

In rodent models of hepatocyte transplantation, the DPPIV system has been used to determine the time course of transplanted hepatocyte integration into the liver cords. Using DPPIV-deficient F344 rats as transplant recipients and congenic DPPIV-positive rats as the source of donor hepatocytes, investigators have shown that immediately after injection into the spleen or portal vein, transplanted hepatocytes are deposited in the portal region and the sinusoidal spaces. The capacity of the sinusoidal spaces limits the number of

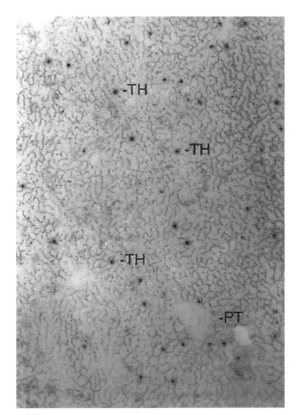

FIG. 28.1. Transplantation of immortalized Gunn rat hepatocytes permanently transduced with the *Escherichia coli* β-galactosidase gene using recombinant retroviral vectors into syngeneic Gunn rats. The cells (2 × 10[7]) were transplanted by injection into the splenic pulp, from which they migrate to the liver. Liver sections were stained for β-galactosidase activity 2 weeks after transplantation. Note that the transplanted cells (dark nuclei) are distributed in both periportal regions and within the liver lobules, are present as single cells rather than as clusters, and are integrated into the liver cords. PT, portal triad; TH, transplanted hepatocytes with β-galactosidase–positive nuclei.

hepatocytes that can be transplanted. It has been estimated that, at any one time, hepatocytes equivalent to up to 10% of the liver mass can be transplanted into livers with normal architecture without long-term deleterious effects.[26] However, immediately after hepatocyte transplantation, there is ischemia of the liver, as indicated by increased expression of γ-glutamyltranspeptidase by both host and donor hepatocytes distal to the hepatocyte deposition sites.[27] Partial occlusion of portal flow also results in transient portal hypertension that resolves with entry of the hepatocytes into the space of Disse and subsequently into the liver cords.[28] The cells that are deposited within the portal triad die within 24 to 48 hours.[27] Some, but not all, hepatocytes that are located within the sinusoidal spaces enter the space of Disse in about 20 hours; the remainder undergo cell death and removal. Studies indicate that less than 30% of transplanted hepatocytes sur-

vive in the liver, although the number of surviving cells increases as more hepatocytes are transplanted.

Passage of hepatocytes into the space of Disse requires retraction of the sinusoidal endothelial cells. Although the mechanism of this process has not been fully elucidated, release of vascular endothelial growth factor by donor and host hepatocytes has been proposed as facilitating entry.[27] Shortly after entering the space of Disse there is a transient disruption of the gap junction and tight junction between adjacent hepatocytes in the vicinity of the transplanted hepatocytes. The transplanted cells then insert themselves between host hepatocytes, with subsequent regeneration of the bile canaliculi and gap junctions in approximately 72 hours.

It takes approximately 3 days for plasma membrane proteins, such as dipeptidyl peptidase IV, to regain their normal localization. Studies in recipient TR⁻ rats, which are deficient in canalicular multispecific organic anion transporter, have shown that following integration of normal donor hepatocytes into the liver cords, newly generated bile canaliculi become functional and begin excreting organic anions. The prolonged time course of donor cell integration into the liver parenchyma may be partially responsible for the delay in full function by transplanted hepatocytes.

In contrast to situations in which hepatocytes are transplanted into livers with normal architecture, hepatocyte transplantation into cirrhotic livers results in a severe and prolonged increase in portal hypertension. Furthermore, there is translocation of a significant number of the transplanted hepatocytes into the pulmonary vascular bed. The cells are cleared from the pulmonary capillaries in a few days, but the initial deposition in the lungs results in transient pulmonary hypertension.[29] Despite this, however, some transplanted hepatocytes do migrate into cirrhotic nodules, although whether these cells can function adequately to improve the metabolic state of the recipient is doubtful. At this time, extrahepatic locations such as the spleen or the peritoneal cavity appear to be the optimal sites for hepatocyte transplantation in cirrhotic recipients.

As previously stated, when transplanted into the splenic pulp, the majority of hepatocytes migrate to the liver.[10] A small percentage of cells, however, implant within the interstices of the spleen and organize into structures resembling hepatic cord in the spaces of Billroth and in the red pulp. These cells then proliferate and can replace up to 40% of the pleen within a matter of months. During the first week following transplantation, engrafted hepatocytes exhibit mitochondrial swelling and accumulate cytoplasmic lipid droplets.[30] However, they gradually recover, and a significant hepatocyte mass starts to develop after about 4 months.[14,31,32] One year after transplantation, subcellular organelles show only minimal ultrastructural abnormalities. Bile canaliculi and junctional complexes form early after transplantation, and sinusoidal structures can be detected about 6 months following transplantation. Endothelial and Ito cells may also appear in these sinusoid-like structures, leading to a histologic appearance that resembles normal hepatic architecture. Because whole-organ liver grafts atrophy

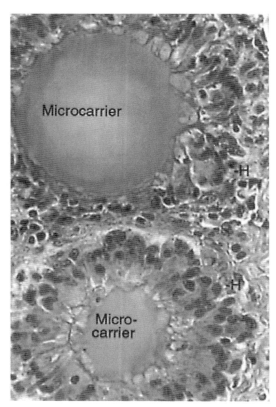

FIG. 28.2. Light microscopic view of sections of conglomerates formed 72 hours after intraperitoneal injection of a slurry of primary rat hepatocytes attached to collagen-coated dextran microcarriers. Note that many hepatocytes are attached to the microcarriers, whereas others are present in the space between the beads.

in the absence of a portal blood supply,[33] the long-term survival and proliferation of hepatocytes in the spleen is intriguing. Injection of hepatocytes into arterial beds leads to rapid cell losses, most likely due to shear injury in the high-pressure circulation and to lack of vessel wall anchorage.[34] This has been the preferred route of intrasplenic hepatocyte transplantation in man, but the likelihood of successful hepatocyte engraftment using this technique is quite low.

Because of its large capacity and easy access, the peritoneal cavity has also been considered an important potential site for hepatocyte transplantation. Isolated hepatocytes do not survive direct injection into the peritoneum; when transplanted with nonparenchymal cells, however, they engraft and survive for months.[35] When attached to microcarriers or placed in hydrogel-based hollow fibers, they also survive for months and may be immunologically protected from rejection.[36,37] Microcarrier-attached hepatocytes rapidly form conglomerates on the anterior surface of the pancreas and are supported by newly formed connective tissue.[38] The mechanism by which microcarriers enhance engraftment is not known, but it may be that they provide a larger surface area for peritoneal neovascularization. Progress in this area has been slowed by the need to optimize the encapsulation de-

vice pore size so as to exclude the macromolecules and cells responsible for allograft rejection without interfering with the formation of a blood supply or the release of cell products important for hepatocyte function (Fig. 28.2).

EVIDENCE OF TRANSPLANTED HEPATOCYTE FUNCTION

Liver Failure

The efficacy of hepatocyte transplantation in altering the mortality associated with acute liver failure has been examined in the laboratory for more than 20 years. Hepatocyte transplantation can rescue rodents with acute liver failure experimentally induced by D-galactosamine, dimethylnitrosamine, liver ischemia, and 90% hepatectomy.[39–42] Intrasplenic transplantation of allogeneic hepatocytes has also been shown to prevent the development of intracranial hypertension in pigs with acute ischemic liver failure.[43]

Using D-galactosamine to induce acute liver failure in rats, transplantation of 30 million hepatocytes into either the spleen, the portal vein, or the peritoneal cavity can produce long-term animal survival rates of 60% to 80% compared with only 10% in saline-treated controls.[44,45] In general, when hepatotoxins have been used to create liver insufficiency, transplantation consistently improves survival when performed after the induction of acute liver failure.

Great variability in the hepatotoxin dose needed to induce hepatic failure and difficulties with reproducibility have led to the development of surgical techniques in the laboratory to induce liver failure. Near-total or 90% hepatectomy produces a reliable model for the study of hepatocyte transplantation. Survival is improved with intraperitoneal transplantation of as few as 10 million microcarrier-attached hepatocytes. However, it is only improved when cells are transplanted 3 days prior to surgical production of acute liver failure. Only recently has it been shown that hepatocyte transplantation can improve survival when performed at the time surgically induced acute liver failure is produced; this required transplantation of 200 million isolated hepatocytes.[46]

Reports have also shown improved animal survival with transplantation of bone marrow cells or injection of hepatocyte lysates. Such studies suggest that hepatocyte engraftment is not necessary for improved survival in these models of acute liver failure and that hepatocyte-derived hepatotrophic factors may be responsible for the effect.[47–49] Because liver regeneration is not significantly inhibited in the experimental models used so far to study hepatocyte transplantation in acute liver failure, the present models may not adequately parallel the clinical situation. Survival may simply result from enhanced liver regeneration or release of substances that may transiently improve the metabolic state of the animal until regeneration is adequate for survival. Thus, direct experimental evidence that hepatocyte transplantation can improve the survival of patients with acute liver failure is lacking.

The role of hepatocyte transplantation in the treatment of chronic liver insufficiency has recently been better defined. Hepatocellular transplantation improves hepatic encephalopathy when liver insufficiency is induced in rats by end-to-side portacaval shunt. Spontaneous activity and certain reflexes are subtly affected in rats following portacaval shunt, and intrasplenic transplantation with 10 million hepatocytes can improve their behavior score and partially correct their amino acid imbalances. It does not, however, produce a lowering of the elevated plasma ammonia level that occurs after portacaval shunt.[50] Cell transplantation can, however, protect portacaval-shunted rats from developing exogenous ammonia-induced hepatic coma.[23] More recently, intrasplenic hepatocyte transplantation in rats with decompensated liver cirrhosis has been shown to stabilize total bilirubin level and to improve albumin level, prothrombin time, ammonia concentration, and encephalopathy score as well as prolong survival.[51]

Liver-Based Metabolic Disease

The efficacy of hepatocyte transplantation in treating liver-based metabolic diseases has also been extensively studied in the laboratory. The most studied animals are the Gunn rat and the Nagase genetically analbuminemic (NAR) rat. The Gunn rat lacks uridine 5′-diphosphate glucuronosyltransferase activity (bilirubin-UGT) and exhibits life-long unconjugated hyperbilirubinemia.[52] A similar enzyme defect in humans, Crigler-Najjar syndrome type 1, causes death from bilirubin-induced brain damage. Several laboratories have shown that intrasplenic or intraportal transplantation of normal donor hepatocytes can lower bilirubin levels toward normal and produce glucuronidation of bilirubin in the bile of Gunn rats.[12,16]

Intrasplenic or intraportal hepatocyte transplantation has also been shown to correct serum albumin levels toward normal in the Nagase rat.[53,54] Unfortunately, transplantation with 30 million hepatocytes raises the serum albumin level in NAR rats to only 1% of that found in normal rats. Somewhat higher albumin levels can be obtained with repeated hepatocyte infusions or by occluding portal vein branches supplying liver lobes that do not contain transplanted cells.[55] Finally, transplanted hepatocytes have also been shown to partially correct the metabolic defect in an animal model of familial hypercholesterolemia, the Watanabe heritable hyperlipidemic (WHHL) rabbit, which lacks cell surface receptors for low density lipoproteins (LDL),[56,57] and in an animal model of Wilson's disease, the Long-Evans cinnamon rat.[58]

Because many biologically active proteins in the liver are present in excess, transplantation of a relatively small number of liver cells would be expected to correct many liver-based metabolic deficiencies. In most animal models, however, only partial correction of the metabolic deficiency has been accomplished. An exception to this rule exists when normal hepatocytes are transplanted into the livers of animals whose own hepatocytes are destroyed as a result of a metabolic abnormality. The repopulating potential of transplanted hepatocytes has been elegantly illustrated in albumin-urokinase transgenic mice.[59] These mice express a hepatotoxic transgene that creates defective hepatocytes. When hepatocytes from normal mice are transplanted into the livers of these mice, more than 80% of the native liver cells become replaced with donor cells.

Similar results have been obtained in fumarylacetoacetate hydrolase (FAH) mutant mice, which express the genetic defect associated with hereditary tyrosinemia type I in man.[60] Serial transplantation of a limiting number of hepatocytes into these mice has been shown to completely repopulate six generations of mouse livers. This corresponds to a minimum of 69 doublings, or an expansion of hepatocytes of 7.3×10^{20} fold.[61] Interestingly, FAH mice are susceptible to the development of hepatocellular carcinomas, and despite extensive liver repopulation with normal cells, they still develop liver cancers. This susceptibility to cancer or recurrent disease will be an important consideration for the clinical application of hepatocyte transplantation in the treatment of virus-induced liver failure, cirrhosis, and liver-based metabolic disease.

Immunogenicity of Transplanted Hepatocytes

Autologous or syngeneic hepatocytes survive indefinitely when placed in the liver or spleen. Allografts, however, are subject to antibody- and cell-mediated rejection. Gene products or antigens of the major histocompatibility complex (MHC) are the major targets of immunologic attack in transplantation; the host response results from presentation of graft antigens on the surface of metabolically active antigen-presenting cells (APC).[62,63] Hepatocytes express low levels of class I MHC antigens that serve as allospecific targets for cytolytic T lymphocytes.[64] Unstimulated hepatocytes do not express class II MHC antigens, but preparations may occasionally be contaminated by immunogenic APC or Kupffer cells.[65] In vivo, transplantation of hepatocytes from animals that differ genetically at the MHC results in sensitization and rapid disappearance of allografts in 4 to 7 days.[66] Conventional immunosuppression with cyclosporine, azathioprine, tacrolimus, and antilymphocyte serum has been shown to prolong hepatocyte survival in laboratory animals.[28,67]

It is interesting that intraportally transplanted hepatocytes can elicit a strong rejection response. Administration of allogeneic or xenogeneic foreign cells through the portal vein has been shown to induce donor-specific tolerance in rodents and pigs.[68-71] It is possible that hepatocytes fail to induce immunologic unresponsiveness because cell preparations do not usually contain large numbers of contaminating APC. Whether cotransplantation of a small number of bone marrow cells that contain APC or the use of transient immunosuppression, which has been needed to induce tolerance in some studies, will allow intraportally transplanted hepatocytes to induce tolerance is not known.

Because antigen-presenting cells play such a dominant role in allograft rejection, investigators have attempted to modulate graft and APC immunogenicity prior to transplantation. Nowhere has this been investigated more completely than in pancreatic islet transplantation. One approach that has been effective for islet transplantation, ultraviolet B irradiation, has been successfully used to prolong allogeneic hepatocyte survival.[72,73] The efficacy of this approach, however, is somewhat confusing because the presumed mechanism of tolerance induction is physical or functional depletion of putative antigen-presenting cells. Therefore, the precise mechanism of allograft tolerance in this model is not understood.

The immune response to cellular grafts has also been altered by gene transfer using recombinant adenoviruses containing the genes encoding immunosuppressive cytokines. Transduction of donor cells with a number of cytokines has effectively blocked allograft and xenograft rejection. Adenovirus-mediated expression of CTLA-4Ig, a fusion protein of the extracellular domain of cytotoxoic T-lymphocyte antigen 4 (CTLA-4) and the Fc portion of the IgG2a molecule, has been shown to downregulate the immune response to cellular grafts by costimulatory blockade.[74] Transduction of grafts to express viral interleukin 10 (vIL-10); transforming growth factor β1 (TGF-β1); or the adenovirus E3 region, which downregulates MHC expression in transduced cells, has been found to be effective, to some degree, in inhibiting cell-mediated rejection. It is also possible that transplanting hepatocytes with cells expressing Fas ligand, which induces apoptosis of attacking lymphocytes, may be effective in blocking cell-mediated rejection.[75–80] Finally, it has been shown that transplanted hepatocytes that express membrane-bound complement receptor 1 are protected from preformed antibody-mediated rejection. This may be important for cellular xenotransplantation.[81]

Microencapsulation[82] and the use of fetal tissue[83,84] also hold promise for cell transplantation in the future. Encapsulation of hepatocytes in selectively permeable synthetic membranes allows survival of hepatocytes in culture and in vivo. Alginate polylysine–encapsulated hepatocytes that are implanted into the peritoneal cavity are functional, but the synthetic membrane provokes an intense fibrotic reaction that limits their survival. When chitosan is electrostatically bound to anionic sodium alginate, it creates an outer biopolymer membrane that inhibits the development of the fibrous reaction. However, the chitosan fails to prevent rejection. More recently, allogeneic and guinea pig hepatocytes have been recovered from nonimmunosuppressed rats up to 1 month after intraperitoneal transplantation by encapsulation in semipermeable hydrogel-based hollow fibers.[37,85]

One additional approach has been employed to circumvent the problem of allograft rejection. Isolated enzyme deficiencies may be treatable by introducing normal genes into defective hepatocytes. WHHL rabbit hepatocytes have been recovered from their own livers and transduced with a recombinant retrovirus to express the gene encoding a normal LDL receptor.[86] The genetically modified WHHL hepatocytes were then transplanted back into the rabbit from which the cells were harvested. The procedure resulted in 25% to 30% reduction in serum LDL cholesterol levels, and transgene expression was confirmed by in situ hybridization.

This strategy has been evaluated in a clinical trial in which the left lateral segments of the livers of patients with familial hypercholesterolemia were removed to isolate hepatocytes. The cells were then genetically modified in vitro and retransplanted into the patients. This first human trial of liver-directed gene therapy resulted in a modest reduction of hypercholesterolemia; liver biopsies demonstrated that the introduced LDL receptor gene was being expressed at low levels.[87–89]

CLINICAL EXPERIENCE

Acute Liver Failure

Based on the success of laboratory studies, several institutions have used hepatocyte transplantation to treat patients with acute liver failure. In the first study, seven patients with acute liver failure received a single-dose transplant into the peritoneal cavity of approximately 5×10^8 hepatocytes from 26- to 34-week gestational age fetuses. The overall survival of patients receiving hepatocytes was 43%, compared with 33% in matched controls. All patients with grade III hepatic encephalopathy who received hepatocyte transplants survived, whereas only 50% of matched controls did. Recovery from encephalopathy was observed within 48 hours.[90]

In the United States, hepatocyte transplantation has been performed for acute liver failure, sometimes as a bridge to liver transplantation. At the Medical College of Virginia, seven potential transplant candidates received between 10^7 to 10^9 viable cells through the splenic artery; five survived to receive orthotopic liver transplantation.[91] At the University of Colorado, five patients who were not candidates for organ transplantation were treated by transplantation with as many as 2×10^{10} hepatocytes into the liver through the portal vein using a percutaneous transhepatic or transjugular transhepatic approach.[92,93] Soriano has also described an additional three patients, who were treated by intraportal infusion.[94] In general, engrafted hepatocytes could be found in some of the spleens of patients who received intrasplenic cells and could be found in some of the livers of patients who received intraportally transplanted cells. Two patients in this total group recovered spontaneously, and improvements in ammonia concentration, prothrombin time, encephalopathy, cerebral perfusion pressure, and cardiovascular stability have been described in abstracts. Reported complications included transient hemodynamic instability during intraportal hepatocyte infusion, overwhelming sepsis (which may or may not be related to the transplant procedure), and embolization of hepatocytes into the pulmonary circulation without clinical evidence of pulmonary embolism.[95] Portal hypertension as a result of transplantation through the portal vein has been transient, but significantly prolonged elevation of cyclosporine and tacrolimus levels has occurred because of poor clearance of these drugs in the presence of liver failure. Whether immunosuppressive medications are needed to control rejection in these patients is unknown.

Although there is some suggestion that the transplanted hepatocytes provided a benefit, convincing evidence for the engraftment and function of the transplanted cells has not been obtained. Part of the problem could be that relatively small numbers of hepatocytes were transplanted in many of the patients. In addition, because patients with acute liver failure can survive without transplantation, survival is difficult to use as a definitive marker of functional hepatocyte engraftment.

Chronic Liver Disease

In Japan, ten patients with either chronic hepatitis or cirrhosis received transplanted hepatocytes recovered from their own left lateral liver segment. Four of these patients underwent hepatic artery ligation in addition to hepatocyte transplantation to control ascites. Patients received from 10^7 to 6×10^8 hepatocytes into their spleen, either by direct splenic puncture or via the splenic artery or portal vein. In one patient, hepatocyte engraftment and survival was detected in the spleen 11 months after transplantation by ^{99m}PMT-radioisotope uptake. This patient eventually resolved his ascites and encephalopathy. Unfortunately, even the authors of this study do not feel that the improvement was necessarily a consequence of the transplant procedure.[96]

In the United States, eight patients with decompensated chronic liver disease have been treated by transplantation with up to 10^{10} hepatocytes through the splenic artery. One of the three patients who was a candidate for organ transplantation successfully underwent liver transplantation. Patients appeared to tolerate the infusions well, and abstracts report improvement in encephalopathy, as well as synthetic and renal function. In two patients, scanning for transplanted hepatocytes using uptake of glycosylated albumin with ^{99m}Tc indicated the presence of engrafted hepatocytes in the spleen.[95]

If hepatocyte transplantation proves to be effective in improving some of the physiologic abnormalities associated with chronic liver disease, portal hypertension will need to be controlled by surgery or placement of a transjugular intrahepatic portosystemic shunt, and surveillance for the development of hepatocellular carcinoma will be needed. It is not clear how rejection will be diagnosed, although it is possible that nuclear scanning of the spleen will prove useful.

Liver-Based Metabolic Disease

The first patients to undergo hepatocyte transplantation for a metabolic deficiency were those with familial hypercholesterolemia who were part of the *ex vivo* gene therapy trial described previously. Patients with ornithine transcarbamylase (OTC) deficiency, α_1-antitrypsin deficiency, and

Crigler-Najjar syndrome type 1 have undergone transplantation with allogeneic hepatocytes. At least one child with OTC deficiency showed some evidence of enzyme activity on a liver biopsy, but died from hyperammonemia following cell transplantation.[9] An additional child received hepatocytes at birth via the umbilical vein and had transient clinical evidence of enzyme activity, maintaining a normal ammonia and glutamine level without administration of phenylbutyrate and phenylacetate while receiving more than 2 g of protein per kg per day. The child probably rejected the cells because of inadequate immunosuppression and is awaiting retransplantation. An 18-week-old child with α_1-antitrypsin deficiency also received a few million hepatocytes through the portal vein; however, a liver biopsy obtained at the time of portal vein catheter placement demonstrated cirrhosis that was not present on an earlier biopsy. The cell infusions were stopped, and the child later underwent orthotopic liver transplantation.[95]

Unequivocal evidence of transplanted human hepatocyte function has been obtained only in a single patient with Crigler-Najjar syndrome type 1 (bilirubin-UGT deficiency) who had a partial correction of her hyperbilirubinemia after transplantation.[97] The patient, a 10-year-old girl, required 10 to 12 hours of phototherapy daily before transplantation to keep her serum unconjugated bilirubin level between 24 and 27 mg/dL. Approximately 7 billion hepatocytes were infused into her portal vein through a percutaneously placed catheter. The child was awake during the cell infusion and was discharged 20 hours after it was completed. After the transplant procedure, the serum bilirubin level fell to between 10.6 and 14 mg/dL and has remained at that level for more than a year even though she receives less phototherapy. Hepatic bilirubin-UGT activity increased from barely detectable (0.4%) levels to 5.5% of mean normal enzyme activity, and more than 30% of the child's bile pigments became bilirubin glucuronides. Standard tacrolimus-based immunosuppression has been successfully used to control rejection. Rejection has been assessed during transient episodes of unconjugated hyperbilirubinemia by analysis of bile for bilirubin conjugates and by biopsy with measurement of enzyme activity.

FUTURE PROSPECTS

A number of issues hamper further development of the field. The number of livers available for hepatocyte isolation and later transplantation is limited. Residual segments from reduced liver transplants and organs with traumatic damage and excess macrovesicular fat, which are not suitable for transplantation, are the usual source of hepatocytes. Unfortunately, fatty livers do not consistently yield cells of good quality or provide cells of sufficient number to transplant. Although hepatocytes can be cryopreserved for storage and transportation, the efficacy of preservation is variable and depends on a variety of known and unknown factors.[8] Finally, human hepatocyte isolation is expensive, time-consuming, and inefficient. Research on cell isolation and cryopreservation techniques, on *in vitro* expansion of human hepatocytes using growth factors or immortalizing genes,[23,46,98,99] and on the feasibility of transplanting hepatocytes from other species may help address these issues.[100]

In addition to the problem of hepatocyte availability, there is a physiologic limit on the number of hepatocytes that can be transplanted at any one time. Less than 30% of transplanted cells engraft in the liver; thus, improvement in isolation and cryopreservation will not overcome the need for repeated cell infusion.[27] A better understanding of the factors that allow hepatocyte integration may lead to techniques for transplanting a larger number of hepatocytes at any one time.

In some diseases, such as hereditary tyrosinemia, transplanted cells will have a selective growth advantage over native liver cells. In most situations, however, a significantly larger number of cells than originally anticipated will need to be transplanted. Alternatively, transplanted hepatocytes will need to be selectively expanded after engraftment. Experimentally, this has been accomplished by inhibiting native liver cell growth using liver-directed radiation therapy,[101] recombinant virus-mediated delivery of suicide genes to the liver,[102] and drugs that block the hepatocyte cell cycle[103] while inducing selective proliferation of transplanted cells by ligation of portal vein branches, partial liver resection, and hepatocyte growth factors.

Because gene therapy is likely to supplant hepatocyte transplantation for the treatment of liver-based metabolic disease, the future of hepatocyte transplantation most likely resides in the treatment of liver failure. Hepatocyte transplantation may not be able to reverse portal hypertension or the development of hepatocellular carcinoma, but improvement in liver physiology and patient survival may be possible. It is not clear, at this time, what factors regulate engraftment, survival, and function of transplanted cells in the presence of liver disease. Further questions relate to the safest way to deliver hepatocytes in the face of cirrhosis, since arterial delivery results in significant cell destruction and poor engraftment. It is possible that techniques similar to those used for a splenoportography may be useful if adequate hemostasis can be achieved.

Liver disease can also recur in transplanted tissue; however, it may be possible to engineer hepatocytes to be resistant to recurrent disease. Transplantation of nonhuman hepatocytes may also accomplish this goal. Recently, using standard cyclosporine-based immunosuppression, pig hepatocytes have been successfully transplanted through the portal vein of WHHL rabbits. In immunosuppressed animals, serum cholesterol levels fell by nearly 40% for at least 100 days, and 1% to 5% of the infused cells could be found at the time of sacrifice by *in situ* RNA hybridization and PCR.[104] Whether nonhuman hepatocytes will engraft and function adequately in patients with liver failure is not known at this time.

Although clinical evidence of hepatocyte function can be used to indicate function of transplanted hepatocytes, defin-itive histologic evidence is difficult to obtain. Distinguishing donor from host hepatocytes in the liver is difficult at best. For liver-based metabolic disease, biopsy measurement of enzyme activity in the liver can be useful; however, to assess whether rejection is taking place in a timely fashion, less cumbersome ways of detecting donor hepatocytes will be needed.

CONCLUSION

The future is difficult to predict. Until effective gene therapy becomes available, hepatocyte transplantation offers more immediate hope to children with debilitating metabolic disease. At this time it is too early to know what percentage of the millions of patients with acute and chronic liver disease could benefit from hepatocyte transplantation.

REFERENCES

1. Berry M, Friend D. High yield preparation of isolated rat liver parenchymal cells: a biochemical and fine structural study. *J Cell Biol* 1969;43:506–520.
2. Seglen P. Preparation of isolated rat liver cells. *Methods Cell Biol* 1976;13:29–83.
3. Strom SC, Jirtle RL, Jones RS, et al. Isolation, culture, and transplantation of human hepatocytes. *J Natl Cancer Inst* 1982;68:771–778.
4. Grundmann R, Koebe HG, Waters W. Transplantation of cryopreserved hepatocytes or liver cytosol injection in the treatment of acute liver failure in rats. *Res Exp Med* 1986;186:141–149.
5. Loretz LJ, Li AP, Flye MW, et al. Optimization of cryopreservation procedures for rat and human hepatocytes. *Xenobiotica* 1989;19:489–498.
6. Lawrence JN, Benford DJ. Development of an optimal method for the cryopreservation of hepatocytes and their subsequent monolayer culture. *Toxicol In Vitro* 1991;5:39–51.
7. Rijntes PJM, Moshage HJ, Van Gemert PJL, et al. Cryopreservation of adult human hepatocytes. The influence of deep freezing storage on the viability, cell seeding, survival, fine structure and albumin synthesis in primary cultures. *J Hepatol* 1986;3:7–18.
8. Moshage HJ, Rijntjes PJ, Hafkenscheid JC, et al. Primary culture of cryopreserved adult human hepatocytes on homologous extracellular matrix and the influence of monocytic products on albumin synthesis. *J Hepatol* 1988;7:34–44.
9. Reyes J, Rubenstein W, Mieles L, et al. The use of cultured hepatocyte infusion via the portal vein for the treatment for ornithine transcarbamylase deficiency by transplantation of enzymatically competent ABO/Rh-matched cells [Abstract]. *Hepatology* 1996;24:308A.
10. Ponder KP, Gupta S, Leland F, et al. Mouse hepatocytes migrate to liver parenchyma and function indefinitely after intrasplenic transplantation. *Proc Natl Acad Sci U S A* 1991;88:1217–1221.
11. Gupta S, Aragona E, Vemuru R, et al. Permanent engraftment and function of hepatocytes delivered to the liver: implications for gene therapy and liver repopulation. *Hepatology* 1991;14:144–148.
12. Groth C, Arborgh B, Bjorken C, et al. Correction of hyperbilirubinemia in glucoronyltransferase-deficient rats by intraportal hepatocyte transplantation. *Transplant Proc* 1977;9(1):313–316.
13. Mito M, Ebata H, Kusano M, et al. Morphology and function of isolated hepatocytes transplanted into rat spleen. *Transplantation* 1979;28:499–505.
14. Kusano M, Mito M. Observations on the fine structure of long survived isolated hepatocytes inoculated into rat spleen. *Gastroenterology* 1982;82:616–628.
15. Jirtle R, Biles C, Michalopoulos G. Morphologic and histochemical analysis of hepatocytes transplanted into syngeneic hosts. *Am J Pathol* 1980;101:115–126.
16. Matas AJ, Sutherland DE, Steffes MW, et al. Hepatocellular transplantation for metabolic deficiencies: decrease of plasma bilirubin in Gunn rats. *Science* 1976;192:892–894.

17. Soriano HE, Lewis D, Legner M, et al. The use of DiI-marked hepatocytes to demonstrate orthotopic, intrahepatic engraftment following hepatocellular transplantation. *Transplantation* 1992;54:717–723.
18. Fujioka H, Hunt PJ, Rozga J, et al. Carboxyfluorescein (CFSE) labelling of hepatocytes for short-term localization following intraportal transplantation. *Cell Transplant* 1994;3:397–408.
19. Gupta S, Lee C-D, Vemuru R, et al. 111Indium-labeling of hepatocytes for analyzing biodistribution of transplanted cells. *Hepatology* 1994;19:750–757.
20. Gupta S, Vasa S, Rajvanshi P, et al. Analysis of hepatocyte distribution and survival in vascular beds with cells marked by 99m-Tc or endogenous dipeptidyl peptidase IV activity. *Cell Transplant* 1997;6:377–386.
21. Vroemen J, Van der Linden C, Buurman W, et al. *In vivo* dynamic 99M Tc-HIDA scintigraphy after hepatocyte transplantation: a new method for monitoring graft function. *Eur Surg Res* 1987;19:140–150.
22. Gupta S, Chowdhury NR, Jagtiani R, et al. A novel system for transplantation of isolated hepatocytes utilizing HBsAg-producing transgenic donor cells. *Transplantation* 1990;50:472–475.
23. Schumacher IK, Okamoto T, Kim BH, et al. Transplantation of conditionally immortalized hepatocytes to treat hepatic encephalopathy. *Hepatology* 1996;24:337–343.
24. Krishna Vanaja D, Sivakumar B, Jesudasan R, et al. *In vivo* identification, survival, and functional efficacy of transplanted hepatocytes in acute liver failure mice model by FISH using Y-chromosome probe. *Cell Transplant* 1998;7:267–273.
25. Gupta S, Rajvanshi P, Lee C-D. Integration of transplanted hepatocytes in host liver plates demonstrated with dipeptidylpeptidase IV deficient rats. *Proc Natl Acad Sci U S A* 1995;92:5860–5864.
26. Rajvanshi P, Kerr A, Bhargava K, et al. Efficacy and safety of repeated hepatocyte transplantation for significant liver repopulation in rodents. *Gastroenterology* 1996;111:1092–1102.
27. Gupta S, Gorla G, Irani A. Hepatocyte transplantation: emerging insights into mechanisms of liver repopulation and their relevance to potential therapies [Abstract]. *J Hepatol* 1999;30:162–170.
28. Benedetti E, Kirby JP, Asolati M, et al. Intrasplenic hepatocyte allotransplantation in dalmation dogs with and without cyclosporine immunosuppression. *Transplantation* 1997;63:1206–1209.
29. Rajvanshi P, Fabrega A, Bhargava K, et al. Rapid clearance of hepatocytes from pulmonary capillaries in rats allows development of surrogates for testing safety of liver repopulation. *J Hepatol* 1999;30(2):299–310.
30. Maganto P, Cienfuegos J, Santamaria L, et al. Effect of cyclosporin on allogeneic hepatocyte transplantation: a morphological study. *Eur Surg Res* 1988;20:248–253.
31. Darby H, Selden C, Hodgson H. Prolonged survival of cyclosporine-treated allogeneic hepatocellular implants. *Transplantation* 1986;42:325–326.
32. Woods R, Fuller B, Attenburro V, et al. Functional assessment of hepatocytes after transplantation into rat spleen. *Transplantation* 1982;33:123–126.
33. Halgrimson C, Marchiorio R, Faris T, et al. Auxiliary liver transplantation: effect of host portacaval shunt. *Arch Surg* 1966;93:107–118.
34. Mito M, Kusano M, Ohnishi T, et al. Hepatocellular transplantation. *Gastroenterol Jpn* 1978;13:480–490.
35. Selden C, Calnan D, Morgan N, et al. Histidinemia in mice: a metabolic defect treated using a novel approach to hepatocellular transplantation. *Hepatology* 1995;21:1405–1412.
36. Dixit V, Darvasi R, Arthur M, et al. Restoration of liver function in Gunn rats without immunosuppression using transplanted microencapsulated hepatocytes. *Hepatology* 1990;12:1342–1349.
37. Roger V, Balladur P, Honiger J, et al. Internal bioartificial liver with xenogeneic hepatocytes prevents death from acute liver failure: an experimental study. *Ann Surg* 1998;228:1–7.
38. Demetriou AA, Levenson SM, Novikoff PM, et al. Survival, organization, and function of microcarrier-attached hepatocytes transplanted in rats. *Proc Natl Acad Sci U S A* 1986;83:7475–7459.
39. Sutherland DER, Numate M, Matas AJ, et al. Hepatocellular transplantation in acute liver failure. *Surgery* 1977;82:124–132.
40. Sommer B, Sutherland D, Matas D, et al. Hepatocellular transplantation for treatment of D-galactosamine induced acute liver failure in rats. *Transplant Proc* 1977;11:578–584.
41. Makowka L, Rotstein LE, Falk RE, et al. Reversal of toxic and anoxic induced hepatic failure by syngeneic, allogeneic, and xenogeneic hepatocyte transplantation. *Surgery* 1980;88:244–253.
42. Contini S, Pezzarossa A, Sansoni P, et al. Hepatocellular transplantation in rats with toxic induced liver failure: results of iso-, allo- and xenografts. *Ital J Surg Sci* 1983;13:25–30.
43. Arkadopoulos N, Chen SC, Khalili TM, et al. Transplantation of hepatocytes for prevention of intracranial hypertension in pigs with ischemic liver failure. *Cell Transplant* 1998;7:357–363.
44. Demetriou A, Reisner A, Sanchez J, et al. Transplantation of microcarrier-attached hepatocytes into 90% partially hepatectomized rats. *Hepatology* 1988;8:1006–1009.
45. Demetriou A, Whiting J, Feldman D, et al. Replacement of liver function in rats by transplantation of micro-carrier attached hepatocytes. *Science* 1986;233:1190–1192.
46. Nakamura J, Okamoto T, Schumacher IK, et al. Treatment of surgically induced acute liver failure by transplantation of conditionally immortalized hepatocytes. *Transplantation* 1997;63:1541–1547.
47. Makowka L, Rotstein LE, Falk RE, et al. Studies into the mechanism of reversal of experimental acute hepatic failure by hepatocyte transplantation. 1. *Can J Surg* 1981;24:39–44.
48. Miyazaki M, Makowka L, Falk R, et al. Reversal of lethal, chemotherapeutically induced acute hepatic necrosis in rats by regenerating liver cytosol. *Surgery* 1983;94:142–150.
49. Baumgartner D, LaPlante-O'Neill P, Sutherland D, et al. Effects of intrasplenic injection of hepatocytes, hepatocyte fragments, and hepatocyte culture supernatants on D-galactosamine-induced liver failure in rats. *Eur Surg Res* 1983;15:129–135.
50. Ribeiro J, Nordlinger B, Ballet F, et al. Intrasplenic hepatocellular transplantation corrects hepatic encephalopathy in portacaval-shunted rats. *Hepatology* 1992;15:12–18.
51. Kobayashi N, Ito M, Nakamura H, et al. Hepatocyte transplantation improves liver function and prolongs survival in rats with decompensated liver cirrhosis. *Transplant Proc* 1999;31:428–429.
52. Rugstad H, Robinson S, Yamoni C, et al. Transfer of bilirubin uridine-5-diphosphate-glucuronyltransferase to enzyme deficient rats. *Science* 1970;170:553–555.
53. Fabrega A, Bommineni V, Blanchard J, et al. Amelioration of analbuminemia by transplantation of allogeneic hepatocytes in tolerized rats. *Transplantation* 1995;59:1362–1364.
54. Holzman MD, Rozga J, Neuzil DF, et al. Selective intraportal hepatocyte transplantation in analbuminemic and Gunn rats. *Transplantation* 1993;55:1213–1219.
55. Rozga J, Holzman M, Moscioni AD, et al. Repeated intraportal hepatocyte transplantation in analbuminemic rats. *Cell Transplant* 1995;4:237–243.
56. Wilson J, Roy Chowdhury N, Grossman M, et al. Transplantation of allogeneic hepatocytes into LDL receptor deficient rabbits leads to transient improvement in hypercholesterolemia. *Clin Biotechnol* 1991;3:21–26.
57. Wiederkehr J, Kondos G, Pollak R. Hepatocyte transplantation for the low-density lipoprotein receptor-deficient state. A study in the Watanabe rabbit. *Transplantation* 1990;50:466–471.
58. Yoshida Y, Tokusashi Y, Lee G, et al. Intrahepatic transplantation of normal hepatocytes prevents Wilson's disease in Long-Evans cinnamon rats. *Gastroenterology* 1996;111:1654–1660.
59. Rhim J, Sandgren E, Degen J, et al. Replacement of diseased mouse liver by hepatic cell transplantation. *Science* 1994;263:1149–1153.
60. Overturf K, Al-Dhalimy M, Tanguay R, et al. Hepatocytes corrected by gene therapy are selected *in vivo* in a murine model of hereditary tyrosinaemia type I [published erratum appears in *Nat Genet* 1996;12:458]. *Nat Genet* 1996;12:266–273.
61. Overturf K, Al-Dhalimy M, Ou C, et al. Serial transplantation reveals the stem-cell-like regenerative potential of adult mouse hepatocytes. *Am J Pathol* 1997;151:1273–1280.
62. Lafferty K, Prowse S, Simeonovic C. Immunobiology of tissue transplantation: a return to the passenger leukocyte concept. *Ann Rev Immunol* 1983;1:143–173.
63. Baumgardner G, Li J, Apte S, et al. Effect of tumor necrosis factor alpha and intercellular adhesion molecule-1 expression on immunogenicity of murine liver cells in mice. *Hepatology* 1998;28:466–474.
64. So S, Wilkes L, Platt JL, et al. Purified hepatocytes can stimulate allospecific cytolytic T lymphocytes in a mixed lymphocyte-hepatocyte culture. *Transplant Proc* 1987;19:251–252.
65. Brent L, Bain A, Butler R, et al. The antigenicity of purified liver parenchymal cells. *Transplant Proc* 1981;13:860–862.

66. Makowka L, Lee G, Cobourn C, et al. Allogeneic hepatocyte transplantation in the rat spleen under cyclosporine immunosuppression. *Transplantation* 1986;42:537–541.

67. Kokudo N, Horimoto H, Ishiday K, et al. Allogeneic hepatocyte and fetal liver transplantation and xenogeneic hepatocyte transplantation for Nagase's analbuminemic rats. *Cell Transplant* 1996;5:S21–S31.

68. Morita H, Sugiura K, Inaba M, et al. A strategy for organ allografts without using immunosuppressants or irradiation. *Proc Natl Acad Sci U S A* 1998;95:6947–6952.

69. Morita H, Nakamura N, Sugiura K, et al. Acceptance of skin allografts in pigs by portal venous injection of donor bone marrow cells. *Ann Surg* 1999;230:114–119.

70. Qian J, Hashimoto T, Fujiwara H, et al. Studies on the induction of tolerance to alloantigens. I. The abrogation of potentials for delayed-type-hypersensitivity response to alloantigens by portal venous inoculation with allogeneic cells. *J Immunol* 1985;134:3656–3661.

71. Goss J, Flye M, Lacy P. Induction of allogeneic islet survival by intrahepatic islet preimmunization and transient immunosuppression. *Diabetes* 1996;45:144–147.

72. Patel A, Hardy M, Chowdhury N, et al. Long term correction of genetic defect of liver function in rat by transplantation of liver cells after ultraviolet irradiation. *Mol Biol Med* 1989;6:187–196.

73. Kawai Y, Price J, Hardy M. Reversal of liver failure in rats by UV-irradiated hepatocyte transplantation. *Transplant Proc* 1987;19:989–991.

74. Feng S, Quickel R, Hollister-Lock J, et al. Prolonged xenograft survival of islets infected with small doses of adenovirus expressing CTLA4Ig. *Transplantation* 1999;67:1607–1613.

75. Qin L, Chavin KD, Ding Y, et al. Multiple vectors effectively achieve gene transfer in a murine cardiac transplantation model. Immunosuppression with TGF-beta 1 or vIL-10. *Transplantation* 1995;59:809–816.

76. Drazan K, Wu L, Olthoff K, et al. Transduction of hepatic allografts achieves local levels of viral IL-10 which suppress alloreactivity *in vitro*. *J Surg Res* 1995;59:219–223.

77. Ilan Y, Sauter B, Roy Chowdhury N, et al. Expression of adenoviral E3 gene production in normal rat hepatocytes prevents their rejection upon transplantation into allogeneic Gunn rats {Abstract}. *Hepatology* 1997;26: 251A.

78. Drazan K, Olthoff K, Wu L, et al. Adenovirus-mediated gene transfer in the transplant setting: early events after orthotopic transplantation of liver allografts expressing TGF-beta. *Transplantation* 1996;62:1080–1084.

79. Lenschow DJ, Zeng Y, Thistlethwaite JR, et al. Long-term survival of xenogeneic pancreatic islet grafts induced by CTLA4Ig. *Science* 1992;257:789–792.

80. Lau H, Yu M, Fontana A, et al. Prevention of islet allograft rejection with engineered myoblasts expressing FasL in mice. *Science* 1996; 273:109–112.

81. Hammel J, Elfeki S, Kobayashi N, et al. Transplanted hepatocytes infected with a complement receptor type 1 (CR1)-containing recombinant adenovirus are resistant to hyperacute rejection. *Transplant Proc* 1999;31:939.

82. Bosman D, de Hann J, Smit J, et al. Metabolic activity of microcarrier attached liver cells after intraperitoneal transplantation during severe liver insufficiency in the rat. *J Hepatol* 1989;9:49–58.

83. Ebata H, Oikawa I, Mito M. Rejection of allogeneic hepatocytes and fetal hepatic tissue transplanted into the rat spleen. *Transplantation* 1985;39:221–223.

84. Hullett D, Falany J, Love R, et al. Transplantation of interim hosted and murine fetal pancreatic tissue. *Fed Proc* 1986;45:267.

85. Wen L, Calmus Y, Honiger J, et al. Encapsulated xenogeneic hepatocytes remain functional after peritoneal implantation despite immunization of the host. *J Hepatol* 1998;29:960–968.

86. Chowdhury JR, Grossman M, Gupta S, et al. Long-term improvement of hypercholesterolemia after *ex vivo* gene therapy in LDLR-deficient rabbits. *Science* 1991;254:1802–1805.

87. Grossman M, Raper SE, Kozarsky K, et al. Successful *ex vivo* gene therapy directed to liver in a patient with familial hypercholesterolaemia. *Nat Genet* 1994;6:335–341.

88. Grossman M, Rader DJ, Muller DW, et al. A pilot study of *ex vivo* gene therapy for homozygous familial hypercholesterolaemia. *Nat Med* 1995;1:1148–1154.

89. Raper SE, Grossman M, Rader DJ, et al. Safety and feasibility of liver-directed *ex vivo* gene therapy for homozygous familial hypercholesterolemia. *Ann Surg* 1996;223:116–126.

90. Habibullah C, Syed I, Qamar A, et al. Human fetal hepatocyte transplantation in patients with fulminant hepatic failure. *Transplantation* 1994;58:951–952.

91. Strom SC, Fisher RA, Thompson MT, et al. Hepatocyte transplantation as a bridge to orthotopic liver transplantation in terminal liver failure. *Transplantation* 1997;63:559–569.

92. Bilir B, Durham J, Krystal J, et al. Transjugular intra-portal transplantation of cryopreserved human hepatocytes in a patient with acute liver failure [Abstract]. *Hepatology* 1996;24:308A.

93. Bilir B, Guenette D, Ostrowska A, et al. Percutaneous hepatocyte transplantation (PHT) in liver failure [Abstract]. *Hepatology* 1997; 26:252A.

94. Soriano H, Wood R, Kang D, et al. Hepatocellular transplantation (HCT) in children with fulminant liver failure (FLF) [Abstract]. *Hepatology* 1997;26:239A.

95. Strom S, Roy Chowdhury J, Fox IJ. Hepatocyte transplantation for the treatment of clinical disese. *Semin Liver Dis* 1999;19:39–48.

96. Mito M, Kusano M. Hepatocyte transplantation in man. *Cell Transplant* 1993;2:65–74.

97. Fox IJ, Roy Chowdhury J, Kaufman S, et al. Treatment of Crigler-Najjar syndrome type I with hepatocyte transplantation. *N Engl J Med* 1998; 338:1422–1426.

98. Tada K, Roy-Chowdhury N, Prasad V, et al. Long-term amelioration of bilirubin glucuronidation defect in Gunn rats by transplanting genetically modified immortalized autologous hepatocytes. *Cell Transplant* 1998;7:607–616.

99. Block G, Locker J, Bowen W, et al. Population expansion, clonal growth, and specific differentiation patterns in primary cultures of hepatocytes induced by HGF/SF, EGF and TGF alpha in a chemically defined (HGM) medium. *J Cell Biol* 1996;132:1133–1149.

100. Platt JL. Xenotransplanting hepatocytes: the triumph of a cup half full. *Nat Med* 1997;3:26–27.

101. Guha C, Vikram B, Gupta S, et al. Hepatocyte transplantation increases survival after partial hepatectomy and whole liver irradiation in F344 rats [Abstract]. *Gastroenterology* 1998;114:A1250.

102. Vrancken Peeters M, Patijn G, Lieber A, et al. Expansion of donor hepatocytes after recombinant adenovirus-induced liver regeneration in mice. *Hepatology* 1997;25:884–888.

103. Laconi E, Oren R, Mukhopadhyay DK, et al. Long-term, near-total liver replacement by transplantation of isolated hepatocytes in rats treated with retrorsine. *Am J Pathol* 1998;153:319–329.

104. Gunsalus J, Grady D, Coulter S, et al. Reduction of serum cholesterol in Watanabe rabbits by xenogeneic hepatocellular transplantation. *Nat Med* 1997;3:48–53.

Transplantation of the Liver, edited by Willis C. Maddrey, Eugene R. Schiff, and Michael F. Sorrell. Lippincott Williams & Wilkins, Philadelphia © 2001.

CHAPTER 29

The Role of the Clinical Transplant Coordinator

Laurel Williams-Todd

The clinical transplant coordinator (CTC) is a professional nurse who has the unique opportunity to act as the liaison among patients, families, the transplant team, and referring physicians. As an educator, advocate, counselor, confidante, and collaborator, the transplant coordinator is positioned to ensure high-quality, cost-effective care by decreasing the fragmentation and duplication of medical care and diagnostic testing, enhancing quality nursing care, ensuring efficient use of resources, and contributing to strategies for cost containment.[1–4]

In 1976, 22 clinical and procurement transplant coordinators from across the country met for the first time in Dr. Paul Terasaki's laboratory. Their goal was to learn from each other, share strategies for care of both recipient and donor families, and lend support to each other in the evolving field of organ transplantation. This group went on to organize the North American Transplant Coordinator's Organization (NATCO). With more than 2,000 members, NATCO is the largest organization of transplant professionals in the United States. As the field of organ transplantation has evolved, so has the role and responsibilities of the transplant coordinator.

Since that meeting, a number of significant events affecting the role of the CTC have occurred. With the development of new immunosuppressive medications and the improvement in survival rates, more people are seeking transplantation as an option for treatment, while the number of organ donors remains stagnant. New programs continue to open across the country, allowing patients, their physicians, and health care providers more choices in transplant care. The continued growth of managed care and the move to integrated delivery networks is constantly challenging transplant programs to deliver quality care at the lowest cost.[1] Under managed care and capitated reimbursement systems, transplant coordinators are strategically placed to facilitate both quality and cost containment. In collaboration with many other health care professionals, including physicians, social workers, dietitians, pharmacists, and financial counselors, the nurse coordinator evaluates, coordinates, and monitors options to meet patient and family needs throughout the phases of transplantation. Although the phases of transplantation remain the same—pretransplantation, hospitalization, immediate posttransplantation, and long-term follow-up care—the challenges are ever-changing in the current health care arena.

PRETRANSPLANTATION AND EVALUATION

The initial contact between the patient and the transplant team is made through a variety of sources. The CTC is often the first person to receive and respond to initial inquiries. Requests for information and referrals for transplantation have come from patients and family members, their local hepatologists, internists, primary care physicians, and third-party payers. New technology has also brought a number of inquiries from the Internet.

A comprehensive liver transplant program provides a full range of services for patients with all types and degrees of severity of liver disease. These services include medical alternatives, such as the most current licensed or investigational medications, and a wide variety of surgical options, such as liver resection, cryoablative surgery, and orthotopic, split-liver, reduced-size liver, living-related liver, and hepatocyte transplantation. The CTC in collaboration with a transplant physician is able to discuss treatment options with patients, family members, referring physicians, and insurers and provide them with educational materials as requested. Based on the patient's medical condition, the CTC will make arrangements for the patient to undergo an appropriate and timely evaluation. The patient is requested to obtain medical records from the referring physician so that duplication of tests is kept to a minimum. Detailed medical information about the patient's past medical history guides the transplant team in its review of treatment options.

L. Williams-Todd: Department of Surgery, University of Nebraska Medical Center, Omaha, Nebraska 68198.

The majority of liver transplant evaluations are done in the outpatient setting unless the patient meets medical criteria for an admission to the hospital. The scheduling for the evaluation is done in a manner that ensures the appropriate tests and secondary consultations are completed in a timely fashion. The nurse coordinator contacts patients by telephone prior to their arrival, to review their schedule. Patients then receive a written itinerary that includes the time and location of all tests and appointments. The CTC meets patients at their first appointment to welcome them to the center and ensure that they have a copy of their schedule. Any immediate questions or concerns can be addressed promptly at this time. This initial introduction allows the patient and family to establish a critical connection with the CTC, who will be their contact person throughout the evaluation should problems or questions arise. The CTC is the facilitator for the patient during the evaluation process, coordinating the scheduling of any additional testing that may be required once the patient is seen and communicating any changes to the patient and family. In addition, the CTC meets with the patient and family to discuss the various aspects of transplantation (Table 29.1).

The verbal information is reinforced by written patient education materials that patients can take home and use as a reference for themselves, other family members, or friends. Patients who require an inpatient evaluation are scheduled in a similar manner and are seen by the CTC and members of the transplant team during daily patient rounds.

Once the initial evaluation has been completed, the patient is presented at a multidisciplinary team meeting to ascertain the patient's candidacy. At this meeting, the CTC is able to provide unique insights about medical and social issues faced by the patient and family, which assists the team in their decision making. Because the majority of patients return to their home after completion of the evaluation, the team recommendations are relayed to the patient through the CTC by phone. A summary of the data from the evaluation, as well as the team recommendations, is sent to the referring physician. If additional tests need to be completed, the CTC coordinates this with the referring physician. In conjunction with the financial counselor, the CTC ensures that the appropriate information for insurance approval is

completed and notifies both the patient and the referring physician when the patient becomes an active candidate on the waiting list.

In many regions of the country, the waiting times for locating suitable donor organs are prolonged. Because of the uncertainty of finding a suitable donor organ in the face of progressive liver disease, patients and family members have described the waiting period as one of the most stressful periods of the transplant process. All patients on the waiting list carry a pager in case they are not at home when a donor organ becomes available. The pager, usually provided free of charge, usually has a 30-mile radius, thus limiting the patient's ability to travel freely, further increasing the level of stress.

During the waiting period the CTC remains in contact with patients by monthly phone calls or letters. This contact reassures the patients that they have not been forgotten during the waiting process. The telephone contact provides the coordinator and transplant team with critical, updated medical information about the patient that may affect the patient's status on the waiting list. It also allows the CTC to identify other areas of concern or stress that the family may be experiencing. The CTC is often the most knowledgeable member of the transplant team readily available to answer questions from patients, local physicians, or third-party payers. The CTC is often in the best position to facilitate physician-to-physician contact when needed.

SURGERY AND HOSPITALIZATION

When a donor organ becomes available, the transplant surgeon in conjunction with the nurse coordinator will select the appropriate patient based on the United Network for Organ Sharing (UNOS) guidelines. The CTC notifies the patient and makes the other necessary arrangements at the transplant center to facilitate the arrival of the patient and family, such as notifying the admissions department, appropriate hospital staff, and patient care units and arranging housing for the accompanying family members. The CTC monitors the progress of the surgery and ensures that the family is informed about progress in the operating room. If problems or complications arise during the operation, the CTC is once again the liaison between the surgeons and the family, continuously updating family members on the events in the operating room.

Once the operation is completed, the patient is transported to the intensive care unit and the CTC notifies the referring physician by phone that the transplant has occurred. Subsequently, weekly letters or phone calls are initiated to the referring physician to update him or her on the patient's progress.

The use of critical pathways and oversight by managed care companies has had an impact on the length of stay post-transplantation, with the majority of adult patients leaving the hospital within 7 to 14 days. During this time, the physicians, CTC, and nursing staff are constantly focused on discharge

---

TABLE 29.1. *Issues discussed by the coordinator with the patient and family during evaluation*

Waiting time and the national organ allocation system
Donor criteria
Candidate selection
The operative procedure
Monitoring equipment, care, and visitation in the intensive care unit
Postsurgical floor or transplant unit routines
Estimated length of stay and discharge criteria
Risks and benefits of transplantation
Survival, rehabilitation, and long-term follow-up care

planning. The CTC participates in patient rounds daily as part of the transplant team, assessing individual patient's needs and coordinating support services to facilitate discharge activities. The CTC also sees the patient and family members on a one-to-one basis, clarifying individual questions or concerns about the patient's medical condition.

The time spent with patients and family members gives the coordinators the opportunity to know their unique personal needs and fears based on individual cultural and psychosocial backgrounds. Combined with the advanced assessment skills of the coordinator, the information obtained influences the daily care provided by all team members. The patient and family members often see the CTC as their primary advocate and ally. Formal and informal meetings between the CTC, physicians, staff nurses, and other health care professionals ensure communication of information that addresses the unique needs of each family member. These meetings also promote continuity of care in and out of the hospital.

Once patients leave the hospital setting, they remain locally as outpatients for several weeks, depending on their medical condition, if they do not already live nearby. The time spent in the area allows close monitoring of the patient's medications, laboratory tests, and physical condition. This time period allows the patient to develop physical strength and self-confidence in following the daily medical regimen. When it is determined that the patient may return home, the CTC notifies the referring physician and sends a detailed letter regarding follow-up care. If problems arise, the CTC is available on a 24-hour basis to triage and facilitate rapid access to other members of the transplant team.

Pediatric Issues

Many aspects of the postoperative care of children are similar to those of the adult population. However, some issues are specific to pediatric patients. Many transplant programs have developed specialized pediatric teams to address the unique needs of the child. The CTC addresses a number of these issues during discharge teaching, including immunizations, risk of communicable disease, school, and limit setting for the chronically ill child.

Immunizations

Ideally, children will have received routine, age-appropriate vaccinations prior to transplantation. Because of young age and the severity of the underlying illness, this is not always possible, and children are often behind on their vaccinations following transplant surgery. Initiation or resumption of vaccinations following surgery is desirable. However, historically there have been three concerns about vaccinating children after transplantation. First, immunosuppression may impair the immune response. Second, vaccination may promote rejection of the transplanted organ. Third, and

most important as relates to the live attenuated viruses, vaccination may actually result in disease in the immunocompromised patient.

Concerns about promoting rejection and about the adequacy of response have been largely dispelled. Thus, the use of killed vaccines, including the influenza, pneumococcus, hemophilus, and hepatitis vaccines, is no longer controversial.[5] Controversy remains concerning the role of live attenuated vaccines, notably MMR (measles, mumps, rubella) and Varivax (varicella). Of the two, the safety and effectiveness of the MMR has been best established in pediatric liver transplant recipients.[6] Although given sporadically to liver transplant recipients, the safety and effectiveness of Varivax has been demonstrated only in pediatric kidney transplant patients.[7] Because the killed poliovirus vaccine (IPV) is both safe and effective, the live attenuated poliovirus vaccine (OPV) is virtually never given to immunosuppressed patients. Currently, we administer MMR to children receiving alternate-day or no prednisone who have been stable for 6 months to a year after surgery; we use Varivax under similar circumstances on an individual basis.

Communicable Disease

Varicella (chickenpox) seems to be most problematic virus among the school-age population. If a child has never acquired chickenpox or has not received Varivax before transplantation, the recommendation following a close exposure is to administer varicella-zoster immune globulin (VZIG) within 48 to 72 hours. If a child contracts varicella despite having received a dose of VZIG, the standard recommendation is for administration of intravenous acyclovir. In practice, however, milder cases of chickenpox are often treated at home with daily oral acyclovir.

Rubeola (measles) may also be a concern in a posttransplantation child. If exposed, the child may benefit from a dose of immune globulin within 6 days in an attempt to boost the immune system and limit the effects of the virus.[8]

In general, all communicable diseases in the school should be reported to the parents so they are able to monitor for any signs and symptoms of the disease and take any necessary medical actions. Additional questions or concerns may be further addressed by the CTC and other members of the transplant team.

School

During hospitalization, every effort is made to assist the child in meeting age-appropriate educational goals and objectives. Good communication between the hospital teacher and the teacher at home is important so that the child is able to keep pace with the class and experience support during hospitalization. This communication will help the child reintegrate into the school system upon return home. Most children are able to return to a normal classroom following transplantation and to participate in all age-appropriate activities. Some transplant centers recommend that children avoid contact sports such as football.

Limit Setting

Children with life-threatening illness may have experienced little or no limit setting. Following transplantation, discipline strategies should be consistently implemented for all children, whether in the school or home. A child ultimately feels more secure in an environment in which discipline is used fairly and consistently. Discipline for any child is directed at creating a safe, predictable environment in which the child is aware of limits, expectations, and outcomes.

HOME CARE AND LONG-TERM CARE

Written communication from transplant physicians to referring physicians throughout a patient's hospitalization facilitates the return of the patient to his or her local community. After returning home, the primary care or referring physician resumes the care of the transplant patient. In conjunction with the local physician, the transplant team maintains its involvement with the care of the transplant recipient. The CTC is often the central figure in maintaining communications among the primary care physician, patients, families, and transplant center. Laboratory studies performed at varying intervals are monitored by the CTC. A transplant physician reviews any abnormalities, and a plan is devised and communicated through the CTC to the patient and primary care physician.

Often the transplant recipient will call the transplant program with specific problems or concerns. The CTC has 24-hour responsibility for screening these problems and pursuing the appropriate course of action. In addition, the CTC focuses on routine health maintenance issues such as nutrition, growth and development, readjustment to the home setting, and screening exams. The primary care physician can manage most of these issues at home. If major problems arise, such as rejection, sepsis, lymphoproliferative disease, other suspected cancers, or the need for additional surgery, the CTC, after consulting with the transplant physician and referring physician, may ask the patient to return to the transplant center.

PROFESSIONAL RESPONSIBILITIES

The CTC assumes other responsibilities besides the direct care of transplant patients. Collaborative and independent research activities ensure that the care provided to patients is state of the art and that a high quality of care is maintained. Formal presentations to a variety of professional and lay or-

ganization groups allow the dissemination of information about transplantation and organ donation. Consultation with other nurses and hospital administrators promotes changes in care practices that are necessary in an ever-changing health care environment. Participation with national organizations allows the CTC to be current with advances at other centers and with national health care issues.

SUMMARY

The role of the CTC has evolved over the past 20 years to accommodate changes in the severity of patient illness, increased patient volume, growing numbers of transplant teams and referral sources, and the demands of the external environment, such as managed care and the disparity of organ distribution. However, the CTC continues to play a pivotal role as a resource to patients and families, referring physicians, other members of the transplant team, and the community at large. Through advanced physical assessment and communication skills, the CTC constantly strives to ensure that patients and families have the knowledge and support necessary to achieve the highest quality of care throughout all phases of transplantation. This involves effecting collaboration and consultation with the many disciplines involved in the care of the transplant patient. Although all the members of the health care team are vital components to the success of an effective transplant program, the nurse coordinator is the critical link that ensures rapid access to consistent, compassionate, and capable care.

ACKNOWLEDGMENTS

I acknowledge the editorial assistance of Dr. Michael F. Sorrell, Dr. Stuart S. Kaufman, Dr. Geri Wood, and Joyce Rogge and thank Christine Hall for her secretarial assistance.

REFERENCES

1. Taylor P. Comprehensive nursing case management: an advanced practice model. *Nursing Case Management* 1999;4(1):2–10.
2. Heyl AK, Staschak S, Folk P, et al. The patient coordinator in a liver transplant program. *Gastroenterol Clin North Am* 1988;17:195–206.
3. Ribka JP. Building systems to measure continuity of care. *Nursing Case Management* 1999;3(4):151–154.
4. Fuzard B. *Case management: a challenge for nurses.* Kansas City, MO: American Nurses Association, 1988.
5. Mauch TJ, Crouch NA, Freese DK, et al. Antibody response of pediatric solid organ transplant recipients to immunization against influenza virus. *J Pediatr* 1995;127:957–960.
6. Rand EB, McCarthy CA, Whitington PF. Measles vaccination after orthotopic liver transplantation. *J Pediatr* 1993;123:87–89.
7. Zamora I, Simon JM, Da Silva ME, et al. Attenuated varicella virus vaccine in children with renal transplants. *Pediatr Nephrol* 1994;8:190–192.
8. American Academy of Pediatrics. *The red book: report of the Committee on Infectious Diseases,* 23rd ed. Elk Grove Village, IL: American Academy of Pediatrics, 1994.

Transplantation of the Liver, edited by Willis C. Maddrey, Eugene R. Schiff, and Michael F. Sorrell. Lippincott Williams & Wilkins, Philadelphia © 2001.

CHAPTER 30

Survival following Liver Transplantation

Jorge Rakela, David D. Douglas, Sumodh Kalathil, and David C. Mulligan

Liver transplantation has become a well-established therapeutic option in patients with acute or chronic liver disease. Since the 1980s, complications associated with immunosuppression, rejection, and infections that are unique to the immunosuppressed host have become better diagnosed and more effectively treated. These developments have led to the current outstanding results in terms of patient and graft survival.

As liver transplant patients live longer, the overwhelming cause of graft dysfunction and, in some patients, organ failure is recurrence of the disease that was the indication for liver transplantation in the first place. The clinical expression and tempo of the recurrent disease may be different because it occurs in an immunosuppressed host. This chapter reviews the current status of patient and graft survival by major etiologic groups.

HEPATITIS B

There are an estimated 1.25 million individuals in the United States who are chronically infected with the hepatitis B virus (HBV). Approximately 15% of these individuals with chronic hepatitis B infections will progress to cirrhosis. The lifetime risk of developing hepatocellular carcinoma in a patient with cirrhosis from chronic hepatitis B approaches 40%. Currently, hepatitis B is the sixth most common indication for liver transplantation and constitutes about 5% of the total number of liver transplantations performed in this country.

Historically, in the absence of immunoprophylaxis and antiviral therapy, liver transplantation for patients with hepatitis B yielded dismal results. Cumulative results from liver transplantations performed in the 1970s and 1980s for hepatitis B show that 55% of these recipients died within 60 days

of transplantation. Those recipients who did survive had a high rate of allograft loss due to recurrent HBV infection. Because of these initial poor results many insurance carriers refused to reimburse for liver transplantations performed for hepatitis B, and many transplant centers considered this diagnosis a contraindication for transplantation.

Immunoprophylaxis with hepatitis B immune globulin (HBIG) revolutionized the treatment of patients with hepatitis B undergoing liver transplantation. In 1993, Samuel et al.[1] reported the results of a multicenter European trial utilizing HBIG immunoprophylaxis and showing the potential for better survival in patients undergoing liver transplantation for hepatitis B. This study involved 17 European transplant centers and evaluated 372 consecutive patients who were positive for hepatitis B surface antigen (HBsAg) and who underwent liver transplantation between 1977 and 1990. Participants were divided into three groups: no treatment, short-term HBIG therapy, or long-term HBIG therapy. The average time to recurrence of hepatitis B in the short-term HBIG treatment group was about 3 months, compared with 8 months in the long-term HBIG treatment group. Survival at 2 years in the short-term HBIG treatment group was about 65%, compared with 80% in the long-term HBIG treatment group.

Another important part of this trial was the stratification of risk of recurrence of hepatitis B, based on the pretransplantation replication status of the recipient. The recipients with the highest risk of recurrence were those who were chronically infected with HBV and were HBV DNA positive prior to transplantation, whereas recipients with the lowest risk of recurrence were those with fulminant hepatitis B or coinfections with hepatitis D (groups that were more likely to be HBV DNA negative prior to transplantation). This observation led many transplant centers to accept only nonreplicative (hepatitis B e antigen–negative or HBV DNA–negative) hepatitis B patients as potential candidates for liver transplantation, even with the use of immunoprophylaxis.

J. Rakela, D. D. Douglas, S. Kalathil, and D. C. Mulligan: Department of Medicine and Department of Surgery, Mayo Clinic Scottsdale, Scottsdale, Arizona.

Antiviral treatments for hepatitis B have also made an impact on graft and patient survival rates. Interferon, although effective in patients with noncirrhotic hepatitis B, is of limited use in the pretransplantation setting because of the high complication rate seen in treating patients with decompensated cirrhosis secondary to chronic hepatitis B. Interferon has also been shown to be relatively ineffective in the posttransplantation setting once HBV infection has already become reestablished in the allograft. A better understanding of the role of immunosuppression in recurrent HBV infection and more targeted immunosuppression protocols have contributed to better survival posttransplantation in this group of patients. Newer antiviral agents such as nucleoside analogues have shown promise when they are used preemptively either alone or in combination with HBIG to lower pretransplantation HBV DNA levels and prevent recurrent hepatitis B posttransplantation.

The most promising of the currently available nucleoside analogues has been lamivudine. Recent reports have shown that lamivudine at a dose of 100 mg per day effectively suppresses hepatitis B replication in almost all chronically infected patients and also in liver transplant recipients infected with HBV.[2,3] Long-term therapy with lamivudine can improve liver function test results and lead to loss of hepatitis B e antigen (HBeAg) and occasionally HBsAg in some patients. Improvement in clinical parameters, including jaundice, ascites, and coagulopathy, in some patients with decompensated cirrhosis has also been described. The main problem with long-term lamivudine therapy has been the development of resistant virus variants. Newer nucleoside analogues such as adefovir have shown promise in preliminary trials and seem to be effective in patients who have developed lamivudine resistance. Future studies using combinations of nucleoside analogues in conjunction with HBIG will likely improve the control of recurrent HBV replication even further.

A recent symposium reviewing the latest United Network for Organ Sharing (UNOS) survival data on patients undergoing liver transplantation for hepatitis B found that survival rates among recipients treated with long-term HBIG have increased dramatically over the past decade; most major centers are reporting 1-year survival rates of between 75% and 90% in these patients. In an analysis of data from the University of Pittsburgh–UNOS Scientific Liver Transplant Registry collected from over 23,000 liver transplant recipients in 117 liver transplant centers in the United States and divided into three time-related patient cohorts (1988–1990, 1991–1993, and 1994–1996), a significant increase in patient survival for the most recent time period was demonstrated for all transplant patients. The results for patients with acute hepatitis B were dramatic, with 2-year survival in the earliest cohort (1988–1990) being 56% and increasing to 80% by the most recent time period (1994–1996). This increase was greater than that seen in other transplant recipients presenting with acute liver failure not caused by hepatitis B as an indication for transplantation. Similarly, patients with chronic hepatitis B showed a dramatic improvement in survival over these time periods, and the current 2-year survival rate in these patients is comparable with the survival rates in transplant recipients with end-stage liver disease from other etiologies.

The conclusions of the symposium were as follows: (a) among liver transplant recipients with hepatitis B, irrespective of viral replicative status pretransplantation, the long-term use of passive immunization (HBIG) has brought about an increase in liver transplantation survival from 50% in 1993 to 80% in 1998; (b) transplant outcomes for hepatitis B are now comparable with the outcomes for other indications for liver transplantation; and (c) given these advances, hepatitis B patients today are universally considered appropriate candidates for liver transplantation, and no chronic hepatitis B patient should be excluded from liver transplantation due to replicative status.

Rarely, transplant recipients who are HBsAg negative pretransplantation can develop de novo hepatitis B after transplantation. This has been most commonly described in recipients of a donor liver that was positive for antibody to hepatitis B core antigen (anti-HBc). Transmission rates between 50% and 80% have been described from donor livers that are HBsAg negative but positive for anti-HBc either alone or in conjunction with antibody to HBsAg (anti-HBs).[4,5] Compared with patients with recurrent hepatitis B posttransplantation, de novo infected patients tend to have lower levels of HBV replication and better long-term outcomes and survival rates. This observation has prompted some transplant centers to increase the use of donors positive for anti-HBc for highly selected recipient populations, such as chronic hepatitis B patients or patients exhibiting pretransplantation immunity (anti-HBs positive) to hepatitis B and possibly even UNOS status 1 or 2A patients. Recipients who are HBsAg negative but have antibody evidence of prior hepatitis B exposure (either anti-HBc positive or anti-HBs positive) do not usually reactivate their hepatitis B posttransplantation, even though 29% of these recipients may have detectable HBV DNA by polymerase chain reaction (PCR) assay in their native explanted liver.

HEPATITIS C

Over 4 million individuals in this country are estimated to be chronically infected with the hepatitis C virus (HCV), and over time 25% to 30% of these patients will develop cirrhosis. Hepatitis C is currently the most common indication for liver transplantation in the United States and Europe. Serologic testing for the hepatitis C virus first became commercially available in 1990; thus, the statistics on posttransplantation outcomes are based on data collected over the past decade. Recurrent HCV replication as measured by detectable HCV RNA is present in almost all hepatitis C patients after liver transplantation, although the amount of allograft dysfunction is variable.

Recent reports on the long-term outcome of HCV infection after liver transplantation have shown good results with up to 10 years of follow-up. The King's College group in England reported the cumulative survival rates in 149 patients with hepatitis C as 79% after 1 year, 74% at 3 years, and 70% at 5 years.[6] These survival rates were comparable with the survival rates in recipients without hepatitis C. Serial follow-up biopsies showed 12% of recipients had no evidence of chronic hepatitis, 54% had mild chronic hepatitis, 27% had moderate chronic hepatitis, and 8% had cirrhosis. This study found an increased incidence of genotype 1b associated with severe allograft injury, which has not been substantiated by other reports.

The clinical outcome of 183 liver transplant recipients with end-stage liver disease (ESLD) secondary to HCV infection (HCV group) was compared with a contemporary cohort of 556 patients with HCV infection who underwent transplantation for nonviral, nonmalignant ESLD (control group) at the Thomas E. Starzl Transplantation Institute.[7] All patients were prospectively screened for anti-HCV antibodies and HCV RNA by reverse transcriptase PCR. All transplant recipients received low-dose tacrolimus immunosuppression. Cumulative patient survival rates for the HCV group were 80% after 1 year and 75% after 3 years, compared with rates of 84% and 78%, respectively, in the control group ($P = 0.452$). Primary graft survival rates for the HCV group and the control group were 72% and 77.5% at 1 year and 67% and 72% at 3 years, respectively ($P = 0.144$). The incidence of retransplantation was 12.6% in the HCV group and 10.4% in the control group ($P = 0.42$). Patients whose indication for transplantation was chronic HCV infection and who were treated with a lower dose of tacrolimus immunosuppression (0.05 mg/kg per day or less intravenously and 0.1 mg/kg per day or less orally) had patient and graft survival rates similar to those seen in transplant recipients without HCV infection.

Although these reports are encouraging that the short- to intermediate-term survival in hepatitis C patients is no different from that of other etiologies of end-stage liver disease, a significant number of patients may develop significant fibrosis and even cirrhosis with long enough follow-up. Since the natural history of hepatitis C in the nontransplantation setting usually requires 20 years or longer to progress to cirrhosis, even longer-term follow-up studies of patients who undergo transplantation for chronic hepatitis C will be needed to better define the natural history of this disease after liver transplantation.

Because of the increasing disparity between the number of available donor organs and the number of candidates awaiting liver transplantation, the use of donor organs positive for anti-HCV in recipients already chronically infected with hepatitis C is becoming more common in most liver transplant centers. Vargas et al.[8] recently reported the outcome of chronically infected hepatitis C patients who received donors organs that were also positive for hepatitis C. The recipients of HCV-infected organs had cumulative survival rates of 89% and 72% at 1 and 5 years, respectively, which did not differ from the control group. There were no differences in graft survival, incidence of cirrhosis, mean hepatitis activity index score, fibrosis, or mean activity of

serum transaminases in this group of recipients. There was a trend toward a lower incidence of recurrent hepatitis C in the study group compared with controls. Patients in whom the donor strain of hepatitis C became predominant after transplantation had significantly longer disease-free survival than patients who retained their own hepatitis C strain. This report supports the practice of expanding the donor pool to include HCV-positive donors for recipients with chronic hepatitis C and even suggests a protective effect in those patients in whom the donor strain predominates after transplant.

Rarely, *de novo* hepatitis C can occur after transplantation in recipients who were negative for HCV prior to transplantation. Those recipients who develop *de novo* infections with hepatitis C tend to have favorable outcomes similar to those found in patients with recurrent infection. This transmission is usually from the donor organ. The incidence of *de novo* HCV infections in transplant recipients has dropped dramatically with second-generation hepatitis C antibody testing of blood and tissue donors.[9]

HEPATOCELLULAR CARCINOMA

Hepatocellular carcinoma is one of the most common malignant tumors occurring worldwide, with an estimated annual incidence of 1 million cases. In the United States, hepatocellular carcinoma is the twenty-second most common malignancy, with an annual incidence of about 2 in 100,000. Hepatocellular carcinoma is associated with aflatoxin exposure as well as all forms of cirrhosis, especially hemochromatosis, alcohol-related cirrhosis, and hepatitis B and C.

Historically, malignancy was one of the primary indications for liver transplantation; in fact, the first successful liver transplantation by Starzl was performed in an 18-month-old infant with hepatocellular carcinoma. The results initially were very disappointing. A series from Pittsburgh reported a 75% recurrence rate and a 3-year survival rate of 25%, UCLA reported a 48% recurrence rate and a 3-year survival rate of 31%, and the Cincinnati Transplant Tumor Registry reported a 5-year survival rate of only 18%. More recent reports have shown that individuals with early operative-stage disease have excellent long-term survival rates. In three separate series evaluating patients with early-stage hepatocellular carcinomas (stage I or II), Ringe et al.[10] reported a 56% five-year survival, Iwatsuki et al.[11] reported a 68% to 75% five-year survival, and Mazzaferro et al. found a recurrence-free survival rate of 83% at 4 years of follow-up.[12]

One of the growing concerns about performing transplantations in patients with hepatocellular carcinoma is the ever-lengthening waiting time for liver transplantation. The estimated doubling time for hepatocellular carcinoma ranges between 27 and 605 days, with mean values around 200 days and shorter doubling times reported in larger tumors. Another limitation is the underestimation of tumor involvement by current imaging studies. This has led many to the use of adjunctive treatment protocols in the pretransplantation period to try to slow tumor growth and prevent metastasis prior to transplantation. Preoperative hepatic artery chemoembolization has shown some promise in early uncontrolled trials. Venook et al.[13] used this technique in a limited number of selected patients and reported a 100% disease-free survival rate at 40 months. Harnois et al.[14] reported 1- and 2-year disease-free survival rates of 91% and 84%, respectively, in 24 patients with various stages of hepatocellular carcinoma (8% stage I, 54% stage II, 8% stage III, and 29% stage IVa). Further studies are needed to find the best technique available to control tumor growth and spread prior to liver transplantation and possibly down-stage the tumor.

At the present time, patients with Child's class A cirrhosis and hepatocellular carcinoma are still considered appropriate candidates for hepatic resection, but unfortunately only about 20% have anatomically resectable disease. Patients with Child's class B or C cirrhosis and early-stage tumors (a single lesion less than 5 cm in diameter or no more than three lesions, each less than 3 cm) are considered appropriate candidates for liver transplantation and should have survival rates comparable with patients having other forms of benign liver disease, at least out to 5 years.

ACUTE LIVER FAILURE

A recent publication on acute liver failure (ALF) in the United States has provided useful information regarding this entity.[15] Demographic data were collected retrospectively for a 2-year period from July 1994 to June 1996 on all cases of ALF from 13 hospitals (12 liver transplant centers). Among 295 patients, 74 (25%) survived spontaneously, 121 (41%) underwent transplantation, and 99 (34%) died without undergoing transplantation. Ninety-two (76%) of 121 patients survived 1 year after transplantation. Acetaminophen overdose was the most frequent cause of ALF (60 patients; 20%), followed by cryptogenic non-A, non-B, non-C hepatitis (15%), idiosyncratic drug reactions (12%), hepatitis B (10%), and hepatitis A (7%). Spontaneous survival rates were highest for patients with acetaminophen overdose (57%) and hepatitis A (40%) and lowest for those with Wilson's disease (no survivors of 18 patients). The transplantation rate was highest for Wilson's disease (17 of 18 patients; 94%) and lowest for autoimmune hepatitis (29%) and acetaminophen overdose (12%). Age did not differ between survivors and nonsurvivors, perhaps reflecting a selection bias for patients transferred to liver transplant centers. Coma grade on admission was not a significant determinant of outcome, but showed a trend toward affecting both survival and transplantation rate.

Acute liver failure represents one of the most challenging conditions in hepatology. In most cases, there is no effective therapy, and aggressive intensive care continues to be the most important management approach. These patients frequently develop multiorgan failure, placing them at risk of systemic infections, cerebral edema, hemodynamic instability, coagulopathy, and various renal and metabolic complications. A report from the American Society of Transplantation defined minimum listing criteria for patients with end-stage liver diseases, including ALF. These included the onset of stage 2 hepatic encephalopathy as a sole minimal criterion for patients with fulminant hepatic failure regardless of etiology.[16]

Cerebral edema is one of the most serious complications of ALF and could determine the outcome after liver transplantation. During orthotopic liver transplantation (OLT) for fulminant hepatic failure, some patients develop cerebral injury secondary to intracranial hypertension. Detry et al.[17] monitored intracranial pressure (ICP) and cerebral perfusion pressure (CPP) before and during OLT in 12 patients with fulminant hepatic failure undergoing transplantation. All 4 patients who had normal ICP preoperatively maintained normal ICP and CPP throughout the transplant procedure. During OLT, 4 of the 8 patients with pretransplantation intracranial hypertension had six episodes of ICP elevation. These episodes of intracranial hypertension occurred during difficult liver dissections (n = 3) and graft reperfusions (n = 3). At the end of the anhepatic phase, the ICP was lower than the preoperative ICP in all patients, and was below 15 mm Hg in all but one patient. The authors suggested that in patients with ALF who develop intracranial hypertension before OLT, dissection of the native liver and graft reperfusion are associated with a risk of brain injury resulting from intracranial hypertension and cerebral hypoperfusion.

The majority of patients who present with ALF continue to have an indeterminate etiology for their hepatic failure.[15] It is presumed that in many patients the ALF has been caused by a virus or viruses not yet characterized. An interesting observation is that follow-up biopsies in these patients showed that chronic hepatitis was present in 29 patients (71%) who underwent transplantation for fulminant seronegative hepatitis (23 mild, 3 moderate, and 3 severe) compared with 5 patients (31%, all mild) who underwent transplantation for other causes of fulminant hepatic failure. Twenty-five patients (61%) grafted for seronegative fulminant hepatic failure had fibrosis (13 mild, 9 moderate, and 3 severe), in contrast to 4 cases of fibrosis (25%; all mild) in the comparison group. Excluding early allograft failure because of primary graft nonfunction or vascular complications, 6 patients with seronegative fulminant hepatic failure required retransplantation (2 for chronic rejection, 1 for severe hepatitis with panacinar necrosis resembling the original liver histology, and 3 for chronic hepatitis with precirrhotic fibrosis and prominent cholestasis of unknown cause). One patient in the comparison group required a second graft because of chronic rejection. Posttransplantation chronic hepatitis is more frequent and severe in patients who undergo transplantation for seronegative hepatitis.[18]

The selection of patients with ALF to undergo liver transplantation is a major clinical challenge. If these patients recover spontaneously, they do so without significant clinical and pathological sequelae. One of the first attempts to define early prognostic criteria came from the King's College Liver Unit. Univariate and multivariate analyses were performed on 588 patients with acute liver failure managed medically between 1973 and 1985. In acetaminophen-induced fulminant hepatic failure, survival correlated with arterial blood pH, peak prothrombin time, and serum creatinine concentration. A pH less than 7.30, a prothrombin time greater than 100 seconds, and a creatinine concentration greater than 300 μmol/L indicated a poor prognosis. In patients with viral hepatitis (non-A, non-B hepatitis) and drug reactions as the cause of their hepatic failure, age younger than 11 years or older than 40 years, duration of jaundice before the onset of encephalopathy greater than 7 days, serum bilirubin level greater than 300 μmol/L, and prothrombin time greater than 50 seconds indicated a poor prognosis.[19] A more recent publication found that these criteria, although useful, are not as accurate as initially suggested;[20] application of King's College Hospital criteria at the time of admission to 145 patients admitted with acetaminophen-induced ALF had a positive predictive value of 88%, a negative predictive value of 65%, and a predictive accuracy of 71%. The positive predictive value, negative predictive value, and predictive accuracies of these criteria for non–acetaminophen-induced fulminant hepatic failure were 79%, 50%, and 68%, respectively. Multivariate analysis identified prothrombin time, serum creatinine concentration, white blood cell count, and abnormal serum potassium levels as independent predictors of mortality in acetaminophen-induced fulminant hepatic failure, and prothrombin time alone as a predictor in fulminant hepatic failure induced by other etiologies.

Renal failure present prior to liver transplantation has been associated with a worse prognosis after this procedure.[21] This observation also seems to hold true in patients with ALF.[22] One hundred eighty-one consecutive patients with ALF were reviewed to assess the impact of pretransplantation renal failure on mortality and morbidity following liver transplantation. Renal failure was present in 14 patients, 7 of whom died, whereas there was 100% survival in patients without renal failure. Pretransplantation renal failure was associated with prolonged mechanical ventilation (13 days versus 6 days for the control group, $P = 0.05$), prolonged intensive care stay (17 days versus 8 days, $P = 0.01$) and prolonged hospital stay (27 versus 21 days, P not significant). The authors concluded that renal failure prior to transplantation strongly predicted poor outcome with significantly greater consumption of resources.

The management of patients with ALF continues to evolve, and progress is being made in the development of a liver assist device. Several prototypes are undergoing clinical evaluation. These basically consist of a dialysis cartridge with human or animal hepatocytes in an attempt to provide temporary and sufficient liver function until the native liver regenerates or a donor becomes available.[23–25]

Another approach that seems promising is the use of an auxiliary graft in an orthotopic position while the right lobe of the native liver is left in place. As a result of this approach, the patient has temporary liver function support while the native liver regenerates. After regeneration occurs, immunosuppression can be discontinued and the loss of the graft goes unnoticed.[26–28]

ALCOHOLIC LIVER DISEASE

In 1988, Starzl et al.[29] demonstrated that patients with alcoholic cirrhosis who underwent liver transplantation had a 1-year survival of 73.2%; after 1 to 3 years, 28 (68%) of the recipients were alive. Only 2 patients returned to alcohol abuse. Social and vocational rehabilitation was the rule in these recipients. This seminal publication allowed liver transplantation to be considered among patients with alcoholic liver disease (ALD). Access to transplantation is usually regulated by the patient's demonstration of a commitment to long-term rehabilitation and abstinence.

The percentage of patients with ALD receiving liver transplantation has increased in recent years in almost every program. Combined ALD and hepatitis C are the leading indications for liver transplantation today. Rates of graft and patient survival are excellent and are not different from those observed among patients with other etiologies. The 7-year survival rate after liver transplantation is 60% according to data provided by UNOS. The rate of relapse to alcohol use has been estimated to be between 10% to 15% during the first year and 25% to 30% at 2 to 3 years after transplantation. The overall rate of relapse appears to level off at 3 to 5 years. These rates are much lower than those observed after a 1-year rehabilitation program.[30]

This optimistic outlook has to be tempered by the experience of a European group.[31] Seventy patients with ALD received transplants, and 59 survived more than 3 months; 56 of these were interviewed. Of the 56 patients interviewed, 28 (50%) had consumed alcohol after transplantation. There was no significant difference in episodes of acute rejection or compliance with medication between those who were abstinent and those who drank alcohol. Histologic evidence of liver injury was common in ALD patients who had returned to drinking. Mild fatty change was found in 1 of 11 biopsy specimens from abstinent patients, but moderate to severe fatty change and ballooned hepatocytes were seen in all the specimens from patients who drank. Two patients who drank heavily had early fibrosis. Return to alcohol consumption after liver transplantation in this series was associated with rapid development of histologic liver injury, including fibrosis.

An attempt to correlate the length of sobriety before transplantation with outcome after this procedure failed to show any correlation.[32] A total of 183 adults who had alcohol-related liver disease and underwent liver transplantation were studied at the Thomas E. Starzl Transplantation Institute. These patients had a better, though not statistically significant, 5-year survival rate compared with all other patients. Seventy-eight of these patients were UNOS status IIA (critically ill) at the point of transplantation. Although there was a trend toward poorer survival in patients with the shortest length of sobriety (1 month or less), pre-OLT length of sobriety or alcohol rehabilitation did not predict survival. Twenty-four percent of these patients used alcohol at some point after OLT. The minimal listing criteria[16] considered a requirement of 6 months' abstinence from alcohol to be appropriate before placing most patients with alcoholic liver disease on the transplant waiting list.

Patients who present with alcoholic hepatitis on top of chronic ALD have a very high fatality rate, and liver transplantation may seem the only option for many of them. However, many cannot fulfill the criteria of abstinence that is in place in most programs, and many of these patients die before they reach transplantation.[33] The group from the Thomas E. Starzl Transplantation Institute studied 9 liver transplant recipients in whom severe acute alcoholic hepatitis was retrospectively diagnosed; 8 had underlying cirrhosis, and 1 had advanced fibrosis. All had Maddrey's discriminant function greater than 32, and most had hepatic encephalopathy and hepatorenal syndrome. History regarding abstinence was unreliable in some patients. Episodes of acute cellular rejection responded quickly to therapy, and despite recidivism in some patients, the long-term survival rate was comparable with that of patients receiving transplants for alcoholic cirrhosis alone and with that of patients with a milder degree of alcoholic hepatitis and cirrhosis. This was a small, retrospective series, however, and should not be used to change current criteria of eligibility in this patient population.

There is a common association between chronic hepatitis C and alcoholic liver disease. A limited number of studies have assessed the outcome of these patients after liver transplantation.[34] Liver function tests 1 and 4 years after OLT showed aspartate aminotransferase and alanine aminotransferase values that were significantly higher in anti-HCV–positive patients, and histologically proven chronic hepatitis was found in 45% and 61% of these patients at 1 and 4 years posttransplantation, respectively. Pretransplantation HCV infection in patients with ALD did not affect survival after liver transplantation. However, the high incidence of posttransplantation chronic hepatitis secondary to recurrence of HCV infection may lead to more progressive disease in the long term.

AUTOIMMUNE HEPATITIS

Liver transplantation has a definite role in the management of autoimmune hepatitis.[35] When a series of patients who failed medical therapy were compared with a group of patients who underwent liver transplantation for severe autoimmune hepatitis, the former group had significantly lower survival rates. Successive biopsies in that early experience did not disclose evidence of disease recurrence.

When patients are followed for longer periods, recurrence of autoimmune hepatitis after liver transplantation may be seen. There is little information about its time of onset, risk factors, and response to treatment and prognosis. In a recently published series, 9 (33%) of 27 patients evaluated fulfilled criteria for recurrence of autoimmune hepatitis, with a mean time of recurrence after OLT of 2.6 ± 1.5 years.[36] Patients with recurrence had a longer follow-up time after transplantation (5.1 versus 2.5 years, $P = 0.0012$) and were receiving less immunosuppressive treatment. The estimated risk of recurrence of autoimmune hepatitis in the graft increased over time: from 8% in the first year to 68% at 5 years after transplantation. Fifty percent of the patients failed to respond or responded only partially to therapy, although none of the patients has deteriorated clinically after 2.4 ± 1.06 years of follow-up after recurrence. Although response to treatment was suboptimal, patient and graft survival rates were not decreased during the period of observation.

Another transplant center observed that despite triple immunosuppressive therapy, 3 (20%) of 15 patients developed chronic hepatitis with histologic and serologic features of autoimmune hepatitis in the absence of any other identifiable cause. The disease was severe in 2 patients, leading to graft failure, and asymptomatic in another despite marked histologic abnormalities. In one of these 3 patients, autoimmune hepatitis recurred in the second liver graft as well.

These observations have led to the suggestion that patients who undergo transplantation for autoimmune hepatitis should be kept on at least double immunosuppressive therapy and that special attention should be given to avoid tapering immunosuppressive drugs too quickly. This approach will probably need to be evaluated in a randomized, controlled trial to assess its efficacy.

PRIMARY BILIARY CIRRHOSIS

Primary biliary cirrhosis (PBC) clearly recurs after orthotopic liver transplantation. In a series from Mayo Clinic, 60 consecutive patients with PBC with at least 1 year of follow-up after liver transplantation were studied.[37] All patients were treated with triple-drug immunosuppression (cyclosporine, prednisone, and azathioprine). Forty-one of the 60 patients had near-normal histologic liver appearance. Of those with abnormal histologic appearance, 5 patients had histologic features typical of a florid bile duct lesion, suggesting recurrent primary biliary cirrhosis, 2 to 6 years after OLT. All 5 patients with portal granulomas had normal hepatic biochemical values and were clinically asymptomatic. Two of the 5 patients had persistent antimitochondrial antibody titers. The authors considered the histologic changes highly suggestive of recurrence of PBC after liver transplantation.[37]

In another series, the authors reviewed the most recent and the 1-year protocol liver biopsies of 69 patients who received transplants for PBC and of 53 control patients. They defined histologic features consistent with PBC recurrence as the presence of nonsuppurative destructive cholangitis, mixed portal infiltrates, fibrosis, and ductopenia. These histologic features were present in 6 patients who received transplants for PBC (8.7%, versus 0% in the control group) and occurred between 1 and 8 years after transplantation. In 5 of the 6 patients, antimitochondrial antibody 2 (anti-M2) antibodies remained at high titers. Cholestasis was present in 4 patients, and clinical symptoms in 2 patients. The investigators also found that the presence of plasma cells in the portal infiltrate at 1 year after transplantation was predictive of the risk of recurrence.[38]

PBC has been a suitable condition for studies of survival and for timing models because of its slowly progressive nature. In an attempt to define the optimal timing for liver transplantation, 143 patients with PBC undergoing liver transplantation were followed prospectively.[39] Disease severity was measured immediately before transplantation by a summary score ("risk score") used in the Mayo natural history model and based on the factors of age, bilirubin level, albumin level, prothrombin time, and the presence or absence of edema. Proportional hazards analyses were performed to assess patient survival following transplantation. Following transplantation, patient survival probabilities at 1, 2, and 5 years were 93%, 90%, and 88%, respectively. In the proportional hazards analysis, the risk of death following transplantation remained low until a risk score of 7.8 was reached. Risk scores greater than 7.8 were associated with a progressively increased mortality. Resource utilization, measured by the days in the intensive care unit (ICU) and hospital and the requirement for intraoperative blood transfusions, was significantly greater for recipients who had higher risk scores before transplantation. This study suggests that an optimal timing for liver transplantation, as determined by patient survival and resource utilization, appears to be at a risk score around 7.8 in patients with PBC. The current situation with donor availability makes the usefulness of these studies more theoretical than practical.

An intriguing observation was provided by the European trial comparing tacrolimus (FK506) and cyclosporine-based immunosuppression.[40] During the 2-year period, histologic features characteristic of primary biliary cirrhosis, including bile duct damage, ductopenia, bile duct proliferation, and portal granulomas, were found more commonly and earlier after transplantation in patients receiving tacrolimus (7 of 16 patients) than in those receiving cyclosporine (1 of 11). These findings suggest that the incidence of disease recurrence may be affected by the immunosuppressive regimen used.

PRIMARY SCLEROSING CHOLANGITIS

The outcomes of 436 patients with primary biliary cirrhosis or primary sclerosing cholangitis (PSC) who underwent orthotopic liver transplantation were studied at three major liver transplant centers.[41] Univariate predictors of outcome included age, Karnofsky score; Child's class; Mayo risk score; UNOS status; nutritional status; serum albumin level; serum bilirubin level; prothrombin (international normalized ratio); and the presence of ascites, encephalopathy, renal failure (serum creatinine concentration above 2 mg/dL), and edema refractory to diuretics. Using these predictors, a four-variable mathematical prognostic model was developed to help the liver transplant physician predict the following: the amount of

intraoperative blood loss, the number of days in the ICU, and the occurrence of severe complications after surgery. This study is the first to model the outcome of liver transplantation in patients with a specific etiology of chronic liver disease (PBC or PSC). The model may be used to help select patients for OLT and to plan the timing of their transplantation.

The results of liver transplantation in patients with PSC are excellent, and patient quality of life is markedly improved. Indeed, liver transplantation is the therapy of choice for patients with end-stage PSC. Liver transplantation should be offered to PSC patients who have (a) a Mayo risk score greater than 4.8 in whom malignancy is ruled out; (b) cirrhosis and complications of portal hypertension such as variceal bleeding, refractory ascites, or portosystemic encephalopathy; or (c) disabling symptoms such as fatigue, pruritus, or recurrent bacterial cholangitis.[42]

Recurrence of PSC following liver transplantation has been more difficult to establish because what are considered typical bile duct abnormalities for this condition may have different mechanisms in the transplant setting. Between March 1985 and June 1996, 150 patients with PSC underwent liver transplantation at the Mayo Clinic; the mean follow-up period was 55 months. The definition of recurrent PSC was based on characteristic cholangiographic and histologic findings that occur in nontransplant PSC patients. By using strict criteria, 30 patients with other known causes of posttransplantation nonanastomotic biliary strictures were excluded, leaving 120 patients for analysis of recurrence of PSC. The authors found evidence of PSC recurrence after liver transplantation in 24 patients (20%). Of these, 22 patients showed characteristic features of PSC on cholangiography, and 11 had compatible hepatic histologic abnormalities, with a mean time to diagnosis of 360 and 1,350 days, respectively. Both cholangiographic and hepatic histologic findings suggestive of PSC recurrence were seen in 9 patients. Therefore, up to 20% of patients may have recurrent disease after liver transplantation. None of these patients has required retransplantation so far.[43]

METABOLIC LIVER DISORDERS

Hereditary Hemochromatosis

Although experience with OLT for genetic hemochromatosis is limited, the survival rates at 1 year and 5 years have been reported to be 54% and 43%, respectively, which are inferior to the rates observed in other liver conditions. Posttransplantation deaths are usually related to infectious or cardiac complications.[44] Because the genetic defect resides in the enterocyte, patients with genetic hemochromatosis reaccumulate iron in the liver after transplantation.

A candidate gene, HFE, was recently described in patients with hereditary hemochromatosis and found to contain a missense mutation leading to a cysteine-to-tyrosine substitution (C282Y). A second mutation, H63D, was also found in the gene. A recently published study was conducted to determine the HFE genotype in liver transplant recipients clinically diagnosed with hereditary hemochromatosis and those incidentally found to have increased iron deposition in their explanted livers and to evaluate whether biochemical or histologic hepatic iron indices (HIIs) correlated with homozygosity for the C282Y mutation.[45] Among 918 adult patients who underwent liver transplantation from 1988 to 1995, increased liver iron was found in 15 patients clinically diagnosed with various liver disorders other than hereditary hemochromatosis. Four additional patients were clinically diagnosed as having hereditary hemochromatosis. Two of 4 patients with clinically suspected hereditary hemochromatosis were homozygous for C282Y, and 2 patients had neither mutation. One of the 15 patients not suspected to have hereditary hemochromatosis was homozygous for C282Y, 1 was heterozygous for C282Y, 6 were heterozygous for H63D, and 7 had neither mutation. Surprisingly, among patients fulfilling established clinical criteria for hereditary hemochromatosis, only a minority were homozygous for the C282Y mutation. Therefore, hepatic iron overload clearly may result from other causes, and in end-stage liver disease, an elevated HII may not necessarily establish the diagnosis of hereditary hemochromatosis.

It is necessary to continue to accumulate data in this patient population and establish whether this diagnosis entails a worse outcome, as initially was suggested. These patients may also provide insight into the mechanisms of excessive iron deposition and better define the interaction between the hepatocyte and enterocyte in determining excessive systemic iron deposition.

Wilson's Disease

The recent discovery that the gene for Wilson's disease encodes a copper-transporting adenosine triphosphatase has greatly improved our understanding of the pathophysiology of this disorder and of copper metabolism in humans.[46–48] The heterogeneity of disease-specific mutations and their location at multiple sites across the genome have limited molecular genetic diagnosis to the kindred of known patients. Chelation therapy with penicillamine and trientine remains effective treatment for most symptomatic patients with hepatic and neurologic Wilson's disease. Liver transplantation is the only treatment for patients who present with acute liver failure and also for those in whom pharmacotherapy is ineffective.[49]

Liver transplantation has also been shown to improve the neurologic symptoms of Wilson's disease, although this has not been a general observation.[50–52] More recently, a group from Germany reported their experience from 1988 until 1995, during which 13 (1.9%) of 700 liver transplantations were performed for Wilson's disease. The indications for liver transplantation were intractable neurologic impairment with normal liver function (n = 4, including 1 patient with Child's class A cirrhosis), ALF (n = 3), and end-stage liver cirrhosis (n = 6, with 1 patient having Child's class B cirrhosis and the other 5 having Child's class C cirrhosis). The patient group

with Wilson's disease included 8 women and 5 men with a mean age of 27 years (range, 15–34 years). All patients with neurologic involvement required continuous nursing care before transplantation, in spite of pretreatment with penicillamine and zinc. The most frequent symptoms were dysphagia, dysarthria, tremor, sialorrhea, ataxia, dystonia, and handwriting difficulties. All patients with ALF presented with hemolytic anemia. The survival rate was 100%, and all patients were doing well after a mean follow-up period of 32.8 months (range, 8–68 months). Neurologic symptoms began to improve 4 to 6 weeks after transplantation. Therefore, in some patients transplantation may be considered in hopes of stabilizing the neurologic manifestations.[53]

On the other hand, some patients do not show significant posttransplantation improvement of their neuropsychiatric symptoms. A 22-year-old man with advanced neurologic impairment and prominent psychiatric manifestations due to Wilson's disease who underwent liver transplantation showed a slow and incomplete neurologic improvement, and his behavioral and personality disorder was entirely unaffected. He committed suicide 43 months posttransplantation.[54]

In conclusion, liver transplantation is the treatment of choice for patients with Wilson's disease presenting with acute liver failure or decompensated cirrhosis. Patients with neurologic symptoms show improvement in many instances. Copper metabolism parameters improve rapidly, and Kayser-Fleischer rings disappear rapidly.[55]

CONCLUSION

Survival after liver transplantation improved remarkably after the advent of cyclosporine-based immunosuppression, and further improvement has been observed after tacrolimus became the immunosuppressive drug of choice. Both patient and graft survival rates have improved steadily. The vast majority of patients also enjoy a better quality of life. As these patients live longer, we are beginning to face recurrence of disease as the preeminent factor that will ultimately determine graft function and patient survival or the need for retransplantation.

REFERENCES

1. Samuel D, Muller R, Alexander G, et al. Liver transplantation in European patients with the hepatitis B surface antigen. *N Engl J Med* 1993; 329:1842–1847.
2. Dienstag JL, Schiff ER, Wright TL, et al. Lamivudine as initial treatment for chronic hepatitis B in the United States. *N Engl J Med* 1999; 341:1256–1263.
3. Perrillo R, Rakela J, Dienstag J, et al. Multicenter study of lamivudine therapy for hepatitis B after liver transplantation. Lamivudine Transplant Group. *Hepatology* 1999;29:1581–1586.
4. Douglas DD, Rakela J, Wright TL, et al. The clinical course of transplantation-associated *de novo* hepatitis B infection in the liver transplant recipient. *Liver Transplant Surg* 1997;3:105–111.
5. Dodson SF, Issa S, Araya V, et al. Infectivity of hepatic allografts with antibodies to hepatitis B virus. *Transplantation* 1997;64:1582–1584.
6. Gane EJ, Portmann BC, Naoumov NV, et al. Long-term outcome of hepatitis C infection after liver transplantation. *N Engl J Med* 1996; 334:815–820.

7. Casavilla FA, Rakela J, Kapur S, et al. Clinical outcome of patients infected with hepatitis C virus infection on survival after primary liver transplantation under tacrolimus. *Liver Transplant Surg* 1998;4:448–454.

8. Vargas HE, Laskus T, Wang LF, et al. Outcome of liver transplantation in hepatitis C virus-infected patients who received hepatitis C virus-infected grafts. *Gastroenterology* 1999;117:149–153.

9. Everhart JE, Wei Y, Eng H, et al. Recurrent and new hepatitis C virus infection after liver transplantation. *Hepatology* 1999;29:1220–1226.

10. Ringe B, Canelo R, Lorf T. Liver transplantation for primary liver cancer. *Transplant Proc* 1996;28:1174–1175.

11. Iwatsuki S, Marsh JW, Starzl TE. Survival after liver transplantation in patients with hepatocellular carcinoma. *Princess Takamatsu Symp* 1995;25:271–276.

12. Mazzaferro V, Regalia E, Doci R, et al. Liver transplantation for the treatment of small hepatocellular carcinomas in patients with cirrhosis. *N Engl J Med* 1996;334:693–699.

13. Venook AP, Ferrell LD, Roberts JP, et al. Liver transplantation for hepatocellular carcinoma: results with preoperative chemoembolization. *Liver Transplant Surg* 1995;1:242–248.

14. Harnois DM, Steers J, Andrews JC, et al. Preoperative hepatic artery chemoembolization followed by orthotopic liver transplantation for hepatocellular carcinoma. *Liver Transplant Surg* 1999;5:192–199.

15. Schiodt FV, Atillasoy E, Shakil AO, et al. Etiology and outcome for 295 patients with acute liver failure in the United States. *Liver Transplant Surg* 1999;5:29–34.

16. Lucey MR, Brown KA, Everson GT, et al. Minimal criteria for placement of adults on the liver transplant waiting list: a report of a national conference organized by the American Society of Transplant Physicians and the American Association for the Study of Liver Diseases. *Liver Transplant Surg* 1997;3:628–637.

17. Detry O, Arkadopoulos N, Ting P, et al. Intracranial pressure during liver transplantation for fulminant hepatic failure. *Transplantation* 1999;67:767–770.

18. Mohamed R, Hubscher SG, Mirza DF, et al. Posttransplantation chronic hepatitis in fulminant hepatic failure. *Hepatology* 1997;25:1003–1007.

19. O'Grady JG, Alexander GJ, Hayllar KM, et al. Early indicators of prognosis in fulminant hepatic failure. *Gastroenterology* 1989;97:439–445.

20. Anand AC, Nightingale P, Neuberger JM. Early indicators of prognosis in fulminant hepatic failure: an assessment of the King's criteria. *J Hepatol* 1997;26:62–68.

21. Rimola A, Gavaler JS, Schade RR, et al. Effects of renal impairment on liver transplantation. *Gastroenterology* 1987;93:148–156.

22. Mendoza A, Fernandez F, Mutimer DJ. Liver transplantation for fulminant hepatic failure: importance of renal failure. *Transpl Int* 1997;10:55–60.

23. Kamohara Y, Rozga J, Demetriou AA. Artificial liver: review and Cedars-Sinai experience. *J Hepato-Biliary-Pancreatic Surg* 1998;5:273–285.

24. Bismuth H, Samuel D, Castaing D, et al. Liver transplantation in Europe for patients with acute liver failure. *Semin Liver Dis* 1996;16:415–425.

25. McCarthy M, Ellis AJ, Wendon JA, et al. Use of extracorporeal liver assist device and auxiliary liver transplantation in fulminant hepatic failure. *Eur J Gastroenterol Hepatol* 1997;9:407–412.

26. van Hoek B, de Boer J, Boudjema K, et al. Auxiliary versus orthotopic liver transplantation for acute liver failure. EURALT Study Group. European Auxiliary Liver Transplant Registry. *J Hepatol* 1999;30:699–705.

27. Inomata Y, Kiuchi T, Kim I, et al. Auxiliary partial orthotopic living donor liver transplantation as an aid for small-for-size grafts in larger recipients. *Transplantation* 1999;67:1314–1319.

28. Rosenthal P, Roberts JP, Ascher NL, et al. Auxiliary liver transplant in fulminant failure. *Pediatrics* 1997;100:E10.

29. Starzl TE, Van Thiel D, Tzakis AG, et al. Orthotopic liver transplantation for alcoholic cirrhosis. *JAMA* 1988;260:2542–2544.

30. Hoofnagle JH, Kresina T, Fuller RK, et al. Liver transplantation for alcoholic liver disease: executive statement and recommendations. Summary of a National Institutes of Health workshop held December 6–7, 1996, Bethesda, Maryland. *Liver Transplant Surg* 1997;3:347–350.

31. Tang H, Boulton R, Gunson B, et al. Patterns of alcohol consumption after liver transplantation. *Gut* 1998;43:140–145.

32. DiMartini A, Jain A, Irish W, et al. Outcome of liver transplantation in critically ill patients with alcoholic cirrhosis: survival according to medical variables and sobriety. *Transplantation* 1998;66:298–302.

33. Shakil AO, Pinna A, Demetris J, et al. Survival and quality of life after liver transplantation for acute alcoholic hepatitis. *Liver Transplant Surg* 1997;3:240–244.

34. Pera M, Garcia-Valdecasas JC, Grande L, et al. Liver transplantation for alcoholic cirrhosis with anti-HCV antibodies. *Transpl Int* 1997;10:289–292.

35. Sanchez-Urdazpal L, Czaja AJ, van Hoek B, et al. Prognostic features and role of liver transplantation in severe corticosteroid-treated autoimmune chronic active hepatitis. *Hepatology* 1992;15:215–221.

36. Prados E, Cuervas-Mons V, de la Mata M, et al. Outcome of autoimmune hepatitis after liver transplantation. *Transplantation* 1998;66:1645–1650.

37. Balan V, Batts KP, Porayko MK, et al. Histological evidence for recurrence of primary biliary cirrhosis after liver transplantation. *Hepatology* 1993;18:1392–1398.

38. Sebagh M, Farges O, Dubel L, et al. Histological features predictive of recurrence of primary biliary cirrhosis after liver transplantation. *Transplantation* 1998;65:1328–1333.

39. Kim WR, Wiesner RH, Therneau TM, et al. Optimal timing of liver transplantation for primary biliary cirrhosis. *Hepatology* 1998;28:33–38.

40. Dmitrewski J, Hubscher SG, Mayer AD, et al. Recurrence of primary biliary cirrhosis in the liver allograft: the effect of immunosuppression. *J Hepatol* 1996;24:253–257.

41. Ricci P, Therneau TM, Malinchoc M, et al. A prognostic model for the outcome of liver transplantation in patients with cholestatic liver disease. *Hepatology* 1997;25:672–677.

42. Wiesner RH. Liver transplantation for primary biliary cirrhosis and primary sclerosing cholangitis: predicting outcomes with natural history models. *Mayo Clin Proc* 1998;73:575–588.

43. Graziadei IW, Wiesner RH, Batts KP, et al. Recurrence of primary sclerosing cholangitis following liver transplantation. *Hepatology* 1999;29:1050–1056.

44. Poulos JE, Bacon BR. Liver transplantation for hereditary hemochromatosis. *Dig Dis* 1996;14:316–322.

45. Fiel MI, Schiano TD, Bodenheimer HC, et al. Hereditary hemochromatosis in liver transplantation. *Liver Transplant Surg* 1999;5:50–56.

46. Tanzi RE, Petrukhin K, Chernov I, et al. The Wilson disease gene is a copper transporting ATPase with homology to the Menkes disease gene. *Nat Genet* 1993;5:344–350.

47. Petrukhin K, Fischer SG, Pirastu M, et al. Mapping, cloning and genetic characterization of the region containing the Wilson disease gene. *Nat Genet* 1993;5:338–343.

48. Bull PC, Thomas GR, Rommens JM, et al. The Wilson disease gene is a putative copper transporting P-type ATPase similar to the Menkes gene [Published erratum appears in *Nat Genet* 1994;6:214]. *Nat Genet* 1993;5:327–337.

49. Schilsky ML, Scheinberg IH, Sternlieb I. Liver transplantation for Wilson's disease: indications and outcome. *Hepatology* 1994;19:583–587.

50. Polson RJ, Rolles K, Calne RY, et al. Reversal of severe neurological manifestations of Wilson's disease following orthotopic liver transplantation. *Q J Med* 1987;64:685–691.

51. Rothfus WE, Hirsch WL, Malatack JJ, et al. Improvement of cerebral CT abnormalities following liver transplantation in a patient with Wilson disease. *J Comput Assist Tomogr* 1988;12:138–140.

52. Guarino M, Stracciari A, D'Alessandro R, et al. No neurological improvement after liver transplantation for Wilson's disease. *Acta Neurol Scand* 1995;92:405–408.

53. Schumacher G, Platz KP, Mueller AR, et al. Liver transplantation: treatment of choice for hepatic and neurological manifestation of Wilson's disease. *Clin Transplant* 1997;11:217–224.

54. Kassam N, Witt N, Kneteman N, et al. Liver transplantation for neuropsychiatric Wilson disease. *Can J Gastroenterol* 1998;12:65–68.

55. Song HS, Ku WC, Chen CL. Disappearance of Kayser-Fleischer rings following liver transplantation. *Transplant Proc* 1992;24:1483–1485.

Transplantation of the Liver, edited by Willis C. Maddrey, Eugene R. Schiff, and Michael F. Sorrell. Lippincott Williams & Wilkins, Philadelphia © 2001.

CHAPTER 31

Economic, Actuarial, and Contracting Perspectives on Liver Transplantation

Roger W. Evans

Liver transplantation remains one of the most expensive medical and surgical procedures performed in the United States today.[1–3] For this and other reasons, it has often been the subject of intense controversy.[4–14] Fortunately, the level of debate has subsided somewhat as public and private insurers have developed increasingly favorable coverage and reimbursement policies.[1,15–17] Today, liver transplantation is routinely paid for as an established therapy, instead of rejected on grounds that it is an experimental treatment.[18–22]

Many attempts have been made to better understand, and more fully appreciate, the economics of organ transplantation.[23–30] To date, virtually all analyses are deficient in many different respects. These shortcomings reflect neither a lack of intelligence nor profound ignorance on behalf of the investigators. More often than not, the data available for analysis are inconsistent with the concepts that accountants, actuaries, and economists use to address health care financing issues.[31–34]

This chapter does nothing to dramatically improve on the current state of the art; however, it approaches what I sometimes refer to as "transplant economics" in a systematic manner. In the course of doing so, all the major concepts used are carefully defined. Most important, it avoids the all too common pitfall of using the term *cost* to describe anything with which one can associate a dollar value. In general usage, the term *cost* is used incorrectly more often than it is applied appropriately.

In reading this chapter, it is important to recognize that, over the past 20 years, I have written extensively on economic, social, ethical, legal, and public policy issues as these relate to the financing of organ transplanta-

R. W. Evans: 2251 Baihly Hills Drive SW, Rochester, Minnesota 55902–1311.

tion.[1–3,15,16,23,24,26,35–37] Some people consider me an expert, whereas others prefer to think of me less favorably.

CONCEPTUAL FRAMEWORK

Nearly every paper I write on the economics of organ transplantation begins with a conceptual framework.[23,24,26,35–37] Once I have cleared the rubble from the financial landscape, I then feel I can make some headway in helping people understand the complexity of these economic issues.

Elsewhere, various colleagues and I have presented and refined a framework within which organ transplant-related expenses should be considered.[23,24,26,35–37] The word *expenses* is preferred to avoid the inappropriate use of the word *costs*. With this in mind, we have also found it helpful to distinguish between the *components* and the *elements* of expense. This framework is shown in Table 31.1. Without a clear specification of what we are trying to analyze, it would be difficult, if not impossible, to reach reasonable conclusions as to what the data actually represent. Inconsistent comparisons naturally offer little basis for valid interpretation.

As will become apparent later, the framework presented in Table 31.1, applying the definitions that follow, has been frequently used to develop actuarial estimates of the charges associated with liver transplantation.[38–40] *Pretransplantation expenses* are incurred in caring for the patient prior to a possible transplant procedure. At the time these expenses are incurred, a patient may *not* be recognized as in need of a transplant. *Evaluation expenses* are those associated with working up a patient in an effort to determine if he or she is suitable for transplantation. *Candidacy expenses* are incurred by a patient immediately following his or her acceptance as a transplant candidate, up through the period immediately before the transplantation procedure is performed. *Transplant expenses* are

TABLE 31.1. *A conceptual framework for the analysis of liver transplantation expenses*

Components of expense
Pretransplantation period
Evaluation
Candidacy
Transplantation
Posttransplantation period
Elements of expense
Hospital
Professional
   Surgeon
   Physician
   Other
Donor organ

Adapted from Evans RW. Liver transplantation in a managed care environment. *Liver Transplant Surg* 1995;1:61–75; Evans RW. Organ transplantation in an era of economic constraint: liver transplantation as a case study. *Semin Anesthesiol* 1995;14:127–135; and Evans RW, Kitzmann DJ. Contracting for services: liver transplantation in the era of mismanaged care. *Clin Liver Dis* 1997;1:287–303.

accumulated from the time of surgery until the date of initial discharge. Finally, *posttransplantation expenses* are usually summarized according to the year since transplantation. The major problem here is determining which expenses are related to, or coincident with, the transplant per se.

The definitions of the elements of expense, displayed in Table 31.1, may be self-evident. *Hospital expenses* are incurred in an inpatient setting. For purposes of assessment, professional fees associated with services provided in the inpatient setting are intentionally excluded. Thus, in effect, hospital expenses are equated with *facility fees,* or *Part A services* as they are often denoted by the Health Care Financing Administration (HCFA) in relationship to the Medicare program.

Professional services are of three types—physician, surgeon, and other. These services may be provided in the inpatient, as well as the outpatient, setting. Either way, HCFA has typically denoted these services as *Part B services.*

Of course, *donor organ acquisition expenses* are also an essential element of the transplant recipient's inpatient experience. Donor organ acquisition is never considered to be an outpatient expense. In the United States, organ procurement organizations often bill transplant centers a "standard acquisition cost" or fee for the donor organ.[41]

Therefore, a complete assessment of the hospital expenses associated with liver transplantation will include Part A (facility fees), Part B (professional fees), and donor organ acquisition fees. As expected, these fees, or expenses, constitute the most significant portion of the transplant recipient's financial experience. Outpatient expenses, in comparison, are relatively small.

Unfortunately, a transplant recipient's outpatient experience is more difficult to assess and quantify. It is largely composed of physician services and clinic visits. Complicating matters is the fact that follow-up care is not always provided by the center where the patient received his or her transplant. In other words, physicians unassociated with the transplant team, and clinics unaffiliated with the transplant hospital, may be the source of follow-up care. Therefore, because it is often next to impossible to obtain complete data from multiple geographically dispersed providers of health care services, the postoperative expenses associated with transplantation are, at best, crudely assessed, if estimated at all.

No conceptual framework is complete without the precise definition of those concepts essential to a standard economic analysis. Table 31.2 identifies and defines some of the more critical economic concepts to be used in the following discussion.[23,24,26,35–37]

Often, many of the terms displayed in Table 31.2 are used in a very confusing manner. For example, the terms *cost* and

TABLE 31.2. *Economic concepts in health care*

Concept	Definition
Cost	The economic value of both the labor and resource inputs required to provide a service or perform a procedure, excluding markup (i.e., production cost).
Charge	The amount a patient or third-party payer is actually billed by a health care organization or provider of health care services (i.e., list price).
Reimbursement	The amount a patient or third-party payer actually pays based on billed charges, determined retrospectively or prospectively. There is often a substantial difference between what is charged and what is reimbursed.
Price	The amount a third-party payer, usually a managed care plan, has determined in advance (i.e., prospectively) that it will pay for a service or procedure individually or in the aggregate (i.e., capitation).
Margin	The difference between the amount it actually costs to provide a service or procedure and the amount ultimately reimbursed or paid. Margin is sometimes referred to as *profit.*
Discount	The difference between what is charged for a service or a procedure and what is paid, expressed as a percent.

Adapted from Evans RW. Liver transplantation in a managed care environment. *Liver Transplant Surg* 1995;1:61–75; Evans RW. Organ transplantation in an era of economic constraint: liver transplantation as a case study. *Semin Anesthesiol* 1995;14:127–135; and Evans RW, Kitzmann DJ. Contracting for services: liver transplantation in the era of mismanaged care. *Clin Liver Dis* 1997;1:287–303.

charge are typically used interchangeably, as are the terms *coverage* (what is paid for) and *reimbursement* (how much is paid).[15–17,42,43] In some cases, under contractual relationships, a *price* may in fact be equal to a *charge*, which, in turn, may be equal to the amount reimbursed. However, in many circumstances, this is not the case.

Of the concepts listed in Table 31.2, *cost* is undoubtedly the most deceptive. Despite managed care, with its capitated and contracted payment arrangements, most health care providers are not even close to being in a position to understand, let alone quantify, their actual production costs.[44,45] Most organizations simply try to price their services in hopes that they will be able to achieve a favorable margin. However, as you might expect, if you do not know what it costs, it is next to impossible to determine if you have made a profit.

CONTRACTING FOR TRANSPLANT SERVICES

Today, the health care marketplace in the United States is littered with a variety of payment methodologies, most of which are intended to exploit the ignorance of health care providers.[35–37] Payers, who are in the best position to associate dollars with services, are ideally situated to manipulate pricing strategies to their advantage. Thus, as the enthusiasm for capitation has waned, it has been replaced with per diem rates, case rates, and strange variations on discounted fee-for-service arrangements. The name of the game here is simple—shift as much risk as possible to the other party, namely, the provider. Historically, the provider has been contemptuously viewed as the dealer holding all the cards.

As I have noted elsewhere, contracting with insurers is a complex undertaking.[44,45] There is little by way of a scientific basis for negotiating the most satisfactory payment arrangements. Nonetheless, billed charges typically serve as the source for contracted prices, since both insurers and providers possess these data. Major insurers have access to such data based on their historical experience with large numbers of patients and transplant centers. Of course, the provider knows what has been billed. Thus, the negotiation usually revolves around reaching an agreeable price, which is typically nothing more than a discounted charge. This situation is frequently disadvantageous to transplant centers, since they are widely perceived as high-cost purveyors of relatively dubious procedures.

Negotiated prices vary depending on the level of risk a transplant center is willing to assume.[35–37,46,47] At one time, contracts covered the transplant period only (see Table 31.1). Increasingly, however, the window covered by the contracted price has become much wider. Some insurers now expect transplant centers to include candidacy expenses in their contracted price. Others have even larger expectations, assuming transplant centers will include candidacy expenses, plus all expenses up to and through 1 year (12 months) posttransplantation.

Global, or *bundled,* prices are no longer optional; they are a market expectation. Transplant centers should be prepared to offer a single price for all services—hospital (Part A), professional (Part B), and organ procurement—as shown in Table 31.1. A global fee window often includes not only the procedure itself, but also all related services and visits that occur within a designated time frame. In some cases, separate payment may be permitted for the initial evaluation, for services necessary to treat unrelated problems, and, more rarely, for return trips to the operating room to resolve complications. In some situations, outlier payments may be made when a transplant center justifiably incurs excess expense relative to the contracted price for services. In reality, however, add-on payments have become an exception. In effect, assuming risk means precisely that.

As alluded to earlier, insurers shift risk to providers through a variety of reimbursement methods, with discounted fee-for-service payments becoming less prevalent over time.[35–37] For example, under *per diem contracts,* hospital reimbursement is nothing more than a previously agreed-upon dollar amount for each patient bed day. These contracts often cover hospital expenses only, although they sometimes include physician services. This fixed-payment approach shifts the risk that actual expenses per day will be more or less than expected from the insurance carrier to the provider.

Medicare uses a *per case* approach in reimbursing hospitals for their services, making a single payment based on the diagnosis. This approach not only shifts the risk to the hospital when the level of charges (that is, the intensity of care provided) is greater than expected, but also shifts the risk when the length of stay is longer than expected. Unlike the per diem approach, which pays more money for a long length of stay, the per case approach yields the same reimbursement for a long or a short length of stay.

Capitation payments, which are based on a per member per month fee for each enrollee in a health plan, shift from insurance carriers to hospitals the risk that (a) the frequency of admissions will be more than expected, (b) the level of charges or intensity of services will be more than expected, and (c) the case mix will be more severe than expected. Under a capitation contract, the hospital essentially underwrites the risk for the scope of services that fall under its contract with the carrier.

Clearly, as described here, capitation per se is not well suited to transplantation. However, some transplant centers have considered the possibility of extending to insurers an exclusive capitated arrangement for transplant services based on a per member per month payment for enrolled members. The center would then perform all transplants required by the insurer's enrollees. If no patients undergo transplantation, the financial benefit to the transplant center could be considerable. However, if a large number of transplants are performed, and the use or frequency rate on which the per member per month payment amount was based proved too low, the transplant center would necessarily lose money.

As noted, all of the foregoing methods have been used for transplant contracting. In reality, there is probably no single ideal method that would generalize to all transplant centers. Thus, each center should carefully evaluate its situation and pursue the reimbursement methodology that minimizes its risk. Of course, third-party payers are intent on doing likewise.

DATA

Data relevant to the economic analysis of organ transplantation are hard to come by. Over the years, I have had to rely on both published and unpublished sources. In some instances, the data I use are proprietary and therefore not readily accessible in the public domain. Other data have been derived from various licensed databases made available through vendors that often have access to an enormous number of health insurance claims. Still other data are clearly in the public domain and can generally be accessed accordingly.

Fortunately, as the number of transplantations performed each year has increased, both the reliability and the validity of the financial data available through commercial vendors have improved. Historically, much of the financial data in the public domain have had little more than an anecdotal quality about them, primarily because people have made far-reaching conclusions based on a mere handful of cases.

It should also be noted that many of these data are not particularly useful for research purposes, although they have considerable merit in helping transplant centers meet their business and contracting objectives. Therefore, as is true of most data, many proprietary databases are far from ideal.

Other data currently available in the public domain, such as those often released by the HCFA or the Agency for Healthcare Quality and Research (AHRQ), have limited utility and often serve as the basis for some rather misleading generalizations. These data are almost exclusively limited to billed hospital charges only. The HCFA data represent Medicare beneficiaries, whereas the AHCPR data are essentially a concatenation of state-level databases.

Physician and surgeon fee data can be obtained from a variety of commercial vendors. These data are reported at the Current Procedural Terminology (CPT) level and are expressed in percentiles. Not surprisingly, fee information is simply unavailable for many rarely provided services, including some transplant procedures. In some cases, vendors attempt to estimate fees based on other services of comparable complexity.

Given current trends and pricing strategies, it could be argued that all the foregoing data have very limited utility. For example, in the era of global pricing, fees for individual services may have minimal value. Thus, the fee for liver transplant surgery in Los Angeles may be of little interest to competing transplant centers, either regionally or nationally, because the real issue is the overall contracted price. In other words, transplant centers are not competing on the basis of prices for individual services any longer.

Alternatively, for what should be obvious antitrust reasons, it is totally inappropriate for transplant centers to be trading contracted pricing information, such as case rates or package prices. Only payers, such as the United Resource Network or the national Blue Cross Blue Shield Association, are in a position to directly compare contracted prices across numerous competing transplant centers. Nonetheless, this does not preclude transplant centers from advertising their prices, as is often done for cosmetic surgery in major urban markets. Once again, however, because transplant procedures are performed in such small numbers, it probably makes little sense to advertise package prices. In fact, I would argue that to do so could have deleterious consequences, since such data would favorably advantage competitors.

For all of these reasons, the data reported here are deficient. In dealing with this issue, I often tell users that such data provide perspective, serve an educational function, and sensitize people to some serious issues that are easily glossed over in typical business and, worse yet, academic, discourse.

RESULTS

There are many different approaches one can take in analyzing the financial aspects of organ transplantation. Actuaries, accountants, and economists all approach the topic from a variety of noncompeting perspectives. The data presented here reflect, in part, the diversity of these perspectives. Although this may add to the confusion, it also helps to enhance our appreciation of how very complex transplant financing has become.

The presentation begins with actuarial data, followed by an assessment of surgical fees. Next, attention is directed to aggregate hospital charges and surgical fees. Then some center-specific data focusing on charges, reimbursement, costs, and margins are examined. Finally, the presentation concludes with a review of insurance underwriting data intended to address the issue of per person per month costs.

Actuarial Estimates

Since 1993, the actuarial firm Milliman & Robertson, with offices located in Brookfield, Wisconsin, has published three reports on organ transplantation.[38-40] These reports have been intended to meet the needs of the health insurance industry.

Actuaries are persons who assess risks and then derive rates and premiums for insurance companies and managed care organizations. Like most analysts, actuaries rely primarily on billed charge data. Therefore, all of the Milliman & Robertson reports are based on billed charges derived from administrative, or claims, databases. Because actuaries function as consultants, selling their services, most of their source data are proprietary. As a result, the data are not in the public domain and therefore cannot be considered as "public use."

TABLE 31.3. *Average billed charges per liver transplantation from candidacy through the first posttransplantation year: 1993, 1996, and 1999*

Component or element of expense	1993	1996	1999	Percentage change, 1993 to 1999
Evaluation	$9,500	$11,000	$15,000	58
Candidacy (per month)	9,200	10,600	8,900	−3
Organ procurement	21,500	24,700	25,100	17
Hospital	194,800	188,900	107,600	−45
Physician, including surgeon	37,200	42,600	30,300	−19
Follow-up	23,000	26,400	45,000	96
Immunosuppressants	7,700	10,300	12,700	65
Totals	$302,900	$314,500	$244,600	−19

Data are from Hauboldt RH. *Cost implications of human organ transplantation, an update: 1993.* Brookfield, WI: Milliman & Robertson, 1993; Hauboldt RH. *Cost implications of human organ and tissue transplantation, an update: 1996.* Brookfield, WI: Milliman & Robertson, 1996; and Haubloldt RH, Courtney TD. *Cost implications of human organ and tissue transplantation, an update: 1999.* Brookfield, WI: Milliman & Robertson, 1999.

Table 31.3 summarizes the average billed charges for liver transplantation, from evaluation through the first year following transplant surgery, as reported by Milliman & Robertson.[38–40] As indicated, between 1993 and 1999, total charges have actually decreased by 19%, from $302,900 to $244,600. Hospital charges decreased by 45%, and professional fees decreased by 19%. Candidacy charges per month decreased by 3%. Meanwhile, follow-up charges increased by 96%, immunosuppressive drugs by 65%, evaluation by 58%, and organ procurement by 17%.

Table 31.4 summarizes the Milliman & Robertson data for the initial inpatient hospital stay only, during which transplantation surgery was performed. As indicated, for this period, total charges decreased 36%, from $253,500 to $163,000. Much of this decrease Milliman & Robertson attributes to a significant reduction in the hospital length of stay.

Table 31.5 explicitly focuses on the period after the patient's discharge from the hospital, following the transplant surgery. In the 1999 report Milliman & Robertson did not itemize these data. Nevertheless, between 1993 and 1996, there was a substantial increase in follow-up

charges, with the largest percentage increase associated with immunosuppressive drugs. Overall, during this same period, there was a 33% increase in the total charges associated with follow-up care.

Table 31.6 provides some additional data, although, once again, two of the estimates are not provided in the 1999 report. In the past, Milliman & Robertson attempted to derive estimated annual follow-up charges for the year after transplant surgery occurred. In 1999 they did not do so because of "the lack of data and interest in cost [actually *charges*] after one year."[40]

Milliman & Robertson have also previously estimated a total charge for the first 5 years, adjusted for patient survival. According to Milliman & Robertson, the "total charges for the first five years after transplantation were calculated as the sum of the estimated first-year charge and four times the estimated annual follow-up charge, adjusted for survival. The average of the one- and five-year survival rates was used as the survival adjustment factor, based on a simplifying assumption that survival rates decrease linearly with time."[39] In 1999, Milliman & Robertson chose not to provide this estimate.[40]

TABLE 31.4. *Average billed charges per liver transplantation for the surgical procedure hospital stay only: 1993, 1996, and 1999*

Component or element of expense	1993	1996	1999	Percentage change, 1993 to 1999
Hospital	$194,800	$188,000	$107,600	−45
Physician, including surgeon	37,200	42,600	30,300	−19
Organ procurement	21,500	24,700	25,100	17
Totals	$253,500	$256,200	$163,000	−36

Data are from Hauboldt RH. *Cost implications of human organ transplantation, an update: 1993.* Brookfield, WI: Milliman & Robertson, 1993; Hauboldt RH. *Cost implications of human organ and tissue transplantation, an update: 1996.* Brookfield, WI: Milliman & Robertson, 1996; and Haubloldt RH, Courtney TD. *Cost implications of human organ and tissue transplantation, an update: 1999.* Brookfield, WI: Milliman & Robertson, 1999.

TABLE 31.5. *Average billed charges for follow-up care per liver transplantation per year following surgery:*
1993, 1996, and 1999

Component or element of expense	1993	1996	1999	Percentage change, 1993 to 1999
Follow-up medical care	$16,100	$18,500	NA	15
Immunosuppressants	5,800	10,600	NA	83
Totals	$21,900	$29,100	NA	33

NA, not available. Milliman & Robertson no longer provides this estimate.
Data are from Hauboldt RH. *Cost implications of human organ transplantation, an update: 1993.* Brookfield, WI: Milliman & Robertson, 1993; Hauboldt RH. *Cost implications of human organ and tissue transplantation, an update: 1996.* Brookfield, WI: Milliman & Robertson, 1996; and Haubloldt RH, Courtney TD. *Cost implications of human organ and tissue transplantation, an update: 1999.* Brookfield, WI: Milliman & Robertson, 1999.

The foregoing data must be put in perspective relative to overall national inflation. During the period covered by the Milliman & Robertson reports, overall medical inflation was 26.3%, hospital inflation was 32.0%, and inflation associated with physicians' services was 25.8%. Therefore, taking general medical inflation into account, the total first-year liver transplant charges in 1999 were 45.3% *below* expected, hospital charges were 77.0% *below* expected, and charges for physician services were 44.8% *below* expected. Clearly, these figures are remarkable.

In reality, liver transplantation charges vary enormously across transplant centers, as do payments on behalf of insurers. As described at length previously, significant discounts, based on billed charges, are often possible due to contracted prices through transplant "centers of excellence" agreements.[46-47] Under such agreements, patients are referred to selected networked centers that are contracted to the payer. These centers offer discounts off billed charges of at least 30%, if not much more, depending on the market wherein the services are provided. Prices are often based on a global case rate. This price, as noted previously, encompasses all services, including organ procurement and, in many cases, some medical care the patient may require prior to transplant surgery. In other words, the candidacy charges are often incorporated directly into the contracted price.

Surgical Fees

As described previously, professional fees are primarily of two types: those associated with physician services and those related to the transplant surgical procedure. Both types of fees are readily identifiable according to CPT codes. Thus, each physician and surgical service has a unique code.

Unfortunately, physician fees accumulate over the patient's transplant experience and, as a result, it is difficult to precisely estimate the dollar value of all physician services the patient may require either in or out of the hospital. Because surgeon's services tend to be largely confined to the transplant procedure itself, there is at least a reasonable basis for comparing surgeon fees across transplant centers.

Table 31.7 shows private-payer fees for orthotopic liver transplantation by percentile for 1997, 1998, and 1999. These are the type of data that can be obtained from a variety of proprietary sources, and are readily available in the public domain. In addition, the Medicare fee schedule for orthotopic liver transplant surgery is provided in Table 31.7.

TABLE 31.6. *Summary of estimated charges per liver transplantation: 1993, 1996, and 1999*

Time period covered	1993	1996	1999	Percentage change, 1993 to 1999
Estimated first-year charge	$302,900	$314,500	$244,600	−19
Estimated annual follow-up charge	$21,900	$29,100	NA	33
Estimated total charge for first 5 years, adjusted for survival	$364,200	$393,900	NA	8

NA, not available. Milliman & Robertson no longer provides this estimate.
Data are from Hauboldt RH. *Cost implications of human organ transplantation, an update: 1993.* Brookfield, WI: Milliman & Robertson, 1993; Hauboldt RH. *Cost implications of human organ and tissue transplantation, an update: 1996.* Brookfield, WI: Milliman & Robertson, 1996; and Haubloldt RH, Courtney TD. *Cost implications of human organ and tissue transplantation, an update: 1999.* Brookfield, WI: Milliman & Robertson, 1999.

TABLE 31.7. *Surgeon fees for orthotopic liver transplantation: 1997–1999*

Surgeon fees[a]	1997	1998	1999
Private payer			
50th percentile	$13,076	$14,160	$14,284
75th percentile	18,072	19,285	19,285
90th percentile	23,181	24,525	24,397
Medicare fee schedule	5,494	5,053	4,981

[a]Current Procedural Terminology (CPT-4) code 47135.
The data displayed here have been compiled from various proprietary sources.

As is apparent from Table 31.7, for the fiftieth and the ninetieth percentiles during the period 1997 to 1999, there have been very modest (5.2% to 9.2%) increases in the fees private insurers pay for liver transplant surgical services. Interestingly, the seventy-fifth percentile has remained unchanged. Meanwhile, between 1997 and 1999 there has been a 9.3% decrease in the fees Medicare pays for the same surgical services.

Data on surgical fees are suggestive, giving some idea of the variability in the marketplace. However, due to contracted pricing, these fees are simply rolled into the total global price for which the transplant center offers its services. As a result, in large measure, transplant centers are competing based on global prices as opposed to individual surgeon fees.

Hospital and Surgeon Fees

It is possible to combine data from various sources to get a more complete, but less than perfect, perspective on the charges associated with liver transplantation. In this regard, Table 31.8 may serve to confuse matters to some extent, but let me explain.

The data in Table 31.8 are similar to those developed by Milliman & Robertson and presented previously (see Table 31.4). They represent the initial hospital stay only, include surgeon's fees, but exclude all physician services. As indicated, in 1997 the fiftieth percentile for liver transplant

charges was $118,088, and the seventy-fifth percentile was $172,564. In 1998, the fiftieth percentile was $115,969, and the seventy-fifth percentile was $172,801. Thus, consistent with the Milliman & Robertson reports, these data suggest that liver transplant charges have moderated, and even decreased to some extent.

Center-Specific Hospital Charges and Reimbursement

Table 31.9 presents center-specific data on hospital charges and surgeon fees for ten major liver transplant programs in the United States (see columns 1 through 4). These data depict the transplant period only. The surgeon's fees reflect the usual, customary, and reasonable (UCR) fee in the market where the transplant center is located (see column 3). As already discussed, exact center-specific data on professional fees are unavailable. Fee schedules are not in the public domain, although private payers have the ability to reconstruct them based on billed charges filed as claims on behalf of individual providers.

Once again, it is noteworthy that the average total charges shown in Table 31.9 exclude all fees for physician services (see column 4) These, as already noted, are simply unavailable on a per admission, or per encounter, basis.

Depending on the level of managed care market penetration, discounts throughout the United States are highly variable. This is apparent from Table 31.9. Discounts available from various sources (see column 5) are typically described as *gross deductions from revenue*. To derive an estimate of reimbursement expected (see column 6), one merely subtracts the average percent discount in the market (see column 5) from 1 and multiplies the average total charges (see column 4) by the resulting number. This then gives an estimate of the average total reimbursement (see column 6).

Not surprisingly, Table 31.9 is the source of several critical observations. First, as shown, there is an enormous variation in the average total charges for liver transplantation (see column 4), with a nearly 200% difference in the range of charges (lowest to highest) at ten major programs in the United States. Second, the UCR surgeon's fees range between $18,224 and $21,734—a 19.3% difference between

TABLE 31.8. *Liver transplantation charges by type of service for the hospital stay when the transplant procedure was performed: 1997 and 1998*

Charges according to percentile by year	Hospital charges ($)	Surgeon fees ($)	Total charges ($)
1997			
50th percentile	105,102	13,076	118,088
75th percentile	154,492	18,072	172,564
1998			
50th percentile	101,809	14,160	115,969
75th percentile	153,516	19,285	172,801

Charges exclude all inpatient physician fees.
The data displayed here have been compiled from various proprietary sources.

TABLE 31.9. *Average charges and estimated reimbursement for liver transplant procedures performed at ten major liver transplantation programs in the United States, 1999*

(1) Transplant center	(2) Average billed charges for hospital services ($)	(3) Average billed charges for surgeon's fees ($)	(4) Average total charges ($)	(5) Average percent discount in market (%)	(6) Average total reimbursement ($)
1	274,228	21,157	295,385	46	159,508
2	268,008	21,156	289,164	47	153,257
3	267,697	18,668	286,365	43	163,228
4	225,981	18,437	244,418	61	90,435
5	215,801	20,886	236,687	53	111,243
6	129,604	18,224	147,828	21	116,784
7	125,372	21,734	147,106	31	101,503
8	122,375	21,542	143,917	33	96,424
9	109,612	20,693	130,305	40	78,183
10	80,041	19,189	99,230	21	78,392

Charges exclude all inpatient physician fees.
The data displayed here have been compiled from various proprietary sources.

the lowest and the highest (see column 3). Finally, it is obvious that those programs with the highest charges (see columns 2 and 3) typically have more favorable reimbursement (see column 6), although this depends on the size of the market discount (see column 5). For example, Center 4 has reasonably high charges, but an equally substantial market discount.

Once again, from a managed care contracting perspective, data such as those displayed in Table 31.9 may appear to have questionable utility. However, recent marketplace dynamics suggest otherwise. For example, some insurers are now pursuing a "lesser of" reimbursement policy. Under this policy, the insurer pays whichever is lowest—the contracted global price the center offers, or the total billed charges the center claims—for the transplantation procedure.

The "lesser of" reimbursement policy typically advantages those transplant centers with historically high charges, while seriously handicapping centers with low charges caused by small markups. Thus, for example, let us assume Center 10 offers a per procedure contracted price for liver transplantation of $150,000. After adding crudely estimated physician's fees to the total billed charges in Table 31.9, the result would likely be about $120,000. Therefore, under the "lesser of" reimbursement policy, the transplant center would be paid $30,000 less than their contracted price.

Assuming that a patient has serious complications, actual experience suggests that the billed charges for a liver transplantation could easily exceed $300,000. Yet, under the "lesser of" reimbursement policy this same center would only be paid the contracted price of $150,000. Under these circumstances, the net loss would exceed $150,000.

Overall, based on the data and analysis presented here, there are obvious advantages associated with excessively marking up the charges for all transplantation services. Such an approach allows centers to offer substantial discounts and still achieve a very favorable margin. Mean-

while, these same centers are unlikely to be penalized by the "lesser of" reimbursement policy.

Charges, Reimbursement, Cost, and Margin

Although the foregoing analyses are intuitively appealing, intellectually challenging, and operationally helpful, it is obvious that some of the economic concepts presented in Table 31.2 have yet to be addressed, namely, cost and margin. In this regard, Table 31.10 provides the required perspective.

The charges listed in Table 31.10 (see column 2) are the same as those listed in Table 31.9 (see column 2). They exclude all professional fees. The reimbursement column in Table 31.10 (see column 3) is based on hospital charges only; for this reason, it differs from the reimbursement data provided in Table 31.9 (see column 6). The cost data are derived, in part, from the Medicare cost report submitted annually to the Health Care Financing Administration by each transplant hospital (see column 4). These data reflect true accounting costs, as defined in Table 31.2. Finally, the margin (see column 5) is also based on the Medicare cost report, and is defined as the difference between the amount it costs to provide the procedure (see column 4) and the amount reimbursed (see column 3)

As was true of Table 31.9, Table 31.10 indicates that there is considerable variability across all centers, with some centers having very high costs as well as sizable margins. Other centers have relatively low costs and equally narrow margins. As shown, Center 1 has the highest costs, followed by Centers 3 and 2. Meanwhile, Center 3 has the largest margin, followed by Centers 2 and 1. Percentage-wise, Center 5 has the largest margin, followed by Centers 2, 3, and 1 (see column 6). However, Center 9, which has the lowest cost, does not, at 37%, have the largest percentage margin.

Overall, some of the "highest cost" centers also have the most substantial percentage margins. Thus, Table 31.10,

TABLE 31.10. *Comparison of hospital charges, reimbursement, actual costs, and margins for liver transplant procedures performed at ten major programs in the United States, 1999*

(1) Transplant center	(2) Charges ($)	(3) Reimbursement ($)	(4) Cost ($)	(5) Margin ($)	(6) Percent margin (%)
1	274,228	147,672	100,751	46,921	47
2	268,008	140,651	89,005	51,646	58
3	267,697	151,731	99,476	52,255	53
4	225,981	87,161	77,624	9,537	12
5	215,801	101,729	54,986	46,743	85
6	129,604	102,426	78,397	24,029	31
7	125,372	87,033	86,933	100	0
8	122,375	81,710	58,238	23,472	40
9	109,612	66,249	48,295	17,954	37
10	80,041	63,120	53,563	9,557	18

Hospital or Part A charges only.
The data displayed here have been compiled from various proprietary sources.

like Table 31.9, underscores the merit of high markups in the managed care era. In effect, the centers with the highest costs can subsidize their inefficiency through high markups, which, in turn, yield large margins. Alternatively, centers with low costs and low markups tend to suffer accordingly with small margins.

From a management perspective, one could argue as to which centers in Table 31.10 are truly the most attractive. If one is interested in margin only, Center 3 would appear to be the winner. Alternatively, if a transplant center is trying to respond to generalized societal concerns about the overall cost of health care, Centers 8 and 9 would seem to be the clear-cut winners—they have minimized their actual costs, maximized their reimbursement, and, thus, generated a healthy margin.

In my opinion, in today's marketplace, Centers 8 and 9 have the preferable business strategy. The reason should be clear: in a straight competition for transplant contracts, they would certainly appear to be in the most favorable position to both compete and to make a profit. Centers 3, 2, 1, and 5 would undoubtedly be signing contracts yielding substantial losses.

Unfortunately, although Center 10 is currently achieving a reasonable margin, it is extremely vulnerable to the "lesser of" reimbursement policy described earlier. Therefore, as it now stands, Center 10 is financially unstable; as a result, its future is uncertain.

Per Person Per Month Costs

Premiums remain a serious concern for public and private insurers. Therefore let us return, once again, to the reports prepared by Milliman & Robertson, the actuarial firm that has served as a major resource for the insurance industry.[38–40]

In evaluating the implications of medical technology, such as organ transplantation procedures, insurance underwriters typically want to understand the impact the technology is likely to have on insurance premiums. For example, a very expensive procedure with a high use, or frequency rate, can have extraordinary financial implications. In other words, insurance premiums would have to be increased substantially to cover the costs of the new technology. Alternatively, if a new technology is very expensive, but the frequency rate is projected to be low, the direct impact on insurance premiums can actually be minuscule.

It is also important to consider the premium impact relative to the size of the health plan membership. For example, because persons 65 years old and older are likely to have a low frequency rate for most organ transplant procedures, the premium impact will be much smaller than it would be for the typical private insurer with younger beneficiaries.

Of course, the number of covered lives must also be factored into all of the foregoing calculations. Small health plans often have a hard time incorporating high-cost, low-frequency technologies because their premiums can easily be put out of reach of their beneficiaries.

Table 31.11 summarizes data relevant to this discussion for persons younger than 65 years. As shown, in 1993 the per capita cost per month for liver transplantation was estimated to be 45 cents. In 1996, this figure increased to 50 cents but, by 1999, the cost had been reduced to 34 cents.[38–40] For persons 65 years and older, the per capita costs (not shown) are somewhat lower because of a lower transplant incidence or frequency rate. In 1999, Milliman & Robertson estimated that the per capita per month costs for liver transplantation for persons 65 years and older were 19 cents.[40]

As noted in the Milliman & Robertson reports, patient cost sharing, maximum benefit limitations, and provider discounts would all combine to further reduce these costs. However, they also note that administrative costs and margins for variation and profit would need to be considered. The Milliman & Robertson actuaries further note that, although the per member per month amount is relatively small in relation to total per capita health care expenditures in the United States, liver transplant procedures remain expensive, with average charges and reimbursement exceeding $100,000.[40] Thus, we can expect insurers to remain vigilant in their efforts to monitor overall transplant expenditures.

TABLE 31.11. *Projected U.S. liver transplantation monthly costs per person under age 65: 1993, 1996, and 1999*

Estimate	1993	1996	1999	Percentage change, 1993 to 1999
Estimated charges for first five years	$364,200	$393,900	NA	8
Estimated number of transplants annually	3,280	3,780	$3,910	19
Estimated cost per person per month	0.45	0.50	0.34	−24

NA, not available. Milliman & Robertson no longer provides this estimate.
Data are from Hauboldt RH. *Cost implications of human organ transplantation, an update: 1993.* Brookfield, WI: Milliman & Robertson, 1993; Hauboldt RH. *Cost implications of human organ and tissue transplantation, an update: 1996.* Brookfield, WI: Milliman & Robertson, 1996; and Haubloldt RH, Courtney TD. *Cost implications of human organ and tissue transplantation, an update: 1999.* Brookfield, WI: Milliman & Robertson, 1999.

DISCUSSION

Although liver transplantation remains an expensive surgical procedure, the evidence presented here suggests that expenses, however measured, have, at the very least, moderated. The same cannot be said for all other transplantation procedures. For example, available data indicate that the total first-year charges for heart transplantation have increased by 45% between 1993 and 1999.

The substantial increases associated with follow-up care and immunosuppression for liver transplantation are not surprising, but they are a source of concern. Many analyses have concluded that superior immunosuppressive agents have the potential to reduce the cost of post-transplantation patient care. Unfortunately, the data do not seem to be consistent with the rhetoric. Clearly, objective pharmacoeconomic studies are necessary to substantiate the relative cost-effectiveness of new immunosuppressive drugs in comparison with established agents.

The remarkable variation in charges across liver transplant centers is also noteworthy, but it is understandable. In markets with a high managed care penetration, there is clear evidence of business strategies based on high markups. This, in turn, gives rise to high charges, which lead to favorable contract negotiation. Transplant centers with conservative pricing policies are clearly vulnerable as third-party payers continue their aggressive and relentless efforts to shift risk to providers. Obviously, centers must address their actual costs, even if excessive markups offer temporary financial protection. In the long run, the market is unlikely to subsidize provider inefficiencies.

Despite many years of study, it is evident that transplant economics remains largely a descriptive field. Only in the past 5 years or so have we begun to see published multivariate analyses of liver transplant costs and resource utilization.[48–53] Unfortunately, although these studies are critical, they often tell us relatively little. By and large, these studies underscore the fact that the sickest patients tend to be the most expensive to treat and, in turn, have the poorest outcomes. This is hardly consistent with the overall goal of cost-effective health care.

Thus, it remains unfathomable why the Department of Health and Human Services has chosen to endorse a policy for donor organ distribution that guarantees achieving the poorest outcome at the greatest expense.[54–57] Even simple descriptive analyses tell us what we need to know and what we should avoid.

Unfortunately, public health policy is not currently evidence based. Instead, it is politically motivated, with the interests of selected transplant centers being given favored status in the policy development process. Clearly, these centers have made institutional interests their primary consideration, and they are now committed to patient care as an inconvenient secondary issue.

With these thoughts in mind, it should be obvious that the sociopolitical climate surrounding liver transplantation over the past several years has hardly been devoid of controversy. Transplantation has never been, nor will it ever be, the most significant health care issue in the United States. Perhaps it is time a few cowboys got off their horses, took a look around, and realized that the goals they have in mind do not reflect real world considerations. Until public health policies begin to recognize the fragile economic climate that surrounds transplantation, the field itself will continue to struggle with its own survival as a reputable discipline.

REFERENCES

1. Evans RW. Organ transplantation and the inevitable debate as to what constitutes a basic health care benefit. In: Terasaki PI, Cecka JM, eds. *Clinical transplants, 1993.* Los Angeles: UCLA Tissue Typing Laboratory, 1994:359–391.
2. Evans RW. Effect of liver transplantation on local, regional, and national health care. In: Busuttil RW, Klintmalm GB, eds. *Transplantation of the liver.* Philadelphia: WB Saunders, 1996:869–879.
3. Evans RW, Manninen DL, Dong FB. An economic analysis of liver transplantation: costs, insurance coverage, and reimbursement. *Gastroenterol Clin North Am* 1993;22:451–473.
4. Evans RW. Health care technology and the inevitability of resource allocation and rationing decisions [First of two parts]. *JAMA* 1983;249:2047–2053.
5. Evans RW. Health care technology and the inevitability of resource allocation and rationing decisions [Second of two parts]. *JAMA* 1983;249:2208–2219.

6. Dean M. Is your treatment economic, effective, and efficient? *Lancet* 1991;337:480–481.

7. Caplan AL. *If I were a rich man could I buy a pancreas?* Bloomington, IN: Indiana University Press, 1992.

8. Ubel PA. Can we continue to afford organ transplants in an era of managed care? *Am J Managed Care* 1996;2:293–297.

9. Asch DA, Ubel PA. Rationing by any other name. *N Engl J Med* 1997;336:1668–1671.

10. Robinson R. Rationing health care: a national framework and local discretion. *J Health Serv Res Policy* 1997;2:67–70.

11. Lamm RD. Marginal medicine. *JAMA* 1998;280:931–933.

12. Feek CM, McKean W, Henneveld L, et al. Experience with rationing health care in New Zealand. *Br Med J* 1999;318:1346–1348.

13. Smith R, Hiatt H, Berwick D. Shared ethical principles for everybody in health care: a working draft from the Tavistock Group. *Br Med J* 1999;318:248–249.

14. Dolan P, Cookson R, Ferguson B. Effect of discussion and deliberation on the public's views of priority setting in health care: focus group study. *Br Med J* 1999;318:916–919.

15. Evans RW. Organ transplantation costs, insurance coverage, and reimbursement. In: Terasaki PI, ed. *Clinical transplants, 1990.* Los Angeles: UCLA Tissue Typing Laboratory, 1990:343–355.

16. Evans RW. Third party payment and the cost of transplantation. *J South Carolina Med Assoc* 1991;87:345–352.

17. Wilensky GR. Medicare program: criteria for Medicare coverage of adult liver transplants: final notice. *Federal Register* 1991;58:15006–15018.

18. Steinberg EP, Tunis S, Shapiro D. Insurance coverage for experimental technologies. *Health Affairs* 1995;14(4):143–158.

19. Finkelstein BS, Silvers JB, Marrero U, et al. Insurance coverage, physician recommendations, and access to emerging treatments. *JAMA* 1998;279:663–668.

20. Sabin JE, Daniels N. Making insurance coverage for new technologies reasonable and accountable. *JAMA* 1998;279:703–704.

21. Priester R, Gervais KG, Vawter DE. A model for improving coverage policy decisions. *Am J Managed Care* 1999;5:981–991.

22. Frick KD, Lyles A, Powe NR. To cover or not to cover: how to decide? *Am J Managed Care* 1999;5:1064–1066.

23. Evans RW. The socioeconomics of organ transplantation. *Transplant Proc* 1985;17(suppl 4):129–136.

24. Evans RW. Cost-effectiveness analysis of organ transplantation. *Surg Clin North Am* 1968;66:603–616.

25. Schersten T, Byringer H, Karlberg I, et al. Cost-effectiveness analysis of organ transplantation. *Int J Tech Assess Health Care* 1986;2:545–552.

26. Evans RW. A catastrophic disease perspective on organ transplantation. In: Ginzberg E, ed. *Medicine and society: clinical decisions and societal values.* Boulder, CO: Westview Press, 1987:61–95.

27. Kankaanpaa J. Cost-effectiveness of liver transplantation. *Transplant Proc* 1987;19:3864–3866.

28. Williams JW, Vera S, Evans LS. Socioeconomic aspects of hepatic transplantation. *Am J Gastroenterol* 1987;82:1115–1119.

29. Sabesian SM, Williams JW, Evans LS. Ethical and economic issues. In: Maddrey WC, ed. *Transplantation of the liver.* New York: Elsevier, 1988:331–343.

30. Eggers PW, Kucken LE. Cost issues in transplantation. *Surg Clin North Am* 1994;74:1259–1267.

31. Finkler SA. The distinction between cost and charges. *Ann Intern Med* 1982;96:102–109.

32. Finkler SA, ed. *Issues in cost accounting for health care organizations.* Gaithersburg, MD: Aspen Publications, 1994.

33. Clement JP. Dynamic cost shifting in hospitals: evidence from the 1980s and 1990s. *Inquiry* 1998;34:340–350.

34. Balas EA, Kretschmer RAC, Gnann W, et al. Interpreting cost analyses of clinical interventions. *JAMA* 1998;279:54–57.

35. Evans RW. Liver transplantation in a managed care environment. *Liver Transplant Surg* 1995;1:61–75.

36. Evans RW. Organ transplantation in an era of economic constraint: liver transplantation as a case study. *Semin Anesthesiol* 1995;14:127–135.

37. Evans RW, Kitzmann DJ. Contracting for services: liver transplantation in the era of mismanaged care. *Clin Liver Dis* 1997;1:287–303.

38. Hauboldt RH. *Cost implications of human organ transplantation, an update: 1993.* Brookfield, WI: Milliman & Robertson, 1993.

39. Hauboldt RH. *Cost implications of human organ and tissue transplantation, an update: 1996.* Brookfield, WI: Milliman & Robertson, 1996.

40. Haubloldt RH, Courtney TD. *Cost implications of human organ and tissue transplantation, an update: 1999.* Brookfield, WI: Milliman & Robertson, 1999.

41. Evans RW. Organ procurement expenditures and the role of financial incentives. *JAMA* 1993;269:3113–3118.

42. Towery OB, Perry S. The scientific basis for coverage decisions by third-party payers. *JAMA* 1981;245:59–61.

43. Schaffarzick RW. Technology assessment: perspective of a third party payer. In: Lohr KN, Rettig RA, eds. *Quality of care and technology assessment.* Washington, DC: Institute of Medicine, National Academy of Sciences, 1987:98–105.

44. Conrad D, Bonney R, Sachs M, et al. *Managed care contracting: concepts and applications for the health care executive.* Chicago: Health Administration Press, 1996.

45. Todd MK. *The managed care contracting handbook.* Burr Ridge, IL: McGraw Hill, 1997.

46. Ascher NL, Evans RW. Designation of liver transplant centers in the United States. *Transplant Proc* 1987;19:2405.

47. Evans RW. Public and private insurer designation of transplantation programs. *Transplantation* 1992;53:1041–1046.

48. Kim WR, Therneau TM, Dickson ER, et al. Preoperative predictors of resource utilization in liver transplantation. In: Cecka JM, Terasaki PI, eds. *Clinical transplants, 1995.* Los Angeles: UCLA Tissue Typing Laboratory, 1996:315–322.

49. Brown RS Jr, Ascher NL, Lake JR, et al. The impact of surgical complications after liver transplantation on resource utilization. *Arch Surg* 1997;132:1098–1103.

50. Brown RS Jr, Lake JR, Ascher NL, et al. Predictors of the cost of liver transplantation. *Liver Transplant Surg* 1998;4:170–176.

51. Russo MW, Sandler RS, Mandelkehr L, et al. Payer status, but not race, affects the cost of liver transplantation. *Liver Transplant Surg* 1998;4:370–377.

52. Showstack J, Katz PP, Lake JR, et al. Resource utilization in liver transplantation: effects of patient characteristics and clinical practice. *JAMA* 1999;281:1381–1386.

53. Russell PS. Understanding resource use in liver transplantation. *JAMA* 1999;281:1431–1432.

54. Steinbrook R. Allocating livers—devising a fair system. *N Engl J Med* 1997;336:436–438.

55. Neuberger J, Lake J. Allocating donor livers. *Br Med J* 1997;314:1140–1141.

56. Evans RW, Kitzmann DJ. The "arithmetic" of donor liver allocation. In: Terasaki PI, Cecka JM, eds. *Clinical transplants, 1996.* Los Angeles: UCLA Tissue Typing Laboratory, 1997:338–342.

57. Institute of Medicine. *Organ procurement and transplantation.* Washington, DC: National Academy of Sciences, 1999.

Subject Index